OXFORD MEDICAL PUBLICATIONS

Shorter Oxford
Textbook of
Psychiatry

Shorter Oxford
Textbook of
Psychiatry

FOURTH EDITION

Michael Gelder

Emeritus Professor of Psychiatry
University of Oxford

Richard Mayou

Professor of Psychiatry, University of Oxford

and

Philip Cowen

Professor of Psychopharmacology, University of Oxford

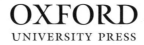

OXFORD
UNIVERSITY PRESS

OXFORD
UNIVERSITY PRESS

Great Clarendon Street, Oxford OX2 6DP

Oxford University Press is a department of the University of Oxford.
It furthers the University's objective of excellence in research, scholarship,
and education by publishing worldwide in

Oxford New York

Auckland Cape Town Dar es Salaam Hong Kong Karachi Kuala Lumpur
Madrid Melbourne Mexico City Nairobi New Delhi Shanghai Taipei Toronto

With offices in

Argentina Austria Brazil Chile Czech Republic France Greece Guatemala
Hungary Italy Japan South Korea Poland Portugal Singapore Switzerland
Thailand Turkey Ukraine Vietnam

Published in the United States
by Oxford University Press Inc., New York

© Oxford University Press, 2001

The moral rights of the authors have been asserted

Database right Oxford University Press (maker)

First edition published (as the Oxford Textbook of Psychiatry) 1983
Second edition 1989
Third edition 1996; reprinted 1996, 1998
Fourth edition (as the shorter Oxford Textbook of Psychiatry) 2001
Reprinted 2002, 2004 (with corrections), 2005 (with corrections)

British Library Cataloguing in Publication Data
Data available

Library of Congress Cataloguing in Publication Data

Gelder, Michael G.
Shorter Oxford textbook of psychiatry / Michael Gelder, Richard Mayou and Philip Cowen.—4th ed.
p. ; cm.
Rev. ed. of: Oxford textbook of psychiatry / Michael Gelder ... [et al.]. 3rd ed. 1996.
Includes bibliographical references.
1. Psychiatry. I. Mayou, Richard. II Cowen, Philip. III Oxford textbook of psychiatry. IV. Title.
[DNLM: 1. Mental Disorders. 2. Psychiatry. WM 140 G315s 2001]
RC454 G42 2001   616/.89—dc 21   2001021818

ISBN 0 19 263241 8 (pbk)
ISBN 0 19 263242 6 (hbk)

10 9 8 7 6 5 4

Typeset in Garamond 3
by Florence Production Ltd, Stoodleigh, Devon
Printed in Italy
by Legoprint S.p.A.

Preface to the fourth edition

This book is the fourth edition of the *Oxford Textbook of Psychiatry*. The name of the book has been changed in this edition to take account of the publication of the longer and more comprehensive two volume *New Oxford Textbook of Psychiatry*. The present volume provides a more concise account of clinical psychiatry and is intended as a basic text for trainees in psychiatry and as an advanced text for students of medicine and clinical psychology, general practitioners, and others whose work requires knowledge of psychiatry.

The complete text and the references have been extensively revised. There are new chapters on Evidence-Based Psychiatry and on Ethics and the Law. The latter contains new material on ethics and revised material on the law, previously in another chapter. The related topics of dissociative disorders and somatoform disorders, previously in different chapters, have been brought together in a new chapter. Chapter Two has been renamed Assessment and broadened to take account of assessment in community psychiatry as well as in hospital practice. We have tried throughout to maintain the style of the previous editions while making more use of lists, tables, and other means of presenting the material more concisely.

This is the first edition that has been prepared without the contribution of Dr Dennis Gath who has retired. We pay tribute to the important part that he played in the success of the previous editions, through his scholarship and the high quality of his writing.

It is increasingly difficult for three authors to keep pace with the rapid increase in the psychiatric literature. In this edition special advisors have helped to revise several chapters. Their names are listed overleaf. Other colleagues who gave us valuable advice include: Dr Sidney Crown, Professor Richard Green, Dr David Julier, Dr Frank Margison, Professor Robin Jacoby, and Mr Mark Underwood. We also thank Mrs Wendy Swift for considerable help in the preparation of the manuscript.

Finally, we draw our readers' attention to our use of words he and she, explained at the foot of page 3.

Oxford
2001

M.G.
R.M.
P.C.

Chapter advisors

We wish to thank the following colleagues who advised us about the revision of major parts of the book:

Gwen Adshead
Consultant and Honorary Senior Lecturer in Forensic Psychotherapy, Broadmoor Hospital, and St George's Hospital Medical School, and Consultant Psychiatrist, Traumatic Stress Clinic, UCL & Middlesex Hospitals

Michael Crawford
Senior Lecturer in Psychiatry, Imperial College, London

Anke Ehlers
Professor of Experimental Psychopathology, Institute of Psychiatry, London

Christopher Fairburn
Wellcome Principal Research Fellow and Professor of Psychiatry, University of Oxford

Nick Fox
Dementia Research Group, Institute of Neurology, UCL, London

John Geddes
Senior Clinical Research Fellow, University of Oxford

Richard Harrington
Professor of Child and Adolescent Psychiatry, University of Manchester

Paul Harrison
Professor of Psychiatry, University of Oxford

Tony Hope
Professor of Medical Ethics, University of Oxford, and Director of Ethox

Matthew Hotopf
Clinical Senior Lecturer, Guy's King's and St Thomas School of Medicine, King's College London

Max Marshall
Reader in Community Psychiatry, University of Manchester

Jenny McCleery
Clinical Lecturer in Psychiatry, University of Oxford

Eugene Paykel
Professor of Psychiatry, University of Cambridge

Dermot Rowe
ConsultantPsychiatrist, Oxfordshire Learning Disability NHS Trust

Hugh Series
Consultant in Psychiatry of Old Age, Oxfordshire Mental Healthcare NHS Trust

Gregory Stores
Professor of Developmental Neuropsychiatry, University of Oxford

Jason Warren
Dementia Research Group, Institute of Neurology, UCL, London

Sarah Welch
Consultant Psychiatrist and Honorary Senior Lecturer, Bethlem Royal and Maudsley NHS Trust

Kevan Wylie
Consultant Psychiatrist, Sheffield Community Health NHS Trust

Preface to the third edition

This third edition has been revised extensively to take account of new knowledge and advances in practice reported since the publication of the second edition. It includes the latest revisions of the *International Classification of Diseases* (ICD10) and of the *Diagnostic and Statistical Manual for Mental Disorders* (DSMIV). Least change has been made in Chapters 1 and 2, on signs and symptoms and the clinical method respectively; most revision has been made in Chapter 6 which is now concerned with stress-related and adjustment disorders, and Chapter 19 in which the account of psychiatric services has been revised extensively. In other chapters, necessary changes have been made to bring them up to date while preserving the original clinical descriptions. In this revision the authors of the second edition have been joined by Dr Philip Cowen.

In preparing this third edition we have been greatly helped by Dr R. S. Abell, Dr Gwen Adshead, Professor David Barlow, Dr Jennifer Barraclough, Professor Sidney Bloch, Dr David Clark, Dr Robert Cloninger, Professor John Cooper, Dr Tim Crow, Dr Christopher Fairburn, Dr Ray Fitzpatrick, Dr Bill Fulford, Dr David Geaney, Dr Guy Goodwin, Dr Paul Harrison, Dr Keith Hawton, Dr Tony Hope, Dr Robin Jacoby, Dr David Julier, Professor Eve Johnstone, Dr Harold Koenig, Professor Alwyn Lishman, Professor Joseph LoPiccolo, Dr Marie-Anne Martin, Dr Max Marshall, Professor Gethin Morgan, Professor William Parry-Jones, Dr Phil Robson, Professor Gene Paykel, Professor John Rush, Dr David Schaffer, Dr Michael Sharpe, Dr Alan Stein, Dr Greg Stores, Dr Eric Taylor, and Professor Peter Tyrer.

Oxford
1995

M.G.
D.G.
R.M.
P.C.

Preface to the second edition

In this edition the main aims and general approach are the same as in the first edition, but the text has been extensively revised. This revision has been undertaken with three aims: to incorporate the latest systems of classification, namely the draft ICD10 and DSMIIIR, in the sections dealing with clinical syndromes; to introduce advances in knowledge and practice; and to correct errors.

In preparing this second edition we have been greatly helped by:

Dr D. H. Clark	Dr I. B. Glass
Dr P. J. Cowen	Dr A. Hope
Dr K. E. Hawton	Mr H. C. Jones
Dr D. Jones	Professor D. Shaffer
Professor P. McGuffin	Professor Sir David
Dr G. Stores	Weatherall

We acknowledge with gratitude the permission of the World Health Organization to quote material from the 1988 Draft of Chapter V of ICD10, Categories F00–F99, Mental, Behavioural and Developmental Disorders; Clinical Descriptions and Diagnostic Guidelines, World Health Organization, Division of Mental Health, Geneva, 1988 (MNH/MEP/87.1, Rev.2). The copyrights of ICD and the trial drafts are held by WHO. The authors wish to make it clear that the trial drafts are provisional and subject to alteration in the final version.

Oxford
1988

M.G.
D.G.
R.M.

Preface to the first edition

This book is written primarily as an introductory textbook for trainee psychiatrists, and also as an advanced textbook for clinical medical students. We hope that the book will also be useful, for purposes of revision and reference, to psychiatrists who have completed their training and to general practitioners and other clinicians.

The subject matter of this book is the practice of clinical psychiatry. Recent years have seen the increasing development of sub-specialties such as child and adolescent psychiatry, forensic psychiatry, and the psychiatry of mental retardation. This book is mainly concerned with general psychiatry, but it also contains chapters on the sub-specialties. Throughout the whole book, our purpose has been to provide an introduction to each subject, rather than a fully documented account. It is assumed that the trainee psychiatrist will go on to consult more comprehensive works such as the *Handbook of Psychiatry* (Shepherd 1983), the *Comprehensive text-book of psychiatry* (Kaplan *et al*. 1980), and special-ized textbooks dealing with the sub-specialties. In some chapters references are made to basic sciences such as psychology, genetics, biochemistry, and pharmacology. Discussion of these subjects is based on the assumption that the reader already has a working knowledge of them from previous study.

The chapters dealing with psychiatric treatment fall into two groups. First, there are three chapters wholly devoted to treatment and concerned only with general issues. In this group, Chapter 17 deals mainly with drug treatment and electroconvulsive therapy; Chapter 18 deals with psychological treat-ments; and Chapter 19 discusses the organization of services for the rehabilitation and care of patients with chronic psychiatric disorders. Second, there

are the various chapters on individual syndromes, which include sections on the treatments specific to those syndromes. In these chapters, treatment is usually discussed in two parts. The first part exam-ines the evidence that a particular treatment is effective for a particular syndrome; the second part discusses (under the heading of management) practical issues in treatment, such as ways of using various treatments singly or in combination at different stages of a patient's illness. The separation of chapters on general issues from those on specific issues means that the reader has to consult more than one chapter for complete information on the treatment of any disorder. None the less this arrangement is preferred because a single treatment may be used for several syndromes. For example, antipsychotic drugs are used to treat mania and schizophrenia, and supportive psychotherapy is part of the treatment of many disorders.

In this book there is no separate chapter on the history of psychiatry. Instead certain chapters on specific topics include brief accounts of their history. For example, the chapter on psychiatric services contains a short historical review of the care of the mentally ill; and the chapter on abnormal personality includes some information about the development of ideas about the subject. This arrangement reflects the authors' view that, at least in an introductory text, historical points are more useful when related to an account of modern ideas. The historical references in this book can be supplemented by reading a history of psychiatry such as that by Ackerknecht (1968) or Bynum (1983).

The use of references in this book also needs to be explained. As this is an introductory postgraduate text, we have not provided references for every statement that could be supported by evidence. Instead we have generally followed two principles: to give references for statements that may be controversial; and to give more references for issues judged to be of topical interest. In an introductory text it also seemed appropriate to give references mostly to the Anglo-American literature. For all these reasons the coverage of the literature may seem uneven; but – as explained above – the book is written in the expectation that the trainee psychiatrist will progress to other works for more detailed literature surveys. Suggestions for further reading are given at the end of each chapter.

Oxford
May 1983

M.G.
D.G.
R.M.

Contents

1

CHAPTER 1

Signs and symptoms
of mental disorder

CHAPTER 1

Signs and symptoms of mental disorder

Psychiatrists require two distinct capacities. One is the capacity to collect clinical data objectively and accurately by history taking and examination of the mental state, and to organize the data in a systematic and balanced way. The other is the capacity for intuitive understanding of each patient as an individual. When the psychiatrist exercises the first capacity, he draws on his clinical skills and knowledge of clinical phenomena; when he exercises the second capacity, he draws on his knowledge of human nature and experience with former patients to gain insights into the feelings and behaviour the patient he is now seeing, and the ways in which he has been influenced by past experiences. Both capacities can be developed by listening to patients, and by learning from more experienced psychiatrists. A textbook can provide the information and describe the procedures necessary to develop the first capacity. The focus of the chapter on the first capacity does not imply that intuitive understanding is unimportant, but simply that it cannot be learnt directly or solely from a textbook.

Skill in examining patients depends on a sound knowledge of how symptoms and signs are defined. Without such knowledge, the psychiatrist is liable to misclassify phenomena and thereby make inaccurate diagnoses. For this reason, definitions are considered in the first part of this chapter before history taking and mental state examination are described.

Having elicited a patient's symptoms and signs, the psychiatrist needs to decide how far these phenomena fall into a pattern that has been observed in other psychiatric patients. In other words, he decides whether the clinical features conform to a recognized syndrome. He does this by combining observations about the patient's present state with information about the history of the condition. The value of identifying a syndrome is that it helps to predict prognosis and to select an effective treatment. It does this by directing the psychiatrist to the relevant body of accumulated knowledge about the causes, treatment, and outcome of similar patients. Diagnosis is discussed in Chapter 4 along with classification, and also in each of the chapters dealing with the various psychiatric syndromes.

Since much of the present chapter consists of definitions and descriptions of symptoms and signs, it may be less easy to read than those that follow. It is suggested that the reader might approach it in two stages. The first reading would be applied to the introductory sections and to a general understanding of the more frequently observed phenomena. The second reading would focus on details of definition and the less common symptoms and signs. This second reading is usually done best in conjunction with an opportunity to interview a patient with the relevant signs or symptoms.

There are numerous examples in this chapter and almost all apply as much to women as to men. The question arises, how this fact should be reflected in the use of personal pronouns. We have decided that throughout the book, the pronoun 'he' will be used with the meaning 'he or she'. This long-established, but currently somewhat unfashionable, convention has been chosen because the alternative he/she seems clumsy, and the device of writing he in some places and she in others seems artificial. We hope that our readers will accept this usage which does not reflect any lack of concern for the rights and special needs of women, as patients or as professionals.

General issues

Before individual phenomena are described, some general issues will be considered concerning the methods of studying symptoms and signs, and the terms used to describe them

Psychopathology

The study of abnormal states of mind is known as psychopathology. The term embraces three distinct approaches to the subject.

Descriptive psychopathology

This approach, also called *phenomenology*, is the objective description of abnormal states of mind avoiding, as far as possible, preconceived ideas or theories. Its aim is to elucidate the essential qualities of morbid mental experiences and to understand each patient's experience of illness. This approach to psychopathology is concerned solely with the description of conscious experiences and observable behaviour. Its most important exponent was the German psychiatrist and philosopher, Karl Jaspers, and his classical work, *Allgemeine Psychopathologie* (*General psychopathology*), first published in 1913, still provides the most complete account of the subject. The seventh (1959) edition is available in an English translation by Hoenig and Hamilton (Jaspers 1963). This chapter is concerned with descriptive or phenomenological psychopathology.

Psychodynamic psychopathology

This approach originated in psychoanalytical investigations. Like phenomenological psychopathology, it starts with the patient's description of his mental experiences and the doctor's observations of his behaviour. Unlike phenomenological psychopathology, however, this approach goes beyond description and seeks to explain the causes of abnormal mental events which it does in terms

---

Box 1.1 The psychodynamic approach to depression

The psychodynamic approach to depression starts with the observation that mourning is a normal response to loss. Depression without an objectively confirmed loss is thought to be due to the loss of an internal mental representation of a person or the loss of a hoped-for outcome (the loss of an 'object'). Freud explained the self-blame of depressed people in the following way. He suggested that the depressed person has mixed feelings toward this person or object and that when love and anger are combined, it is difficult to blame the lost person (e.g. for going away) and the anger is converted into self-reproach. The psychodynamic approach is sometimes taken further to explain how the current response to loss developed in childhood years. For example, Melanie Klein traced this response back to an early stage of childhood when an infant first experiences anger towards the mother that he loves, while she is temporarily absent. Klein suggested that failure to reconcile the conflicting feelings at this early stage of development could lead to vulnerability to depression in adult life.

---

of mental processes of which the patient is unaware (they are 'unconscious'). The difference between the two approaches can be illustrated in relation to persecutory delusions. In descriptive psychopathology, delusions are described and differences noted between delusions and normal beliefs or other forms of abnormal thinking such as obsessions. At the same time, the experience of the deluded person is described: for example, the accompanying feeling of dread and apprehension. By contrast, the psychodynamic approach views delusions as evidence in the conscious mind of activities in the unconscious mind including the mechanisms of repression and projection (see p. 189). The psychodynamic approach to abnormal states of depression is summarized in Box 1.1 as an example of this approach to psychopathology.

Experimental psychopathology

This approach also seeks to explain abnormal phenomena as well as to describe them. The explanations are in terms of experimentally verifiable psychological processes, rather than the unconscious processes referred to in psychodynamic psychopathology. The methods used to investigate abnormal phenomena are those of neuroscience, including brain imaging and cognitive psychology. Although experimental psychopathology is concerned with the causes of symptoms, these have been investigated, necessarily, in the context of the syndromes in which they occur. For this reason, the findings of experimental psychopathology are presented in the chapters on the relevant clinical syndromes. For example, since the experimental psychopathology of anxiety has been studied mainly in patients with anxiety disorders, it is described in the chapter on these disorders. The single exception is the experimental psychopathology of memory which extends across several disorders and will be outlined later in this chapter as an example of the experimental approach.

Terms used to describe symptoms

The form and content of symptoms

When psychiatric symptoms are described, it is useful to distinguish between form and content, a distinction that can be best explained by an example. If a patient says that, when he is alone, he hears voices calling him a homosexual, the *form* of the experience is an auditory hallucination (a sensory perception in the absence of an external stimulus – see below) whilst the *content* is the statement that he is homosexual. A second person might hear voices saying that he is about to be killed; again the form is an auditory hallucination but the content is different. A third person might experience repeated obsessional thoughts that he is homosexual but realizes that these are untrue. The content is the same as that of the first example (concerning homosexuality) but the form is

different – an obsessional thought. Form assists in making a diagnosis. Content is less useful in diagnosis but often highly important in management; for example, the content of a delusion may suggest that the patient could attack a supposed persecutor.

Primary and secondary symptoms

The terms primary and secondary are often used to describe symptoms but unfortunately with two different meanings. The first meaning is *temporal*, primary means occurring first, and secondary means subsequent. The second meaning is *causal* primary means arising directly from the pathological process, and secondary means arising as a reaction to a primary symptom. The two meanings often coincide since symptoms that arise directly from the pathological process usually appear first. However, although subsequent symptoms are often a reaction to the first symptoms, they are not always of this kind, for they, too, may arise direct from the pathological process. The terms primary and secondary are used more often in the temporal sense because this usage does not involve an inference about causality. However, many patients cannot say in what order their symptoms appeared. In such cases, when it seems likely that one symptom is a reaction to another, for example, that a delusion of being followed by persecutors is a reaction to hearing accusing voices, it is called secondary (using the word in the causal sense).

The significance of individual symptoms

Psychiatric disorders are diagnosed when a defined group of symptoms (a syndrome) is present. Almost any single symptom can be experienced by a healthy person; even hallucinations, which are often regarded as a hallmark of mental disorder, are sometimes experienced occasionally and transiently by healthy people. An exception is that an isolated delusion is generally considered to be evidence of psychiatric disorder if it is definite and persistent – see paranoid disorders (Chapter 13). In general, however, the finding of a single symptom is not evidence of psychiatric disorder but an indication for a thorough and, if necessary repeated, search for other symptoms and signs of psychiatric disorder.

The patient's experience

Symptoms and signs are only part of the subject matter of psychopathology. It is concerned also with the patient's experience of illness, and the way in which psychiatric disorder changes his view of himself, his hopes for the future, and his view of the world. A depressive disorder may have a very different effect on a person who has lived a satisfying and happy life and has fulfilled his major ambitions, and a person who has had many previous misfortunes but has lived on hopes of future success. To understand this aspect of the patient's experience of psychiatric disorder, the psychiatrist has to understand him in the way that a biographer understands his subject. This way of understanding is sometimes called the life-story approach. It is not something that can be learnt easily from textbooks; it can be learnt best by taking time to listen to patients. The psychiatrist may be helped by reading biographies or works of literature which can provide useful insights into the ways in which experiences in childhood and throughout life shape the personality, and account for many of the differences in the ways in which different people respond to the same events.

Cultural variations in psychopathology

Symptoms are similar in their form in widely different cultures. However, there are cultural differences in the symptoms that are revealed to doctors; for example, people from the Indian subcontinent are less likely than Europeans to report low mood when they have a depressive disorder, and more likely to report somatic symptoms. The content of symptoms also differs between cultures. For example, people from some African cultures may have delusions concerned with evil spirits, a subject that is observed infrequently among Europeans. Cultural differences

also affect the person's experience of illness. In some cultures, the effects of psychiatric disorder are ascribed to witchcraft, a belief that adds to the patient's distress. In some cultures, mental illness is so greatly stigmatized that it is a bar to marriage. In such a culture the effect of illness on the patient's view of himself and his future will be very different from the effect on a patient living in a society that is more tolerant of mental disorder.

Descriptions of symptoms and signs

Disorders of mood

In psychiatry two terms are used to refer to an emotional state – mood and affect. The words have often been used interchangeably, but mood is now in more general use because it has been adopted in the major classifications. In psychiatric disorders, mood may be abnormal in three ways:

- its nature may be altered;
- it may fluctuate more or less than usual; and
- it may be inconsistent with the patient's thoughts or actions or with his current circumstances.

Changes in the nature of mood

These can be towards anxiety, depression, elation, or irritability and anger. Any of these changes may be associated with events in the person's life, but they may arise without an apparent reason. Change in mood is usually accompanied by other symptoms and signs. For example, an increase of anxiety is accompanied by autonomic overactivity and increased muscle tension, and depression is accompanied by gloomy preoccupations and psychomotor slowness.

Changes in the way that mood varies

Normal mood varies in relation to the person's circumstances and preoccupations. In abnormal states, mood may continue to vary with circumstances but the variations may be greater or less than normal. Increased variation is called *lability* of mood; extreme variation is sometimes called *emotional incontinence*. Reduced variation of mood is called *blunting* or *flattening*. Severe flattening is sometimes called *apathy* (note the difference from the layman's meaning of the word).

Mood can also vary in a way that is not in keeping with the person's circumstances and thoughts. For example, a normal person feels sad when thinking about a loss. In some psychiatric disorders, mood is *incongruous*, that is, it does not match the patient's circumstances and thoughts. For example, a patient may appear to be in high spirits and may laugh when talking about the death of his mother. Such incongruity of mood must be distinguished from the embarrassed laughter that indicates that the person is ill at ease. Sometimes, patients show no emotion in circumstances which would normally elicit an emotional response. This condition is called *flattening* of mood.

Clinical associations Disorders of mood are found in many psychiatric disorder. They are the central feature of the mood disorders and anxiety disorders. They are common also in obsessional disorders, eating disorders, substance-induced disorders, delirium, dementia, and schizophrenia.

Anxiety

Anxiety is a normal response to danger. Anxiety is abnormal when its severity is out of proportion to the threat of danger or when it outlasts the threat. Anxious mood is closely coupled with somatic and autonomic components, and with psychological ones. All can be thought of as equivalent to the preparations for dealing with danger seen in other mammals, ready for flight from, avoidance of, or fighting with a predator. Mild-to-moderate anxiety enhances most kinds of performance, but very high levels interfere with it.

The components of the anxiety response are considered further in Chapter 9; here they can be summarized as follows.

Psychological components The essential feelings of dread and apprehension are accompanied by restlessness, narrowing of attention to focus on the source of danger, worrying thoughts, increased alertness (with insomnia) and irritability (that is a readiness to become angry).

Somatic components Muscle tension and respiration increase. If these changes are not followed by physical activity, they may be experienced as muscle tension tremor, or the effects of hyperventilation (e.g. dizziness – see p. 220).

Autonomic components Heart rate and sweating increase, the mouth becomes dry, and there may be an urge to urinate or defecate.

Avoidance of danger The term *phobia* is used to describe the habitual avoidance of a situation to an extent that exceeds the extent of the danger. A phobia is a persistent irrational fear of, and wish to avoid, a specific object or situation. The fear is out of proportion to the objective threat, and is recognized as such by the person experiencing it. The objects that provoke fear include animate ones such as dogs, snakes, and spiders, and natural phenomena such as thunder. The situations include high places, crowds, and open spaces. Phobic people feel anxious not only in the presence of the object or situation but also when thinking about them (*anticipatory anxiety*).

Clinical associations

Phobias are common among healthy children, becoming less frequent in adolescence and adult life. Phobic symptoms occur in all kinds of anxiety disorder but are the major feature in the phobic disorders (see p. 226).

Readers should note that the term phobia is sometimes used to denote excessive fears without avoidance as the terms phobia of illness (see p. 227) and dysmorphophobia (see p. 259). Phobias are discussed further in relation to anxiety disorders on p. 226–37.

Depression

Depression is a normal response to loss or misfortune. Depression is abnormal when it is out of proportion to the misfortune or unduly prolonged. Depressive mood is closely coupled with other changes, notably a lowering of self-esteem, self-criticism, and pessimistic thinking. A sad person has a characteristic expression with turned corners of the mouth, a furrowed brow, and a hunched, dejected posture. The level of arousal is reduced in some depressed patients but increased in others with a consequent feeling of restlessness. Depression occurs in many psychiatric disorders. It is the defining feature of the depressive disorders (see Chapter 11) and it occurs commonly in schizophrenia, anxiety and obsessional disorders, and in eating disorders.

Depressive mood and associated changes are discussed further in relation to mood disorders on p. 272–74.

Elation

Happy moods have been studied less than depressed mood. Elation is an extreme degree of happy mood which, like depression, is coupled with other changes including increased feelings of self-confidence and well-being, increased activity, and increased arousal. The latter is usually experienced as pleasant but sometime as an unpleasant feeling of restlessness. Elation occurs most often in mania and hypomania.

Irritability and anger

Irritability is a state of increased readiness for anger. Both irritability and anger may occur in many kinds of disorder so that they are of little value in diagnosis. They are, however, of great importance in management and, if present, they should prompt an assessment of the risk of violence (see p. 55). Irritability and depression may occur in anxiety disorders, mood disorders, schizophrenia, dementia and intoxication with alcohol or drugs. In some cases they may result not only in harm to others but also in self-harm.

Disorders of perception

Perception and imagery

Perception is the process of becoming aware of what is presented through the sense organs. It is not a direct awareness of data from the sense organs because these data are acted on by cognitive processes that reassemble them and extract patterns. Perception can be attended to or ignored, but it cannot be terminated by an effort of will.

Imagery is the awareness of a percept that has not arisen from the sense organs but has been generated within the mind. Imagery can be called up and terminated by an effort of will. Images are experienced as lacking the sense of reality that characterizes perception so that a healthy person can distinguish between images and percepts. A few people experience *eidetic imagery* that is visual imagery so intense and detailed that it has a 'photographic' quality akin to a percept, though in other ways it differs from a percept. Imagery is generally terminated when perception starts. Occasionally, imagery persists despite the presence of percept (provided this is weak and unstructured). This sort of imagery is called *pareidolia*.

Changes in the intensity and quality of perception

Percepts may alter in intensity and in quality. Anxious people may experience sensations as more intense than usual; for example, a person may be unusually sensitive to noise. In mania, perceptions seem more intense and vivid than usual. Depressed patients may experience perceptions as dull and lifeless. Some schizophrenic patients experience sensations as unpleasant (for example, food tastes bitter), or as distorted in unusual ways, (for example, a flower smells like burning flesh).

Illusions

Illusions are misperceptions of external stimuli. They occur when the general level of sensory stimulation is reduced and when attention is not focused on the relevant sensory modality. For example, at dusk the outline of a bush may be perceived at first as the that of a man, though not when attention is focused on the outline. Illusions occur also when the level of consciousness is reduced, as in delirium. Thus delirious patients may experience illusions even when the level of illumination is normal, though they do so more readily when lighting is poor. In both a healthy state and in delirium, illusions are more likely when the person is anxious. Thus in a dark lane a frightened person is more likely than a calm person to misperceive the outline of a bush as that of a man.

Hallucinations

A hallucination is a percept experienced in the absence of an external stimulus to the corresponding sense organ. It differs from an illusion in being experienced as originating in the outside world or from within the person's body (rather than as imagined). Hallucinations cannot be terminated at will.

Although hallucinations are generally indications of a psychiatric disorder, they occur occasionally in healthy people, usually when falling asleep (hypnagogic hallucinations) or on waking (hypnopompic hallucinations). These two types of hallucination may be either visual or auditory, the latter sometimes as the experience of hearing one's name called. Such hallucinations are common in narcolepsy (see p. 440). Some recently bereaved people experience hallucinations of the dead person. Hallucinations can occur after sensory deprivation, in people with blindness or deafness of peripheral origin, occasionally in neurological disorders affecting the visual pathways, in temporal lobe seizures and the fortification spectra of epilepsy, and in the Charles Bonnet syndrome (visual hallucinations associated with disease of the visual pathways).

Pseudohallucinations

This term refers to experiences that are similar to hallucinations but do not meet all the requirements of the definition. The word pseudohallucination has two distinct meanings, which correspond to two of the ways in which an experience can fail to meet the criteria for a hallucination. In the first meaning, pseudohallucination is a sensory experience that differs from a hallucination in not seeming to the patient to represent external reality. Instead, the percepts seem to be located within the mind rather than in external space. In this way pseudohallucinations resemble imagery though, unlike imagery, they cannot be dismissed by an effort of will. In the second meaning of pseudohallucination, the sensory experience appears to originate in the external world, but it seems unreal. Taylor (1981) suggested separate terms for these two kinds of experience:

◆ 'imaged' pseudohallucinations for those experienced within the mind; and

◆ 'perceived' pseudohallucinations for those experienced as located in external space but recognized as unreal.

Though logical, these terms are not used widely.

Both definitions of pseudohallucination are difficult to apply to a particular case because patients can seldom describe their experiences in sufficient detail. In everyday clinical work, however, failure to identify pseudohallucinations is not particularly important since neither kind is significant in diagnosis. It is enough to decide whether an experience is a hallucination or not. If it is not a hallucination, the experience should be described but need not be labelled as one or other kind of pseudohallucination. For a more detailed discussion see Hare (1973), Taylor (1981), Jaspers (1963, pp. 68–74), and Sedman (1966).

Types of hallucination

Hallucinations can be described in terms of their complexity and their sensory modality (Table 1.1). The term *elementary hallucination* refers to experiences such as bangs, whistles, and flashes of light; *complex hallucination* refers to experiences such as hearing voices or music, or seeing faces and scenes.

Hallucinations may be auditory, visual, gustatory, olfactory, tactile, or of deep sensation. *Auditory hallucinations* may be experienced as noises, music, or voices. (Hallucinatory 'voices' are sometimes referred to as *phonemes*.) Voices may be heard clearly or indistinctly; they may seem to speak words, phrases, or sentences. They may seem to address the patient directly (*second-person hallucinations*) or talk to one another referring to the patient as 'he' or 'she' (*third-*

Table 1.1 Description of hallucinations

According to complexity
    Elementary
    Complex
According to sensory modality
    Auditory
    Visual
    Olfactory and gustatory
    Somatic (tactile and deep)
According to special features
    Auditory
        second-person
        third-person
        Gedankenlautwerden
        écho de la pensée
    Visual
        extracampine
Autoscopic hallucinations
Reflex hallucinations
Hypnagogic and hypnopompic

person hallucinations). Sometimes patients say that the voices anticipate what they are about to think a few moments later. Sometimes the voices seem to speak the patient's thoughts as he is thinking them (*Gedankenlautwerden*) or to repeat them immediately after he has thought them (*écho de la pensée*).

Visual hallucinations may also be elementary or complex. The content may appear normal or abnormal in size; if the latter, they are more often smaller than the corresponding real percept. Visual hallucinations of dwarf figures are sometimes called *lilliputian*. Occasionally, patients describe the strange experience of visual hallucinations located outside the field of vision, usually behind the head (*extracampine hallucinations*).

Olfactory and gustatory hallucinations are frequently experienced together. The smells and tastes are often unpleasant.

Tactile hallucinations, sometimes called *haptic* hallucinations, may be experienced as sensations of being touched, pricked, or strangled. Sometimes they are felt as movements just below the skin, which the patient may attribute to insects, worms, or other small creatures burrowing through the tissues. *Hallucinations of deep sensation* may be experienced as feelings of the viscera being pulled upon or distended, or of sexual stimulation or electric shocks.

An *autoscopic hallucination* is the experience of seeing one's own body projected into external space, usually in front of oneself, for short periods. The experience is reported occasionally by mentally healthy people in situations of sensory deprivation, when it is called an out-of-body experience, or after a near-fatal accident or heart attack when it has been called a near-death experience. Autoscopic hallucinations occur occasionally in a psychiatric disorder, usually associated with temporal lobe epilepsy or an organic brain disorder (see Lukianowicz 1958 and Lhermitte 1951 for detailed accounts). Rarely, the experience is accompanied by the conviction that the person has a double (*Doppelganger*).

The term *reflex hallucination* is used to describe the rare condition in which a stimulus in one sensory modality results in a hallucination in another; for example, music may provoke visual hallucinations. Reflex hallucinations may occur after taking drugs such as LSD or, rarely, in schizophrenia.

Hypnagogic and *hypnopompic* hallucinations occur at the point of falling asleep and of waking, respectively. When they occur in healthy people, they are brief and elementary – for example, hearing a bell ring or a name called. Usually the person wakes suddenly and recognizes the nature of the experience. In narcolepsy, such hallucinations are common and may last longer and be more elaborate than those experienced by healthy people who are falling asleep or waking.

Abnormalities in the meaning attached to percepts

People ascribe meaning to the things they perceive. In some psychiatric disorders an abnormal meaning or significance is attached to a normal percept. When this happens we speak of *delusional perception*.

Delusional perception is a disorder of thinking, not of perception, and it is considered with other disorders of thinking (see p. 15).

Diagnostic associations

Hallucinations may occur in severe affective disorders, schizophrenia, organic disorders, and dissociative states, and at times among healthy people. Therefore, the finding of hallucinations does not itself help much in diagnosis. However, the following kinds of hallucination do have important implications for diagnosis.

Auditory hallucinations Both the form and content of auditory hallucinations can help in diagnosis. Of the various types – noises, music, and voices – the only ones of diagnostic significance are voices heard as speaking clearly to or about the patient. As already explained, voices that appear to be talking to each other, referring to the patient as he or she, are called *third-person hallucinations*. They are associated strongly with schizophrenia. Such voices may be experienced as commenting on the patient's intentions (e.g. 'he wants to make love to her') or actions (e.g. 'she is washing her face').

Second-person auditory hallucinations appear to address the patient (e.g. 'you are going to die') or give commands (e.g. 'hit him'). In themselves they do not point to a particular diagnosis, but their content and especially the patient's reaction may do so. Thus voices with derogatory content (e.g. 'you are a failure, you are wicked'), suggest severe depressive disorder, especially when the patient accepts them as justified. In schizophrenia the patient more often resents such comments. Voices which *anticipate, echo, or repeat* the patient's thoughts also suggest schizophrenia.

Visual hallucinations should always suggest the possibility of an organic disorder, although they occur also in some severe affective disorders, schizophrenia, and dissociative disorder. The content of visual hallucinations is of little significance in diagnosis.

Hallucinations of taste and smell are infrequent. They may occur in schizophrenia, severe depressive disorders, and temporal lobe epilepsy, and in tumours affecting the olfactory bulb or pathways.

Tactile and somatic hallucinations are not of much diagnostic significance, although a few special kinds are weakly associated with particular disorders. Thus hallucinatory sensations of sexual intercourse suggest schizophrenia, especially if interpreted in an unusual way (e.g. as resulting from intercourse with persecutors). The sensation of insects moving under the skin occurs in people who abuse cocaine and occasionally among schizophrenics.

Disorders of thinking

The term disorder of thinking covers four separate kinds of phenomena (Table 1.2):

- particular kinds of abnormal thinking, namely delusions and obsessional thoughts;
- disorders of the stream of thought, that is, the amount and the speed of thinking;
- disorders of the form of thought, that is, abnormalities of the way that thought are linked together;
- abnormal beliefs about the 'possession' of thoughts, that is, of the normal awareness that one's thoughts are one's own.

The second and third of these four kinds of phenomena are considered next.

Table 1.2 **Disorders of thinking**
Particular kinds of abnormal thoughts
Delusions
Obsessions (see p. 19)
Disorders of the stream of thought (speed and pressure)
Disorder of the form of thought (linking of thoughts together)
Abnormal beliefs about the possession of thoughts

Disorders of the stream of thought

In disorders of the stream of thought, the amount and the speed of thinking are changed. In *pressure of thought*, ideas arise in unusual variety and abundance and pass through the mind rapidly. In *poverty of thought*, the patient has a few thoughts, and these lack variety and richness and seem to move slowly through the mind. Pressure of thought occurs in mania; poverty occurs in depressive disorders. Either may be experienced in schizophrenia.

Thought block

Sometimes the stream of thought is interrupted suddenly. The patient feels that his mind has gone blank, and an observer notices a sudden interruption in the patient's speech. In a minor degree this experience is common, particularly among people who are tired or anxious. In thought blocking, the interruptions are sudden, striking, and repeated, and experienced by the patient as an abrupt and complete emptying of his mind. Thought blocking is an important symptom since it strongly suggests schizophrenia, so it is important to record it only if it is certainly present. Other reasons for a sudden interruption in speech should be excluded, namely sudden distraction, tiredness, and anxiety. The diagnostic association with schizophrenia is stronger when the patient interprets the experience in an unusual way, for example, when he says that his thoughts have been removed by another person.

Disorders of the form of thought

Disorder of the form of thought (also known as *formal thought disorder*) is usually recognized from speech and writing but is sometimes evident from the patient's behaviour; for example, he may be unable to file papers under appropriate category headings. Disorders of the form of thought can be divided into perseveration, flight of ideas, and loosening of associations. Each kind has associations with a particular mental disorder, but none of the associations is strong enough to be diagnostic.

Perseveration is the persistent and inappropriate repetition of the same thoughts. The disorder is detected by examining the person's words or actions. Thus, in response to a series of simple questions, the person may give the correct answer to the first but continue to give the same answer inappropriately to subsequent questions. Perseveration occurs in dementia but is not confined to this condition.

In *flight of ideas*, thoughts and speech move quickly from one topic to another so that one train of thought is not carried to completion before another takes its place. The normal logical sequence of ideas is generally preserved, although ideas may be linked by distracting cues in the surroundings and by distractions arising from the words that have been spoken. These verbal distractions are of three kinds: *clang associations* (a second word with a sound similar to the first), *puns* (a second meaning of the first word), and *rhymes*. In practice, the distinction between flight of ideas and loosening of associations (see below) is difficult, especially when the patient speaks rapidly. When this happens it is often helpful to record a sample of speech and listen to it several times. Flight of ideas is characteristic of mania.

Loosening of associations denotes a loss of the normal structure of thinking. To the interviewer the patient's discourse seems muddled and illogical and it does not become clearer when the patient is questioned further. Several specific features of this muddled thinking have been described (see below), but they are difficult to identify with certainty and the most striking clinical impression is often a general lack of clarity. This lack of clarity differs from that of people who are anxious or of low intelligence. Anxious people give a more coherent account when they have been put at ease, and people with low intelligence usually express their ideas more clearly when the interviewer simplifies the questions and allows more time for the reply. When there is loosening of associations, the interviewer has the experience that the more he tries to clarify the patient's thinking, the less he understands it. Loosening of associations occurs most often in schizophrenia.

Three kinds of loosening of associations have been described:

- *Knight's move or derailment* refers to a transition from one topic to another, either between sentences or in mid-sentence, with no logical relationship between the two topics and no evidence of the associations described above under flight of ideas.

- In *talking past the point* (Vorbeireden) the patient seems always about to get near to the matter in hand but skirts round it and never reaches it.

- *Verbigeration* is said to be present when speech is reduced to the senseless repetition of sounds, words, or phrases. This abnormality can occur with severe expressive aphasia and occasionally in schizophrenia. When this abnormality is extreme the disorder is called *word salad*.

Related disorders of thinking include overinclusion and neologisms. *Overinclusion* refers to a widening of the boundaries of concepts, such that things are grouped together that are not normally regarded as closely connected. *Neologisms* are words or phrases, invented by the patient, often to describe a morbid experience. Neologisms must be distinguished from incorrect pronunciation, the wrong use of words by people with limited education, dialect words, obscure technical terms, and the 'private words' that some families invent to amuse themselves. Before deciding that a word is a neologism, the interviewer should ask the patient what he means by it. Neologisms occur most often in chronic schizophrenia.

Delusions

The definition

A delusion is a belief that is firmly held on inadequate grounds, is not affected by rational argument or evidence to the contrary, and is not a conventional belief that the person might be expected to hold given his educational and cultural background. This definition is intended to separate delusions, which are indicators of mental disorder, from other kinds of strongly held belief found among healthy people.

Problems with the definition

Delusions are firmly held despite evidence to the contrary The hallmark of a delusion is that it is held with such conviction that it cannot be altered by presenting evidence to the contrary. For example, a patient who holds the delusion that there are persecutors in the adjoining house will not be convinced by evidence that the house is empty; instead he may suggest that the persecutors left the house shortly before it was searched. The problem of this criterion for delusions is that some of the ideas of normal people are equally impervious to contrary evidence; for example, the beliefs of a convinced spiritualist are not undermined by the counter-arguments of a non-believer. Such strongly held non-delusional beliefs are called *over-valued ideas* (see below).

A further problem about this part of the definition of delusion relates to *partial delusions*. Although delusions are usually held strongly from the start, sometimes they are at first held with a degree of doubt. Also during recovery from a delusional disorder it is not uncommon for patients to pass through a stage of increasing doubt about their delusions before finally rejecting them. The term partial delusion refers to both these situations of doubt. It should be used during recovery only when it is known that the beliefs were preceded by a full delusion, and applied to the development of a delusion only when it is known in retrpspect that a full delusion developed later. Partial delusions are not helpful in diagnosis though they should prompt a search for other evidence of mental disorder.

Delusions are held on inadequate grounds Delusions are not arrived at by the ordinary processes of observation and logic. Some delusions appear suddenly without any previous thinking about the subject (primary delusions – see below). Other delusions appear to be attempts to explain another abnormal experience, for example, the delusion that hallucinated voices are those of people who are spying on the patient. (Delusions that fail to meet this criterion, are nevertheless not corrected by evidence so they meet the first criterion.)

Delusions are not beliefs shared by others in the same culture This criterion is important when the patient is a member of a culture or subculture because healthy people in such a group may hold beliefs that are not accepted outside it. Like delusions, such cultural beliefs are generally impervious to contrary evidence and reasoned argument, for example, beliefs in evil spirits. Therefore, before deciding that an idea is delusional, it is important to determine whether other members of the same culture share the belief.

Delusions as false beliefs Some definitions of delusion indicate that they are false beliefs but this criterion was not included in the definition given above. This omission is because in exceptional circumstances a delusional belief can be true or subsequently become true. A well-recognized example relates to pathological jealousy (p. 389). A man may develop a jealous delusion about his wife in the absence of any reasonable evidence of infidelity. Even if the wife is secretly being unfaithful at the time, the belief is still delusional if there is no rational ground for holding it. It is not falsity that determines whether the belief is delusional, but the nature of the mental processes that led up to it. (The difficulty of this statement is that we cannot define these mental processes precisely.) There is a further practical problem about the use of falsity as a criterion for delusion. It is that if the criterion is used, it may be assumed that because a belief is highly improbable, it is false. This is certainly not a sound assumption because improbable stories of, for example, persecution by neighbours, or of attempts at poisoning by a spouse, sometimes turn out to be true and arrived at through sound observations and logical thought. Ideas should be investigated thoroughly before they are accepted as delusions.

Beliefs and behaviour

Strongly held normal beliefs usually affect the feelings and actions of the person who holds them. The same is generally true of delusions but not always. Sometimes a patient is wholly convinced that a delusional belief is true, but this conviction does not influence all his feelings and actions. This separation of belief from feeling and action is known as *double orientation*. It occurs most often in chronic schizophrenia. For example, a patient may believe that he is a member of a Royal Family while living contentedly in a hostel for discharged psychiatric patients.

Types of delusion

Delusions are of many kinds, which will now be described. Readers may find it helpful to refer to the summary in Table 1.3. as a guide to the account that follows.

Table 1.3 **Descriptions of delusions**
According to fixity
Complete
Partial
According to onset
Primary
Secondary
Other delusional experiences
Delusional mood
Delusional perception
Delusional memory
According to theme
Persecutory (paranoid)
Delusions of reference
Grandiose (expansive)
Delusions of guilt and worthlessness
Nihilistic
Hypochondriacal
Religious
Jealous
Sexual or amorous
Delusions of control
Delusions concerning possession of thought
Thought insertion
Thought withdrawal
Thought broadcasting
According to other features
Shared delusions

Primary delusions A primary or *autochthonous* delusion is one that appears suddenly and with full conviction but without any mental events leading up to it. For example, a schizophrenic patient may be suddenly and completely convinced that he is changing sex, without ever having thought of it before and without any preceding ideas or events which could have led in any understandable way to this conclusion. The belief arrives in the mind suddenly, fully formed, and in a totally convincing form as if it were a direct expression of the pathological process causing the mental illness.

Not all primary delusional experiences start with an idea. Sometimes the first experience is a delusional mood (see below) or a delusional perception (see below), either of which can arise suddenly and without any antecedent to account for it. Because patients do not find it easy to remember the exact sequence of such unusual and distressing mental events, it is often difficult to be certain which experience came first. Primary delusions are given considerable weight in the diagnosis of schizophrenia, and they should be recorded only when it is certain that they are present.

Secondary delusions These are delusions apparently derived from a preceding morbid experience. The latter may be of several kinds, including hallucinations (e.g. someone who hears voices may believe that he is being followed), a change of mood (e.g. a person who is profoundly depressed may believe that people think he is worthless), or an existing delusion (e.g. a person with the delusion that he has lost all his money may come to believe he will be put in prison for failing to pay debts). Some secondary delusions seem to have an integrative function, making the original experiences more comprehensible to the patient, as in the first example above. Others seem to do the opposite, increasing the sense of persecution or failure, as in the third example.

Secondary delusions may accumulate until there is a complicated delusional system. When this happens the delusions are said to be *systematized*.

Shared delusions As a rule, other people recognize delusions as false and argue with the patient in an attempt to correct them. Occasionally, a person who lives with a deluded patient comes to share his delusional beliefs. This condition is known as shared delusions or *folie à deux*. Although the second person's delusional conviction is as strong as the partner's while the couple remain together, it often recedes quickly when they are separated. The condition is described more fully on p. 394.

Delusional mood When a patient first experiences a delusion, he responds emotionally. For example, a person who believes that a group of people intend to kill him is likely to feel afraid. Occasionally, the change of mood precedes the delusion. This preceding mood is often a feeling of foreboding that some as yet unidentified sinister event is about to take place. When the delusion follows, it appears explain this feeling. For example, the sense of unexplained foreboding may be followed by the delusion that the people are plotting to harm the patient. In German this change of mood is called Wahnstimmung. This term usually translated as *delusional mood* although it is really the mood from which a delusion arises.

Delusional perception Sometimes the first abnormal experience is the attaching of a new significance to a familiar percept without any reason to do so. For example, the position of a letter left on the patient's desk may be interpreted as a signal that he is to die. This experience is called delusional perception. The abnormality is, presumably, in the later stages of perception in which meaning is ascribed to a percept.

Delusional misinterpretation In this rare disorder, a patient has the delusional belief that a familiar person has been replaced by an impostor who is the exact double of the original. This symptom is sometimes referred to by the French term *l'illusion de sosies* (translated as the *illusion of doubles* although it is a delusion, not an illusion). The symptom is the central feature of Capgras' syndrome – see

p. 393. The opposite kind of misinterpretation occurs when a patient sees several different people, one after the other, and believes that he has seen a single person in multiple disguises. This rare delusion, which is called the *Fregoli delusion*, is described further on p. 394.

Delusional memory In delusional memory, a new significance is attached to past events. For example, a patient who believes that there is a current plot to poison him, may remember that he vomited after a meal, eaten long before his present delusional system began, and conclude that he was poisoned on that occasion. This experience has to be distinguished from the accurate recall of a delusional idea already present on the previous occasion. The term delusional memory is unsatisfactory because it is not the memory that is delusional but the significance attached to it.

Delusional themes

For the purposes of clinical work, it is useful to group delusions according to their main themes. This grouping is useful because there is some correspondence between these themes and the major forms of mental illness. Some important associations are described next but there are many exceptions to them. Before considering delusional themes we need to consider the term paranoid.

The term paranoid The term paranoid is often used as if it were equivalent to persecutory. Strictly interpreted, however, paranoid has a wider meaning. The word was used in ancient Greek writings to mean the equivalent of 'out of his mind'; for example, Hippocrates used it to describe patients with febrile delirium. Many later writers applied the term to grandiose, erotic, jealous, and religious delusions as well as to persecutory delusions. Although, for historical reasons, it is preferable to retain the broader meaning of paranoid, the narrower usage is current. This usage is sanctioned, in the nomenclature, in the term paranoid personality disorder, which is characterized by suspicion, sensitivity and mistrust – see p. 166. Until recently, the wider use of the term paranoid was also approved in the nomenclature by the use of the term paranoid syndromes. However, these syndromes are now referred to by the term delusional disorder (see Chapter 13). Because the term paranoid has two possible meanings, the term persecutory is preferable when the narrow sense of paranoid is required.

Persecutory delusions These are most commonly concerned with persons or organizations that are thought to be trying to inflict harm on the patient, damage his reputation, or make him insane. Such delusions are common but of little help in diagnosis, because they can also occur in organic states, schizophrenia, and severe affective disorders. However, the patient's attitude to the delusion may point to the diagnosis. In a severe depressive disorder, a patient with persecutory delusions characteristically accepts the supposed activities of the persecutors as justified by his own wickedness. In schizophrenia, however, he resents these activities as unwarranted. In assessing persecutory ideas, it is essential to remember the warning, given above, that apparently improbable accounts of persecution are sometimes true, and that it is normal in some cultures to ascribe misfortunes to the malign activities of other people, for example through witchcraft.

Freud's theory of persecutory delusions is of interest as it was important in the history of psychiatry. It is, however, unsupported by evidence (see Box 1.2).

Delusions of reference These are concerned with the idea that objects, events, or people, unconnected with the patient, have a personal significance for him. For example, the patient may believe that an article in a newspaper or a remark on television, is directed specifically to himself, either as a message to him or to inform others about him. Delusions of reference may also relate to actions or gestures made by other people which are thought to convey a message about the patient; for example, a person who touches his hair may be thought by the patient to be signalling that he, the patient, is turning into a woman. Although most delusions of reference

Box 1.2 Freud's theory of persecutory delusions

Freud expressed his theory as follows (see Freud 1958):

'the study of a number of cases of delusions of persecution has led me as well as other investigators to the view that the relation between the patient and his persecutor can be reduced to a simple formula. It appears that the person to whom the delusion ascribes so much power and influence is either identical with someone who played an equally important part in the patient's emotional life before illness, or an easily recognizable substitute for him. The intensity of the emotion is projected in the shape of external power, whilst its quality is changed into the opposite. The person who is now hated and feared for being a persecutor was at one time loved and honoured. The main purpose of the persecution asserted by the patient's delusion is to justify the change in his emotional attitude.'

Freud went on to summarize his view as follows:

'delusions of persecution are the result of the sequence "I do not love him – I hate him, because he persecutes me".' (Freud 1958, p. 63–4)
Freud's theory has not been supported by evidence.

have persecutory associations, some relate to grandiose or reassuring themes.

Grandiose or expansive delusions These are beliefs of exaggerated self-importance. The patient may think himself wealthy, endowed with unusual abilities, or a special person. Such ideas occur in mania and in schizophrenia.

Delusions of guilt and worthlessness These are found most often in depressive illness, and for this reason are sometimes called *depressive delusions*. Typical themes are that a minor infringement of the law in the past will be discovered and bring shame upon the patient, or that his sinfulness will lead to retribution on his family.

Nihilistic delusions These are beliefs that some person or thing has ceased, or is about to cease, to exist. Examples include a patient's delusion that he has no money, that his career is ruined or that the world is about to end. Nihilistic delusions are associated especially with very severe depressive disorder. Occasionally, nihilistic delusions concern failures of bodily function, often that the bowels are blocked. When this delusion occurs in a severe depressive disorder, the condition is known as *Cotard's syndrome* (see p. 275).

Hypochondriacal delusions These are concerned with illness. The patient believes, wrongly and in the face of all medical evidence to the contrary, that he is suffering from a disease. Such delusions are more common in the elderly, reflecting the increasing concern with health among the people of this age group. Other hypochondriacal delusions are concerned with cancer or venereal disease, or with the appearance of parts of the body, especially the nose. Patients with delusions of the last kind sometimes request plastic surgery. The delusions of a patient with Cotard's syndrome, described above under nihilistic delusions, can also be regarded as hypochondriacal.

Religious delusions When a member of a religious group holds firmly to seemingly abnormal religious beliefs, it is important to speak to another member of the group to determine whether they are in fact abnormal within the group. Normally held religious beliefs are shared by others of the same faith, have been acquired through teaching, and may be subject to periods of doubt. Delusions with a religious content were much more frequent in the nineteenth century than they are today (Klaf and Hamilton 1961), presumably because religion played a greater part in the lives of ordinary people at that time.

Delusions of jealousy These are more common among men than women. Not all jealous ideas are delusions; less intense jealous preoccupations are common, and some obsessional thoughts are concerned with doubts about the spouse's fidelity. Jealous delusions are important because they may lead to dangerously aggressive behaviour towards the person thought to be unfaithful. Special care is needed if the patient acts on the beliefs, for example, by following the partner, examining clothes for marks of semen, or searching for letters or other evidence of infidelity. A patient with delusional jealousy is not satisfied if he fails to find evidence supporting his beliefs; his search will continue. These important and potentially dangerous problems are discussed further in Chapter 13.

Sexual or amorous delusions These are rare. When they occur, they are more frequent among women. Sexual delusions may be primary, or secondary to somatic hallucinations felt in the genitalia. A person with amorous delusions believes that she is loved by a man who is usually inaccessible to her, and often of higher social status. In many cases she has never spoken to the person. Erotic delusions are the most prominent feature of De Clérambault's syndrome which is described in Chapter 13.

Delusions of control A patient who has a delusion of control believes that his actions, impulses, or thoughts are controlled by an outside agency. Because the symptom strongly suggests schizophrenia, it is important not to record it unless it is definitely present. The symptom may be confused with:

- voluntary obedience to commands from hallucinatory voices; and
- religious beliefs that God controls human actions.

By contrast, a patient with a delusion of control firmly believes that his movements or actions are brought about by an outside agency (other than the divine), and not willed by himself.

Delusions concerning the possession of thoughts Healthy people take it for granted that their thoughts are their own. They know also that thoughts are private experiences that become known to other

people only if spoken aloud, or revealed in writing or through facial expression, gesture, or action. Patients with delusions concerning the possession of thoughts lose these normal convictions in one or more of three ways, all of which are strongly associated with schizophrenia:

- *Delusions of thought insertion* are beliefs that certain thoughts are not the patient's own but implanted by an outside agency. Often there is an associated explanatory delusion, for example, that persecutors have used radio waves to insert the thoughts. This experience must not be confused with that of the obsessional patient who may be distressed by thoughts that he feels are alien to his nature but who never doubts that these thoughts are his own. The patient with a delusion of thought insertion believes that the thoughts are not his own but have been inserted into his mind.

- *Delusions of thought withdrawal* are beliefs that thoughts have been taken out of the mind. The delusion usually accompanies thought blocking: the patient experiences a sudden break in the flow of thoughts and believes that the 'missing' thoughts have been taken away by some outside agency. Often there are associated explanatory delusions comparable to those accompanying delusions of thought insertion (see above).

- *Delusions of thought broadcasting* are beliefs that unspoken thoughts are known to other people through radio, telepathy or in some other way. Some patients also believe that their thoughts can be heard by other people [a belief which also accompanies the experience of hearing one's own thoughts spoken (Gedankenlautwerden), described above]. Delusions of thought broadcasting are often accompanied by explanatory delusions.

Overvalued ideas

An overvalued idea is an isolated preoccupying belief, neither delusional nor obsessional in nature, which comes to dominate a person's life for many years and may affect his actions. The preoccupying belief may be understandable when the person's background is known. For example, a person whose mother and sister suffered from cancer one after the other may become convinced that cancer is contagious. Overvalued ideas were first described by Wernicke (1900). They differ from religious beliefs in that the latter are shared by a wider group, arise from religious instruction, and are subject to periodic doubts. Although the distinction between delusions and overvalued ideas is not always easy to make, this difficulty seldom leads to practical problems because diagnosis depends on more than the presence or absence of a single symptom. Overvalued ideas concerning shape and weight are a prominent feature of anorexia nervosa. For further information about overvalued ideas the reader is referred to McKenna (1984).

Intrusive thoughts

Intrusive thoughts appear spontaneously in the mind, interrupting the train of thought. Intrusive thoughts can usually be terminated before long by an effort of will. According to their content, the thoughts may provoke an emotional response of anxiety, depression, anger, or sexual arousal. The latter may be experienced as pleasurable and the thoughts encouraged, but others are resisted. Although efforts to suppress may succeed in the short term, they may make recurrence more likely in the longer term (Salkovskis and Campbell 1994), suggesting that distraction may be a better way of coping with such thoughts. Intrusive thoughts do not have diagnostic value. They occur in depressive, anxiety, and many other psychiatric disorders, and occur after substance abuse when they are associated with craving.

Obsessional and compulsive symptoms

Obsessions

Obsessions are recurrent persistent thoughts, impulses, or images that enter the mind despite efforts to exclude them. One characteristic feature is the subjective sense of a struggle – the patient resists the obsession, which nevertheless intrudes into his awareness. Another characteristic feature is a conviction that to think something is to make it more likely to happen. Obsessions are recognized by the person as his own and not implanted from elsewhere (in contrast to delusions of thought insertion – see p. 18). Obsessions are regarded as untrue or senseless – an important point of distinction from delusions. They are generally about matters which the patient finds distressing or otherwise unpleasant.

The presence of resistance is important because, together with the lack of conviction about the truth of the idea, it distinguishes obsessions from delusions. However, when obsessions have been present for a long time, the amount of resistance may diminish. This change seldom causes diagnostic difficulties because, by the time it happens, the nature of the symptom has usually been established. Also, when the obsessions are very intense, patients may become less certain that they are false. However, the former lack of conviction returns when the intensity grows less.

The various forms of obsessions (Table 1.4)

Obsessional thoughts These are repeated and intrusive words or phrases which are upsetting to the patient, for example, repeated obscenities or blasphemous phrases coming into the awareness of a religious person.

Obsessional ruminations These are repeated worrying themes of a more complex kind, for example, about the ending of the world.

Obsessional doubts These are repeated themes expressing uncertainty about previous actions, for example, whether or not the person turned off an electrical appliance that might cause a fire. Whatever the nature of the doubt, the person realizes that the degree of uncertainty and consequent distress is unreasonable.

Table 1.4 Obsessional and compulsive symptoms
Obsessions
Thoughts
Ruminations
Doubts
Impulses
Obsessional phobias
Compulsions (rituals)
Obsessional slowness

Obsessional impulses These are repeated urges to carry out actions, usually actions that are aggressive, dangerous, or socially embarrassing. Examples are the urge to pick up a knife and stab another person, to jump in front of a train, or to shout obscenities in church. Whatever the urge, the person has no wish to carry it out, resists it strongly, and does not act on it.

Obsessional phobia This term denotes an obsessional symptom associated with avoidance as well as anxiety; for example, the obsessional impulse to injure another person with a knife may lead to consequent avoidance of knives. Sometimes obsessional fears of illness are called *illness phobias*.

The content of obsessions

Although the content (or themes) of obsessions are various, most can be grouped into one or other of six categories:

- dirt and contamination
- aggression
- orderliness
- illness
- sex
- religion.

Thoughts about *dirt and contamination* are usually associated with the idea of harming others through the spread of disease. *Aggressive thoughts* may be about striking another person or shouting angry or obscene remarks in public. Thoughts about *orderliness* may be about the way objects are to be arranged or work is to be organized. Thoughts about *illness* are usually of a fearful kind, for example, a dread of cancer or venereal disease. Obsessional ideas about *sex* usually concern practices that the individual would find shameful, such as anal intercourse. Obsessions about *religion* often take the form of doubts about the fundamentals of belief (e.g. 'does God exist?') or repeated doubts about whether sins have been adequately confessed ('scruples').

Compulsions

Compulsions are repetitive and seemingly purposeful behaviours, performed in a stereotyped way (hence the alternative name of compulsive rituals). They are accompanied by a subjective sense that the behaviour must be carried out and by an urge to resist. Like obsessions, compulsions are recognized as senseless. A compulsion may be understandably associated with an obsession. For example, a compulsion to wash the hands repeatedly is usually associated with obsessional thoughts that the hands are contaminated. Sometimes obsessional ideas concern the consequences of failing to carry out the compulsion in the 'correct' way, for example, that another person will suffer an accident.

Compulsive acts are of many kinds, but four are particularly common:

- *Checking rituals* are often concerned with safety, for example checking over and over again that a gas tap has been turned off.
- *Cleaning rituals* often take the form of repeated handwashing but may involve household cleaning.
- *Counting rituals* usually involve counting in some special way, for example in threes, and are frequently associated with doubting thoughts such that the count must be repeated to make sure that it was carried out adequately in the first place. The counting is often silent so that an onlooker may be unaware of the ritual.

♦ In *dressing-rituals* the person lays out clothes in a particular way or puts them on in a special order. The ritual is often accompanied by doubting thoughts that lead to seemingly endless repetition. In severe cases, patients may take an hour or more to dress in the morning.

Obsessional slowness

Many obsessional patients perform actions slowly because their compulsive rituals or repeated doubts take time and distract them from their main purpose. Occasionally, however, the slowness does not seem to be secondary to these other problems but a primary feature of unknown origin.

Depersonalization and derealization

Depersonalization is a change of self-awareness such that the person feels unreal, detached from his own experience and unable to feel emotion. *Derealization* is a similar change in relation to the environment, such that objects appear unreal and people appear as lifeless, two-dimensional 'cardboard' figures. Despite the complaint of inability to feel emotion, both depersonalization and derealization are described as highly unpleasant experiences.

These central features are often accompanied by other morbid experiences. There is some disagreement as to whether these other experiences are part of depersonalization and derealization or separate symptoms since they do not occur in every case. These accompanying features include changes in the experience of time, changes in the body image such as a feeling that a limb has altered in size or shape, and occasionally a feeling of being outside one's own body and observing one's own actions, often from above.

Because patients find it difficult to describe the feelings of depersonalization and derealization, they often resort to metaphor and this can lead to confusion between depersonalization and delusional ideas. For example, a patient may say that he feels 'as if part of my brain had stopped working', or 'as if the people I meet are lifeless creatures'.

Such statements should be explored carefully to distinguish depersonalization and derealization from delusional beliefs that the brain is no longer working or that people have really changed. Sometimes it is difficult to make the distinction.

Depersonalization and derealization are experienced quite commonly as transient phenomena by healthy adults and children, especially when tired. The experience usually begins abruptly and in normal people seldom lasts more than a few minutes (Sedman 1970). The symptoms have been reported after sleep deprivation and sensory deprivation, and as an effect of hallucinogenic drugs. The symptoms occur in generalized and phobic anxiety disorders, depressive disorders, schizophrenia, and temporal lobe epilepsy, as well as in the rare depersonalization disorder (see p. 265). Because depersonalization and derealization occur in so many disorders, they do not help in diagnosis.

Motor symptoms and signs

Abnormalities of social behaviour, facial expression, and posture occur frequently in mental disorders of all kinds. They are considered in Chapter 2 where the examination of the patient is described. Motor slowing and agitation, which are important features of depressive disorder, are discussed in Chapter 11. With the exception of tics, other specific symptoms are mainly observed among schizophrenic patients. The following are recognized most often:

♦ *Tics* are irregular repeated movements involving a group of muscles, for example, sideways movement of the head or the raising of one shoulder.

♦ *Mannerisms* are repeated movements that appear to have some functional significance, for example, saluting.

♦ *Stereotypies* are repeated movements that are regular (unlike tics) and without obvious significance (unlike mannerisms), for example, rocking to and fro.

♦ *Posturing* is the adoption of unusual bodily postures continuously for a long time. The posture may appear to have a symbolic meaning, for example, standing with both arms outstretched as if being crucified, or may have no apparent significance, for example, standing on one leg.

- *Grimacing* has the same meaning as in everyday speech. The term *Schauzkrampf* (snout cramp or spasm) is used occasionally to denote pouting of the lips to bring them closer to the nose.
- *Negativism.* Patients are said to show negativism when they do the opposite of what is asked and actively resist efforts to persuade them to comply.
- *Echopraxia* is the imitation of the interviewer's movement automatically even when asked not to do so.
- *Mitgehen* (going along with) describes another kind of excessive compliance in which the patient's limbs can be moved into any position with the slightest pressure.
- *Ambitendence.* Patients are said to exhibit ambitendence when they alternate between opposite movements, for example, putting out the arm to shake hands, then withdrawing it, extending it again, and so on repeatedly.
- *Catatonia* is a state of increased muscle tone affecting extension and flexion and abolished by voluntary movement.
- *Waxy flexibility* is a term to describe the tonus in catatonia. It is detected when a patient's limbs can be placed in a position in which they then remain for long periods whilst at the same time muscle tone is uniformly increased. Patients with this abnormality sometimes maintain the head a little way above the pillow in a position that a healthy person could not maintain without extreme discomfort (*psychological pillow*).

Disorders of the body image

The body image or body schema is a person's subjective representation against which the integrity of his body is judged and the movement and position of its parts assessed. Specific abnormalities of the body image arise in neurological disorders. These abnormalities include the awareness of a *phantom limb* after amputation, *unilateral lack of awareness or neglect* (usually following stroke), *hemisomatognosia* (the person feels, incorrectly, that a limb is missing), and *anosognosia* (lack of awareness of loss of function often of hemiplegia). These abnormalities are described in textbooks of neurology and in the textbook of neuropsychiatry by Lishman (1998).

Distorted awareness of size and shape of the body occurs occasionally in healthy people when they are tired or falling asleep. The experience, which includes feelings that a limb is enlarging, becoming smaller, or otherwise being distorted, occurs also in migraine, as part of the aura of epilepsy, and after taking LSD. Changes of shape and size of body parts are described by some schizophrenic patients. Except for some schizophrenics, the person is aware that the experience is unreal. *Coenestopathic states* are localized distortions of body awareness, for example, the nose feels as if it is made of cotton wool.

A *general distortion of the body image* occurs in anorexia nervosa: the patient is convinced that he is fat when in fact he is underweight, sometimes to the point of emaciation.

The *reduplication phenomenon* is the experience that the body has doubled, or that part of the body has done so, for example, that there are two left arms. The experience is reported very occasionally in migraine, temporal lobe epilepsy, and schizophrenia. The related experience of autoscopic hallucinations is described on p. 10.

Disorders of the self

The experience of self has several aspects. It is more than the awareness of the body; we have a feeling of unity between the various aspects of the self; we recognize our activities as our own; we recognize a boundary between the self and the outside world; and we have a feeling of continuity between our past and present selves. The concept of self overlaps with that of the *body image*. Although the body image is usually experienced as part of the self, it can also be experienced in a more objective way, as when we say 'my leg hurts'. Some of these aspects of the self are changed in certain psychiatric disorders. The experiences are often associated with other abnormal phenomena, so that the account of abnormalities of the self overlaps with several other parts of this chapter.

Disorders of the self can be divided into those concerned with activities, with the unity of the self, with identity, and with the boundaries of the self.

Disorders concerned with activities

We take it for granted that our actions are our own. Patients with delusions of control (see p. 18) lose this awareness. They have the experience that thoughts are not their own and believe instead that they have been inserted from outside. Some patients lose the conviction that their actions are their own and believe instead that they have been imposed by an outside agency.

Disordered awareness of the unity of the self

Some patients lose the normal experience of existing as a unified being. Patients with *multiple personality disorder* (see p. 264) have the experience of existing as two more selves, alternating at different times. In the experience of *autoscopy* (see p. 10) and the related experience of the *Doppelganger* (see p. 10), the person experiences two selves, present at the same time, but with the conviction that each is a version of the self.

Disorders of the unity of the self

Although we recognize that we change over time, we retain a conviction of being the same person. Rarely, this feeling of continuity is lost in schizophrenia; a patient may say that he is a different person from the one existing before the disorder began, or that a new self has taken over from the old.

Disorders of the boundaries of the self

This type of disorder is experienced by some people after taking LSD or other drugs, who may say that they feel as if they were dissolving. Hallucinations can be regarded as involving a loss of awareness of what is within the self and what is located outside. The same inability to determine what is part of the self, and what is not, is seen in passivity phenomena in which actions willed by the patient are experienced as initiated from outside.

Disorders of memory

Failure of memory is called *amnesia*. The related term *dysmnesia* is occasionally used, principally in the name of the dysmnesic syndrome, more often called the amnestic syndrome (see p. 412). *Paramnesia* is distortion of memory. Several kinds of disordered memory occur in psychiatric disorders, and it is usual to describe them in terms of two stages which approximate to the scheme of memory derived from psychological research but omit many of the details (see Box 1.3).

Immediate memory concerns the retention of information over a short period measured in minutes. It is tested clinically by asking the patient to remember a name and address (which they did not know before the test) and to recall it about 5 minutes later.

Recent memory concerns events in the last few days. It is tested clinically by asking about events in the patients daily life which are known also to the interviewer directly or via an informant (for example, what they have eaten) or in the wider environment (for example, well known news items).

Long term (remote) memory concerns events over longer periods of time. It is tested by asking about events before the presumed onset of memory disorder.

In testing any state of memory, a distinction is made between spontaneous *recall* and *recognition* of information. In some conditions, patients who cannot recall information can recognize it correctly.

Memory loss caused by organic conditions usually affects recall of recent events more than

Box 1.3 Some aspects of the experimental psychopathology of memory

Anatomy Lesions in specific brain area have profound effects on memory. These areas are thought to be involved in adding to, and retrieving from, memory: it is still not known which areas are involved in the storage of memories. The first area important for memory includes parts of the medial temporal lobe including the hippocampus, amygdala, parahippocampal gyrus, and entorhinal cortex. The second area important for memory is the fornix system comprising the mamillary bodies, the dorsomedial thalamus and the cingulate gyri. Bilateral damage to any part of this system can cause severe amnesia such that new information can be remembered for a few minutes only. Motor and perceptual skills (implicit memory – see below) can still be learnt but the person cannot remember learning them.

Physiology Physiological research suggests that short-term memory is mediated by changes in electrical activity of neurons, whilst long-term storage involves changes in the synaptic connections between neurons. Several neurotransmitter systems, including cholinergic ones, are involved, but the detailed mechanisms have not been worked out.

Psychology Psychological research indicates that the stages of memory are more complex than those generally recognized in the clinical practice. Memory passes through the stages of *encoding*, *storage*, and *retrieval*. Retrieval can take place in two ways, through *recall*, that is, an effort to find an item of information, and through *recognition*, that is, matching a presented item with an item that has been stored. Recall varies from one time to another even with well-learned material, as in the inability to recall the name of a person but remembering it a few minutes later. Recognition is less demanding than recall both for healthy people and for amnesics.

Several memory stores have been identified:

- *Sensory stores* receive information from the sense organs and retain it for about a quarter of a second while it is processed. Damage to this system leads to perceptual disorders rather than disorders of memory in the everyday sense.

- *Working memory* holds information for only 15–20 seconds, though this period can be extended if the information is rehearsed repeatedly. This store has

a limited capacity. Working memory has an executive function, keeping to allocating resources between tasks. There are separate short-term stores for verbal and for visual information.

- *Long-term memory* receives information that has been selected for more permanent storage. Unlike short-term memory, it has a large capacity and holds information for a long time. Information in this store has been processed and is stored according to either verbal characteristics (meaning or sound), or as visual images. Long-term memory, as understood by psychologists, includes events that happened within minutes and days (the clinician calls this recent memory) and events that took place years ago (the clinician's concept of long-term memory). Because it covers such a large span, long-term memory is sometimes divided into (i) *delayed memory* for items added within minutes, (ii) *recent memory* for items added within days or weeks, and (iii) *remote memory* for the rest.

- *Prospective memory* is concerned not only with past events but also with actions to be carried out in the future, for example to take medication at a prearranged time. Failures of prospective memory are evident in many patients with amnesia.

Memory can also be classified according to type of information stored:

- *Semantic memory* is concerned with factual information, the meaning of words, and the attributes of objects. Memory-disordered patients have difficulty in adding to this store of knowledge though they usually retain most of what they have stored already.

- *Episodic memory* is for experiences such as a meeting with a friend or an item seen on television.

- *Procedural memory* is for skills such as riding a bicycle. This kind of memory is also called *implicit memory*, in contrast to *explicit memory*, in which the learned information can be recalled. (We may remember how to ride a bicycle, but cannot say what we learnt.) Procedural memory is preserved in amnesic patients, though they may forget the occasion on which the skill was learnt (they have lost the corresponding episodic memory).

recall of distant ones, and it is not a total loss. Total loss of all memory including that of personal identity strongly suggests psychogenic causes (see below) or malingering. Some organic conditions give rise to an interesting partial effect known as *amnestic disorder*, in which the person is unable to remember events occurring a few minutes before, but can recall remote events (see p. 412). Some patients with memory disorder recall more when given cues. When this happens, it suggests that the disorder is concerned at least in part with retrieval.

After a period of unconsciousness, memory is impaired for the interval between the ending of complete unconsciousness and the restoration of full consciousness (*anterograde amnesia*). Some causes of unconsciousness (e.g. head injury and electroconvulsive therapy) lead also to inability to recall events before the onset of unconsciousness (*retrograde amnesia*).

Several *disorders of recognition* occur occasionally in neurological and psychiatric disorders:

◆ *jamais vu* is the failure to recognize events that have been encountered before;

◆ *déjà vu* is the conviction that an event repeats one that has been experienced in the past when in fact it is novel;

◆ *confabulation* is the reporting as memories of events at one time, of events that took place at another time, or never involved the person.

Recall of events can be *biased by the mood* at the time of recall. Importantly, in depressive disorders, memories of unhappy events are recalled more readily than other events, a process which adds to the patient's low mood.

Psychogenic amnesias

Psychogenic amnesia is thought to result from an active process of repression which prevents the recall of memories that would otherwise evoke unpleasant emotions. The ideas arose from the study of dissociative amnesia (see p. 264), but the same factors may play a part in some cases of organic amnesia, helping to explain why the return of some memories is delayed longer than others.

False memory syndrome

It is a matter of dispute whether memories can be repressed completely but return many years later. The question arises most often when memories of sexual abuse are reported during psychotherapy by a person who had no recollection of the events before the psychotherapy began, and the events are strongly denied by the alleged abusers. Many clinicians consider that these recollections have been 'implanted' by overzealous questioning, others contend that they are true memories that have previously been completely repressed. Those who hold the latter opinion point to evidence that memories of events other than child abuse can sometimes be completely lost and then regained and also that some recovered memories of child abuse are corroborated subsequently by independent evidence (see Brewin 2000 for a review of the evidence). Although the quality of the evidence has been questioned, the possibility of complete and sustained repression of memories has not been ruled out. However, it seems likely that only a small minority of cases of 'recovered memory syndrome' can be explained in this way (see also p. 36).

Disorders of consciousness

Consciousness is awareness of the self and the environment. The *level* of consciousness can vary between the extremes of alertness and coma. The *quality* of consciousness can also vary: sleep differs from unconsciousness, as does stupor (see below).

Coma is the most extreme form of impaired consciousness. The patient shows no external evidence of mental activity and little motor activity other than breathing. He does not respond even to strong stimuli. Coma can be graded by the extent of the remaining reflex responses and by the type of EEG activity.

Clouding of consciousness refers to a state which ranges from barely perceptible impairment to definite drowsiness in which the person reacts incompletely to stimuli. Attention, concentration, and memory are impaired to varying degrees and orientation is disturbed. Thinking seems muddled, and events may be interpreted inaccurately.

Stupor, in the sense used in psychiatry, refers to a condition in which the patient is immobile, mute, and unresponsive but appears to be fully conscious in that the eyes are usually open and follow external objects. If the eyes are closed, the patient resists attempts to open them. Reflexes are normal and resting posture is maintained. (Note that in neurology the term stupor is used differently and generally implies an impairment of consciousness.)

Confusion means inability to think clearly. It occurs characteristically in states of impaired consciousness but it can occur when consciousness is normal. In delirium, confusion occurs together with partial impairment of consciousness, illusions, hallucinations, delusions, and a mood change of anxiety or apprehension. In the past, the resulting syndrome has been called a confusional state with the result that the term confusion was also used to mean impairment of consciousness as well as muddled thinking. The term delirium is now preferred.

Other terms used to describe states of impaired consciousness include:

- *oneiroid state*, in which there is dream like imagery although the person is not asleep;
- *twilight state*, which is a prolonged oneiroid state; and
- *torpor*, in which the patient appears drowsy, readily falls asleep, and shows evidence of slow thinking and narrowed range of perception.

Disorders of attention and concentration

Attention is the ability to focus on the matter in hand. *Concentration* is the ability to maintain that focus. The ability to focus on a selected part of the information reaching the brain is important in many everyday situations, for example, when conversing in a noisy place. It is also important to be able to attend to more than one source of information at the same time, for example, when conversing while driving a car.

Attention and concentration may be impaired in a wide variety of psychiatric disorders including depressive disorders, mania, anxiety disorders, schizophrenia, and organic disorders. Therefore, the finding of abnormalities of attention and concentration does not assist in diagnosis. Nevertheless, these abnormalities are important in management; for example, they affect patients' ability to give or receive information when interviewed, and can interfere with a patient's ability to work, drive a car, or take part in leisure activities.

Insight

In psychopathology, the term insight refers to awareness of morbid change in oneself and a correct attitude to this change including, in appropriate cases, a realization that there is a mental disorder. This awareness is difficult for a patient to achieve, since it involves some knowledge of what are the limits of normal mental functioning (a matter on which doctors do not always agree). Also, insight has to be assessed against the background of knowledge of, and beliefs about, mental disorder; it is not the same as complete agreement with the views of the doctor. Although in the past lack of insight was said to be a distinguishing feature between psychosis (where it was said to be absent) and neurosis (where it is present), this distinction is no longer thought to be reliable or useful.

Insight is not simply present or absent, it is a matter of degree which is best determined by asking four questions:

- Is the patient aware of phenomena that others have observed (e.g. that he is unusually active and elated)?
- If so, does he recognize the phenomena as abnormal (rather than, for example, maintaining that his unusual activity and cheerfulness are normal high spirits)?

◆ If so, does he consider that they are caused by mental illness (as opposed to, say, a physical illness or poison administered by enemies)?

◆ If so, does he think that he needs treatment?

The answers to these questions are more informative and more reliable than those of the single question, is insight present or not? The value of determining the degree of insight is that it helps to predict whether a patient is likely to comply with treatment

In discussions of psychotherapy, insight has a meaning different from the one considered so far which is used in general psychiatry. In psychotherapy, insight is the capacity to understand one's own motives and to be aware of previously unconscious aspects of mental activity. The term *intellectual insight* is sometimes used to denote the capacity to formulate this understanding, whereas *emotional insight* is the term for the capacity to feel and respond to the understanding.

Further reading

Jamison, K. R. (1996) *An unquiet mind*. Knopf, New York. (Provides a valuable insight into the experience of manic-depressive disorder).

Jaspers, K. (1963) *General psychopathology* (trans. from the 7th German edition by J. Hoenig and M. W. Hamilton), Chapter I, Phenomenology. Manchester University Press. (The most important classic work on the subject. Chapter 1 (read in whole or in part) shows Jasper's approach to the subject).

Schneider, K. (1949) *The concept of delusion*. Reprinted and translated in *Themes and variations in European psychiatry* (eds S. R. Hirsch and M. Shepherd). John Wright, Bristol, 1974. (A classical account that is valuable background reading.)

Sims, A. (1995). *Symptoms in the mind; an introduction to descriptive psychopathology*, 2nd edn. Baillière Tindall, London. (A comprehensive modern text.)

Wing, J. K., Cooper, J. E., and Sartorius, N. (1974). *The measurement and classification of psychiatric symptoms.* Glossary of definitions, pp.141–88. Cambridge University Press, Cambridge. (Illustrates how definitions considered in this chapter can be used to develop the standardized assessments considered in the next chapter.)

2

CHAPTER 2

Assessment

Assessment

The assessment of a patient who may have a psychiatric disorder has several stages. The interviewer will usually need to decide whether there is a disorder, and if so of what kind; whether the patient disabled, and if so in what way; whether there is danger to the patient or to others; and what sort of person has become ill, and what are his social circumstances. To make these decisions, the clinician needs to take a history from the patient and other informants, examine the mental state, carry out a physical examination, and formulate a plan of action; and he will need to write case notes, letters, and sometimes reports. Increasingly, assessment is carried out by a multidisciplinary team in which the psychiatrist has the important role of constructing an integrated assessment.

This chapter begins with an account of interviewing and mental state examination. It is assumed that readers are already competent in physical examination and this matter is considered only briefly. Readers who need more information should consult a textbook of medicine.

Readers who require more information about psychiatric assessment than is contained in this chapter are referred to the account by Cooper and Oates (2000). The chapter is long and the table of contents (Table 2.1) may help the reader.

Collecting information

Interviewing the patient

The interview described here is comprehensive and may take upwards of an hour to complete. In many clinical situations, time is limited and a shorter

---

Table 2.1 Contents of Chapter 2

interview is required. This shorter interview can be achieved by using a problem-solving approach in which the interviewer repeatedly evaluates the information obtained and considers what further items are most relevant. When time is short, it may be necessary to deal only with matters of immediate relevance and to see the patient on a second occasion to complete the history. However, brief interviews can be carried out effectively only when the interviewer has practised the complete interview schedule many times.

Preparing for the interview

Interviews have to be carried out in many settings. The following recommendations should be followed as far as is practicable, but they cannot always be achieved completely. Arrangements in the patient's home are likely to be less ideal than those in an out-patient department, and those in a general hospital ward, an emergency department, or a police station may be still less ideal. It is important, nevertheless, to do what is possible to make arrangements to put the patient at ease, to ensure privacy, and to ensure the safety of the interviewer. The steps in arranging an interview are as follows.

Put the patient at ease The interview should be carried out, as far as possible, in a place that is free from interruptions and where the interview cannot be overheard. The patient should be comfortable and the interviewer should not face the patient directly but arrange his chair at an angle; nor, if possible, should he sit at a much higher level.

Arrange to take notes Whenever possible the interviewer should make notes during the interview; attempts to memorize the interview and write notes afterwards, are time consuming and not always wholly accurate. However, it is usually better to delay note taking for some minutes until the patient feels that he has the interviewer's undivided attention. The patient should be placed at the left side of a right-handed interviewer. With this arrangement, the interviewer can attend to the patient and maintain an informal atmosphere while writing. Occasionally, when a patient is very anxious or agitated, note taking may be deferred until after the interview.

Ensure safety Only a small minority of patients are potentially dangerous, but the need for precautions should be considered before every interview. Whenever there is a possibility of violence, the interviewer should:

- make sure that another person knows where and when the interview is taking place and how long it is expected to last. This is especially relevant to interviews in the community, but applies also to certain hospital situations such as interviews at the end of clinic when other staff have left.

- ensure that help can be called if it is needed. In hospital, check for an emergency call button and its position, and otherwise try to arrange for another person to be within earshot.

- ensure that neither the patient nor any physical obstruction is between himself and exit.

- remove from sight any objects that could be used as weapons.

If the risk is thought to be high, it may be necessary to defer the interview until appropriate additional helpers are close by.

Starting the interview

The interviewer should welcome the patient by name, give his own name and explain in a few words why he wishes to interview the patient. If the patient is accompanied, the interviewer should greet the companions and explain how long they should expect to wait and whether they will be interviewed. It is usually better to see the patient alone and interview others afterwards, having obtained the patient's consent. If the patient is unable to give an account of the problems, informants are seen at an earlier stage of the assessment. If the patient is being seen at the request of another doctor, the interviewer should indicate this. He can indicate the general lines of any referral letter but it is not usually necessary to reveal the details.

The interviewer should explain that he will take notes (see above), which will be confidential. If the interview is for the purposes of a report to an outside agency (e.g. a court report) this should be made clear. The general structure of the interview should be explained (e.g. present problems will be considered first, before past events are reviewed) and the time available. The interview should begin with an open question (one that cannot be answered yes or no) such as: 'Tell me about your problems.' The patient should be allowed to talk freely for several minutes before further questions are asked. As the patient describes his problems, the interviewer should observe how he is responding, for example, is he reticent or unduly circumstantial.

The following techniques have been shown to improve the results of the interview (Goldberg *et al.* 1980). The interviewer should:

◆ adopt a relaxed posture and appear unhurried – even when time is short;

◆ maintain appropriate eye contact with the patient and not appear engrossed in note taking;

◆ be alert to verbal and non-verbal cues of distress as well as to the factual content of the interview;

◆ control an over-talkative or discursive patient.

Some problems in starting the interview

Anxious patients Although anxiety may be part of the patient's disorder, it may relate also to the interview. If the person seems unduly anxious, the interviewer can say that many people feel anxious when they first take part in a psychiatric interview and go on to find out the patient's concerns.

The uncooperative patient Some patients are reluctant to be interviewed and have come at the insistence of the spouse or general practitioner. When the patient seems unwilling to collaborate, the interviewer should talk over the circumstances of the referral, and try to persuade the patient that the

interview will be in his own interests. Some depressed, schizophrenic, or confused patients are uncooperative because they do not realize that they are ill. In such cases it may be necessary to interview an informant before returning to the patient.

Other problems Some patients try to dominate the interview, especially when the interviewer is younger than themselves. Others adopt an unduly friendly approach that threatens to convert the interview into a social conversation. In either case, the interviewer should explain why he needs to guide the patient to relevant issues.

Continuing the interview

The first step is to obtain a clear account of the patient's problems, separating symptoms from impairment, handicap and disability. From the start, the interviewer considers possible diagnoses and as the interview progresses, questions are selected to confirm or reject these diagnoses. The interviewer considers also what information is relevant to prognosis and treatment. Thus interviewing is not simply the asking of a routine set of questions. *Interviewing is an active and iterative process* in which the focus of attention is directed by hypotheses formed from the information elicited already, and modified repeatedly as more information is collected. This active process of interviewing is particularly necessary when time is short, as in an emergency where a decision has to be made about immediate treatment.

It is important to allow the patient, as far as possible, to describe his problem spontaneously. In this way, unexpected material may be revealed that might not be revealed by the answers to questions. This spontaneous account can be encouraged by prompting, for example, by repeating in an enquiring tone the last few words of the patient's last statement. Questions may be needed to bring the patient back to the point after a digression, and to elicit specific information, for example, about the relationship between symptoms and stressful events. Whenever possible, the interviewer should use open rather than leading or closed questions (a leading question suggests the answer; a closed question allows only the answers yes or no). Thus instead of the closed question: 'Are you happily married?' the interviewer might ask: 'How do you and your wife get on with one another?' When there is no alternative to a closed question, the answer should be followed by a request for an example. Before ending the interview, it is good practice to ask a general question such as: 'Is there anything that I have not asked you about, that you think I should know?'

It is generally better to establish clearly the nature of the symptoms before asking how and when they developed. If there is any doubt about the nature of the symptoms, the patient should be asked to describe specific examples. When all presenting symptoms have been explored suffi-ciently, direct questions are asked about others that have not come to light but may be relevant. In doing this, the interviewer uses his knowledge of psychiatric syndromes to decide what further questions to ask. For example, a person who com-plains of feeling depressed would be asked about ideas concerning the future, and about suicidal ideas (see p. 315). When suicidal thought are described, further specific questions should be asked (see p. 526).

The onset and course of the symptoms is clari-fied next, together with their relationship to any stressful events or physical illness. Exacerbations and periods of complete or partial remission should be included in this enquiry. Considerable persis-tence may be needed to date the onset or an exac-erbation of symptoms accurately. It sometimes helps to ask how the onset related to an event that the patient is likely to remember, such as a birthday or public holidays. The patient's attempts to cope with the symptoms are noted, for example, increased drinking of alcohol to relieve distress. If treatment has been was received, the nature, timing, and effects are noted.

The interviewer completes the relevant parts of the full interview schedule described below. If time is short it may be better to examine the mental state after the present complaints have been clari-fied. This can make it easier to select the points to be asked about in the rest of the history, in order to make the decisions needed immediately. When time is adequate, the mental state is usually exam-ined at the end of the interview, together with any relevant physical examination.

Some problems in continuing the interview:

Taciturn patients Taciturn patients can often be encour-aged to speak more freely if the interviewer shows non-verbal expressions of concern (e.g. leaning forward a little in the chair with an expression of interest) additional to those that are part of any good interview.

Garrulous patients It is less easy to curb an over-talkative patient. If efforts to focus the interview are unsuccessful, the interviewer should wait for a natural break in the flow of speech. He should then explain that, because time is limited, he proposes to interrupt the patient from time to time to help him focus on issues that are important for planning treatment. If this proposal is made tactfully, most garrulous patients are relieved to receive it.

Disturbed patients When patients are disturbed, rest-less or aggressive, it may be difficult to follow a preset plan of interviewing. In these cases it is espe-cially important to have diagnostic possibilities in mind and to take what opportunities arise to ask relevant questions.

Interviewing informants

Whenever possible, the history from the patient should be supplemented by information from a close relative or another person who knows him well. This is much more important in psychiatry than in the rest of medicine, because some psychi-atric patients are unaware of the extent of their symptoms or their abnormal behaviour. Other patients are aware of their problems but do not wish to reveal them; for example, alcoholics often conceal the extent of their drinking. When person-ality is being assessed, patients and relatives may give quite different accounts of characteristics such as irritability, obsessional traits, and jealousy.

As explained above, informants should be seen separately unless the patient refuses this arrangement.

Interviews with a partner or relative are used to obtain additional information about the patient's condition, to assess their attitudes to the patient and the illness, and to involve them in the treatment plan. It is also an opportunity to learn what burdens the illness has placed on them, and how they have tried to cope. A history from an informant is essential when the patient is unable to give an accurate account of his condition, for example, because of impaired memory. In every case the views of a partner or relative concerning patient's illness and personality are likely to be informative. A relative may be more able than the patient to date the onset of illness accurately, especially if it was gradual. A relative can also indicate how disabling the illness is and how it affects other people. Finally, when it is important to know about a patient's childhood, an interview with a parent or older sibling may reveal important information.

With few exceptions, the patient's permission should be obtained before interviewing a relative. Exceptions occur when the patient is a child, and when adult patients are mute, stuporous, confused, violent, or extremely retarded. In other cases, the doctor should explain to the patient the reasons for interviewing the informant, while emphasizing that confidential information given by the patient will not be passed to the relative. If any information needs to be given to a relative, for example, about treatment, the patient's permission should be obtained. Questions from relatives should be dealt with in the same way.

The interviewer begins by explaining the purpose of the interview. Relatives may fear that the interviewer will make demands on them. For example, a daughter may think that she will be asked to take her demented mother into her own home. Some relatives expect to be blamed for the patient's illness; for example, the parents of a young schizophrenic may expect the doctor to imply that they have failed as parents. It is important for the interviewer to be sensitive to such ideas and, when appropriate, to discuss them in a reassuring way. The interviewer should be sensitive to the relatives point of view but should not become involved in their problems to an extent that conflicts with his primary duty to his patient.

After the interview, the psychiatrist should not tell the patient what the relative has said unless the latter has given permission. This is important even when the relative has revealed something that should be discussed with the patient, for example, an account of excessive drinking previously denied by the patient. If the relative is unwilling that information should be passed on, this wish must be respected; for example, a wife may fear violent retaliation from her husband. If the relative refuses permission, the interviewer can only try to elicit the relevant information from the patient in a further interview. Since, in most places, patients are generally entitled to read at least part of their medical notes, interviews with relatives should be noted on separate sheets and kept in a way that safeguards their wishes about confidentiality.

Sometimes it is necessary to speak to *employers, friends, or police* who have been involved in some way in the effects of the patient's illness. They should be seen only with the patient's permission and the psychiatrist should collect information from them but not discuss the patient's problems unless he has the patient's permission to do so.

Information about the patient should not normally be given *over the telephone*, unless the doctor is certain of the caller's identity and the patient has agreed that they can be informed. Even then it is usually better to arrange an interview with the enquirer after informing the patient and confirming the permission. The psychiatrist must not allow a conspiratorial atmosphere to develop in which he conceals conversations with family members or takes sides in their disputes.

The psychiatric history

Although, as explained above, it is not possible to take a full history on every occasion, the information that has been elicited should always be recorded systematically and in a standard order. This practice helps the interviewer to remember all potentially important topics and, if necessary, to add further information on another occasion. The practice also makes it easier for colleagues who need to refer to the notes at a later time. This order can be followed in the written record, even when it was not possible to elicit the information in the desired sequence. This and all other entries in the notes should be dated and signed.

A commonly used scheme for history taking is given below. For ease of reference, this scheme is presented as a list of headings and items. More detail is provided, for readers who require it, in the subsequent notes. The notes on personality are especially important since this is generally the most difficult topic in history taking. As well as obtaining factual information, the interviewer should try to understand how the patient experienced the illness, the way in which it has interfered with his present life and his plans for the future, what he thinks is wrong, and what are his concerns about the future effects of the illness on himself and his family.

Checking memory for events

All parts of a history may be distorted by the patient's failure to distinguish accurately between true and false memories. For this reason, additional information is often collected to check important points. Some events cannot be checked in this way because there is no reliable informant to consult. This problem is greatest in relation to memories of sexual abuse. In recent years concern has been expressed about accounts of abuse, often by parents, 'recovered' by patients, usually in the course of questioning during counselling or during psychotherapy.

Memory is never a completely accurate record of the details of past events, and memories that previously seemed lost can come to mind. Events which were highly unpleasant and aversive are generally less accessible than others so that the patient has only a partial recollection – a process that Freud called repression (see p. 189). It is unusual, however, for memories of important events to be lost completely in this way and then recovered. Extreme caution should be taken in evaluating 'recovered' memories, especially when they are a response to directed questioning, or in the context of heightened suggestibility. This caution should, of course, be balanced by the recognition that many people who were abused in childhood have been unable to obtain help because they were not believed, or because they feared disbelief (see also p. 25).

A scheme for history taking

Information is grouped under the headings shown in Table 2.2, which are expanded in note form below. For readers who require it, further information appears in the subsequent section. Assessment of personality is important but difficult. It is suggested that all readers consider the part of the section that deals with this topic. For brevity, the scheme is written in the style of short notes.

Informant(s)

- Usually the principal informant is the patient. If not, state the reason.
- The name(s), relation to patient, and length of acquaintance of any other person interviewed.

Table 2.2 **Outline of the psychiatric history**
Name, age, and address of the patient
Name of any informants and their relationship to the patient
History of present condition
Family history
Personal history
Past illness
Personality
Use of drugs, alcohol, tobacco

- The interviewer's impression of the reliability of each informant.
- The name of the referrer and a brief statement of the reasons for referral.

Present condition

- Symptoms with duration and mode of onset of each.
- The time relations between symptoms and any physical disorder, or psychological or social problems.
- The nature and duration of any impairment, disability and handicap.
- Any treatment received.

Family history

- *Parents* age now or at death (if dead, the cause), health, occupation, personality, quality of relationship with patient.
- *Siblings* names, ages, marital status, occupation, personality, psychiatric illness, and quality of relationship with patient.
- *Social position* of family.
- *Atmosphere* in the home.
- Any *disorders in the family*, including psychiatric disorder, personality disorder or alcoholism. Epilepsy or other neurological or medical disorders.

When the family history is complex and relevant, it can be summarized diagrammatically as a family tree. The following symbols are in general use:

- squares for males, circles for females, crossed through if the person is deceased;
- marriages or liaisons leading to the birth of a child indicated by a line joining the partners, crossed through with two oblique lines after divorce or other permanent separation (see the example of a 'genogram' on p. 760).

Table 2.3 **The personal history**
Mother's pregnancy and the birth
Early development
Childhood
Separations
Emotional problems
Illnesses
Schooling and higher education
Occupations
Menstrual history
Sexual relationships
Marriage
Children
Social circumstances
Past medical history
Past psychiatric history
Forensic history

Personal history (Table 2.3)

- *Pregnancy and birth* abnormalities, especially brain damage or conditions that might cause this, for example difficult labour.
- *Early development* delay in walking, talking, sphincter control, etc.
- *Childhood* any prolonged separation from parents and the patient's reaction to it. Any emotional problems – age of onset, course, and treatment. Excessive fears, temper tantrums, shyness, stammering, blushing, food fads, sleep-walking, prolonged bed-wetting, and frequent nightmares, occurring at an age when these behaviours are not found in most children. Any serious illness in childhood, especially disease affecting the central nervous system, such as febrile seizures; Whether hospitalized and if so for how long.
- *Schooling and higher education* age of starting and finishing each stage; character of the school, college or university. Academic record;

sporting and other extracurricular achievements; relationships with teachers and other students.

- *Occupations:* chronological list of jobs, with reasons for changes; present financial circumstances, satisfaction in work. Any service or war experience, with information about achievements and problems.

- *Menstrual history:* age of menarche, attitude to periods, regularity, and amount, dysmenorrhoea, premenstrual tension, age of menopause, and any symptoms at the time, date of last menstrual period.

- *Marriage and cohabitation:* age at marriage; or start of the cohabitation; how long partner known; quality of present and previous relationships; personality, occupation, and health of partner.

- *Sexual history:* attitude to sex; heterosexual and homosexual experience; current sexual practices, contraception. Any experience of sexual abuse.

- *Children:* names, sex, and age of children; date of any abortions or stillbirths; temperament, emotional development, and mental and physical health of children.

- *Social circumstances:* accommodation, household composition and any financial problems

- *Past medical history:* illnesses, operations, and accidents.

- *Past psychiatric illness:* nature and duration of each illness. Include any episodes of self-harm. Date, duration, and nature of any treatment. Names of hospitals and of doctors. Outcome.

- *Current medication* for physical as well a psychiatric illness; also the contraceptive pill and self-medication. Any allergic or other adverse reactions.

- *'Substance' use:* alcohol, 'street' drugs, and tobacco.

- *Forensic history:* arrests, convictions, imprisonment. Nature of the offences, especially regarding dangerousness.

Table 2.4 Assessment of personality
Relationships
Leisure activities
Prevailing mood
Character
Attitudes and standards
Habits, including alcohol/drug use

Personality (see Table 2.4)

- Relationships: friendships, few or many, superficial or close, with own or opposite sex; relations with workmates and superiors.

- *Use of leisure:* hobbies and interests; membership of societies and clubs.

- *Predominant mood:* anxious, worrying, cheerful, despondent, optimistic, pessimistic, self-depreciating, overconfident; stable or fluctuating; controlled or demonstrative.

- *Character:* sensitive, reserved; timid; shy; suspicious; jealous; resentful; quarrelsome; irritable; impulsive; selfish; self-centred; self-conscious, lacking in confidence; dependent; strict; fussy; rigid; meticulous; punctual; excessively tidy.

- *Attitudes and standards:* moral and religious; attitude towards health and the body.

Notes on history taking

The scheme just outlined lists the items to be considered when a full history is taken, but gives no indication as to why these items are important or what sort of difficulties may arise in eliciting them. These issues are discussed in this section, which is written in the form of notes referring to the headings used above.

The reason for referral

Only a brief statement need be given, for example, 'severe depression, failing to respond to drug treatment'.

The present illness

Record the severity and duration of each symptom, how it began, and what course it has taken (increasing gradually or stepwise, staying the same, intermittent). Indicate which symptoms co-vary and which take an independent course. Note any treatment, the response, and any adverse effects. When a drug was ineffective, ask whether the patient took it in the required dosage.

Family history

Mental disorder among parents or siblings may indicate genetic or environmental influences. Because the family is the environment in which the patient grew up, the personality and attitudes of the parents are relevant. If there have been separations from the parents, ask the reasons. Ask about the parents' relationship with one another, for example, whether there were frequent quarrels. Enquire about separations, divorce, and remarriage or a new partner. Rivalry between siblings may be important, as may favouritism towards one child by the parents. The occupation and social standing of the parents reflect the material circumstances of the patient's childhood.

Recent events in the family may have been stressful to the patient, for example, the serious illness or divorce of a family member. Events in the family may throw light on the patient's concerns about himself. For example, the death of an older brother from a brain tumour may partly explain a patient's extreme concern about headaches.

Personal history

Pregnancy and birth Events in pregnancy and delivery are most likely to be relevant when the patient is mentally retarded or physically handicapped. An unwanted pregnancy may be followed by a poor relationship between mother and child.

Early development Few patients know whether they have passed through developmental stages normally. However, this information is more important if the patient is a child or adolescent, in which case the parents are likely to be available for interview. This information is important also in cases of mental retardation. (Developmental stages are outlined on pp. 798–9.)

The effects of separation from the mother vary considerably. They depend in part on the age of the child at the time, the duration, and the reason (see Chapter 24).

Health in childhood There is little point in recording minor childhood ailments, but disorders of the nervous system such as encephalitis or convulsions are potentially important and so is any illness leading to a long admission to hospital, or prolonged disability.

Early 'neurotic traits' Fears, sleep-walking, shyness, stammering, and food fads are all normal at certain stages of development. The may be significant during childhood if they outlast the normal period (see p. 817) but even then they are rarely important for disorders of adult life.

Education The school record not only gives an indication of intelligence, scholastic achievements, and social development. Ask whether the patient made friends and got on well with teachers, and about success at games and other activities. Similar questions are relevant to higher education.

Occupational history Information about the present job helps the interviewer to understand the circumstances of the patient's life and to judge whether he is under stress at work. A list of previous jobs and reasons for leaving is relevant to the assessment of personality. Repeated dismissals may reflect an awkward, aggressive, or otherwise abnormal personality (though there are many other reasons for repeated dismissals). If the status of jobs has declined, consider declining efficiency caused by chronic mental illness or by alcohol abuse. Information about relationships with colleagues, senior and junior, helps to assess personality. Service in the armed forces is enquired into in the same way.

Menstrual history Questions about current menstrual function should be asked in all relevant cases.

Dysmenorrhoea, menorrhagia, and premenstrual tension should be identified, and amongst women in middle life the menopause should be noted. Enquiries about the age of menarche and how the patient first learnt about menstruation used to be routine, but are less relevant now that health education is widespread. The date of the last period should be noted.

Sexual history The interviewer should use common sense in deciding how much to ask the individual patient. For example, a detailed account of masturbation and sexual techniques may be essential when the patient is seeking help for sexual impotence, but more often the interviewer is concerned to establish generally whether the patient's sexual life is satisfying or not. Only if there are problems need he enquire into all the details under this heading. Judgement must also be used about the optimal timing and amount of detail of questions about experience of sexual abuse. The interviewer should ask about methods of contraception and, when relevant, a woman's wishes about bearing children. Questions relevant to sexual disorders are considered further in Chapter 19.

Marital history This heading includes lasting relationships outside marriage. Ask about the present and any previous lasting relationships. Frequent broken relationships may reflect abnormalities of personality. A previous relationship may determine the patient's attitude to the present one; for example, when a previous partner was unfaithful, the patient may over-react to minor difficulties. The spouse's occupation, personality, and state of health are relevant to the patient's circumstances. Present difficulties can often be understood better by enquiring about each partner's original expectations of the relationship.

Children Pregnancy, childbirth, miscarriages, and induced abortions are important events which are sometimes associated with adverse psychological reactions in the mother. Information about the patient's children is relevant to present worries and the pattern of family life. Since children may be affected by the parent's illness, it is important to know, for example, whether a seriously depressed woman has the care of a baby, or whether a violent alcoholic man has children in the home. If admission to hospital is being considered for a patient who has the care of children, it is important to find out their needs and, if necessary, arrange for their care. This is obvious but is sometimes overlooked.

Previous illness Previous medical or surgical treatment should always be asked about, and particularly careful inquiries should be made about previous mental illness. Patients or relatives may be able to recall the general nature of the illness and treatment but it is nearly always appropriate to request information from others who have treated the patient.

Social circumstances Questions about housing, finances, and the composition of the household help the interviewer to understand the patient's circumstances. Assets and resources are assessed as well as problems and sources of stress. Find out also what informal carers are available who might agree to assist in the plan of management. There can be no general rule about the amount of detail to elicit, and this must be left to common sense.

'Substance' use This includes past as well as present use. Answers may be evasive or misleading and may need to be checked with other informants. See p. 551 for further information about interviewing about alcohol use.

Personality

Aspects of personality can be judged by asking for a self-assessment, by asking others who know the patient well, and by observing behaviour at interview. Mistakes can arise from paying too much attention to the patient's own assessment of his personality. Some people give an unduly favourable account of themselves; for example, antisocial people may conceal the extent of their aggressive behaviour or dishonesty. Conversely, depressed patients often judge themselves too severely, for example as being ineffectual, selfish, or unreliable, an impression that is not confirmed by other people. Therefore it is essential to interview other informants whenever possible.

Good indications of personality can often be obtained by asking the patient or others how he has behaved in particular circumstances. For example, if a patient says he is self-confident, it is useful to enquire how he behaves in particular situations when he has to convince other people or speak in public. Similarly, personality can often be assessed by asking about occasions when social roles are changing, such as leaving school, starting work, marrying, or becoming a parent.

When assessing personality from behaviour at interview, it is essential to allow for the possible effects of psychiatric illness. Thus, when depressed, a person who is normally self-possessed and sociable may appear reserved and lacking in self-confidence. Whatever the source of information, it is important to assess the strengths as well as the weaknesses of personality.

Enquiries about personality are most fruitful when they are systematic. The scheme outlined on p. 38 is widely used, and covers the most important areas of enquiry in clinical work. The points given below refer to patient interviews but can be adapted to informant interviews.

Relationships Is the person shy or does he make friends easily? Are his friendships close and are they lasting? Relationships at work, as well as those with friend and relatives, are significant Leisure activities can throw light on personality, by reflecting a person's interests and preferences for company or solitude, as well as levels of energy and resourcefulness.

Mood The interviewer enquires whether the patient is generally cheerful or gloomy and whether he has marked changes of mood, and if so, how quickly they appear, how long they last, and if they follow life events. The interviewer asks also whether the patient shows emotions or hides them.

Character It is possible to gain some impression of this while taking the personal history. Further information about the patient's character should be sought, by asking questions that help to reveal whether he is reserved, timid, shy, or self-conscious, sensitive or suspicious, resentful or jealous, irritable, impulsive, or quarrelsome, selfish or self-centred, lacking in confidence, and strict, fussy, rigid, meticulous, punctual, or excessively tidy.

These are chiefly negative attributes of character but, as mentioned above, it is also important to ask about positive ones including resilience to adversity. It is not appropriate to go though a complete list of questions with every patient; common sense will indicate what to enquire about as the picture of the patient gradually builds up.

Answers should not always be taken at face value. Thus, if a patient says that he never feels angry, the interviewer might respond that everyone feels angry at times and go on to ask what makes the patient angry. The interviewer should also find out whether the patient expresses anger or bottles it up, and if the former, whether through angry words or violent acts. If the patient bottles up anger, he should be asked how he feels when he does so.

Attitudes and standards This part of the assessment is concerned with attitudes to the body, health, and illness, as well as religious and moral standards. The personal history will usually have provided general indications about these matters so that extensive questioning is seldom necessary.

Mental state examination

The history records symptoms up to the time of the interview. The mental state examination is concerned with the symptoms and behaviour at the time of the interview. If the patient is being seen by nurses and other professional staff in hospital or in the community, their observations of mental state are important and sometimes more revealing than the small sample of behaviour observed during the mental state examination. On the other hand, mental state examination may reveal

Table 2.5 **Summary of the mental state examination**

Behaviour

Speech

Mood

Depersonalization, derealization

Obsessional phenomena

Delusions

Hallucinations and illusions

Orientation

Attention and concentration

Memory

Insight

information not disclosed at other times, for example suicidal intentions, and details of hallucinations.

The symptoms and signs referred to in the following account are described in Chapter 1 and, with a few exceptions, will not be repeated. Mental state examination is a practical skill that should be learned by watching experienced interviewers and by practising repeatedly under supervision, as well as by reading.

Mental state examination follows the headings in Table 2.5.

Appearance and behaviour

Much can also be learnt from the patient's appearance and behaviour. The patient's *general appearance* repays careful observation. A dirty, unkempt look and crumpled clothing may indicate self-neglect. Manic patients may wear bright colours, or dress incongruously. Occasionally an oddity of dress may provide the clue to diagnosis; for example, a rainhood worn on a dry day may be the first evidence of a patient's belief that rays are being shone on her head by persecutors. An appearance suggesting recent weight loss should alert the observer to the possibility of physical illness, or of anorexia nervosa, depressive disorder, or a chronic anxiety disorder.

Facial appearance provides information about mood. In depression, the corners of the mouth are turned down, and there are vertical furrows on the brow. Anxious patients have horizontal creases on the forehead, widened palpebral fissures, and dilated pupils. Facial expression may reflect elation, irritability, and anger, or the fixed 'wooden' expression due to drugs with parkinsonian side-effects. The facial appearance may also suggest physical thyrotoxicosis or myxoedema.

Posture and movement also reflect mood. A depressed patient characteristically sits with hunched shoulders, the head and gaze inclined downwards. An anxious patient may sit on the edge of the chair with hands gripping its sides. Anxious people and patients with agitated depression may be tremulous and restless, touching jewellery, adjusting clothing, or picking at the fingernails. Manic patients are overactive and restless. Other abnormalities of movement include tardive dyskinesia, and the disorders of motor behaviour seen mainly in schizophrenia. Tardive dyskinesia is characterized by chewing and sucking movements, grimacing, and choreoathetoid movements affecting the face, limbs, and respiratory muscles (see p. 668). The motor disorders of schizophrenia include stereotypies, posturing, negativism, echopraxia, ambitendence, and waxy flexibility (see pp. 21–2).

Social behaviour may provide further clues to diagnosis. Manic patients may be unduly familiar. Demented patients may behave as if they were elsewhere than in a medical interview. Schizophrenic patients may be overactive and socially disinhibited, or withdrawn and preoccupied, or aggressive. Patients with antisocial personality disorders may behave aggressively. If social behaviour is highly unusual, the interviewer should note what exactly is unusual, rather than use imprecise terms such a 'bizarre'.

Speech

The *rate and quantity* of speech are assessed first. Speech may be unusually fast, as in mania, or slow, as in depressive disorders. Depressed or demented patients may pause for a long time before replying to questions and then give short answers, producing little spontaneous speech. The same may be observed among shy people or those of low intelligence. The amount of speech is increased in manic patients and in some anxious patients.

The *content* of speech is observed next, keeping in mind some unusual disorders found mainly in schizophrenia (see p. 13). There may be neologisms, i.e. private words invented by the patient, often to describe morbid experiences. Before assuming that a word is a neologism it is essential to make sure that it is not merely mispronounced or a word from another language.

The *flow of speech* is considered next. Sudden interruptions may indicate thought blocking, but are more often the effects of distraction (see p. 12). Rapid shifts from one topic to another suggest flight of ideas, while a general diffuseness and lack of logical thread may indicate the kind of thought disorder characteristic of schizophrenia (see p. 12). It can be difficult to be certain about these abnormalities at interviews, and it is often helpful to record a sample of speech and listen to it several times.

Mood

The assessment of mood begins with the observations of behaviour described already, and continues with direct questions such as 'What is your mood like?' or 'How are you in your spirits?'

To assess *depression*, questions should be asked about a feeling of being about to cry (actual tearfulness is often denied), pessimistic thoughts about the present, hopelessness about the future, and guilt about the past. Suitable questions are 'What do you think will happen to you in the future?' or 'Have you been blaming yourself for anything?'

Some inexperienced interviewers are wary of asking about *suicide* in case they should suggest it to the patient. There is no evidence to warrant this caution although questions should be in stages, starting with the question such as 'Have you thought life is not worth living?' and, if appropriate, going on to ask 'Have you wished you could

die?' or 'Have you considered any way in which you might end your life?' (Questions about suicide are considered further on p. 515.)

Anxiety is assessed further by asking about physical symptoms and thoughts. These enquiries are described further in Chapter 9, and only the main questions are noted here. The interviewer should start with a general question such as 'Have you noticed any changes in your body when you feel upset?', and then go on to specific enquiries about palpitations, dry mouth, sweating, trembling, and the various other symptoms of autonomic activity and muscle tension. To detect anxious thoughts, one can ask: 'What goes through your mind when you are feeling anxious?' Possible replies include thoughts of fainting, losing control, and going mad. Many of these questions overlap with enquiries about the history of the disorder.

Questions about *elation* correspond to those about depression; for example, 'How are you in your spirits?' followed, if necessary, by direct questions such as: 'Do you feel in unusually good spirits?' Elated mood is often accompanied by ideas reflecting excessive self-confidence, inflated assessment of one's abilities, and extravagant plans. Note that the mood in mania can be irritable as well as cheerful.

As well as assessing the prevailing mood, the interviewer should find out *how mood varies*. When mood varies excessively, it is said to be labile; for example, the patient appears dejected at one point in the interview but quickly changes to a normal or unduly cheerful mood. Any persisting lack of affective response, usually called blunting or flattening, should also be noted.

Incongruity of mood

Normally, mood varies during an interview in parallel with the topics discussed. The patient appears sad while talking of unhappy events, angry while describing things that have annoyed him, and so on. When the mood is not suited to the context, it is recorded as incongruent, for example, if a patient giggles when describing the death of his mother. Apparent incongruity may have another explanation; for example, giggling when speaking of sad events may result from embarrassment.

Depersonalization and derealization

Patients who have experienced depersonalization and derealization usually find them difficult to describe. Patients who have not experienced them may say that they have because they have misunderstood the questions. Therefore it is particularly important to obtain specific examples of the patient's experiences. It is useful to begin by asking 'Do you ever feel that things around you are unreal?' and 'Do you ever feel unreal or that part of your body is unreal?' Patients with derealization often describe things in the environment as seeming artificial and lifeless. Patients with depersonalization may say that they feel detached, unable to feel emotion, or as if acting a part. Some patients use illustrations to describe their experience, for example 'as if I were a robot'; such descriptions should be distinguished carefully from delusions. A patient who has described these experiences should be asked to explain them. Most cannot suggest a reason, but a few give a delusional explanation, for example, that the feelings are caused by a persecutor.

Obsessional phenomena

Obsessional thoughts

An appropriate question is: 'Do any thoughts keep coming into your mind, even though you try hard to stop them?' If the patient says 'yes', he should be asked for an example. Patients are often ashamed of obsessional thoughts, especially those about violence or sexual themes, so that persistent but sympathetic questioning may be required. Before recording thoughts as obsessional, the interviewer should be certain that the patient accepts them as his own (and not implanted by an outside agency).

Compulsive rituals

Some can be observed, but others are private events (such as repeating phrases silently), which may be detected only because they interrupt the patient's conversation. Appropriate questions are: 'Do you have to keep checking activities that you know you have completed?' 'Do you have to do things over and over again when most people would have done them only once?' 'Do you have to repeat exactly the same action many times?' If the patient answers 'yes' to any of these questions, the interviewer should ask for specific examples.

Delusions

A delusion is the one symptom that cannot be asked about directly, because the patient does not recognize it as differing from other beliefs. The interviewer may be alerted to the possibility of delusions by information from other people or by events in the history. In searching for delusional ideas, it is useful to begin by asking what might be the reason for other symptoms, or unpleasant experiences that the patient has described. For example, a patient who says that life is no longer worth living may believe without any objective evidence that he is thoroughly evil and that his career is ruined. Many patients hide delusions skilfully, and the interviewer needs to be alert to evasions, changes of topic, or other hints of information being withheld. However, once the delusion has been uncovered, patients often elaborate on it without much prompting.

When ideas are revealed that could be delusional, the interviewer should find out how strongly they are held. To do this without antagonizing the patient requires patience and tact. The patient should feel that he is having a fair hearing. If the interviewer expresses contrary opinions to test the strength of the patient's beliefs, his manner should be enquiring rather than argumentative. On the other hand, the interviewer should not agree with the patient's delusions.

The next step is to decide whether the beliefs are culturally determined convictions rather than delusions. This judgement may be difficult if the patient comes from another culture or is a member of a religious group whose beliefs are not known to the interviewer. In such cases any doubt can usually be resolved by finding a healthy informant from the same country or religion, and by asking this person whether the patient's ideas would be shared by others from that background.

Some *special types of delusion* present particular problems of recognition. Delusions of thought broadcasting must be distinguished from the belief that other people can infer a person's thoughts from his expression or behaviour. In eliciting such delusions an appropriate question is: 'Do you ever feel that other people know what you are thinking, even though you have not spoken your thoughts aloud?' If the patient says 'yes', the interviewer should ask how other people know this. (Some patients answer 'yes' when they mean that others can infer their thoughts from their facial expression.) A corresponding question about delusions of thought insertion is: 'Have you ever felt that some of the thoughts in your mind were not your own but were put there from outside?' A suitable question about delusions of thought withdrawal is: 'Do you ever feel that thoughts are being taken out of your head?' In each case, if the patient answers 'yes', detailed examples should be sought.

Delusions of control present similar difficulties to the interviewer. It is appropriate to ask 'Do you ever feel that some outside force is trying to take control of you?' or 'Do you ever feel that your actions are controlled by some person or thing outside you?' Some patients misunderstand the question and answer 'yes' when they mean that they have a religious or philosophical conviction that man is controlled by God or the devil. Others think that the questions refer to the experience of being 'out of control' during extreme anxiety; some schizophrenic patients say 'yes' when they have heard commanding voices. Therefore positive answers should be followed by further questions to eliminate these possibilities.

Finally, the reader is reminded of the various categories of delusion described in Chapter 1, namely persecutory, grandiose, nihilistic, hypochondriacal, religious, and amorous delusions, together with delusions of reference, guilt, unworthiness, and jealousy. The interviewer should also distinguish between primary and secondary delusions, and should look out for the experiences of delusional perception and delusional mood that may precede or accompany the onset of delusions.

Illusions and hallucinations

When asked about hallucinations, some patients take offence because they think that the interviewer regards them as insane. Therefore enquiries should be made tactfully, and common-sense judgement used to decide when it is safe to omit them altogether. Questions can be introduced by saying 'Some people find that, when their nerves are upset, they have unusual experiences'. This can be followed by enquiries about hearing sounds or voices when no one else is within earshot. Whenever the history makes it relevant, corresponding questions should be asked about visual hallucinations, or those of taste, smell, touch, and deep bodily sensations.

If the patient describes *auditory hallucinations*, certain further questions are required depending on the type of experience. Has the patient heard a single voice or several and, if the latter, did the voices appear to talk to each other about the patient in the third person. The latter experience must be distinguished from that of hearing actual people talking and believing that they are discussing the patient (a delusion of reference). If the patient says that the voices are speaking to him (second-person hallucinations), the interviewer should find out what the voices say and, if the words are experienced as commands, whether the patient feels that they must be obeyed. It is important to record examples of the words spoken by hallucinatory voices.

Visual hallucinations should be distinguished carefully from visual illusions. Unless the hallucination is experienced at the time of the interview, this distinction may be difficult because it depends on the presence or absence of a visual stimulus which has been misinterpreted.

The interviewer should also distinguish dissociative experiences from hallucinations. The former are described by the patient as the feeling of being in the presence of another person or a spirit with whom he can converse. Such experiences are reported by people with histrionic personality, though not confined to them; they are encouraged by some religious groups and have little importance in diagnosis.

Orientation

This is assessed by asking about the patient's awareness of time, place, and person. If the question of orientation is kept in mind throughout the interview, it may not be necessary to ask specific questions at this stage of the examination because the interviewer will already know the answers.

Specific questions begin with the day, month, year, and season. In assessing the replies, it is important to remember that many healthy people do not know the exact date and that, understandably, patients in hospital may be uncertain about the day of the week, particularly if the ward has the same routine every day. When enquiring about orientation in place, the interviewer asks what sort of place the patient is in (such as a hospital ward or an old people's home). Questions are then asked about other people such as the spouse or the ward staff; for example, who they are and what is their relationship to the patient. If the patient cannot answer these questions correctly, he should be asked about his own identity.

Attention and concentration

Attention is the ability to focus on the matter in hand. Concentration is the ability to sustain that focus. Whilst taking the history, the interviewer should look out for evidence of attention and concentration. In this way he will already have formed a judgement about these abilities before reaching the mental state examination. Formal tests add to this information and provide a semi-quantitative indication of changes between occasions. It is usual to begin with the serial sevens test. The patient is asked to subtract seven from 100 and then subtract seven from the remainder repeatedly until this is less than seven. The time taken is recorded, together with the number of errors. If poor performance seems to be due to lack of skill in

arithmetic, the patient should be asked to do a simpler subtraction or to say the months of the year in reverse order. If mistakes are made with these, he can be asked to give the days of the week in reverse order.

Memory

Whilst taking the history, the interviewer should compare the patient's account of past events with that of any other informant, and be alert to gaps or inconsistencies. If memory is impaired, any evidence of confabulation or false memory should be noted. During the examination of mental state, tests are given of short-term, recent, and remote memory. Since none is wholly satisfactory, the results should be assessed alongside other information about memory and, if there is doubt, supplemented by standardized psychological tests.

Short-term memory can be assessed by asking the patient to memorize a name and a simple address, to repeat it immediately (to make sure it has been registered correctly), and to retain it. The interview continues on other topics for 5 minutes before recall is tested. A healthy person of average intelligence should make only minor errors. In another test, the patient is told he is to remember a flower, a colour, and a town, and then given specific items (for example, rose, blue, York). After checking that he has heard correctly, recall is tested after 5 minutes without prompting. If recall is imperfect, memory can be prompted by naming the categories. The number of items can be increased by adding new categories such as months, or common makes of car.

Memory for recent events can be assessed by asking about news items from the last few days, or personal events provided that the latter are known to the interviewer either directly or through information supplied by relatives or others. Questions about news items should be adapted to the patient's interests, and should have been reported widely.

Remote memory can be assessed by asking the patient to recall personal events or well-known items of news from former years. Personal items could be the birth dates of children or the names of grandchildren (provided these are known to the interviewer); news items could be the names of well-known former political leaders. Awareness of the sequence of events is as important as the recall of individual items.

When a patient is in hospital, important information about memory is available from observations made by nurses and occupational therapists. These observations include how fast the patient learns the daily routine and the names of staff and other patients, and whether he forgets where he has put things, or where to find his bed, the sitting room, and so on. When at home, comparable observations made by relatives are valuable.

For elderly patients, the questions about memory in the clinical interview discriminate poorly between those who have a cerebral pathology and those who do not. For these patients it is more informative to use a standard set of questions that lead to a rating. One widely used rating, the Mini-Mental State Examination, is reproduced in the appendix to this chapter. A useful extended scheme (reproduced from Jacoby 2000b), is shown in Table 2.6. Assessment of the elderly is considered further in Chapter 20.

Standardized psychological tests of learning and memory can help in diagnosis and provide a quantitative assessment of the progression of memory disorder. One useful example is the Wechsler Logical Memory Test (Wechsler 1945) in which the patient has to recall the contents of a short paragraph immediately and after 45 minutes. The score is based on the number of items recalled. This test is a good discriminator between patients with organic brain disease on the one hand, and healthy controls and patients with depressive disorder on the other. (Kopelman 1986).

Insight

A note that merely records 'insight present' or 'no insight' is of little value. Instead the interviewer should enquire about the patient's appraisal of his difficulties and prospects, and whether he ascribes them to illness or to some other cause (such as persecution). If the patient recognizes that he is ill, does he think that the illness is physical or mental, and does he think that he needs treatment or care? The interviewer should also find out whether the patient thinks that stressful life experiences or his actions have played a part in causing his illness. The patient's views on these matters are a guide to his likely collaboration with treatment.

Some common difficulties in mental state examination

Unresponsive patients

If a patient is mute or stuporous (that is conscious but not speaking or responding) it is essential to interview an informant who can describe the onset and course of the condition. When it comes to the mental state, the interviewer can only observe behaviour, but this can be informative. Because some stuporous patients change rapidly from inactivity to violent overactivity, it is wise to have help at hand when seeing such a patient.

Before deciding that a patient is mute, the interviewer should allow adequate time for reply, and try several topics. If the patient still fails to respond, the interviewer should attempt to persuade him to communicate in writing. Apart from observations of behaviour, the interviewer should note whether the patient's eyes are open or closed. If open, he should note whether they follow objects, move apparently without purpose, or are fixed. If the eyes are closed, he should find out whether the patient opens them on request, and, if not, whether he resists attempts at opening them. A physical examination including neurological assessment is essential in all such cases. Also, certain signs found in catatonic schizophrenia should be sought, namely waxy flexibility of muscles and negativism (see Chapter 12).

Overactive patients

Some patients are so active and restless that systematic questioning about mental state is difficult. The interviewer then has to limit his questions to a few that seem particularly important, and observe the patient's behaviour and any spontaneous utterances. However, if the patient is being seen in an

Table 2.6 Schema for testing cognitive function based on an extended Mini-Mental State Examination

Function	Subfunctions	Examples
Orientation	Time	Year, month, date, day, season
	Place	Own address or that of hospital, city, county/state, country
	Person	Own name (married women sometimes cannot give married name; (recognize others by name or function (e.g. you are a doctor)
Memory	Immediate recall	Immediate repetition of three objects or a name and (local) address
	Delayed recall	Repetition as per above but after a distractor task
	Long-term recall	Give historical or personal events (that can be verified)
	General information	Names of politicians or other VIPs
Concentration		Months of the year in reverse order, counting back from 20, spelling 'WORLD' forward then backwards
Praxis	Constructional	
	Ideomotor	
	Dressing	
Sensory recognition (gnosis)	Visual including prosopagnosia	Show photos taken from unusual angles and of familiar faces
	Auditory	Recognize the doorbell
	Tactile	Recognize objects placed in palm, e.g. coins
	Reading	Any sample but *use large print*
	Olfactory	Recognize something from kitchen, e.g. coffee
Language	Expressive	Repeat 'no ifs and or buts'
	Understanding	Carry out a three-stage command
	Naming	Naming objects of increasing complexity
Verbal fluency		List as many items from a category as possible in one minute, such as boys and girls forenames; or as many words beginning with a specified letter.
Writing		Write an ordinary English sentence.
Calculation		Not too complex – subtraction of serial sevens from 100 is too difficult for many. A simple sum involving money is better.
Left/right orientation		Face/hand test (e.g. left hand to left ear, right hand to left ear); finger recognition on own and examiner's hand.
Abstract reasoning		'In what way are an apple and a banana alike?'
		'In what way are a boat and a car similar?'
		Interpretation of simple proverbs

Testing one function usually depends on one or more others, for example, most tests depend on understanding of language. Examples are neither prescriptive nor exhaustive.

Reproduced with permission from Jacoby (2000b).

emergency, some of his overactivity may be a reaction to other people's attempts to restrain him. In such a case, a quiet but confident approach by the interviewer may calm the patient enough to allow more adequate examination.

Confused patients

When the patient gives a history in a muddled way, or appears perplexed or frightened, the interviewer should test cognitive functions early in the interview. If there is evidence of impaired consciousness, the interviewer should try to orientate the patient and to reassure him before starting the interview again in a simplified form. In such cases every effort should be made to interview another informant.

Physical examination

With day- or in-patients, the psychiatrist is generally responsible for their physical as well as their mental health, and he should conduct a thorough physical examination. Many out-patients have been referred by another doctor who may have reported the results of an appropriate physical examination. The care of many patients is shared between the psychiatrist and the referring doctor, but the psychiatrist should still decide what physical examination is relevant and carry it out himself if it has not been done by the referring doctor, or in certain cases ask that another doctor complete it.

The extent of the physical examination has to be judged case by case, on the basis of diagnostic possibilities. However, the psychiatrist is most likely to be concerned with examination of the central nervous system (including its vascular supply) and the endocrine system. Physical examination should not, of course, be limited to these systems and, as indicated above, all in-patients should have a full routine examination. For readers who require it, neuropsychiatric examination is summarized in Box 2.1.

Special investigations

These vary according to the nature of the patient's symptoms and the differential diagnosis. No set of routine investigations is essential for every case.

Investigations most relevant to suspected specific psychiatric disorders are reviewed in the chapters on individual syndromes, particularly the section on delirium, dementia, and related disorders. If there is any reason to suspect co-morbid physical ill-health, relevant investigations should be carried out.

Psychological assessment

Many standardized tests are available. The most useful for the clinician are tests of intelligence and of higher neurological functions. Other tests are still in use but have less general value, for example, those of personality and 'brain damage'. In this section, a knowledge of the principles of psychological testing is assumed and no detailed account will be attempted. When psychological testing is an important part of assessment, it will be mentioned in the chapters on clinical syndromes. At this stage only a few general points will be considered.

Tests of intelligence In general adult psychiatry it is not necessary to have an accurate assessment of every patient's intelligence. However, if a patient seems to be of borderline or low subnormal intelligence, intelligence tests are indicated. Intelligence tests and standard tests of reading ability are important also in child and adolescent psychiatry (see Chapter 24) and essential in the assessment of patients with learning disability (see Chapter 25).

Neuropsychological tests Computerized axial tomography is generally the best way of assessing diffuse cerebral pathology, but specific neuropsychological tests are of some value as pointers to dysfunction of the frontal or parietal cortex. Such tests are also valuable in measuring the progression of deficits caused by disease. Further discussion of these issues will be found in Chapter 14.

Personality tests Personality tests have some value in clinical research, but they are not useful in clinical practice as they do not measure aspects of personality that are most relevant to psychiatric disorder.

Box 2.1 The neuropsychiatric examination

Language abilities

Dysarthria is difficulty in the production of speech by the speech organs. *Dysphasia* is partial failure of language function of cortical origin. Dysphasia may be expressive or receptive, or both, and may involve either spoken or written language. Testing for dysphasia and tests for dysarthria should be done by giving difficult phrases such as 'West Register Street' or a tongue twister.

Receptive dysphasia can be detected by asking the patient to read a passage of appropriate difficulty or, if he fails in this, individual words or letters. If he can read the passage, he is asked to explain it. Comprehension of spoken language is tested by asking a patient to listen to a spoken passage and explain it (first checking that memory is intact), or to respond to simple commands, for example, to point at named objects.

Expressive dysphasia is detected by asking patients to name common objects such as a watch, key, and pen, and some of their parts (for example, the face of a watch), and parts of the body. They are asked also to talk spontaneously (for example, about hobbies) and to write a brief passage, first to dictation, and then spontaneously on a familiar topic (for example, the members of the family). A patient who cannot do these tests should be asked to copy a short passage.

Language disorders point to the left hemisphere in right-handed people. In left-handed patients localization is less certain, but in many it is still the left hemisphere. The type of language disorder gives some further guide to localization: expressive dysphasia suggests an anterior lesion, receptive dysphasia suggests a posterior lesion, mainly auditory dysphasia suggests a lesion towards the temporal region, and mainly visual dysphasia a more posterior lesion.

Construction abilities

Apraxia is inability to perform a volitional act even though the motor system and sensorium are sufficiently intact for the person to do so. Apraxia can be tested in several ways.

- *Constructional apraxia* is tested by asking the patient to make simple figures with matchsticks (a square, triangle, and cross) or to draw them. He can also be asked to draw a bicycle, house, or clock face.
- *Dressing apraxia* is tested by asking the person to put on some of his clothes.

- *Ideomotor apraxia* is tested by asking him to perform increasingly complicated tasks to command, usually ending with a three-stage sequence such as: (i) touch the right ear with (ii) the left middle finger while (iii) placing the right thumb on the table.

Constructional apraxia, especially if the patient fails to complete the left side of figures, suggests a right-sided lesion in the posterior parietal region. It may be associated with other disorders related to this region, namely sensory inattention and anosognosia. Dressing apraxia also suggests a non-dominant parietal lobe lesion.

Agnosia is the inability to understand the significance of sensory stimuli even though the sensory pathways and sensorium are sufficiently intact for the patient to be able to do so. Agnosia cannot be diagnosed until there is good evidence that the sensory pathways are intact and consciousness is not impaired.

- *Astereognosia* is failure to identify three-dimensional form; it is tested by asking the patient to identify objects placed in his hand while his eyes are closed. Suitable items are keys, coins of different sizes, and paper clips.
- *Atopognosia* is failure to know the position of an object on the skin.
- In *finger agnosia* the patient cannot identify which of his fingers has been touched when he has his eyes shut. Right-left confusion is tested by touching one hand or ear and asking the patient which side of the body has been touched.
- *Agraphognosia* is failure to identify letters or numbers 'written' on the skin. It is tested by tracing numbers on the palms with a closed fountain pen or similar object.
- *Anosognosia* is failure to identify functional deficits caused by disease. It is seen most often as unawareness of left-sided weakness and sensory inattention after a right parietal lesion.

Agnosias point to lesions of the association areas around the primary sensory receptive areas. Lesions of either parietal lobe can cause contralateral astereognosia, agraphognosia, and atopognosia. Sensory inattention and anosognosia are more common with right parietal lesions. Finger agnosia and right-left disorientation are said to be more common with lesions of the dominant parietal region.

Projective tests such as the Rorschach test are not recommended.

Standardized rating scales of behaviour These are often useful in everyday clinical practice. When no ready-made rating scale is available, a clinical psychologist can often devise *ad hoc* ratings that are sufficiently reliable to chart the effects of treatment in the individual patient. For example, in measuring the progress of a depressed in-patient, a scale could be devised for the nurses to show how much of the time he was active and occupied. This could be a five-point scale, in which the criteria for each rating refer to behaviour (such as playing cards or talking to other people) relevant to the individual patient.

Psychological principles are also used to make a *behavioural assessment*. This is a detailed account of the component elements of a patient's disorder (for example, in a phobic state the elements of anticipatory anxiety, avoidance behaviour, and coping strategies) and their relationship to stimuli in the environment (for example, heights), or more general circumstances (for example, crowded places), or internal cues (for example, awareness of heart action). Behavioural assessment is a necessary preliminary to cognitive–behaviour therapy (see p. 734).

Special kinds of interview

Interviews in an emergency

If the patient is brought by another person, such as a member of the police, the interview should find out how long that person is able to stay so as to be sure that he obtains any necessary information from the informant before he has to leave.

Since time is limited and an immediate decision is required about diagnosis and management, it is usually possible to obtain only an outline history. However short the time, it is essential to obtain a clear account of the presenting symptoms, including their onset, course, and severity. Knowledge of the major clinical syndromes will then guide the interviewer to enquiries about other relevant symptoms, remembering always the possibility of an organic brain syndrome. Recent stressful events should always be asked about, together with any previous physical or mental illness. A brief account of previous personality is important, though it may be difficult to obtain unless there are relatives or close friends present. Habits regarding alcohol and drugs are especially important. The family and personal history will often have to be covered quickly by asking a few salient questions. Throughout the interview the psychiatrist should be thinking which questions need to be asked immediately and which can be deferred until later. Any relevant physical examination should be carried out unless it has been performed by another doctor

If the patient has been treated before, by the same health team or elsewhere, strenuous efforts should be made to contact a professional who knows the patient.

Interviews in a patient's home

It is often appropriate to add to information about the patient's social circumstances by visiting the home, or arranging for another member of the psychiatric team to do so. Such a visit often throws new light on the patient's home life. It can sometimes lead to a more realistic evaluation of the relationship between family members than can be obtained from interviews in hospital. Before arranging a visit the psychiatrist should, if possible, talk to the general practitioner, who often has first-hand knowledge of the family and their circumstances from home visits over the years. If another member of the psychiatric team is to make the visit, the psychiatrist should discuss the purpose of the visit with him. Such visits are especially important in the assessment of older patients (see Chapter 20).

Interviews with the family

Sometimes an interview is carried out with several family members together to find out their attitudes to the patient and the illness and the nature of any conflicts within the family. The interviewer should remember that the family has usually tried to help the patient but failed and may feel demoralized, frustrated, or guilty, and should be careful not to add to these feelings.

The interviewer should then ask:

◆ How has the family tried to cope with the illness and its consequences?

◆ How has the illness affected family life?

◆ Are the members willing to try new ways of helping the patient?

◆ What are the relationships within the family? For example, alliances across the generations such as father and daughter taking sides against mother. Are there important differences of opinion between the members of the family?

The interviewer should be alert for cues in the interview. Sometimes one person repeatedly answers for another. If so, the interviewer might ask whether this happens at home and what the second person feels about it. However, such questions should be asked cautiously for, unless the family is to be seen again soon, they may lead to conflict after the family has left the interview.

Useful further information about these and other aspects of family interviews will be found in Goldberg (1997).

Interviewing a patient from another culture

If the patient and interviewer do not speak the same language, an interpreter will obviously be needed. However, accurate interpretation is not the only requirement, and the interviewer may not know the patient's culture as well as he knows the language. Also, female patients from another culture may be reluctant to describe personal matters to a male interviewer. Even when these problems are absent, the presence of a third person, and the process of translation, affect the interview. If possible the interpreter should be a health professional (if appropriately qualified he may conduct the interview himself if he is briefed appropriately about the points that are most important). If the only available interpreter is a family member, the patient may not speak freely, and the interpretation may be influenced by the interpreter's opinions.

Certain events may be more stressful to a patient from another culture than they would be in the interviewer's culture. The stigma of mental illness may be greater and may be added to by the stigma attached to membership of a minority group. Priorities within the family may be different, with the well-being of the family outweighing that of its individual members. Differences in religion within a wider culture are likely to be important, for example, in attitudes to marriage. Emotional disorder may be experienced more in terms of physical than mental symptoms. Expectations and fears about treatment may be based on knowledge of less developed services in the country of origin. Behaviours that suggest illness in one culture may be socially sanctioned ways of expressing distress in others, for example, extreme displays of emotion. Ideas about causation may differ; for example, distress may be ascribed to the actions of evil spirits. Also it may be difficult to decide whether strongly held ideas are delusional or normal within the culture or subculture. These and other cultural differences are usually understood best by asking a healthy person from the same cultural group.

Interviewing a patient with learning disability

The procedures for interviewing people with learning disability are similar to those for people with normal intelligence but certain points should receive particular attention. Questions should be brief and worded in a simple way, avoiding structures such as subordinate clauses, passive verb constructions, and figures of speech. It may be difficult to avoid closed questions, but if they are used, the answers should be checked; for example, if the question 'Are you sad?' is answered 'yes', the question 'Are you happy?' should not be answered in the same way. Some people with learning disability repeat the interviewer's last word, and such a response should not be accepted as agreement unless checked. (For example, Interviewer: Do you feel sad? Patient: Feel sad.)

People with learning disability may have difficulty in timing the onset of symptoms or describing their sequence, and to obtain this and other information it is important to interview an informant. Nevertheless, an attempt should always be made to obtain from patients an account of their symptoms and their concerns.

Interviewing the elderly

Interviewing and assessment of the elderly are considered on pp. 638–9.

Interviewing children and adolescents

Interviewing and assessment of children and adolescents are considered on pp. 808–12.

Assessment

General principles

Symptoms and disablement

When patients describe their problems, they usually include matters which, for the purpose of assessment, can be usefully divided into symptoms and disablement. Symptoms were discussed in Chapter 1. Disablement has three components:

- *impairment*, which is interference with the functioning of a psychological or physical system, such as memory;

- *disability*, which is interference with the activities of the whole person, for example, inability to dress oneself;

- *handicap*, which is the social disadvantage consequent upon impairment and disability, for example, inability to work or to fulfil the role of a parent.

There is some overlap between the concepts – for example, deficient memory is both a symptom and an impairment – but generally the distinctions are useful. Disablement is usually caused by a disorder (e.g. schizophrenia) that also causes symptoms. However, symptoms are sometimes the consequence of disablement, for example, depression

that is consequent upon inability to work caused by the effects of a stroke (see p. 88).

Although social disadvantage (handicap) is usually a consequence of symptoms or disablement, it can result from the negative opinions of other people about the patient and the disorder. This process by which a patient is judged not as a person but as a member of a group, is an aspect of *stigma*. For example, the widely held opinion that schizophrenics, as a group, are unpredictable and dangerous, makes it difficult for an individual schizophrenic patient to obtain work (a handicap) even though he may have neither impairment nor disability. The tendency of people to assume that everyone with the same diagnosis shares all the same attributes has led some writers to assert that diagnoses should not be assigned to patients. However, diagnosis is an essential stage in evaluation and stigma will be reduced by public education about psychiatric disorder, not by pretending that psychiatric disorders do not exist.

Disease and illness

These concepts are considered in Chapter 4 but some discussion is required here. *Illness* refers to a patient's experience and *disease* to the pathological cause for this experience. Patients can be diseased without feeling ill (as in the early stages of cancer) or feel ill without having a disease. Patients tell doctors about their experience of illness and doctors seek to discover the disease that is causing the illness since this will guide treatment. Patients and their relatives also want to find a cause and a treatment for their illness but they do not always understand how a medical diagnosis helps in finding them. Native healers and practitioners of alternative medicine are aware of the wishes of patients' relatives and owe much of their success to the naming of a cause and the provision of a treatment, both explained in terms that patients understand.

Psychologists and social workers are also concerned with a patient's experience (that is with illness) but they prefer to explain this in terms other than disease; for example, psychologists may explain it as an extreme variation from the norm, and social workers may explain it as a reaction to circumstances. In psychiatry all three approaches – disease, extreme variation, and reaction to circumstances – should be considered in every case. There is therefore no fundamental difference between the approach of psychiatrists and other members of the psychiatric team, though there is sometimes a difference of emphasis. Such a difference can lead to apparent disagreements during a multidisciplinary assessment, and it is important that psychiatrists are aware of this possibility, so that they can help to resolve the differences.

The stages of assessment

The stages of a full assessment of a patient requires decisions about the factors shown in Table 2.7.

In a textbook, a description of assessment necessarily follows a description of the ways in which information is collected. However, in clinical practice experienced assessors undertake the two processes in parallel. From the start of the inter-

Table 2.7 **The nature and severity of the problem**
The problem
• diagnosis
• severity
• risk of suicide
• disablement
• effects on others
• the risk of dangerousness to others
The person who has the problem and his circumstances
• personality
• social circumstances
• life story
Aetiology
A plan of management incorporating
• prognosis
• treatment

view, they have in mind the questions that will need to be answered in the assessment, and collect information accordingly. This approach to interviewing is especially important when time is limited and questioning has to be selective. Nevertheless, even when time is short it is essential to allow adequate time for the patient to describe the problems spontaneously before the interviewer starts to direct questions to the topics that appear to be most relevant for assessment. If this is not done, important leads may be overlooked and wrong conclusions drawn. For example, if a patient describes depression and anxiety, premature questioning directed to the possibility of a mood disorder might cut short a patient's account of his problems before he has expressed concerns about the behaviour of neighbours which could lead the interviewer to persecutory delusions.

Assessing the problem and the risks

The first step is to make a *diagnosis* using information about the nature and time course of symptoms gained from the history and mental state examination and, in relevant cases, from physical examination. Sometimes this diagnosis has to be provisional until further information becomes available. The diagnosis of particular psychiatric disorders is discussed in subsequent chapters; here we are concerned with the general approach to assessment. Diagnosis is accompanied by an assessment of the severity of the disorder into categories of mild, moderate, and severe. Generally, this will be done solely on clinical grounds but sometimes a standard method – such as the Beck depression inventory (Beck *et al.*, 1961) – may be used to supplement, though never to replace, the clinical evaluation. An important aspect of severity is the assessment of *suicide risk*, which should always be considered. This assessment is considered on p. 515.

Sometimes no psychiatric disorder can be found. This negative finding does not necessarily remove the need for treatment, but it helps to determine what help is required. For example, a patient who has taken an overdose of drugs may have no psychiatric disorder, but still requires help with social and interpersonal problems.

Disablement is considered next, dividing the problems into impairment, disability, and handicap. When a patient is seen for the first time, this part of the assessment may have to be incomplete but it will still be possible to decide what additional information will be needed to complete the assessment.

The effect on others is considered next. For example, in assessing an elderly patient, the effect of the patient's illness on the health of the spouse may be an important factor in deciding whether admission to hospital is required.

Risk assessment

Risk assessment is an important part of the evaluation. Three kinds of information are used to assess the risk that a patient will behave in a way that may endanger others: personal factors (derived mainly from population studies), factors related to illness, and factors in the mental state (see Table 2.8).

The most important of the *personal factors* is previous violence towards others (starred in the table). It is important to seek full information on this and other factors not only by questioning the patient but, in appropriate cases, from additional sources including relatives and close acquaintances, previous medical and social services records, and in certain cases the police. Antisocial, impulsive, or irritable features in the personality are a further risk factor, and men are more at risk then women. Other personal factors are listed in Table 2.8. Social circumstances at times of any previous episodes of violence may reveal *provoking factors*, and should be compared with the patient's current situation (see below). Men are more often violent than are women, and personality traits of impulsivity and irritability should be taken into account. Social isolation and a recent life crisis also increase the risk.

Among the *illness factors*, psychotic disorder and drug or alcohol misuse are important, especially when present together. Failure to continue treatment in the past is a guide to the possible protective effect of further treatment, as is previous resistance to treatment.

Factors in the *mental state* listed in Table 2.7 require careful consideration. Thoughts of violence

Table 2.8 Risk factors for harm to others

Personal factors
- Previous violence to others*
- Antisocial, impulsive, or irritable personality traits
- Male and young
- Recent life crisis
- Poor social network
- Divorced or separated
- Unemployed
- Social instability

Illness-related factors
- Pychotic symptoms (see below)*
- Substance abuse*
- Treatment resistant
- Poor compliance with treatment
- Stopped medication recently

Factors in the mental state
- Irritability, hostility, anger
- Suspiciousness
- Thoughts of violence towards others
- Threats to people to whom patient has access*
- Planning of violence*
- Persecutory delusions
- Delusions of jealousy
- Delusions of influence
- Hallucinations commanding violence to others
- Suicidal ideas with severe depression
- Clouding of consciousness
- Lack of insight about illness

Situational factors
- Confrontation and provocation by others
- Situations associated with previous violence
- Ready availability of weapons*

to others are very important, especially if concerned with a specific person to whom the patient has access. The entry concerning suicidal ideas refers to the occasional killing, usually of family members, by a patient with severe (usually psychotic) depression (see p. 909).

Situational factors are highly important. Actual or perceived confrontational behaviour towards the patient by others may trigger violence, as may a return to situations in which violence has been expressed in the past. Enquiries should always be made about the *availability of weapons*.

Clinical experience and common sense judgement have to be used to combine the risk factors into an overall assessment. Risk assessment schedules have been developed but to date they cannot replace thorough and repeated clinical assessment. Risk assessment is considered further on pp. 924–5.

The assessment of risk should be shared among the members of the team treating the patient, or if the patient is in individual treatment, may need to be discussed with a colleague. In certain circumstances the assessment may need to be made known to an individual at risk (see p. 78). Risk assessments should be *reviewed regularly*, combining information from the members of the clinical team. See Mullen (2000) for further information.

Assessing the person and his circumstances

Social circumstances are assessed from the same sources of information and should include supportive aspects as well as social disadvantages.

The assessment of personality is described on pp. 40–1. The assessment does not end with a decision whether there is a co-morbid personality disorder. Instead the personality should be described, noting its strengths and weaknesses. When there is time – usually after the first assessment interview – the psychiatrist should gain an understanding of the patient's life story. This is an understanding of the person's previous experiences, hopes, and plans. The life story often helps to explain how a patient has responded to current

events and how he is likely to respond in future. For example, when a suicide attempt follows an apparently minor setback, this may be the last in a long series of losses and frustrated hopes.

Assessing aetiology

Aetiological models are discussed in Chapter 5. Here we are concerned with the general approach. The general approach is chronological: causes are divided into predisposing, precipitating, and perpetuating factors. Predisposing factors may be genetic or related to temperament, or to damage to the brain in early life. Precipitating factors are often stressful events. Perpetuating factors may be continuing stressors, or related to the way that the patient attempts to cope with stressors. Perpetuating factors are highly relevant to treatment.

A *life chart* is a tool for evaluating the role of life events in aetiology. It helps to reveal the time relations between episodes of physical and mental disorder and potentially stressful events in the patient's life. It is often useful when the history is long and complicated. The chart has three columns – one for life events, and one each for physical and mental disorder. Its rows represent the years in the patient's life. In principle there is one line per year, but in practice it is easier to allocate this amount of space to periods of most interest, and attenuate the years between.

Completion of a life chart requires detailed enquiry into the timing of events, and this may clarify the relationships between stressors and the onset of illness, and also between physical and mental disorders. For example, in the case of a recurrent illness previously thought to be provoked by stressful events, the chart may show that it has run a regular course and that comparable events have occurred at other times without consequent illness. In another case the chart may provide convincing evidence of a relationship between stressful events and illness

Assessing prognosis and planning management

Factors determining the prognosis and approaches to management of the various psychiatric disorders are considered in other chapters.

Explaining the assessment

The assessment should be discussed with the patient, but many patients are too anxious to remember much of this explanation and are helped by a written note to refer to later. If a relative is present and the patient agrees, it is often helpful to ask this person to join the discussion. If the plan includes a contribution by a relative, this presence is essential.

Assessment in primary care

General practitioners have to identify minor psychiatric disorders in a brief interview and among patients who often have an associated physical illness. The latter requirement is reflected in the finding (Goldberg and Huxley 1980) that general practitioners who diagnose mental disorder accurately, as compared with a standard assessment, have a good knowledge of general medicine. Psychiatrists often work in primary care and need to understand how assessments are made by general practitioners.

In the very brief interviews used in general practice, the first few minutes are especially important. However, little time is available, and the patient should always be allowed enough time to describe the complaint in his own words, before any questions are asked. The interview technique is broadly similar to that described on pp. 31–4, using prompts and clarifying questions and with attention to non-verbal behaviour. In general practice, the presenting complaint is often physical when the disorder is psychiatric. While a physical cause should always be sought for such symptoms, questions directed to this possibility should not be allowed to stifle the full spontaneous description that is needed if psychiatric causes are to be assessed.

The assessment of a patient whose complaint that may have a psychological cause has four elements (Goldberg and Huxley 1980):

- *general psychological adjustment* fatigue, irritability, poor concentration, and the feeling of being under stress;
- *anxiety and worries* physical symptoms of anxiety and tension, phobias, and persistent worrying thoughts;
- *symptoms of depression* persistent depressive mood, tearfulness, crying, hopelessness, self-blame, thoughts that life is unbearable, ideas about suicide, early morning waking, diurnal variation of mood, weight loss, and loss of libido;
- *the psychological context* although often known to the general practitioner from previous contacts, this should be reviewed and brought up to date.

Although it may not be possible to reach a conclusion by the end of the brief interview that is possible during a busy clinic in primary care (unless the problem is an emergency when more time must be found), a preliminary plan can usually be made and a longer interview arranged for a later time.

Recording information

The importance of case notes

Good case records are important in every branch of medicine. In psychiatry they are vital because a large amount of information has to be collected from a variety of sources, often by more than one member of the psychiatric team. Unless material is recorded clearly, with facts separated from opinions, it will be difficult to make appropriate decisions about treatment. It is important to summarize the information in a way that allows essential points to be grasped readily by someone new to the case, especially a colleague called to deal with an emergency. Case notes are not just an aide mémoire for the writer, they are essential for others concerned with the patient and should be legible and well organized.

Case notes are also of medico-legal importance. If a psychiatrist is called upon to justify his actions in the coroner's court, at a trial, or after a complaint has been made by a patient, he will be greatly assisted by good case notes. In writing notes, it should be remembered that in many places patients are permitted to read their own notes and that they may be called in evidence by lawyers. It is important also that information given confidentially by informants should be separated from the rest of the record (see p. 35).

Admission notes

When a patient is admitted to hospital urgently, the doctor often has limited time so that it is then particularly important to record the right topics. The admission note should contain at least:

- the reasons for admission
- any information required for a decision about immediate treatment
- any other relevant information that will not be available later such as details of the mental state on admission, and information from any informant who may not be available again. The account of the mental state should include verbatim extracts to illustrate phenomena such as delusions or flight of ideas.

If there is time, a systematic history can be added. However, inexperienced interviewers sometimes spend too much time on details that are not essential to the immediate decisions, while failing to record details of mental state that may be transitory and yet of great importance in diagnosis. The admission note should end with a brief provisional plan of management, agreed with the senior nurses caring for the patient at the time

Progress notes

Progress notes need to contain specific information if they are to be of value when the case is reviewed later. Instead of recording merely that the patient feels better or is behaving more normally, the note should state in what ways he feels better (for example, less preoccupied with thoughts of suicide) or is less disturbed in behaviour (for example, no longer so restless as to be unable to sit at table throughout a meal).

Progress notes should record treatment. Although details of drug treatment appear on the prescription sheet, when progress is reviewed, it is usually convenient to have this information, together with any non-drug treatments, alongside the record of changes in mental state and behaviour. Sessions of counselling or psychotherapy need not be recorded in full, but notes should be made of the main themes, together with any relevant observations of the patient's response. It is often useful to add an occasional note summarizing progress over several sessions. Also a note should be made of the conclusions of team meetings.

A careful note should also be made of any information or advice given by the doctor to the patient or his relatives. This should be sufficient to make it clear whether the patient was appropriately informed when consenting to any new treatment. Also it should enable anyone giving advice later to know whether or not it differs from what was said before, so that any necessary explanation can be given.

Observations of progress are made not only by psychiatrists but also by nurses, occupational therapists, clinical psychologists, and social workers. Often, these other members of staff keep separate notes for their own use, but it is desirable that important items of information are written in the medical record. These may be incorporated in a note of a team meeting, though separate entries may be required as well. A note should also be kept of formal discussions between the consultant or named worker and other members of the team. It is particularly important to set out clearly the plans made for the patient's further care on discharge from hospital.

The case summary

This section can best be understood by referring to the summary of a hypothetical case in Box 2.2. The case summary is often written in two parts. The first, completed soon after the patient's admission, serves to highlight the salient features of the case. The second part of the summary is prepared when the assessment has been completed and plans for discharge have been considered. This second part contains information obtained since the first part was written, a resumé of treatment received, and

---

Box 2.2 Example of a case summary

Patient Mrs AB. Date of birth 7.2.70

Consultant Dr C. Summary complied by Dr D

Admitted 27.6.01

Discharged 4.8.01

Reason for referral Severe depression increasing despite out-patient treatment.

Family history Father 66, retired gardener, good physical health, mood swings, poor relationship with patient. Mother 57, housewife, healthy, convinced spiritualist, distant relationship. Sibling Joan, 35, divorced, healthy. Home materially adequate, little affection. Mental illness father's brother in hospital four times – 'manic depression'.

Personal history Birth and early development normal. Childhood health good. School 6–16 uneventful; made friends. Worked 16–22 shop assistant. Several boyfriends; married at 22, husband 2 years older, lorry driver. Unhappy in last year following husband's infidelity. Children Jane, 7, well; Paul, 4, epileptic. Sexual relations satisfactory until last year. Menses no abnormality. Circumstances council house, financial problems.

Previous illness Aged 20, appendicectomy. Aged 24, (postnatal) depressive illness lasting 3 weeks.

Previous personality Few friends, interests within the family, variable mood, worries easily, lacks self-confidence, jealous, no obsessional traits, no conventional religious beliefs but shares mother's interest in the supernatural. Drinks occasionally, non-smoker, denies drugs.

History of present illness For 6 weeks, since learning of husband's infidelity, increasingly low-spirited and tearful, waking early, inactive, neglecting children. Eating little. Low libido. Believes herself to be in contact with dead grandmother through telepathy. Progressive worsening despite fluoxetine 20 mg daily for 3 weeks.

On examination Physical n.a.d. Mental dishevelled and distraught. Talk slow, halting, normal form. Preoccupied with her unhappy state and its effect on her children. Mood depressed, with self-blame, hopelessness, but no ideas of suicide. Delusions none. Hallucinations none. Compulsive phenomena none. Orientation normal. Attention and concentration poor. Memory not impaired. Insight thinks she is ill but believes she cannot recover.

Special investigations Haemoglobin and electrolytes n.a.d.

Treatment and progress Medication changed to amitriptyline, progressively increased to 175 mg per day, graded activities, joint interviews with husband to improve marital relationship. Advice to husband about management of financial problems. Gradual improvement in hospital with three weekends at home before final discharge. Amitriptyline reduced to 100 mg per day at time of discharge.

Condition on discharge Not depressed but remains uncertain about future of marriage.

Diagnosis Depressive disorder.

Prognosis Depends on outcome of marital problems. If these improve, the short-term prognosis is good but will be at risk of further depressive illness in the long term.

Further management

◆ Continue amitriptyline 100 mg per day for 6 months (prescriptions from general practitioner).

◆ Continue marital interviews (first appointment 14.8.01).

◆ Follow-up by GP and community nurse. First review with psychiatrist in one month.

plans for the future. The completed summary is valuable should the patient become ill again, especially if he is under the care of a different team.

Summaries should be brief but comprehensive. They should be written in telegraphic style, using a standard format to help others people to find particular items of information. Particularly confidential details can be omitted and a note made that relevant information appears in the case history. A completed summary should seldom need to be any more than between one and one and a half typewritten pages.

Some of the items in the summary call for comment. The *reason for referral* should state the problem rather than anticipate the diagnosis, for example: 'found wandering at night in an agitated state, shouting about God and the devil', rather than 'for treatment of schizophrenia'. The description of *personality* is important, and the writer should strive hard to find words and phrases which characterize the person. Unless an abnormality has been found, results of *physical examination* can be summarized briefly. However, when the *mental state* is recorded, a comment should be made under each heading whether or not any abnormality has been found. *Diagnosis* should be recorded using terms from ICD-10 or DSM-IV. If the diagnosis is uncertain, alternatives can be listed, with an indication of which is judged more likely. More than one diagnosis may be required in some cases.

The *summary of treatment* should indicate the main treatments used, including the dosage and duration of any medication. The *prognosis* should be stated briefly but as definitely as possible. Statements such as 'prognosis guarded' are of little help to anyone. Unless the assessor commits himself more firmly he will not learn from comparing his predictions with the actual outcome. The writer should note how certain is the prognosis and the reasons for any uncertainty, such as doubt about the patient's future compliance with treatment.

The summary of future treatment should specify not only what is to be done but also who is to do it. The roles of the specialist team and the family doctor should be made clear.

The formulation

Table 2.9 **The formulation**
Statement of the problem
Differential diagnosis
Aetiology
Further investigations
Plan of treatment
Prognosis

A formulation (see Table 2.9) is an exercise in clinical reasoning which helps the writer think clearly about diagnosis, aetiology, treatment, and prognosis. A formulation should not contain speculation, but it may contain hypotheses that can be tested by obtaining further information. By writing formulations of a wide variety of cases, the trainee can learn to analyse the problems of a case. For an experienced psychiatrist, a written formulation remains a valuable aid to the understanding complex cases.

There is more than one way of setting out a formulation A commonly used approach begins with a concise *statement of the problem*, for example: 'Mrs XY is a 60-year-old divorced woman with depressed mood and sleep disturbance which started after an operation for cancer of the bowel and which have not responded to out-patient treatment.'

The *differential diagnosis* comes next with a list of reasonable possibilities in the order of their probability. (The writer should avoid listing every conceivable diagnosis, however remote.) A note is made of the evidence for and against each alternative, followed by the writer's conclusion about the most probable diagnosis.

Disablement and disability are noted where relevant (usually in chronic disorders).

Aetiology comes next. The first step is to identify predisposing, precipitating, and maintaining causes. The reasons for any predisposition are then considered, usually in chronological order to show

how each factor may have added to those that went before.

There follows a list of outstanding problems and any *further information* needed. Next a concise plan of *management* is outlined. This should mention social measures as well as psychological treatment and medication, together with the role of the various members of the psychiatric team.

Finally, a statement is made about *prognosis*. As in the summary (see above), a firm prediction should be made with a note of the uncertainties that may undermine it. The assessor can learn by comparing a failed prediction with the actual outcome, but nothing can be learnt from a non-committal statement. Box 2.3 contains an example of a formulation.

Problem lists

A problem list is a useful in cases with complicated social problems. Such a list makes it easier to identify clearly what can be done to help the patient,

---

Box 2.3 Example of a formulation

(Note: This formulation refers to the hypothetical case summarized in Box 2.2. By comparing the two ways of condensing information, the reader can appreciate the difference between the two approaches.)

Mrs XY is a 31-year-old married woman who for 6 weeks has been feeling increasingly depressed and unable to cope at home, despite out-patient treatment with antidepressant drugs.

Diagnosis
Depressive disorder As well as feeling low-spirited, Mrs XY has woken unusually early, felt worse in the morning, and lost her appetite. She has little energy or initiative. She blames herself for being a bad mother (which she is not) and believes that she cannot recover. Her belief that she is in contact with her dead grandmother is unusual in a depressive disorder. No feature is against the diagnosis.

Schizophrenia Mrs XY's belief that she is in contact with her dead grandmother is an overvalued idea, not a delusion. It was present before she became ill and relates clearly to her own and her mother's interest in spiritualism. She has no first-rank symptom of schizophrenia.

Personality disorder Although Mrs XY has had mood variations for many years, these do not meet the criteria for a cyclothymic personality disorder.

Conclusions Depressive disorder.

Aetiology The symptoms appear to have been *precipitated* by news of the husband's infidelity. Mrs XY was predisposed to react severely to this news by the insecure and jealous traits in her personality. She may be *predisposed* to develop a depressive disorder in relation to stressful events in that (a) she became depressed after the birth of her first child, (b) she is subject to mood variations. Her father suffers similar, but more extreme, mood variations and her uncle has been admitted to hospital four times for treatment of a manic-depressive disorder. This family history could indicate a genetic cause for depression within the family which could be have been inherited by the patient.

The depressive disorder may have been *maintained* by continuing quarrels with the husband and by worry about debts he has incurred. Mrs XY's knowledge of her sister's divorce and subsequent unhappiness has added to her concerns about the future of her own marriage.

Treatment The pattern of symptoms of the depressive disorder suggests that it is likely to respond to an antidepressant drug given in adequate dosage. She has not responded to an SSRI as an out-patient. Amitriptyline may be more effective for severe depressive disorders and should be used now, increasing the dose gradually. Joint interviews with the patient and her husband may resolve or reduce the marital problems. The husband should be advised how to get advice about dealing with his debts.

Prognosis If the marital problems improve, the immediate prognosis is good. However, the several predisposing factors noted above indicate that she may develop further depressive disorder, particularly at future times of stress.

and to monitor progress in achieving agreed objectives of treatment

Table 2.10 shows a problem list that might be drawn up following the initial assessment of a young married women who had taken a small overdose impulsively and had no psychiatric disorder. As progress is made in dealing with problems in this list, new ones may be added or existing ones modified. For example, after a few joint interviews it might appear that the patient's sexual difficulties are a cause of the marital problem rather than a result, and that counselling about sexual matters should be offered. Item 4 in Table 2.10 would then be amended appropriately. Likewise, if the assessment of the child by the general practitioner were to confirm speech delay, an appointment for a specialist opinion might follow.

It is often appropriate to draw up the list with the patient, as a way of helping him to understand which problems can be changed and what he must do himself to bring this about.

Similar lists can be a valuable aid to the review of patient's progress in hospital or the community when the list is used in this way, treatment is listed in the same column as the other actions. Table 2.11 shows a list that might be drawn up for a middle-aged depressed woman.

Communicating with others

Explaining the diagnosis and management plan to the patient

When explaining the assessment to the patient, it is not enough to name the diagnosis. He may misunderstand its meaning or make false assumptions about the implications for prognosis, for example, that all patients with schizophrenia have a rapidly downhill course. The interviewer should explain the significance of the diagnosis in terms of cause, prognosis, and possibilities for treatment. Technical terms should be avoided or, if essential, explained.

When discussing the proposed the plan of management, it is useful to begin by asking what treatment the patient has been expecting. This makes it easier to anticipate objections to the proposed plan, and discuss them. The plan should be explained in an unhurried way, checking from time to time that the patient has understood, and is seeking questions. When drugs are prescribed, the explanation should include appropriate information about:

- why the drug has been chosen
- its name, and the dosage schedule
- the main effects, common side-effects, and any toxic effects, and what, if any, action should be taken if they are experienced

Table 2.10			
Problem	**Action**	**Agent**	**Review**
1 Frequent quarrels with husband	Joint interviews	Dr A	3 weeks
2 3-year old son retarded in speech	Assessment	General practitioner	1 week
3 Housing damp and unsatisfactory	Visit housing department of local authority	Patient	2 weeks
4 Sexual dysfunction (?secondary to 1)	Defer		

Box 2.4 Communicating with patients and relatives

Relevant questions from the following list can be helpful when deciding what information should be given to patients and their relatives:

The diagnosis

- What is the psychiatric diagnosis – if it is uncertain, what are the possibilities?
- Is there a physical diagnosis?
- Is any further information or special investigation required?
- What are the implications of the diagnosis for this patient?
- What may have caused the condition?

The care plan

- What is the plan, and how will it help the patient and the family?
- Are there any legal powers to be used: if so why, and what is their effect?
- What do they need to know about medication? – see list on pp. 62–3
- What do they need to know about psychological treatments?

Who does what?

- Who is the key worker and what will he or she do?
- What is the role of the consultant psychiatrist, and how often will he or she see the patient?
- What is the role of the other members of the psychiatric team?
- What is the role of the general practitioner?
- What can the family do to help the patient?

Emergencies

- Are they likely and how might they be avoided?
- Are there possible early warning signs of a crisis?
- Who should be approached in an emergency, and how can they be found quickly?

Table 2.11

Problem	Action	Agent	Review
Depressive disorder	Prescribe SSRI	Dr A	3 weeks
Loneliness (children grown up)	Seek paid or voluntary work	Patient	5 weeks
Shy and awkward in company	Social skills training	Psychology	6 weeks
Heavy irregular periods	Review and ?refer to gynaecologist	General practitioner	2 weeks

- when signs of improvement are to be expected
- concerns expressed by the patient, for example, that an antidepressant drug may be habit forming
- how long it is planned that the drug should be taken.

If psychological treatment is proposed, the interviewer should explain the purpose, outline what the patient will be asked to do, and indicate the frequency and planned number of sessions.

It is important to set aside enough time for this explanation during the interview, since it is likely to improve compliance with the treatment plan and save time later. If, after full explanation, the patient refuses to accept part of the plan, the interviewer should try to negotiate an acceptable alternative.

Box 2.4 summarizes the points that should be considered when communicating to patients and relatives.

Letters to the general practitioner

When a letter is written to a general practitioner, the first step is to think what the general practitioner already knows about the patient, and what questions he asked when referring the patient. If the family doctor's referral letter outlined the salient features of the case, there is no need to repeat them in the reply. When the patient is less well known to the general practitioner, more detailed information should be given; it is often appropriate to provide this under subheadings (family history, personal history, etc.) so that information can be found readily if needed later. Similarly, if the diagnosis given in the referral letter is correct, it is only necessary to confirm it; otherwise the reasons for the diagnosis should be outlined.

Treatment and prognosis are dealt with next. When discussing treatment, the dosage, timing, and duration of any drug treatment should be stated. The psychiatrist should indicate whether he has issued a prescription, how long a period it covers, and whether he or the general practitioner is to issue any subsequent prescriptions. If

psychotherapy, behaviour therapy, or social work is planned, the letter should name the therapist or agency concerned and indicate the profession involved (for example, supportive counselling from Jane Smith, community psychiatric nurse). The date of the patient's next appointment with the specialist team should be stated, and when the general practitioner should see the patient. These details of collaborative approach should, if possible, be agreed with the general practitioner by phone before the letter is written to confirm them. Alternatively, the letter may be written in a way that encourages the general practitioner to propose alternatives if he wishes.

Standardized methods of interviewing

In research, symptoms and syndromes need to be assessed in a reliable way. In epidemiological research, where large numbers of people have to be examined, interviews are often conducted by interviewers who have not been trained in psychiatry. To achieve reliability, rules are provided for detecting symptoms, and for diagnosing syndromes. Schedules designed for use by interviewers with training in psychiatry can simply give the general rules by which symptoms are to be assessed. The present State Examination is an example of this kind of interview and the extract in the upper part of Box 2.5 illustrates its format. Schedules designed for use by interviewers without formal training in psychiatry use more precise rules. An example of this format is shown in the second part of Box 2.5.

The most frequently used diagnostic schedules will be described next.

Standardized assessments of symptoms

Present State Examination (PSE)

The development of this instrument began in the late 1950s. Early versions were used solely in the

Box 2.5 Standardized assessments of symptoms

Example 1 PSE definition of delusion of thought being read (see Wing et al. 1974)
This is usually an explanatory delusion. Often it goes with delusions of reference or misinterpretation which require some explanation of how other people know so much about the subject's future movements. It may be an elaboration of thought broadcast, thought insertion, auditory hallucinations, delusions of control, delusions of persecution, or delusions of influence. It can even occur with expansive delusions (the subject wishing to explain how Einstein, for example, stole his original ideas). Therefore the symptom is in no way diagnostic. It is most important that it should not be mistaken for diagnostically more important symptoms such as thought insertion or broadcast.

If the subject merely entertains the possibility that his thought might be read but is not certain about it, rate '1'; rate delusional conviction '2'. Exclude those who think that people can read their thoughts as a result of belonging to a group that practices 'thought reading' – this would be rated 1 or 2 on symptom no. 83.

The section on hallucinations in PSE continues with questions about third-person hallucinations and non-verbal hallucinations.

Example 2 SCID questions about delusions (see Spitzer et al. 1987)
Psychotic and associated symptoms This module is for coding psychotic and associated symptoms that have been present at any point in the person's lifetime.

For all psychotic and associated symptoms coded '3', determine whether the symptom is 'not organic', or whether there is a possible or definite organic cause. The following questions may be useful if the overview has not already provided the information: 'When you were experiencing the psychotic symptoms were you taking any drugs or medicine? Drinking a lot? Physically ill?'

If the patient has not acknowledged psychotic symptoms: 'Now I am going to ask you about unusual experiences that people sometimes have.'

If the patient has acknowledged psychotic symptoms: 'You have told me about (psychotic experiences). Now I am going to ask you more about those kinds of things.'

Delusions These are false personal belief(s) based on incorrect inference about external reality and firmly sustained in spite of what almost everyone else believes, and in spite of what constitutes incontrovertible and obvious proof or evidence to the contrary. Code overvalued ideas (unreasonable and sustained belief(s) that is/are maintained with less than delusional intensity) as '2'. Note: a single delusion may be coded '3' on more than one of the following items: 'Did it ever seem that people were talking about you or taking special notice of you?' . . .

Delusions of reference, i.e. personal significance is falsely attributed to objects or events in environment: 'What about receiving special messages from the TV, radio, or newspaper, or from the way things were arranged around you?'
    (Describe: as ?:1:2:3 where 1 = Poss/def organic; and 3 = Not organic.)

Persecutory delusions, i.e. the individual (or his or her group) is being attacked, harassed, cheated, persecuted, or conspired against: 'What about anyone going out of the way to give you a hard time, or trying to hurt you?'
    (Describe: as ?:1:2:3 where 1 = Poss/def organic; and 3 = Not organic.)

Grandiose delusions, i.e. content involves exaggerated power, knowledge, or importance: 'Did you ever feel that you were especially important in some way, or that you had powers to do things that other people could not do?'
    (Describe: as ?:1:2:3 where 1 = Poss/def organic; and 3 = Not organic.)

The section on delusions in SCID continues with questions about other kinds of delusions (somatic, nihilistic, etc.).

authors' own research: the ninth edition (PSE 9) was the first to be published for use by others (Wing *et al.* 1974). It is available in at least 35 languages and has been widely used in many countries. The main principle is that the interview, although clearly structured, retains the features of a clinical examination. A trained interviewer seeks to identify abnormal phenomena that have been present during a defined period of time and to rate their severity. Each of the 140 items is defined in detail in a glossary. Computer programs generate a symptom score, a diagnosis (CATEGO), and a clinically derived measure of the severity of non-psychotic symptoms (the Index of Definition).

Schedules for Clinical Assessment in Neuropsychiatry (SCAN)

The tenth edition of the Present State Examination has been incorporated into this more extensive schedule which can be used to diagnose a broader range of disorders, including eating, somatoform, substance abuse, and cognitive disorders (World Health Organization 1992a). Although the principles are similar to those of PSE 9, there are several differences including a change from three possible ratings to four, an improved system for rating episodes of disorder, and procedures for including information about history and aetiology. The system is compatible with PSE 9, and it allows ICD-10, DSM-IIIR, and DSM-IV diagnoses (Janca *et al.* 1994). A computer-assisted version is available (Glover 1992).

International Personality Disorder Examination (IPDE)

This instrument assesses phenomenology and life experiences so as to enable psychiatric diagnosis according to ICD-10 and DSM-IIIR. It has 153 items and includes open-ended enquiries and questions to determine frequency, duration, and age of onset (Janca *et al.* 1994).

Diagnostic Interview Schedule (DIS)

This schedule was developed in the United States as part of the Epidemiological Catchment Area (ECA) project (Robins *et al.* 1981). The fully structured interview schedule was developed for use by non-clinicians but employs diagnostic criteria used by clinicians. The DIS covers the most common adult diagnoses that can be evaluated by assessing the interview alone (for example, it omits delirium and bulimia). Diagnoses are first made on a lifetime basis. Then the interviewer asks how recently the last symptom was experienced. On the basis of the answer, the disorder is recorded as occurring within the last 2 weeks, the last month, the last 6 months, or the last year. This procedure enables diagnosis of a disorder either within the previous year or at any time during the person's life. Reliability and validity, as determined by a second DIS given by a psychiatrist and by a clinical interview by a psychiatrist, are reasonably satisfactory.

There are problems in making lifetime diagnoses with the DIS (and with all other such instruments) because respondents may have forgotten or denied an illness, and because populations of varying ages have had different durations of time in which to develop a disorder.

Structured Clinical Interview for Diagnosis (SCID)

Soon after the publication of DSM-III, work began on a clinical diagnostic assessment procedure for making DSM diagnoses. The draft instrument was field-tested and then issued for use with DSM-IIIR. It can be used by the clinician as part of a normal assessment procedure to confirm a particular diagnosis or in research or screening as a systematic evaluation of a whole range of medical states. The instrument covers all the criteria of the diagnoses included in the various modules and the interviewer makes a clinical judgement as to whether each criterion is met (Spitzer *et al.* 1990). SCID is available in a patient edition for use with subjects who have been identified as psychiatric patients and in a non-patient edition which is suitable for use in epidemiological studies. In addition the SCID-II is available for making 12 Axis II, i.e. personality disorder, diagnoses in DSM-IIIR.

Composite International Diagnostic Interview (CIDI)

This interview was produced for the WHO and the US Alcohol Drug Abuse and Mental Health Administration. It is a comprehensive and standardized interview derived from the DIS. It is used for the assessment of mental disorders and to provide diagnoses according to ICD and DSM-IV. It is available in 16 languages and is designed to be used by clinicians and non-clinicians in different cultures. The CIDI package includes a core interview in a researcher's version and an interviewer's version (the latter has a diagnostic index that allows linkage of specific CIDI questions to specific diagnostic criteria of ICD-10 and DSM-IIIR), additional modules (concerned, for example, with antisocial personality and post-traumatic stress disorders), as well as training manuals and computer programs. The interview includes questions about symptoms and problems experienced at any time in life, as well as questions about current state (World Health Organization 1989; Essau and Wittchen 1993; Janca *et al.* 1994).

Instruments for measuring symptoms

In research, and at times in clinical practice, it is necessary not only to record whether symptoms are present or absent (in order to make a diagnosis) but also to measure their severity. Some instruments rate a single symptom or a narrow group of symptoms (for example anxiety or depression), others rate a broad group of symptoms as an overall measure of the severity of a disorder. Some diagnostic instruments provide a rating of the severity or (certainty) of symptoms but the instruments to be described next are designed specifically for measurement rather than diagnosis. Some instruments are completed by the patient, and others are filled in by an interviewer who may be allowed to choose the interviewing method or be required to use a standard set of questions.

Ratings of single symptoms and narrow groups of symptoms

Anxiety symptoms

Hamilton Anxiety Scale (HAS) (Hamilton 1959) Although this scale is used widely to measure anxiety, it should be employed solely with anxiety disorders and not for rating anxiety in patients with other disorders. Thirteen items are rated by an interviewer on five-point scales, each on the basis of a brief description. The interviewing method is for the rater to decide. Some depressive symptoms are included so that the scale is in fact a measure of the severity of the anxiety syndrome and not of the symptom of anxiety.

Clinical Anxiety Scale (CAS) (Snaith et al. 1982) This scale was developed from the HAS, to focus more clearly on the symptom of anxiety by leaving out the depressive and somatic symptoms included in the HAS. Its use is not restricted to patients with a diagnosis of anxiety disorder.

The State–Trait Anxiety Inventory (STAI) (Speilberger et al. 1970) This is a self-rating scale with 20 statements, which is completed in two ways: as the person feels when he completed the scale (trait) and how he feels generally (state)

Depressive symptoms

Hamilton Rating Scale for Depression (HRSD) (Hamilton 1967) This scale is filled in by an interviewer who uses an unstructured interview. It measures the severity of the depressive syndrome (p. 271) rather than the symptom of depression.

Beck Depression Inventory (BDI) (Beck et al. 1961) This 21-item inventory is usually completed by the patient: each item has four to six statements, one of which is chosen as best describing the symptom at the time.

Montgomery-Asberg Depression Rating Scale (MADRS) (Montgomery and Asberg 1979) This inventory has 10 items rated on a four-point scale by an interviewer using definitions for each point. Only psychological symptoms of depression are rated.

Obsessional symptoms

Yale–Brown Obsessive Compulsive Scale (YBOCS) (Goodman *et al.* 1989a) This instrument rates obsessive compulsive symptoms in patients diagnosed as having obsessive–compulsive disorder. This scale is rated by a clinician using a four-point scale for each of 10 symptoms. Depressive and anxiety symptoms and obsessional personality traits are not rated.

Other symptoms

- Rating for negative symptoms of schizophrenia, for example the *Positive and Negative Syndrome Scale* (PANSS) (Kay *et al.* 1987) which rates blunted affect, emotional withdrawal, poor rapport, social withdrawal, difficulty in abstract and stereotyped thinking, and lack of spontaneity. A 30 minute interview is required.

- Ratings for extrapyramidal symptoms such as the *Extrapyramidal Symptoms Rating Scale* (ESRS) (Chouinard *et al.* 1980) on which the clinician makes quantitative ratings of the symptoms of parkinsonism, dystonia, and dyskinesia.

Ratings of broad groups of symptoms

General Health Questionnaire (GHQ) (Goldberg 1972) This instrument contains 60 items, but shorter versions have been developed with 30, 28, and 20 items. It is designed for use as a screening instrument in primary care, general medical practice, or community surveys. The full version can be completed within 10 minutes, and the shorter versions even more rapidly. The symptom ratings are added to a score that indicates overall severity, which is expressed by the judgement of whether a psychiatrist would judge the patient to be a 'case' or a 'non-case'. There is also a version with symptom subscales for somatic symptoms, anxiety and insomnia, depression, and social dysfunction (Goldberg and Hillier 1979).

PSE Index of Definition The PSE (Wing *et al.* 1974) and its successors SCAN and CIDI are primarily designed for diagnosis. SCAN requires a clinical training plus a course of training in the use of the instrument. CIDI requires experience in interviewing (for example, in market research) but not clinical training, and a course of training in the use of the instrument. The profile of symptoms obtained from the PSE interview can be used to calculate an overall severity rating, the Index of Definition, which varies from 1 to 8. A rating of 5 or more indicates that the patient probably has a psychiatric disorder.

Brief Psychiatric Rating Scale (BPRS) (Overall and Gorham 1962) This instrument has 16 items, each scored on a seven-point scale. There are criteria to define the symptom items but not for the severity ratings. The time period is not defined and must be decided by the rater. It is suitable for rating severe psychiatric illness but not minor disorders.

Several instruments rate broad groups of symptoms for the purpose of making standard diagnoses. These instruments are described in Chapter 4. For a comprehensive review of rating methods see Thompson 1989 and Task Force on Psychiatric Measures (2000)

Further reading

Blumenthal, S. and Lavender, T. (2000). Violence and mental disorder: a critical aid to the assessment and management of risk. Zito Trust, London.

Cooper, J. E. and Oates, M. (2000). The principles of assessment in general psychiatry. In *The new Oxford textbook of psychiatry* (eds M. G. Gelder, J. J. López Ibor Jr, and N. C. Andreason), Chapter 1.10.1. Oxford University Press, Oxford. (A comprehensive account of assessment procedures with an emphasis on their use in community psychiatry.)

Goldberg, D. (ed.) 1997. *The Maudsley handbook of practical psychiatry.* Oxford University Press, Oxford. (A pocket guide to interviewing and assessment which also

Appendix The Mini-Mental State Examination

(add points for each correct response)

			Score	Points
Orientation				
1	What is the	Year?	____	1
		Season?	____	1
		Date?	____	1
		Day?	____	1
		Month?	____	1
2	Where are we?	State?	____	1
		County?	____	1
		Town or city?	____	1
		Hospital?	____	1
		Floor?	____	1

Registration

3	Name three objects, taking 1 second to say each. Then ask the patient all three after you have said them. Give one point for each correct answer. Repeat the answers until patient learns all three.	____	3

Attention and calculation

4	Serial sevens. Give one point for each correct answer. Stop after five answers. Alternative: Spell WORLD backwards	____	5

Recall

5	Ask for name of three objects learned in Q.3. Give one point for each correct answer.	____	3

Language

6	Point to a pencil and a watch. Have the patient name them as you point.	____	2
7	Have the patient repeat 'No ifs, ands, or buts'.	____	1
8	Have the patient follow a three-stage command: 'Take a paper in your right hand. Fold the paper in half. Put the paper on the floor'.	____	3
9	Have the patient read and obey the following: 'CLOSE YOUR EYES'. (Write it in large letters.)	____	1
10	Have the patient write a sentence of his choice. (The sentence should contain a subject and an object, and should make sense. Ignore spelling errors when scoring.)	____	1
11	Enlarge the design printed below to 1.5 cm per side and have the patient copy it. (Give one point if all sides and angles are preserved and if the intersecting sides form a quadrangle.)	____	1

Total = 30   ____

Reprinted with permission from J. C. Anthony, L. Le Resche, U. Niaz, M. R. Von Korff, and M. F. Folstein (1982). Limits of the 'Mini-Mental State' as a screening test for dementia and delirium among hospital patients. *Psychological Medicine* 12, 397–408.

contains advice about the management of common clinical situations.)

Pincus, J. H. and Tucket, G. J. (1985). *Behavioural neurology*, 3rd edn. Oxford University Press, Oxford. (An account of the neurological disorders most relevant to psychiatry).

Task Force on Psychiatric Measures (2000). *Handbook of psychiatric measures*. American Psychiatric Association Press, Washington, DC. (A reference book containing comprehensive information about instruments for the detection and measurement of psychiatric symptoms and syndromes.)

Taylor, M. A.(1999). *Fundamentals of clinical neuropsychiatry*. Oxford University Press, New York and Oxford. (See, especially, Chapter 2, Neuropsychiatric evaluation, and Chapter 4, The cognitive and behavioural neurologic examination.)

CHAPTER 3

Ethics and civil law

CHAPTER 3
Ethics and civil law

This chapter is concerned with the ways in which general ethical principles, such as those relating to confidentiality and consent, and the civil law are applied to the care of people with mental disorders. It also considers issues about compulsory assessment and treatment. It assumes a basic knowledge of ethical aspects of medicine. In reading the chapter, two important points need to be borne in mind:

◆ There are substantial differences between the laws of different countries. For this reason, the chapter deals with general principles rather than with the details of the law. A psychiatrist called upon to give an opinion on a legal issue should be aware of the relevant legal concepts of the country or region in which he is working and be prepared to seek legal advice.

◆ There are differences between the legal and the psychiatric concepts of mental abnormality. These differences are made more complicated because the concept of mental abnormality varies between different parts of the law.

The increasing *complexity of medical care*, and greater awareness of the *duties of doctors* and *rights of patients* and of the need for them to be explicit is having increasing consequences for medical care. The public is no longer willing to rely on the benevolence and common sense of the medical profession. Psychiatrists need to be aware of the ethical and legal issues in treating their own patients, some of whom may lack the capacity to make judgements about their own care; they also have to be able to respond to requests for advice from colleagues on capacity in relation to physical treatment.

Ethical issues
Two approaches to ethics

There are two principal, and sometimes conflicting, fundamental approaches to ethics. These are the duty-based approaches and utilitarianism.

The duty-based approach

This is the approach most familiar to doctors. It originates from general obligations, often codified by professional organizations, which lay out rules of professional conduct. Whilst this approach provides security and clarity, there may be conflicts in managing particular problems and meeting the individual patient's wishes and needs. Moral theories which emphasize duties are sometimes called deontological (from the Greek deon meaning duty).

Utilitarianism (consequentialism)

Whilst the duty-based approach is focused primarily on the individual patient, the utilitarian approach is 'consequentialist' and concerned with broad judgements of benefit and harm. It assumes the right action is the one that has the best (foreseeable) consequences.

Two examples help to clarify the differences between the two approaches. Utilitarians might conclude that, in those who are dying with distressing symptoms, euthanasia has the best consequences for patients and for the family. By contrast, the duty-based approach might take little or no account of the consequences and see euthanasia as fundamentally ethically wrong. In the same way, a utilitarian psychotherapist might argue that a patient's sexual difficulties could be substantially helped by the patient and therapist having a successful sexual relationship. Again a duty-based approach might state that it is wrong for a therapist to have such relationships in any circumstances.

Ways of applying ethical theories in medical practice

In medical practice, as in everyday life, most people use elements from both theoretical approaches; for example, confidentiality is seen as a duty but public interest exceptions are (as described below) allowed and even encouraged. There are several practical approaches that are useful in considering particular problems.

Applying four widely accepted principles

Current discussion of ethics has been derived from clinical experience and also from the application of general principles of moral philosophy and ethics. These lead to four widely propounded, general principles (Beauchamp and Childress 1994). Although these overlap and may, on occasion, be contradictory, they provide a framework for discussion of particular clinical situations:

◆ respect for the *autonomy* of the patient, the obligation for doctors to respect patients' rights to make their own choices in accordance with their beliefs and responsibilities. This requires the doctor to help patients to come to their own decisions and then to respect and follow those decisions. This principle can clearly be at odds with the principle of beneficence, for example when a patient refuses treatment.

◆ *beneficence* – a fundamental commitment to doing good. When this principle overrules that of autonomy, it is seen as resulting in *paternalism*. One can devive the principle of beneficence either from a duty-based approach (a duty to act in a patient's best interests) or from a utilitarian approach (acting in best

interests produces more welfare than respecting autonomy).

◆ *non-maleficence* – the avoidance of harm, a principle which is largely the reverse side of the coin to the principle of beneficence.

◆ *justice* – the requirement for doctors to act justly and fairly (for example in the allocation of resources).

These principles lie behind the problems of priority setting discussed later in this chapter and elsewhere in this book. However, by themselves they are insufficient to determine medical practice and they need to be interpreted and applied.

Logical analysis

Logical analysis of the clinical problem by setting down premises and issues as the simplest possible statements often helps to clarify what are the key issues on which a decision must be based. It also allows these issues to be separated from the emotions of those involved.

Casuistry

This means achieving consistency and involves comparing the particular clinical problem with other cases that may not be so difficult to resolve. It is useful to ask first whether there are other similar situations in which it is easier to see what the right action should be and, second, to consider whether there are changes to the present situation which would then make it easier to decide what it is right to do.

Application of these varied approaches, alongside legal and professional guidelines, provides a basis for resolution of the practical ethical problems of clinical practice that are discussed in this chapter and elsewhere in this book (see Box 3.1).

Legal and professional statements of duties

Ethical principles have become an important basis of good clinical care and have increasingly made explicit for the benefit of both doctors and patients. Countries differ in the extent to which they impose *statutory requirements* about major ethical issues such as confidentiality and consent or government-enforced *codes of practice*. Most countries have *professional guidelines* prepared and overseen by national medical and psychiatric organizations, for example those of the American Psychiatric Association (1995) in the USA and the General Medical Council (2000) and the Royal College of Psychiatrists (2000) in the United Kingdom. It is important to be aware that other professions involved in psychiatric care also have codes of practice and that these may differ significantly from those of the medical profession. Codes and guidelines may incorporate internationally recommended standards, such as the Hippocratic Oath and the Declaration of Geneva (1948). Although in many countries general ethical statements are accepted as fundamental to everyday medical practice, accumulating evidence of political and other abuse of psychiatry has often led to calls for the widespread adoption of more detailed and prescriptive codes of ethical practice. There are also laws on human rights, for instance the European Convention of Human Rights is incorporated in the national legal process of all member nations in the European Community.

Discussion of ethical issues in this book

In the following sections of this chapter we discuss several general ethical issues and dilemmas:

◆ negligence

◆ misuse of psychiatry

◆ problems of the doctor/patient relationship

◆ confidentiality

◆ consent

◆ compulsory treatment

◆ children

◆ research

◆ setting priorities.

Practical ethical dilemmas, discussed elsewhere in this book, are listed in Box 3.1.

Box 3.1 Some topics relevant to other chapters

Classification (Chapter 4)

Diagnosis on the basis of moral or political judgements.

Evidence-based psychiatry (Chapter 6)

Placebo-controlled trials and randomization (p. 146)

Eating disorder (Chapter 15)

Compulsory treatment in anorexia nervosa (p. 450)

Psychiatry and medicine (Chapter 16)

Factitious disorder: challenging, searching possession, confidentiality (p. 474)

Emergency treatment and consent (p. 484)

Genetic counselling (p. 485)

HIV

Suicide and deliberate self-harm (Chapter 17)

Involuntary treatment following attempted suicide (p. 538)

Physician-assisted suicide (p. 513)

Sexuality and gender (Chapter 19)

Ethical problems in diagnosis and treatment (p. 612)

Psychiatry of the elderly (Chapter 20)

Lack of consent

Confidentiality and carers

Priority setting

Damaging behaviour

Drugs and other physical treatment (Chapter 21)

Drug treatment (p. 652)

ECT and psychosurgery (pp. 713 and 717)

Psychological treatment (Chapter 22)

Autonomy, confidentiality, exploitation (p. 763)

Psychiatric services (Chapter 23)

Ethical problems in the provision of services (p. 793)

Child psychiatry (Chapter 24)

Ethical problems (p. 860)

Learning disability (Chapter 25)

Ethical problems (p. 823)

Forensic psychiatry (Chapter 26)

Acting for third parties

Misuse and abuse of psychiatry

During the twentieth century psychiatry has been misused or, more seriously, abused for political and commercial purposes, both by individual psychiatrists and by the institutions that employ them. Awareness of the ways in which governments could misuse psychiatry was greatly increased by the publicity given by political dissidents, their supporters and a number of Western psychiatrists to the abuse of diagnosis, compulsory treatment, and the role of forensic psychiatry in the former Soviet Union as a means of suppressing opposition and criticism. Some psychiatrists in these countries were willing to classify political dissent as evidence of mental illness. Widespread condemnation led to an acceptance that the World Psychiatric Association should take a lead in setting out ethical rules in that would reduce the risk of further abuses.

Negligence

The most common reason for doctors to be taken to Court is because they are being sued for negligence. This requires the plaintiff to prove three things:

- that the doctor owed a *duty of care* to the particular patient.
- that the doctor was in breach of the appropriate *standard of care* imposed by the law.
- that the breach in duty of care *caused the patient harm*, meriting compensation.

The doctor should have these legal principles in mind, alongside ethical principles of providing information, seeking consent and in the wider aspects of patient care.

Problems in the doctor/patient relationship

Doctors have obligations to respect the patients' wishes and best interests. Unfortunately, psychiatrists have, from time to time, taken personal advantage of their patients in a variety of ways:

- use of the relationship to satisfy the therapist's own psychological needs or self-esteem.

- the imposition of the psychiatrist's own values and beliefs on their patients, for example, in relation to sexual behaviour.

- financial exploitation for the direct benefit of the psychiatrist.

- sexual exploitation.

- putting the interests of third parties who provide or fund medical care above those of the patient. These may be particularly difficult to resolve in the course of multidisciplinary care of complicated medical problems, since those involved may have different obligations to a variety of employers and external interests.

Confidentiality

Confidentiality is fundamental in medical practice because information is collected about private and sometimes highly sensitive matters. In most circumstances, the psychiatrist should not disclose such information or collect information from other informants without the patient's consent. This is a good example of an ethical *rule* with defined exceptions. The Hippocratic Oath states:

. . . whatever, in connection with my professional practice or not in connection with it, I see or hear in the life of men, which ought not to be spoken abroad, I will not divulge as reckoning that all such should be kept secret.

The Declaration of Geneva (1948) states:

I will respect the secrets which are confided in me, even after the patient has died.

There are also national professional guidelines, which may combine ethical codes and legal rules. They may be enforced by law, by contract of employment, or by professional bodies. For example, in the UK the General Medical Council (2000) requires confidentiality and provides professional guidelines that, as described below, allow exceptions. Although these guidelines do not have the force of law, they are taken seriously by the courts as evidence of generally accepted standards of behaviour and health employers expect them to be observed. The General Medical Council guidelines provide an example of the ways in which, even though over recent years the principle of confidentiality has been more explicitly asserted, but at the same time public interest exclusions have become substantially more important.

In a number of countries there are laws of privacy. There are also laws and guidelines that govern the ways in which written and electronic records can be held and give patients rights (with some limitations) to see personal information held on computer or in file notes. In the UK the most important relevant legislation is the Data Protection Act (1998) and the Access to Health Records Act (1990). A doctor must take reasonable precautions to prevent confidential information from falling into the wrong hands (for example, written notes must be kept secure). Similar considerations apply in most other countries, and it is essential that psychiatrists are aware of the ethical and legal requirements in the country in which they are working.

Legal and ethical principles

In the law of England and Wales the general obligation for doctors to maintain confidentiality is a *public*, not a *private* interest. In other words, from the legal perspective, it is in the *public* interest for patients to be able to trust their doctors to maintain confidentiality. The issue, therefore, of when it is lawful and when not lawful for a doctor to breach confidentiality is often a question of balancing public interests (not of balancing a private versus a public interest). No breach of confidentiality has occurred if a patient gives consent (a consent which should be based on full understanding of what will be disclosed, the reason for it, and likely consequences). Whilst confidentiality cannot, in principle, occur when the patient cannot be identified, it is now the usual practice of journals and other publications to publish case history information only if there has been signed consent of the patient, even where the case history is substantially disguised.

Some practical applications of the principles of confidentiality discussed in this section are summarized in Box 3.2.

Box 3.2 Practical applications of the principle of confidentiality

- Disclosure of information should be kept to a minimum and consent should be obtained.

- Wherever possible unidentifiable data should be used.

- Effective measures should be taken to protect personal information.

- Unintentional disclosure should be minimized by avoiding discussions which might be overheard, carrying out consultation in private, and keeping care of records.

- It should be made clear that information will be shared as necessary with the health team and that all members are aware of the principles of confidentiality.

- Information is usually shared with relatives only with the consent of the patient but it may, in special circumstances (for example, dementia), also be shared in the patient's best interests.

- Children over a stated age (usually 16) should enjoy the same rights of confidentiality as adults. For younger children doctors would normally share clinical information with parents. Parents have a legal duty to act in their children's best interests and therefore require to be properly informed. The law with regard to both confidentiality and consent to treatment in children is not entirely clear.

Although there is a general legal obligation for doctors to keep confidential what patients tell them, doctors *may be obliged* to disclose information to a third party in the *public interest* (of the community as a whole or a group or individual with the community). Examples are *statutory obligations* in relation to communicable disease, certain controlled drugs, unfitness to drive, suspicion of child abuse, or by order of a Court (relevant material only), and when there is evidence of *major* crime. The General Medical Council (2000) states:

where a disclosure may assist in prevention, detection or prosecution of a serious crime. Serious crimes, in this context, will put someone at risk of death or serious harm, and will usually be crimes against the person, such as abuse of children.

A widely cited landmark case in the USA is that of Tarasoff in 1976 which illustrates the importance and difficulty of the issues (although it is essential not to generalize to other circumstances in other jurisdictions). A student in therapy at the University of California health service expressed murderous feelings towards Patricia Tarasoff. The therapist informed her supervisor and the police but not Ms Tarasoff. However, the police did not act and the student eventually murdered Patricia Tarasoff. The Californian Supreme Court ruled that therapists do have a duty to take steps to protect third parties and that it is reasonable to inform the victim.

Doctors may also disclose information to a third party in the *patient's best interest* in exceptional circumstances. For example, if the patient is *legally incapable* because of severe physical or mental illness, then information can be disclosed. The patient should, wherever possible, be told before disclosure. A further example is where there is evidence of *severe risk to a third party*; for instance *HIV-positive patients* may be unwilling to disclose information about the diagnosis to sexual partners. The doctor should try to persuade the patient to disclose the information voluntarily but, in the UK and some other countries, he is able to warn the partner of a serious risk without the consent of the patient. The patient should be warned that confidentiality will be breached.

When patients are assessed *on behalf of a third party*, it is essential to make sure at the outset that the patient is aware of the purpose of the assessment and of the obligations of the doctors towards the third party. Written consent should be obtained.

- *Sharing information about patients with other members of the health care team* and for the purpose of providing the best treatment is not generally viewed, by the law, as a breach of confidentiality. It is important that they understand that the information is given to them in confidence and they must respect this. Patients

should be told that information is shared on this basis.

- It is increasingly accepted that patients, or their legal representatives, have a right to read clinical notes that have been made about them, although there are usually restrictions in relation to the possibility of harm to the patient or others. This right, and its limitations, is given legal expression in the UK in the Access to Health Records Act (1990).

- The obligation of confidentiality continues after a patient's death.

If the patient is mentally disordered and unable to give an account of himself, the psychiatrist should use his own discretion about seeking information from someone else without the patient's consent. Sometimes such information is of vital importance to assessment and management. The guiding principle should be to try to act in the patient's best interests, and to obtain information as far as possible from close relatives rather than employers. The same principles apply when the psychiatrist needs to give information or an opinion to relatives or other people regarding a patient who is unable to consent.

Consent to medical treatment

The competent adult

The patient should have a *clear and full understanding* of the nature of a treatment procedure and its probable side-effects, and should *freely agree* to receive the treatment and be *competent* to take decisions, i.e. have legal *capacity*.

In general, competent adults have a right to refuse medical treatment, even if this refusal results in death or permanent disablement. For most treatments, such as established forms of medication, it is sufficient in English law for the psychiatrist to explain the nature of the treatment and probable side-effects. However, there are national differences in the extent of explanation required. For example, the requirement of informed consent involves a more detailed account of side-effects of treatment in the USA than in the UK (see Katz *et al.* 1995 for an account of psychiatric consultation with those refusing medical treatment).

There are several situations in which explicit consent is not needed. The precise nature of these exceptions depends on local law and precedent:

- *implied consent* such as when a patient holds out his arm to have his blood pressure measured.
- *necessity* in which grave harm or death are likely to occur without intervention and there is doubt about the patient's competence (see below).
- *emergency* in order to prevent immediate serious harm to the patient or to others, or to prevent a crime.

If the adult patient does not have the capacity to give, or refuses, consent then no-one can give proxy consent on behalf of the patient. The doctor should act in the patient's best interest.

If a patient refuses medical treatment, the doctor needs to make two judgements before accepting that the patient has the right to refuse:

- Is the patient competent (does he have the mental capacity) to refuse treatment?
- Has the patient been influenced by others to the extent that a refusal has been coerced or is not voluntary?

The doctor should always keep in mind that refusal is often based on misapprehension about the illness and treatment. He should always spend as much time as is needed exploring the medical issues and trying to understand the patient's beliefs and worries. Full, calm discussion may eventually enable agreement about a treatment plan that is medically appropriate and acceptable to the patient.

The incompetent patient

Issues about competence to consent to treatment arise particularly in three groups of patients: people with learning disability, children and adolescents, and patients with mental illness. The judgement of legal *capacity* is usually not defined precisely; it depends upon the patient's *capacity*:

- to comprehend and retain information about the treatment;
- to believe this information;
- to be able to use it to make an informed choice.

Judgements of competence *are specific to the particular decision* that is to be made about treatment. A patient with a severe mental disorder may be incompetent in other respects, but nonetheless may be competent to decide upon a particular treatment. For example, a patient with schizophrenia and paranoid delusions may be capable of deciding on medical treatment of a heart attack.

In the UK, the Mental Health Acts distinguish between consent to medical treatment and consent to psychiatric treatment. They provide for the compulsory treatment of mental disorder, but do not allow compulsory treatment for physical conditions.

In the law of England and Wales no-one can give proxy consent for an adult. However, those with parental responsibility would normally need to give consent for minors. In the UK a minor is a person under the age of 18, although those aged 16–17 can themselves legally consent unless they lack capacity. The situation is less clear for those under 16 years old. Common law does allow a competent minor under 16 years to give consent for medical procedures, but doctors would need to be careful to ensure that the minor had such capacity before proceeding without parental consent. Parents and guardians are under a legal obligation to act in the minor's best interest and occasionally a court may need to rule on this (see p. 860).

Where adult patients do not have the required capacity to consent and have not made an advance directive (see below), others have to decide whether treatment should be given or withdrawn. This decision must be made on the basis of the patient's best interests as determined by the responsible clinicians on the basis of their clinical judgement in accordance with general medical opinion. It is wise to consult relatives (although they cannot give or withhold consent) and to discuss the case with other professional staff. Detailed notes should be kept of the reasons for the decision and the consultations that took place.

Advance directives

Advance directives ('living wills') are accepted in many countries as a means of ensuring that those who previously had the capacity to take decisions but have lost it, for example, because of dementia, are treated in the way that they would have wished. Advance directives can be classified into three main types: an *instruction*, which states what treatment the person would want; a *statement* of general values relevant to medical treatment; and *proxy directives*, which authorize another specified person to take decisions. Proxy directive are allowed in some juristictions but are not valid in the UK which does not have any legal basis for any form of proxy consent for adults.

Advance directives respect the principle of autonomy and are generally seen by doctors and patients as being helpful in treatment decisions. However, there are practical problems. It must be clear that the person was competent and well informed at the time of completing the directive. It may be difficult to interpret general views made in a state of good health in particular medical situations. There is some evidence that the involvement of relatives and other proxies appointed to make the decision is not an entirely satisfactory way of judging what the person would have wanted in a particular clinical situation. The person making the directive should understand that changing circumstances and the need to consider the interests of others may mean that the directive will be interpreted flexibly rather than as a strict instruction to be followed in every detail.

Assessing competence

The assessment of competence requires the full history and examination procedure summarized in Box 3.3.

Box 3.3 Assessment of competence of adult patients

Step 1 *Identify the information relevant to the decision*

- The decision that needs to be made.
- The nature of the alternative reasonable decisions.
- The pros and cons of each reasonable decision.

Step 2 *Assess cognitive ability*

Assess whether the person has the cognitive ability to carry out all three elements of the decision-making process:

- understand the information;
- believe the information;
- weigh up the information and come to a decision.

Consider particularly the following causes of impaired cognitive ability:

- delirium
- dementia.
- other neurological disorders which may impair cognition
- learning disability.

Step 3 *Assess other factors which may interfere with capacity*

Mental illness:

- delusions
- hallucinations
- affective disorder: depression, manic illness

Lack of maturity:

- assessment of emotional and cognitive maturity

Compulsory admission and treatment

In developed countries there are laws to protect mentally disordered persons and to protect society from the consequences of their mental disorder, although the form of these laws differs between countries. Special legal provision is needed for people who are a danger to themselves or others because of mental disorder, and who refuse to accept the treatment that they require. Such people usually have little or no insight into their own psychiatric condition. They present a difficult ethical dilemma: they have a right to be at liberty but they also have a need for care and treatment, and society has a right to be protected.

Countries vary widely in their approach to this dilemma in terms of the definition of mental disorder and in procedures. In some Scandinavian countries, for example, procedures for compulsory care are simple, whilst in some states of the USA, a court hearing may be required. In England and Wales, provisions for compulsory admission and treatment are embodied in the Mental Health Act 1983.

Countries also vary in the ways in which their specialized mental health legislation relates to the larger body of legislation for the whole population. For example, in the UK, mental health laws make no reference to the issue of competence, but this is different in many other countries.

An experienced psychiatrist can often avoid the use of compulsory legal powers by patiently and tactfully discussing with the patient and relatives the reasons why admission is necessary. If this fails and compulsory treatment is justified, a further discussion takes place with family members to seek their support for the patient's admission to hospital. When talking to the family, the doctor should understand their feelings of anxiety and guilt. When the patient is in hospital, restrictions should be kept to the minimum required for safety and adequate treatment. Usually the patient and the family soon realize that compulsory hospital care is little different from that of a voluntary patient, and they may feel relieved that treatment has started. If the hospital staff members are patient, understanding, and adaptable, it is usually possible to establish an effective therapeutic relationship between staff, patient, and relatives. However, a patient admitted under a compulsory order sometimes refuses to accept restrictions or treatment. Such refusal can usually be overcome by skilful nursing with firmness tempered by sympathy, patience, and flexibility. However, when

this fails it may be necessary to proceed with treatment without consent. This should be carefully and clearly explained to the patient and family.

Consent to treatment

Another problem arises when a voluntary patient who is judged to need electroconvulsive therapy (ECT) for a severe and life-threatening psychiatric disorder (for example, extreme depression with dangerous refusal of food and drink) refuses to consent to this treatment. In England and Wales the procedure is to discuss the problem fully with relatives, to seek an independent psychiatric opinion, and to complete a compulsory treatment order with the relatives' agreement.

Appeals

In most mental health legislation, safeguards against unnecessary detention are provided and patients are entitled to easy access to appeal procedures. The type of safeguard varies from country to country.

Children

The application of general ethical principles and of the law to children attempts to strike a balance between increasing autonomy as children grow up, giving parents the right to determine the care of their children, and the duty of the State to protect children whose parents do not act in their best interests. These issues are, in clinical practice and in the law, most difficult to resolve as children near adult life. These issues are discussed more fully in pp. 860–1.

Research

Psychiatric research is bound by the ethical principles that apply to all medical research. These derive from the first internationally agreed guidelines on research involving people, which followed appalling abuse during the Second World War. The principles were incorporated by the medical profession into the Declaration of Helsinki, first published by the World Medical Association in 1964. This has been followed by many, more detailed, national and international guidelines and by the widespread establishment of local ethical committees to oversee medical research.

There are particular problems in consent in relation to those who may not be able to give informed consent and especially in relation to certain forms of treatment. Local ethical procedures need to take a very careful view of any research proposal in terms of the balance of benefits, discomfort, and risk to the individual patient, and the need to advance knowledge so that people with mental disorder can benefit. It is probably wise to consult with relatives or others who may be able to take an informed view of the patient's situation. Juristictions vary in the extent to which this is a legal requirement. Research workers should take great care to follow local ethical procedures.

Setting priorities

Setting priorities is necessary to make the best use of limited resources which are never sufficient to meet all possible clinical needs without regard for cost. Clinicians are often involved in decisions which may affect the doctor/patient relationship. Psychiatrists will be concerned that proper weight is given to the needs of the elderly, those with learning disability and chronic disabling psychiatric disorder, at the same time as providing care for many much more common and less severe psychological problems. This requires a clear framework for evidence-based debate (see p. 793; see also Chapter 23).

Psychiatry and other aspects of civil law

Apart from the issues already discussed in this chapter, civil law is also concerned with property, inheritance, and contracts. In other words, it deals with the rights and obligations of individuals to one another and includes family law (which is a particular concern of child psychiatrists). In this respect civil law differs from criminal law, which is concerned with offences against the state (some of which are directed against an individual, for example, homicide). Proceedings in civil law are undertaken by individuals or groups who believe that they have suffered a breach of the civil law, rather than by an agency of the state as with criminal law.

The psychiatrist may be asked to submit a written report on a patient's state of mind in relation to issues such as those discussed below. The report should be prepared only after full discussion with the patient and only with the patient's full consent. In preparing such a report, the psychiatrist should follow the principles of writing a court report (described on p. 928). As with all psychiatric reports for legal purposes, the report should be concise and factual, and should give the reasons for any opinions.

Since the law on these issues is complicated, it is usually advisable for the psychiatrist to seek legal guidance, particularly in relation to local legal concepts of abnormal mental state relevant to the issue in question. Sometimes international law is relevant. In the European Community the highest court for all members is the European Court of Justice. Other countries may also play a role, for example, the European Court of Human Rights is influential for any country which is a member of the Council of Europe. The following sections are based on the law in England and Wales.

Testamentary capacity

This term refers to the capacity to make a valid will. If someone is suffering from mental disorder at the time of making a will, its validity may be in doubt and other people may challenge it. However, the will may still be legally valid if the testator is of 'sound disposing mind' at the time of making it. Psychiatrists may be asked to report in relation to two issues:

◆ testamentary capacity;

◆ the possibility that the testator was subjected to undue influence.

In order to decide whether or not a testator is of sound disposing mind, the doctor should use four legal criteria:

- whether the testator understands what a will is and what its consequences are;
- whether he knows the nature and extent of his property (though not in detail);
- whether he knows the names of close relatives and can assess their claims to his property;
- whether he is free from an abnormal state of mind that might distort feelings or judgements relevant to making the will (a deluded person may legitimately make a will, provided that the delusions are unlikely to influence it).

In conducting an examination, the doctor should see the testator alone, but should also see relatives and friends to check the accuracy of factual statements.

Assessment of undue influence is more complex and requires assessment of the relationship between testator and beneficiary, the mental state of the testator, and what is known of earlier intentions.

Power of attorney and receivership

If a patient is incapable of managing his possessions by reason of mental disorder, alternative arrangements must be made, particularly if the incapacity is likely to last a long time. Such arrangements may be required for patients living in the community as well as those in hospital. In English law two methods are available – power of attorney and receivership.

Power of attorney is the simpler method, only requiring the patient to give written authorization for someone else to act for him during his illness. In signing such authorization, the patient must be able to understand what he is doing. He may revoke it at any time.

Receivership is the more formal procedure and is likely to be more in the patient's interests. In England and Wales an application is made to the Court of Protection, which may decide to appoint a receiver. The procedure is most commonly required for the elderly. The question of receivership is one that places special responsibility on the psychiatrist. If a patient is capable of managing his affairs on admission to hospital, but later becomes incapable by reason of intellectual deterioration, then it is the doctor's duty to advise the patient's relatives about the risks to property. If the relatives are unwilling to take action, then it is the doctor's duty to make an application to the Court of Protection. The doctor may feel reluctant to act in this way, but any actions taken subsequently are the Court's responsibility and not the doctor's.

Family law

A *marriage contract* is not valid if at the time of marriage either party was so mentally disordered as not to understand its nature. If mental disorder of this degree can be proved, a marriage may be decreed null and void by a divorce court. If a marriage partner becomes of 'incurably unsound mind' later in a marriage, this may be grounds for divorce and a psychiatrist may be asked to make a prognosis. A doctor may also be asked for an opinion about the *capacity of parents or a guardian* to care adequately for a child.

Torts and contracts

Torts are wrongs for which a person is liable in civil law as opposed to criminal law. They include negligence, libel, slander, trespass, and nuisance. If such a wrong is committed by a person of unsound mind, then any damages awarded in a court of law are usually only nominal. In this context the legal definition of unsound mind is restrictive, and it is advisable for a psychiatrist to take the advice of a lawyer on it.

If a person makes a contract and later develops a mental disorder, then the contract is binding. If a person is of unsound mind when the contract is made, a distinction is made between the 'necessaries' and 'non-necessaries' of life. *Necessaries* are legally defined as goods (or services) 'suitable to the condition of life of such person and to his actual requirements at the time' (Sale of Goods Act 1893). In a particular case it is for the court to decide whether any goods or services are necessaries within this definition. A contract made for necessaries is always binding.

In the case of a contract for *non-necessaries* made by a person of unsound mind, the contract is binding unless it can be shown both that he did not understand what he was doing and that the other person was aware of the incapacity.

Personal injury

Psychiatrists may be asked to write reports in relation to claims for compensation by patients with post-traumatic stress disorder or other psychological sequelae of accidents. These conditions are described on p. 191 and p. 496, respectively. Reports should be set out according to the requirements of the relevant local legal and compensation procedures and should clearly state the sources of information, the history of the trauma, the psychiatric and social history, and the post-accident course. They should include a detailed functional assessment and examine the relationship between the trauma and subsequent symptoms and disability.

Fitness to drive

Questions of fitness to drive may arise in relation to many psychiatric disorders, but particularly the major mental disorders. Reckless driving may result from suicidal inclinations or manic disinhibition; panicky or aggressive driving may result from persecutory delusions; and indecisive or inaccurate driving may be due to dementia. Concentration on driving may be impaired in severe anxiety or depressive disorders. The question of fitness to drive also arises in relation to psychiatric drugs, particularly those with sedative effects such as anxiolytic or antipsychotic drugs in high dosage.

Doctors should be aware of and follow the particular legal criteria for fitness to drive in the places in which they are working; these criteria may differ somewhat for drivers of cars and drivers of heavy goods vehicles. In general, a doctor giving an opinion on fitness to drive should consider whether any medical condition or its treatment is liable to cause loss of control, impair perception or comprehension, impair judgement, reduce concentration, or affect motor functions involved in handling the vehicle.

Further reading

General references are listed below. In addition, the National Medical Organisations or Psychiatric Associations of many countries publish guidelines on the applications of the principles discussed in this chapter.

American Psychiatric Association. (2001). *Psychiatric Ethics Primer*. American Psychiatric Publishing Inc. Washington DC.

Bloch, S., Chodoff, P., and Green, S. (eds) (1998). *Psychiatric ethics*, 3rd edn. Oxford University Press, Oxford.
(Contains reviews by leading writers which cover theoretical issues)

Dickenson, D. and Fulford, K. W. M. (2000). *In two minds: a case book of psychiatric ethics*. Oxford University Press, Oxford.
(A readable and practical account based on discussion of case histories representing common clinical problems)

Mason, J. K. and McCall-Smith, R. A. (1999). *Law and medical ethics*, 5th edn. Butterworths, London.
(A useful reference work)

Montgomery, J. (1997). *Health care law*. Oxford University Press, Oxford.
(A useful reference work)

CHAPTER 4

Classification in psychiatry

CHAPTER 4
Classification in psychiatry

In psychiatry, classification attempts to bring order into the great diversity of phenomena met in clinical practice. The purpose of classification is to identify groups of patients who share similar clinical features, so that suitable treatment can be planned and the likely outcome predicted. Psychiatry has favoured a 'medical' model rather than the alternative social and behavioural models for two closely related concepts, disease and illness. The former is defined as referring to medical abnormality based on pathology by signs and symptoms. Illness refers to subjective experiences of pain and incapacity and is the more widely used term and concept in psychiatry.

In general medicine, classification is fairly straightforward. Most physical conditions can be classified on the basis of aetiology (for example, pneumococcal or viral pneumonia) and structural pathology (for example, bronchopneumonia). Some general medical conditions, such as migraine or trigeminal neuralgia, are not yet classifiable in this way; therefore they are classified solely on symptoms. Psychiatric disorders are mainly analogous to this second group. Although some psychiatric disorders have recognized physical aetiology (such as phenylketonuria, Down's syndrome, or Alzheimer's disease), most can be classified only on symptoms.

Concepts of mental illness

In everyday speech the word 'illness' is used loosely. Similarly, in psychiatric practice, the term 'mental illness' is used with little precision. A good definition of mental illness is difficult to achieve. In everyday clinical practice this difficulty is impor-

tant mainly in relation to ethical and legal issues such as compulsory admission to hospital. In forensic psychiatry the definition of mental illness (by the law) is particularly important in relation to the assessment of issues such as criminal responsibility.

Although the major systems of classification refer specifically to *mental disorders* rather than to mental illnesses (World Health Organization 1992b; American Psychiatric Association 1994a), the concept of mental illness is intellectually interesting and (as mentioned above) has ethical and legal implications.

Definitions of mental illness

Many attempts have been made to define mental illness (see Clare 1997). A common approach is to examine the concept of illness in general medicine and to identify any analogies with mental illness. In general medicine there are three types of definition:

- *Absence of health* This approach changes the emphasis of the problem but does not solve it, because health is even more difficult to define. The World Health Organization, for example, defined health as 'a state of complete physical, mental and social well-being, and not merely the absence of disease or infirmity'. As Lewis (1953) rightly commented, 'a definition could hardly be more comprehensive than that, or more meaningless'. Many other definitions of health have been proposed, all equally unsatisfactory.

- *Presence of suffering* This approach has some practical value because it defines a group of people likely to consult doctors. A disadvantage is that the term cannot be applied to everyone who would usually be regarded as ill in everyday terms. For example, patients with mania may feel unusually well and may not experience suffering, though most people would regard them as mentally ill.

◆ *Pathological process* Some extreme theorists, such as Szasz (1960), take the view that illness can be defined only in terms of *physical* pathology. Since most mental disorders do not have demonstrable physical pathology, on this view they are not illnesses. Szasz takes the further step of asserting that most mental disorders are therefore not the province of doctors. This kind of argument can be sustained only by taking an extremely narrow view of pathology. It is also incompatible with the available evidence; thus there are genetic and biochemical grounds for supposing that both schizophrenia and depressive disorders have a physical basis (see pp. 293 and 335), and it is likely that neurobiological pathology processes will be found to underlie other psychiatric disorders.

In psychiatry, abnormalities in psychological function – psychopathology – have been seen as the basis of illness. Because there are considerable difficulties in the definition of mental illness, recent work has focused on the notion of incapacity as a result of a disturbance of function (Hope 2001).

Illness and socially deviant behaviour

Several writers have warned strongly against defining mental illness solely in terms of socially deviant behaviour. For example, the argument is often made that someone must have been mentally ill to commit a particularly cruel murder or grossly abnormal sexual act (the word 'sick' is often used in this context). Although such antisocial behaviour is highly unusual, there is no justification for equating it with mental illness. Moreover, if mental illness is inferred from socially deviant behaviour alone, political abuse may result. For example, opponents of a political system may be confined to psychiatric hospitals simply because they do not agree with the authorities (as happened in the Soviet Union – see p. 76).

A further reason for excluding social criteria from the definition of mental illness (and from diagnostic criteria) is that many behaviours are appraised differently in different countries and at different times. For example, homosexuality was listed as a mental disorder in both DSM-I and DSM-II, but not in DSM-III or IV.

Whilst the antipsychiatry movement of the 1950s, 1960s, and 1970s argued against the concept of mental illness or disease from a variety of perspectives, there are important reasons for maintaining the concept. In addition to the clinical advantages of classification described in the next section, it is useful in understanding the management of mental problems in relation to crime, decisions about health care rationing or other planning, in deciding grounds for insurance claims, and for informed discussion of the abuse of psychiatry for political purposes (Hope and Savelescu 2001).

Impairment, disability, and handicap

It is useful to describe the *consequences* of any disorder, either physical or mental, in terms of *impairment, disability*, and *handicap* (Susser 1990). These concepts, which are derived from medical sociology and social psychology, have been incorporated in the International Classification of Impairment, Disease and Handicap by the World Health Organization (see World Health Organization 1988). The terms are used in the following way:

◆ *impairment*, referring to a pathological defect;

◆ *disability* is the stable persistent limitation of physical or psychological function which results from impairment and the individual psychological reaction to it;

◆ *handicap*, referring to continuing social dysfunction, arising from inability to fill individual and social expectations.

The need for classification

In psychiatry, as in the rest of medicine, classification is needed for three main purposes:

♦ to enable clinicians to communicate with one another about their patients' symptoms, prognosis, and treatment;

♦ to ensure that research can be conducted with comparable groups of patients;

♦ to enable epidemiological studies as a basis for research and planning services.

In the past, the use of psychiatric classification has been criticized as inappropriate or even harmful, especially at the height of the antipsychiatry movement. Three main criticisms were made:

♦ Allocating patients to a diagnostic category distracts from the understanding of their unique personal difficulties. The use of classification can certainly be combined with consideration of a patient's unique qualities; indeed, it is important to combine the two because these qualities can modify prognosis and should be taken into account in treatment. The critics of standard classifications have themselves used idiosyncratic classifications with their own technical terms as a means of summarizing information.

♦ Some sociologists have suggested that to allocate a person to a diagnostic category is simply to label deviant behaviour as illness. They argue that such *labelling* serves only to increase the person's difficulties. There can be no doubt that terms such as epilepsy or schizophrenia attract social stigma, but this does not lessen the reality of disorders that cause suffering and require treatment.

♦ Individuals do not fit neatly into the available categories. Whilst it is not feasible to classify a minority of disorders, this is not a reason for abandoning classification for the majority.

Although these criticisms are important, they are arguments only against the improper use of classification. Disorders such as epilepsy and schizophrenia cannot be made to disappear simply by ceasing to give names to them. Such criticisms have greatly diminished since syndromes have been shown to predict prognosis and to respond to specific treatments, and as familiarity with modern classifications has increased.

The history of classification

The early Greek medical writings contained descriptions of different manifestations of mental disorder, for example, excitement, depression, confusion, and memory loss. This simple classification of mental disorders was adopted by Roman medicine and developed by the Greek physician Galen, whose system of classification remained in use until the eighteenth century.

Interest in the classification of natural phenomena developed in the eighteenth century, partly stimulated by the publication of a classification of plants by Linnaeus, a medically qualified professor of botany who also devised a less well-known classification of diseases in which one major class was mental disorders. Many classifications were proposed. A particularly well-known example was published in 1772 by William Cullen, a Scottish physician. He grouped mental disorders together, though with one exception, delirium, which he classified with febrile conditions. In his scheme, mental disorders were part of a broad class of 'neuroses', a term he used to denote diseases affecting the nervous system (Hunter and McAlpine 1963). Cullen's classification contained an aetiological principle – that mental illnesses were disorders of the nervous system – as well as a descriptive principle for distinguishing individual clinical syndromes within the neuroses. In Cullen's usage, the term neurosis covered the whole range of mental disorders as well as many neurological conditions; the modern narrower usage developed later (see below).

In the early years of the nineteenth century, several French writers published influential classifications of major disorders. Phillipe Pinel's *Treatise on insanity*, which appeared in an English edition in 1806, divided mental disorders into mania with delirium, mania without delirium, melancholia, dementia, and idiocy. One of Pinel's compatriots, Esquirol, wrote another widely read textbook which was published in an English edition in 1845. Esquirol adopted a scheme similar to Pinel's, adding a new category of monomania which was characterized by 'partial insanity', in which there were fixed false ideas that could not be changed by logical reasoning. Esquirol divided the monomanias into subgroups including reasoning monomania, erotic monomania, incendiary monomania, homicidal monomania, and monomania resulting from drunkenness. Like other psychiatrists of the time, Pinel and Esquirol did not discuss neuroses (in the modern sense) or behaviour disorders in their textbooks because these conditions were generally treated by physicians.

Meanwhile, in Germany, Kahlbaum formulated two requirements for research on classification: that the entire course of a mental illness was fundamental to the definition of that illness, and that the total clinical picture must be used in formulating definitions in a system of classification. These ideas were adopted by Kraepelin, who studied the course of mental diseases over many years and thereby made the important distinction between manic-depressive psychosis and schizophrenia. The successive editions of Kraepelin's textbook led to further refinements in the classification of mental illness that are the basis of today's systems.

At the same time, separate developments in the emerging specialty of neurology led to decreasing medical interest in the 'nervous patient', a term used throughout the nineteenth century in Britain and North America (Bynum 1985) to refer to a large group of patients with varied complaints. These were gradually seen as a part of the new specialty of psychiatry alongside the major mental illnesses. The writings of Freud and his contemporaries led to greater recognition of the psychological causes of nervous symptoms and 'neurotic' disorders, and to the modern concepts of hysteria

and anxiety disorder (see Pichot 1994 for a review of nosological models in psychiatry).

Organizing principles

Current classifications are not based on any conceptual model of mental illness but rather on a clincal view of mental disorder.

Neurosis and psychosis

In the past the concepts of psychosis and neurosis were included in most systems of classification. As is explained later in this chapter, neither of these terms is used as an organizing principle in ICD-10 or DSM-IV. In practice, however, these terms are still used widely; hence it is of practical importance to understand their history and usage.

It has been explained above that the term *neurosis* was introduced by Cullen to denote diseases of the nervous system. Gradually the category of neurosis narrowed, first as neurological disorders with a distinct neuropathology (such as epilepsy and stroke) were removed, and later with the development of a separate category of psychosis.

The term *psychosis* was suggested by Feuchtersleben, who, in 1845, published a book entitled *Principles of medical psychology*. This author proposed psychosis as a term for severe mental disorders. He also accepted the term neurosis for mental disorders as a whole; thus he wrote, 'every psychosis is at the same time a neurosis but not every neurosis is a psychosis' (Hunter and MacAlpine 1963, p. 950). As the concept of neurosis was narrowed, psychoses ceased to be subgroups of neuroses and were regarded as independent conditions. Many of the difficulties encountered today in defining the terms neurosis and psychosis are related to these origins.

In modern usage, the term *psychosis* refers broadly to severe forms of mental disorder such as organic mental disorders, schizophrenia, and some affective disorders. Numerous criteria have been proposed to achieve a more precise definition. Greater severity of illness is a common criterion, but the conditions in this group can occur in mild or severe forms.

Lack of insight is often suggested as a criterion for psychosis, but the term insight is itself difficult to define (see p. 26). A more straightforward criterion is the patient's inability to distinguish between subjective experience and reality, as evidenced by hallucinations and delusions. Since none of these three criteria is easy to apply, the term psychosis is unsatisfactory. However, it is not only difficulty of definition that makes the term psychosis unsatisfactory. There are two other reasons: first the conditions embraced by the term have little in common, and second it is less informative to classify a disorder as psychosis than it is to classify it as a particular disorder within the rubric of psychosis (for example, schizophrenia). It is for these reasons that the distinction between neurosis and psychosis, which was a fundamental classificatory principle in ICD-9, was abandoned in DSM-III and subsequently in ICD-10.

Although the term psychosis has little value in a scheme for classifying mental disorders, it is still in everyday use as a convenient term for disorders that cannot be given a more precise diagnosis because insufficient evidence is available, for example, when it is still uncertain whether a disorder is schizophrenia or mania. Similarly, it is useful to retain such terms as 'psychotic disorders not otherwise specified' (as in DSM-IV) and 'acute or transient psychotic disorders' (as in ICD-10). Finally, the adjectival form psychotic is in general use, for example, in the terms psychotic symptom (generally meaning delusions, hallucinations, and excitement) and antipsychotic drug (meaning a drug that controls these symptoms).

The term *neurosis* refers to mental disorders that are generally less severe than the psychoses and characterized by symptoms closer to normal experience (for example, anxiety). The history of the term is referred to on p. 90. Here the value of the term in classification is discussed. The objections to the term neurosis are similar to the objections to the term psychosis. First, neurosis is difficult to define; second, the conditions that it embraces have little in common; and third, more information can be conveyed by using a more

specific diagnosis, such as anxiety disorder or obsessional disorder, than by calling the condition a neurosis. A final objection was put forward in the manual to DSM-III, namely that neurosis has been widely used with an aetiological meaning in psychodynamic writings. It is true that the term has been so used and that such usage is historically unjustified (see p. 90), but if this misuse were the only objection to the term neurosis, it would be appropriate to ensure correct usage rather than to abandon the term. In practice, it has been possible to organize the main groups of disorders in terms of common features without the need to group them as neuroses and psychoses in the classification. The term neurosis is not used in DSM-IV, although it is retained in ICD-10 in the heading of one group of disorders: 'neurotic, stress-related, and somatoform disorders'. Like psychosis, the term neurosis continues to be used in everyday clinical practice as a convenient term for disorders that cannot be assigned to a more precise diagnosis.

Categories, dimensions, and multiple axes

Categorical classification

Traditionally, psychiatric disorders have been classified by dividing them into categories which are supposed to represent discrete entities. Categories have been defined in terms of symptom patterns and of the course and outcome of the different disorders. Such categories have proved useful in both clinical work and research. However, three objections are often raised against them:

- there is uncertainty about the validity of categories as representing distinct entities;

- many systems of classification do not provide adequate definitions and rules of application, and so categories cannot be used reliably;

- many psychiatric disorders do not fall neatly within the boundaries of a category but are intermediate between two categories (for example, cases intermediate between schizophrenia and affective disorder).

Recently, multivariate statistical techniques have been used in attempts to define categories more clearly. The results have been interesting, but so far not conclusive.

Dimensional classification

Dimensional classification rejects the use of separate categories. In the past it was advocated by Kretschmer and other psychiatrists. It has also been strongly promoted by the psychologist Eysenck, who argues that there is no evidence to support the traditional grouping into discrete entities. Instead, Eysenck (1970c) proposed a system of three dimensions: psychoticism, neuroticism, and introversion–extroversion. Patients are given scores, which locate them on each of these three axes. For example, in the case of a person with a disorder that would be assigned to dissociative disorder in a categorical system, in Eysenck's system the person would have high scores on the axes of neuroticism and extroversion, and a low score on the psychoticism axis. Subsequent research has not confirmed specific predictions of this kind, but the example brings out the principles.

Eysenck's three dimensions were established by various procedures of multivariate analysis. They are attractive in theory, but it should be remembered that they depend considerably on the initial assumptions and the choice of methods. The dimension of 'psychoticism' bears little relation to the concept of psychosis as generally used. For example, artists and prisoners score particularly highly on this dimension. The dimensions of neuroticism and introversion–extroversion have been useful in research with groups of patients, but they are difficult to apply to the individual patient in clinical practice.

The multiaxial approach

In one sense, the term multiaxial can be applied to the three dimensions just described. However, the term is usually applied to schemes of classifications in which two or more separate sets of information (such as symptoms and aetiology) are coded. In 1947 Essen-Møller proposed that clinical syn-drome and aetiology should be coded separately. It would then be possible to identify cases with a similar clinical picture on the one hand, and those with a similar aetiology on the other (Essen-Møller 1971). Such a scheme should avoid the unreliability of schemes in which clinical picture and aetiology can be combined in the definition of a single category, such as reactive depression. Multiaxial systems are attractive, but there is an obvious danger that they will be so comprehensive and complicated as to be difficult for everyday use. Several multiaxial systems have been proposed. The introduction of multiaxial classification was a major innovation in DSM-III. The DSM-IV and ICD-10 systems are described on pp. 98 and 96.

Hierarchies of diagnosis

Categorical systems often include an implicit hierarchy of categories. If two or more diagnoses are made, it is often conventional (though not always made explicit) that one takes precedence. For example, organic mental disorders take precedence over schizophrenia. Not only is this convenient, but there is some clinical evidence for an inbuilt hierarchy of significance within the disorders themselves. For instance, affective symptoms occur commonly with schizophrenia and they often improve when the schizophrenia is treated. Similarly, it is well recognized that anxiety symptoms occur commonly with depressive disorders and are sometimes the presenting feature. If the anxiety is treated, there is little response, but if the depressive disorder is treated, there may be improvement in anxiety as well as in the depressive symptoms.

Diagnostic criteria

Diagnostic unreliability can be reduced by providing a clear definition of each category in a diagnostic scheme. Each definition should specify *discriminating symptoms* rather than characteristic symptoms. Discriminating symptoms are those that may occur in the defined syndrome but seldom in other syndromes. Discriminating symptoms are important in diagnosis but may be of little concern to patients and relatively unimportant in treatment. An example is the delusion that thoughts are being inserted into the mind, a symptom that seldom occurs except in schizophrenia. *Characteristic symptoms* occur frequently in the defined syndrome but also occur in other syndromes. Such symptoms may be important to the patient and relevant in planning treatment, but do not help in diagnosis. An example is thoughts of suicide, which occur in depressive disorders but also in other conditions.

Diagnostic criteria can be descriptive statements, as in the ICD-10 clinical criteria, or more precise operational criteria, as in DSM-IV. *Operational definitions* were originally suggested by the philosopher Carl Hempel, and were incorporated in a report to the World Health Organization on ways of overcoming the problems of diverse national classifications (Stengel 1959). The term operational definition in this context means the specification of a category by a series of precise inclusion and exclusion statements.

The first published operational criteria were those devised for a longitudinal study of psychiatric hospital patients. The first detailed set of rules was drawn up by Feighner *et al.* (1972) in the USA, who provided specific inclusion and exclusion criteria. A similar approach was adopted in the Research Diagnostic Criteria (Spitzer *et al.* 1978) and in the American system DSM-III, which is described later in this chapter. When criteria of

---

Table 4.1 The basic classification
Learning disability
Personality disorder
Mental disorder
Adjustment disorder (reaction to stress)
Other disorders
Developmental and learning disorders
Disorders with onset in childhood or adolescence

---

this kind are used, a substantial number of patients may not fit into any of the designated categories and may have to be allocated to an 'atypical' category. In some kinds of research this atypical group may not matter, but it can be a problem in everyday clinical practice.

Other features of schemes of classification

Two other features contribute to the value of a system of classification: *coverage* and *ease of use*. Coverage refers to the extent to which a scheme has categories for all the disorders that are encountered in clinical practice.

The reliability and validity of diagnosis

Diagnosis is the process of identifying disease and allocating it to a category on the basis of symptoms and signs. It involves four main components:

- the interviewing technique of the psychiatrist;
- the perception of the patient's speech and behaviour;
- a complicated series of processes by which the psychiatrist sorts out the available information and decides how to use it and what task to perform next;
- a final stage in which the psychiatrist chooses one or more terms from a stated classification of psychiatric disorders.

The third and fourth stages can be made more objective by agreeing rules or by using a computer programme (see below).

Reliability

Systems of classification are of little value unless psychiatrists can agree with one another in attempting to make a diagnosis. In the past 40 years there has been increasing interest in improving the level of diagnostic agreement between psychiatrists (Kendell 1975). Early studies consistently showed poor diagnostic reliability. For example, in Philadelphia, Ward *et al.* (1962) concluded that overall disagreement was made up of the following elements:

- inconsistency in the patient, 5%;
- inadequate interview technique, 33%;
- inadequate use of diagnostic criteria, 62%.

Interviewing technique

Psychiatrists vary widely not only in the amount of information that they elicit at interview, but also in their interpretation of the information. Thus a psychiatrist may or may not elicit a phenomenon, and he may or may not regard it as a significant symptom or sign. Variations have been found between groups of psychiatrists trained in different countries, and between individual psychiatrists in the same country. When shown filmed interviews, American psychiatrists reported many more symptoms than did British psychiatrists (Sandifer *et al.* 1968). Presumably this reflected differences in training between the two countries.

Criteria for diagnosis

International studies have compared the diagnostic criteria used by different psychiatrists. In the US-UK Diagnostic Project, for example, American and British psychiatrists were shown the same videotaped clinical interviews and were asked to make diagnoses (Cooper *et al.* 1972). Compared with psychiatrists in London, psychiatrists in New York diagnosed schizophrenia twice as often and diagnosed mania and depression correspondingly less often. Further investigation suggested that New York was not typical of North America, and that diagnostic practice in other places in the USA and in Canada was closer to British practice.

A second study, the International Pilot Study of Schizophrenia (World Health Organization 1973) was carried out in nine countries: Colombia (Cali), Czechoslovakia (Prague), Denmark (Aarhus), England (London), India (Agra), Nigeria (Ibadan), Taiwan (Taipei), the USA (Washington), and the USSR (Moscow). The main purposes of this study were first to establish whether standardized interviews could be used in different languages in different cultures, and second to determine whether typical schizophrenic patients could be found in all the different cultures. As a side issue, the study examined some of the differences between the psychiatrists, even though the latter had trained together and had been asked to use the ICD-9 criteria in a standard way. Psychiatrists in all these countries carried out lengthy interviews, which included the Present State Examination (PSE). The psychiatrists made their own diagnoses and these were compared with those of the PSE computer program CATEGO. There was substantial agreement between seven of the centres, but Washington and Moscow differed from the rest. The findings in Washington confirmed the results of the US-UK project described above. The Moscow psychiatrists also appeared to have an unusually broad concept of schizophrenia; this apparently reflected a particular local emphasis on the course of the disorder as a diagnostic criterion.

Despite major developments in the last 30 years in the definition of diagnostic criteria, problems remain. There have been marked differences in the prevalence rates reported in population surveys purportedly using the same diagnostic symptoms. These appear to reflect limitations of diagnostic criteria and of the assessment instrument used. (Regier *et al.* 1998).

Standardized interview schedules

Differences in eliciting and rating symptoms can be reduced when psychiatrists are trained to use standardized interview schedules, such as the Present State Examination (PSE) (Wing *et al.* 1974), which was designed for use by trained clinicians who make judgements about the presence and severity of symptoms. Another example is the Diagnostic Interview Schedule (DIS) which was introduced by the National Institutes of Mental Health for use by non-specialist interviewers who record patients' complaints without making a judgement as to whether these are symptoms. Both types of schedule specify sets of items that must be enquired about, and they also provide definitions and give instructions on rating severity. These and other instruments are listed in Chapter 2.

Diagnosis by computer

Computer diagnosis ensures that the same rules will be applied to every case. Computer programs to generate diagnoses have been based either on a logical decision tree or on statistical models. A decision-tree program evaluates a sequence of yes/no answers, and so successively narrows the diagnosis. Thus it resembles differential diagnosis in clinical practice. Spitzer and Endicott (1968) first used this procedure to develop the program DIAGNO. Later, Wing *et al.* (1974) developed the program CATEGO for use with the PSE. CATEGO has proved valuable in epidemiological studies of major and minor psychiatric disorders, and comparison data are now available from a variety of patient groups and normal populations. Computer programs are available for the major international diagnostic instruments SCAN and CIDI (see p. 65).

In the alternative statistical approach, data are collected from a sample of patients whose diagnoses are known. A system of classification is then devised from this database by statistical methods. Whereas the decision-tree method follows a sequence of arbitrary rules that underlie ordinary clinical practice, this second method estimates the probability that a given patient's symptoms match the symptoms of previously diagnosed patients.

The validity of schemes of classification

Whilst the unreliability of diagnosis can be reduced by the measures just described, a scheme of classification must also be valid. Even if different interviewers can be trained to reach high levels of agreement in making diagnoses, little has been achieved unless the diagnostic categories have some useful relationship to the disorders met in clinical practice. To be valid, a scheme of classification should have categories that fit well with clinical experience (face validity). The categories should also be able to predict the outcome of psychiatric disorders (predictive validity); ideally they should also point to associations between psychiatric disorders and independent variables such as biochemical measures (construct validity).

So far little progress has been made towards establishing the validity of existing schemes of classification. See Spitzer and Williams (1985) for a discussion of reliability and validity in diagnosis.

Systems of classification

During the twentieth century, most nations' systems of classification remained largely within Kraepelin's framework.

In the UK, the approach to classification was more empirical, as was shown by the British glossary to ICD-8, published in 1968 (see below).

In *Scandinavia* much emphasis was placed on the concept of psychogenic or reactive psychoses, which are said to have paranoid, depressive, or confusional symptoms, or sometimes a mixture of all three (Strömgren 1985; Cooper 1986).

In *French* psychiatry, classification was based on a combination of psychopathology and elements of existential philosophy (Pichot 1984, 1994). Certain diagnostic categories in France differed from those in the rest of Europe and North America. They included two special categories: *bouffée délirante* and *délires chroniques*. *Bouffée délirante* is the sudden onset of a delusional state with trance-like feelings, of short duration and good prognosis. Although this condition may develop into schizophrenia, it is clearly separated from acute schizophrenia and acute manic-depressive illness (see Chapter 12). This disorder has been included in ICD-10 in the category of 'acute transient psychotic disorder', which also incorporates features of the Scandinavian concept of reactive psychosis. *Délires chroniques* are conditions which, in the ICD system, would be classified as 'persistent delusional disorders'; they are separated from schizophrenia, a diagnosis used in France only when there is definite evidence of deterioration of personality. The *délires chroniques* are subdivided into the 'non-focused', in which several areas of mental activity are affected, and the 'focused' with a single delusional theme. The latter include several conditions such as erotomania (described on p. 392).

In the 1920s and 1930s, *American* views on psychiatric classification diverged widely from those in Europe. Psychoanalysis and the teaching of Adolf Meyer directed American psychiatry towards a predominant concern with the uniqueness of individuals rather than with their common features. At the same time, diagnostic concepts were increasingly based on presumed psychodynamic mechanisms. Attitudes towards psychiatric classification in the USA have changed considerably. An important first step was the introduction of strict criteria for classification in research, as described above (Feighner *et al*. 1972). This step was followed by the thorough work that led to the new American scheme DSM-III (M. Wilson 1993). Attitudes towards classification in the USA changed considerably after the development and general acceptance of the American Psychiatric Association's classification DSM-III. For example, in the post-war period up to the early 1960s, the concept of schizophrenia was very broad. This has been succeeded by a particularly narrow concept of schizophrenia.

Another example of international variation is the latest *Chinese* national classification (*Chinese classification of mental disorders, second edition revised* – CCMD–2-R) which excludes almost all the somatoform disorders of DSM-IV and ICD-10. However, it does include the category of neurasthenia, which is one of the most frequently used diagnoses in Chinese psychiatry (Kleinman 1982). See Mezzich *et al*. (2000) for a review of international approaches to classification.

International classification

The International Classification of Diseases (ICD)

During the last 40 years, classification has developed largely in terms of the World Health Organization (WHO) international system and the very widely used national classification produced in the USA – DSM. There remain a number of other national classifications which are used locally. Increasingly these have been based directly on ICD or DSM. An example would be the current Chinese classification.

Mental disorders were not included in the ICD until its sixth edition produced by the WHO in 1948. This first scheme for mental disorders was widely criticized. As a preliminary to a major revision of the scheme, a survey of principles of classification in different countries was carried out (Stengel 1959) and wide variations were found. Stengel recommended a new approach based on operational definitions and supported by a glossary, but not linked to any theories of aetiology.

The eighth edition (ICD-8) was published in 1968. It made some progress towards solving the earlier problems but was still unsatisfactory in several ways. It contained too many categories and allowed alternative codings for some syndromes. This probably reflected an endeavour to make the scheme widely acceptable. One major advance was the publication of a glossary, which was largely based on the British version produced by a Working Party chaired by Sir Aubrey Lewis (General Register Office 1968). ICD-9 was very similar to ICD-8 because the WHO believed that national governments would be unwilling to accept many changes. Although the mental health section had asked to be allowed to wait until the publication of ICD-10 before making changes, in the meantime a series of seminars were held which led to a revised and improved glossary (World Health Organization 1978a).

Major changes in the mental health section of ICD-10 have resulted from several initiatives, including the continuing WHO research programme on diagnosis and classification, collaborative studies, and innovations by national organizations, especially the American Psychiatric Association. Public consultation has been achieved through a series of research projects and the work of many advisors. As a result of close collaboration with the American Psychiatric Association and an overlap of the membership of the ICD and DSM working parties, the two systems are now broadly similar.

The aims of the ICD-10 working party were that the scheme should:

- be suitable for international communication about statistics of morbidity and mortality;
- be a reference for national and other psychiatric classifications;
- be acceptable and useful in research and clinical work; and
- contribute to education.

To achieve these aims, the classification has to be acceptable to a wide range of users in different cultures; it also has to be practical in that it is easy to understand and can be translated into many languages. It also has to be versatile; for this reason a policy of 'different versions for different purposes' was used from the start and led to the several versions shown in Table 4.2.

The clinical descriptions and diagnostic guidelines contain descriptions of each of the disorders in the classification; these allow some latitude for clinical judgement in making the diagnosis. The diagnostic criteria for research contain lists of specific criteria that have to be met before a diagnosis can be made. The format resembles that used

Table 4.2 ICD–10 Chapter V

Clinical descriptions and diagnostic guidelines

Diagnostic criteria for research

Primary care version

Multiaspect (axial) systems

Table 4.3 The main categories in ICD–10

F0	Organic, including symptomatic, mental disorders
F1	Mental and behaviour disorders due to psychoactive substance use
F2	Schizophrenia, schizotypal, and delusional disorders
F3	Mood (affective) disorders
F4	Neurotic, stress-related, and somatoform disorders
F5	Behavioural syndromes associated with physiological disturbances and physical factors
F6	Disorders of adult personality and behaviour
F7	Mental retardation
F8	Disorders of psychological development
F9	Behavioural and emotional disorders with onset usually occurring in childhood or adolescence

in DSM-IV for clinical purposes as well as for research.

ICD-10, like DSM-IV, is a descriptive classification. However, aetiology is included in some general categories, namely organic, substance-use-related, and stress-related. Therefore the classification is a mixture of symptoms and aetiology.

Mental disorders are classified in Chapter F of the ICD. The chapter is divided into ten groups, shown in Table 4.3. A decimal system is used in which each group can be subdivided into ten, and each of these into a further ten. Categories are denoted by the letter F (for the mental disorders chapter), followed by a number for the main group (for example, F2 schizophrenia), followed by a further number for the category within the group (for example, F25 schizoaffective disorder). A fourth character is used when it is necessary to subdivide further (for example, F25.1 schizoaffective disorder, depressive type). The traditional division of neurosis and psychosis is no longer an organizing principle.

After wide consultation about a draft of the classification, the WHO carried out an international field trial to evaluate both the clinical descriptions and guidelines and the diagnostic criteria for research, which have been translated into all the widely spoken languages of the world. This trial aimed to assess whether the classification fitted diagnostic practice in different countries, how easy it was to use, and whether psychiatrists could reach agreement about diagnoses after brief training. The trial was carried out at 112 clinical centres in 39 countries. It was found that the classification was generally easy to use and applicable to most common disorders. Reliability was less good for a few conditions, notably personality disorder (Sartorius *et al*. 1993). The field trials of ICD-10 carried out in Canada and the USA showed comparable reliability to the findings world-wide and to DSM (Regier *et al*. 1994).

The Diagnostic and Statistical Manual (DSM)

In 1952 the American Psychiatric Association published the first edition of the *Diagnostic and Statistical Manual* (DSM-I) as an alternative to ICD-6 which, as mentioned above, had been widely criticized. DSM-I was influenced by the views of Adolf Meyer and Karl Menninger, and its simple glossary reflected the prevailing acceptance of psychoanalytic ideas in the USA. DSM-II was published in 1968 as the American National Glossary to ICD-8. It combined psychoanalytic ideas with those of Kraepelin. In 1974, the American Psychiatric Association set up a task force to produce a revised version of DSM to coincide with the publication of ICD-9. The chairman of the task force was a member of the group at Washington University, St Louis, which had published the Feighner criteria for diagnosis, and he had subsequently developed the Research Diagnostic Criteria published in 1975 (Endicott and Spitzer 1978). These developments strongly influenced DSM-III, which was published in 1980. The criteria were prepared with great care. Advisory committees prepared detailed drafts, opinions were obtained from 550 clinicians, and the results were subjected to field tests (American Psychiatric Association 1980). DSM-III was intended to provide a comprehensive classification with clear criteria for each diagnostic category. It contained five main innovations.

1. Precise operational criteria were provided for each diagnosis, with rules for inclusion and exclusion.

2. A multiaxial classification was adopted with five axes: I, clinical syndromes and 'conditions not attributable to mental disorder that are the focus of attention and treatment'; II, personality disorders; III, physical disorders and conditions; IV, severity of psychosocial stressors; V, highest level of adaptive functioning in the last year.

3. The nomenclature was revised and some syndromes were regrouped; for example, the terms neurosis and hysteria were discarded, and all affective disorders were grouped together.

4. Classification relied less on psychodynamic concepts than it had done in previous versions.

5. For some conditions, duration of illness was introduced as one of the criteria for diagnosis.

See Wilson (1993) for an account of the development of DSM-III and a discussion of the consequences for American psychiatry.

The production of DSM-III was an important achievement even though it contained compromises to accommodate different theoretical and clinical viewpoints among American psychiatrists. Not only did it introduce advances in the method of classification and the preparation of diagnostic criteria, but it also marked a major change in attitude to classification in American psychiatry. This revision resulted in many differences between this American national classification and the international classification. The differences are attributable to the different aims of the two classifications, and to unresolved differences in particularly controversial areas of classification (for example, somatoform disorders). In 1987, a further revision of the American classification (DSM-IIIR) was produced as an interim scheme to remedy some of the defects of DSM-III pending the production of a fourth version (DSM-IV) to coincide with the tenth edition of the ICD (American Psychiatric Association 1987).

In 1988, a meeting of the American Psychiatric Association considered how the USA could best fulfil its treaty obligation with the WHO to maintain coding and technological consistency with ICD. The conclusion was that work on DSM-IV and ICD-10 should be closely coordinated. As a result, DSM-IV is technically compatible with ICD-10, although there are a number of specific differences (Table 4.4). Thirteen work groups were established, each responsible for a section of the classification. Each work group carried out a three-stage procedure:

◆ comprehensive reviews of published literature;

◆ analysis of data already collected;

◆ field trials to evaluate proposed changes.

Drafts of DSM-IV were circulated for discussion and comments before publication of the final manual in 1994 (American Psychiatric Association 1994a). The review material has been published in a series of DSM-IV source books.

A new version incorporating minor revisions of the explanatory text – DSM-IV Text Revision (DSM-IV-TR) – was published in 2000. This aimed to update the classification as an educational tool. The changes are mainly small rewordings of the text and there is no alteration to the classification itself or to the criteria (American Psychiatric Association 2000).

Comparison of ICD-10 and DSM-IV

ICD-10 and DSM-IV are closely similar because they are derived from a common base of knowledge and research, and because their authors collaborated closely. The two classifications are complementary rather than competing. Thus DSM has been designed for use in a single country – it is a national classification – whereas ICD has been designed for use in all countries with their varied cultures and needs and was subjected to international field trials (Sartorius *et al* 1995). Table 4.4 summarizes the main differences between the two classifications.

One of the main differences in ICD-10 is the provision of these two sets of criteria – the more flexible ones for clinical purposes and the more precise ones for research. A second difference is the inclusion in ICD-10 of a simplified classification

Table 4.4 Differences between ICD–10 and DSM-IV

	ICD10	DSMIV
Origin	International	American Psychiatric Association
Presentation	Different versions for clinical work, research, and use in primary care	A single document
Languages	Available in all widely spoken languages	English version only
Structure	Part of overall ICD framework Single axis in Chapter V; separate multiaxial systems available	Multiaxial
Content	Guidelines and criteria do not include social consequences of	Diagnostic criteria usually include significant impairment in social,

for use in primary care. This version of the classification contains only broad categories such as dementia, delirium, eating disorders, acute psychotic disorder, chronic psychotic disorder, depression, and bipolar disorder. These categories are not subclassified, and the clinical descriptions are simpler than those in the main classification and are adapted for use in primary care.

Current issues in classification

Cross-cultural issues

Classifications developed in Europe and North America have not proved entirely satisfactory in developing countries where behavioural disturbances can be different. In developing countries acute psychotic symptoms may present particular difficulties of diagnosis; they are often atypical and raise doubt as to whether they represent separate entities or merely variations of syndromes seen in developed countries. Other difficulties arise because ICD and DSM are fundamentally dualist in concept and this has little meaning in many cultures. For example, the concept of somatoform disorder depends upon seeing mind and body aetiologies as alternatives, an approach which causes considerable difficulty in Western medicine and which is not understood at all elsewhere. Investigation of these issues is difficult for outsiders who may not appreciate important cultural factors or the varying use of language to describe emotions and behaviour. For further information about the cultural aspects of classification see Mezzich *et al.* (1999).

Problem categories

Several areas within the current classifications were recognized to be speculative and their value remains uncertain. These include diagnoses which cause particular cross-cultural difficulty. Examples are acute stress disorder and somatoform disorders. (See Widiger and Clark 2000).

Subthreshold disorders

Conditions which do not meet full diagnostic criteria are frequent and associated with considerable costs and disability. This is especially so in primary care and community populations. There remains a lack of information to provide a basis for a nosology which will take adequate account of allegedly subthreshold problems (Pincus *et al.* 1999).

Clinical significance

DSM-IV introduced the criterion of clinical significance into a large proportion of categories in an effort to make definitions more restrictive. However, it may be more logical and more precise to consider modifications to symptom criteria (Spitzer and Wakefield 1999; Regier 2000).

Use in non-specialist settings

DSM is primarily a classification for specialists and this has resulted in the problems described above in relation to clinical significance and subthreshold problems. ICD recognized the problem and the family of versions allows classification in different circumstances. However, the primary care version has not yet been widely adopted.

Co-morbidity

The development of the new classifications has made co-morbidity – subjects whose mental status satisfies several diagnoses – much more conspicuous. It covers several different circumstances:

◆ different and causally unrelated disorder. An example would be the patient with chronic schizophrenia who, in later life, develops dementia as an entirely independent further problem.

◆ disorders with distinctly different, but causally related, psychiatric problems, for example, the patient who has a personality disorder, suffers depressive illness and subsequently an alcohol problem; disorders which are likely to be aetiologically related.

◆ disorders that satisfy more than one set of diagnostic criteria, for example, generalized anxiety disorder and specific phobia. Many clinicians regard the phobic symptoms as within the range of variations of the clinical picture of generalized anxiety disorder such that some clinical problems may satisfy several sets of diagnostic criteria.

Another usage is in epidemiological surveys in which the term lifetime co-morbidity is used. This term refers not to the co-occurrence of two disorders, but to their occurrence in the same person at any time during the lifespan. This relationship may be close in time – for example, panic disorder followed shortly by agoraphobia with panic – or the two disorders may be widely separated by time.

Lifetime diagnosis

The application of the new classifications for the standard criteria of epidemiology led to use of lifetime diagnoses as well as current diagnoses. This has some distinct advantages as compared with the cross-sectional view at one moment of time. However, patient recall and the application of criteria to distance events is difficult. This has been shown by the discrepancies in lifetime rates when surveys are repeated. The problems with lifetime measures (together with a divergence between surveys' assessments and psychiatrists' appraisal of clinical need) have resulted in considerable problems in developing mental heath policy and in planning services (see Cooper and Singh 2000).

Towards DSM-V

This book is published at a time when DSM-IV is in the process of substantial revision. This will be an extended process of review by working groups and of consultation. As an interim stage, DSM-IV-TR introduced more minor changes in the light of experience and new evidence. Despite the powerful political and financial pressures to update classification, there are dangers that changes will once again be made without compelling new evidence to resolve the undoubted problems in the current categories and criteria. (See Widiger and Clark 2000).

Classification in this book

In this book we have generally followed the usage in ICD-10 and DSM-IV by adopting the term mental disorder instead of the term mental illness. The former is defined as:

a clinically significant behaviour or psychological syndrome or pattern that occurs in a person and that is associated with present distress (a painful symptom) or disability (impairment of one or more important areas of functioning) or with a significantly increased risk of suffering death, pain, disability, or an important loss of freedom. In addition, this syndrome or pattern must not be merely an expectable response to a particular event, e.g. the death of a loved one.

In this book both the DSM-IV and the ICD-10 classifications are discussed in the chapters dealing with clinical syndromes. As in other textbooks, disorders are grouped in chapters for convenience and ease of understanding. The headings of the chapters do not always correspond exactly to the terms used in DSM-IV and ICD-10; any difference means that the heading more appropriately summarizes the scope of the chapter.

Further reading

American Psychiatric Association (2000). *Diagnostic and statistical manual of mental disorders – text revision*, 4th edn. American Psychiatric Association, Washington, DC.

Kendell, R. E. (1975). *The role of classification in psychiatry*. Blackwell Scientific Publications, Oxford.

World Health Organization (1992). *The ICD-10 classification of mental and behavioural disorders: diagnostic criteria for research*. World Health Organization, Geneva.

CHAPTER 5

Aetiology

CHAPTER 5
Aetiology

Approaches to aetiology in psychiatry

Psychiatrists are concerned with *aetiology* in two ways. First, in everyday clinical work they try to discover the causes of the mental disorders presented by *individual patients*. Second, in seeking a wider understanding of psychiatry they are interested in aetiological evidence obtained from *clinical studies*, *community surveys*, or *laboratory investigations*. Correspondingly, the first part of this chapter deals with some general issues about aetiology in the assessment of the individual patient, whilst the second part deals with the various scientific disciplines that have been applied to the study of aetiology.

General issues about aetiology

Aetiology and intuitive understanding

When the clinician assesses an individual patient, he draws on a common fund of aetiological knowledge that has been derived from the study of groups of similar patients, but he cannot understand the patient in these terms alone. He also has to use everyday insights into human nature. For example, in assessing a depressed patient, the psychiatrist should certainly know what has been discovered about the psychological and neurochemical changes accompanying depressive disorders, and what evidence there is about the aetiological role of stressful events and about genetic predisposition to depressive disorder. At

the same time he will need intuitive understanding to recognize, for example, that this particular patient feels depressed because he has been informed that his wife has cancer.

Common-sense ideas of this kind are nearly always an important part of aetiological formulation in psychiatry, but they must be used carefully if superficial explanation is to be avoided. Aetiological formulation can be done properly only if certain conceptual problems are clearly understood. These problems can be illustrated by a case history.

For 4 weeks a 38-year-old married man became increasingly depressed. His symptoms started soon after his wife left him to live with another man. In the past the patient's mother had received psychiatric treatment on two occasions, once for a severe depressive disorder and once for mania; on neither occasion was there any apparent environmental cause for the illness. When the patient was 14 years old, his mother went away to live with another man, leaving her children with their father. For several years afterwards the patient felt rejected and unhappy but eventually settled down. He married and had two children aged 13 and 10 at the time of his illness.

Two weeks after leaving home, the patient's wife returned, saying that she had made a mistake and really loved her husband. Despite her return the patient's symptoms persisted and worsened. He began to wake early, gave up his usual activities, and spoke at times of suicide.

In thinking about the causes of this man's symptoms, the clinician would first draw on knowledge of aetiology derived from scientific enquiries. Genetic investigations have shown that, if a parent suffers from mania as well as depressive disorder, a predisposition to depressive disorder is particularly likely to be transmitted to the children. Therefore it is possible that this patient received this predisposition from his mother.

Clinical investigation has also provided some information about the effects of separating children from their mothers. In the present case, the information is not helpful because it refers to people who were separated from their mothers at a younger age than the patient. On scientific grounds there is no particular reason to focus on the departure of the patient's mother, but intuitively it seems likely that this was an important event. From everyday experience it is understandable that a man should feel sad if his wife leaves him; it is also understandable that he is likely to feel even more distressed if this event recapitulates a similar distressing experience in his own childhood. Therefore, despite the lack of scientific evidence, the clinician would recognize intuitively that the patient's depression is likely to be a reaction to the wife's departure. The same sort of intuition might suggest that the patient would recover when his wife came back. In the event he did not recover. Although his symptoms seemed understandable when his wife was away, they seem less so after her return.

This simple case history illustrates some important aetiological issues in psychiatry:

- complexity of causes
- classification of causes
- concept of stress
- concept of psychological reaction
- relative roles of intuition and scientific knowledge in aetiological formulations.

The complexity of causes in psychiatry

In psychiatry the study of causation is complicated by three problems. These problems are met in other branches of medicine, but to a lesser degree.

Lack of temporal association

The first problem is that causes are often *remote in time* from the effects that they produce. For example, it is widely believed that childhood experiences partly determine the occurrence of neuroses in adult life. It is difficult to test this idea because the necessary information can only be gathered either by studying children and tracing them many years later, which is difficult, or by asking adults about their childhood experiences, which is unreliable.

Cause and effect

The second problem is that a single cause may lead to *several effects*. For example, deprivation of parental affection in childhood has been reported to predispose to antisocial behaviour, suicide, depressive disorder, and several other disorders. Conversely, a single effect may arise from several causes. The latter can be illustrated either by different causes in different individuals or by multiple causes in a single individual. For example, learning disability (single effect) may occur in several children, but the cause may be a different genetic abnormality in each child. On the other hand, depressive disorder (single effect) may occur in one individual through a combination of causes, such as genetic factors, adverse childhood experiences, and stressful events in adult life.

Indirect mechanisms

The third problem is that aetiological factors in psychiatry rarely exert their effects directly. For example, the genetic predisposition to depression may be mediated in part through psychological factors which make it more likely that the individual concerned will experience adverse life events. Thus aetiological effects are usually mediated through complex intervening mechanisms which also need to be investigated and understood.

The classification of causes

A single psychiatric disorder, as just explained, may result from several causes. For this reason a scheme for *classifying* causes is required. A useful approach is to divide causes chronologically into *predisposing*, *precipitating*, and *maintaining*.

Predisposing factors

There are factors, many of them operating from early life, that determine a person's *vulnerability* to causes acting close to the time of the illness. They include *genetic endowment* and the *environment in utero*, as well as *physical, psychological, and social factors in infancy and early childhood*. The term *constitution* is often used to describe the mental and physical make-up of a person at any point in his life. This make-up changes as life goes on under the influence of further physical, psychological, and social influences. Some writers restrict the term constitution to the make-up at the beginning of life, whilst others also include characteristics acquired later (this second usage is adopted in this book). The concept of constitution includes the idea that a person may have a predisposition to develop a disorder (such as schizophrenia) even though the latter never manifests itself. From the standpoint of psychiatric aetiology, one of the important parts of the constitution is the *personality*.

When the aetiology of an individual case is formulated, the *personality* is always an essential element. For this reason, the clinician should be prepared to spend considerable time in talking to the patient and to people who know him in order to build up a clear picture of his personality. This assessment often helps to explain why the patient responded to certain stressful events, and why he reacted in a particular way. The obvious importance of personality in the individual patient contrasts with the small amount of relevant scientific information so far available. Therefore, in the evaluation of personality it is particularly important to acquire sound clinical skills through supervised practice.

Precipitating factors

These are events that occur shortly before the onset of a disorder and *appear to have induced it*. They may be physical, psychological, or social. Whether they produce a disorder at all, and what kind of disorder, depends partly on constitutional factors in the patient (as mentioned above). Physical precipitants include cerebral tumours or drugs, for example. Psychological and social precipitants include personal misfortunes such as the loss of a job, and changes in the routine of life such as moving home. Sometimes the same factor can act in more than one way; for example, a head injury can induce psychological disorder either through physical changes in the brain or through its stressful implications to the patient.

Maintaining factors

These factors *prolong the course of a disorder* after it has been provoked. When planning treatment, it is particularly important to pay attention to these factors. The original predisposing and precipitating factors may have ceased to act by the time that the patient is seen, but the perpetuating factors may well be treatable. For example, in their early stages many psychiatric disorders lead to secondary demoralization and withdrawal from social activities, which in turn help to prolong the original disorder. It is often appropriate to treat these secondary factors, whether or not any other specific measures are carried out. Maintaining factors are also called *perpetuating factors.*

The concept of stress

Discussions about *stress* are often confusing because the term is used in two ways. First, it is applied to events or situations, such as working for an examination, which may have an adverse effect on someone. Second, it is applied to the adverse effects that are induced, which may be psychological or physiological change. In considering aetiology it is advisable to separate these components.

The first set of factors can usefully be called *stressors*. They include a large number of physical, psychological, and social factors that can produce adverse effects. The term is sometimes extended to include events that are not experienced as adverse at the time, but may still have adverse long-term effects. For example, intense competition may produce an immediate feeling of pleasant tension, though it may sometimes lead to unfavourable long-term effects.

The effect on the person can usually be called the *stress reaction* to distinguish it from the provoking events. This reaction includes *autonomic responses* (such as a rise in blood pressure), *endocrine changes* (such as the secretion of adrenaline and noradrenaline), and *psychological responses* (such as a feeling of being keyed up). Much current research is involved in studying the effects of stress on the brain, particularly the mechanisms involved in the regulation of mood and processing of emotional information (see Herbert 1997).

The concept of a psychological reaction

As already mentioned, it is widely recognized that psychological distress can arise as a reaction to unpleasant events. Sometimes the association between event and distress is evident, for example, when a man becomes depressed after the death of his wife. In other cases, it is far from clear whether the psychological disorder is really a reaction to an event or whether the two have coincided fortuitously, for example, when a man becomes depressed after the death of a distant relative.

Jaspers (English translation, 1963, p. 392) suggested three criteria for deciding whether a psychological state is a reaction to a particular set of events:

- The events must be adequate in severity and closely related in time to the onset of the psychological state.
- There must be a clear connection between the nature of the events and the content of the psychological disorder (in the example just given, the man should be preoccupied with ideas concerning his distant relative).
- The psychological state should begin to disappear when the events have ceased (unless, of course, it can be shown that perpetuating factors are acting to maintain it).

These three criteria are useful in clinical practice, though they can be difficult to apply (particularly the second criterion).

Understanding and explanation

As already mentioned, aetiological statements about individual patients must combine knowledge derived from research on groups of patients with intuitive understanding derived from everyday experience. Jaspers (1963, p. 302) has called these two ways of making sense of psychiatric disorders 'Erklaren' and 'Verstehen', respectively.

In German, these terms mean 'explanation' and 'understanding', respectively, and they are usually translated as such in English translations of Jaspers' writing. However, Jaspers used them in a special sense. He used 'Erklaren' to refer to the sort of causative statement that is sought in the natural sciences. It is exemplified by the statement that a patient's aggressive behaviour has occurred because he has a brain tumour. He used 'Verstehen' to refer to psychological understanding, or the intuitive grasp of a natural connection between events in a person's life and his psychological state. In colloquial English, this could be called 'putting oneself in another person's shoes'. It is exemplified by the statement, 'I can understand why the patient became angry when his wife was insulted by a neighbour'.

These distinctions are reasonably clear when we consider an individual patient but confusion sometimes arises when attempts are made to generalize from insights obtained in a single case to widely applicable principles. Understanding may then be mistaken for explanation. Jaspers suggested that some psychoanalytical ideas are special kinds of intuitive understanding that are derived from the detailed study of individuals and then applied generally. They are not explanations that can be tested scientifically. They are more akin to insights into human nature that can be gained from reading great works of literature. Such insights are of great value in conducting human affairs. It would be wrong to neglect them in psychiatry, but equally wrong to see them as statements of a scientific kind.

The aetiology of a single case

How to make an aetiological formulation was discussed in Chapter 2 (p. 60). An example was given of a woman in her thirties who had become increasingly depressed. The formulation showed how aetiological factors could be grouped under headings of predisposing, precipitating, and perpetuating factors. It also showed how information from scientific investigations (in this case genetics) could be combined with an intuitive understanding of personality and the likely effects of family problems on the patient. The reader may find it helpful to re-read the formulation on p. 61 before continuing with this chapter.

Aetiological models

Before considering the contribution that different scientific disciplines can make to psychiatric aetiology, attention needs to be given to the kinds of aetiological model that have been employed in psychiatry. A model is a device for ordering information. Like a theory, it seeks to explain certain phenomena, but it does so in a broad and comprehensive way that cannot readily be proved false.

Reductionist and non-reductionist models

Two broad categories of explanatory model can be recognized. *Reductionist models* seek to understand causation by tracing back to simpler and simpler early stages. Examples are the 'narrow' medical model, described below, and the psychoanalytic model. This type of model can be exemplified by the statement that the cause of schizophrenia lies in a disordered neurotransmission in a specific area of the brain.

Non-reductionist models try to relate problems to wider rather than narrower issues. The explanatory models used in sociology are generally of this kind. In psychiatry, this type of model can be exemplified by the statement that the cause of a patient's schizophrenia lies in his family; the patient is the most conspicuous element in a disordered group of people. In the same way it can be asserted that certain depressive states are associated with indices of social deprivation and isolation and can be best understood as being caused by these factors.

The neuroscience approach

The technical and conceptual advances in brain sciences has led to what is often called the *neuroscience approach*. Kandel (1998) has outlined the key assumptions underlying this approach to aetiology:

- All mental processes derive from operations of the brain. Thus all behavioural disorders are ultimately disturbances of brain function even where the original 'cause' is clearly environmental.

- Genes, through their protein products, have important effects on brain function and therefore exert a significant control over behaviour.

- Social and behavioural effects exert their effects on the brain in part through changes in gene expression. Changes in gene expression and the consequent patterns of synaptic connectivity underlie the ability of experiences such learning and psychotherapy to change behaviour.

The latter concept derives from the ability of a wide range of environmental stimuli to *modulate gene expression* by via alterations in *gene transcription factors*. Thus while genes coding for particular proteins are inherited, environmental and developmental influences are involved in determining whether and to what extent a particular gene is expressed. This provides a plausible mechanism by which nature and nurture interact in the production of a behavioural phenotype.

The neuroscience approach therefore seeks to comprehend the role of social, family, and personal factors in behaviour by relating them to changes in brain function. For example, in understanding the effect of childhood neglect on the liability to adult depression, it is important to find out how adverse childhood experiences might alter relevant brain mechanisms (such as the HPA axis response to stress) and how this abnormality might predispose to depression when the individual is exposed to difficulties in adulthood. Thus, although a neuroscience approach encompasses the importance of social and personal factors it seeks to understand their consequences in a *reductionist* way (see Heninger 1999).

Medical models

Several models are used in psychiatric aetiology, but the so-called *medical model* is the most prominent. It represents a general strategy of research that has proved useful in medicine, particularly in studying infectious diseases. A disease entity is identified in terms of a *consistent pattern of symptoms*, a *characteristic clinical course*, and *specific post-mortem findings*. When an entity has been identified in this way, a set of necessary and sufficient causes is sought. In the case of tuberculosis, for example, the tubercle bacillus is the necessary cause, but it is not by itself sufficient. The tubercle bacillus in conjunction with either poor nutrition or low resistance is sufficient cause.

This narrow kind of medical model has been useful in psychiatry, though not for all conditions. It is clearly relevant to syndromes with a well-defined organic aetiology, for example, psychiatric conditions related to obvious cerebral disorder or a general medical condition. It is also applicable to severe psychiatric disorders such as schizophrenia and bipolar disorder. Until recently such disorders were called 'functional' in contrast to 'organic' because the assumption was that brain dysfunction was present but the pathology (with current methods) could not be observed. Recent studies on the aetiology of schizophrenia have shown that this view was essentially correct (see Chapter 12). However, *social and cultural factors* also play a role in the presentation and course of the illness.

The importance of social and cultural factors is now well recognized in general medicine and modern medical models are therefore considerably broader than that based on the elucidation of the mechanism of infectious disease. Modern medical models also recognize that much illness is charac-

terized by quantitative rather than qualitative deviations from normal, for example, high blood pressure. This clearly applies to many disorders in psychiatry, particularly anxiety and milder depressive disorders.

Difficulties with the medical model arise particularly with disorders characterized mainly by *abnormalities of conduct and social behaviour*, for example, antisocial behaviour and substance misuse. As mentioned above, current neuroscience approaches would seek to understand these disorders through changes in relevant brain systems. This is because causal factors in abnormal social behaviour such as environmental hardship and personal deprivation must ultimately express their effects on behaviour through changes in brain mechanisms.

While the latter view is theoretically attractive and increases the aetiological power of the medical model, the key decision for clinician and policy maker is at what level the disorder is best understood and managed. For example, it is possible to understand problems in substance misuse as arising from a defect in brain reward systems which, in a vulnerable individual, results in 'normal' experimentation with illicit substances leading to substance misuse with adverse personal and social consequences. Equally, one can see excessive drug misuse in society as a 'symptom' of social deprivation and family disruption (see Chapter 18). Both kinds of aetiology can be comprehended in a broad medical model, but different forms of intervention would result.

The behavioural model

As explained above, certain disorders psychiatrists treat, particularly those defined in terms of *abnormal behaviour* do not fit readily into the medical model. The latter include some sexual deviations, deliberate self-harm, the misuse of drugs and alcohol, and repeated acts of delinquency. The behavioural model is an alternative way of comprehending these disorders. In this model the disorders are explained in terms of factors that determine normal behaviour: drives, reinforcements, social and cultural influences, and internal psychological processes such as attitudes, beliefs, and expectations. The behavioural model predicts that there will not be a sharp distinction between the normal and the abnormal but a continuous gradation. This model can therefore be a useful way of considering many conditions seen by psychiatrists.

Although the behavioural model is mainly concerned with psychological and social causes, it does not exclude genetic, physiological, or biochemical causes. This is because normal patterns of behaviour are partly determined by genetic factors, and because psychological factors such as reinforcement have a basis in physiological and biochemical mechanisms. Also, the behavioural model employs both *reductionist* and *non-reductionist* explanations. For example, abnormalities of behaviour can be explained in terms of abnormal conditioning (a reductionist model), or in terms of a network of social influences.

Developmental models

Medical and behavioural models incorporate the idea of predisposing as well as precipitating causes, i.e. the idea that past events may determine whether or not a current cause gives rise to a disorder. Some models place even more emphasis on past events in the form of a sequence of experiences leading to the present disorder. This approach has been called the 'life story' approach to aetiology (McHugh and Slavney 1986). One example is Freud's psychoanalysis; another is Meyer's psychobiology. Freud's theories are considered later; Meyer's will be referred to next.

Adolf Meyer and psychobiology

Adolf Meyer was born in Switzerland but spent most of his working life in the USA. Although he practised first as a neuropathologist, he made his most important contribution by emphasizing the role of *psychological and social factors* in the aetiology of psychiatric disorders. He applied the term *psychobiology* to this approach to aetiology, in which a wide range of previous experiences were consid-

ered and then common-sense judgement was used to decide which experiences might have led to the present disorder. Meyer recognized the importance of heredity and brain disorder, but he emphasized that these factors were modified by life experiences, which could increase or decrease a person's basic vulnerability. The clinician was left to decide which experiences were relevant without relying on preconceived ideas or focusing exclusively on scientific findings.

Psychobiology is valuable as an approach to the aetiology of the individual patient rather than as a method of discovering general causes of mental disorder. For the latter purpose it is too general and does not lead to testable hypotheses.

Meyer's approach was influential for a time in the USA, where he was director of the Phipps Clinic at Johns Hopkins University Medical School for 32 years until his retirement in 1942. His ideas had a more lasting impact in Great Britain, where they were disseminated through the teaching of three of his pupils, Sir Aubrey Lewis, Sir David Henderson, and Desmond Curran (Gelder 1991). These three psychiatrists promulgated his ideas after the Second World War, at a time when American psychiatry was increasingly influenced by psychoanalytical teaching. Meyer's approach remains the basis of the evaluation of aetiology for the *individual patient*.

The historical development of ideas of aetiology

From the earliest times, theories of the causation of mental disorder have recognized both *somatic* and *psychological influences*. Greek medical literature referred to the causes of mental disorders, mainly in the Hippocratic writings (fourth century BC). Serious mental illness was ascribed mainly to physical causes, which were represented in the theory that health depended on a correct balance of the four body 'humours' (blood, phlegm, yellow bile, and black bile). Melancholia was ascribed to an excess of black bile. Most of the less severe psychiatric disorders were thought to have supernatural causes and to require religious healing. An exception was hysteria, which was thought to be physically caused by the displacement of the uterus from its normal position. Nowadays hysteria is attributed mainly to psychological causes.

Roman physicians generally accepted the causal theories of Greek medicine and developed them in some respects. Galen accepted that melancholia was caused by an excess of black bile, but suggested that this excess could result either from cooling of the blood or from overheating of yellow bile. Phrenitis, the name given to an acute febrile condition with delirium, was thought to result from an excess of yellow bile.

Throughout the Middle Ages these early ideas about the causes of mental illness were largely neglected, though maintained by some scholars such as Bartholomeus Anglicus. The causes of mental illness were now formulated in theological terms of sin and evil, with the consequence that many mentally ill people were persecuted as witches. It was not until the middle of the sixteenth century that beliefs in the supernatural and witchcraft were strongly rejected as causes of mental disorder, notably by the Flemish writer Johan Weyer (1515–1588) in his book *De praestigiis demonum*, published in 1563. Earlier, Paracelsus (1491–1541), the renowned physician, had emphasized the natural causes of mental illness.

In the seventeenth and eighteenth centuries, a more scientific approach to the causation of mental illness developed as physicians became interested in mental disorders, mainly hysteria and melancholia. The English physician Thomas Willis attributed melancholia to 'passions of the heart', but considered that madness (illness with thought disorder, delusions, and hallucinations) as due to a 'fault of the brain'. Willis realized that this fault was not a recognizable gross structural lesion, but a functional abnormality. In the terminology of the time, he referred to a disorder of the 'vital spirits' that were thought to account for nervous action. Willis also pointed out that hysteria could not be caused by a displacement of the womb because the organ is firmly secured in the pelvis.

Another seventeenth century English physician, Thomas Sydenham, rejected the alternative theory that hysteria was caused by a functional disorder of the womb ('uterine suffocation') because he had observed it in men. Despite this renewed medical interest in the causes of mental disorder, the most influential seventeenth century treatise was written by a clergyman, Robert Burton. This work, *The anatomy of melancholy* (1621), described in detail the psychological and social causes (such as poverty, fear, and solitude) that were associated with melancholia and seemed to cause it.

Aetiology depends on *nosology*. Unless it is clear how the various types of mental disorder relate to one another, little progress can be made in understanding causation. From his observations of patients with psychiatric disorders, the Italian physician, Morgagni, became convinced that there was not one single kind of madness but many (Morgagni 1769). Further attempts at classification followed. One of the best known was proposed by William Cullen, who included a category of neurosis for disorders not caused by localized disease of the nervous system.

The idea that individual mental disorders are caused by lesions of particular brain areas can be traced back to the theory of phrenology proposed by Gall (1758–1828) and his pupil Spurzheim (1776–1832). Gall proposed that the brain was the organ of the mind, that the mind was made up of specific faculties, and that these faculties originated in specific brain areas. He also proposed that the size of a brain area determined the strength of the faculty that resided in it, and that the size of brain areas was reflected in the contours of the overlying skull. Hence the shape of the head reflected a person's psychological make-up. Although the last steps in Gall's argument were false, the ideas of cerebral localization were to develop further. An increased interest in brain pathology led to theories that different forms of mental disorder were associated with lesions in different parts of the brain.

It had long been observed that serious mental illness ran in families, but in the nineteenth century this idea took a new form. In 1809, Morel, a French psychiatrist, put forward ideas that became known as the 'theory of degeneration'. He proposed not only that some mental illnesses were inherited, but also that environmental influences (such as poor living conditions and the misuse of alcohol) could lead to physical changes that could be transmitted to the next generation. Morel also proposed that, as a result of the successive effect of environmental agents in each generation, illnesses appeared in increasingly severe forms in successive generations. It was inherent in these ideas that mental disorders did not differ in kind but only in *severity* – neuroses, psychoses, and mental handicap were increasingly severe manifestations of the same inherited process.

These ideas were consistent with the accepted theories of the inheritance of acquired characteristics, and they were accepted widely. They had the unfortunate effect of encouraging a pessimistic approach to treatment. They also supported the Eugenics Movement, which held that the mentally ill should be removed from society in order to prevent them from reproducing. These developments are an important reminder that *aetiological theories may determine undesirable attitudes to the care of patients*.

Mid-nineteenth century views of the causation of mental illness can be judged from the widely acclaimed textbooks of Esquirol, a French psychiatrist, and of Griesinger, a German psychiatrist. Esquirol (1845) focused on the causes of illness in the individual patient and was less concerned with general theories of aetiology. He recorded psychological and physical factors, which he believed to be significant in individual cases, and he distinguished between predisposing and precipitating causes. He regarded heredity as the most important of the predisposing causes, but he also stressed that predisposition was acted on by psychological causes and by social (at that time called 'moral') causes such as domestic troubles, 'disappointed love', and reverses of fortune. Important physical causes of mental disorder included epilepsy, alcohol misuse, excessive masturbation, childbirth and lactation,

and suppression of menstruation. Esquirol also observed that age influenced the type of illness; thus dementia was not observed among the young, but mania was uncommon in old age. He recognized that personality was often a predisposing factor.

In 'Pathology and therapy of mental disorders', which was first published in 1845, Wilhelm Griesinger maintained that mental illness was a *physical disorder of the brain*, and he considered at length the neuropathology of mental illness. He paid equal attention to other causes, including heredity, habitual drunkenness, 'domestic unquiet', disappointed love, and childbirth. He emphasized the multiplicity of causes when he wrote:

A closer examination of the aetiology of insanity soon shows that in the great majority of cases it was not a single specific cause under the influence of which the disease was finally established but a complication of several, sometimes numerous causes, both predisposing and exciting. Very often the germs of the disease are laid in those early periods of life from which the commencement of the formation of character dates. It grows by education and external influences. . . . (Griesinger 1867, p. 130)

British views on aetiology in the late nineteenth century can be judged from *A manual of psychological medicine* by Bucknill and Tuke (1858), and from *The pathology of mind* by Henry Maudsley (1879). Maudsley described the causes of mental disorder in terms similar to those of Griesinger; thus causes were multiple, whilst *predisposing causes* (including heredity and early upbringing) were as important as the more *obvious proximal causes*. Maudsley held that mistakes in determining causes were often due to

some single prominent event, which was perhaps one in a chain of events, being selected as fitted by itself to explain the catastrophe. The truth is that in the great majority of cases there has been a concurrence of steadily operating conditions within and without, not a single effective cause. (Maudsley 1879, p. 83)

Although these nineteenth-century writers and teachers of psychiatry emphasized the *multiplicity of causes*, many practitioners focused narrowly on the findings of genetic and pathological investigations, and adopted a pessimistic approach to treatment. Meyer's concept of 'psychobiology' (see above) was a reaction to these attitudes.

The nineteenth-century aetiological theories considered so far were mainly concerned with the major mental illnesses. Less severe disorders, particularly those that came to be called neurosis, hysteria, and hypochondriasis, and milder states of depression, were treated mainly by physicians. Pierre Charcot, a French neurologist, carried out extensive studies of patients with hysteria and of their response to hypnosis. He believed that hysteria resulted from a functional disorder of the brain and could be treated by hypnosis. In the USA, Weir Mitchell proposed that conditions akin to mild chronic depression were due to exhaustion of the nervous system – a condition he called *neurasthenia*.

In Austria another neurologist, Sigmund Freud, tried to develop a more comprehensive explanation of nervous diseases, first of hysteria and then of other conditions. After an initial interest in physiological causes, Freud proposed that the causes were psychological, but hidden from the patient because they were in the unconscious part of the mind. Freud took a developmental approach to aetiology, believing that the seeds of adult disorder lay in the process of child development (see below). In France, Pierre Janet developed an alternative psychological explanation which was based on variations in the strength of nervous activity and on narrowing of the field of consciousness.

Interest in psychological explanations of the whole range of mental disorders grew as neuropathological and genetic studies failed to yield new insights. Freud and his followers attempted to extend their theory of the neuroses to explain the psychoses. Although the psychological theory was elaborated, no new objective data were obtained about the causes of severe mental illness. Nevertheless, the theories provided explanations which some psychiatrists found more acceptable than an admission of ignorance. Psychoanalysis became

increasingly influential, particularly in American psychiatry where it predominated until the 1970s. Renewed interest in genetic, biochemical, and neuropathological causes of mental disorder followed – an approach that became known as *biological psychiatry* (Guze 1989).

From the history of ideas on the causation of mental disorder the most important lesson is that each generation bases its theories of aetiology on the scientific approaches most active and plausible at the time. Sometimes psychological ideas prevail, sometimes neuropathological, and sometimes genetic. Throughout the centuries, however, observant clinicians have been aware of the *complexity of the causes of psychiatric disorders*, and have recognized that neither aetiology nor treatment should focus narrowly on the scientific ideas of the day. Instead, the approach should be broader, encompassing whatever psychological, social, and biological factors seem most important in the individual case. Modern psychiatrists are working at a time of rapid development of the neurosciences, and they need to keep the same broad clinical perspective of aetiology whilst assimilating any real scientific advances.

Psychoanalysis

In psychoanalysis the method of investigation differs from the scientific methods reviewed later in this chapter in that it was developed specifically for the study of psychiatric disorders. It arose from clinical experience and not from work in the basic sciences. Psychoanalysis is characterized by a particularly elaborate and comprehensive theory of both normal and abnormal mental functioning. Compared with experimental psychology, it is much more concerned with the *irrational* parts of mental activity. Psychoanalytic theory provides a comprehensive range of explanations for clinical phenomena, and therefore has a wide appeal. However, the features that make it all-embracing also make it difficult to test in a scientific way.

Freud originated psychoanalytical theory, but many other workers contributed to it or developed alternative theories. This section refers only to

Freud's theory and not to the other theories, some of which are mentioned elsewhere in the book. This section focuses on the basic ideas of psychoanalysis; hypotheses about particular syndromes are discussed in other chapters.

Psychoanalytic theories are mainly derived from data obtained in the course of psychoanalytical treatment. These data relate to the patient's thoughts, fantasies, and dreams, together with his memories of childhood experiences. By adopting a passive role, Freud tried to ensure that the material consisted of the patient's free associations and not of Freud's own preconceptions.

However, Freud also made interpretations of the patient's reports, and in some of Freud's writings it is difficult to distinguish clearly between the patient's statements and Freud's interpretations. It is recommended that the reader consult some of Freud's original writings, for example, the Introductory Lectures on Psychoanalysis or the New Introductory Lectures, and the papers listed in the references as Freud (1924a, 1924b). In this way Freud's method of working can be understood better. It is also valuable to study a critical evaluation of psychoanalytic theory (for example, the account by Farrell 1981).

Farrell (1981) pointed out that psychoanalysis is an example of a broad theory of a kind found in other branches of knowledge. Such theories can be useful in science by providing a framework within which other ideas can be developed. These theories should not be judged solely on their ability to generate testable hypotheses; however, to be useful, such theories must be able to incorporate new observations as they arise. Darwin's theory of evolution is an example of a useful theory; it survives because it has proved compatible with later observations from genetics and from the fossil record. Freud envisaged that his ideas would one day be explained on the basis of brain mechanisms but until recently the brain sciences have lacked the necessary conceptual and technical power. It is, however, now possible to begin to understand and test the neurobiological basis of some important psychoanalytic concepts (see below).

As pointed out earlier in this chapter, an important distinction between understanding and explanation can be made in psychiatry. In the sense of this distinction, psychoanalysis is a highly elaborate form of understanding that seeks to make both normal mental processes and psychiatric disorders more intelligible. Psychoanalysis does not lead to explanatory hypotheses that can be tested experimentally, although attempts have been made to test some of the simpler hypotheses. The value of psychological understanding has been discussed earlier, and is repeated here before psychoanalytic ideas are reviewed. These ideas can deepen our understanding of patients, but they are not the only way of doing so.

At this point a summary of the main features of Freud's theory will be presented. It is too short to do full justice to Freud's ideas, but it is long in relation to the space devoted to some other methods of scientific enquiry later in this chapter.

The structure of the healthy mind

Many of the ideas in the theory were current before Freud began his psychological studies, for example, the idea of an *unconscious part of the mind*. However, Freud developed and combined these ideas in an ingenious way. A central feature was his elaborate concept of the unconscious mind. He supposed that all mental processes originated there. Some of these processes were allowed to enter the conscious mind freely (for example, sensations), some not at all (the unconscious proper), and some occasionally (most memories, which made up the 'preconscious'). According to Freud, the unconscious mind had three characteristics that were important in the genesis of neurosis:

- it was divorced from reality;
- it was dynamic in that it contained powerful forces;
- it was in conflict with the conscious mind.

These three characteristics will be discussed in turn.

The *unconscious mind* was held to be divorced from reality in several ways. It contained flagrant contradictions and paradoxes, and it tended to tele-scope situations and fantasies that were widely sep-arated in time. In Freud's view, these features were well illustrated by dream analysis. Freud believed that the manifest content of a dream (what the dreamer remembered) could be traced back through analysis to a 'latent' content, which was an infantile wish. The sleeper was thought to perform 'dream work' to translate the latent to the manifest content. This translation was effected by a series of mechan-isms, such as condensation (several images fused into one), displacement (of feelings from an essen-tial feature to non-essential features of an object), and secondary elaboration (rearrangement of the assembled elements). Freud attached importance to this dream theory because he supposed the compo-sition of neurotic symptoms to be like that of dreams, though with greater secondary elaboration.

Second, the unconscious mind was *dynamic*, i.e. it contained impulses that were kept in equilibrium by a series of checks and balances. In Freud's early writings, these impulses were regarded as entirely sexual. Later, he placed more emphasis on aggres-sive impulses. Sexual impulses were supposed to be active even in infancy, receding by about the age of 4 years and then remaining latent until re-emer-gence at puberty. In Freud's view, psychosexual development not only began early, but was long and complicated. The first stage of organization was oral, i.e. the sexual drive was activated by stim-ulation of the mouth by sucking and touching with the lips. The second stage was anal, i.e. the drive was activated by expelling or retaining faeces. Only in the third stage did the genital organs become the primary source of sexual energy. Sometimes these stages were not passed through smoothly. The libido (the energy of the sexual instincts) could become fixated (partially arrested) at one of the early stages. When this happened, the person would engage in infantile patterns of behaviour or regress to such patterns under stress. In this way the point of fixation determined the nature of any neurosis that developed later in life.

As libido developed, not only was it activated in these three successive ways, but its object was

supposed to change. Self-love came first, to be followed in both boys and girls by love of the mother. Next, still in infancy, boys focused their sexual wishes more intensely upon the mother while developing hostile feelings towards the father (the Oedipus complex). Girls developed the reverse attachments. These attachments came to an end through repression of sexual impulses. As a result, the capacity to feel shame and disgust devel-oped, and the child passed into the latency period. Finally, the sexual impulses emerged again at puberty and were directed into relationships with other adults.

The third aspect of the unconscious mind was its *struggle against the conscious mind*. This conflict was regarded as giving rise to anxiety that could persist throughout life and generate neurotic symptoms. One of Freud's lasting contributions was his idea that anxiety could be reduced by a variety of defence mechanisms, which could be discerned at times in the behaviour of healthy people. These mechanisms are considered on pp. 188–90.

Applications to psychiatric disorder

The application of psychoanalytic theory to psychi-atric aetiology can be illustrated by summarizing the development of Freud's ideas about the aeti-ology of neurosis (for a longer account see Freud 1935). These ideas originated in Freud's work with Breuer on the causes of hysteria. This work led Freud to conclude that hysteria was caused by a disorder of sexual function.

Initially, writing in 1895, Freud (1895a, 1895b) postulated two kinds of disturbance that caused separate kinds of neurosis. First, he suggested that suppression of sexual function had direct toxic effects that caused anxiety neurosis and neuras-thenia. He referred to these conditions as 'aktuell', a term that means 'contemporary' and refers to their direct and current causes. Suppressed sexual function was thought to have other indirect psychological effects, including the causation of hysteria, anxiety hysteria (agoraphobia), and obses-sional neurosis. Before long, the idea of aktuell neurosis was abandoned, and instead all neuroses were thought to be psychologically caused by suppressed memories of disturbing sexual events.

Freud had difficulty in eliciting the supposed suppressed memories, and this problem led him to postulate an active process keeping the memories from consciousness. He named this process 'repression'. He developed a method of overcoming repression that reportedly led to revelations by the patient of childhood sexual trauma. Freud later concluded that some of these accounts were not true memories but fantasies. Nevertheless, he maintained that these fantasies were important in aetiology. Thus he wrote, 'neurotic symptoms were not related directly to actual events but to phantasies embodying wishes and psychical reality was of more importance than material reality' (Freud 1935, p. 61).

In general, there are three components in all later versions of Freud's theory of the aetiology of the neuroses. First, it is proposed that *anxiety* is the central symptom of all neuroses; other symptoms arise secondarily through mechanisms of defence (see p. 188–90) which act to reduce this anxiety. Second, anxiety arises when the *ego* fails to deal on the one hand with the mental energy reaching it from the *id,* and on the other hand with the demands of the *superego*. Third, the predisposition to develop neurosis in adult life originates in childhood from a failure to pass normally through one or other of three postulated stages of development – oral, anal, and genital.

Psychoanalysis and psychiatry

Freud's ideas have been of considerable influence in psychiatry and his proposal that developmental processes play an important role in the aetiology of adult psychopathology is widely accepted. However, many of the details of Freud's theories, for example, the importance of unconscious homosexuality in the causation of paranoid states (see p. 383) have been not been found helpful, either as an aetiological explanation of clinical syndromes or as a guide to practice. The question for the future is whether or not psychoanalysis will develop as a scientific discipline. As noted above, it is now possible to explore the brain mechanisms that may underlie some psychoanalytical concepts. This area has been reviewed recently by Kandel (1999) and Gabbard (2000). Kandel (1999) outlined a number of points of convergence:

- The importance of infant attachment to a caregiver for development has been consistently supported by animal experimental and human studies. Disruptions of attachment result in irreversible changes in HPA axis function and impaired physiological and behavioural adaptation to stress in adult life.

- The delineation of a procedural (implicit, unconscious) memory system working together with a declarative (explicit, conscious) memory system has important implications for the way in which traumatic experiences can influence behaviour through non-conscious mechanisms.

- The prefrontal cortex has the task of selecting preconscious material from explicit memory stores and holding it in working memory for conscious evaluation, planning, and action. The prefrontal cortex therefore can be regarded as the brain region that coordinates the activities associated with the 'executive function' of the ego.

The contribution of scientific disciplines to psychiatric aetiology

The main groups of disciplines that have contributed to the knowledge of psychiatric aetiology are shown in Table 5.1. In this section each group is discussed in turn, and the following questions are asked:

- What sort of problem in psychiatric aetiology can be answered by each discipline?

- How, in general, does each discipline attempt to answer the questions?

- Are any particular difficulties encountered in applying its methods to psychiatric disorders?

Table 5.1 Scientific disciplines contributing to psychiatric aetiology
Clinical descriptive studies
Epidemiology
Social sciences
Experimental and clinical psychology
Genetics
Biochemical studies
Pharmacology
Endocrinology
Physiology
Neuropathology

Clinical descriptive studies

Before reviewing more elaborate scientific approaches to aetiology, attention is drawn to the continuing value of simple *clinical investigations*. Psychiatry was built on such studies. For example, the view that schizophrenia and the mood disorders are likely to have separate causes depends ultimately on the careful descriptive studies and follow-up enquiries carried out by earlier generations of psychiatrists.

Only two examples can be given here of the many clinical investigations that have contributed in important ways to knowledge. Both are from the British literature, but similar examples could have been chosen from the literature of continental Europe or America.

Anyone who doubts the value of clinical descriptive studies should read the paper by Aubrey Lewis on 'melancholia' (Lewis 1934). The paper describes a detailed investigation of the symptoms and signs of 61 cases of severe depressive disorder. It provided the most complete account in the English language and it remains unsurpassed. It is an invaluable source of information about the clinical features of depressive disorders untreated by modern methods. Lewis's careful observations drew attention to unsolved problems, including the nature of retardation, the relation of depersonalization to affective changes, the presence of manic symptoms, and the validity of the classification of depressive disorders into reactive and endogenous groups. None of these problems has yet been solved completely, but the analysis by Lewis was important in focusing attention on them.

A second classic example is a clinical follow-up study by Roth (1955). Elderly psychiatric patients were classified on the basis of their symptoms into five diagnostic groups: affective (mood) disorder, late paraphrenia, acute or subacute delirious states, senile dementia, and arteriosclerotic dementia. These groups were found to differ in their course. Two years later, about two-thirds of the patients with affective psychoses had recovered, about four-fifths of those with senile dementia and almost as many with arteriosclerotic dementia had died, over half the patients with paraphrenia were alive but still in hospital, and of those with acute confusional states, half had recovered and half had died. These findings confirmed the value of the original diagnoses, and refuted the earlier belief that affective and paranoid disorders in old age were part of a single degenerative disorder that could also present as dementia. This investigation clearly illustrates how careful clinical follow-up can clarify issues of aetiology.

Although many opportunities for this kind of research have been taken already, it does not follow that clinical investigation is no longer worthwhile. For example, the study of Judd *et al.* (1998) described in Chapter 6 (p. 154) is a recent example of how a clinical follow-up study can provide important insight into the aetiology of milder depressive disorders in relation to major depression. Well-conducted clinical enquiries are likely to retain an important place in psychiatric research for many years to come.

Epidemiology

Epidemiology is the study of the distribution of a disease in space and time within a population, and of the factors that influence this distribution. Its concern is with disease in groups of people, not in the individual person.

Aims of epidemiological enquiries

In psychiatry, *epidemiology* attempts to answer three main kinds of question:

- What is the prevalence of psychiatric disorder in a given population at risk?
- What are the clinical and social correlates of psychiatric disorder?
- What factors may be important in aetiology?

Prevalence can be estimated in community samples or among people attending general practitioners or hospital cases. Studies of prevalence in different locations, social groups, or social classes can contribute to aetiology. Studies of associations between a disorder and personal and social variables can do the same and may be useful for clinical practice; for example, epidemiological studies have shown that the risk of suicide is increased in elderly males with certain characteristics, such as living alone, misusing drugs or alcohol, suffering from physical or mental illness, and having a family history of suicide.

Epidemiological studies of aetiology have been concerned with *predisposing and precipitating* factors, and with the social correlates of mental illness. Amongst *predisposing factors*, the influence of *heredity* has been examined in studies of families, twins, and adopted people, as described in the later section on genetics. Other examples are the influence of maternal age on the risk of Down's syndrome, the psychological development of premature babies in later life, and the psychological effects of parental loss during childhood. Studies of *precipitating factors* include life-events research, which is described in the following section on the social sciences.

There have been numerous studies of the social correlates of psychiatric disorder. For example, in an influential study, Hollingshead and Redlich (1958) in the USA found that schizophrenia was 11 times more frequent in social class V than in social class I. In itself, this finding throws no light on aetiology, but it suggests studies of other factors associated with social class (for example, poor housing). It also raises questions about the interpretation of associations. For example, do people with schizophrenia drift into the lower social classes when they become disabled, or were they in the lower social classes before the disorder began?

Concepts and methods of epidemiology

The basic concept of epidemiology is that of *rate*, or the ratio of the number of instances to the numbers of people in a defined population. Instances can be episodes of illness, or people who are or have been ill. Rates may be computed on a particular occasion (*point prevalence*) or over a defined interval (*period prevalence*).

Other concepts include *inception rate*, which is based on the number of people who were healthy at the beginning of a defined period but became ill during it, and *lifetime expectation or risk*, which is based on an estimate of the number of people who could be expected to develop a particular illness in the course of their whole life. In *cohort studies*, a group of people are followed for a defined period of time to determine the onset or change in some characteristic with or without previous exposure to a potentially important agent (for example, lung cancer and smoking).

Three aspects of method are particularly important in epidemiology:

- defining the population at risk;
- defining a case;
- finding cases.

It is essential to define the *population at risk* accurately. Such a population can be all the people living in a limited area (for example, a country, an island, or a catchment area), or a subgroup chosen by age, gender, or some other potentially important defining characteristic.

Defining a case is the central problem of psychiatric epidemiology. It is relatively easy to define a condition such as Down's syndrome, but until recently the reliability of psychiatric diagnosis has not been satisfactory. The development of standardized techniques for defining, identifying, rating, and classifying mental disorders (see p. 63–9) has greatly improved the reliability and validity of epidemiological studies.

Two methods are used for *case finding*. The first is to enumerate all cases known to medical or other agencies (*declared cases*). Hospital admission rates may give a fair indication of rates of major mental illnesses, but not, for example, of most mood or anxiety disorders. Moreover, hospital admission rates are influenced by many variables, such as the geographical accessibility of hospitals, attitudes of doctors, admission policies, and the law relating to compulsory admissions.

The second method is to search for both *declared and undeclared cases in the community*. In community surveys, the best technique is often to use two stages: preliminary screening to detect potential cases with a self-rated questionnaire such as the General Health Questionnaire (Goldberg 1972), followed by detailed clinical examination of potential cases with a standardized psychiatric interview.

Causes in the environment

Epidemiological approaches to aetiology can be illustrated by the results of studies of environmental causes of mental disorders. It is commonly supposed that *poor living conditions* can predispose to mental disorder, either directly or through their effects on family life. If this supposition is correct, people who move from poor to better housing should experience fewer disorders. Two well-known studies examined this possibility. Taylor

and Chave (1964) investigated people moving from poor urban conditions to a new town; Hare and Shaw (1965) studied people moving from an old to a new housing estate in the same town. In neither investigation was the rate of mental disorder reduced after the move.

A possible explanation is that the beneficial effect of better housing was cancelled by the adverse effect of greater social isolation in new surroundings. (The epidemiological relationship between mental health and indices of social deprivation including housing is considered by Kendrick 1999.)

It has been suggested that some kinds of *working conditions* cause mental disorder. This possibility was studied extensively during the Second World War, when it was concluded that work requiring constant attention but little initiative or responsibility (such as repetitive machine work) can cause mental disorder. More recent studies have focused on the role of *work stress*. Studies have confirmed a relationship between stressful working conditions and psychological symptomatology in many working groups including doctors in training and general practitioners (see, for example, Appleton *et al.* 1998).

Social sciences

Many of the concepts used by sociologists are relevant to psychiatry (see Table 5.2). Unfortunately, some of these potentially fruitful ideas have been used uncritically, for example, in the suggestion that mental illness is no more than a label for

Table 5.2 Some applications of social theory to psychiatry	
Concept	**Application**
Social class and subculture	Epidemiology of substance misuse
Stigma and labelling	Analysis of handicaps of seriously mentally ill in community
Institutionalization	Negative behavioural effects of institutions
Social deviance	Delinquent behaviour
Abnormal illness behaviour	Psychological consequences of physical illness

socially deviant people, the 'myth of mental illness'. This development points to the obvious need for sociological theories to be tested in the same way as other theories by collecting appropriate data.

Some of the concepts of sociology overlap with those of social psychology, for example, attribution theory (which deals with the way in which people interpret the causes of events in their lives, and ideas about self-esteem). An important part of research in sociology, the study of life events, uses epidemiological methods (see below).

Transcultural studies

Studies in different societies help in making an important causal distinction. Biologically determined features of mental disorder are likely to be similar in different cultures, whilst psychologically and socially determined features are likely to be dissimilar. Thus the 'core' symptoms of schizophrenia have a similar incidence in people from widely different societies, suggesting that a common neurobiological abnormality is likely to be important in aetiology (see Chapter 12).

By contrast, depressive disorders often present differently in different cultures. For example, Kim *et al.* (1999) found that depression in Chinese was more likely to manifest a somatic presentation relative to Koreans who experienced more psychological symptomatology.

The study of life events

Epidemiological methods have been used in social studies to examine associations between *illness and certain kinds of events in a person's life*. In an early study, Wolff (1962) studied the morbidity of several hundred people over many years and found that episodes of illness clustered at times of change in the person's life. Holmes and Rahe (1967) attempted to improve on the highly subjective measures used by Wolff. They used a list of 41 kinds of life event (e.g. work, residence, finance, and family relationships) and weighted each according to its apparent severity, for example,

100 for the death of a spouse and 13 for a spell of leave for a serviceman.

As these last two examples show, the changes could be desirable or undesirable, and within or outside the person's direct control. In latter developments the study of the psychological impact of life events has been approached in a number of ways:

- to reduce memory distortion, limits are set to the period over which events are to be recalled;
- efforts are made to date the onset of the illness accurately;
- attempts are made to exclude events that are not clearly independent of the illness, for example, losing a job because of poor performance;
- events are characterized in terms of their nature (for example, losses or threats) as well as their severity;
- data are collected with a semi-structured interview and rated reliably.

Although significant, life events taken in isolation may be less important than at first appears. For example, in one study (Paykel *et al.* 1969), events involving the loss or departure of a person from the immediate social field of the respondent ('exit events') were reported in 25% of patients with depressive disorders but in only 5% of controls. This difference was significant at the 1% level and appears impressive, but Paykel (1978) has questioned its real significance and carried out the following calculation.

The incidence of depressive disorder is not accurately known, but if it is taken to be 2% for new cases over a 6-month period, then a hypothetical population of 10 000 people would yield 200 new cases. Paykel's study showed that exit events occurred to 5% of people who did not become cases of depressive disorder; therefore, in the hypothetical population, exit events would occur to 490 of the 9800 people who were not new cases. Amongst the 200 new cases, exit events would occur to 25%, i.e. 50 people. Thus the total number of people experiencing exit events would be 490 plus

50, or 540, of whom only 50 (less than 1 in 10) would develop depressive disorders. Hence the greater part of the variance in determining depressive disorder must be attributed to something else. That is, life events trigger depression largely in *predisposed individuals*.

In developing this theme, Rutter (1999) has pointed out that acute life events are usually part of long-standing psychosocial difficulties and it is these difficulties that are important in determining the psychological impact of life events on the individual over time. Moreover follow-up studies show that the individual is not a passive recipient of experiences but tends to gravitate towards environments that serve to accentuate previous maladaptive behavioural patterns and carry an increased risk of adverse life events.

Studies of genetic epidemiology have taken this argument a stage further by showing that the tendency to experience adverse life events is partly genetically determined. For example, part of the liability of an individual to 'select' environments which put them at relatively higher risk of experiencing adverse life events is genetically determined. Presumably this is one way in which the genetic vulnerability to depression may be expressed (see Kendler *et al*. 1999). It should be noted that the fact that genetic factors might be involved in individual selection of high-risk environments does not imply that social intervention will not be useful in clinical management. Indeed, helping such individuals find better psychosocial environment can produce significant benefits in mental health (Rutter 1999).

Vulnerability and protective factors

People may differ in their response to life events for three reasons. First, the same event may have different meanings for different people, according to their previous experience. For example, a family separation may be more stressful to an adult who has suffered separation in childhood.

The other reasons are that certain contemporary factors may increase vulnerability to life events or protect against them. Ideas about these last two factors derive largely from the work of Brown and Harris (1978) who have found evidence that, among women, vulnerability factors include having the care of small children and can be decreased by having a confidant who can share problems. The idea of protective factors has been used to explain the observation that some people do not become ill even when exposed to severe adversities – a finding that is particularly evident in studies of the effects of adverse family factors on children (see Rutter 1999).

Causes in the family

It has been suggested that some mental disorders are an expression of emotional disorder within a whole family, not just a disorder in the person seeking treatment (the 'identified patient'). Although family problems are common among people with psychiatric disorder, their general importance in aetiology is almost certainly overstated in this formulation since emotional difficulties in other family members may be the result of the patient's problems rather than its cause. In addition, emotional difficulties in close relatives may result from shared genetic inheritance. For example, the parents of children with schizophrenia have an increased risk of schizotypal personality disorder (see p. 349).

Migration

Moving to another country, or even to an unfamiliar part of the same country, is a life change that has been suggested as a cause of mental disorder. A number of possible mechanisms have been identified:

- *Selective migration* People in the early stages of an illness such as schizophrenia may migrate because of failing relationships in their country of origin (see for example, Mortensen *et al*. 1997).

- *Process of migration* Events around the process of migration itself for example, prolonged waiting periods, exhaustion, and social deprivation and isolation may cause several different kinds of stress-related disorder.

◆ *Post-migration factors* Many factors come into play post-migration which could influence the risk of developing mental illness. These include *social adversity*, caused, for example, by racial discrimination and *acculturation* in which the breakdown of traditional cultural structures results in loss of self-esteem and social support. In addition, immigrants may be exposed to unfamiliar viruses, which could conceivably affect intrauterine development and predispose to psychiatric disorder in the next generation.

While some groups of immigrants experience higher rates of psychiatric disorder (for example, Afro-Carribeans in the UK), others do not and some experience a relative improvement in mental health compared with their native populations. This suggests that there is not a simple relationship between immigration and psychiatric disorder (see Cheng and Chang 1999, for a review).

Experimental and clinical psychology

There are a number of characteristic features of the psychological approach to psychiatric aetiology:

◆ the idea of a *continuity between the normal and abnormal*. This idea leads to investigations that attempt to explain psychiatric abnormalities in terms of processes determining normal behaviour.

◆ concern with the *interaction between the person and his environment*. The psychological approach differs from the social approach in being concerned less with environmental variables and more with the person's ways of processing information coming from the external environment and from his own body.

◆ an emphasis on factors *maintaining abnormal behaviour*. Psychologists are less likely to regard behaviour disorders as resulting from internal disease processes, and more likely to assume that persisting behaviour is maintained, for

example, by anxiety-reducing avoidance strategies.

Neuropsychology

Neuropsychological approaches share common ground with biological psychiatry in attempting to identify the neurobiological substrates for psychological phenomena. Various methodologies are employed but the aim is to understand psychopathology in the context of brain science. Investigations may therefore involve animal experimental work or a range of human studies including neurological patients with defined brain lesions and patients with psychiatric disorders.

For example, animal experimental models have shown that there is a crucial role for the *amygdala* in fear conditioning. Furthermore, because of its connections to the thalamus, the amygdala is activated by threatening stimuli and can produce autonomic fear responses before any conscious awareness of threat. LeDoux (1998) has related this circuitry to traumatic anxiety by proposing an imbalance in the *implicit (unconscious) emotional memory system* involving the thalamus and amygdala and the *explicit (conscious) declarative memory system* in the temporal lobe and hippocampus (see below).

As well as animal experimental studies, neuropsychological investigations also involve different groups of human subjects. Valuable information may be gained from subjects who have suffered *well-defined brain lesions*. For example, Adolphs *et al.* (1994) found that a patient with bilateral *amygdala lesions* could recognize the personal identity of faces but not the facial expression of fear. This supports the notion that the amygdala is important in the processing of fear-related stimuli.

Current neuropsychological approaches also make extensive use of *brain imaging techniques*. This allows localization of the brain regions and circuits involved in specific psychological processes and facilitates comparisons with patients who experience abnormalities in the processes concerned. For example, in a magnetic resonance imaging investigation it was found that when patients with schizophrenia listened to externally generated speech, the presence of *auditory hallucinations* was linked to reduced activity of the temporal regions that normally process external speech. This may represent competition by the hallucinations and external speech for a common neural substrate (see David and Busatto 1999).

Information processing

The *information theory approach* to psychology proposes that the brain can be regarded as an information channel, which receives, filters, processes, and stores information from sense organs, and retrieves information from memory stores. This approach, which compares the brain to a computer, suggests useful ways of thinking about some of the abnormalities in psychiatric disorders. There are various mechanisms involved at different stages of information processing and therefore different points at which dysfunctional processing could give rise to psychiatric disorder. Two of these mechanisms are *attention* and *memory*, changes in which have been linked to psychiatric symptomatology.

Attention

Attention is viewed as an active process of selecting, from the mass of sensory input, the elements that are relevant to the processing that is being carried out at the time. One method of limiting incoming information to a manageable level is *latent inhibition*, which excludes information that past experience has shown to be irrelevant to the task in hand. It has been suggested that latent inhibition might be defective in schizophrenia, and this defect could contribute to the disruption of other psychological processes in this condition. However, recent studies have indicated that latent inhibition is preserved in unmedicated patients with schizophrenia but it is altered by antipsychotic drug treatment (Williams *et al*. 1998). This shows the importance of devising studies to test psychological theories and of the relevance of drug treatment as a confounding variable.

It is generally agreed that anxiety states are associated with abnormalities in attention in that patients with anxiety disorders attend selectively to threat stimuli. A key question is whether this effect is a cause or consequence of the anxiety disorder (see van den Hout *et al*. 2000).

Memory

The *information-processing model* has been applied fruitfully to the study of memory. It suggests that there are different kinds of memory store: sensory stores in which sensory information is held for short periods while awaiting further processing, a short-term store in which information is held for only 20 seconds unless it is continually rehearsed, and a long-term store in which information is retained for long periods. There is a mechanism for retrieving information from this long-term store when required, and this mechanism could break down while memory traces are intact. This model has led to useful experiments. For example, patients with the amnestic syndrome (see p. 412) score better on memory tests requiring recognition of previously encountered material than on tasks requiring unprompted recall; this finding suggests a breakdown of information retrieval rather than of information storage.

It is well established that low mood facilitates recall of unhappy events. This can be demonstrated in healthy subjects undergoing a negative mood induction as well as depressed patients. Once again it is not clear whether in depressed patients this phenomenon is a manifestation of depressed mood. However, it is possible that it could play a role in maintaining the depressive state (Teasdale 1983). More recent research has focused on the tendency of depressed patients to produce general rather than specific autobiographical memories. Williams (1992) has suggested that a memory problem of this kind might make problem solving difficult and thereby perpetuate the depressed state.

As noted above, there is increasing interest in how *explicit declarative* and *implicit emotional* memories might be involved in the processing of traumatic events. It has been suggested that during highly traumatic experiences explicit memory of the event is relatively poor while implicit (unconscious emotional memory) is vivid. This could give rise to the automatic intrusions and poor explicit memory seen in post-traumatic stress disorder (see van den Hout *et al.* 2000).

Beliefs and expectations

The information processing model also predicts that responses to information, including the emotional response, are determined by *beliefs and expectations*. This idea proposes that behaviour of all individuals is guided by their beliefs and that psychopathology is associated with altered *content of beliefs* about the self and the world. Cognitive psychology assumes that such beliefs are organized into *schemas*. Schemas have important properties in relation to different kinds of psychopathology:

- they influence information processing, conscious thinking, emotion, and behaviour;

- though not necessarily accessible to direct introspection, their content can usually be reconstructed in verbal terms (known as *assumptions or beliefs*);

- in patients with psychiatric disorders, these beliefs are dysfunctional, resistant to refutation, and play a part in the aetiology and maintenance of the disorder.

These ideas have been used in the development of *cognitive therapy* where researchers aim to identify the dysfunctional beliefs associated with particular disorders and apply techniques which help the patient re-evaluate and change them. For example, experimental work has shown that patients with panic disorder (p. 237) have inaccurate expectations that sensory information about rapid heart action predicts an imminent heart attack. This expectation results in anxiety when the information is received, with the result that the heart rate accelerates further and a vicious circle of mounting anxiety is set up. Changing these expectations can alleviate panic attacks (see also p. 246). (For a review of how experimental psychology can inform studies of psychiatric aetiology, see van den Houte *et al.* 2000).

Ethology and evolutionary psychology

Many psychological studies involve quantitative observations of behaviour. In some of these investigations use is made of methods developed originally in the related discipline of ethology. Complex behaviour is divided into simpler components and counted systematically. Regular sequences are noted as well as interactions between individuals, for example, between a mother and her infant. Such methods have been used, for example, to study the effects of separating infant primates from their mothers, and to compare this primate behaviour with that of human infants separated in the same way.

More recent applications of ethology have used insights from the field of *evolutionary psychology* to understand both normal and abnormal behaviour in an evolutionary context. This approach attempts to explain why various behaviours might have arisen in terms of evolutionary *adaptation*.

For example, because depressive states are ubiquitous in human societies, it is reasonable to ask what their adaptive value may be. One suggestion is that depression may reflect a form of subordination in animals who have lost rank in a social hierarchy. Rather than fighting a losing battle, the depressed individual withdraws and conserves emotional resources for another day (see Williams 1998).

Such ideas are not readily testable experimentally but can give rise to hypotheses concerning possible brain mechanisms. One theoretical difficulty is that psychiatric disorders often appear to represent *maladaptive* rather than adaptive behaviours. Wolpert (1999), for example, has drawn an analogy with cancer in which the consequences of abnormal cell growth are clearly maladaptive and injurious to the individual. As cancer can be regarded as normal cell division 'gone wrong', so depression might be normal emotion 'gone wrong'. From this viewpoint the question is not what is the adaptive value of the abnormal behaviour but rather the adaptive value of the normal behaviour to which the abnormal state is related.

Genetics

Genetic investigations are concerned with three issues:

- the relative contributions of genetic and environmental factors to aetiology;
- the mode of inheritance of disorders that have a hereditary basis;
- identification of relevant genes and their mutations and polymorphisms.

In psychiatry, important advances have been made with the first issue, but so far little progress has been made with the other two. Methods in genetics are of three broad kinds: *population and family studies (genetic epidemiology), cytogenetics*, and *molecular genetics*. Population and family studies are mainly concerned with estimating the contribution of genetic factors and the mode of inheritance, whilst cytogenetics and molecular genetics provide information about mechanisms of inheritance. To date, genetic research in psychiatry has relied mainly on methods of population genetics. For reviews of the topics in this section, see Henderson and Blackwood (1999) and Owen *et al.* (2000).

Extent of genetic contribution

Methods of population genetics (*genetic epidemiology*) are used to assess risk in three groups of people: families, twins, and people who have been adopted. In *family risk studies*, the investigator determines the risk of a psychiatric condition among the relatives of affected persons and compares it with the expected risk in the general population. (The affected persons are usually referred to as *index cases* or *probands*.) Such studies require a sample selected in a strictly defined way. Moreover, it is not sufficient to ascertain the current prevalence of a psychiatric condition among the relatives because some of the population may go on to develop the condition later in life. For this reason, investigators use corrected figures known as expectancy rates (or morbid risks). However, caution is needed in interpretation of results from studies of this nature for a number of reasons, as follows.

Family studies

Family risk studies have been used extensively in psychiatry. Examples will be found in the chapters on mood disorders and schizophrenia (see pp. 287 and 348). Since these studies by themselves cannot distinguish between inheritance and the effects of family environment, they are the least satisfactory way of determining the genetic contribution. They are useful chiefly in pointing to the need for other kinds of investigation.

Twin studies

In twin studies the investigator seeks to separate genetic and environmental influences by comparing *concordance rates* in uniovular (monozygous, MZ) and binovular (dizygous, DZ) twins. Such studies depend crucially on the accurate determination of zygosity. If concordance for a psychiatric disorder is substantially higher in MZ twins than in DZ twins, a major genetic component is presumed. More precise estimates of the relative importance of heredity and environment can be made by comparisons of MZ twins reared together and MZ twins reared apart from early infancy. In addition, twin studies allow an estimate of the environmental contribution that is unique to the individual ('non-shared') to be distinguished from the common ('shared') family environment. Examples of twin studies will be found in Chapter 12 on schizophrenia (see p. 349).

Twin studies make a number of assumptions, mainly that when twins are raised together, they *share the same environment* and this degree of environmental sharing is similar between MZ and DZ twins. This may not be true, especially if the concept is broadened to include the prenatal (intrauterine) environment. In addition, MZ pairs may not, in fact, be genetically identical because of factors such as genetic imprinting and mitochondrial inheritance.

Heritability Twin studies allow estimates of *heritability* which is the proportion of the liability to a particular disorder that is accounted for by genetic effects. It should be noted that estimates of

Table 5.3 Heritability estimates for selected psychiatric disorders

Disorder	Heritability estimate (%)
Schizophrenia	80
Bipolar disorder	80
Major depression	40
Generalized anxiety disorder	30
Panic disorder	40
Phobia	35
Alcohol problem or dependence	60

From Owen *et al.* (2000).

heritability are not fixed but apply to particular populations under the environmental conditions prevailing during the study concerned. In addition, they cannot be applied to individual cases (see Rutter and Plomin 1997). Many psychiatric disorders show a high heritability (Table 5.3).

It should be noted that gene and environment effects often *interact* with each other and so their effects are not simply additive. For example, parents with antisocial personality disorder may pass on genes increasing the risk that children will inherit a liability to conduct disorder but may also produce a family environment that itself increases the risk of behavioural disturbance.

Adoption studies

Adoption studies provide another useful method of separating genetic and environmental influences. These studies are concerned with children who, since early infancy, have been reared by non-related adoptive parents. Two main comparisons can be made. First, the frequency of the disorder can be compared between two groups of adopted people: those whose biological parents had the illness, and those whose biological parents did not have it. If there is a genetic cause, the rate will be greater in the former. Second, in the case of adopted people

who have a psychiatric disorder, the frequency of the disorder can be compared between the biological parents and the adoptive parents. If there is a genetic cause, the rate will be greater in the former.

Adoption studies may be affected by a number of biases, such as the reasons why the child was adopted, non-random assignment of the children on socioeconomic status, and the effects on adoptive parents of raising a difficult child. (An example is provided by the studies of schizophrenia reviewed on p. 350.)

Boundaries of the phenotype

The studies of genetic epidemiology described above can lead to clearer identifications of the limits of the *clinical phenotype* associated with inheritance of particular genes. For example, such studies have established that *schizotypal personality* can be inherited as part of a genetic predisposition to schizophrenia (p. 349). Similarly, major depression and generalized anxiety disorder appear to share many of the same genes. These observations have implications for the classification of psychiatric disorders and for establishing phenotypes for molecular genetic and pathophysiological studies.

The mode of inheritance

This is assessed by using special statistical methods to test the fit of pedigree or family data with alternative models of inheritance. Traditionally, four models have been considered: *the single major locus model*, which may be *dominant*, *recessive*, or *sex-linked*, and a *mixed model of major genes operating together*. This approach has been successful in studies of certain dementias such as early-onset Alzheimer's disease and Huntington's chorea. Attempts to study other psychiatric disorders in this way have generally led to equivocal results despite considerable research, particularly on schizophrenia and mood disorder.

The common psychiatric disorders do not show classic Mendelian patterns of inheritance. Moreover, linkage studies using molecular genetic techniques have made it unlikely that genes of major effect are involved in aetiology. It seems likely that common psychiatric disorders involve the combined action of several genes of moderate effect, none of which by themselves is *sufficient* to cause the disorder. In this model there are additive and interactive effects of both genes and environmental influences and the illness will be clinically manifest only when a certain susceptibility threshold is crossed. This kind of mechanism makes it difficult to specify the mode of inheritance of clearly (Gelernter 1999).

Cytogenetic studies

These studies are concerned with identifying structural abnormalities in chromosomes and associating them with disease. The most important example in psychiatry concerns *Down's syndrome*. In this condition two kinds of abnormality have been detected: in the first kind there is an additional chromosome (trisomy); in the second kind the chromosome number is normal but one chromosome is unusually large because a segment of another chromosome is attached to it (translocation) (see p. 881). Other examples involve the X and Y chromosomes. In *Turner's syndrome* there is only one sex chromosome (XO), whereas in three other syndromes there is an extra one – XXY (Klinefelter's syndrome), XXX, and XYY.

Molecular genetics

Goal of molecular genetic studies

The aims of molecular genetic studies are:

- to identify the particular genes implicated in the inheritance of a phenotype, in this case a psychiatric disorder;
- to find out why the gene is functioning abnormally.

Polymorphic variations

An important key to the study of molecular genetics is the presence of variations in DNA sequences between individuals. These are called *polymorphisms or allelic variants*. Many genes show this kind of variation and their identification is

necessary both for *molecular linkage analysis* and for more direct *candidate gene studies*.

Polymorphic variations are caused by *DNA mutation*. There are various kinds of mutation from changes in a single nucleotide (*single nucleotide polymorphism*, or *SNPs*) to insertion or deletions of many base pairs. Not all mutations cause functional consequences because they may occur in noncoding regions of DNA. However, sometimes mutations in non-coding regions can have phenotypic effects because, for example, they affect the efficiency of gene transcription (see Blackwood and Muir 1998).

The usual factor involved in a malfunctioning gene will be a change in its nucleotide sequence. If one is searching for abnormalities related to psychiatric disorder, therefore, it is sensible to identify DNA sequences that show this kind of variation. This is called *mutational analysis*. Mutational analysis usually involves the polymerase chain reaction (PCR) to amplify a DNA region of interest, which might harbour variation in some individuals. Mutations in PCR products are identified by electrophoretic methods that take advantage of the fact of that differences in nucleotide sequence will induce different DNA conformations and thereby different migration patterns on a suitable medium. A number of techniques are currently employed (Box 5.1).

It is worth noting that that the allelic variant of a gene that contributes to the expression of a particular disorder may be common in the healthy population. For example, a large candidate gene association study (see below) showed that a polymorphism in the 5-HT_{2A} receptor gene (T102C), while making a small contribution to the risk of schizophrenia was also present in 80% of the normal population (Williams *et al.* 1996).

Identification of predisposing genes

Classical linkage studies Classical ('Mendelian') linkage studies seek to identify the locus of a gene on the chromosomes by studying the extent to which it *co-segregates with a* 'marker' gene. Genetic markers are readily identifiable characters with known single

---

> ### Box 5.1 Techniques for identifying mutations
>
> - Single-stranded conformational polymorphisms (SSCP). Electrophoresis of single-stranded (denatured) DNA molecules on a gel matrix.
> - Denaturing gradient gel electrophoresis (DGGE). DNA segments are separated by electrophoresis through an acrylamide gel with a denaturing gradient.
> - Short tandem repeats (STRs). Varying repeats of 2–4 base pair units widely dispersed through genome. Electrophoresis identifies alleles of different length.
> - Restriction fragment length polymorphisms (RFLPs). Restriction enzymes of bacterial origin cut DNA at specified points, allowing recognition of polymorphisms. Different polymorphisms identified by electrophoresis on agarose gel.
>
> See Gelernter 1999

modes of inheritance and two or more allelelic variants. They include blood groups, human leucocyte antigens (HLAs), and certain physiological abnormalities (e.g. colour blindness).

Large family pedigrees are studied to determine to what extent two genes 'stick together', departing from Mendel's law of independent assortment. In this way, by using appropriate mathematical techniques, it can be estimated how closely the gene loci are likely to be linked on a chromosome. Many such studies have been carried out with psychiatric disorders, but so far no linkage has been found with a marker of this kind.

Classical linkage studies work best when:

- there is an established mode of inheritance for the disorder;
- there is a single gene of major effect;
- diagnosis is reliable and supported by pathological findings.

Common psychiatric disorders are not of this kind and the value of linkage studies thus far has

been limited (see below). Among disorders of interest to psychiatrists, this method has so far been applied successfully only to Huntington's chorea and certain forms of early-onset Alzheimer's disease.

Molecular genetic linkage studies As noted above, human DNA shows many variations in its base sequences which can be detected by the methods outlined in Box 5.1. These variations are scattered through the human genome and can be used to carry out a *systematic search for genetic linkage* even if knowledge of the pathological process is lacking and the mode of inheritance uncertain. The clinical material required depends on the study design but could include affected and discordant sibling pairs (usually with their biological parents) or large extended multiply-affected pedigrees. Once linkage has been established, the disease gene can be located and its mutation identified. This approach has proved useful in Huntington's chorea where the disease gene and its mutations have been characterized (Ross *et al.* 1993), though the nature of the resulting pathophysiological process is still obscure.

However, linkage analyses in common psychiatric disorders have not yet proved decisive although there are some suggestive findings for schizophrenia and bipolar disorder with a number of different loci being implicated (see Owen *et al.* 2000). The major problem in this work is the lack of replication of positive findings. There are a number of reasons why linkage analysis in common psychiatric disorders may be problematic:

- Linkage studies are more difficult to undertake and may not be feasible when the disorder concerned arises through the interplay of many genes of small effect.
- Inappropriate mathematical models based on Mendelian inheritance may give false positives.
- Common psychiatric conditions may be genetically heterogeneous. In addition, some cases may be phenocopies lacking a significant genetic element. Lumping these cases together

in the same linkage analysis might obscure a gene effect even if one were present.

Quantitative trait loci Many human qualities, such as intelligence or personality traits, are complex phenotypes, that can be regarded as existing on a dimension rather than simply present or absent. Genes contributing to the amount of variation in the trait concerned are called *quantitative trait loci* (QTL). QTL mapping may be particular useful for identifying a personality trait that may predispose to the aetiology of a disorder, for example, neuroticism in the case of depression (see Rutter and Plomin 1997). In addition, where a disorder can be seen as existing on a dimension (rather than being present or absent), QTL mapping may be the correct method to identify relevant genes (Henderson and Blackwood 1999).

Association studies In *association studies* it is necessary to have a *candidate gene*, that is, a gene which could be plausibly involved in aetiology from what is known about the pathophysiology of the disorder. In this approach the frequencies of different alleles for a particular gene are examined in patients and a control population A successful use of this approach involves apolipoprotein E (ApoE), a polymorphic protein found in the plaques associated with Alzheimer's disease. Association studies have shown that individuals with a particular genetic variant of ApoE (the $\epsilon4$ allele) have a high risk of developing late-onset Alzheimer's disease. Possession of one copy of the $\epsilon4$ allele moderately increases the risk of developing Alzheimer's disease (odds ratio 2.2–4.4) whereas possession of two copies increases it further (odds ratio 5.1–17.9). However, the $\epsilon4$ allele is neither necessary nor sufficient to cause the disease (see Owen *et al.* 2000).

The applicability of association studies in psychiatric disorders is limited by the fact that there is little definite information on pathophysiology. We do, however, have some effective drug treatments and, accordingly, genes that code for their target proteins are reasonable candidates. Thus far few replicated findings have emerged. Box 5.2 demon-

---

Box 5.2 Mutations in serotonin transporter gene

Serotonin transporter (5-HTT) gene – single gene on chromosome 17

Polymorphisms

♦ Tandem repeat in exon 2 (no known effect on amino acid coding)

♦ Deletion/insertion polymorphism in transcriptional control region (long and short variant). Population frequency: L = 55%, S = 45%

   (a) Long variant: increased transcriptional efficiency; increased expression of 5-HTT in cell model systems and increased 5-HT uptake

   (b) Short variant: compared to L form, less expression of 5-HTT and decreased 5-HT uptake

Short variant of 5-HTT gene may be more common in mood disorder but results are contradictory

---

strates how this approach has been applied to a polymorphic variant in the serotonin transporter gene. The abundance of single nucleotide polymorphisms (which are usually bi-alleleic) could theoretically be used to perform automated genome wide association studies in the future (Gelernter 1999).

Gene expression in psychiatric disorders

A defective gene may manifest itself at one or more of the points that lead to the synthesis of a particular protein. In general, the end result is either a structurally abnormal protein or a protein product that is present in reduced amounts or is entirely absent. Therefore, to understand the phenotypic presentation of psychiatric disease, it is necessary to study gene expression and protein synthesis in the human brain.

Molecular genetic techniques can be readily adapted for this purpose. Thus cDNA libraries made from neuronal tissue can be used to determine whether the complementary mRNAs are expressed differently in patients with psychiatric disorders and in controls. The technique of *in situ* hybridization employs labelled DNA or RNA probes to hybridize to complementary RNA coding for a particular protein. Using autoradiographic methods it is possible to study gene expression in individual neurons in a quantitative manner. Other techniques used for studying gene expression include reverse transcription-polymerase chain reaction (RT-PCR) and gene expression chip arrays.

Of course, these techniques can be used to study acquired changes in gene expression caused by environmental changes, brain injury, drugs, or hormones. Most information on the nature and localization of a neuronal abnormality is likely to come from studies that combine molecular biology techniques with established neurochemical methods (see Owens and Ritchie 1999).

Biochemical studies

These studies can be directed either to the causes of diseases or to the mechanisms by which disease produces its effects. The methods of biochemical investigation are too numerous to consider here, and it is assumed that the reader has some knowledge of them. The main aim here is to consider some of the problems of using biochemical methods to investigate psychiatric disorder.

It will be clear from the above account that the scope for molecular genetic studies is greatly enhanced by the presence of a *biochemical abnormality* that reliably distinguishes patients with a particular psychiatric disorder. The value of such an abnormality would be greater still if the biochemical abnormality concerned played a significant role in the cause of the illness or its pathophysiology. However, the nature of the biochemical changes associated with most psychiatric disorders remains unknown. This is due both to our lack of knowledge about the biochemical complexities of the normal brain and to the difficulty of investigating the biochemistry of the living human brain directly. Moreover, because most psychiatric disorders do not lead to death (other than by suicide), post-mortem material is not widely available except among the elderly.

Because of these problems, workers have adopted a variety of *indirect methods* involving sampling of peripheral tissues and fluids such as cerebrospinal fluid, blood cells, and urine. These studies, whilst more feasible to carry out, are not always easy to interpret. For example, concentrations of neurotransmitters and their metabolites in lumbar cerebrospinal fluid have an uncertain relationship to the corresponding functionally active neurotransmitter in the brain. Equally, neurotransmitter receptors and their second messengers in blood platelets and lymphocytes often appear to be regulated in a different way to their brain counterparts. Finally, measures in plasma and urine are very susceptible to confounding dietary and behavioural changes (see below).

The reader will find accounts of the results of biochemical research in subsequent chapters, especially those on mood disorders and schizophrenia. At this point a few examples will be given of the different kinds of investigation.

Post-mortem studies

Post-mortem studies of the brain can provide direct evidence of chemical changes within it. Unfortunately, interpretation of the findings is difficult because it must be established that any changes in the concentrations of neurotransmitters or enzymes did not occur after death. Moreover, because psychiatric disorders do not lead directly to death, the ultimate cause of death is another condition (often bronchopneumonia or the effects of a drug overdose) that could have caused the observed changes in the brain.

Even if this possibility can be ruled out, it is still possible that the chemical findings are the results of treatment rather than of disease. For example, the increases in density of dopamine receptors in the nucleus accumbens and caudate nucleus in patients with schizophrenia might be interpreted as supporting the hypothesis that schizophrenia is caused by changes in dopamine function in these areas of the brain. The finding could equally be the result of long-term treatment with antipsychotic drugs which block dopamine receptors and might lead to a compensatory increase of receptors (see Owens and Ritchie 1999).

As mentioned above, *molecular genetic techniques* can be used to complement biochemical investigations in post-mortem brain. For example, *in situ hybridization* provides information about the gene expression of neurotransmitter receptors of interest. Using this technique it was shown that the mRNA for glutamate receptors is decreased in the hippocampus of patients with schizophrenia, a finding that complements ligand-binding studies of the glutamate receptors in this area of the brain (see Harrison 2000a). An important development in post-mortem studies is the combined use of gene expression, neurochemical and neuropathological techniques to investigate abnormalities in neurotransmitter function in carefully defined brain regions.

Brain biochemistry and brain imaging

Novel methods of studying biochemical events in the living brain have recently become available and have been used in some studies of psychiatric disorders. These methods include:

◆ magnetic resonance imaging (MRI)

◆ single-photon emission tomography (SPET)

◆ positron emission tomography (PET).

The use of these techniques to measure cerebral structure and blood flow is discussed below under the relevant headings. However, brain imaging can also be employed to measure aspects of brain biochemistry. For example, it is possible to carry out *in vivo* receptor binding in different groups of psychiatric patients using positron-labelled ligands and PET or SPET imaging.

Receptor binding with PET and SPET

Using PET imaging in conjunction with a positron-labelled 5-HT_{1A} receptor antagonist, two groups have found that the binding of 5-HT_{1A} receptors in the brain is decreased in patients with major depression. Interestingly, quite contrary findings have been reported in post-mortem studies of depressed suicide victims, showing that the *in vivo* and *in vitro* methods can obtain very different results (see Sargent *et al* 2000).

For reasons of cost, studies employing PET are likely to remain restricted to a small number of specialist research centres. However, SPET imaging is more widely available and increasing numbers of specific receptor ligands suitable for SPET studies are being developed. For example, there are already several studies using SPET in conjunction with specific dopamine receptor ligands examining dopamine receptor binding in mood disorders and schizophrenia (see Verhoeff 1999).

Neurotransmitter release *in vivo*

Recent studies using PET and SPET in conjunction with specific dopamine receptor ligands have enabled estimation of *dopamine release in vivo*. The principle is to scan subjects on two occasions, one after administering a drug that modulates endogenous dopamine release, such as amphetamine, and once after placebo. Amphetamine increases dopamine release presynaptically and the increased levels of endogenous dopamine compete with the tracer ligand for access to post-synaptic receptors. Therefore, the specific binding of the tracer is reduced and the difference in tracer signal between the amphetamine and placebo scans provides a measure of how much dopamine was released by the amphetamine.

A similar approach can be taken with drugs that lower endogenous dopamine release, such as the tyrosine hydroxylase inhibitor α-methyl-para-tyrosine (AMPT). Use of these models has led to the conclusion that dopamine release is increased in patients with acute schizophrenia (for a review see Harrison 2000b). Current studies are investigating how these techniques can be applied to the release of other neurotransmitters.

MRI

MRI has the advantage over SPET and PET that subjects are not exposed to radiation. Whilst MRI has proved an excellent tool for structural brain imaging and more recently for the examination of

Table 5.4 Neuronal metabolites and transmitters measured by MRS

^{1}H-NMR	^{31}P-NMR
N-Acetyl-aspartate (NAA)	ATP
Creatinine	Phosphocreatine
Myoinositol	Inorganic phosphate
GABA	Phosphodiesters
Glutamate	Phosphomonoesters

cerebral blood flow, its application to the study of brain biochemistry (magnetic resonance spectroscopy, MRS) has been somewhat limited by lack of sensitivity. However, proton (^{1}H) MRS can be used to detect a number of compounds of neurobiological interest (Table 5.4). MRS can also be used to identify the spectrum of phosphorus-containing compounds and thereby can provide information about *energy metabolism and intracellular pH*. A number of psychotropic drugs possess fluorine atoms, which can be imaged by MRS; this provides a means of imaging the distribution of such drugs at their specific receptor sites in the brain. MRS has also been used to image *lithium* in the human brain where it appears that brain levels of lithium are about half those seen in plasma.

One reasonably consistent finding from proton MRS is that the patients with schizophrenia have decreased levels of N-acetyl-aspartate (NAA) and the ratio of NAA to creatinine. This could reflect decreases in neuronal populations or the density of their projections (for a review, see Seibyl *et al.* 1999).

Peripheral measures

There have been long-standing doubts as to whether changes in the composition of neurotransmitters in the cerebrospinal fluid (CSF) reflect functionally significant changes in the brain. However, there are strong links between lowered CSF levels of 5-hydroxindoleacetic acid (5-HIAA) and impulsive aggressive behaviour in both human

and non-human primates (see Linnoila and Charney 1999). This suggests that CSF 5-HIAA does correlate with certain defined aspects of behaviour. The major limitation of CSF studies is that it is often ethically and practically difficult to obtain CSF samples from psychiatric patients. In addition, it is not feasible to monitor time-dependent changes in neurotransmitter metabolism through repeated sampling.

Ingenious attempts have been made to infer biochemical changes in the brain from measurements of substances in the blood. For example, it is known that the rate of synthesis of 5-HT depends on the concentration of the 5-HT precursor tryptophan in the brain. Several studies have shown that *plasma tryptophan is decreased in patients with major depression*, a finding which supports the hypothesis that brain 5-HT function may be impaired in depressive disorders. However, it cannot be assumed that a modest reduction in concentrations of plasma tryptophan will necessarily be associated with impaired brain 5-HT neurotransmission. Furthermore, the same reduction in plasma tryptophan concentrations is found when healthy people lose weight through dieting. Therefore, it is quite possible that the decrease in plasma tryptophan found in depressed patients is a consequence of concomitant weight loss (see Anderson *et al.* 1990).

In general, investigations of biochemical abnormalities in blood and urine have not proved particularly fruitful in understanding the aetiology of psychiatric disorders. The real advances from such studies are in the field of learning disability, where measurement of metabolites in blood and urine have sometimes provided a useful picture of the abnormalities present in the brain as well as valuable diagnostic tests. A good example is phenylketonuria (see p.878).

Peripheral blood cells such as platelets and lymphocytes possess receptors for neurotransmitters that often resemble the analogous receptor binding sites in the brain. There have been many studies of monoamine receptors in platelets of depressed patients, but the findings tend to be inconsistent and easily confounded by factors such as drug treatment. In addition, it is far from clear that abnormalities found in these peripheral binding sites will necessarily also be present in the brain. Indeed, those studies that have looked simultaneously at peripheral receptor binding and *in vivo* receptor imaging have not found correlations (see, for example, Yatham *et al*. 2000). Similar comments apply to the use of blood cells to investigate neurotransmitter-linked second messengers and ion flux processes such as calcium entry.

Pharmacology

The study of effective treatment of disease can often throw light on aetiology. In psychiatry, because of the great problems of studying the brain directly, research workers have examined the *actions of effective psychotropic drugs* in the hope that the latter might indicate the biochemical abnormalities in disease. Of course, such an approach must be used cautiously. If an effective drug blocks a particular transmitter system, it cannot be concluded that the disease is caused by an excess of that transmitter. The example of parkinsonism makes this clear; anticholinergic drugs modify the symptoms, but the disease is due to a deficiency in dopaminergic transmission and not an excess of cholinergic transmission.

It is assumed here that the general methods of neuropharmacology are familiar to the reader, and attention is focused on the particular difficulties of using these methods in psychiatry. There are two main problems. First, most psychotropic drugs have more than one action and it is often difficult to decide which is relevant to the therapeutic effects. For example, although lithium carbonate has a large number of known pharmacological effects, it has so far been impossible to explain its remarkable effect of stabilizing the mood of manic-depressive patients.

The second difficulty arises because the therapeutic effects of many psychotropic drugs are slow to develop, whereas most pharmacological effects identified in the laboratory are quick to appear. For example, it has been suggested that the beneficial effect of antidepressant drugs depends on alterations in the re-uptake of transmitter at pre-synaptic neurons. However, changes in re-uptake occur quickly, whereas the therapeutic effects are usually delayed for about 2 weeks.

Recent studies in animals have concentrated on changes that occur in brain neurotransmitter receptors during *long-term psychotropic drug treatment*. These changes are interesting because the time course is similar to that of the development of therapeutic effects. Also, antidepressant treatments that have different pharmacological effects when first given may, after repeated administration, produce similar effects on neurotransmitter receptors. Thus it appears that the late effects of both antidepressant drugs and electroconvulsive shock are to produce in somewhat different ways facilitation of neurotransmission of post-synaptic 5-HT_{1A} receptors (see Blier and de Montigny 1994).

The introduction of new drugs with different pharmacological actions from conventional compounds can often be used to generate hypotheses about the mode of action of beneficial treatments and the pathophysiology of the disorder concerned. For example, with the introduction of *selective serotonin re-uptake inhibitors* (SSRIs), it has become clear that only drugs with potent 5-HT re-uptake inhibitor properties are effective in the pharmacological treatment of obsessive–compulsive disorder. Conventional tricyclic antidepressants (with the exception of clomipramine) are not useful (Insel 1991). This suggests that the pathophysiology of obsessive–compulsive disorder differs from that of major depression, for which both classes of compounds are equally effective.

The SSRIs may be effective for obsessive–compulsive disorder because they produce larger overall increases in 5-HT neurotransmission than conventional tricyclic antidepressants, or because they activate particular 5-HT receptor subtypes which are not affected by tricyclics. Specific experiments can be designed to test these hypotheses (see Sargent *et al*. 1998).

Another drug that has stimulated research in this way is *clozapine*, an antipsychotic drug which is effective in a significant proportion of patients who are unresponsive to traditional antipsychotic agents. Most antipsychotic drugs are believed to produce their therapeutic effects through blockade of dopamine D_2 receptors, but clozapine has a weak affinity for this binding site. In fact, clozapine binds potently to certain 5-HT receptor subtypes, particularly the 5-HT_{2A} receptor.

This has led to development of numerous 'atypical' antipsychotic agents that have combined 5-HT_2 and dopamine D_2 receptor antagonist properties. Whilst these agents have some advantages over conventional antipsychotic drugs, they do not seem to be as effective as clozapine in patients with treatment-resistance illness (see p. 664).

Endocrinology

Changes in circulating concentrations of hormones can have profound effects on mood and behaviour, whilst abnormalities in endocrine function are responsible for a number of well-defined clinical syndromes, some of which have characteristic neuropsychiatric presentations, for example, depression in *Cushing's disease*.

Measurement of plasma hormone levels in psychiatric disorders has not, in general, shown consistent abnormalities in psychiatric patients or thrown much light on aetiology. The exception is major depression, in which a significant proportion of patients *hypersecrete cortisol*. There is increasing evidence that in some depressed patients elevated cortisol levels may play a role in the pathophysiology of depression.

Hormones and gene expression

Recently, knowledge of how hormones may alter brain function has increased, which makes it possible to see pathophysiological links between altered hormone secretion and changes in relevant brain mechanisms. Hormones can alter both intracellular and extracellular signalling, usually by altering *gene expression*.

For example, corticosteroids act on the cell nucleus to alter the expression of receptors for various neurotransmitters. In animal experimental studies, the density of 5-HT_{1A} receptors is modulated by circulating corticosterone levels, and it has been proposed that excessive cortisol secretion may predispose to a depressive disorder through an attenuation of 5-HT_{1A} receptor function in limbic brain regions (see Dinan 1994). Animal studies have also indicated that corticosteroid administration can cause cell loss in the hippocampus. This finding has led to the hypothesis that the cognitive impairment seen in elderly depressed patients may be a consequence of neuronal damage produced by excessive cortisol secretion (O'Brien 1997).

Peptide releasing factors

Hormones such as thyroid stimulating hormone (TSH) and adenocorticotropic hormone (ACTH) are regulated by peptide releasing factors that have additional signalling roles in other brain regions, often those involved in the regulation of emotion. These peptides often coexist with classical neurotransmitters; for example, thyrotropin releasing hormone (TRH) is co-localized with 5-HT in 5-HT neurons. There is growing interest in the development of drugs that act on peptide receptors. An example is the possible use of corticotropic releasing hormone (CRH) antagonists in depression (see p. 298).

Neuroendocrine tests

Another use of plasma hormone measurement is to monitor the functional activity of brain neurotransmitters. The secretion of pituitary hormones is controlled by a variety of neurotransmitters. Under certain circumstances, changes in the concentration of a plasma hormone can be used to assess the function of the neurotransmitters involved in its release. For example, stimulating brain 5-HT function with a specific drug gives rise to an increase in plasma prolactin levels; accordingly, the rise in prolactin concentration that accompanies administration of a standard dose of the drug gives a measure of the functional state of brain 5-HT pathways.

These *neuroendocrine challenge tests* provide dynamic functional measures of brain neurotransmitter pathways, and in certain psychiatric disorders they have yielded consistent evidence of impairments in neurotransmitter function. For example, in depressed patients there is good evidence that the prolactin response to 5-HT stimulation is blunted.

This suggests that depressive disorders are associated with a deficit in brain 5-HT neurotransmission. However, as with other biological measures, great care must be taken to control for possible confounding effects such as weight loss and impaired sleep. In fact, weight loss does alter brain 5-HT function but causes the opposite change in p5-HT-mediated prolactin release as is seen in depressed patients. Thus in 5-HT neuroendocrine studies of depressed patients it is important to assess and control for concomitant weight loss, otherwise the impairment in 5-HT-mediated prolactin release may be obscured (for a review of this field see Cowen 1998b).

Neuroendocrine challenge tests can also be used to assess the effect of psychotropic drugs on brain neurotransmitter function. For example, the cortisol response to the 5-HT receptor agonist *m*-chlorophenylpiperazine is blocked in patients receiving treatment with the atypical antipsychotic drug clozapine, but not in patients receiving a conventional antipsychotic agent such as fluphenazine (Owen *et al*. 1993). This suggests that clozapine treatment attenuates neurotransmission at a specific subpopulation of 5-HT receptors, and this action may relate to its unusual therapeutic efficacy or perhaps to aspects of its side-effect profile such as excessive weight gain.

Physiology

Physiological methods can be used to investigate the cerebral and peripheral disorders associated with disease states. Several methods have been used:

♦ psychophysiological methods including measurements of pulse rate, blood pressure, blood flow, skin conductance, and muscle activity;

♦ studies of cerebral blood flow;

♦ electroencephalographic (EEG studies).

Psychophysiological measures

Psychophysiological measures can be interpreted in at least two ways. The first interpretation is straightforward. The data are used as information about the activity of peripheral organs in disease, for example, to determine whether electromyographic (EMG) activity is increased in the scalp muscles of patients who complain of tension headaches. The second interpretation depends on the assumption that peripheral measurements can be used to infer changes in the state of *arousal of the central nervous system*. Thus increases in skin conductance, pulse rate, and blood pressure are taken to indicate greater arousal.

Measurement of cerebral blood flow and metabolism

Advances in brain imaging methods have led to increasing sophistication in the measurement of cerebral blood flow in psychiatric disorders. Studies using PET and SPET have largely replaced older techniques using xenon inhalation because the addition of tomographic techniques allows a three-dimensional measurement of regional cerebral blood flow to be achieved.

Functional MRI (fMRI)

Another important recent development is the demonstration that *MRI techniques using the water proton signal* are sufficiently sensitive to define regional increases in cerebral blood flow following neuronal activation. This technique is usually referred to as *functional MRI (fMRI)*. The principal method of fMRI is *blood oxygenation-level-dependent (BOLD) imaging*. The use of BOLD depends on the fact that *deoxyhaemoglobin* is paramagnetic; it therefore aligns with an applied magnetic field, making the local magnetic field stronger. By contrast, oxygenated haemoglobin is only slightly diamagnetic and creates weak local field disturbances.

Increases in neuronal activity are associated with increases local cerebral blood flow, which causes *decreases in deoxyhaemoglobin.* This is because under normal conditions of activation there is a relatively greater increase in blood flow than neuronal oxygen consumption. The change in local deoxy-haemoglobin levels can be imaged and measured. It will be seen from this that fMRI can measure *changes* in activation but not baseline local cerebral blood flow. Accordingly, it has to be used with an 'activation' paradigm. Such paradigms are usually those that can be readily repeated in an 'off–on' manner over time, for example, a simple test of cognitive function. The advantages of fMRI is that it *has greater spatial and temporal resolution* than other imaging techniques and does not require the use of radioactivity (see Seibyl *et al.* 1999).

fMRI has been used widely to map the neuronal representation of psychological functions in healthy subjects and many interesting findings have emerged. For example, Pantev *et al.* (1998) were able to show that in trained musicians, musical tones activated a greater area of sensory cortex than in non-musical subjects. This study is a good demonstration of how the cortex is able to re-organize itself during learning, presumably via alterations in gene expression. Conceivably, aberrant effects of this nature could be important in the development of certain psychiatric disorders. fMRI is being increasingly used in studies in different groups of psychiatric patients. For a discussion of the use of fMRI in psychiatric disorders see Longworth *et al.* (1999).

PET

PET imaging can be used to measure either *cerebral metabolism or cerebral blood flow.* Usually the two measures are closely correlated. In the adult brain, functional activity is almost entirely dependent on oxidative metabolism, which requires glucose and oxygen as substrates. Hence rates of metabolism can be determined by measuring the utilization of oxygen or accumulation of *deoxyglucose.* Measurement of regional cerebral blood flow can be made by assessing the accumulation of radioactivity in the brain during inhalation of suitably labelled CO_2 or H_2O (Seibyl *et al.* 1999).

SPET

Measurement of blood flow with SPET employs lipophilic radiotracers such as technetium-labelled hexamethyl propyleneamine oxime (^{99m}Tc-HMPAO). Following intravenous administration, these compounds are retained in the brain in a stable form for several hours. This enables high-resolution images to be obtained with the use of a conventional detector such as a rotating gamma camera. The uptake of ^{99m}Tc-HMPAO is linearly related to cerebral blood flow. However, unlike PET, SPET cannot provide an absolute measure of regional cerebral blood flow; therefore, the results of SPET studies are often expressed by comparing the radioactive counts in each brain region of interest with a reference area, usually either whole brain or cerebellum.

Baseline blood flow in psychiatric disorders

There have been many studies of *basal blood flow* in various psychiatric disorders, but the results of different investigations have often been contradictory. To a large extent the conflicting data may result from the considerable methodological difficulties in standardizing the imaging conditions and the patient population. It is possible that resting conditions are not ideal for the detection of differences between patients and controls because the resting state is inherently physiologically and psychologically variable (see Berman and Weinberger 1999).

Despite these difficulties, more recent, carefully controlled investigations in rigorously assessed drug-free patients are reaching a greater level of consensus. For example, both PET and SPET studies of patients with obsessive–compulsive disorder have revealed increased metabolic activity and blood flow in the frontal cortex, notably in orbitofrontal regions (Saxena *et al.* 1998). In addition, further information can be gained by correlating basal regional cerebral blood flow with the psychopathology of the patients at the time of scanning. This approach has been successful in mapping symptom clusters in patients with schizophrenia to specific brain regions (see p. 354).

Activation paradigms

As with fMRI, *psychological activation paradigms* have been widely used in PET studies of healthy volunteers to map the brain regions and distributed neuronal circuits involved in fundamental processes such as memory and language. Activation paradigms can also be applied to patients with psychiatric disorders with perhaps more consistent results emerging than with baseline blood flow studies.

For example, when normal control subjects undertake the Wisconsin Card Sort Test, there is an increase in blood flow in the prefrontal cortex. On this test, patients with schizophrenia perform less well than controls, and produce a much smaller change in blood flow in the corresponding cortical area. This suggests that some patients with schizophrenia may have a dysfunction of the *prefrontal cortex*, which is associated with poor performance on tasks that depend on increased neuronal activity in this brain region. Another explanation is that the lesser increase in blood flow during the task simply represents poor performance, which is actually caused by some other factor. Disentangling these possibilities is methodologically challenging (see Berman and Weinberger 1999).

Electroencephalography

Methods

The electroencephalograph (EEG) provides a measure of *cortical neuronal activity* through detection of potential differences across the scalp. A number of different techniques are relevant to studies of aetiology in psychiatry:

◆ standard (analogue) EEG

◆ quantified (digital) EEG

◆ sleep EEG (polysomnogram)

◆ magnetoencephalography (MEG)

◆ evoked potentials.

Standard EEG

The standard clinical EEG is a qualitative assessment of a paper trace by a trained observer using visual inspection. These kind of recordings have been most helpful in studying the relationships between *epilepsy* and psychiatric disorders but otherwise have not been particularly informative about aetiology. About 30% of psychiatric patients referred for an EEG are reported as having an abnormal recording but the relevance of this has proved elusive. Artefacts from drug treatment are probably common (see Hughes 1995).

Quantified EEG

The EEG signal can also be examined *quantitatively* using a number of different mathematical approaches. The most commonly used method employs power spectral analysis with Fourier transformation. Characteristic spectral patterns have been reported for certain disorders, although relating these to underlying brain mechanisms is not straightforward. Statistical removal of EEG artefact is also problematic. Thus far the main clinical research application has been in the analysis and detection of the effects of different drugs with the hope of developing an objective method of screening for novel psychotropic compounds (Saletu and Anderer 2000).

Sleep EEG (polysomnogram)

During sleep the EEG shows a characteristic recurrent pattern of waves which can be divided into stages. The fundamental distinction is between *rapid eye movement* (REM or dream sleep) and *non-REM* (or quiet) sleep. The sleep EEG or polysomnogram shows fairly consistent abnormalities in depressed patients, notably a decrease in the *latency to the onset of REM sleep*. Some of these abnormalities may persist into clinical remission and may indicate vulnerability to mood disorder.

The main disadvantage of polysomnography has been the need for a specialized facility (a 'sleep laboratory'). However, the development of home-based monitoring with ambulatory equipment has been helpful in this respect (see Sharpley *et al* 2000). The polysomnogram has also been useful in measuring the effects of drugs on sleep quality and architecture (for a review of the use of the polysomnogram in psychiatric research see Nofzinger *et al*. 1999).

Magnetoencephalography

Magnetoencephalography (MEG) is able to measure changes in extracranial magnetic fields to detect ion fluxes in cortical neurons. Like EEG, MEG has the ability to detect changes in physiological signals over millisecond time intervals. MEG can provide better localization of signals than EEG, but the most useful information may come from using the techniques in combination or by combining MEG with functional imaging. In this way superior temporal and spatial resolution of cortical processing can be obtained. Neither MEG nor EEG is generally helpful in identifying changes in subcortical neuronal activity. In some studies of psychiatric patients, MEG has been used to measure evoked potentials (for a review of the use of the MEG in psychiatry see Reite *et al.* 1999).

Evoked potentials

EEG techniques can also be used to detect changes in brain electrical activity in response to environmental stimuli. These evoked (or event-related) potentials can be detected by computerized averaging methods, and can be identified as waveforms occurring at particular times after the stimulus. For example, the P300 response is a positive deflection that occurs 300 ms after a subject identifies a target stimulus embedded in a series of irrelevant stimuli.

The P300 wave probably corresponds to the cognitive processes required for the recognition, retrieval from memory, and evaluation of a specific stimulus. In patients with schizophrenia, the amplitude of the P300 wave is reduced. It is notable that the same abnormality can be found in first-degree relatives of schizophrenic patients and those with schizotypal personalities.

In these subjects, the change in the P300 response is likely to stem from an abnormality in information processing, and may represent a vulnerability trait marker factor for the development of schizophrenia. However, these changes are not specific in that they can also be found in patients with other disorders such as alcohol misuse (see Blackwood 2000). In addition, interpretation of evoked potentials in terms of brain mechanism is

not easy because the potential recorded from the scalp is far from its generational source and reflects the activity of many different neural systems operating in parallel (see Boutros and Braff 1999).

Neuropathology

Neuropathological studies attempt to answer the question as to whether a *structural change* in the brain (localized or diffuse) accompanies a particular kind of mental disorder. Such studies have an obvious application to the aetiology of dementia and other psychiatric disorders in which organic lesions can readily be found. In the past, many post-mortem studies were carried out on the brains of patients who had suffered from schizophrenia and mood disorders. Consistent changes were not identified and therefore it was assumed that these psychiatric conditions were disorders of function rather than of structure (hence the name *functional psychoses* was sometimes used as a collective name for these conditions).

Structural imaging

Improved methods of *structural brain imaging* have played an important role in the resurgence of interest in the neuropathology of psychosis. For example, Johnstone *et al.* (1976) showed that computerized tomography (CT) scanning could be used to demonstrate enlargement of the lateral ventricles in schizophrenia. More recently, *structural MRI* has allowed the examination of cortical and subcortical structures with a high degree of resolution. These studies have shown that medial temporal structures are often reduced in volume in patients with schizophrenia (Wright *et al.* 2000).

Post-mortem investigations have confirmed several of the abnormalities detected by structural imaging, whilst detailed neuropathological studies have identified neuronal loss and architectural disarray in the temporal lobe and other cortical regions. These findings have stimulated post-mortem neurochemical and molecular pathological studies on temporal lobe structures and the brain regions with which they are closely connected (see p. 357).

The recent discovery of consistent brain neuro-pathological changes in patients with schizophrenia is a useful reminder that methods of investigation available at a particular time may fail to detect relevant biological abnormalities even when the latter are undoubtedly present. In addition, as neuropathological investigations embrace the molecular level, drawing distinctions between 'functional' and 'structural' disorders becomes somewhat arbitrary. Finally, the recent neurobiological studies in schizophrenia emphasize that progress in determining aetiology is most likely to be made through *the integration of different kinds of pathological and biochemical investigation*, so that the various approaches can be used to inform and guide each other.

Relationship of this chapter to those on psychiatric syndromes

This chapter has reviewed several diverse approaches to aetiology. It may be easier for the reader to put these approaches into perspective when reading the sections on aetiology in the chapters on the different psychiatric syndromes, especially those on mood disorders (pp. 287–302) and schizophrenia (pp. 347–62).

Further reading

Charney, D. S., Nestler, E. J., and Bunney, B. S. (1999). *Neurobiology of mental illness*. Oxford University Press, Oxford. (Comprehensive overview of the developing methods and concepts in biological psychiatry.)

Freud, S. (1916–17). *Introductory lectures on psychoanalysis*. Reprinted in Penguin Freud Library, Vol. 1. Penguin, Harmondsworth. (Lucid account of psychoanalytic theory by its original proponent.)

Gelder, M. G., Lopez-Ibor, J. J., and Andreason, N. C. (2000) *New Oxford Textbook of Psychiatry*. Oxford University Press. (Part 2. The scientific basis of psychiatric epidemiology contains 22 chapters on various aspects of and scientific approaches to aetiology. Part 3 is concerned with psychodynamic approaches.)

Jaspers, K. (1963). *General psychopathology* (trans. J. Hoenig and M. W. Hamilton), pp. 301–11, 355–64, 383–99. Manchester University Press, Manchester. (The classical text: these pages explain the concepts of meaningful connections and psychological reactions.)

Strachan, T. and Read, A. P. (1996). *Human molecular genetics*. Bios Scientific publishers, Oxford. Comprehensive and well-illustrated introduction to molecular genetics.

6

CHAPTER 6

Evidence-based approaches to psychiatry

CHAPTER 6
Evidence-based approaches to psychiatry

What is evidence-based medicine?

Evidence-based medicine (EBM) is a systematic way of obtaining clinically important information about aetiology, diagnosis, prognosis, and treatment. The evidence-based approach is a *process* in which the following steps are applied:

◆ formulation of an answerable clinical question;

◆ identification of the best evidence;

◆ critical appraisal of the evidence for validity and utility;

◆ implementation of the findings;

◆ evaluation of performance.

The principles of EBM can be applied to a variety of medical procedures. For psychiatry, the main use of EBM at present is assessing the value of *therapeutic interventions*. For this reason, in the following sections the application of EBM will be linked to studies of treatment. Applications to other areas such as diagnosis and prognosis are discussed later.

Why do we need evidence-based medicine?

There are two main related problems in clinical practice which can be helped by the application of EBM:

◆ the difficulty in keeping up to date with clinical and scientific advances;

◆ the tendency of practitioners to work in idiosyncratic ways that are not justified by available evidence.

With the burgeoning number of clinical scientific journals, the most assiduous clinician is unable to keep up to date with all relevant articles even in his own field. Clinicians therefore have to rely on information gathered from other sources which might include, for example, unsystematic expert reviews, opinions of colleagues, information from pharmaceutical representatives, and their own clinical experiences and beliefs. This can lead to wide variations in practice, for example, those described for the use of electroconvulsive therapy and various kinds of drug treatment (Pippard 1992; Lehman and Steinwachs 1998).

Kinds of evidence

The fundamental assumption of EBM is that some kinds of evidence are *better* (that is, more valid and of greater clinical applicability) than others. This

Table 6.1 **Hierarchy of research for treatment studies**	
Ia	Evidence from a systematic review of randomized controlled trials
Ib	Evidence from at least one randomized controlled trial
IIa	Evidence from at least one controlled study without randomization
IIb	Evidence from at least one other type of quasi-experimental study
III	Evidence from non-experimental descriptive studies, such as comparative studies, correlation studies, and case control studies
IV	Evidence from expert committee reports or opinions and/or clinical experience of respected authorities

view is most easily elaborated for questions about therapy. A commonly used 'hierarchy' is shown in Table 6.1.

In this hierarchy, *randomized evidence* is regarded as more *valid* than non-randomized evidence with *systematic review of randomized trials* seen as the gold standard for answering clinical questions in the most objective way possible (see Geddes and Harrison, 1997). This assumption has itself yet to be tested systematically but at present seems likely to be true. It is important that clinicians are trained in critical evaluation of systematic reviews before applying them to their clinical practice (see below and Greenhalgh, 1997).

Individual treatment studies

Validity

The key criterion for validity in treatment studies is *randomization*. In addition, clinicians entering patients into a therapeutic trial should be unaware of the treatment group to which their patients are being allocated. This is usually referred to as *concealment of the randomization list*. Without concealed randomization, the validity of a study is questionable and its results may be misleading .

Other important points when assessing the *quality* of a study are:

◆ Were all the patients who entered the trial accounted for at its conclusion?

◆ Were patients analysed in the groups to which they were allocated (so-called 'intention to treat' analysis)?

◆ Were patients and clinicians blind to the treatment received (a different question to that of blind *allocation*)?

◆ Apart from the experimental treatment, were the groups treated equally?

◆ Did the randomization process result in the groups being similar at baseline?

Presentation of results

Odds ratios

When the outcome of a clinical trial is an event (for example, admission to hospital), a commonly used measure of effectiveness is the *odds ratio*. The odds ratio is the odds of an event occurring in the experimental group divided by the odds of it occurring in the control group. The odds ratio is given with 95% confidence intervals (which indicate the range of values within which we have a 95% certainty that the *true* value falls). The narrower the confidence intervals the greater the precision of the study.

If the odds ratio of an event such as admission to hospital is 1.0, this means the rates of readmission do not differ between control and experimental groups. Therefore if the confidence interval of the odds ratio of an individual study includes the value of 1.0, the study has failed to show that the experimental and control treatments differ from each other.

Effect sizes

In many studies the outcome measure of interest is a continuous variable, such as a mean score on the Hamilton Rating Scale for Depression. It is possible to use the original measure in the meta-analysis although more often an estimate of *effect size* is made because it is more statistically robust.

Effect sizes are obtained by dividing the difference in effect between the experimental group and the control group by the standard deviation of their difference. The clinical interpretation of the effect size is discussed below.

Clinical utility of interventions

Risk reduction and number needed to treat

An important part of EBM is using randomized trials to derive the impact of an intervention at the level of the individual patient. A useful concept when assessing the value of a treatment is that of *absolute risk reduction*. This compares the proportion

Box 6.1 Indices for translating research results into clinical practice

	Experimental treatment, X	Control treatment, Y
Positive outcome	a	b
Negative outcome	c	d

Control Event Rate (CER) = b/(b + d)

Experimental Event Rate (EER) = a/(a + c)

Absolute Risk Reduction (ARR)

The difference in the proportions with a positive outcome on treatments X and Y = (CER − EER)

Odds ratio (OR)

The ratio of the odds of a positive outcome on treatments X and Y = (a/c)/(b/d) = ad/bc

Number Needed to Treat (NNT) – how many patients need to be treated with treatment X to get one more positive outcome than would be expected on treatment Y (= 1/AAR)

From Geddes and Harrison (1997)

of patients receiving the experimental treatment who experienced a clinically significant adverse outcome (for example, clinical relapse) compared to the rate in patients receiving the comparison treatment. These are known as the *experimental event rate (EER)* and *control event rate (CER)*, respectively, and

are calculated as percentages. The difference between these two outcome rates is *the absolute risk reduction (ARR)*.

The ARR can be converted into a more clinically useful number, the *number needed to treat (NNT)*. The NNT is the reciprocal of the ARR and tells us how many patients would need to be treated to experience one less adverse outcome event (Box 6.1). Like odds ratios, NNTs are usually given with 95% confidence intervals (see Geddes and Harrison 1997).

Example

Paykel *et al.* (1999) randomized 158 patients with residual depressive symptoms following an episode of major depression to either clinical management or clinical management with 18 sessions of cognitive behaviour therapy (CBT). Over the following 68 weeks the relapse rate in CBT-treated group (29%) was significantly less than that of the clinical management group (47%; *P* = 0.02).

The absolute risk reduction (ARR) in relapse with CBT is 47 − 29 = 18%. The number needed to treat (NNT) is the reciprocal of this number, which is approximately 6 (usually the NNT is rounded up to the next highest integer). This means that six patients with residual depressive symptoms have to be treated with CBT to avoid one relapse. In general, an NNT of less than 10 denotes a useful treatment effect. However, interpretation of the NNT will also depend on the

Table 6.2 Examples of number needed to treat (NNT) for intervention in psychiatry

Intervention	Outcome	NNT
Cognitive therapy in bulimia nervosa	Remission	2
Light treatment in winter depression	Clinical response	2
Lithium augmentation in resistant depression	Clinical response	4
Chlorpromazine in schizophrenia	Relapse prevention	4
Family therapy in schizophrenia	Relapse at 1 year	7
SSRIs compared with TCAs in acute depression	Remain in treatment at 6 weeks	33

SSRIs, selective serotonin re-uptake inhibitors; TCAs, tricyclic antidepressants.

nature of the treatment together with the extent of its therapeutic and adverse effects. The NNT for some common psychiatric treatments are shown in Table 6.2.

If the outcome measure of an intervention is a beneficial event (such as recovery) rather than avoidance of an adverse one, the effect of the intervention is calculated as the *absolute benefit increase (ABI)* in the same way as the ARR (see above) with the NNT being similarly computed. A related concept to NNT is the *number needed to harm (NNH)* which describes the adverse risks of particular therapies, for example, extrapyramidal symptoms with antipsychotic drugs.

Computing the NNT from odds ratios.

If a study or meta-analysis provides an odds ratio it is possible to compute an NNT that may be more relevant to the clinical circumstances of the practitioner and his patient. For example, in the example given above, relapses occurred in 35 of 78 subjects in the clinical management group compared with 23 of 80 in the CBT group. This gives an odds ratio in the risk of relapse between the two treatments of 0.49. To obtain an NNT from the odds ratio it is necessary to know, or estimate, the expected relapse rate in the control group. This is known as the *patient expected event rate (PEER)*. The PEER is combined with the odds ratio (OR) in the following formula:

$$NNT = \frac{1 - PEER(1 - OR)}{(1 - PEER) \times PEER(1 - OR)}$$

If we take the relapse rate in the patients given clinical management in the above study (45%) we have:

$$NNT = \frac{1 - [0.45 \times (1 - 0.49)]}{(1 - 0.45) \times 0.45 \times (1 - 0.49)}$$

This gives an NNT of about 6, which we also derived from the other method of calculation involving the ARR. If however, from a local audit, we know that the relapse rate in our own service of patients with residual depressive symptoms is about 20% (rather than the 45% of Paykel *et al.*), using the formula above, the NNT becomes about

11. This means in our own service we would need to treat 11 patients with CBT to obtain one less relapse. In this way odds ratios can be used to adjust NNTs to local clinical conditions, thereby helping decisions over the applicability of interventions (see Freemantle and Geddes, 1998).

Clinical relevance of effect size

Like the odds ratio, the *effect size* is not easy to interpret clinically. A useful approach is to use the effect size to estimate the degree of overlap between the control and experimental populations. In this way we obtain the proportion of control group scores that are lower than those in the experimental group. (A negative effect size simply means that scores in the control group are *higher* than those in the experimental group.)

For example, in a review of the effects of benzodiazepines and zolpidem on total sleep time relative to placebo, Nowell *et al.* (1997) found an overall effect size of 0.71. From normal distribution tables this means that 76% of controls had less total sleep time than the average sleep time in the hypnotic-treated patients. Effect sizes have been classified in the following way:

- 0.2 = small
- 0.5 = moderate
- 0.8 or more = large.

The effect size of antidepressant medication relative to placebo is about 0.4–0.5. Furukawa (1999) has devised a tabular method of converting effect sizes to NNT values. At the sort of response levels seen in antidepressant-treated patients (about 30% response rate in the placebo group and 60% in the experimental group) an effect size of 0.2 is equivalent to an NNT of about 10. With an effect size of 0.5, the NNT falls to 5.

Ethical aspects of therapeutic trials

Randomization

As we have seen, *randomization* is a key process in the conduct of an evidence-based clinical trial because it is best way of avoiding bias due to chance and random error. However, a clinician may feel uncomfortable about randomization when, for example, he has a strong belief in the efficacy of one of the treatments being assessed. Randomization is ethical where there is genuine *uncertainty* about the best treatment for the individual concerned. In fact, EBM suggests that this situation is more common than clinicians may realize, in that many strongly held beliefs about efficacy of therapeutic interventions are based on anecdotal experience rather than systematic evidence.

Use of placebo

The use of drug placebo in trials of psychotropic agents is controversial. However, such studies are required by many drug-licensing authorities before, for example, a new antidepressant drug is licensed. The arguments for the use of placebo in antidepressant drug trials have been summarized (see Miller 2000):

- The placebo response in major depression is variable and unpredictable, and is not infrequently equivalent in therapeutic effect to active treatment.

- Placebo is required to establish efficacy of new antidepressants. Comparison against an active treatment is not methodologically sufficient.

- The lack of placebo-controlled design in antidepressant drug development might lead to the marketing of a drug that is ineffective, thereby harming public health.

These arguments have to be weighed against the knowledge that antidepressants are generally somewhat more effective than placebo in the treatment of depression. Therefore, a patient treated with placebo in a randomized trial is not receiving the best available therapy. One way of trying to deal with this is to ensure that patients in such trials receive particularly close clinical monitoring which will result in their being withdrawn from the study if they are not doing well.

Informed consent

The role of informed consent is crucial to the ethical conduct of randomized and placebo-controlled trials. This raises difficulties with some psychiatric disorders where the judgement and decision-making abilities of patients may be impaired. Miller (2000) has outlined a number of important factors:

- Patients must be made specifically aware that the trial is not being conducted for their individual benefit.

- With placebo treatment there needs to be clear specification of the probability of receiving placebo, the lack of improvement that might result, and the possibility of symptomatic worsening.

- Patients must be free from any coercion or inducement.

- Patients have right to withdraw from the study at any time without any kind of penalty.

- In addition to the investigator, a family member or other suitable person should be encouraged to monitor the patient's condition and report to the investigator if there are concerns.

The key issues therefore are *open and explicit* information sharing with patient and family, and all necessary measures to avoid placebo treatment leading to *harm to the subject*. The issue, however, remains controversial (see Lavori 2000).

Systematic reviews

Validity

The aim of a systematic review is to obtain all available *valid* evidence about a specific procedure or intervention and from this to provide a more precise quantitative assessment of its efficacy. Two advances have greatly increased the feasibility of systematic reviews: first, the availability of electronic databases such as Medline and Embase, and second, new statistical techniques through which results from different studies can be combined in a quantitative manner. Because a meta-analysis uses all available valid data, its *statistical power* is greater than that of an individual study; it may therefore demonstrate moderate but clinically important effects of treatment that were not apparent in individual randomized studies.

Systematic reviews of treatment, like single therapeutic studies, have to be tested for *validity* and *quality*. The following questions should be posed.

Is it a systematic review of relevant and randomized studies?

We have already seen that the first task in the EBM process is to ask a clearly formulated question. It is therefore necessary to determine whether the subject of the systematic review is truly relevant to the therapeutic question that needs to be answered. The next step is to make sure that only randomized studies have been included. Systematic reviews that contain a mixture of randomized and non-randomized studies may give misleading results.

Do the authors describe the methods by which relevant trials were located?

Whilst electronic searching greatly facilitates identification of clinical trials, up to half the relevant studies may be missed because of miscoding. It is therefore important for authors to make clear whether they supplemented electronic searching with hand-searching of appropriate journals. They may also, for example, have contacted authors of trials, as well as relevant groups in the pharmaceutical industry. In general, negative studies are less likely to be published than positive ones, which can lead to falsely optimistic conclusions about the efficacy of particular treatments.

How did the authors decide which studies should be included in the systematic review?

In a systematic review, authors have to decide which of the various studies they identify should be included in the overall analysis. This means defining *explicit measures of quality*, which will be based on the factors outlined above. Because these judgements are in part subjective, it is desirable for them to be made independently by at least two of the investigators.

Were the results of the therapeutic intervention consistent from study to study?

It is common to see differences in the size of the effect of a therapeutic intervention from study to study. However, if the effects are mixed, with some studies showing a large clinical effect while others find none at all, the trials are said to show *heterogeneity*. Sometimes heterogeneity can be accounted for by factors such as lower doses of a drug treatment or differences in patient characteristics. If there is no likely explanation for it, the results of the review must be considered tentative.

Presentation of results

Combining odds ratios

Results of meta-analyses are often presented as a 'forest plot' in which the findings of the various studies are shown in diagrammatic form (Figure 6.1). As noted above, studies in which the outcome is an event are presented as odds ratios with 95% confidence intervals.

The aim of meta-analysis is to obtain a *pooled estimate* of the treatment effect by combining the odds ratios or effect sizes of all the studies. This is not simply an average of all the odds ratios but is *weighted* so that studies with more statistical information and greater precision (with narrower confidence intervals) contribute relatively more to the final result. The pooled odds ratio also has a 95% confidence interval. Once again, if this interval overlaps with value of 1.0, the experimental intervention does not differ from the control.

In Figure 6.1 some of the studies show a significant effect of assertive community treatment (ACT) to decrease readmission, whilst others do not. The two pooled analyses are difficult to inter-

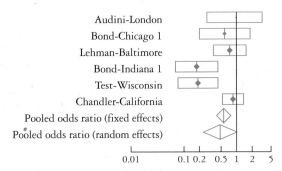

Figure 6.1 Effect of active community treatment on the odds of admission to hospital. (From Freemantle and Geddes 1998)

pret because the confidence intervals of one of them (*the fixed effects model*) do not overlap with 1.0, making ACT significantly different from control, whereas the other (*the random effects model*) just overlaps with 1.0 and is therefore of marginal statistical significance.

We have already seen that the studies in a meta-analysis may indicate *heterogeneity*. This can be tested statistically with a modification of the chi-squared test. If significant heterogeneity is present the most appropriate meta-analytic technique is a *pooled random effects model*. This model assumes that different treatment effects will occur in different studies and takes this into account in the pooled estimate. This usually results in wider confidence intervals as in the pooled random effect odds ratio in the ACT studies. If the studies suggest a single underlying population treatment effect (that is, lack of heterogeneity) then the pooled treatment analysis should use a *fixed effects model*. This estimate has narrower confidence intervals that may, however, be misleading in the presence of significant heterogeneity.

In Figure 6.1 there is statistically significant heterogeneity between the studies, and inspection of the data shows that the majority of the benefit is contributed by two of the studies, which are not the largest. The random and fixed effects models find a similar mean benefit of ACT in preventing readmission but the random effects model has a wider confidence interval and, as noted above, just

overlaps with 1.0. Because of the heterogeneity of the studies, the random effects model is the more appropriate way of analysing the data. Overall therefore we would be cautious about accepting the efficacy of ACT in lowering readmission rates, unless we were able to find a convincing reason for the variation in study results (see Freemantle and Geddes, 1998).

Effect sizes

As noted above, where the outcome measure is a continuous variable, the usual method of calculating results is to use effect sizes. As with odds ratios, the effect sizes can be combined to give a pooled estimate of greater precision.

Clinical utility

The clinical utility of meta-analyses is assessed as described for individual studies above. Meta-analyses will often provide figures for the NNT. As shown above, however, it is also possible to calculate NNT values from meta-analysis data using ARR or odds ratios.

Problems with meta-analysis

Biased conclusions

Apart from a systematic location of evidence, the aim of meta-analysis is to combine data from multiple studies into a single estimate of treatment effect. There are a number of ways in which results of such an exercise can be misleading:

◆ *Publication bias* Evidence indicates that studies showing positive treatment effects are more likely to be published than negative studies. If negative studies are not included in the meta-analysis the effect of treatment will be inflated.

◆ *Duplication of publication* Just as negative treatment studies may go unpublished, positive studies may be published several times in different forms, sometimes with different authors! This, again, will falsely elevate treatment effects if the same study is included more than once.

- *Heterogeneity of studies* As noted above, individual studies may vary widely in the results obtained because of quite subtle differences in study design, quality, and patient population. If such heterogeneity is not recognized and accounted for in the meta-analysis, misleading conclusions will be drawn.

How accurate is meta-analysis?

There are some well-known examples where results of meta-analyses have been contradicted subsequently by single, large randomized trials. For example, a meta-analysis which showed that intravenous magnesium improved outcome in patients with myocardial infarction was later decisively refuted by a single, large randomized trial of 58 000 patients. The misleading result of the meta-analysis was later explained on the basis of publication bias, poor methodological quality in the smaller trials, and clinical heterogeniety (see Greenhalgh, 1997).

Reviews of this area have generally found that about 80% of meta-analyses agree with single large trials in terms of direction of effect of treatment, but the size and statistical significance of the effect often differs between the two methods. Also, separate meta-analyses of the same therapeutic intervention may come to quite different conclusions (see Naylor, 1997).

Funnel plots

One way of improving the reliability of meta-analyses is by the use of 'funnel plots'. The funnel plot is based on the assumption that the precision (confidence interval) of the estimated treatment effect will be greater in studies with a larger sample size. Therefore, the effect sizes of larger studies should cluster around the overall mean difference between experimental and control groups. By contrast, results from smaller studies should be more dispersed around the mean. This means that when the precision of individual studies is plotted against their odds ratios or effect sizes, the resulting graphical plot should resemble a symmetrical inverted funnel (the funnel plot). Statistically significant devations from this plot

suggest that that the meta-analysis may be biased and should be received with caution (see Egger *et al.* 1997).

Large-scale randomized trials

As noted above, the advantage of meta-analysis is that by combining individual studies it can assemble sufficient patient numbers to allow detection of moderate-sized, but clinically important, therapeutic effects. Another way of detecting moderate-sized treatment effects is to randomize very large numbers of patients to a single study. These large-scale randomized trials (or *mega-trials*) have advantages over meta-analysis in that all patients can be allocated to a single study design. Such studies need numerous collaborators and therefore require a *simple study design* and a *clear end point*.

This metholodology has been most successfully applied to areas of medicine, such as cardiovascular disorders, where interventions can sometimes be simple (for example, one dose of aspirin daily) and end points (cardiac infarction, or death) clearly identified (see Collins *et al.* 1996). The challenge for psychiatric trials is to adapt such methodology to conditions where interventions are more complex and end points more subtle.

Applicability

A general problem of applying evidence from randomized trials and meta-analysis to routine clinical work is that clinical trials are often carried out in rather 'ideal' conditions which in a number of respects may not match routine clinical work:

- *Patient population* Patients in controlled trials may differ systematically from those in routine clinical care in being less severely ill and having fewer co-morbid difficulties. Thus trials may be carried out on patients who are, in fact, rather unrepresentative of a usual patient population.

- *Level of supervision* In drug trials concordance is regularly monitored by frequent review and supervision. Thus drugs that in routine practice may be less likely to be taken for a significant length of time (for example, tricyclic antidepressants), may appear better tolerated than they are in a routine setting.

◆ *Therapist variables* Particularly in psychotherapy trials, treatment may be administered by skilled and experienced therapists. In routine practice such individuals may be few and far between; hence results from psychotherapy trials may not transfer well to routine clinical settings.

Pragmatic trials

To overcome these limitations, it has been suggested that *pragmatic trials* might be a more appropriate to study the effect of certain psychiatric interventions. Such studies aim to carry out randomized trials in 'real-life' situations. Methodologically they have much in common with the mega-trials described earlier in that they are designed to answer simple and important clinical questions. As far as possible, pragmatic trials are carried out in a *routine clinical setting*.

Pragmatic trials need large numbers of subjects to produce accurate estimates of benefit, and simple, relevant end points to maximize follow-up rates and clinical applicability. For example, in a trial of a therapeutic intervention in schizophrenia, a rating by patient and family member on a simple scale of well-being may carry more clinical relevance than a score on a standardized rating scale (see Hotopf *et al.* 1999).

Implementation of EBM

Implementing EBM for the individual patient

Having obtained the best evidence on a therapeutic intervention and decided that it is valid and therapeutically useful, it is necessary to decide how applicable it is to the individual patient you are considering. In large measure this depends on the answers to the questions on 'applicability' listed above. The key issues are :

◆ How similar is the patient to those in the randomized trials?

◆ Can the local service deliver the intervention successfully? (It is no use recommending interpersonal therapy if there are no trained therapists available to carry it out.)

In making the decision about implementation it may be useful to adjust the NNT for local clinical conditions if the relevant information is available (see above).

Implementing EBM at a service level

We have already seen there are different kinds of randomized trials which are suitable for different purposes. Haynes (1999) proposed the following classification:

◆ *Efficacy* Does the intervention work under carefully controlled ('ideal') conditions?

◆ *Effectiveness* Does the intervention work when provided under the usual circumstances of health care practice?

◆ *Efficiency* What is the effectiveness of the intervention in relation to the resources it consumes (cost-effectiveness or cost-benefit)?

Ideally, the full implementation of EBM would involve all these processes and only interventions that have satisfied the three criteria of efficacy, effectiveness, and efficiency would be used. In practice many therapeutic interventions in psychiatry (particularly drug treatment and cognitive–behaviour therapy) are of proven *efficacy* but we lack clear evidence on *effectiveness* and *efficiency*. For example, lithium treatment is *efficacious* in the prophylaxis of bipolar disorder but has disappointing *effectiveness*, mainly because under standard clinical conditions relatively few patients take lithium reliably (see Goodwin, 1999).

Clinical practice guidelines

In some medical fields there is a substantial amount of evidence of different kinds but still considerable clinical uncertainty about the best therapeutic management. In this situation it may be worth developing *clinical practice guidelines*, which are explicitly evidence-based.

Such guidelines are best developed in the following way:

◆ A guideline development group, composed of a multidisciplinary group and patient representatives, decide the precise clinical questions to be answered.

◆ The available evidence is systematically reviewed and classified according to the hierarchy shown in Table 6.1.

◆ The guideline development group make recommendations, explicitly demonstrating how their recommendations are linked to the available evidence.

Clinical guidelines are best developed at national level by appropriate professional organizations but usually require modification to take local clinical conditions into account. Guidelines will only be effective if they are actively disseminated and implemented. There is some evidence from randomized studies that guidelines can improve patient outcome (see Geddes 2000).

Evaluation of EBM

EBM needs to evaluated through randomized trials of effectiveness as described above for the guidelines on treating depression. Individual practitioners can also evaluate their EBM performance by:

◆ auditing what proportion of their clinical decisions are evidence-based;

◆ recognizing gaps in practice that require a search and appraisal of relevant evidence;

◆ auditing the effectiveness of evidence-based practice changes.

In this way the process of EBM can become an integral part of continuing professional development and the audit cycle.

Other applications of EBM

The foregoing account has focused on the use of EBM in the assessment of therapeutic interventions in psychiatry. Other applications of EBM include assessment of evidence relating to diagnosis, prognosis, and aetiology. These applications require rather different methodologies from the randomized trials previously considered and diagnosis and prognosis will be discussed in the remainder of the chapter. Approaches to aetiology have been discussed in Chapter 5. All these applications start with a focused question which, as with treatment-related questions, must:

◆ be directly relevant to the identified problem;

◆ be constructed in a way that facilitates searching for a precise answer (see Geddes 1999, Table 6.3).

Diagnosis

If we are trying to assess the value of a particular study assessing a diagnostic test, the practitioner needs to consider a number of questions (see Sackett *et al.* 1997):

◆ Was there an independent, blind comparison of the test with a diagnostic gold standard?

◆ Did the sample include the range of patients to whom the test is likely to be applied in clinical practice?

◆ What is the sensitivity and specificity of the test?

◆ Will it help the management of my patients?

Example
Question

How useful is the CAGE questionnaire in detecting problem drinking in medical and surgical in-patients?

The CAGE questionnaire is a simple four-item questionnaire designed to detect patients with alcohol misuse (see Chapter 18, p. 551). Sackett (1996) describes a study in a community-based teaching hospital in Boston where the CAGE

Table 6.3 Common types of clinical question

Form of the question	Most reliable study architecture
How likely is a patient who has a particular symptom, sign, or diagnostic result to have a specific disorder?	A *cross-sectional study* of patients suspected of having the disorder comparing the proportion of the patients who *really have the disorder and have a positive test with the proportion of patients who do not have the disorder and have a positive test result*
Is the treatment of interest more effective in producing a desired outcome than an alternative treatment (including no treatment)?	Randomized evidence in which the patients are randomly allocated to receive either the treatment of interest or the alternative (Table 6.1)
What is the probability of a specific outcome in this patient?	A study in which an *inception cohort* patients at a common stage in the development of the illness – especially first onset) are followed up for an adequate length of time
What has caused the disorder (or, how likely is a particular intervention to cause a specific adverse effect)?	A study comparing the frequency of an exposure in a group of people with the disease (cases) of interest with a group of people without the disease (controls) – this may be a randomized controlled trial, a case control study, or a cohort study

From Geddes (1999).

---

questionnaire was administered to 518 patients. The gold standard to which the CAGE questionnaire was compared was an extensive social history and clinical examination supplemented by liver biopsy where indicated. We can be reasonably confident therefore that cases of alcohol misuse were reliably identified.

On clinical ('gold standard') grounds, 117 patients met criteria for alcohol misuse or dependence. Of the 61 patients who scored positively on the CAGE questionnaire (scores of 3 or 4), 60 were found to have independent evidence of alcohol misuse. The CAGE is therefore highly specific (Figure 6.2). However the remaining 57 patients with alcohol misuse were not identified by the CAGE. The CAGE therefore has only a modest sensitivity (Figure 6.2).

These results show that the CAGE is a useful screening instrument for problem drinking in a general hospital setting, in that a positive response

		Alcohol abuse or dependency		
		Yes	No	
Number of positive answers to the 4 CAGE questions	3 or 4	60 (true +) a	1 (false +) b	61 $a+b$
	2, 1, or none	57 (false −) c	400 (true −) d	457 $c+d$
		$a+c$ 117	$b+d$ 401	$a+b+c+d$ 518

Sensitivity = a/(a + c) = 60/117 = 0.51 or 51%
Specificity = d/(b + d) = 400/401 = 0.998 or 99.8%

Figure 6.2 The CAGE questions for alcohol abuse/dependency. (From Sackett 1996)

is highly predictive of alcohol problems. However, the test would have to be applied in the knowledge that a negative CAGE response does not rule out alcohol misuse, particularly if there is other evidence of problem drinking.

Prognosis

Studies relating to prognosis should be assessed in the following way (see Sackett *et al.* 1997):

- ◆ Was a defined, representative sample of patients identified at a common point, early in the course of the disorder?
- ◆ Was the follow-up sufficiently long and was it complete?
- ◆ Were objective outcome criteria applied in a blind fashion?
- ◆ Are these follow-up data likely to apply my own patients?

A common problem with prognostic studies is lack of complete follow-up. As a rule of thumb, less than 5% drop-out is ideal and more than 20% makes the study of questionable validity. As with treatment trials, the applicability of the study will depend critically on the how far the patients in it resemble those whom the practitioner is considering.

Example

Question How much of the time are patients troubled by depressive symptomatology following a first episode of depression ?

Judd *et al.* (1998) recruited 122 patients with a first episode of major depression from five tertiary care centres in the USA. They were followed up with interviews every 6 months for the first 5 years and annually thereafter. At interview, depressive symptoms were elicited using Psychiatric Status Rating Scales linked to the Research Diagnostic criteria. Depressive symptoms were classified in four ways: subsyndromal depression, minor depression, dysthymia, and major depression.

The mean follow-up period was 8.5 years and 92% of subjects were followed up for more than 2 years. Of the patients, 61% experienced depressive symptoms at all four levels; only a minority (3%) experienced symptoms at a single diagnostic level. On average patients were symptom-free 54% of the time.

This study suggests that patients who are referred to a tertiary centre with a first episode of depression will have some depressive symptoms about half the time over the next few years. These symptoms are not experienced at a consistent level of severity but wax and wane, meeting criteria for different diagnostic categories over time. This study also has some aetiological implications because it suggests that major depression and other milder depressive syndromes are different expressions of the same underlying disorder. In terms of applicability, we would note that the patients in the study are tertiary referrals, so the findings might not apply, for example, to patients in primary care (see Persons 1999).

Further reading

Sackett, D. L., Richardson, W. S., Rosenberg, W., and Haynes, R. B. (1997). *Evidence-based medicine*. Churchill Livingstone, New York. (Concise handbook with clear exposition of principles of EBM.)

CHAPTER 7

Personality and personality disorder

Personality and personality disorder

Personality

The term personality refers to enduring qualities of an individual that are shown in his ways of behaving in a wide variety of circumstances. Personality therefore differs from mental disorder in that the behaviours which define it have been present throughout adult life, whereas the behaviours that define mental disorder differ from the person's previous behaviour. The distinction is easy to make when behaviour changes markedly over a short period of time (as in a manic disorder), but difficult when behaviour changes slowly over a longer time (as in some early cases of schizophrenia).

The importance of personality

Variations in personality are important because they may predispose to psychiatric disorder, they may account for unusual features in a psychiatric disorder (they are 'pathoplastic' factors) – and they may affect the way that patients approach psychiatric treatment.

Personality as predisposition

Personality can predispose to psychiatric disorder by increasing the response to stressful events. For example, adverse circumstances are more likely to induce an anxiety disorder in a person who has always worried about minor problems.

Personality as a pathoplastic factor

Personality can account for unusual features of a disorder. This usually occurs when features of personality have become exaggerated in response to stressful events associated with illness. For example, histrionic features suggesting a diagnosis of dissociative disorder may arise from histrionic personality traits. When such unusual features are marked, diagnosis is difficult if the psychiatrist has not made an accurate assessment of personality.

Personality in relation to treatment

Personality is an important determinant of a person's approach to treatment. For example, people with obsessional traits may become angry if treatment does not follow their expectations exactly; anxiety-prone people may be overcautious when asked to do more during rehabilitation; and people with antisocial traits may be uncooperative with treatment or aggressive with the staff who are caring for them.

Personality types

A first step in understanding personality is to identify basic types. Clinicians generally derive these types from their collective experience, which suggests several generally recognizable categories such as a sociable and outgoing type and a solitary and self-conscious type. Psychologists have attempted to produce a more scientific set of categories by using personality tests to measure certain aspects of personality ('traits'), and then employing statistical methods to discover which traits cluster together as 'factors'. Examples of personality traits include: anxiety, energy, flexibility, hostility, impulsiveness, moodiness, orderliness, and self-reliance. The various investigators have derived rather different personality factors from such traits: Cattell (1963) identified five factors, while Eysenck (1970b) proposed a scheme that originally had only two 'dimensions' (high-level factors) labelled extraversion–introversion and neuroticism.

Subsequently a third dimension, psychoticism, was added (Eysenck and Eysenck 1976). Eysenck used this term in a special way to denote a constellation of traits of coldness, aggressivity, cruelty, and a propensity to antisocial behaviour.

It is now generally agreed that personality can be described by five factors. These have been variously named but can be referred to usefully as openness to experience (or novelty seeking), conscientiousness, extraversion/introversion, agreeableness (or affiliation), neuroticism. (The initial letters of these factors form the mnemonic OCEAN.) Widiger and Costa (1994) have proposed a scheme in which each of these five factors is made up from scores on six traits. Assessment inventories for these factors have been developed based on self-report and report from informants (Costa and McCrae 1992), as well as a semi-structured interview (Trull and Widiger 1997).

Cloninger (1986) and Cloninger et al. (1993) developed an alternative scheme with three 'basic behavioural dispositions' which are expressed as four basic temperaments. The behavioural dispositions are behavioural activation, behavioural inhibition, and behavioural maintenance. According to Cloninger, behavioural activation is associated with the basic temperament of novelty seeking; behavioural inhibition is associated with harm avoidance; and behavioural maintenance is associated with reward dependence. The fourth basic temperament is persistence. Cloninger's scheme also includes three character traits of self-directedness, cooperativeness, and transcendence. These character traits originate in experiences during childhood and adolescence rather than from the biologically determined behavioural dispositions. The various types of personality and personality disorder are constructed from these four basic temperaments and three character traits. For example, novelty seeking may be expressed as curiosity, readiness to boredom, enthusiasm, and unconventional behaviour. Although going beyond the present evidence, Cloninger's scheme is noteworthy for its attempt to identify basic behavioural dispositions which can account for the observable behaviours that characterize personality, and for its inclusion of both inherited differences in brain function and the effects of experience.

Despite these scientific findings, clinicians continue to use other terms to describe the positive and negative features of normal personality. Positive attributes include outgoing, self-confident, stable, and adaptable. Negative attributes include shy, reserved, lacking in confidence, sensitive, jealous, irritable, impulsive, self-centred, rigid, and aggressive. In addition, two terms are in general use to describe sets of attributes which are often found together. These terms are as follows.

Obsessional traits These traits include positive qualities such that people who possess them are reliable, dependable, persistent, and precise. They set high standards, observe social conventions, and keep to the law. When these traits are more marked they include negative qualities of obstinacy, preoccupation with unimportant detail, bigotry, and lack of a sense of fun.

Histrionic traits In a minor form these traits are socially advantageous. People with such traits are lively and engaging company, they are popular as guests and party-goers, successful in amateur dramatics, and entertaining as public speakers. When the traits are rather more intense they carry some disadvantages. These people are easily moved to tears and dramatize situations. They react to illness in the same demonstrative way, sometimes described as a 'hysterical overlay', which makes it difficult to assess the severity of their suffering. As patients they may be demanding or flirtatious.

The origins of personality

The biological basis of personality types

Genetic influences

Everyday observation suggests that children often resemble their parents in personality. Such similarities could be inherited, or acquired through social learning. Three kinds of scientific study have been used to study the inheritance of personality.

Studies of body build and personality It is commonly thought that personality is linked to body build. If this is true, a possible link between the two could be that they are genetically determined. Kretschmer (1936) described three types of body build: pyknic (stocky and rounded), athletic, and asthenic (lean and narrow). He suggested that the pyknic body build was linked to the cyclothymic personality type (sociable, with variable moods), whereas the asthenic build was related to the 'schizotypal' personality type (cold, aloof, and self-sufficient). Kretschmer's ideas were based on subjective judgements. Sheldon et al. (1940) repeated the studies using quantitative methods for assessing physique and more objective ratings of personality. The results did not support any simple relationship between body build and personality type (Sheldon *et al.* 1940).

Studies of twins More direct evidence of a genetic basis of personality has been obtained by studying the degree of similarity between the scores on personality tests of identical twins reared together or reared apart. The scores, on several measures of personality, of pairs of twins reared apart are as similar as those of pairs of twins reared together (Shields 1962; Pedersen *et al.* 1988), suggesting genetic inheritance. The general conclusion from these and other studies is that the heritability for traits of extraversion and neuroticism is 35–50% (McGuffin and Thapar 1992). The heritability of other traits is uncertain.

Linkage studies Methods of molecular genetics have been used to seek for linkages with measures of novelty seeking and of neuroticism. Linkage has been reported between novelty seeking and the dopamine D_4 receptor gene on the short arm of chromosome 11 (Benjamin *et al.* 1996; Ebstein *et al.* 1996), accounting for about 10% of the variance. However, subsequent studies failed to replicate the finding (see Jönson *et al.* 1997). Linkage has been reported in humans between harm avoidance, neuroticism and a region of the q12 segment of chromosome 17 related to a transporter for serotonin (Lesch *et al.* 1996); and, in mice, between emotional reactivity and a marker on chromosome 1 (Flint *et al.* 1995). These studies are important because they suggest biological bases for aspects of personality. However, more research is needed before the importance of the findings can be evaluated.

Childhood temperament and adult personality

Young infants differ in patterns of sleeping and waking, approach or withdrawal from new situations, intensity of emotional responses, and span of attention. These differences, which are described further in Chapter 24, could be a basis from which differences in personality develop. However, whilst the differences persist into the later years of childhood, they have not been shown to be related to specific features of adult personality (Berger 1985).

Childhood experience and personality development

Everyday experience suggests that experiences in childhood shape personality. It is not easy, however, to produce objective evidence to test this impression. Experiences that seem relevant are difficult to quantify or even to record reliably, and it is difficult to arrange prospective studies that span the long interval between childhood events and adult personality. Retrospective studies are easier to arrange but recall by adults of childhood experiences is unreliable. The difficulties in producing objective evidence have left the field open for subjective accounts based on selective observations and unconfirmed theories. The most influential of these theories are the psychodynamic theories of Freud and others.

Freudian theory Freud's scheme of personality development emphases events in the first five years of life. It is proposed that crucial stages of development of the libido (oral, anal, and genital) must be passed through successfully if personality development is to proceed normally. Failure at particular stages is thought to account for certain features of adult personality, for example, difficulties at the anal stage are said to lead to obsessional personality traits. The scheme allows for some modification of personality at later stages of development through identification with people other than the parents, but this influence is thought to be less important than the earlier ones. The scheme is comprehensive and flexible so that it is possible to explain many features of personality in terms of earlier experience. However, the same features of the theory make it impossible to test it scientifically.

Jung's theory This theory of personality development resembles Freud's in recognizing the importance of psychic events in early life. Unlike Freud, however, Jung thought of personality development as a life-long process. He referred to events in the first part of life as merely 'fulfilling one's obligations' and applied this term to events such as severing ties with parents, finding a spouse, and starting a family. Jung's account is useful in drawing attention to the adjustments in personality that occur throughout life but in other ways it has not been as influential as Freud's theory and it is equally impervious to scientific testing.

Adler and the neo-Freudians Adler rejected Freud's ideas of libido development, proposing instead that personality develops through efforts to compensate for basic feelings of inferiority. The 'neo-Freudians' (Fromm, Horney, and Sullivan) emphasized social factors in development rather than the biologically determined stages of Freud's scheme, though they differed amongst themselves in the details of these social factors. The details of these theories have not been widely accepted but their general emphasis of social factors has been influential.

Erikson The theory proposed by Erikson is essentially similar to Freud's though the nomenclature is different. Erikson referred to the oral stage as the stage of trust versus mistrust, to indicate that this is the period in which feelings of security develop. He referred to the anal stage as the stage of autonomy versus doubt, to indicate that it is the period in which the child learns self-control, social rules, and self-confidence. Erikson referred to the genital stage as the stage of initiative versus guilt, to indicate that it is the stage at which children develop an image of themselves as people. If this stage goes well, the child emerges with confidence and initiative; otherwise, the child emerges insecure and inhibited. Erikson adopted Freud's idea of a latency period but extended it into adolescence. He called this last stage the period of industry versus inferiority. In it the child learns the value of achievements in work and at school, and in social relationships outside the family. Erikson's scheme has been influential in the study of adolescents, largely because it recognizes the importance of this period of life while Freud gave it little attention.

The assessment of personality

The assessment of personality is discussed in Chapter 2, but two points need to be mentioned again. The first is that the means of assessment of personality used in everyday life cannot be applied reliably in clinical practice. In everyday life, we assume that current behaviour reflects the person's habitual ways of behaving (the personality) and generally this assumption is correct. The same assumption is often misleading when patients are assessed because the current behaviour of an ill person reflects the effects of the illness as well as the personality. The personality of an ill person can be judged effectively only from reliable accounts of past behaviour, obtained wherever possible from informants as well as from the patient.

Some assessment instruments for personality were mentioned in the section on personality types (p. 158). It might be supposed that these and similar standardized tests would give better information about personality than the clinician could obtain. However, although personality tests are more reliable in healthy people, their results can be affected by the presence of mental disorder. Also, they do not measure the traits that are most relevant to clinical practice. For this reason, tests of personality, although useful in research, are seldom used in clinical practice. (Some standardized assessment instruments for personality disorder are considered on p. 65.)

For a review of methods of assessment of personality see Skodol and Oldham (1991) and Westen (1997).

The importance of personality assessment

As explained in the introduction to this chapter, the assessment of personality is important in decisions about aetiology, diagnosis, and treatment. In aetiology, knowledge of personality helps to explain why certain events are stressful to the patient. In diagnosis, an understanding of personality may explain the presence of unusual features in a disorder, which would otherwise cause uncertainty. In treatment, an assessment of personality helps understanding of the way that patients react to illness and to its treatment. Personality should be assessed in every case and not just in those where there is a disorder of personality (i.e. an extreme deviation from the normal – see below).

The assessment is recorded best with a series of descriptive terms. This is because the personality factors are too general to convey the information that is important to the clinician. Examples of such descriptions are sensitive, lacking in self-confidence, and prone to worry unreasonably; or abnormally aggressive with little remorse or concern for others. Descriptions of this kind are useful in constructing a picture of the unique features of each patient, an activity which is at the basis of good clinical practice.

Personality disorder
The concept of abnormal personality

Some personalities are obviously abnormal, for example, paranoid personalities characterized by extreme suspiciousness, sensitivity, and mistrust. It is, however, impossible to draw a sharp dividing line between normal and abnormal personalities. Indeed, it is even difficult to decide what criterion should be used to make this distinction. Two kinds of criteria have been suggested, the first statistical and the second social.

On the *statistical criterion*, abnormal personalities are quantitative variations from the normal and the dividing line is decided by a cut-off score on an appropriate measure. In principle, this scheme is attractive as it parallels the approach used successfully in defining abnormalities of intelligence, and it has obvious value in research. However, it is of limited value in clinical work with individual patients.

When a *social criterion* is used, abnormal personalities are those that cause the individual to suffer, or cause suffering to other people. For example, an abnormally sensitive and gloomy personality causes suffering for the individual, and an emotionally cold and aggressive personality causes suffering for others. Although such criteria are subjective and lack the precision of the first approach, they correspond well to the realities of clinical practice and they have been adopted widely.

Given the conceptual problems, it is not surprising that it is difficult to frame a satisfactory definition of abnormal personality. In ICD-9, personality disorders were described as follows:

severe disturbances in the personality and behavioural tendencies of the individual, not directly resulting from disease, damage or other insult to the brain, or from another psychiatric disorder. They usually involve several areas of the personality and are nearly always associated with considerable personal distress and social disruption. They are usually manifest since childhood or adolescence and continue throughout adulthood.

ICD-10 has a somewhat different definition in terms of enduring patterns of behaviour, but the ICD-9 definition is more concise, and still valuable.

It can be added that the personal distress referred to in the ICD-9 definition may become apparent only late in the course of the condition (for example, when a long-standing supportive relationship is lost), and that there are usually, though not always, significant problems in occupational and social performance.

Whilst definitions naturally focus on abnormal features, it is important to recognize that people with abnormal personalities generally have favourable as well as unfavourable traits. The clinician should always assess positive as well as unfavourable features, since it may be possible to build on the former in a plan of management.

Personality change

In some circumstances during adult life, there may be a profound and enduring change in personality, distinct from the temporary changes in behaviour that may accompany stressful events or illness. These lasting changes may result from:

- injury to or organic disease of the brain;

- severe mental disorder, especially schizophrenia;

- exceptionally severe stressful experiences, for example, those experienced by hostages or prisoners undergoing torture.

In ICD-10, *change in personality due to organic disease of the brain* is classified with the organic mental disorders in section F00, which contains a category for personality and behavioural disorders due to brain disease, damage, and dysfunction. Examples include the changes in personality following encephalitis and head injury. In DSM-IV this condition is diagnosed as personality change due to a general medical condition.

In ICD-10 the other two forms of personality change listed above are classified in section F60, disorders of adult personality and behaviour. To diagnose *enduring personality change after psychiatric illness*, the change of personality must have

lasted for at least 2 years, be clearly related to the experience of the illness, and not present before it. The person with this condition may, for example, be dependent, passive, and demanding, or socially withdrawn and isolated because of the (non-delusional) conviction of being changed or stigmatized. The authors of ICD noted that the change must be understandable in terms of the person's experiences during the illness, and his previous attitudes, adjustment, and life situation. However, it is generally thought that schizophrenic illness can change personality directly as well as in these indirect ways.

In ICD10, *enduring personality change after a catastrophic experience* must also have lasted for at least 2 years. The stressful experience must have been extreme, for example, a disaster, prolonged captivity with the imminent possibility of being killed, being the victim of terrorism, torture, or confinement in a concentration camp. The person with this condition is hostile, irritable, distrustful, and socially withdrawn, and feels empty, hopeless, estranged, and on edge. These features were not present before the experience and, although the condition may follow post-traumatic stress disorder, it is separate from it.

How ideas about abnormal personality developed

In psychiatry the concept of abnormal personality can be traced to the beginning of the nineteenth century, when the French psychiatrist Pinel described *manie sans délire*. Pinel applied this term to patients who were prone to outbursts of rage and violence but were not deluded (at that time delusions were regarded as the hallmark of mental illness, and *délire* is the French term for delusion). Presumably this group of patients included not only those who would now be regarded as having an antisocial personality, but also some who were mentally ill but not deluded, for example, some manic patients. (See Kavka 1949 for a translation of the relevant section of the second edition of Pinel's book, first published in 1801.)

Although other writers, such as the American Benjamin Rush, were interested in similar clinical problems, it was an English physician who took the next important step forward. In 1835, J. C. Prichard, senior physician to the Bristol Infirmary, published his *A treatise on insanity* and other disorders of the mind. After referring to Pinel's *manie sans délire*, he suggested a new term, moral insanity, which he defined as a

morbid perversion of the natural feelings, affections, inclinations, temper, habits, moral dispositions and natural impulses without any remarkable disorder or defect of the intellect or knowing or reasoning faculties and in particular without any insane delusion or hallucination. (Prichard 1835, p. 6)

Although this description included the violent patients described by Pinel, Prichard clearly had a wider group in mind, since he added:

a propensity to theft is sometimes a feature of moral insanity and sometimes it is its leading if not sole characteristic. (p. 27)

Prichard's category of moral insanity, like Pinel's *manie sans délire*, seems to have included some affective disorders, for he wrote:

a considerable proportion among the most striking instances of moral insanity are those in which a tendency to gloom or sorrow is the predominant feature. (p. 18)

He added:

a state of gloom and melancholy depression occasionally gives way to the opposite condition of preternatural excitement. (p. 19)

Prichard's moral insanity included conditions we would now diagnose as personality disorder. However, he did not confine the term to people who had always behaved in these ways:

When however such phenomena are observed in connection with a wayward and intractable temper, with a decay of social affections, an aversion to the nearest relatives and friends formerly beloved – in short, with a change in the moral character of the individual, the case becomes tolerably well marked.

In this passage the reference to change in character indicates that Prichard had in mind not only conditions we would classify as personality disorder but also some that we would classify as mental disorder.

Later in the nineteenth century, it was recognized that mental illness could occur without delusions and the concept of moral insanity took on a more restricted meaning. Thus, Henry Maudsley applied the term to someone whom he described as having

no capacity for true moral feeling – all his impulses and desires, to which he yields without check, are egoistic, his conduct appears to be governed by immoral motives, which are cherished and obeyed without any evident desire to resist them. (Maudsley 1885, p. 171)

Maudsley commented on the current dissatisfaction with the term moral insanity, which he referred to as

a form of mental alienation which has so much the look of vice or crime that many people regard it is an unfounded medical invention. (p. 170)

The next step towards modern ideas was the introduction by Koch (1891) of the term psychopathic inferiority to denote this same group of people who have marked abnormalities of behaviour in the absence of mental illness or intellectual impairment. (Later, the word inferiority was replaced by personality to avoid judgemental overtones.) Kraepelin was, at first, uncertain how to classify these people, and it was not until the eighth edition of his textbook that he finally adopted the term psychopathic personality and devoted a long chapter to it. He included not only the antisocial type but also six others: the excitable, unstable, quarrelsome, and eccentric, together with liars and swindlers.

Kurt Schneider broadened the concept of psychopathic personality. Whereas Kraepelin's seven types of psychopathic personality applied to people causing inconvenience, annoyance, or suffering to other people, Schneider included as well people who suffered themselves. For example, he included people with markedly depressive or insecure characters. Thus, in Schneider's usage, psychopathic personality covered the whole range of abnormal personality, not just antisocial personality. In this way the term came to have two meanings: the wider meaning of abnormal personality of all kinds, and the narrower meaning of antisocial personality.

Confusion about the term psychopathic personality does not end with Schneider's broader definition. Two other usages call for attention. The first originated in the work of the Scottish psychiatrist, Sir David Henderson, who in 1939 published the influential book *Psychopathic states*. He defined psychopaths as people who, although not mentally subnormal,

throughout their lives or from a comparatively early age, have exhibited disorders of conduct of an antisocial or asocial nature, usually of a recurrent or episodic type which in many instances have proved difficult to influence by methods of social, penal and medical care or for whom we have no adequate provision of a preventative or curative nature.

So far this definition corresponds to the previous narrow concept of psychopathic personality. However, Henderson extended his definition by referring to three groups of psychopaths:

- *predominantly aggressive* personalities, including not only those who are repeatedly aggressive, but also those prone to suicide, drug addiction, and alcohol abuse;

- *passive and inadequate* personalities, included unstable, hypochondriacal, and sensitive people, pathological liars, and those with a schizoid nature;

- *creative psychopaths*, a group so wide that it is of little value. Henderson gave as examples T. E. Lawrence and Joan of Arc who, though both creative, had little else in common.

Henderson's main contribution was to draw attention to the group of inadequate personalities.

Yet another variation in the meaning of the term psychopathic was introduced in the 1959 Mental Health Act for England and Wales. In this Act, psychopathic disorder was defined in Section 4(4) as

a persistent disorder or disability of mind (whether or not including subnormality of intelligence) which results in abnormally aggressive or seriously irresponsible conduct on the part of the patient, and requires or is susceptible to medical treatment.

This definition was a return to the narrow concept of aggressive or irresponsible behaviour causing suffering to other people. However, the definition is unsatisfactory because it includes the criterion of requirement for or response to treatment, which may be administratively convenient but certainly illogical. Not surprisingly, many difficulties have attended the use of this definition. (In Britain new mental health legislation is under discussion at the time of writing).

The two meanings of psychopathic personality – the wider meaning of all abnormal personality, and the narrower meaning of antisocial personality – persist to the present day. Because the term psychopathic personality is ambiguous, the preferred terms are personality disorder and antisocial personality disorder to denote the wide and narrow senses, respectively.

The classification of abnormal personalities

General issues

The use of categories

Personality is a continuous variable but systems for the classification of psychiatric disorders use categories that require cut-off points. Categories are useful when cases have to be counted in epidemiological studies and clinical audit. However, the chosen criterion – distress to the person or to others – is both arbitrary and imprecise, and cases that just fall short of it (subthreshold cases) are frequent and often present clinical problems similar to those of definite cases.

Co-morbidity

It is not only the boundary between normal and abnormal personality that is imprecise and arbitrary; the boundaries between different types of personality are also ill defined. In addition, many patients have features contained among the criteria for more than one personality disorder (see Fyer *et al.* 1988). When more than one personality diagnosis can be made in a single patient, the term co-morbidity is used. The same term is used when a patient meets the criteria for both a mental disorder and a personality disorder. In the latter case, it can be argued that two separate conditions are present but when two personality disorders can be diagnosed, the same cannot be maintained convincingly. It seems more likely, that the patient has a single personality disorder which has features which overlap two of the arbitrary sets of criteria used in the current systems of diagnosis.

Conditions related to personality disorder and classified elsewhere

Cyclothymia and schizotypal disorder were previously classified as personality disorders on the grounds that they are long-lasting patterns of behaviour that can cause distress. In ICD-10 both have been removed from the personality disorders and classified instead with the mental disorders: cyclothymia with affective disorders, schizotypal disorder with schizophrenia. This arrangement takes account of the fact that these two conditions may begin in adult life, after the time when personality has developed fully. In DSM-IV, cyclothymic disorder is classified with mood disorders, but schizotypal disorder is retained as a personality disorder. In both classifications, multiple personality disorder is classified with dissociative disorders (see p. 264).

Classification of personality disorders in ICD-10 and DSM-IV

In Table 7.1, the classification of personality disorders in ICD-10 is compared with that in DSM-IV. The two schemes are broadly similar but the following differences should be noted.

The use of Axis II

In DSM-IV, personality disorders are classified on a different 'axis' (Axis II) from mental disorders (classified on Axis I). This arrangement recognizes the different nature of the two diagnoses and it

Table 7.1 Classification of personality disorders

ICD–10	DSM-IV
Paranoid	Paranoid
Schizoid	Schizoid
(Schizotypal, see text)	Schizotypal
Dissocial	Antisocial
Emotionally unstable Impulsive type Borderline type	Borderline
Histrionic	Histrionic
–	Narcissistic
Anankastic (obsessive-compulsive)	Obsessive–compulsive
Anxious (avoidant)	Avoidant
Dependent	Dependent
–	Passive–aggressive

encourages a search for personality disorder in every case. This convention is not adopted in ICD-10. (If no personality disorder is present, the normal personality should still be assessed for the reasons given earlier in this chapter and recorded in the formulation even though it cannot be included among the diagnoses).

Grouping into clusters

In DSM-IV, but not in ICD-10, personality disorders are grouped into three 'clusters':

- *cluster A* paranoid, schizoid, schizotypal;
- *cluster B* antisocial, borderline, histrionic, narcissistic;
- *cluster C* avoidant, dependent, obsessive–compulsive.

This useful convention is adopted later in this chapter.

Different names for the same personality disorder:

- In ICD-10 the term dissocial is used for the personality disorder referred to as antisocial in

DSM-IV (the term antisocial is used in this book).

- In ICD-10 anankastic is the preferred term for the personality disorder called obsessive–compulsive in DSM-IV.
- In ICD-10 anxious is the preferred term for the personality disorder called avoidant in DSM-IV.

Categories included in one system only:

Present in ICD-10 but not in DSMIV

- Emotionally unstable impulsive personality disorder.
- Enduring personality change, not attributable to brain damage or disease (see above).

Present in DSM-IV but not in ICD-10

- Narcissistic personality disorder.
- Passive aggressive personality disorder (listed as a category for further study).

Conditions classified differently in DSM-IV and ICD-10

As noted above, schizotypal personality disorder is classified with schizophrenia in ICD-10 (and named schizotypal disorder). In DSM-IV it is classified as a personality disorder.

Descriptions and diagnostic criteria

This section contains an account of the abnormal personalities listed in the ICD-10 and DSM-IV (see Table 7.1). The criteria for diagnosis are lengthy and differ somewhat in wording and emphasis in the two systems. The following description refers to the main common features of the two sets of definitions and, where appropriate, has simplified or paraphrased the criteria to present a more general description of the personality disorder.

In each case the condition must meet the general criteria for personality disorder for which the ICD-10 criteria for research (see p. 97) can be summarized as follows:

- the person's characteristic and enduring patterns of behaviour deviate markedly from the cultural norm, with deviation in more than one of the areas of cognition (i.e. attitudes and ways of perceiving and interpreting), affectivity, control of impulses and gratification, and ways of relating to others;
- the deviation is pervasive, and the behaviour is inflexible, and maladaptive or dysfunctional in a broad range of situations;
- there is personal distress or an adverse impact on others;
- the deviation is stable and long-lasting, beginning usually in late childhood or adolescence;
- the deviant behaviour is not caused by another mental disorder;
- the deviant behaviour is not caused by brain injury, disease, or dysfunction.

There are several diagnostic instruments (see Appendix, p. 184). They are of value in research, but less useful in clinical practice

Cluster A personality disorders

Paranoid personality disorder (Table 7.2)

People with this kind of abnormal personality are suspicious and sensitive. They have a marked sense of self-importance, but easily feel shame and humiliation. They are suspicious and constantly on the lookout for attempts by others to deceive them or play tricks on them. As a result, other people

Table 7.2 **Features of a paranoid personality disorder**
Suspicious
Mistrustful
Jealous
Sensitive
Resentful
Bears grudges
Self-important

find them difficult and unreasonable. These people are mistrustful and jealous. They doubt the loyalty of other people and do not trust them. Sexual jealousy is common. They do not make friends easily and avoid involvement in groups. They appear secretive, devious, and self-sufficient to a fault. They take offence easily and see rebuffs where none is intended. Presented with a new proposal, they look for ways in which it might be designed to harm their interests.

These people are *sensitive* to rebuff, prickly, and argumentative. They read demeaning or threatening meanings into innocent remarks. Kretschmer described how such people's sensitivity leads to feelings of humiliation and to suspicious ideas so intense that they can be mistaken for persecutory delusions. These '*sensitive ideas of reference*' are considered further in Chapter 13. These people are also *resentful and bear grudges*, and they do not forgive real or perceived insults. They have a strong sense of their rights and may engage in litigation, with which they may persist long after others would have abandoned the case.

Paranoid personalities have a strong sense of *self-importance*. They believe that they are unusually talented and capable of great achievements. This unrealistic idea is maintained, despite modest accomplishments, by beliefs that others have prevented them from fulfilling their potential.

Schizoid personality disorder (Table 7.3)

The name schizoid was suggested by Kretschmer (1936), who believed that this type of personality is related to schizophrenia but the idea has not been confirmed (see Chapter 12) People with this disorder are emotionally cold, detached, aloof, humourless, introspective, and prone to engage in fantasy.

These people are emotionally cold and incapable of expressing either tender feelings or anger. They show little interest in sexual relationships. When the disorder is extreme, they appear cold and callous. They are *detached and aloof* and show little concern for the opinions of other people. They are ill at ease in company, do not make intimate relationships, and show little satisfaction in membership of a family group. They are seclusive, following a solitary course through life, and often remain unmarried. These people also *lack a sense of enjoyment,* have little sense of humour, and take little pleasure in activities that most people enjoy. These qualities contribute to their separation from other people.

These people are *introspective and prone to fantasy.* They are more interested in intellectual matters than in people. They have a complex inner world of fantasy, although this lacks emotional content.

Schizotypal personality disorder

People with schizotypal personality disorder are socially anxious, experience cognitive and perceptual distortions, show oddities of speech and inappropriate affective responses, and behave eccentrically. This personality disorder appears to be related to schizophrenia, and in ICD-10 (but not DSM-IV) it is not classified as a personality disorder but placed with schizophrenia and called schizotypal disorder.

These people have *social anxiety*. They feel anxious in company so that they have difficulty in making relationships and lack friends and confidants. They feel different from other people and do not fit in. *Cognitive and perceptual distortions* include ideas (but not delusions) of reference, suspicious ideas, odd beliefs, and magical thinking (for example, belief in clairvoyance, mind reading, and telepathy), and unusual perceptual experiences (for example, awareness of a presence, or experiences bordering on hallucinations). They also show *oddities of speech* such as unusual constructions, words and phrasing, as well as vagueness, and a tendency to digression.

Table 7.3 **Features of schizoid personality disorder**
Emotionally cold
Detached
Aloof
Lacking enjoyment
Introspective

Their *affective responses are unusual* and they appear stiff, odd, and constricted in their emotions. Their *behaviour is eccentric* with odd mannerisms, unusual choices of clothing, disregard of conventions, and awkward social behaviour.

Cluster B personality disorders

Antisocial (dissocial) personality disorder

The term antisocial is used in DSM-IV; dissocial is the term in ICD-10. In this book, the term antisocial is preferred. People with this disorder show a callous lack of concern for the feelings of others. They disregard the rights of others, act impulsively, lack guilt, and fail to learn from adverse experiences (Table 7.4). Often their abnormal behaviour is made worse by the abuse of alcohol or drugs. An influential description of this type of personality disorder was written in 1941 by Cleckley in his book *The mask of sanity* (see Cleckley 1964).

The criteria for diagnosis differ slightly in the two classifications; the following are taken from ICD-10. The DSM-IV criteria include the requirement of conduct disorder before the age of 15 years.

These people have a *callous lack of concern for others*. Their sexual activity is without tender feelings. They may inflict cruel or degrading acts on other people, including the sexual partner and any children, who may be physically or sexually abused. Their *relationships are shallow and short-lived* despite their superficial charm. They are *irresponsible and depart from social norms*. They do not obey rules and may repeatedly break the law, often committing violent offences. Their offending typically begins in adolescence.

These people are *impulsive*. They lack goals, do not plan ahead, and typically have an unstable work record marked by frequent dismissals. They take risks, disregarding their own safety and that of other people. They are *irritable* and when angry sometimes assault others in a violent way. These features of personality are accompanied by a striking *lack of guilt or remorse* and a failure to change their behaviour in response to punishment or other adverse outcomes. They *avoid responsibility*, transferring blame onto other people, and rationalizing their own failures. They are also deceitful and irresponsible about finances.

Borderline personality disorder

The term borderline personality was used originally to describe people who show marked 'instability'. This instability was originally described in psychodynamic terms, notably by Kernberg (1975), as involving (a) ego weakness, with poor control of impulses, (b) 'primary process' (i.e. irrational) thinking despite intact reality testing, (c) use of less 'mature' defence mechanisms such as projection and denial, and (d) diffuse personal identity.

When this type of personality disorder was recognized in the classification systems, more objective criteria were developed, but it proved difficult to isolate a few core features. Also, different names have been adopted in the two systems of classification: in DSM-IV the term is borderline personality disorder, whereas in ICD-10 the term is emotionally unstable personality disorder. The latter is divided into a borderline type and an impulsive type. In DSM-IV borderline personality disorder is characterized by nine features, of which five are required to make a DSM-IV diagnosis. In ICD-10 there are five criteria for each subtype and four are required for diagnosis. The criteria are shown in summary form in Table 7.5 using terms that summarize those in the published criteria but do not repeat the exact wording. Table 7.5 shows that several features of the ICD-10 impulsive type are

Table 7.4 Features of antisocial personality disorder
Callous
Transient relationships
Irresponsible
Impulsive and irritable
Lack guilt and remorse
Fail to accept responsibility

Table 7.5 Abbreviated criteria for emotionally unstable and for borderline personality disorders

ICD–10 **Emotionally unstable personality disorder**	DSM-IV **Borderline personality disorder**
Borderline type	
Disturbed or uncertain self-image	Identity disturbance
Intense and unstable relationships	Intense and unstable relationships
Efforts to avoid abandonment	Efforts to avoid abandonment
Recurrent threats or acts of self-harm	Recurrent suicidal behaviour
Chronic feelings of emptiness	Chronic feelings of emptiness
–	Transient stress-related paranoid ideation
Impulsive type	
Impulsive	Impulsive
Liability to anger and violence	Difficulty controlling anger
Unstable, capricious mood	Affective instability
Quarrelsome	–
Difficulty maintaining a course of action	–

among the criteria for borderline personality disorder in DSM-IV.

Despite these attempts to define a borderline personality disorder, it is uncertain whether it exists as a separate entity. Many people who meet the criteria for borderline personality disorder in DSM-IV also meet the criteria for histrionic, narcissistic, and antisocial personality disorder (Pope *et al.* 1983; Oldham *et al.* 1992).

Impulsive personality disorder

As explained above, this disorder is recognized in ICD-10 as a subtype of emotionally labile personality disorder. It is not included separately in DSM-IV though several of its features are listed as criteria for borderline personality disorder. Diagnostic criteria are shown in Table 7.5; three are required to make the diagnosis People with impulsive personality disorder cannot control their emotions adequately. They are liable to sudden unrestrained anger, which they regret subsequently. These outbursts are not always confined to words, but may include physical violence, which may at times cause serious harm. Unlike people with antisocial personality disorder, who also exhibit explosions of anger, the impulsive group does not have other difficulties in relationships.

Histrionic personality disorder

Although histrionic personality disorder is included in both ICD-10 and DSM-IV, the criteria adopted are somewhat different. Table 7.6 shows the features that are diagnostic criteria in ICD-10 and notes also the criteria which differ between the two systems.

Self-dramatization is a striking feature of this personality disorder. It may extend to emotional 'blackmail', angry scenes, and demonstrative suicide attempts. These people are *suggestible* and easily influenced by others, especially by figures of

Table 7.6 **Features of histrionic personality disorder**
Self dramatization
Suggestibility
Shallow, labile affect
Seeks attention and excitement
Inappropriately seductive
Over-concern with physical attractiveness
Note DSM-IV has two additional criteria: • speech excessively impressionistic; and • considers relationships more intimate than they are

Table 7.7 **Features of narcissistic personality disorder**
Grandiose self-importance
Fantasizes unlimited success, power, etc.
Believes himself special
Requires excessive admiration
Sense of entitlement to favours and compliance
Exploits others
Lacks empathy
Envious; believes others envy him
Arrogant and haughty

authority. They follow the tastes and opinions of others, and adopt the latest fads and fashions. These people *seek attention and excitement*. They crave new experiences, are easily bored, and have short-lived enthusiasms.

These people have a *shallow labile affect*. They display their emotions in a dramatic manner, and may exhaust others with tantrums of rage or unrestrained expressions of despair. There is little depth to these emotional outpourings and they recover quickly, and seem surprised that other people have not forgotten the scenes as quickly as they have done. They are flirtatious and *inappropriately seductive*, but their sexual feelings, like their other emotions, are shallow and they may fail to reach orgasm despite elaborate displays of passion.

These people are *overconcerned with physical attractiveness*. In an attempt to impress others they spend excessive amounts of time and money on clothes, and personal grooming, and they are unreasonably upset by even minor criticism of their appearance.

As well as the above features, which are used as diagnostic criteria, two other aspects of the histrionic personality disorder deserve mention. These people are *self-centred*. They lack consideration for others, and put their own interests and enjoyment first. They appear vain, inconsiderate, and demanding, and may go to extreme lengths to force other people to fall in with their wishes. They also have a marked capacity for *self-deception*. They

believe their own lies, however elaborate and improbable, even when other people have seen through the deceit. This pattern of behaviour is observed in its most extreme form in 'pathological liars' and swindlers.

Since some of the above qualities are normal in children (for example, transient enthusiasms, and make-believe), some psychiatrists have applied the term 'immature' to this type of personality disorder. However, the term should be avoided because it is imprecise and pejorative.

Narcissistic personality disorder

This personality disorder is listed in DSM-IV but not in ICD-10 where it is one of the disorders coded in the residual category 'other specific personality disorder'. The DSM-IV criteria are summarized and paraphrased in Table 7.7.

People with this disorder have a grandiose sense of self-importance and are boastful and pretentious. They are preoccupied with fantasies of unlimited success, power, beauty, or intellectual brilliance. They think themselves special and expect others to admire them and offer special services and favours. They feel entitled to the best and seek to associate with people of high status. They exploit people and do not empathize with, or show concern for, their feelings. They envy the possessions and achievements of others, and expect that others will envy them in the same way. They appear arrogant,

Table 7.8 **Features of avoidant (anxious) personality disorder**
Feelings of tension*
Feels socially inferior
Preoccupied with rejection
Avoids involvement
Avoids risk
Avoids social activity
Note DSM-IV has two additional criteria: • restraint in intimate relationships because of fear of being shamed or ridiculed; and • inhibited in new personal situations because of feelings of inadequacy. *Not a DSM-IV criterion.

Table 7.9 **Features of dependent personality disorder**
Allows others to take responsibility
Unduly compliant
Unwilling to make reasonable demands*
Feels unable to care for himself
Fear of being left to care for himself
Needs excessive help to make decisions
Note Three additional criteria are used in DSM-IV. They can be summarized as: • difficulty in initiating projects; • goes to excessive lengths to obtain support; and • urgently seeks a supportive relationship. *Not a criterion in DSM-IV.

disdainful, and haughty, and behave in a patronizing or condescending way.

Cluster C personality disorders

Avoidant (anxious) personality disorder

In DSM-IV the term avoidant is used to denote this kind of personality disorder, whilst in ICD-10 the term anxious personality is preferred, with 'avoidant' as an accepted alternative. Slightly different features are used as diagnostic criteria in the two classifications, as shown in Table 7.8 in which the features are summarized. Liability to tension is a criterion only in ICD-10.

People with this disorder are *persistently tense*. They feel insecure and lack self-esteem. They feel *socially inferior*, unappealing, and socially inept. They are *preoccupied with the possibility of rejection*, disapproval, or criticism, and worry that they will be embarrassed or ridiculed. They are cautious about new experiences and *avoid involvement* with unfamiliar people. They are timid in the face of everyday hazards and *avoid risk*. They are ill at ease in company and *avoid social activity*. They have few close friends, are inhibited in new personal situations, and their intimate relationships are constrained by fears of being shamed or ridiculed. Unlike people with schizoid personalities, they are

not emotionally cold; indeed, they crave the social relationships that they cannot attain.

Dependent personality disorder

Table 7.9 shows that the features used as diagnostic criteria differ slightly in ICD-10 and DSM-IV. People with this disorder *allow others to take responsibility* for important decisions in their lives. They appear weak-willed and *unduly compliant* with the wishes of others. Nevertheless, they are *unwilling to make direct demands* on other people, but do this indirectly by appearing unable to help themselves. They lack vigour and *feel unable to care for themselves* and fear that they may have to do so. They lack self-reliance, avoid responsibility, and need *excessive help to make decisions*, asking repeatedly for advice and reassurance.

If married, such people may be protected from the full effects of their personality by support from a more energetic and determined spouse who is willing to make decisions and arrange activities. Their difficulties come to medical attention only when the spouse leaves or dies. Left to themselves, some drift down the social scale and are found among the long-term unemployed and the homeless. In the past this type of personality was called asthenic, inadequate, or passive.

Table 7.10 **Features of obsessive–compulsive (anankastic) personality disorder**

Preoccupied with details, rules, etc.

Inhibited by perfectionism

Overconscientious and scrupulous

Excessively concerned with productivity

Rigid and stubborn

Expects others to submit to his ways

Excessively pedantic and bound by convention*

Excessively doubting and cautious*

Note DSM-IV has two additional criteria:
- cannot discard worthless or worn out objects; and
- miserly; hoards money.

* These are not included in the DSM-IV criteria.

Obsessive–compulsive personality disorder

The term obsessive–compulsive personality disorder is used in DSM-IV. In ICD-10 the term anankastic (originated by Kahn 1928), is used to avoid the false implication that this type of personality is directly linked to obsessional-compulsive disorder (see p. 243–4). Table 7.10 shows that slightly different features are used as diagnostic criteria in ICD-10 and DSM-IV.

These people are *preoccupied with details and rules*, order and schedules. They have an *inhibiting perfectionism* that makes ordinary work a burden and leaves the person immersed in trivial detail. They lack imagination and fail to take advantage of opportunities. They have high moral standards evident as *excessive conscientiousness and scruples*, and a judgemental approach. These characteristics stifle enjoyment so that these people seem humourless and are ill at ease when others are enjoying themselves. They are *unduly concerned with productivity at work* to the exclusion of relationships.

These people lack adaptability to new situations. They are *rigid and inflexible*; they dislike change and prefer a safe and familiar routine. They are and *stubborn and controlling*, expecting others to submit to their ways They are mean, sometimes to the point of being miserly, and they do not enjoy giving or receiving gifts. They do not like throwing things away and may hoard objects and money.

They are *pedantic and unduly concerned with social conventions*. Such people display *excessive doubt and caution* and they are indecisive. They find it hard to weigh up the advantages and disadvantages of new situations; they delay decisions, and often ask for more and more advice. They fear making mistakes, and after coming to a decision, they worry lest the choice was wrong.

Two other features are important, though they are not used as diagnostic criteria. *Sensitivity to criticism* is shown in an undue concern about other people's opinions, and an expectation of being judged harshly. These people show little emotion. They are, however, given to smouldering and unexpressed *feelings of anger and resentment*, often directed to people who have interfered with their routine of life. Such angry feelings may be accompanied by obsessional thoughts and images of an aggressive kind, even in those who do not develop the full syndrome of an obsessional disorder.

Passive–aggressive personality disorder

This term is applied to a person who, when demands are made upon him for adequate performance, responds with some form of passive resistance, such as procrastination, dawdling, stubbornness, deliberate inefficiency, pretended forgetfulness, and unreasonable criticism of people in authority. The category does not appear among the personality disorders in ICD-10 or DSM-IV.

Affective personality disorders

Some people have lifelong disorders of mood regulation. They may be persistently gloomy (depressive personality disorder) or habitually in a state of inappropriate elation (hyperthymic personality disorder). A third group alternates between these two extremes (cycloid or cyclothymic personality disorder). These types of personality disorder have been described for many years and are readily recognized in clinical practice. However, they do not appear in either the ICD-10 or DSM-IV systems of classification. The reason is that in both systems these disorders are classified under disorders of mood and not under disorders of personality. Thus they are classified under 'persistent mood (affective) states' (cyclothymia or dysthymia) in ICD-10, and under cyclothymia or dysthymia in DSM-IV. Nevertheless, it is convenient to describe them briefly here.

People with *depressive personality disorder* always seem to be in low spirits. They take a persistently gloomy view of life, anticipating the worst outcome of every event. They brood about their misfortunes and worry unduly. They often have a strong sense of duty. They show little capacity for enjoyment and they express dissatisfaction with their lives. Some are irritable and bad-tempered.

People with *hyperthymic personality disorder* are habitually cheerful and optimistic, and show a striking zest for living. If they have these traits to a moderate degree, they are often effective and successful. If they have these traits to an extreme degree, they show poor judgement and may be uncritical and hasty in coming to conclusions. Their habitual cheerfulness is often interrupted by periods of irritability, especially when their aims are frustrated. In the past, exceptionally contentious people in this group were called pseudoquerulant.

People with *cycloid personality disorder* alternate between the extremes of depressive and hyperthymic states described above. This instability of mood is much more disruptive than either of the persisting conditions. People with this disorder are periodically extremely cheerful, active, and productive. At such times they take on additional commitments in their work and social lives. Eventually their mood changes. Instead of confident optimism, they have a gloomy defeatist approach to life. Their energy is reduced. Whereas in the elated phase they took up activities with much relish, now they find them a burden. They make different but equally unwise decisions, and they refuse opportunities that could be managed. Eventually they return to a normal mood or to further elation.

Terms to avoid

It has been explained above that the term psychopathic personality is unsatisfactory (see pp. 163–4). Two other commonly used terms are also unsatisfactory and should be avoided. Both tend to be used when the doctor has not thought clearly enough about the precise nature of his patient's difficulties. The first, inadequate personality, is often used pejoratively. In place of this term, it is better to specify precisely the ways in which the person is inadequate to the demands of life. Such a specification will lead to more constructive ideas about helping the person to cope better.

The second term, immature personality, is often used vaguely to denote a non-specific discrepancy between the patient's behaviour and his chronological age, such that the behaviour is more appropriate to a younger person than to a person of the patient's age. To avoid the vagueness of the term immature, it is better to specify the exact nature of the problem, whether it is in social relationships, the control of emotions, willingness to take responsibility, or elsewhere. Such specification of the patient's problems is more likely to lead to a constructive approach than is the mere labelling of the personality as immature. It also avoids the implication of an unsubstantiated cause, namely a failure of maturation.

Epidemiology

Epidemiological research into personality disorders in the general population began after the development of standardized instruments using DSM-III criteria. The studies require large samples because the prevalence rates of some personality disorders are low. Also, it is difficult to identify personality disorder reliably in community surveys in which interviewers seldom have access to information from informants. Data come mainly from eight studies in the USA, the UK, and Germany (reviewed by de Girolamo and Gotto 2000).

Estimates of the *total prevalence* (i.e. the sum of all types) of personality disorders vary from about 6 to 15% in the eight studies. Rates are generally higher in urban than in rural populations (see, for example, Casey and Tyrer 1986). The overall rates of personality disorder are about the same in men and women and decrease with age.

Higher overall rates of personality disorder have been reported in *patients with psychiatric symptoms.* Among those attending a general practitioner the rate is similar to that in the general population, about 5–8%. The rate rises to 30% in those with conspicuous psychiatric morbidity (Casey *et al.* 1984). Among psychiatric out-patients and in-patients, overall rates of personality disorders of up to 50% have been reported (see de Girolamo and Gotto 2000).

Estimates of the prevalence of the various types of personality disorder are shown in Table 7.11. In these studies sample sizes ranged from 200 to 1600. Some of these estimates have a substantial range, reflecting, among other sources of variation, the use of different assessment instruments. Rates of some disorders vary between men and women: antisocial personality disorder is more common among men (estimated ratios vary between 2.1 and

7.1). Although borderline and histrionic personality disorders are often described as more frequent among women, this was not a consistent finding in these studies.

Aetiology

General issues

The causes of personality disorder are largely unknown. Genetic factors have been proposed, together with various kinds of early life experience. Some personality disorders have been linked aetiologically with the psychiatric disorders which they resemble.

Genetic causes are considered below, where the aetiology of particular kinds of personality disorder is outlined. The study of the influence of *early life experiences* is made difficult by the long interval between these experiences and diagnosis of personality disorder in adult life. This lack of scientific studies has allowed the growth of theories based on the retrospective accounts of adults, or on psychoanalytic interpretations. Such theories are

Table 7.11 Median prevalence rates of personality disorders in epidemiological surveys

Personality cluster	Personality disorder	Number of studies	Rate (%)
Cluster A	Paranoid	8	0.6
	Schizoid	9	0.4
	Schizotypal	8	0.6
Cluster B	Antisocial	18	1.9
	Borderline	9	1.6
	Histrionic	8	2.0
Cluster C	Obsessive–compulsive	8	1.7
	Avoidant	7	0.7
	Dependent	8	0.7
	Passive–aggressive	7	1.7

Data from de Girolamo and Dotto (2000).

mentioned in the account that follows because they have been influential in the recent past. However, they are not supported by evidence.

Despite the scientific weakness of psychoanalytic theories, most clinicians accept that there is some aetiological link between childhood experience and personality disorder. It is agreed good practice to assess childhood experiences and use common-sense judgement to decide whether any of these experiences could be a cause of the abnormalities of personality. For example, extreme and repeated rejection by the parents might explain low self-esteem.

The relationship between some *personality disorders and mental disorder* has already been considered. The similarity between schizoid personality disorder and some features of schizophrenia led to the suggestion that the former is a partial expression of the latter. A similar relationship was proposed between cyclothymic personality and manic–depressive disorder, and between obsessional personality disorder and obsessive–compulsive disorder. Until more is known about the causes of these three psychiatric disorders, these theories about their relationship to personality disorders do not add to knowledge of the latter.

Since rather different causes have been suggested for the various types of personality disorder, they are considered separately below. Antisocial personality disorder is considered first because more research has been reported on this than on the other disorders. The rest are considered in the order in which they were described earlier in the chapter.

Antisocial personality disorder

Genetic causes

Twin studies The much quoted early twin studies by Lange (1931) and Rosanoff (1934) were concerned with probands with repeated conviction for criminal offences, rather than antisocial personality disorder, so that their relevance to the latter is uncertain. More recent twin studies have confirmed the heritability of antisocial behaviour in adults and shown that genetic factors are more important in adults than in antisocial children or adolescents where shared environmental factors are more important (Lyons *et al.* 1995).

Adoption studies Cadoret (1978) found that adoptees separated at birth from a parent who had persistent antisocial behaviour, had higher rates of antisocial personality disorder, than did adoptees whose parents were not antisocial. This finding held whether the biological father or biological mother had shown antisocial behaviour. Among the offspring, however, antisocial personality disorder was diagnosed more often in men than women, although the women had an increased rate of hysteria. Cadoret suggested that hysteria is an expression in women of the genetic endowment that causes antisocial personality disorder in men. Although this study had the shortcoming of a refusal rate of almost 30% among those approached for interview, another study reached similar conclusions (Crowe 1974). A small study of the biological parents of adoptees with antisocial behaviour found an excess of antisocial behaviour compared with the biological parents of children who were not antisocial (Schulsinger 1982).

Cadoret *et al.* (1995) studied the family environment as well as the parentage of adoptees. Again antisocial personality disorder in the biological parents predicted antisocial disorder in the adopted-away children. However, adverse factors in the adoptive environment (for example, marital problems or substance abuse) independently predicted adult antisocial behaviours.

Chromosomal abnormalities In an early study the XYY karyotype was found in about 3% of patients in a maximum security hospital (Jacobs *et al.* 1965). Subsequent studies suggest that the true figure is not greatly in excess of the rate in the general population.

Linkage studies These are beginning to be reported but at the time of writing it is too early to assess their significance.

Cerebral pathology and cerebral maturation

The observation that some brain-injured patients show aggressive behaviour suggested that minor degrees of brain injury might be a cause of antisocial personality. However, there is no convincing evidence to support of this idea. A report of evidence from MRI of reduced prefrontal grey matter in the absence of gross brain lesions in people with antisocial personality disorder (Raine *et al.* 2000) could indicate some kind of prefontal dysfunction. However, the findings need confirmation before their significance can be assessed. A related idea is that antisocial personality disorder results from delay in the maturation of the brain. Weak evidence for this hypothesis exists in EEG abnormalities consistent with maturational delays, found in aggressive offenders, some of whom are likely to have had antisocial personalities (Hill 1952; Williams 1969).

5-Hydroxytryptamine and aggression

Abnormalities in brain 5-hydroxytryptamine (5-HT) neurotransmission have been reported in patients with impulsive and aggressive behaviour, though not specifically in relation to antisocial personality disorder. Low levels of the 5-HT metabolite, 5-hydroxyindoleacetic acid (5-HIAA), have been found in the cerebrospinal fluid of subjects who have committed acts of unpremeditated violence (Linnoila and Virkkunen 1992); and 5-HT-mediated prolactin release is lower in subjects with histories of impulsive aggressiveness (Coccaro *et al.* 1989). Although not specific, it has been suggested that the same abnormalities may be relevant to antisocial personality disorder.

Developmental theories

Separation Bowlby (1944, 1946) studied 44 'juvenile thieves' and concluded that separation of a young child from its mother can lead to antisocial behaviour and failure to form close relationships. This work stimulated much research into the effects of separating children from their mothers (see p. 806) and this research showed that the effects of separation are more varied than Bowlby had originally supposed. Not all separated children are affected adversely and the effects of separation depend on many factors, including the child's age, the previous relationship with the mother and father, and the reasons for separation.

Parental causes Separation from a parent usually follows a long period of tension and arguments between parents that could itself affect the child's development. For example, Rutter (1972) showed that marital disharmony partly accounts for the association between separation and antisocial disorder in sons. As antisocial behaviour in childhood is linked to antisocial behaviour disorder in adult life (see below), these findings suggest a relationship between parental factors and antisocial personality disorder.

Social learning in childhood Eysenck (1970a) suggested that antisocial personality results from failure to learn normal social behaviour, due to slow conditioning. Although attractively simple, this suggestion does not explain why people with antisocial personality learn other behaviour patterns normally. Scott (1960) proposed four ways in which antisocial behaviour could develop through learning:

♦ by growing up in an antisocial family;

♦ through lack of consistent rules in the family;

♦ learnt as a way of overcoming an emotional problem (for example, aggressive behaviour to hide feelings of inferiority);

♦ from poor ability to sustain attention and other impediments to learning.

Although unproven, the scheme provides a useful framework for the clinical assessment of possible causes in an individual patient with antisocial personality.

Childhood behaviour problems and antisocial personality An important 30-year follow-up study of children attending a child guidance clinic found an association between behaviour problems in childhood and antisocial personality disorder in adult life (Robins 1966). Although only a minority of those even with the more serious antisocial behaviour in childhood went on to persistent antisocial behaviour in adult life, most of the adults with antisocial personality disorder had behaviour problems in childhood.. This outcome was particularly likely if, in childhood, there was more than one kind of antisocial behaviour and if antisocial acts were repeated. Stealing among boys and sexual delinquency among girls were especially likely to be followed by antisocial behaviour in adult life.

Paranoid personality disorder

Little is known about the causes of this disorder. Some investigators have reported that paranoid personality disorder is more frequent among first-degree relatives of probands with schizophrenia than among the general population (Kendler *et al.* 1984), but others have not confirmed this finding (Coryell and Zimmerman 1989). Cameron (1963) suggested that one of the central features of the disorder, an absence of trust, results from a lack of consistent parental affection and protection, but this idea has not been confirmed.

Schizoid personality disorder

The cause of this disorder is unknown. As noted above, schizoid personality does not appear to be closely related genetically to schizophrenia (Fulton and Winokur 1993). Psychoanalytic ideas focus on the inability to give or receive love. This inability is thought to be a defence that developed early in life in response to inadequate mother–child relationships. Klein (1952) suggested that all infants pass through a stage of development, which she called 'schizoid position', in which oral and sadistic impulses are experienced as dangerous and are projected on to the parent. According to this theory, most children pass through this stage, but people with a schizoid personality have retained some of the projective defences. These ideas are unsupported by scientific evidence.

Schizotypal personality disorder

Some studies have found increased rates of schizotypal personality disorder amongst relatives of probands with this disorder compared with controls,

both among co-twins (Torgersen 1984) and among other family members (Baron *et al.* 1985), findings that suggest a genetic aetiology for the disorder. It has been suggested that schizotypal personality disorder is related genetically to schizophrenia since it has been reported to be more frequent among biological relatives of probands with schizophrenia than among adopted relatives or controls (Kendler *et al.* 1981). When investigations have begun with probands with schizotypal personality disorder, rates of schizophrenia have not been found to be increased in the same way (Soloff and Millward 1983; Schulz *et al.* 1986), but the groups may have been too small to exclude an effect. Questionnaire studies in normal subjects of the personality trait called 'schizotypy' have shown an inherited component (Claridge and Hewitt 1987). However, it is not certain how far the scores of normal subjects on this questionnaire are related to schizotypal personality disorder

Borderline personality disorder

Conflicting results have come from studies of the prevalence of borderline personality disorder among the relatives of probands with this disorder (Dahl 1993), although a high rate of affective disorder has been reported in the relatives (Stone 1980). Taken together, these results are not convincing evidence for an important genetic component of aetiology. Psychoanalytic theories propose a disturbed relationship with the mother at the stage of individuation of the child (Kernberg 1975). In keeping with this idea, people with the borderline personality are more likely than controls to report physical and sexual abuse in childhood (Berelowicz and Tarnopolsky 1993), although prospective studies have not been reported. Paris (1994) has suggested a multifactorial aetiology, with adverse childhood experiences acting on a so-far-unconfirmed genetic predisposition.

Histrionic personality disorder

There have been few objective studies of the causes of this personality disorder. The genetics of histrionic personality disorder has not been studied with standardized methods of assessment, and the few reported investigations have yielded inconsistent findings (McGuffin and Thapar 1992). Psychoanalytic explanations relate this disorder either to failure to resolve Oedipal conflicts (Fenichel 1945) or to oral conflicts (Marmor 1953),

Obsessional personality disorder

Obsessional personality appears to have a substantial genetic aetiology (Murray and Reveley 1981), although its nature is unknown. Psychoanalytic theory suggests that obsessional personality disorder originates in problems at the anal stage of development. The clinical features of the disorder are explained as the result of the defence mechanisms of regression, reaction formation, and isolation (see p. 189). Neither explanation is supported by scientific evidence.

Anxious (avoidant) personality disorder

The genetics of anxious-avoidant personality disorder has not been studied separately from anxiety disorder. This pesonality category was introduced recently and there are no well-established psychological theories to account for the disorder. A cognitive model has been proposed by Beck and Freeman (1990) in which the central features are fear of rejection, self-criticism, and inaccurate evaluations of the reactions of other people, and the other features of the personality derive from them.

Dependent and passive aggressive personality disorders

The cause of these personality disorders is unknown. No genetic causes have been identified. Psychoanalytic ideas suggest that both disorders originate in problems at the oral stage of development.

The prognosis of personality disorder

Personality disorders are defined as lifelong conditions, so little change would be expected with time. There is little reliable evidence about their outcome. A review of nine follow-up studies showed that only two were over periods of more that 4 years. The studies varied widely in methods of sampling and assessment, and most were concerned with rather small groups. A large-scale ongoing study by the US National Institute of Mental Health should provide better information.

Clinical impressions suggest that minor improvement may take place slowly, especially in *aggressive and antisocial* behaviour. The study by Robins, mentioned above, supports this impression. About a third of people with persistent antisocial behaviour in early adult life improved later, as judged by the number of arrests and contacts with social agencies. However, they still had problems in relationships, as shown by hostility to wives and neighbours, as well as an increased rate of suicide.

Studies of the outcome of *borderline personality disorder* have yielded varying results. Stone *et al.* (1987) found that only about one in four people with this diagnosis in their twenties still met criteria for the same diagnosis in middle age, although most met the criteria for another personality disorder (including histrionic, avoidant, and obsessive types). People who continued to meet the criteria for the original diagnosis more often had co-morbid substance abuse or a criminal record. Another study found that about 60% of people with borderline personality disorder still met diagnostic criteria for this diagnosis at follow-up (Berelowicz and Tarnopolsky 1993, p. 99). A high rate of suicide was found in some studies (8.5% in the study by Stone *et al.* 1987) but not in others.

Mehlum *et al.* (1991) reported a 3–5-year follow-up in which *schizotypal personality disorder* had a worse outcome than borderline personality disorder, whilst 'cluster C' personality disorders (see p. 171) had the best outcome (see Stone 1993 for a review of the outcome of borderline personality disorder).

The management of personality disorders

Assessment

As well as deciding the diagnosis, the *strengths and weaknesses* of the individual should be assessed. Strengths are important because treatment should build on favourable features as well as to attempt to modify unfavourable ones. The patient's *circumstances* should be assessed next. Detailed observations over several weeks should be made to discover any circumstances that provoke undesirable behaviour, such as aggression. Patients generally appreciate the value of this practical approach and collaborate in the assessment. If such enquiries reveal factors that worsen the abnormal behaviour, attempts should be made to change or avoid them. Sometimes the enquiries suggest a new approach to treatment. For example, a man who is aggressive to women may become angry when he is rejected, and this rejection may be provoked by his clumsy approach to women. He might be helped by counselling and social skills training directed to this clumsiness.

Evidence for the effectiveness of treatment

There is little evidence to guide the clinician in the choice of treatment for personality disorders. Few studies have met the basic requirements of randomization, blind assessment, and an appropriate control treatment. Tyrer and Davidson (2000) have identified other reasons for the lack of clinically relevant research, as follows.

Co-morbidity

Co-morbidity is common between personality disorders and other disorders, especially mood disorders and substance abuse. Few trials have ruled out the possibility that changes following treatment are due to improvement in a co-morbid condition rather than in the personality disorder.

Ideally, two kinds of trial are required: trials with pure personality disorder to show whether treatment has an effect independent of any co-morbid condition; and pragmatic trials, each with one of the co-morbid disorders, to show the treatment effect that can be expected in clinical practice where co-morbidity is common.

Duration of treatment and follow-up

Most clinical trials report changes over periods that are too short when judged against the natural course of personality disorders. Tyrer and Davidson suggest 2 years as the necessary minimum. At the time of writing, no trials have met this criterion.

Compliance

Personality disorder is often associated with poor compliance with treatment but clinical trials have to study patients who are compliant enough to agree to take part. Even with the more compliant patient, the size of the drop-out rates makes it difficult to generalize from the results. The problem is made worse by the long follow-up period required – see above.

Outcome measures

Assessments of personality disorder reflect change in mental state as well as change in personality (and change in mental state may be due to change in a co-morbid disorder – see above). Also, personality disorder is defined by suffering to the self or others but it is difficult to measure change in these variables. In trials of treatment of antisocial personality, easily counted events such as reoffending have been used as an outcome measure but changes in these measures may be due to factors other than change in personality.

Psychological treatments

At the time of writing only two controlled trials of psychological treatment of personality disorder have met reasonable criteria. Winston *et al.* (1991) compared short-term dynamic psychotherapy and short-term psychotherapy directed to better adaptation. Both were superior to a waiting list condition, but they did not differ from one another. The second by Linehan *et al.* (1991) concerns dialectic behaviour therapy, a treatment designed for borderline personality disorder. This trial is considered below, in the section on borderline personality disorder (p. 183). Although good short-term results were obtained, they were measured by the effect on self-harm and not by direct measures of the personality disorder, and they were not maintained on longer follow-up. See Perry, J.C et al. (1999) for a review

Drug treatments

Antipsychotic drugs have been evaluated as a treatment for borderline personality disorder. Early reports suggested a positive effect but subsequent reports have not confirmed this conclusion (see Tyrer and Davidson 2000). These drugs have been used also for antisocial personality but no satisfactory controlled comparisons have been reported..

Antidepressant drugs

Amitriptyline has been tested against placebo as a treatment for borderline personality disorder (Soloff *et al*. 1986; Soloff 1994). Some patients responded well, others not at all, a finding that could be due to an effect on associated depressive disorder. Fluoxetine has also been reported to be more effective than placebo in reducing anger in people with borderline personality disorder (Salzmann *et al*. 1995; Coccaro and Kavoussi 1997). More trials are needed before the effect of antidepressants can be evaluated.

Mood stabilizers

In one study, lithium reduced anger and impulsiveness in antisocial personalities (Sheard *et al*. 1976) but the finding has not been convincingly replicated (see Nilsson 1993 for a review). In any case, there is a practical difficulty that people with aggressive behaviour may not comply with the strict regimen required for the safe use of lithium.

General aims of management

Although there has been some progress in finding ways of effecting change in personality disorders, management still consists largely of helping the person to find a way of life that conflicts less with his character. Whatever treatment is used, aims should be modest and considerable time should be allowed to achieve them. The relationship with the patient is important. When the personality disorder includes traits of dependency, patients should not be seen frequently, otherwise they may become excessively dependent. These patients readily exploit inconsistencies in the treatment plan, using them to divert attention from their own problems. Usually, more than one professional is involved in the care of patients with personality disorder, and close collaboration is needed to avoid inconsistencies of approach. Many of these patients react badly to changes in staff which may re-enact painful losses, rejections, or separations in their earlier life.

The treatment plan should include attempts to help the patient have less contact with situations that provoke difficulties, and more opportunity to develop assets in the personality. Patients should be helped to avoid adding to their problems by misusing drugs or alcohol, or by entering into unsatisfactory relationships. They should be encouraged to develop leisure interests, pursue further education, or join clubs. Even if no improvement is achieved, these basic steps may stabilize the situation until some fortuitous change in the patient's life brings about improvement. When progress is achieved, it is often as a series of small steps whereby the patient gradually moves nearer to a satisfactory adjustment. Setbacks are common and they can be used constructively since it is at these times that patients are most likely to confront their problems. Although the therapist should try hard and long to help these patients, it should be recognized that, however skilful the therapist, some patients will not benefit.

Psychological treatment: general considerations

Supportive therapy

Psychological support often helps people with personality disorder. For some personality disorders, modest but useful progress can be achieved over a period of months, but for antisocial personality disorders support may be required for years.

Support may be provided by a doctor, a social worker, a psychiatric nurse, or a probation officer. A probation order can be a useful external control for people with antisocial behaviour when their initial motivation for treatment is poor.

Counselling

Problem-solving counselling (see p. 728) can help patients deal with stressful circumstances that provoke abnormal behaviour or painful feelings. The approach is less likely than other forms of counselling to lead to dependency and transference problems in patients with cluster C disorders. Its practical step-by-step aspects are also valuable for patients with cluster B disorders.

Counselling which links past experiences to present difficulties should be used selectively for personality disorders. It is most likely to help young people who lack confidence, have difficulty in making relationships, and are uncertain about the direction that their lives should take. It is important that they be highly motivated to work at solving their problems by examining their attitudes and emotions. Problem-solving counselling is generally more helpful than a non-directive approach, especially with borderline and antisocial personalities.

Dynamic psychotherapy

Psychodynamic treatment of personality disorders differs only in emphasis from other forms of psychodynamic treatment. With personality disorders the approach is more directive and there is less emphasis on the reconstruction of past events and more on the ways in which the person relates to others, copes with external difficulties, and deals with feelings. The analysis of transference and counter-transference is important as a way of identifying problems in relationships. For a review of dynamic psychotherapy for severe personality disorder see Kernberg (1993).

Cognitive therapy

Beck and Freeman (1990) adapted cognitive therapy methods for use with personality disorders. Therapists focus on modes of thinking and beliefs that characterize the personality disorder and underlie the problematic emotions and behaviour. They attempt to change these cognitions with the usual cognitive therapy techniques (see p. 733). Good results have been claimed but the methods have not been evaluated in controlled trials. *Cognitive–analytic therapy* is an amalgam of techniques chosen from cognitive therapy and analytic psychotherapy. The approach has been applied to borderline personality disorder (Ryle 1997), but its value has not been established in clinical trials.

The management of specific personality disorders

The type of personality disorder is not a good guide to the choice of effective treatment. Nevertheless, some associations have been claimed, mainly on the basis of clinical experience, and these will be considered next.

Paranoid personality disorder

Patients with this disorder do not engage well in treatment because they are touchy and suspicious. If this problem can be overcome, supportive treatment may prevent the accumulation of problems caused by the patient's suspicious or angry responses to other people.

Schizoid personality disorder

Patients with schizoid personality avoid close personal contact and often drop out after a few sessions of treatment. If they can be persuaded to continue, they tend to intellectualize their problems and question the value of their treatment. The therapist should try to help patients become more aware of their problems, and respond in ways that cause fewer difficulties. At best, the process is slow and the results are limited. Exploratory psychotherapy is unlikely to succeed, and medication is generally unhelpful.

Antisocial (dissocial) personality disorder

Treatment usually consists of the general measures discussed above. Medication has little value except that an antipsychotic drug may have a temporary effect of calming aggressive behaviour arising in response to increased stress, and antidepressant medication may be needed for a co-morbid depressive disorder. Fluoxetine has been found to reduce measures of aggression in patients with personality disorder (Coccaro and Kavoussi 1997). Lithium has been claimed to reduce aggressive behaviour in some patients (see p. 180). It should not be prescribed unless it is reasonably certain that the patient will comply strictly with the dosage regimen and the other requirements for safety (see p. 700). Anxiolytic drugs should be avoided because they may cause for disinhibition and dependency.

If resources are available, individual or group psychotherapy can be considered but the results are uncertain. The following points should be considered.

Individual psychotherapy

Good results have been reported with a modified form of dynamic psychotherapy in which people are confronted repeatedly and directly with evidence of their own abnormal behaviour. The method, derived from the work of Schmideberg (1947), requires a therapist with a particularly forceful and robust personality. The claims for good results are so far unproved.

Small-group therapy

People with antisocial personality disorder seldom benefit from the usual kind of small-group therapy, and often disrupt the treatment of the others in the group. Groups composed entirely of antisocial patients can sometimes be more constructive but they are difficult to conduct. The therapist needs considerable general skills in psychotherapy, and special training with this group of patients.

The therapeutic community

Jones (1952) was the first to apply the principles of the therapeutic community (see Chapter 22) to the treatment of antisocial personalities. The approach has not been adopted widely but has continued in a few specialized units such as the Henderson Hospital in England. In such a unit antisocial patients live and work together. They meet several times a day for group discussions in which there is frank discussion of each person's behaviour and feelings, and the effects that these have on the others. These discussions often provoke strong emotions, which have to be contained. It is hoped that by repeatedly facing these issues, patients will gradually learn to control their antisocial behaviour and adopt more acceptable ways of dealing with feelings and relationships. Rapoport (1960) identified four therapeutic factors at work in these special communities:

- permission to act out feelings within the community;
- sharing of tasks and responsibilities;
- participation in making rules; and
- confrontation with the effects of ones actions on other people.

No controlled evaluation of this treatment has been carried out, and there is no consensus about its value. Follow-up studies of 1–2 years have reported improvement rates of 40–60%, depending on whether the criterion for improvement was general social functioning, employment, or reconviction (Taylor 1966), but these rates may reflect factors other than the specific treatment.

Other group regimens

Group methods have been applied in a more authoritarian setting to prisoners with personality disorder. At Grendon Prison in England this approach has been applied to the care and rehabilitation of prisoners who have not responded well in other prison environments.

Histrionic personality disorder

These patients make many demands on their carers. Frequent problems include attempts to impose impractical conditions on treatment, requests for inappropriate medication, and demands for help at unreasonable times. Other problems include seductive behaviour, threats of self-harm, and attempts to prolong interviews unreasonably. It is important to identify these problems early because, once established, they cannot easily be controlled. The behaviours should be discussed with the patient, and clear limits set by offering appropriate help while explaining which behaviours cannot be accepted. Exploratory psychotherapy should be avoided, and treatment should focus on developing more adaptive ways of responding to stressful situations. Medication has little value unless there is a co-morbid depressive disorder.

Borderline personality disorder

The general problems in managing borderline personality disorders are similar to that encountered with histrionic personality disorder (described above). However, there are more therapeutic options. Problem-solving counselling (see p. 728) is sometimes helpful, with a focus on dealing with everyday problems. Anxiolytic medication should be avoided because of its potential for disinhibition and dependence. Small doses of an antipsychotic drug may reduce aggressive behaviour in the short term. A selective serotonin re-uptake inhibitor (SSRI) can be tried since these drugs appear to reduce impulsive behaviour in some patients (Salzmann *et al.* 1995), though at the time of writing the evidence for this effect is not convincing.

Several kinds of psychological treatment can be tried when resources are available, though none has been proved to have a substantial and reliable effect. The following points should be considered.

Dynamic psychotherapy

People with borderline personality disorder do not respond well to the usual forms of dynamic psychotherapy, and unskilled treatment may result in reduced emotional control and increased impulsiveness. Kernberg (1984) described an alternative approach for these patients, which is less likely to have these adverse effects but still deals with what is thought to be the core psychopathology. This approach, called *expressive psychotherapy*, is claimed to give good results (see, for example, Stone *et al.* 1987), but to date no randomized controlled trials have been reported. For a review of psychotherapy for borderline personality disorder see Higgitt and Fonagy (1993).

Group psychotherapy

This treatment has the advantages that transference relationships are spread over the group instead of focused on the therapist, and that the group's comments on acting out behaviour may be accepted more readily than those of the therapist. The therapist needs considerable skill if the borderline patient is to be helped without disrupting the treatment of the other group members. It is seldom practicable to treat more than one borderline patient in a group. For a review of group treatment see Clarkin *et al.* (1991).

Dialectic behaviour therapy

This type of therapy was developed by Linehan. The treatment combines weekly individual sessions, psychoeducation, and behavioural skills training in a group, with telephone consultation when necessary. Patients are taught ways of dealing with distress without losing control of emotions, and encouraged to react by doing what will be effective rather than what feels right to them at the time. As noted above, this treatment is one of the few that have been evaluated in a controlled trial – with borderline personalities who had made repeated suicide attempts. Dialectic behaviour therapy was more effective than the control treatment in reducing self-harm but the effect on the personality disorder was not assessed directly. Also, the benefits diminished on longer follow-up (Linehan *et al.* 1991, 1993).

Obsessional personality disorder

People with this personality disorder do not respond well to psychotherapy. Unskilled treatment can lead to excessive morbid introspection, which leaves the person worse rather than better. Treatment should be directed to avoiding situations that increase the patient's difficulties, and to developing better ways of coping with stressful situations. Patients often seek help during an associated depressive disorder, and it is important to identify and treat this co-morbid condition.

Avoidant (anxious) personality disorders

These patients generally have low self-esteem and fear disapproval and criticism. They can be helped by a therapeutic relationship in which they feel valued and able to consider their perception of themselves. Some leave treatment, fearing criticism or rejection, and such feelings should be anticipated and discussed constructively as soon as they appear. The therapist should be alert to the possibility of a co-morbid depressive disorder, requiring treatment.

Dependent personality disorder

Dynamic psychotherapy may increase these patients' dependence. They are usually helped more by problem-solving counselling, in which they are encouraged to take increasingly more responsibility for themselves. Medication should be avoided unless there is an associated depressive disorder.

Further reading

Dolan, B. and Cord, J. (1993). *Psychopathic and antisocial personality disorders; treatment and research issues.* Gaskell, London.

Gelder, M. G., López-Ibor, J. J. Jr, and Andreasen, N.C. (eds) (2000). *The new Oxford textbook of psychiatry*, Section 4.12: Personality disorder. Oxford University Press, Oxford. (The seven chapters in this section provide a comprehensive review of personality disorder.)

Schneider, K. (1950). *Psychopathic personalities* (trans. M. W. Hamilton). Cassell, London. (A classic text of great importance in the development of ideas about personality disorder.)

Tyrer, P. (ed.) (2000). *Personality disorders: diagnosis, management and course*, 2nd edn.Butterworth-Heinemann, Oxford. (Contains systematic reviews of the subject, and an account of the editor's Personality Assessment Schedule.)

Appendix

Box 7.1 Some instruments for diagnosing personality disorders

International Personality Disorders Examination (Loranger et al. 1994)

◆ Assesses DSM-IV and /or ICD-10 personality disorders categorically and/or dimensionally

◆ Semi-structured clinical interview in two versions: a DSM-IV version with 99 sets of questions and an ICD-10 version with 67 sets of questions. There is a screening questionnaire for each version which can be used to identify people who are unlikely to have a personality disorder

Structured Clinical Interview for DSM-IV Axis II Personality Disorders (SCID-II) (First et al. 1995)

◆ Assesses DSM-IV personality disorders either categorically or dimensionally

◆ Semi-structured clinical interview with 119 sets of questions. There is a screening interview to identify people unlikely to have a personality disorder

Structured Interview for DSM-IV Personality (SIDP-IV) (Pfohl et al. 1997)

◆ Assesses DSM-IV and ICD-10 personality disorders either categorically or dimensionally

◆ A semi-structured clinical interview with 101 questions in a thematic version and 107 questions in a disorder-by-disorder version

For further information on these and other instruments for personality assessment see Task Force for Psychiatric Measures (2000), Chapter 32.

CHAPTER 8

Reactions to stressful experiences

Reactions to stressful experiences

Stressful events frequently provoke psychiatric disorders. Such events can also provoke emotional reactions that are distressing but not of the nature or severity required for the diagnosis of an anxiety disorder or a mood disorder. These less severe reactions are the subject of this chapter. With the exception of normal grief reactions, the conditions described in this chapter are listed as disorders in ICD-10 and DSM-IV.

The chapter begins with a description of the several components of the response to stressful events, including coping strategies and mechanisms of defence. The classification of reactions to stressful experience is discussed next. The various syndromes are then described, including acute stress reactions, post-traumatic stress disorder, special forms of response to severe stress, and adjustment disorders. The chapter ends with an account of special forms of adjustment reaction, including adjustment to bereavement (grief), and to terminal illness, and the problems of adults who experienced sexual abuse in childhood.

The response to stressful events

The response to stressful events has three components:

♦ an emotional response, with somatic accompaniments;

♦ a coping strategy;

♦ a defence mechanism.

Coping strategies and defence mechanisms are overlapping concepts but they originated from different schools of thought and for this reason they are described separately in the following account.

Emotional and somatic responses

These responses are of two kinds. *Anxiety* responses with autonomic arousal leading to apprehension, irritability, tachycardia, increased muscle tension, and dry mouth. *Depressive* responses with poor appetite and reduced physical activity. Anxiety responses are generally associated with events that pose a *threat*, whilst depressive responses are usually associated with events that involve separation or *loss*. These features of these responses are similar to, but less intense than, the symptoms of anxiety and depressive disorders (described in Chapters 10 and 11, respectively).

Coping strategies

Coping strategies serve to reduce the impact of stressful events, thus attenuating the emotional and somatic responses and making it more possible to maintain normal performance at the time (though not always in the longer term, see below). The term coping strategy is derived from research in social psychology; it is applied to activities of which the person is aware, for example, deliberately avoiding stressors. (Responses of which the person is unaware are called mechanisms of defence, described below.)

Coping strategies are of two kinds: problem-solving strategies, which can be used to make adverse circumstances less stressful, and emotion-reducing strategies, which alleviate the response to the stressors.

Problem-solving strategies include:

♦ *seeking help* from another person;

♦ *obtaining information* or advice that would help to solve the problem;

- *solving problems* – making and implementing plans to deal with the problem;
- *confrontation* – defending one's rights, and persuading other people to change their behaviour.

Emotion-reducing strategies include:

- *ventilation* of emotion – talking to another person and expressing emotion;
- *evaluation* of the problem – to assess what can be changed and try to change it (by problem solving), and what cannot be changed and to accept it;
- *positive reappraisal* of the problem – recognizing that it has led to some good, for example, that the loss of a job is an opportunity to find a more satisfying occupation;
- *avoidance* of the problem by refusing to think about it, avoiding people who are causing it, or avoiding reminders of it.

Coping strategies are generally useful in reducing the problem or in lessening the emotional reaction. However, they are not always adaptive. For example, avoidance may not be adaptive in the early stages of physical illness because it can lead to delay in seeking appropriate treatment. Hence a person needs not only the ability to use coping strategies but also the ability to judge which strategy should be used in particular circumstances.

Maladaptive coping strategies

These strategies reduce the emotional response to stressful circumstances in the short term, but lead to greater difficulties in the long term. Maladaptive coping strategies include the following:

- *use of alcohol or unprescribed drugs* to reduce the emotional response or to reduce awareness of stressful circumstances.
- *deliberate self-harm* either by drug overdose or self-injury. Some people gain relief from tension by cutting the skin with a sharp instrument to induce pain and draw blood. Others take overdoses to withdraw from the situation or to show their need for help (see p. 522).

- *unrestrained display of feelings* can reduce tension, and in some societies such behaviour is sanctioned in particular circumstances, for example, grieving. In other circumstances, such behaviour can damage relationships with people who would otherwise have been supportive.
- *aggressive behaviour* – aggression provides immediate release of feelings of anger. In the longer term, it may increase the person's difficulties by damaging relationships.

Coping styles

When particular coping mechanisms are used repeatedly by the same person in different situations, they are said to constitute a coping style. Some people change their coping strategies according to the circumstances; for example, they use problem-solving strategies at work but employ avoidance when unwell. Some people habitually use maladaptive strategies; for example, they repeatedly abuse alcohol or take overdoses of drugs when under stress. For a review of coping strategies see Lazarus (1993).

Mechanisms of defence

Mechanisms of defence (Table 8.1) are unconscious responses to external stressors as well as to anxiety arising from internal conflict. They were described originally by Sigmund Freud and later elaborated by his daughter Anna Freud (1936). In response to stressful circumstances, the most frequent mechanisms are repression, denial, displacement, projection, and regression. Defence mechanisms are unconscious processes, i.e. people do not use them deliberately and are unaware of their own real motives, although they may become aware later through introspection or through another person's comments. Freud identified defence mechanisms in his study of the 'psychopathology of everyday life', a term that he applied to slips of the tongue and lapses of memory. The concept of defence

Table 8.1 **Mechanisms of defence**
Repression
Reaction formation
Denial
Rationalization
Displacement
Sublimation
Projection
Identification
Regression

mechanisms has proved useful in understanding many aspects of the day-to-day behaviour of people under stress, notably those with physical or psychiatric illness. Freud also used the concept of mechanisms of defence to explain the aetiology of mental disorders, but this extension of his original observations has not proved useful.

The main mechanisms of defence can be illustrated by the following examples.

Repression

This is the exclusion from consciousness of impulses, emotions, or memories that would otherwise cause distress. For example, especially painful aspects of the memory of distressing events such as sexual abuse in childhood may be kept out of awareness for many years.

Denial

This is a related concept: it is inferred when a person behaves as if unaware of something that he may reasonably be expected to know. For example, on learning that he is dying of cancer, a patient may continue to live normally as if unaware of the diagnosis. In this example, denial is adaptive since it can help to reduce depression. However, in the early stage of illness denial may delay seeking help or lead to refusal of necessary investigations and treatment. In this second example, denial is maladaptive.

Displacement

This is the transfer of emotion from a person, object, or situation with which it is properly associated, to another source. For example, after the recent death of his wife, a man may blame the doctor for failure to give adequate care, and may thus avoid blaming himself for putting his work before her needs in the last months of her life.

Projection

This is the attribution to another person of thoughts or feelings similar to one's own, thereby rendering one's own thoughts or feelings more acceptable. For example, a person who dislikes a colleague may attribute reciprocal feelings of dislike to him; it is then easier to justify his own feelings of dislike for the colleague.

Regression

This is the adoption of behaviour appropriate to an earlier stage of development, for example, dependence on others. Regression often occurs among physically ill people. In the acute stages of illness it can be adaptive, enabling the person to acquiesce passively to intensive medical and nursing care. If regression persists into the stage of recovery and rehabilitation, it can be maladaptive because it reduces the patient's ability to make efforts to help himself.

Reaction formation

This is the unconscious adoption of behaviour opposite to behaviour that would reflect true feelings and intentions. For example, excessively prudish attitudes to sex are sometimes (but not always) a reaction to the person's own sexual urges that he cannot accept.

Rationalization

This is the unconscious provision of a false but acceptable explanation for behaviour that has a less acceptable origin. For example, a husband may leave his wife at home because he does not enjoy her company, but he may reassure himself falsely that she is shy and would not enjoy going out.

Sublimation

This is the unconscious diversion of unacceptable impulses into more acceptable outlets, for example, turning the need to dominate others into the organization of good works for charity. (There are, of course, many other motives for charitable work.)

Identification

This is the unconscious adoption of the characteristics or activities of another person, often to reduce the pain of separation or loss. For example, a widow may undertake the same voluntary work that her husband used to do.

Present circumstances, previous experience, and response to stressful events

Brown and Harris (1978) showed that the response to a stressful life event is modified by present circumstances and by past experience. Some current circumstances make a person more vulnerable to stressful life events, for example, the lack of a confidant with whom to share problems. Such circumstances are called *vulnerability factors*. Previous experience can also increase vulnerability; for example, the experience of losing a parent in childhood may make a person more vulnerable in adult life to stressful events involving loss. It is difficult to examine these more remote associations scientifically. (Life events and vulnerability factors are considered further on p. 121.)

Classification of reactions to stressful events

Although included within the classifications of diseases, not all reactions to stressful events are abnormal. Grief is a normal reaction to the stressful experience of bereavement, and only a minority of people have a very severe or abnormally prolonged reaction. There is also a normal pattern of reaction to a dangerous or traumatic event such as a car accident. Most people have an immediate feeling of great anxiety, are dazed and restless for a few hours afterwards, and then recover; a few people have more severe and prolonged symptoms – an abnormal reaction. It is difficult to decide where to make a separation between normal and abnormal reactions to stressful events in terms of severity or of duration, and in practice the division is arbitrary.

Table 8.2 Classification of reactions to stressful experience	
ICD–10	**DSM-IV**
Acute stress reaction	Acute stress disorder
Post-traumatic stress disorder	Post-traumatic stress disorder
Adjustment disorder	Adjustment disorder
Brief depressive reaction	With depressed mood
Mixed anxiety and depressive reaction	With mixed anxiety and depressed mood
Predominant disturbance of other emotions	With anxiety
Predominant disturbance of conduct	With disturbance of conduct
Mixed disturbance of emotions and conduct	With mixed disturbance of emotions and conduct
Other specified symptoms	Unspecified

The order of the subgroups has been changed to show similarities and differences between the two systems.

Similarly, amongst patients in hospital for medical or surgical treatment, most are anxious but a few are severely anxious and show extreme denial or other defence mechanisms that impair cooperation with treatment.

ICD-10 and DSM-IV reactions to stressful experiences are classified into three groups (Table 8.2).

Acute reactions to stress

This category is for immediate and brief responses to sudden intense stressors in a person who does not have another psychiatric disorder at the time. The ICD-10 definition of acute stress reaction requires that the response should start within an hour of exposure to the stressor and begins to diminish after not more than 48 hours. The DSM-IV definition of acute stress disorder states that the onset should be while or after experiencing the distressing event and requires that the condition lasts for at least 2 days and for no more than 4 weeks. These two definitions capture different phases of the anxiety response as the different terms, reaction and disorder, suggest. ICD refers to the short-lived normal response. DSM-IV refers to the more prolonged response, which is less common.

Post-traumatic stress disorder

This is a prolonged and abnormal response to exceptionally intense stressful circumstances such as a natural disaster or a sexual or other physical assault.

Adjustment disorder

This is a more gradual and prolonged response to stressful changes in a person's life. In both ICD-10 and DSM-IV, adjustment disorders are subdivided, according to the predominant symptoms, into depressive, mixed anxiety, and depressive, with disturbance of conduct, and with mixed disturbance of emotions and conduct. DSM-IV has an additional category of adjustment disorder with anxiety. ICD-10 has an additional category of 'predominant disturbance of other emotion', which

includes not only adjustment disorder with anxiety but also adjustment disorder with anger.

In ICD-10 the three types of reaction to stressful experience are classified together under 'reactions to stress and adjustment disorders', which is a subdivision of section F4, 'neurotic, stress related and somatoform disorders'. The defining characteristics of this group of reactions to stress and of adjustment disorders are:

◆ they arise as a *direct consequence* of either acute stress or continued unpleasant circumstances;

◆ it is judged that the disorder would not have arisen without these factors.

A different organizing principle is used in DSM-IV: acute stress disorder and post-traumatic stress disorder are classified as anxiety disorders, whilst adjustment disorders have their own place in the classification, separate from the anxiety disorders.

Additional codes in ICD-10

If any of these reactions is accompanied by an act of deliberate self-harm, another code can be added to record this fact (codes X60-X82 list 23 methods of self-harm). It is also possible to specify certain kinds of stressful event by adding a code from Chapter Z; for example, Z58 problems related to employment and unemployment, and Z63 problems related to family circumstances.

Coding grief reactions

In ICD-10, abnormal grief reactions are coded as adjustment disorders. Reactions to bereavement that are appropriate to the person's culture are not included. If it is appropriate to code them as part of the description of the patient's condition, code Z63.4 (death of a family member) can be used.

Acute stress reaction and acute stress disorder

Clinical picture

The *core symptoms* of an acute psychological response to stress are anxiety or depression. Anxiety is the response to threatening experiences; depression is the response to loss. Anxiety and depression often occur together, because stressful events often combine danger and loss; an extreme example is a road accident in which a companion is killed. Other symptoms include feelings of being numb or dazed, difficulty in remembering the whole sequence of the traumatic event, insomnia, restlessness, poor concentration, and physical symptoms of autonomic arousal, especially sweating, palpitations, and tremor. Anger or histrionic behaviour may be part of the response. Occasionally there is a flight reaction, for example, when a driver runs away from the scene of a road accident.

Coping strategies and defence mechanisms are also part of the acute response to stressful events. Avoidance is the most frequent coping strategy; the person avoids talking or thinking about the stressful events, and avoids reminders of them. The most frequent defence mechanism is denial, which is experienced as a feeling that the events have not really happened, or as inability to remember them. Usually avoidance and denial recede as anxiety diminishes: memories of the events return and the person is able to think or talk about them with less distress. This sequence allows working through and coming to terms with the stressful experience, though there may be continuing difficulty in recalling details of highly stressful events.

Variations in the clinical picture

Not all responses to acute stress follow this orderly sequence, in which coping strategies and defences are maintained long enough to allow the person to function until anxiety and depression subside and are then abandoned so that working through can occur. Not all coping strategies are adaptive; an example is excessive use of alcohol or drugs to reduce distress. Defence mechanisms may also be of the less adaptive types such as regression, displacement, or projection. Sometimes defence mechanisms persist longer than is adaptive; for example, denial may persist so long that 'working through' is delayed. Sometimes vivid memories of the stressful events intrude into awareness as images

and flashbacks or disturbing dreams. When this state persists, the condition is called a post-traumatic stress disorder (see p. 194).

Diagnostic conventions

The names and the definitions of this condition differ in ICD-10 and DSM-IV. In ICD-10 the term acute stress reaction is defined as a response to severely stressful events that starts within an hour of exposure and begins to diminish within no more than 8 hours if the stressor is transient, or 48 hours if it continues. In DSM-IV, acute stress disorder is defined as starting while experiencing or after experiencing the distressing event, and lasting at least 2 days to at most 4 weeks. Thus the ICD-10 definition captures an earlier stage of the reaction than that described in DSM-IV. Conditions lasting less than 48 hours would be diagnosed as acute stress reaction in ICD-10 but would fail the minimum duration criterion in DSM-IV. In either scheme, a reaction that lasts longer than the arbitrary limit is classified as either a post-traumatic stress disorder (p. 194) or an adjustment disorder (p. 201). The DSM definition refers to cases of more clinical importance and it is widely used. It was hoped that the DSM-IV definition would identify people who were more likely than others to develop post-traumatic stress disorder. However, around 40% of those who develop PTSD 6 months after a trauma do not meet criteria for acute stress disorder soon after it (Harvey and Bryant 1998).

Both systems of classification describe typical symptoms of the disorder. In DSM-IV the diagnosis of acute stress disorder requires marked symptoms of anxiety or increased arousal; three from a list of five 'dissociative' symptoms, namely:

- a sense of numbing or detachment;
- reduced awareness of the surroundings ('being in a daze');
- derealization;
- depersonalization; and
- dissociative amnesia.

There must be avoidance of stimuli that arouse recollections of the trauma, and significant distress or impaired social functioning. ICD-10 requires that the symptom criteria for generalized anxiety disorder are met.

In ICD 10 dissociative and other symptoms are not required to diagnose the disorder in its mild form (F43.00) but two are required for the moderate form (F43.01) and four for the severe form (F43.02) from a list of seven, namely:

- withdrawal from expected social interaction;
- narrowing of attention;
- apparent disorientation;
- anger and verbal aggression;
- despair and hopelessness;
- inappropriate or purposeless activity; and
- uncontrollable and excessive grief.

The terms acute stress reaction and acute stress disorder are used only when the person was free from these symptoms immediately before the impact of the stressful event; otherwise the response is classified as an exacerbation of pre-existing psychiatric disorder.

Epidemiology

Rates in the population are unknown. The rate of acute stress disorder reported among survivors of motor vehicle accidents is 13% among survivors (Harvey and Bryant 1998), among victims of violent crime 19% (Brewin *et al.* 1999), and among the witnesses of a mass shooting 33% (Classen *et al.* 1998).

Aetiology

Many kinds of event can provoke an acute reaction to stress. Examples are involvement in a significant but brief event such as a motor accident or a fire, an event that involves actual or threatened injury such as a physical assault or rape, or the sudden discovery of serious illness. Some of these stressful events involve life changes to which further adjustment is required, for example, the serious injury of a close friend involved in the same accident. Not all people exposed to the same stressful situation develop the same degree of response (see epidemiology, above); this variation suggests that differences in constitution, previous experience, and coping styles may play a part in aetiology. However, there is little factual information since research has focused on the more severe and lasting post-traumatic stress disorder.

Treatment

The treatment of acute reactions to stressful events has two generally agreed elements: to reduce the emotional response, and to help with more effective coping with residual problems. The value of a third component, recall of the traumatic events (debriefing), is disputed. By definition, acute stress reactions are brief and most are dealt with by general practitioners, physicians, or surgeons caring for the patient (for example, after a road accident) or by nurses or counsellors attached to medical teams. Psychiatrists seldom treat these acute and transitory reactions, though they may be called upon to advise others about care.

Debriefing

After a major incident, counselling often takes the form known as debriefing, provided individually or in a group. In debriefing the victim goes through the following stages after the counsellor has first explained the procedure (Mitchell 1983):

- facts – the victims relate what happened;
- thoughts – they describe their thoughts immediately after the incident;
- feelings – they recall the emotions associated with the incident;
- assessment – they take stock of their responses;
- education – the counsellor offers information about stress responses and how to manage them.

Debriefing is used widely but with little evidence that it is effective. A review of the few randomized controlled studies of debriefing found that although most recipients thought it helpful, psychological symptoms were not reduced more than in the control procedures (Rose and Bisson 1998). Two studies included in this review and two subsequent ones have found that the debriefed group had either a worse outcome than the control group, or one that was no better (Hobbs *et al.* 1996; Bisson *et al.* 1997; Carlier *et al.* 1998; Rose *et al.* 1999; Mayou *et al.* 2000; Raphael and Wilson 2000).

Management

Since acute stress reactions and disorders are transient conditions, supportive treatment is usually appropriate. After a traumatic event, many people talk informally to a sympathetic relative or friends, or to a member of the professional staff dealing with any physical injuries originating during the incident.

More formal counselling may be needed if there is no friend or professional who can assist, or if the stressful circumstances cannot easily be discussed with a relative or friend (for example, in some cases of rape), or if the response is prolonged or severe. The victim can be reassured that the condition is frequent, and often short lived. Advice may be needed about ways of dealing with the consequences of the traumatic events. If anxiety is severe, an anxiolytic drug may be prescribed for a day or two, and when sleep is severely disrupted a hypnotic drug may be given for one or two nights. There is evidence that cognitive behavioural methods are more effective than supportive counselling (Bryant *et al.* 1998; see also p. 198).

Although large-scale debriefing is unlikely to reduce the symptomatic response to traumatic events (see above), the other components of counselling have a place in the response to events which have had a major impact on a whole community so that few people are left to act as unaffected, supportive listeners. It seems, however, that attention should be focused on improving coping rather than working through traumatic events. In some circumstances victims need help to deal with feelings of anger.

Although 78% of people who meet the criteria for acute stress disorder in DSM-IV go on to develop PTSD, so do 60% of those who fail to meet

these criteria (Harvey and Bryant 1998), so the diagnosis is of limited value in deciding who should have extra help.

The prevention of post-traumatic stress disorder is considered further in the next section.

Post-traumatic stress disorder

This term denotes an intense, prolonged, and sometimes delayed reaction to an intensely stressful event. The essential features of a post-traumatic stress reaction are hyperarousal, re-experiencing of aspects of the stressful events, and avoidance of reminders. Examples of extreme stressors that may cause this disorder are natural disasters such as floods and earthquakes, man-made calamities such as major fires, serious transport accidents, or the circumstances of war, and rape or serious physical assault on the person. The original concept of post-traumatic stress disorder was of a reaction to such an extreme stressor that any person would be affected. Epidemiological studies have shown that not everyone exposed to the same extreme stressor develops post-traumatic stress disorder; hence personal predisposition plays a part. In many disasters the victims suffer not only psychological distress but also physical injury, which may increase the likelihood of a post-traumatic stress disorder. Other predisposing factors are reviewed below under aetiology.

The condition now known as post-traumatic stress disorder has been recognized for many years, though under other names. The term post-traumatic stress disorder originated in the study of American servicemen returning from the Vietnam War. The diagnosis meant that affected servicemen could be given medical and social help without being diagnosed as suffering from another psychiatric disorder. Similar psychological effects have been reported (under other names) among servicemen in both world wars, and amongst survivors of peacetime disasters such as the serious fire at the Coconut Grove nightclub in America (Adler 1943). (For a historical review see Gersons and Carlier 1992.)

Other reactions to severe stress

Post-traumatic stress disorder occurs only after exceptionally stressful events, but not every response to such events is a post-traumatic stress disorder. Combat veterans have high rates of depression, somatization disorder, and alcohol and drug abuse as well as post-traumatic stress disorder (see Rundell *et al.* 1989). After road accidents, anxiety disorders are actually more frequent than post-traumatic stress disorder (Mayou 1992). Survivors of concentration camps may develop post-traumatic stress disorder, but also persistent irritability and poor memory (Eitinger 1960), and survivors of disasters may develop marital problems (Raphael 1986). These other conditions may occur instead of, but also as well as, post-traumatic stress disorder. For example, whilst 90% of Vietnam war veterans met diagnostic criteria for post-traumatic stress disorder, 43% had at least one other diagnosis. The most frequent were atypical depression, alcohol dependence, anxiety disorder, substance abuse, and somatization disorder (MacFarlane 1985).

Clinical picture of PTSD

The clinical features of post-traumatic stress disorder can be divided into three groups (Table 8.3). The first group of symptoms are related to *hyperarousal* persistent anxiety, irritability, insomnia, and poor concentration. The second group of symptoms centres round *intrusions* despite difficulty in recalling stressful events at will, there is intense intrusive imagery of the events, sudden flashbacks, and recurrent distressing dreams. The third group of symptoms is concerned with *avoidance:* avoidance of reminders of the events, a feeling of detachment, inability to feel emotion ('numbing'), and diminished interest in activities. The most characteristic symptoms are flashbacks, nightmares, and intrusive images, sometimes known collectively as *re-experiencing symptoms.*

Maladaptive coping responses may occur, including persistent aggressive behaviour, the excessive use of alcohol or drugs, and deliberate self-harm

---

Table 8.3 The principal symptoms of post-traumatic stress disorder

Hyperarousal
  Persistent anxiety
  Irritability
  Insomnia
  Poor concentration

Intrusions
  Difficulty in recalling stressful events at will
  Intense intrusive imagery ('flashbacks')
  Recurrent distressing dreams

Avoidance
  Avoidance of reminders of the events
  Detachment
  Inability to feel emotion ('numbness')
  Diminished interest in activities

(Davidson *et al.* 1991) and suicide (Hendin and Haas 1991).

Other features

Depressive symptoms are common, and guilt is often experienced by the survivors of a disaster. After some traumatic events, survivors feel forced into a painful reconsideration of their beliefs about the meaning and purpose of life (Janoff-Bulman, 1985). It has been suggested that dissociative symptoms and depersonalization are important symptoms of the disorder (Foa *et al.* 1995).

Onset and course

Post-traumatic stress disorder may begin very soon after the stressful event or after an interval usually of days, but occasionally of months, though rarely more than 6 months (McFarlane 1988). If the person experiences a new traumatic event, symptoms may return even if the second event is less severe than the original. Most cases resolve within about 3 months but some may persist for years (Blank 1992).

Diagnosis

The diagnostic criteria in ICD-10 and DSM-IV are similar, though the latter assigns rather more importance to numbing. DSM-IV has two criteria not present in ICD-10: symptoms must have been present for at least a month, and must cause significant distress or impaired social functioning. As a result of these differences, the concordance between the diagnosis of PTSD using the two sets of criteria is only 35% (Andrews *et al.* 1999). By convention, post-traumatic stress disorder can be diagnosed in people who have a history of psychiatric disorder before the stressful events.

Differential diagnoses include:

◆ stress-induced exacerbations of previous anxiety or mood disorders;

◆ acute stress disorders (distinguished by the time course);

◆ adjustment disorders (distinguished by the different pattern of symptoms).

PTSD may present as deliberate self-harm or substance abuse which have developed as maladaptive coping strategies (see above).

Epidemiology

Estimates of the prevalence of post-traumatic stress disorder in the general population are mainly from the USA. Rates in other countries are likely to differ somewhat in relation to the frequency of natural and man-made disasters in these places. Using DSM-IV criteria, the 1-month prevalence of PTSD has been found to be 1.2% for men and 2.7% for women (Stein *et al.* 1997b). The lifetime prevalence has been reported as 5–6% among men, and 10–12% among women (Breslau *et al.* 1997a, 1997b, 1998). Studies of groups subjected to unusual stress yield higher rates: for example, to 3.6% in a population affected by a volcanic eruption (Shore *et al.* 1989), about 30% among volunteer firefighters (McFarlane 1989) and victims of torture (Ramsay *et al.* 1993). A rate of 45% has been reported among battered women (Housekamp and Foy 1991).

Aetiology

The stressor

The necessary cause of post-traumatic stress disorder is an exceptionally stressful event. It is not necessary that the person should have been harmed physically or threatened personally; those involved in other ways may develop the disorder, for example, the driver of a train in whose path someone has thrown himself for suicide (Farmer *et al.* 1992), and the bystanders at a major accident. The authors of DSM-IV describe such events as involving actual or threatened death or serious injury or a threat to the physical integrity of the person or others. In a study of people affected by a volcanic eruption, the highest rate of post-traumatic stress disorder was amongst those who experienced the greatest exposure to the stressful events (Shore *et al.* 1989). Even so, not all those most affected by the stressor developed post-traumatic stress disorder, a finding that indicates that some form of personal vulnerability plays a part. Such vulnerability might be genetic or acquired.

Genetic factors

Studies of twins suggest that differences in susceptibility are in part genetic. True *et al.* (1993) studied 2224 monozygotic and 1818 dizygotic male twin pairs who had served in the US armed forces during the Vietnam war. After allowance had been made for the amount of exposure to combat, genetic variation accounted for about one-third of the variance in susceptibility to self-reported post-traumatic stress disorder. Self-reported childhood and adolescent environment did not contribute substantially to this variance.

Other predisposing factors

Vulnerability to developing post-traumatic stress disorder appears to be related to temperament (McFarlane 1989), and in particular to neuroticism. Other factors determining vulnerability are age (children and old people are more vulnerable), gender (women are more vulnerable), a history of psychiatric disorder (Andreasen 1985; Smith *et al.*

1990), previous traumatic experiences, including separation from parents and child abuse, and pre-existing low self-esteem (King *et al.* 1996; Breslau *et al.* 1997a, 1997b). Other possible predisposing factors are differences in the way that threatening events are appraised and encoded in memory (see Ehlers *et al.*, 1998).

Neuroendocrine factors

Several neuroendocrine abnormalities have been reported in patients with PTSD (Charney *et al.* 1993). The findings indicate sensitization of the noradrenergic system, with rather less strong evidence for downregulation of 2-adrenoreceptors, and sensitization of the serotonergic system (see Southwick *et al.* 1997). Cortisol levels increase in response to stress but in PTSD they are reduced (Yehuda *et al.* 1990). This reduction does not seem to be due to a decline in an initially normal response since a study of cortisol levels immediately after a road accident found low cortisol responses at that time in the people who went on to develop PTSD. [People with higher than average cortisol immediately after the accident were more likely to develop depression at follow-up (Yehuda *et al.* 1998).]

Psychological factors

Fear conditioning

Some patients with post-traumatic stress disorder experience vivid memories of the traumatic events in response to smell and sounds related to the stressful situation. This finding suggests that classical conditioning may be involved.

Cognitive theories

These suggest that post-traumatic stress disorder arises when the normal processing of emotionally charged information is overwhelmed, so that memories persist in an unprocessed form in which they can intrude into conscious awareness. In support of this idea, patients with PTSD tend to have incomplete and disorganized recall of the traumatic events (Van Kolk and Fisler 1995). Individual differences in response to the same trau-

matic events are explained as due to differences in the appraisal of the trauma and of its effects. Similarly, difference in the appraisal of the early symptoms may explain why these symptoms persist longer in some people. Negative interpretations of intrusive thoughts (for example, I am going mad) after road accidents predict the continuing presence of PTSD after one year (Ehlers *et al.* 1998). The cognitive model of PTSD has been reviewed by Ehlers and Clark (2000).

Psychodynamic theories

These emphasize the role of previous experience in determining individual variations in the response to severely stressful events (see, for example, Horowitz 1986). The general approach is plausible, but it is not supported by scientific evidence.

Maintaining factors

As noted above, symptoms of PTSD may be maintained in part by negative appraisals of the early symptoms. Other suggested maintaining factors include avoidance of reminders of the traumatic situation (which prevents deconditioning and cognitive reappraisal), and suppression of anxious thoughts which is known to make them more likely to recur (Wegner *et al.*, 1989).

Prognosis

In general, about half those developing PTSD recover during the first year whilst the rest may continue for long periods (see Ehlers 2000). Recovery is less likely if the initial symptoms are severe.

Assessment

This should include enquiries about the nature and duration of symptoms, previous personality, and psychiatric history. When the traumatic events have included head injury (for example, in an assault or transport accident), a neurological examination should be carried out.

Treatment

Planning for disaster

Planning is needed to ensure an immediate and appropriate response to the psychological effects of a major disaster. Such a response can be achieved by enrolling and training helpers who can support victims and are willing to be called on at short notice, and by agreeing procedures for contacting these helpers promptly. At the time of the disaster, priorities have to be decided between the needs of the victims of the disaster, those of relatives (including children), and those of members of the emergency services who may be severely affected by their experiences.

Immediate measures

The initial treatment of post-traumatic stress disorder is the same as that described already for acute reactions to stress, namely sympathetic support and help with any practical problems. A few doses of a benzodiazepine drug may be needed when anxiety is very severe, and a hypnotic drug may be required for a few nights to restore sleep. This simple early care is best carried out by personnel treating any physical injury resulting from the traumatic events, or by other emergency workers (see below). As explained on p. 193, debriefing is widely offered to the victims of disasters and to people involved in their rescue and care. Debriefing has not been shown to help; the majority of victims recover as quickly without it. Recall of events is a component of cognitive therapy but in this treatment memories are not just recalled but also processed and integrated (see below).

Later treatment

Counselling

The treatment of established post-traumatic stress disorder is difficult. The general approach is to provide emotional support, to encourage recall of the traumatic events to integrate them into the patient's experience, and to facilitate working through the associated emotions. Treatment may also need to deal with the person's feelings of guilt about perceived shortcomings in responding during the events, grief, and guilt about surviving when others have died. There may be existential concerns about the meaning and purpose of life and death (Horowitz 1986). Victims of personal assault or rape have additional concerns (see p. 199).

Cognitive–behavioural treatment

This treatment has several components:

- information about the normal response to severe stress, and the importance of confronting situations and memories related to the traumatic events;
- self-monitoring of symptoms;
- *exposure* to situations that are being avoided;
- *recall of images* of the traumatic events, to integrate these with the rest of the patient's experience. When first recalled these images are often fragmentary and are not related clearly in time to the other contents of memory;
- *cognitive restructuring* through the discussion of evidence for and against the appraisals and assumptions;
- *anger management* for people who still feel angry about the traumatic events and their causes.

A meta-analysis suggests that cognitive behavioural treatments have an effect size of 1.89 for ratings made by observers, and 1.27 for ratings made by patients, compared with ratings for placebo of 0.77 for observer-rated and 0.51 for patient-rated symptoms (Van Etten and Taylor 1998). An effect size of 1 corresponds with improvement of one standard deviation on the relevant measure.

Eye movement and desensitization reprocessing was designed for the treatment of post-traumatic stress disorder (see p. 738). When compared with a wait list control, the method was significantly more effective (Rothbaum 1997). When compared with exposure plus stress inoculation in a study with 23 patients with PTSD, the latter was more effective (Devilly and Spence 1999). Further studies are needed before the method can be evaluated. For a review see Shepherd *et al.* (2000).

Psychodynamic psychotherapy aims to modify unconscious conflicts, which are thought to have been reactivated by the traumatic events (see Marmar 1991). In the meta-analysis referred to above, the single study of psychodynamic treatment had an effect size of 0.90 for self-rated symptoms.

Medication

Anxiolytic drugs should be avoided for established post-traumatic stress disorder because prolonged use may lead to dependence. Specific serotonin re-uptake inhibitors had an effect size of 1.38 in the meta-analysis referred to above. Monoamine oxidase inhibitors have been recommended for post-traumatic symptoms, but their effect size was not significantly greater than placebo in the meta-analysis referred to above. Clinical trials of tricyclics have shown only a modest effect even with high doses (Davidson *et al.* 1990). Without clearer guidance from clinical trials, the clinician can try the effect of a specific serotonin uptake inhibitor such as paroxetine or a sedative antidepressant, if drug treatment seems an appropriate part of management.

For a review of the treatment of medication for post-traumatic stress disorder see Davidson (1997) and for psychological treatments see Ehlers (2000). For treatment guidelines see Foa *et al.* (1999b) and Foa *et al.* (2000).

Response to special kinds of severe stress

Rape and physical assault

Victims of rape or physical assault experience acute reactions to stress, post-traumatic stress disorder, anxiety and depressive disorders, and psychosexual dysfunction. Post-traumatic stress disorder is the most frequent of these consequences. In one study of women victims of rape, 94% had post-traumatic stress disorder immediately after the assault, and 47% had the symptoms 3 months later (Rothbaum *et al.* 1992). In another study of rape victims, two-thirds of women reported reduced sexual activity, whilst 40% gave up intercourse or had impaired orgasm for 6 months after the rape (Burgess and Holmstrom 1979a).

As well as experiencing symptoms of post-traumatic stress disorder, victims of rape and assault feel humiliated, ashamed, and vulnerable to further attack. They lose confidence and self-esteem, question why they were chosen as victims, and blame themselves for putting themselves in unnecessary danger (Janoff-Bulman and Frieze 1983). To these problems are added issues of betrayal and secrecy when the rapist is a family member or a friend (Nadelson 1989). The victims may have problems in trusting, persistent anger and irritability, and excessive dependence. These problems were described first among women victims of rape but similar difficulties have been described among victims of male sexual assault (Mezey and King 1989).

Problems are more likely to persist when there has been an actual or perceived threat to life, previous psychological and social problems, past victimization, particularly abuse in childhood, past psychiatric illness or substance abuse, or a lack of social support (see Mezey and Robbins 2000).

Treatment

Social support is important in providing opportunities for the victim to talk over the problem and to regain self-esteem (Burgess and Holmstrom 1979b). Specific treatment is similar to that of other kinds of post-traumatic stress disorder, including prolonged exposure by reliving the events in imagination (Foa *et al.* 1991), with additional emphasis on overcoming feelings of vulnerability and self-blame. Since half the victims of rape no longer have symptoms 3 months after the assault; early treatment should be focused on those who are most distressed or have the risk factors noted above.

War and other armed conflict

Shell shock, battle fatigue, or war neurosis are terms used during the First World War, to describe psychological reactions to battle in British and

American servicemen. Most of the reactions appear to resemble cases now diagnosed as post-traumatic stress disorder; others seem to have resembled panic disorder or depressive disorders. Cases with panic attacks and concerns about the heart, now diagnosed as panic disorder (see p. 238), were known then as Da Costa's syndrome or disorderly action of the heart. Army psychiatrists were few in number, and were unable to deal with the many cases. In any case, their experience of mental hospital work with severely ill patients did not equip them to treat these reactions to battle. Therefore, patients with shell shock were treated mainly by neurologists or psychologists. W. H. Rivers, William Brown, and William McDougall were British psychologists who treated shell shock during the war, and used this experience to write influential books on medical psychology in the years after the war (Rivers 1920; McDougall 1926; Brown 1934).

Treatment

At first, shell shock was treated with the methods in use at the time for neurasthenia (see p. 469), namely rest, isolation, massage, and diet, but these methods had a low success rate. Hypnosis achieved some dramatic cures but was not generally effective. Medical psychologists tried psychotherapeutic methods advocated by Freud, including the recall of stressful events to remove repression and the expression of associated emotion. There was an increasing emphasis on early treatment, and it became evident that psychotherapy had to be combined with military drill to maintain general fitness and morale. This combined treatment led to improved results.

These general principles of early treatment, abreaction, and maintenance of fitness and morale were adopted in the Second World War and in subsequent conflicts. Abreaction with anxiolytic drugs was used widely in the Second World War (see Sargant and Slater 1940). In subsequent conflicts it has been reported that, with immediate counselling (without drug-induced abreaction), about 70% of 'battle shock' personnel can be returned to

their units within 5 days (Brandon 1991). Recently, patients have been treated along the lines described above for PTSD.

The treatment of shell shock in the British army in the First World War has been described by Stone (1985).

Problems of refugees and victims of torture

Refugees may have experienced a wide range of traumatic events, including: the conditions of war, loss of home and possessions, loss by death or separation of relatives and friends, physical injury (including brain injury) either from the actions of war or from assault, rape or torture, and the witnessing of violence to others. Those involved may develop any of the reactions to stressful events, especially post-traumatic stress disorder and depressive disorders, These conditions have been identified in refugees from many cultures, though the presenting complaints may differ somewhat in people from different cultures, with more emphasis on physical than on psychological symptoms among people from non-Western countries. Victims of torture often experience post-traumatic stress disorder as well as the physical consequences of the experience. Factors increasing a person's resistance to the psychological effects of torture are said to be strong political convictions, and strong religious faith (see Mollica 2000).

Treatment

Treatment should combine physical and psychiatric care. The latter should be introduced carefully since it may be resisted as stigmatizing, not only by the refugee but also by aid workers. Special care is needed to establish a trusting relationship. Many refugees have problems related to separation, bereavement, and loss of material possessions, so that it is important not to focus narrowly on post-traumatic stress disorder. Victims of torture may need additional help to cope with feelings of personal humiliation and of remorse for the suffering of others.

Care is needed in working through interpreters. If possible, they should not be family members, community elders, or others to whom the refugee is unlikely to speak of shameful experiences. This point is especially important in situations in which women may have experienced sexual assaults, for these may bring shame to the whole family. Ideally, such problems should be dealt with by a female mental health professional who understands the patient's language and culture, but this may be very difficult to arrange.

For further information about the psychiatric problems of refugees see Mollica (2000). For a review of the treatment of victims of torture see Allodi (1991).

Adjustment disorders

This term refers to the psychological reactions arising in relation to adapting to new circumstances. Such circumstances include divorce and separation, a major change of work and abode, such as transition from school to university or migration, and the birth of a handicapped child. Bereavement, the onset of a terminal illness, and sexual abuse involve special kinds of adjustment which are discussed below.

Clinical features

The symptoms of an adjustment disorder include anxiety, worry, poor concentration, depression, and irritability, together with physical symptoms caused by autonomic arousal such as palpitations and tremor. There may be outbursts of dramatic or aggressive behaviour, single or repeated episodes of deliberate self-harm, or the abuse of alcohol or drugs. The onset is more gradual than that of an acute reaction to stress, and the course is more prolonged. Usually social functioning is impaired.

Stressful life events may precipitate depressive, anxiety, schizophrenic, and other psychiatric disorders; for this reason the diagnosis of adjustment disorder is not made when diagnostic criteria for another psychiatric disorder are met. In prac-

tice, therefore, the diagnosis is usually made by excluding an anxiety or depressive disorder. A further requirement for diagnosis is that the disorder starts soon after the change of circumstances. Both ICD-10 and DSM-IV require that the disorder starts within 3 months, and ICD-10 indicates that it usually starts within 1 month. An essential point is that the reaction is understandably related to, and in proportion to, the stressful experience when account is taken of the patient's previous experiences and personality.

Diagnostic conventions

As explained on p. 191, in ICD-10 adjustment disorders are divided into depressive reactions, mixed anxiety and depressive reactions, reactions with disturbance of other emotions, and reactions with disturbed conduct with or without emotional disturbance. DSM-IV lists six types of adjustment disorder:

- with depressed mood;
- with anxious mood;
- with mixed anxiety and depressed mood;
- with disturbance of conduct;
- with mixed disorder of emotions and conduct; and
- unspecified.

Epidemiology

The prevalence of adjustment disorder in the community is unknown. Prevalence in hospital attenders has been estimated as 5% by Andreasen and Wasek (1980). However, this finding is from the USA and it is possible that the rates would be different in countries, such as the UK, in which a greater proportion of these disorders are treated in primary care.

Aetiology

Stressful circumstances are the necessary cause of an adjustment disorder, but individual vulnerability is also important because not all people exposed to the same stressful circumstances develop an adjustment disorder. The nature of this vulnerability is unknown; it seems to vary from person to person, and may relate in part to previous life experiences.

Prognosis

Clinical experience suggests that most adjustment disorders last for several months and a few persist for years. There is little systematic follow-up information though Andreasen and Hoenck (1982) reported that while the prognosis is good for adults, some adolescents with adjustment disorder develop psychiatric disorders in adult life.

Treatment

Treatment is designed to help the patient resolve the stressful problems if this is possible, and to aid the natural processes of adjustment. The latter is done by reducing denial and avoidance of the stressful events, encouraging problem solving, and discouraging maladaptive coping responses. Anxiety can usually be reduced by encouraging the patient to talk about the problems and to express feelings. Occasionally, an anxiolytic or hypnotic drug is needed for a few days.

Problem-solving counselling (see p. 728) encourages the patient to seek solutions to stressful problems, and to consider the advantages and disadvantages of various kinds of action. The patient is then helped to select and implement a course of action to solve the problem. If this action succeeds, another problem is considered. If the first attempt fails, another approach to the original problem is tried. If problems cannot be resolved, the patient is encouraged to come to terms with them. The effectiveness of this treatment is not known.

Special kinds of adjustment

Adjustment to physical illness and handicap

Appraisal of illness

Adjustment to illness cannot be understood simply in terms of the facts about the disease and its objective consequences. Adjustment depends on patients' beliefs about their disorder and its effects on their lives – on their appraisal of their illness. This appraisal may be similar to that of the professionals who are treating them, or it may be very different because it is based on false information or on emotions rather than facts. The appraisal may be reinforced by members of the family who share the patient's views, or it may be contradicted by them, thus adding to the patient's distress. Three terms are much used in the discussions of adjustment to illness and handicap: illness behaviour, the sick role, and quality of life. These terms are considered next.

Illness behaviour

Mechanic (1978) suggested the term illness behaviour for behaviour associated with adjustment to physical or mental disorder, whether adaptive or not. Illness behaviour includes consulting doctors, taking medicines, seeking help from relatives and friends, and giving up inappropriate activities. These behaviours are adaptive in the early stages of illness, but may become maladaptive if they persist into the stage of convalescence when the patient should be becoming independent. Illness behaviour results from the person's conviction that he is ill rather than from the objective presence of disease, and it may develop when no disease is present. Illness behaviour without disease is an important problem in general practice, and once firmly established it is difficult to treat. The concept of illness behaviour overlaps with that of the sick role (described next) but the two are described separately because they have different origins.

The sick role

Society bestows a special role for people who are ill. Parsons (1951) called this the sick role, which is made up of two privileges and two duties:

- exemption from certain social responsibilities;
- the right to expect help and care from others;
- the obligation to seek and cooperate with treatment; and
- the expectation of a desire to recover.

While the person is ill, the sick role is adaptive. If people continue in the sick role after the illness is over, recovery is delayed since they continue to avoid responsibilities and depend on others instead of becoming independent.

Quality of life

Quality of life is a general term applied to the totality of physical, psychological, and social functioning. It is determined by physical impairment, emotional reaction, personality, illness behaviour, and sick role. Illness usually impairs quality of life but occasionally enhances it, for example, as a result of changing excessive commitments to work or excessive use of alcohol. Quality of life is difficult to measure since it covers so many aspects of functioning that rating scales must be either very lengthy or, if brief, very general in their questioning. For a review of measures of quality of life see Fitzpatrick *et al.* (1992) and Fletcher *et al.* (1992).

Adjustment to the onset of physical illness

When people become physically ill, they may feel anxious, depressed, or angry. Usually this emotional reaction is transient, subsiding as the patient comes to terms with the new situation. As in other adjustment reactions, denial or minimization can protect the patient against overwhelming anxiety when the diagnosis is first known. Although helpful in this way, denial can be maladaptive: in the early stage of illness it may lead to delay in seeking help; at a later stage it may lead to poor compliance with treatment. Other coping strategies can be divided into emotion-reducing and problem-solving groups (see p. 187). Coping strategies that reduce emotion are often appropriate in the early stages of illness but should give way to problem-solving coping. Coping may fail when demands are very great, or when coping resources are limited either in the long term, or as a temporary result of disease of, or trauma to, the brain.

Physical illness as a direct cause of psychiatric symptoms

As well as acting as a stressor, physical illness may induce psychiatric symptoms directly. Anxiety, depression, fatigue, weakness, weight loss, or abnormal behaviour may all be caused directly by physical disorders; common examples are listed in Table 8.4. Similarly, sexual dysfunction may be impaired by physical illness or its treatment (see pp. 590–1). Any of these symptoms may be the reason for referral, and psychiatrists should always be alert to the possibility of undetected physical illness in their patients.

Psychiatric symptoms due to treatments for physical illness

Some drugs used in the treatment of physical illness may affect mood, behaviour, and consciousness. The drugs most likely to have these effects are listed in Table 8.5.

Help for people adjusting to physical illness

Most people adjust well to physical illness, but when adjustment is slow and incomplete, psychological treatment may be needed. This treatment need not be complicated and can usually be provided effectively by the general practitioner or the hospital doctors or nurses dealing with the physical illness. Generally, the psychiatrist has a role in treating only the most severe problems or in supporting the medical and nursing staff.

Table 8.4 Physical illness as a direct cause of psychiatric symptoms

Depression	Carcinoma, infections, systemic lupus erythematosus, neurological disorders (including dementias), thyroid disorder, diabetes, Addison's disease
Anxiety	Hyperventilation, hyperthyroidism, hypoglycaemia, neurological disorders, phaeochromocytoma, drug withdrawal
Fatigue	Anaemia, sleep disorders, chronic infection, carcinoma and radiotherapy, diabetes, hypothyroidism, Addison's disease, Cushing's syndrome
Weakness	Myasthenia gravis and other muscle disorder, peripheral neuropathy, other neurological disorders
Episodes of disturbed behaviour	Epilepsy, hypoglycaemia, early dementia,, transient global amnesia, phaeochromocytoma, porphyria, toxic states
Headache	Migraine, giant-cell arteritis, space-occupying lesions
Loss of weight	Carcinoma, diabetes, tuberculosis, hyperthyroidism, malabsorption, chronic infections including tuberculosis and HIV

Table 8.5 Drugs that may cause psychiatric symptoms

Delirium	Central nervous system depressants (hypnotics, sedatives, alcohol, antidepressants, neuroleptics, anticonvulsants, antihistamines), anticholinergic drugs, beta-blockers, digoxin, cimetidine
Psychotic symptoms	Hallucinogenic drugs, appetite suppressants, sympathomimetic drugs, beta-blockers, corticosteroids, L-dopa, indomethacin
Depression	Antihypertensive drugs, oral contraceptives, neuroleptics, anticonvulsants, corticosteroids, L-dopa
Elation	Antidepressants, corticosteroids, anticholinergic drugs, isoniazid
Behavioural disturbance	Benzodiazepines, neuroleptics

The first step is to identify patients who are adjusting badly (failing to cope). This is generally done by the professional staff who are caring for the physical illness. They can do this most easily by looking out for patients who are progressing less well than would be expected from the severity of the disease. Mood disorders are a common cause of slow progress, but some are dismissed as normal responses to the problems of the illness. Screening questionnaires can be used to detect mood disorders among this group, but the results should be checked at least by a brief interview, carried out, if possible, in surroundings in which the replies will not be overheard. Generally, one or more members of the family should be interviewed to obtain information about the patient's previous adjustment to problems and illness, and to discover how the family views the illness.

Some patients require medication but for many counselling is more appropriate. Counselling requires a trusting relationship with the patient and this in turn requires adequate time for the interviews. Counselling begins with an explanation of the nature of the illness and its treatment; the patient is then helped to accept the implication of the diagnosis, to adjust to illness, and to give up any maladaptive behaviours such as excessive dependence on others or denial of the need for treatment. Graded activities, motivational interviewing, and anger management may be useful in some cases.

If the reaction to physical illness is an anxiety or a depressive, treatment appropriate to the disorder should be given (see Chapters 9 and 11).

Adjustment to terminal illness

Amongst patients dying in hospital, about half have emotional symptoms of anxiety, depression, anger, or guilt. Determinants of emotional reactions include the patient's personality, and the amount and quality of support from family, friends, and carers. Understandably, emotional reactions are more common among young dying patients than among the elderly. They are less common among patients who believe in an afterlife.

Anxiety

Anxiety may be provoked by the prospect of severe pain, disfigurement, or incontinence, by fear of death, and by concerns about the future of the family. Families and carers sometimes try to spare the patient anxiety by concealing the truth about the condition. Since most patients become aware of the diagnosis, attempts at concealment only increase their fear of possible consequences of the disease such as pain or incontinence.

Depression

Depression may be provoked by the prospect of separation from family and friends and the loss of valued activities. Changes in physical appearance caused by the illness, the effects of surgery, and the debilitating effects of radiotherapy are other causes of low mood. Depressive disorders develop in 5–15% of patients (Cody 1990).

Guilt and anger

Some patients experience guilt because they believe that they are making excessive demands on rela-

tives or friends. Patients with religious beliefs may believe that illness is a punishment for previous wrongdoing. Anger may be felt about the unjustness of impending death; this anger may be displaced onto doctors, nurses, and relatives, making care more difficult (see below).

Defence mechanisms

Defence mechanisms observed in dying patients are most often denial, dependency, and displacement:

- *Denial* is usually the first reaction to the news of fatal illness. It may be experienced as a feeling of disbelief and may lead to an initial period of calm. Denial diminishes as the patient becomes reconciled to the illness. Denial may return as the disease progresses, and the patient may again behave as if unaware of the nature of the illness.

- *Dependency* is adaptive in the early stages of severe physical illness when the patient needs to comply passively with treatment. Excessive or prolonged dependency makes subsequent treatment more difficult, and increases the burden on the family. A further stage of dependency may be appropriate as the patient nears death.

- *Displacement* is often of anger, which may be directed to staff and relatives, who may not understand this reaction so that they find it difficult to tolerate. As a result they may spend less time with the patient, thereby increasing his feelings of despair.

Denial, dependency, and displacement are usually followed by *acceptance*. The doctor's aim should be to help the patient to reach this acceptance before the final stage of the illness. This aim is more likely to be achieved when there is good communication between patients, the staff caring for them, and relatives.

Psychological symptoms

Psychological symptoms induced by the disease or its treatment may add to the patient's distress. The more frequent associations between disease and psychological symptoms are summarized in Table 8.4. There is a particularly strong association between dyspnoea and anxiety. The associations between drug treatment and psychological symptoms are summarized in Table 8.5.

Treatment

Usually dying patients are helped to adjust by the staff who are caring for the physical illness. Psychiatrists are called upon only when there are special problems (see below), or to assist with staff support and training.

The aims of treatment

According to Hackett and Weissman (1962), the aim of treating the dying patient should be to achieve an 'appropriate death'. By this they meant that

the person should be relatively free from pain, should operate on as effective a level as possible, should recognize and resolve remaining conflicts, should satisfy as far as possible remaining wishes, and should be able to yield control to others in whom he has confidence.

Kubler-Ross (1969) formulated the aims in different terms and described five phases of psychological adjustment to death. The phases do not necessarily occur in the same sequence, and some may not occur at all, but they are a useful guide for professionals helping dying patients. The phases are:

- denial and isolation,
- anger,
- partial acceptance ('bargaining for time'),
- depression, and
- acceptance.

Reducing symptoms

Adequate control of pain and breathlessness and the reduction of confusion due to delirium are particularly important. Anxiety and depression may diminish as pain and breathlessness are controlled. The causes of delirium are listed on p. 404. Among dying patients, important remediable causes are dehydration, the side-effects of drugs, secondary infection, cardiac or respiratory failure, and hypercalcaemia (Stedeford and Regnard 1991).

Helping the patient to adjust

It is essential to establish a good relationship with the patient so that he can talk about his problems and ask questions. The nature of the illness should be explained honestly and in simple language. Sometimes doctors are apprehensive that such an explanation will increase patients' distress. Although excessive detail given unsympathetically can have this effect, it is seldom difficult to decide how much to say about diagnosis and prognosis provided that patients are allowed to lead the discussion, express their worries, and say what they want to know. If patients ask about the prognosis, they should be told the truth; evasive answers undermine trust in the carers. If patients do not seem to wish to know the full extent of their problems, it is usually better to save this information until later. At an appropriate stage patients should be told what can be done to make their remaining time as comfortable as possible. Whilst the whole account should be truthful, the amount disclosed on a single occasion should be judged by patients' reactions and by their questions. If necessary, the doctor should be prepared to return for further discussion when patients are ready to continue. It is important to bear in mind that most dying patients become aware of their prognosis whether or not they are told directly, because they infer the truth from the behaviour of those who are caring for them. They notice when answers to questions are evasive and when people avoid talking to them. Patients who are anxious, angry, or despairing need to be able to express these feelings and to discuss the ideas that induce them.

Informing the staff

The information given to the patient should be known to all the staff, otherwise conflicting advice and opinions may be given. If all those involved know what has been said, they will feel more at ease in talking to the patient. Otherwise they will draw back from the patient, isolating him, and increasing his difficulty in adjusting.

Informing and supporting relatives

Relatives need to know what has been said to the patient so that they will feel less ill at ease when talking to him. Relatives may need as much help as the patient. They may become anxious and depressed, and they may respond with guilt, anger, or denial. Such reactions make it difficult for them to communicate helpfully with the patient or the staff. Relatives need information, and opportunities to talk about their feelings, and to prepare for the impending bereavement. Without these the patient and the family may become increasingly distant and alienated.

Special services

In many hospitals, *specialist nurses* work with the family doctor and with the hospital staff caring for dying patients. These nurses are trained in the psychological as well as the physical care of the dying. Sometimes care is provided in *hospices* where it is possible to provide close attention to the details of care that improve quality of life for the dying person. These hospices care for patients when home care is impractical, and provide periods of respite care to relieve those who are caring for the patient at home.

Referral to a psychiatrist

Referral to a psychiatrist is appropriate when psychiatric symptoms or behaviour disturbance are severe. About 10–15% of patients in terminal care units are referred to a psychiatrist (Stedeford and Bloch 1979; Ramsay 1992). The referrals are concerned with the assessment and management of:

- *depressed patients*, to decide the cause and whether they require medication;
- *uncommunicative patients* who will not talk about the illness;
- *uncooperative patients* who do not accept the social restrictions imposed by the illness, will not make appropriate plans, or take necessary decisions;
- *long-standing problems made worse by the illness* and related to personality or family conflicts;

- *other symptoms.* Although anxiety and delirium are common, these problems are more often dealt with appropriately by medical staff, than referred to a psychiatrist The exception is delirium with paranoid symptoms (Ramsay 1992).

Management of depressive disorders

Depressive disorders may be caused by pain, breathlessness, or delirium, all of which should be treated appropriately. Any drugs that can cause depression (see Table 8.5) should be reviewed and, if possible, given in lower dose or replaced. Some symptoms of depressive disorder are difficult to evaluate in patients with advanced cancer; thus weight loss, anorexia, insomnia, loss of interest, and fatigue may be caused by the physical illness. Early morning wakening, extreme hopelessness, and self-blame are surer guides to diagnosis. Suicidal ideation should be assessed carefully. If counselling and improved medical management do not improve the low mood, antidepressant drugs should be prescribed with careful supervision. Among physically ill patients, tricyclic antidepressants may induce side-effects including delirium, nausea, and urinary retention; hence the starting dose should be small, and medication should be changed if necessary to find a compound that is well tolerated (see Block 2000 for treatment guidelines).

Liaison with medical and nursing staff

Liaison with medical and nursing staff is important. Often these staff can provide treatment when the psychiatrist has formulated a plan.

For further information about the care of the dying, see Wiener *et al.* (1996).

Grief and adjustment to bereavement

Terminology

Although the words bereavement, mourning, and grief are sometimes used interchangeably, they have separate meanings which incorporate distinctions that are useful in psychiatry:

◆ *Bereavement* is the loss through death of a loved person.

◆ *Grief* is the involuntary emotional and behavioural response to bereavement.

◆ *Mourning* is the voluntary expression of behaviours and rituals that are socially sanctioned responses to bereavement. These behaviours and rituals differ between societies and between religious groups both in their form and in their duration.

The systems of classification do not make these distinctions in consistent ways. In ICD-10, bereavement is coded appropriately as Z63.4, that is as one of the 'factors influencing health status and contact with health services'. In DSM-IV, however, bereavement is coded as a 'condition that may be the focus of clinical attention'; thus, the term is used to denote the response to bereavement rather than the event itself. ICD-10 codes grief under adjustment disorders, but uses the term grief reaction. Mourning – a form of social behaviour – is not a disorder and, appropriately, is not listed in the index to either classification. In this chapter the term bereavement reaction is used to denote all responses to bereavement, normal and abnormal. Normal reactions are called grief, abnormal reactions include abnormal (or pathological) grief, and depressive disorders.

Grief

Grief is a continuous process, but it can be described conveniently as having three stages (Table 8.6).

The first stage lasts from a few hours to several days. There is denial, which is manifested as a lack of emotional response ('numbness'), often with a feeling of unreality, and incomplete acceptance that the death has taken place. The bereaved person may be restless, as if searching for the dead person.

The second stage usually lasts from a few weeks to about 6 months but may be much longer. There may be extreme sadness, weeping, loneliness, and often overwhelming waves of yearning for the dead person. Anxiety is common; the bereaved person is

Table 8.6 **Normal grief reaction**
Stage I: hours to days
Denial, disbelief
'Numbness'
Stage II: weeks to 6 months
Sadness, weeping, waves of grief
Somatic symptoms of anxiety
Restlessness
Poor sleep
Diminished appetite
Guilt, blame of others
Experience of a presence
Illusions, vivid imagery
Hallucinations of the dead person's voice
Preoccupation with memories of deceased
Social withdrawal
Stage III: weeks to months
Symptoms resolve
Social activities resumed
Memories of good times
(Symptoms may recur at anniversaries)

anxious and restless, sleeps poorly, lacks appetite, and may experience panic attacks. Many bereaved people feel guilt that they failed to do enough for the deceased. Some feel anger and project their feelings of guilt, blaming doctors or others for failing to provide optimal care for the dead person. Many bereaved people have a vivid experience of being in the presence of the dead person, and about one in ten experience brief hallucinations (Clayton 1979). The bereaved person is preoccupied with memories of the dead person, sometimes in the form of intrusive images. Withdrawal from social relationships is frequent. Complaints of physical symptoms are common (Parkes and Brown 1972), and widows seek medical care more often than comparable people who are not bereaved (Stein and Susser 1969).

In the third stage, these symptoms subside and everyday activities are resumed. The bereaved person gradually comes to terms with the loss and recalls the good times shared with the deceased in the past. Often there is a temporary return of symptoms on the anniversary of the death.

Although these stages are a useful guideline, individual responses are not all the same and no one feature is universal (Schuchter and Zisook 1993).

Abnormal or pathological grief

Grief is considered abnormal if it is unusually intense, unusually prolonged, delayed, or inhibited or distorted. The criterion for abnormal intensity is that the symptoms meet the criteria for a depressive disorder. The criterion for abnormal duration is that the response lasts more than 6 months. The usual criterion for delay is that the first stage of grief has not occurred by 2 weeks after the death of the loved person. In all these forms of grief, persistent avoidance of situations and of other reminders of death are common.

Abnormally intense grief Depressive symptoms are a frequent component of normal grief and up to 35% of bereaved people meet the criteria for a depressive disorder at some time during their grieving (Clayton *et al.* 1974; Zisook and Schuchter 1993). Most of these depressive disorders resolve within 6 months but about 20% persist for longer (Jacobs 1993). It might be argued that if about a third of bereaved people meet the criterion for depressive disorder at some time, the threshold has been set too low. However, people who meet the criteria for a depressive disorder are more likely to have poor social adjustment, to visit doctors frequently (Zisook and Shuchter 1993), and to use alcohol (Clayton and Darvish 1979). Therefore, it is of practical value to use the criterion and to record the additional diagnosis of a depressive disorder in these cases. When there is doubt whether depressive disorder should be recorded, particular attention should be paid to symptoms of retardation and

global loss of self-esteem (clearly greater than regret about omissions of care during the terminal illness), because these features are seldom present in uncomplicated grief (Clayton *et al.* 1974; Jacobs *et al.* 1989).

Suicidal thoughts may occur when grief is intense. The rate of suicide is increased most in the year after bereavement, but continues to be high for 5 years after the death of a spouse or parent. Young widows and elderly widowers are at higher risk than other bereaved people (MacMahon and Pugh 1965; Bunch 1972). The presence of suicidal ideas should prompt appropriate assessment of suicide risk (see p. 515).

Prolonged grief As explained above, prolonged (or chronic) grief is often defined as grief lasting for more than 6 months. Instead of the normal progression, symptoms of the first and second stages persist. However, it is difficult to set a precise limit to normal grief, and complete resolution may take much longer. One study found that only a minority of widows had ceased to grieve a year after the death (Parkes 1971). Prolonged grief may be associated with a depressive disorder but can occur without it.

Delayed grief By convention, delayed grief is said to occur when the first stage of grief does not appear until more than 2 weeks after the death. It is said to be more frequent after sudden, traumatic, or unexpected deaths (Jacobs 1993, p. 175).

Inhibited and distorted grief The term inhibited grief refers to a reaction which lacks some normal features. Distorted grief refers to features (other than depressive symptoms) that are either unusual in degree, for example, marked hostility, overactivity, and extreme social withdrawal, or else unusual in kind, for example, physical symptoms that were part of the last illness of the deceased. These distorted presentations were described by Lindemann (1944) in a study of survivors of a fire in a nightclub. Whilst the idea has some value, it has not led to clear criteria by which to judge a particular case.

In all these forms of grief, persistent avoidance of situations and of other reminders of death are common.

Causes of abnormal grief

Abnormal grief is generally thought to be more likely when:

- the death was sudden and unexpected;
- the bereaved person had a very close, or dependent, or ambivalent relationship with the deceased;
- the survivor is insecure, or has difficulty in expressing feelings, or has suffered a previous psychiatric disorder;
- the survivor has to care for dependent children and so cannot show grief easily.

It might be expected that lack of social support would be a cause of abnormal grief, but the available research evidence does not support this idea (Jacobs 1993, Chapter 6) even though social support certainly assists people who are bereaved (see Parkes 1985 or Stroebe and Stroebe 1993 for a review).

Mortality after bereavement

Several studies (reviewed by Stroebe and Stroebe 1993) have shown an increased rate of mortality among bereaved spouses and other close relatives, with the greatest increase being in the first 6 months after bereavement. Most studies report increased rates of death from heart disease, and some have reported increased rates of death from cancer, liver cirrhosis, suicide, and accidents. The reasons for these associations are uncertain, and are likely to be different for different conditions. Increased rates of suicide have been reported (Bunch 1972).

Management of grief

Grief is a normal response and most people pass through it with the help of family, friends, spiritual advisors, and the rituals of mourning. In some Western societies, many people may not have links with a religion, the rituals of mourning may be attenuated, and family may not be close at hand. For these and other reasons, family doctors have an important part to play in helping the bereaved. Psychiatrists may be asked to help people with abnormal grief.

Although bereaved people have some problems in common, they also have problems that are individual. For example, a young widow with small children has many difficulties that are not shared by an elderly widow whose adult children can support her. A mother grieving for a stillborn child will have special problems (discussed below). In planning management it is important to take into account the individual circumstances of the patient as well as the general guidelines outlined below.

Counselling

When counselling is appropriate, it is similar to counselling for other kinds of adjustment reaction. The bereaved person needs to talk about the loss, to express feelings of sadness, guilt, or anger, and to understand the normal course of grieving. It is helpful to forewarn a bereaved person about unusual experiences such as feeling as if the dead person were present, illusions, and hallucinations; otherwise these experiences may be alarming. Help may be needed to:

- accept that the loss is real;
- work through the stages of grief;
- adjust to life without the deceased.

The bereaved person may need help to progress from the first stage of denial of loss to the acceptance of reality. Viewing the dead body and putting away the dead person's belongings help this transition, and a bereaved person should be encouraged to perform these actions. Practical problems may need to be discussed, including funeral arrangements and financial difficulties. A young widow may need help in maintaining and caring for young children, and in supporting them without inhibiting her own grief excessively. As time passes, the bereaved person should be encouraged to resume social contacts, to talk to other people about the loss, to remember happy and fulfilling experiences that were shared with the deceased, and to consider positive activities that the latter would have wanted survivors to undertake. (For further information about grief counselling see Worden 1991.)

Parents grieving for a stillborn child need special help. They should be encouraged to name the dead baby and to view the body. If they do not feel able to take these steps, it is often helpful to obtain a photograph of the body, which the parents can see later if they wish. If these steps are combined with counselling, the mothers of stillborn children experience less distress than those not given this help (Forrest and Standish 1984).

Medication

Drug treatment cannot remove the distress of normal grief, but it may be needed in specific circumstances. In the first stage of grief, a hypnotic or anxiolytic drug may be needed for a few days to restore sleep or to relieve any severe anxiety. In the second stage, antidepressant drugs may be beneficial if the criteria for depressive disorder are met, though such usage has not been evaluated in this special group Medication may be needed for a short period in the second stage to relieve severe anxiety.

Support groups

Support groups have been developed to help recently bereaved people, particularly young widows. One such organization in the UK is known as CRUSE. By sharing their experience with others who have dealt successfully with bereavement, recently bereaved people can share grief, obtain practical advice, and discuss ways of coping. In one study a support group was found to be as effective as brief psychotherapy, although more people dropped out of the support group (Marmar *et al.* 1988); in another study of support groups the benefit was small (Barrett 1978).

Psychotherapy

It is not practical, nor is there evidence that it is helpful, to provide psychotherapy for all bereaved persons. There is some evidence that crisis intervention may be helpful for people who are at high risk of an abnormal grief reaction (Raphael 1977), though not for unselected grieving people (Polak *et al.* 1975). Marmar *et al.* (1988) studied brief dynamic psychotherapy and they found it no more effective than a mutual support group. Similarly, Lieberman and Yalom (1992) found no significant difference in outcome between bereaved spouses treated with group psychotherapy and a control group who were not treated.

Guided mourning

Guided mourning is the name given to a procedure which reduces avoidant behaviours that are thought to prolong grief. The bereaved person is helped to confront memories of the dead person and to enter situations that provoke these memories (it is a form of exposure treatment, see p. 735). In a controlled evaluation, this approach produced modest benefit (Mawson *et al.* 1981; Foa *et al.* 1991).

For a fuller description of the psychological treatment of grief, see Worden (1991) or Jacobs (1993).

Long-term adjustment to sexual abuse in childhood

When sexually abused, children may experience anxiety, depression, and post-traumatic stress disorder (see p. 858). These effects usually subside during childhood, but people who have been abused in childhood appear to be more vulnerable than others to psychiatric disorder in adult life. Also, sexual abuse in childhood may be followed by persistent low self-esteem and psychosexual difficulties whether or not a psychiatric disorder develops.

Some adults who were previously unaware that they had been sexually abused in childhood suddenly recall the abuse in a vivid and disturbing way. Sometimes this recall occurs spontaneously, often when the person has encountered a reminder of the events. It may occur also during counselling or psychotherapy, at a time when childhood experiences are being discussed. Some of these recollections are confirmed by other evidence, but many are vigorously denied by the alleged abuser, who is often one of the parents. It has been suggested that some, perhaps most, of these unconfirmed reports of abuse are not accurate memories and that some have been induced by questions, suggestions, or interpretations from the therapists. This phenomenon has been called the false memory syndrome.

Recovered memory and false memory

Many victims of sexual abuse, and of other severe stressful events, have partial amnesia for the most stressful parts of the experience, even though they have suffered no head injury that could lead to post-traumatic amnesia. Indeed, partial amnesia is part of the clinical picture of post-traumatic stress disorder. However, complete amnesia is less frequent and, to many psychiatrists, complete amnesia for repeated stressful events followed by their recall, is improbable, especially when there is no supporting evidence for the events from another source. This doubt is increased by evidence that 'memories' of single non-abusive childhood events can be implanted by suggestion in about a quarter of subjects (see Lindsay and Read 1995; Brewin 2000).

Evidence for the proposition that true memories can be inaccessible for many years and then recovered, comes mainly from clinical reports (see Brewin 2000). These reports suggest that between about a quarter and a half of people reporting childhood sexual abuse describe long periods in which they did not remember the abuse. Also, clinicians have reported that up to 40% of memories recovered in therapy are confirmed by other evidence.

In the absence of conclusive evidence about the status of memories recovered in counselling or psychotherapy, the clinician who is carrying out these procedures should:

◆ take special care not to suggest memories of sexual abuse; and

◆ consider most carefully apparent recovered memories arising for the first time in therapy, before concluding that they are true memories of actual events.

It seems reasonable to conclude that many of the 'recovered memories' elicited without these precautions are likely to be false, and that true recovered memories of repeated sexual abuse are uncommon.

Epidemiology

There have been no satisfactory prospective studies of people who were sexually abused as children, but adults who report sexual abuse in childhood appear to have higher rates of psychiatric disorder in adult life (Beitchman *et al.* 1992). Most of the retrospective information is about the effects on women. Female psychiatric patients are more likely than healthy controls to report sexual abuse in childhood; such reporting is particularly frequent in those with eating disorders (Palmer *et al.* 1992), somatization disorder (Morrison 1989), borderline personality disorder (Bryer *et al.* 1987), multiple personality disorder (Putnam *et al.* 1986), and sexual dysfunction (Briere 1988). It is not clear what proportion of women who were sexually abused in childhood develop these disorders in adult life, but some make a good adjustment.

Aetiology

There could be three explanations for an association between the reporting of childhood sexual abuse and the symptoms of psychiatric disorder in adult life. First, people with psychiatric disorder may be more likely than controls to report childhood sexual abuse, perhaps because they have been asked questions about their childhood in the course of psychiatric assessment. Second, childhood sexual abuse may be a direct cause of vulnerability to adult psychiatric disorder. Third, sexual abuse may be a marker of some other factor, such as disturbed relationships within the family, which is the real cause of the excess psychiatric disorder in adult life. These three possible causes will now be considered in turn.

It seems unlikely that the association can be explained solely by the greater recall of sexual abuse by women who have psychiatric disorder because community studies have also found an association between the reporting of childhood sexual abuse and the reporting of psychiatric symptoms (Bushnell *et al.* 1993).

There is some evidence in favour of the second explanation (a direct causal relationship). Thus, in another community survey, Mullen *et al.* (1993) found higher rates of psychiatric disorder among women reporting severe abuse involving penetration than among women reporting less severe abuse, a finding that suggests a causal relationship between abuse and subsequent disorder.

It appears that, whilst extreme forms of abuse can increase vulnerability, in other cases an association between childhood abuse and adult psychiatric disorder may be explained in part by disturbed relationships in the family of the abused child (Neumann *et al.*, 1996). Clinical observations suggest that effects are more severe when the abusing person is a parent. Also, people who have been abused as children are more likely to report to others that their parents were uncaring or emotionally distant (Alexander and Lupfer 1987). Mullen *et al.* (1993) found that, with less severe forms of abuse, the relationship between abuse and subsequent disorder could be accounted for by the family factors alone, but when abuse was severe, it had an independent effect.

Treatment

The late effects of childhood sexual abuse have been treated with counselling, dynamic psychotherapy, cognitive therapy, and group treatments. The various methods have several common features:

- the general aim is to help the patient understand the earlier experiences and their effects on her life, in order to improve present adjustment;
- the therapeutic relationship is used to help the patient feel trusted, understood, and respected, and to increase self-esteem;
- the patient is allowed to set the pace at which she talks about the experience of being abused. (Otherwise she may be overwhelmed by an

extreme emotional response to the memories of abuse, and withdraw from treatment);

- present problems of adjustment are identified, especially any avoidance of problems and difficulties in expressing anger. Help is given to overcome these difficulties;
- some patients need help with psychosexual problems.

The main difference between the dynamic and cognitive behavioural approaches is the greater emphasis given in the former to understanding the effects of the trauma on self-esteem and emotional expression, and the greater emphasis given in the latter to more precise specification of ways in which current patterns of thinking affect present behaviour.

For a review of psychological treatment of the long-term effects of sexual abuse see Hobbs (1994) and Paddison (1993).

Further reading

Calhoun, K. S. and Atkeson, B. M. (1991). *Treatment of rape victims. Facilitating psychosocial adjustment.* Pergamon Press, New York.

Foa, E. B., Keane, T. M. and Friedmand, M. J. (2000). *PTSD treatment guidelines.* Guilford, New York.

Fullerton C. S. and Ursano, R. J. (eds) (1997). *Posttraumatic stress disorder: acute and long term responses to trauma and disaster.* American Psychiatric Press, Washington, DC and London.

Gelder, M. G., López-Ibor, J. J. Jr, and Andreasen, N. C. (eds) (2000). *The new Oxford textbook of psychiatry*, Section 4.6: Stress related and adjustment disorders. Oxford University Press, Oxford. (The four chapters in this section contain systematic reviews of acute stress reactions, post-traumatic stress disorder, recovered and false memories, and adjustment disorders.)

Parkes, C. M. (1996). *Bereavement: studies of grief in adult life*, 3rd edn. Penguin Books, Harmondsworth. (A brief but comprehensive review, written for the layman but containing useful information for the professional, including a scientific appendix.)

9

CHAPTER 9

Anxiety and obsessive–compulsive disorders

CHAPTER 9
Anxiety and obsessive–compulsive disorders

Terminology and classification

The symptom of anxiety is found in many disorders. In the anxiety disorders, it is the most severe and prominent symptom, and it is also prominent in the obsessional disorders though these are characterized by their striking obsessional symptoms. In DSM-IV, obsessional disorders are classified as a type of anxiety disorder, but in ICD-10 the obsessional symptoms are given more weight and the disorders are classified separately. Because anxiety and obsessional disorders are related, whether closely as in DSM-IV or less closely as in ICD-10, they are considered together in this chapter.

Anxiety disorders

Anxiety disorders are abnormal states in which the most striking features are mental and physical symptoms of anxiety, occurring in the absence of organic brain disease or another psychiatric disorder. The symptoms of anxiety are described on p. 7 and are listed for convenience in Table 9.1. Although all the symptoms can occur in any of the anxiety disorders, there is a characteristic pattern in each disorder which will be described later. In addition there are characteristic differences in the time course of anxiety in the various disorders:

- In generalized anxiety disorders, anxiety is continuous – though it may fluctuate somewhat in intensity.
- In phobic anxiety disorders, anxiety is intermittent, arising only in particular circumstances.

- In panic disorder, anxiety is intermittent but its occurrence is unrelated to any particular circumstances.

These differences will be explained further when the various anxiety disorders are described.

The development of ideas about anxiety disorders

Anxiety has long been recognized as a prominent symptom of many psychiatric disorders. Anxiety and depression often occur together and, until the last part of the nineteenth century, anxiety disorders were not classified separately from other mood disorders. It was Freud (1895b) who first suggested that cases with mainly anxiety symptoms should be separated under the name of anxiety neurosis.

Freud's original anxiety neurosis included patients with phobias and panic attacks, but subsequently he divided it into two groups. The first, which retained the name anxiety neurosis, was for cases with mainly psychological symptoms of anxiety; the second group, which he called anxiety hysteria, was for cases with mainly physical symptoms of anxiety and with phobias. Thus anxiety hysteria included the cases we now diagnose as agoraphobia. Freud originally proposed that the causes of anxiety neurosis and anxiety hysteria were related to sexual conflicts, though he later accepted a rather wider range of causes. By the 1930s most psychiatrists considered that a very wide range of stressful problems could cause anxiety neurosis (see, for example, Henderson and Gillespie 1930, pp. 416–17).

Table 9.1 Symptoms of anxiety

Psychological arousal

Fearful anticipation
Irritability
Sensitivity to noise
Restlessness
Poor concentration
Worrying thoughts

Autonomic arousal

Gastrointestinal
    Dry mouth
    Difficulty in swallowing
    Epigastric discomfort
    Excessive wind
    Frequent or loose motions
Respiratory
    Constriction in the chest
    Difficulty inhaling
Cardiovascular
    Palpitations
    Discomfort in chest
    Awareness of missed beats
Genitourinary
    Frequent or urgent micturition
    Failure of erection
    Menstrual discomfort
    Amenorrhoea

Muscle tension

Tremor
Headache
Aching muscles

Hyperventilation

Dizziness
Tingling in the extremities
Feeling of breathlessness

Sleep disturbance

Insomnia
Night terror

Phobic disorders have been recognized since antiquity, but the first systematic medical study of these conditions was probably that of Le Camus in the eighteenth century (Errera 1962). The early nineteenth century classifications assigned phobias to the group of monomanias, which were disorders of thinking rather than emotion. However, when Westphal (1872) first described agoraphobia, he emphasized the importance of anxiety in the condition. Later, in 1895, Freud divided phobias into two groups: common phobias, in which there was an exaggerated fear of something that is commonly feared (for example, darkness or high places), and specific phobias, that is, fears of situations not feared by healthy people, such as open spaces (Freud 1895a, pp.135–6). As explained later, the term specific phobia now has a rather different meaning.

In the 1960s, the different responses of certain phobias to behavioural methods suggested a grouping into simple phobias, social phobia, and agoraphobia, and these groups were found to differ also in their age of onset. Simple phobias generally begin in childhood, social phobia in late adolescence, and agoraphobia in early adult life (Marks and Gelder 1966). At about the same time, it was observed that when phobias were accompanied by marked panic attacks, they responded poorly to behaviour therapy and better to imipramine (Klein 1964). These cases were subsequently classified separately under the rubric of panic disorder. This led to the present scheme of classification into generalized anxiety disorder, phobic anxiety disorder (simple, social, and agoraphobic), and panic disorder.

The relationship between obsessive–compulsive disorders and anxiety disorders has been and remains uncertain. Freud thought at first that phobias and obsessions were closely related (see Freud 1895a). He proposed later that anxiety is the central problem in both conditions and that their characteristic symptoms – phobias and obsessions – resulted from different kinds of defence mechanisms against anxiety. Others considered that obsessional disorders were a separate group of neuroses of uncertain aetiology. As explained above, this division of opinion is reflected today in the two major classification systems. As explained above, obsessive–compulsive disorders are classified as a subgroup of the anxiety disorders in DSM-IV, whilst in ICD-10, anxiety disorders and obsessive–compulsive disorders have separate places in the classification.

The classification of anxiety disorders

The classification of anxiety disorders in DSM-IV and ICD-10 is broadly similar (Table 9.2), but there are four important differences:

◆ in ICD-10, anxiety disorders are divided into two named subgroups: (a) phobic anxiety disorder (F40) and (b) other anxiety disorder (F41), which includes panic disorder and generalized anxiety disorder;

◆ panic disorder is classified differently in the two schemes (the reasons are explained on p. 238);

◆ in DSM-IV, obsessive–compulsive disorder is classified as one of the anxiety disorders, but in ICD-10 it has a separate place in the classification;

◆ ICD-10 contains a category of mixed anxiety-depressive disorder, but DSM-IV does not.

Generalized anxiety disorders

Clinical picture

The symptoms of generalized anxiety disorder (Table 9.3) are persistent and are not restricted to, or markedly increased in, any particular set of circumstances (in contrast to phobic anxiety disorders; see p. 226). All the symptoms of anxiety (see Table 9.1) can occur in generalized anxiety disorder but there a characteristic pattern comprised of the following features:

◆ *worry and apprehension*, which are difficult to control and more prolonged than the ordinary worries and concerns of healthy people. The worries are widespread and not focused on a specific issue such as the possibility of having

Table 9.2 **Classification of anxiety disorders**		
	ICD–10	**DSM-IV**
F4	Anxiety disorders	Anxiety disorders*
F40	Phobic anxiety disorder	
	Agoraphobia	Agoraphobia
	Without panic disorder	Without a history of panic disorder
	With panic disorder	Panic disorder with agoraphobia
	Social phobia	Social phobia
	Specific phobia	Specific phobia
F41	Other anxiety disorders	
	Panic disorder	Panic disorder without agoraphobia
	Generalized anxiety disorder	Generalized anxiety disorder
	Mixed anxiety and depressive disorder	–

*The order of presentation has been altered to facilitate comparison of the schemes.

Table 9.3 Symptoms of generalized
Worry and apprehension
Muscle tension*
Autonomic overactivity*
Psychological arousal*
Sleep disturbance*
Other features
Depression
Obsessions
Depersonalization
*See also Table 9.1.

a panic attack (as in panic disorder) or of being embarrassed (as in social phobia) or contaminated (as in obsessive–compulsive disorder).

◆ *psychological arousal*, which may be evident as irritability, poor concentration, and sensitivity to noise. Some patients complain of poor memory but this is due to poor concentration. If true memory impairment is found, a careful search should be made for a cause other than anxiety.

◆ *autonomic overactivity*, which is experienced most often as sweating, palpitations, dry mouth, epigastric discomfort, and dizziness. However, patients may complain of any of the symptoms listed in Table 9.1. Some patients ask for help with any of these symptoms without mentioning spontaneously the psychological symptoms of anxiety.

◆ *muscle tension*, which may be experienced as restlessness, trembling, inability to relax, headache (usually bilateral and frontal or occipital) and aching in the shoulders and back.

◆ *hyperventilation*, which may lead to dizziness, tingling in the extremities and, paradoxically, a feeling of shortness of breath.

◆ *sleep disturbances*, which include difficulty in falling asleep and persistent worrying thoughts. Sleep is often intermittent, unrefreshing, and accompanied by unpleasant dreams Some patients have night terrors in which they wake suddenly feeling intensely anxious. Early morning waking is not a feature of generalized anxiety disorder and its presence strongly suggests a depressive disorder.

◆ *other features* These include tiredness, depressive symptoms, obsessional symptoms, and depersonalization. These symptoms are never the most prominent feature of a generalized anxiety disorder. If they are prominent, another diagnosis should be considered (see differential diagnosis below).

Clinical signs

The face appears strained, the brow is furrowed, and the posture is tense. The patient is restless and may tremble. The skin is pale and sweating is common, especially from the hands, feet, and axillae. Readiness to tears, which may at first suggest depression, reflects the generally apprehensive state.

Diagnostic conventions

There is no clear dividing line between generalized anxiety disorder and normal anxiety. For this reason, diagnostic criteria are arbitrary, and they differ in several ways between DSM-IV and ICD-10. Both DSM-IV and the research version of ICD-10 require the presence of a minimum number of symptoms from a list. However, the ICD-10 list contains 22 physical symptoms of anxiety, whilst there are only 6 in the DSM-IV list. Both systems specify a minimum duration for symptoms. In DSM-IV and the research version of ICD-10 symptoms must have been present for 6 months. However, the rule ICD-10 criteria for clinical practice is more flexible; symptoms should have been present on 'most days for at least several weeks at a time, and usually several months'.

Co-morbidity

Anxiety and depression

The two classifications differ in their approach to cases which fulfil the diagnostic criteria for both depressive disorder and generalized anxiety disorder. ICD-10 has a separate category for these cases, namely mixed anxiety and depressive disorder. This category is not included in DSM-IV (though it is included among 'criteria sets for further study') and both diagnoses are made.

Intermittent exacerbations of continuous anxiety

The guidance differs in DSM-IV and ICD-10 about the circumstances in which two diagnoses should be made:

- *in ICD-10*, generalized anxiety disorder is not diagnosed when the disorder meets the criteria for phobic anxiety disorder (F40), panic disorder (F41), or obsessive compulsive disorder (F42).
- *in DSM-IV*, generalized anxiety disorder can be diagnosed in addition to one of these other diagnoses When this rule is used, concurrent anxiety disorders are frequent: social phobia in 23% of cases of generalized anxiety disorder, simple phobia in 21% and panic disorder in 11% (Brawman-Mintzer *et al.* 1993).

Differential diagnosis

General anxiety disorder has to be distinguished not only from other psychiatric disorders but also from certain physical conditions. Anxiety symptoms can occur in nearly all the psychiatric disorders, but there are some in which particular diagnostic difficulties arise.

Depressive disorder

Anxiety is a common symptom in depressive disorder, and generalized anxiety disorder often includes some depressive symptoms. The usual convention is that the diagnosis is decided on the basis of the severity of two kinds of symptom and the order in which they appeared. Information on these two points should be obtained, if possible, from a relative or other informant as well as from the patient. Whichever type of symptoms appeared first and is more severe is considered primary. An important diagnostic error is to misdiagnose the agitated type of severe depressive disorder for generalized anxiety disorder. This mistake will seldom be made if anxious patients are asked routinely about symptoms of a depressive disorder including depressive thinking and, when appropriate, suicidal ideas.

Schizophrenia

Schizophrenic patients sometimes complain of anxiety before other symptoms are recognized. The chance of misdiagnosis can be reduced by asking anxious patients routinely what they think caused their symptoms. Schizophrenic patients may give an unusual reply, which leads to the discovery of previously unexpressed delusional ideas.

Dementia

Anxiety may be the first abnormality complained of by a person with presenile or senile dementia. When this happens, the clinician may not detect an associated impairment of memory or may dismiss it as the result of poor concentration. Therefore, memory should be assessed in middle-aged or older patients presenting with anxiety.

Substance misuse

Some people take drugs or alcohol to relieve anxiety. Patients who are dependent on drugs or alcohol sometimes believe that the symptoms of drug withdrawal are those of anxiety and take anxiolytic drugs to control them. The clinician should be alert to this possibility, particularly when anxiety is particularly severe on waking in the morning (the time when alcohol and drug withdrawal symptoms tend to occur). Anxiety that is worst in the morning also suggests a depressive disorder.

Physical illness

Some physical illnesses have symptoms that can be mistaken for those of an anxiety disorder. This possibility should be considered in all cases but especially when there is no obvious psychological cause for anxiety or no history of past anxiety. The following conditions are particularly important:

- *thyrotoxicosis* in which the patient may be irritable and restless with tremor and tachycardia. Physical examination may reveal characteristic signs of thyrotoxicosis, such as enlarged thyroid, atrial fibrillation, and exophthalmos. If there is doubt, thyroid function tests should be arranged.

- *phaeochromocytoma and hypoglycaemia* usually cause episodic symptoms and are therefore more likely to mimic a phobic disorder or panic disorder. However, they should be considered also as a differential diagnosis of generalized anxiety disorder. When there is doubt, appropriate physical examination and laboratory tests should be carried out.

Anxiety secondary to the symptoms of physical illness

Sometimes the first complaint of a physically ill person is anxiety caused by worry that certain physical symptoms portend a serious illness. If the physical symptoms are non-specific, they may be dismissed as related to anxiety. Also some patients do not mention all the physical symptoms unless questioned. This is particularly likely when the patient has a special reason to fear serious illness, for example, if a relative or friend died of cancer after developing similar symptoms. It is good practice to ask anxious patients with physical symptoms, whether they know anyone who has had similar symptoms.

Generalized anxiety disorder mistaken for physical illness

When this happens, extensive investigations may be carried out which increase the patient's anxiety. While physical illness should be considered in every case, it is also important to remember the diversity of the anxiety symptoms. Palpitations, headache, frequency of micturition, and abdominal discomfort can all be the primary complaint of an anxious patient. Correct diagnosis requires systematic enquiries about other symptoms of generalized anxiety disorder, and about the order in which the various symptoms began.

Epidemiology

Estimates of incidence and prevalence vary according to the diagnostic criteria used in the survey. Thus in one study, ICD-10 criteria gave rates at least twice as large as those obtained with DSM-IIIR criteria (Wacker *et al.* 1992). In the US Epidemiological Catchment Area Study, the one year prevalence of generalized anxiety disorder, using DSM-IIIR criteria was 3.8% (Blazer *et al.* 1991). The US National Comorbidity Survey, produced one-year prevalence rates from 2.5 to 6.4% according to the site (Weissman and Merikangas 1986), whilst in another study the one-year rate was 2% in men and 4.3% in women (Kessler *et al.* 1994). In the National Co-morbidity Survey, the life-time prevalence was 5.1% using DSM-IIIR criteria and 8.9% using ICD-10 criteria while the male to female ratio was about 2 to 1 (Wittchen *et al.* 1994).

Aetiology

In general terms, generalized anxiety disorder appears to be caused by stressors acting on a personality predisposed by a combination of genetic factors and environmental influences in childhood. However, evidence for the nature and importance of these causes is incomplete.

Stressful events

Clinical observations indicate that generalized anxiety disorders often begin in relation to stressful events, and some become chronic when stressful problems persist. Stressful events involving threat are particularly related to anxiety disorder (loss events are associated more with depression (Finlay-Jones and Brown 1981). In the Epidemiological Catchment Area Study, men who reported four or more stressful life events in the preceding year were eight times more likely to meet DSM-IIR criteria for generalized anxiety disorder than were men reporting three or fewer such events in that period (Blazer *et al.* 1991).

Genetic causes

Family studies Early studies showed that anxiety disorders are more frequent among the relatives of patients with anxiety disorder than among the general population (for example, Brown 1942) A study using DSM-IIR criteria confirmed that generalized anxiety disorders were more frequent (19.5%) among the first-degree relatives of probands with generalized anxiety disorder than among first-degree relatives of controls (3.5%).

Twin studies Early twin studies (for example, Slater and Shields (1969) showed a higher concordance for anxiety disorder between monozygotic than dizygotic pairs, suggesting that the familial association has a genetic cause. However, the study did not distinguish between different kinds of anxiety disorder. A study of a population sample of 1033 female twins confirmed that generalized anxiety disorder has genetic causes but showed that the hereditability is only about 30% with the remaining variance related to environmental factors that were not shared by the twins (Kendler *et al.* 1992b). (Note that, to increase the sample size, the authors required a duration of only 1 month instead of the 6 months specified in DSM-IV.) The hereditability was shared with mood disorders, suggesting that, at least in women, environmental factors may also determine how the inherited vulnerability is expressed (Kendler *et al.* 1992a).

Early experience

Objective studies Accounts given by anxious patients of their experience in childhood suggest that early adverse experiences is a cause of generalized anxiety disorder. Brown and Harris (1993) studied the relation between such experience and anxiety disorder in adult life in 404 working-class women living in an inner city. Adverse early experience was assessed from patients' accounts of parental indifference and of physical or sexual abuse. Women reporting early adversity had increased rates of generalized anxiety disorder (and also agoraphobia, and depressive disorder, but not mild agoraphobia or simple phobia). Also Kendler *et al.* (1992b) found that the rates of several psychiatric disorders were greater in women separated from the mother before the age of 17 years.

Psychoanalytic theories According to psychoanalytical theory, anxiety arises from intrapsychic conflict. It is when the ego is overwhelmed by excitation from any of three sources:

- the outside world (realistic anxiety);
- the instinctual levels of the id, including love, anger, and sex (neurotic anxiety);
- the superego (moral anxiety).

In generalized anxiety disorder, anxiety is experienced directly unmodified by the defence mechanisms that are thought to be the basis of phobias or obsessions (see pp. 235 and 245).

Psychoanalytical theory proposes that in generalized anxiety disorders, the ego is readily overwhelmed because it has been weakened by development failure in childhood. Separation and loss are thought to be particularly important causes of this failure (Bowlby 1969) because in early childhood anxiety is linked to separation from the mother. Normally, children overcome this anxiety through secure relationships with loving parents. If they do not achieve this security, they will be liable, as adults, to anxiety when experiencing separation. Freud suggested that, at a later stage of childhood, anxiety is linked to rivalry with the father. He used the term castration anxiety, and described the rivalry as the Oedipal conflict (see p. 116). Failure to surmount this stage of development successfully is thought to be another cause of vulnerability to anxiety in adult life.

Cognitive–behavioural theories

Conditioning theories propose that generalized anxiety disorders arise when there is an inherited predisposition to excessive responsiveness of the autonomic nervous system, together with generalization of the responses through conditioning of anxiety to previously neutral stimuli. Although this is a plausible explanation, it has not been shown convincingly that patients with generalized anxiety disorder differ from controls on measures of conditioning.

Cognitive theories propose that generalized anxiety disorders arise as the result of a tendency to worry unproductively about problems and to focus attention on potentially threatening circumstances. These theories provide a plausible explanation of the role of thinking in generalized anxiety disorder and complement the conditioning theory. They are supported directly by studies of thinking in anxious patients and controls, and indirectly by the efficacy of cognitive–behavioural treatments (see p. 225). (For a review of research on the cognitive aspects of generalized anxiety disorder see Wells and Butler 1997.)

Personality

Anxiety as a symptom is associated with neuroticism. Generalized anxiety disorder occurs in people with anxious-avoidant personality disorders, but also in people with other personality disorders. Generalized anxiety disorder is also associated with anxious personality traits but it has not been shown that these traits preceded the disorder (Nestadt *et al.* 1992).

Neurobiological mechanisms

The neurobiological mechanisms involved in general anxiety disorders are presumably those which mediate normal anxiety in man and other animals. These mechanisms are complex, involving several brain systems and several neurotransmitter systems. Noradrenergic neurons originating in the locus ceruleus increase arousal and anxiety. Serotonergic neurons originating in the raphe nuclei appear to have complex effects, some inhibitory, others anxiogenic. Gamma-aminobutyric acid (GABA) receptors, which are widely distributed in the brain, are inhibitory. (For a review of the neurobiological basis of anxiety see Noyes and Hoehn-Saric 1998, Chapter 1.)

These mechanisms are certainly involved in generalized anxiety disorder but it is not known whether they are themselves abnormal or responding normally to an abnormality of another kind, for example, to abnormal cognitive processes (see above). Indirect evidence for increased noradrenergic function in generalized anxiety disorder includes subnormal response to stimulation and blockade of α-2-receptors (Charney *et al.* 1989), and to blocking these receptors (Abelson *et al.* 1991). Both findings could result from downregulation of 2-receptors due to high levels of noradrenaline. There is insufficient evidence to decide about the role of serotonergic and GABA receptors in generalized anxiety disorder.

Functional scanning of the brain has not yet revealed any specific regional differences in blood flow between patients with generalized anxiety disorder and controls.

For a review of aetiological theories of generalized anxiety disorder see Noyes and Hoehn-Saric 1998, Chapter 2.

Prognosis

The DSM definition excludes the many states of high anxiety that improve within 6 months. (One of the DSM-IV criteria for generalized anxiety disorder is that the symptoms should have been present for 6 months.) Research carried out before the present DSM criteria were available indicated that anxiety disorders lasting for longer than 6 months have a poor prognosis. In one study, 80% were still present after 3 years (Kedward and Cooper 1966). In a study of medical patients with anxiety disorder, two-thirds improved substantially or recovered within 6 years (Yonkers *et al.* 1996).

On follow-up, episodes of major depression occur frequently among patients with anxiety disorders (Clancy *et al.* 1978). (The relationship between anxiety and depression is considered further on p. 241.) The rates of schizophrenia and manic–depressive disorder found in patients with anxiety disorders are no greater than in the general population (Greer 1969; Kerr *et al.* 1974).

Treatment

Counselling

In the absence of a sufficient number of satisfactory controlled trials carried out with formally diagnosed general anxiety disorders, guidance has to be based on clinical experience. In the early stages of a generalized anxiety disorder (before symptoms have been established for the 6 months necessary for a DSM-IV diagnosis), simple methods of counselling are often effective. Some patients with more severe or persistent generalized anxiety disorders respond to counselling, but others need either cognitive–behavioural therapy or medication (both described below). Counselling for generalized anxiety disorder follows the general lines described on p. 728 emphasizing the following:

- *a clear plan* of management agreed with the patient and, when appropriate, a relative or partners.

- an *explanation* of the nature of the disorder and *reassurance* that any physical symptoms of anxiety are not caused by physical disease. (Since anxious people often concentrate poorly, it is useful to provide an information leaflet that contains the same points.)

- *problem solving* or help in adjusting to problems.

- advice about the use of *caffeine*. Patients with generalized anxiety disorder are more sensitive than normal subjects to the anxiogenic effects of caffeine (Bruce *et al.* 1992). Although many patients discover this for themselves and reduce their caffeine intake, those who have not done so may be helped by avoiding excessive caffeine intake.

Relaxation training

Without controlled trials with patients with formally diagnosed generalized anxiety disorder, advice has to be based on clinical experience. If practised regularly, relaxation can reduce anxiety in all the less severe disorders. However, many patients fail to persevere with the relaxation exercises. Practice in a group sometimes improves motivation, and some patients do better when relaxation is part of a programme of yoga exercises which engage their interest.

Cognitive–behaviour therapy

This treatment combines relaxation with cognitive procedures designed to help patients to control worrying thoughts. The method is described on p. 740. A review of clinical trials by Barlow *et al.* (1997) concluded that the severity of anxiety is reduced by about 50%. Drop-out rate was low.

Medication

Medication should be used selectively for generalized anxiety disorders. It can be used to bring symptoms under control quickly, while the effects of psychological treatment are awaited. Medication is helpful also in the minority of patients who do not improve with psychological measures. However, there is a general tendency to prescribe drugs too often and for too long. There have been many clinical trials of the various anxiolytic drugs but few with patients meeting present criteria for generalized anxiety disorder. The placebo response rate with generalized anxiety disorder is about 40%, indicating that non-specific factors are important (Fossey and Lydiard 1990). Anxiolytic drugs are described further on pp. 655–9.

Benzodiazepines One of the longer acting benzodiazepines is appropriate for the short-term treatment of generalized anxiety disorders, for example, diazepam in a dose from 5 mg twice daily in mild cases to 10 mg three times a day in the most severe. Anxiolytic drugs should seldom be prescribed for more than 3 weeks because of the risk of dependence when given for longer.

Buspirone An azapirone, buspirone is as effective as the benzodiazepines in the short-term management of generalized anxiety disorder and is much less likely to cause dependency (Cowen 1992).

Beta-adrenergic antagonists These have been used to control severe palpitations that have not responded to short-term treatment with an anxiolytic. Generally, however, it is more appropriate to treat the cause with psychological measures. If one of this group of drugs is used, care should be taken to observe the contraindications and to follow the advice given on p. 658 and in the manufacturer's literature.

Antidepressants Most antidepressants have anxiolytic as well as antidepressant effects. They act more slowly than benzodiazepines but their effect is equivalent or greater (Kahn *et al.* 1986; Rickels *et al.* 1993). They are much less likely to cause dependence than benzodiazepines. One of the more sedative antidepressants, such as amitriptyline or trazodone, can be used to treat generalized anxiety disorder, though imipramine (which is less sedating) appears to have a comparable effect (Rickels *et al.* 1993). If imipramine is used, the initial dosage should be low and should be increased gradually as described on p. 240. Of the newer antidepressants, venlafaxine appears to be effective.

Monoamine oxidase inhibitors Monoamine oxidase inhibitors (see p. 685) have been used to treat generalized anxiety disorders. This usage was described many years ago (Sargant and Dally 1962) but has not been widespread because the drugs interact with some drugs and foodstuffs (see p. 688).

Management

In primary care, many patients are seen in the early stage of an anxiety disorder before a formal diagnosis of generalized anxiety disorder can be made. These patients often respond to counselling. If anxiety is severe, a short course of a benzodiazepine can bring rapid relief. Psychiatrists are more likely to encounter established cases, some of which may already be chronic. The diagnosis should be checked, especially to exclude a depressive disorder, substance abuse, or a physical cause such as thyrotoxicosis. Maintaining factors should be evaluated, including persistent social problems and marital conflict, and concerns that physical symptoms of anxiety are evidence of serious physical disease. Treatment often begins with counselling, sometimes with short-term benzodiazepine medication. In chronic cases, one of the antidepres-

sant drugs will carry less risk of dependency than would a benzodiazepine. Problem-solving counselling (see p. 728) is indicated if social problems appear to be maintaining the condition. Cognitive–behaviour therapy should be tried when anxiety is maintained by unwarranted concerns about the symptoms, or about other aspects of the patient's life.

Phobic anxiety disorders

Phobic anxiety disorders have the same core symptoms as generalized anxiety disorders, but these symptoms occur only in particular circumstances. In some phobic disorders these circumstances are few and the patient is free from anxiety for most of the time. In other phobic disorders many circumstances provoke anxiety, with the result that anxiety is more frequent, but even so there are situations in which no anxiety is experienced. Two other features characterize phobic disorders: the person avoids circumstances that provoke anxiety, and experiences anticipatory anxiety when there is the prospect of encountering these circumstances. The circumstances provoking anxiety include *situations* (for example, crowded places), '*objects*' (for example, spiders), and *natural phenomena* (for example, thunder). For clinical purposes, three principal phobic syndromes are recognized: specific phobia, social phobia, and agoraphobia. These syndromes will be described next.

Classification of phobic disorders

Phobic disorders are classified in slightly different ways in DSM-IV and ICD-10. In both systems, phobic disorders are divided into specific phobia, social phobia, and agoraphobia. In DSM-IV, agoraphobic patients who experience more than four panic attacks in 4 weeks, or one attack followed by a month of persistent fear of having another attack, are classified as having a type of panic disorder. The reasons why panic attacks are given this importance in DSM-IV are explained on p. 238.

Specific phobia

Clinical picture

A person with a specific phobia is inappropriately anxious in the presence of one or more objects or situations. The whole range of anxiety symptoms (see Table 9.1) may be experienced in the presence of the object or in the situation. Anticipatory anxiety is common, and so is escape from, and avoidance of, the feared situation. Specific phobias are characterized further by adding the name of the stimulus; for example spider phobia. In the past it was common practice to use terms such as arachnophobia (instead of spider phobia) or acrophobia (instead of phobia of heights), but this practice adds nothing of value to the use of the simpler names.

In DSM-IV, five types of specific phobia are recognized concerned with:

◆ animals

◆ aspects of the natural environment

◆ blood, injection, and injury

◆ situations and

◆ other provoking agents.

The latter includes fears of dental and medical situations and fears of choking.

The following specific phobias merit brief separate consideration.

Phobia of dental treatment

About 5% of adults have fears of the dentist's chair; these fears can become so severe that all dental treatment is avoided and serious caries develops (Gale and Ayer 1969; Kleinknecht *et al.* 1973). For further information see Roy-Byrne *et al.* (1994).

Phobia of flying

Anxiety during aeroplane travel is common. A few people have such intense fear that they are unable to travel in an aeroplane and they seek treatment. This fear occurs occasionally among pilots who have had an accident while flying. Treatment, which is by desensitization, is provided by some airlines, and self-books are available (for example, Greist and Greist 1981).

Blood injury phobia

The sight of blood or injury results in anxiety. However, the accompanying autonomic response differs from that in other phobic disorders. The initial tachycardia is followed by a vasovagal response with bradycardia, pallor, dizziness, nausea, and sometimes fainting. These people are helped by tensing their muscles, rather than the use of relaxation, which is helpful in other phobic responses. There is a high prevalence of the condition among first-degree relatives of affected people. For further information see Marks (1988).

Phobia of choking

These people are intensely concerned that they will choke when attempting to swallow. They have an exaggerated gag reflex and feel intense anxiety. The onset may be in childhood, or after choking on food in adult life. Some of these people also fear dental treatment, others avoid eating in public. Treatment is through desensitization by progressive exposure. For further information see McNally (1994).

Phobia of illness

People with this phobia experience repeated fearful thoughts that they might have cancer, venereal disease, or some other serious illness. When the thoughts are not present, these people recognize that the thoughts are irrational. Moreover, they do not resist the thoughts as obsessional thoughts are resisted. Such fears may be associated with avoidance of hospitals, but are not otherwise specific to situations. If the patient is also convinced that he has the disease, the condition is classified as hypochondriasis (see p. 258); if the thoughts are recognized as irrational and are resisted, the condition is classified as obsessive–compulsive disorder.

Epidemiology

Among adults the lifetime *prevalence* of specific phobias has been estimated, using DSM-IIIR criteria, as 4% in men and 13% in women (Kessler *et al.* 1994). The lifetime rates in the National Comorbidity Survey were 6.7% for men and 15.7% for women (Kessler *et al.* 1994). The *age of onset* of most specific phobias is in childhood: phobias of animals at average age 7 years, blood phobia at 9, dental phobia at 12 (Öst 1987a).

Aetiology

Persistence of childhood fears

Most specific phobias of adult life are a continuation of childhood phobias. Specific phobias are common in childhood (see p. 840). By early teenage years most of these childhood fears have been lost, but a few persist into adult life. Why the few persist is not certain, except that the most severe phobias are likely to last the longest.

Genetic factors

In one study, 31% of first-degree relatives of people with specific phobia also had the condition (Fyer *et al.* 1995). The results of a study of female twins with specific phobia fitted an aetiological model in which a modest genetic vulnerability combined with phobia-specific stressful events (Kendler *et al.* 1992a).

Psychoanalytical theories

These theories suggest that phobias are not related to the obvious external stimulus but to an internal source of anxiety. This internal source is excluded from consciousness by repression and attached to the external object by displacement.

Cognitive–behavioural theories

Conditioning theory suggests that specific phobias arise through association learning. A minority of specific phobias appear to begin in this way in adult life, in relation to a highly stressful experience; for example, a phobia of horses may follow a dangerous encounter with a bolting horse. Some specific phobias may be acquired by observational learning: the child becomes fearful of objects and situations through observing fear responses in the mother or another close person. Cognitive factors include fearful anticipation of phobic situations, and selective attention to the phobic stimuli.

Prepared learning

This term refers to an innate predisposition to develop persistent fear responses to certain stimuli. It occurs in some primates who appear prepared to develop fears of snakes, but it is not certain whether it occurs in human children. Even if it does occur in humans, it is not known whether it is a cause of specific phobias.

Cerebral localization

Positron emission tomography has been used to study blood-flow changes during exposure of patients with specific phobias to the feared stimulus. In one study, significant increases in blood flow were observed mainly in the paralimbic structures (Rauch *et al.* 1995), whilst in a second changes were in the visual association areas and the thalamus (Fredrickson *et al.* 1993). Further studies are required to find the reasons for the differences.

Differential diagnosis

Diagnosis is seldom difficult. The possibility of an underlying depressive disorder should always be kept in mind, since some patients seek help for long-standing specific phobias when a depressive disorder makes them less able to tolerate their phobic symptoms. Obsessional disorders sometimes present with fear and avoidance of specific objects (for example, knives). A systematic history and mental state examination will reveal the associated obsessional thoughts (for example, harming a person with a knife).

Prognosis

The prognosis of specific phobia in adult life has not been studied systematically. Clinical experience suggests that specific phobias that originate in childhood continue for many years, whilst those starting in adult life after stressful events have a better prognosis.

Treatment

The main treatment is the exposure form of behaviour therapy (see p. 735). Usually the phobia can be reduced considerably in intensity and with it the

Table 9.4 Abbreviated diagnostic criteria for social phobia in ICD–10 and DSM-IV*

ICD–10	DSM-IV
Marked fear or avoidance of being the focus of attention or of behaving in an embarrassing or humiliating way – manifested in social situation	Marked fear or avoidance of situations in which the person is exposed to unfamiliar people or to scrutiny with fear of behaving in an embarrassing or humiliating way
Two symptoms of anxiety in the feared situations plus at least one from blushing/shaking, fear of vomiting and fear or urgency of micturition or defecation	–
Significant emotional distress, recognized as excessive or unreasonable	Recognizes that the fear is excessive or unreasonable. Interferes with functioning or causes marked distress
Symptoms restricted or predominate in feared situations or their contemplation	–
Not secondary to another disorder	Not secondary to another disorder
	Duration at least 6 months if the person is under 18 years of age

* To facilitate comparison between the two sets of criteria, the wordings have been paraphrased and the order of some items has been changed.

social disability. However, it is unusual for the phobia to be lost completely. Outcome depends importantly on motivation for the necessary repeated and prolonged sessions of practice. Indeed, drop-out rates of up to 50% have been reported (Schneier *et al.* 1995). Some patients seek help soon before some important engagement that will be made difficult by the phobia. When this happens, a few doses of a benzodiazepine may be prescribed to relieve phobic anxiety until a course of behaviour therapy has been completed.

Social phobia

Clinical picture

In this disorder, inappropriate anxiety is experienced in situations in which the person is observed and could be criticized. Socially phobic people tend to avoid such situations and do not engage in them fully; for example, they avoid making conversation, or they sit in the place where they are least

conspicuous. Even the prospect of encountering the object or situation may cause considerable anxiety. The situations include restaurants, canteens, dinner parties, seminars, board meetings, and other places where the person feels observed by other people. Patients may experience any of the symptoms of an anxiety disorder (see Table 9.3), but complaints of blushing and trembling are particularly frequent. Socially phobic people are often preoccupied with the idea of being observed critically, though they are aware that the idea is groundless (Amies *et al.* 1983). Some patients take alcohol to relieve the symptoms of anxiety, and alcohol misuse is more common in social phobia than in other phobias. Co-morbid depressive disorder is also common, and suicide attempts may be more frequent than in the general population (Schneier *et al.* 1992).

The condition usually begins between the ages of 17 and 30. The first episode occurs in a public place, usually without any apparent reason. Subsequent anxiety occurs in similar places. The episodes gradually become more severe and avoidance increases.

Some patients become anxious in a wide range of social situations (*generalized social phobia*), whilst others are anxious only in specific situations such as public speaking. Some patients experience anxiety in a more limited set of circumstances, for example, writing in front of others, speaking in public, or playing a musical instrument in public (Clark and Agras 1991). These limited or discrete social phobias are classified separately in DSM-IV (but not in ICD-10).

Two discrete social phobias require separate consideration: phobias of excretion and phobias of vomiting.

Phobia of excretion

Patients with these phobias either become anxious and unable to pass urine in public lavatories, or have frequent urges to pass urine and an associated dread of incontinence. Such patients often arrange their lives so as never to be far from a lavatory. A few have comparable symptoms centred around defecation.

Phobias of vomiting

Some patients fear that they may vomit in a public place, often a bus or train; in these surroundings they feel anxious and nauseated. A smaller group have repeated fears that other people will vomit in such places.

Diagnostic conventions

Table 9.4 shows the essential points contained in the criteria for the diagnosis of social phobia in ICD-10 and DSM-IV. Generally, the requirements are similar (although the original wordings differ more than the paraphrased versions in the table). The main difference is the greater emphasis in ICD-10 on symptoms of anxiety: two general symptoms of anxiety and one of three symptoms associated with social phobia. DSM-IV has an additional criterion that symptoms must have been present for at least 6 months if the person is under 18 years of age.

Differential diagnosis

The symptom of social phobia can occur in agoraphobia and panic disorder. When this occurs both diagnoses can be made, but it is more useful for the clinician to decide which symptoms are more severe and which should be given priority in treatment

Social phobia has to be distinguished from *generalized anxiety disorder* (by establishing the situations in which anxiety occurs), *depressive disorder* (by examining the mental state), and *schizophrenia*. Patients with schizophrenia may avoid social situations because of persecutory delusions when anxiety has subsided; patients with social phobia know that their insistent ideas of being observed are untrue. Social phobia has to be distinguished from *avoidant personality disorder* characterized by life-long shyness and lack of self-confidence. In principle, the phobia has a recognizable onset and a shorter history, but in practice the distinction may be difficult since social phobia may often begin in the teenage years and the onset may be difficult to recall. Many cases meet criteria for both diagnoses (Schneier *et al.* 1992). Patients with *body dysmorphic disorder* may avoid social situations but the diagnosis is usually clear from the patient's account of the problem. Finally, a distinction needs to be made between social phobia and *social inadequacy*. The latter is a primary lack of social skills with secondary anxiety; it is not a phobic disorder but a type of behaviour that occurs in personality disorders and schizophrenia, and among people of low intelligence. Its features include hesitant, dull, and inaudible diction, inappropriate use of facial expression and gesture, and failure to look at other people in conversation.

Epidemiology

The 1-year prevalence of social phobia has been estimated as 7% for men and 9% for women (Davidson *et al.* 1993a). Social phobias are about equally frequent among men and women who seek treatment, but in the community surveys they are reported rather more frequently by women (Kessler *et al.* 1994).

Aetiology

Genetic factors

Genetic factors are suggested by the finding that social phobias (but not other anxiety disorders) are more common among the relatives of social phobics than in the population (Fyer *et al.* 1993). The rates of social phobia in first-degree relatives is greater when the probands have generalized social phobia than when they have non-generalized social phobia (Stein *et al.* 1998a). In a population-based sample of over 2000 female twins, the results from probands with social phobia fitted a model in which moderate genetic influences, accounting for less than a third of the variance, interact with non-specific environmental factors (Kendler *et al.* 1992a).

Conditioning

Most social phobias begin with a sudden episode of anxiety in circumstances similar to those which become the stimulus for the phobia, and it is possible that the subsequent development of phobic symptoms is through conditioning and cognitive learning.

Cognitive factors

The principal cognitive factor in the aetiology of social phobia is an undue concern that other people will be critical (often referred to as a 'fear of negative evaluation'). Whether this cognition precedes the disorder or develops with it is unknown, but in either case it is likely to increase and prolong the phobic anxiety. Social phobia usually begins in late adolescence, when young people are expanding their social contacts and are particularly concerned about the impression that they are making on other people. It is possible that social phobias occur particularly among people in whom these concerns are pronounced; however, there is no evidence on which to decide the matter. For a review see Clark (2001).

Course and prognosis

People with social phobia identified in a community survey had experienced the symptoms for an average of almost 20 years (Davidson *et al.* 1993a).

Social phobia generally persists for many years even after treatment that has had an immediate effect (Reich *et al.* 1994). Although there have been reports of an increased rate of deliberate self-harm in these patients, it seems that this behaviour occurs only when there is a co-morbid condition such as depressive disorder and alcohol misuse (Schneier *et al.* 1992).

Treatment

Psychological treatment

Cognitive–behaviour therapy is the psychological treatment of choice for social phobia (this treatment is described on p. 740). Two studies found that the relapse rate is lower after this combined treatment than after exposure alone (Butler *et al.* 1984; Mattick and Peters 1988). Meta-analyses of published studies have reached conflicting conclusions. Two found similar response rates with exposure and exposure plus cognitive procedures (Feske and Chambless 1995; Gould *et al.* 1997), whilst the third found a greater effect for the combined treatment (Taylor 1996). It seems likely that cognitive procedures have an additional effect but that this is too small to be detected in all trials, and possibly too small to be clinically significant for the majority of patients. Cognitive–behaviour therapy can also be given in a group format in which its therapeutic effect appears to be comparable with that of phenelzine (Heimberg *et al.* 1998).

Relaxation training alone appears to be ineffective for social phobia (Alström *et al.* 1984), though it may have greater effect when combined with exposure as 'applied relaxation', though apparently less than that of cognitive therapy (Jerremalm *et al.* 1986).

Dynamic psychotherapy may help some patients, particularly those whose social phobia is associated with pre-existing problems in personal relationships. However, there have been no controlled trials of this form of treatment.

Drug treatment

Benzodiazepines Alprazolam (Gelernter *et al.* 1991) and clonazepam (Davidson *et al.* 1993b) reduce symptoms of social phobia more than does placebo, but there is a risk of dependency if their use is prolonged. The main use of benzodiazepines is to help patients cope with social encounters until another treatment has led to improvement.

Beta-adrenergic blockers Beta-adrenergic blockers such as atenolol help to control tremor and palpitations, which are often the most distressing symptoms, especially in the specific forms of social phobia. However, their overall effect in social phobia is not significantly greater than that of placebo (Liebowitz *et al.* 1992; Turner *et al.* 1994).

Monoamine oxidase inhibitors Phenelzine has been shown to be more effective in the treatment of social phobia than placebo (Liebowitz *et al.* 1988) and atenolol (Liebowitz *et al.* 1992). Moclobemide, the reversible inhibitor of monoamine oxidase, is also effective (Versiani *et al.* 1992), though in one study at dose of 600 mg but not at 300 mg. Reported response rates vary: in a large industry-sponsored trial, 47% were much improved (International Multicenter Clinical Trial Group on Moclobemide in Social Phobia 1997); in a smaller trial, only 17.5% were rated as responders (Schneier *et al.* 1998). However, moclobemide should be less likely than phenelzine to interact with foodstuffs or drugs (see p. 687). At least in the short term, the effects of cognitive–behaviour therapy and phenelzine appear comparable (Gelernter *et al.* 1991; Heimberg *et al.* 1998).

Specific serotonin re-uptake inhibitors Fluvoxamine (van Vliet *et al.* 1994), paroxetine (Stein *et al.* 1998b), and sertraline (Katzelnick *et al.* 1995) have been shown in controlled trials to be effective for social phobia and open studies suggest that fluoxetine may be effective also (Van Ameringen *et al.* 1993).

Management

Having confirmed the diagnosis, the first choice is between medication and psychological treatment. This choice should be discussed with the patient, after explaining the side-effects of medication and the requirements for regular attendance and collaboration with psychological treatment. In many services, psychological treatments have a long waiting period, whilst medication is available immediately. Medication will have to be taken for several months, whilst change after cognitive–behaviour therapy seems more likely to last.

If medication is chosen, the next decision concerns the type of drug. Although benzodiazepines can produce rapid relief of symptoms, they are best reserved for short-term use because of the risk of dependency. When there is co-morbid substance abuse, it is better not to use benzodiazepines at all. The next choice is between a monoamine oxidase inhibitor (MAOI) and a selective serotonin re-uptake inhibitor (SSRI). There is insufficient evidence to make a definite recommendation but the greater side-effects and the risk of interactions with phenelzine suggest the choice of an SSRI. Moclobemide is less likely to cause side-effects and interactions, but the evidence for its effectiveness is not as strong as that for phenelzine.

If psychological treatment is chosen, cognitive–behaviour therapy is supported by the strongest evidence of effectiveness, though it is not certain whether the cognitive component is essential in every case. Psychodynamic treatment is still preferred by some therapists, and may help some patients, though it has not been shown to be as effective as cognitive–behaviour therapy.

For a general review of social phobia see Noyes and Hoehn-Saric (1998, Chapter 4) or den Boer (1997).

Agoraphobia

Clinical features

Anxiety

Agoraphobic patients are anxious when they are away from home, in crowds, or in situations that they cannot leave easily. In these circumstances the symptoms are similar to those of other anxiety disorders (see Table 9.3), though two groups of anxiety symptoms are more marked in agoraphobia. Panic attacks are more frequent, whether in response to environmental stimuli or arising spontaneously. (In DSM-IV, cases with more than four panic attacks in 4 weeks are classified as panic disorder with secondary agoraphobic symptoms; this convention is discussed on p. 234.)

Anxious cognitions about fainting and loss of control are frequent among agoraphobic patients.

Avoidance

Situations that provoke anxiety are avoided. Some people avoid situations so effectively that they experience little anxiety. Others continue to visit the situations even though they experience great distress.

Situations

Many situations provoke anxiety and avoidance. They seem at first to have little in common but, as explained above, there are three common themes of *distance from home*, *crowding*, and *confinement*. The situations include buses and trains, shops and supermarkets, and places that cannot be left suddenly without attracting attention, such as the hairdresser's chair or a seat in the middle row of a place of entertainment. As the condition progresses, patients avoid more and more of these situations until in severe cases they may be more or less confined to their homes (sometimes called the 'housebound housewife syndrome', though not all these patients are housewives). Apparent variations in this pattern are usually due to additional factors that reduce symptoms for a short time. For example, most patients are less anxious when accompanied by a trusted companion and some are helped even by the presence of a child or pet dog. The variability in anxiety produced in this way may suggest erroneously that the patient is exaggerating symptoms when they are said to be severe, rather than that the symptoms have been alleviated at times when less severe.

Anticipatory anxiety

This is common. In severe cases this anxiety appears hours before the person enters the feared situation, adding to the patient's distress and sometimes misleading doctors into thinking that the anxiety is generalized rather than phobic.

Other symptoms

These include depressive symptoms, depersonalization, and obsessional thoughts. Depressive symptoms are common, and often seem to be consequent upon the limitations to normal life caused by anxiety and avoidance. Depersonalization was at one time thought to signify a special subgroup of agoraphobia, the phobic anxiety depersonalization syndrome (Roth 1959), but this has not been confirmed.

Onset and course

The onset and course of agoraphobia differ in several ways from those of other phobic disorders. Most cases begin in the early or middle twenties, though there is a further period of high onset in the mid-thirties. Both these ages are later than the average ages of onset of simple phobias (childhood) and social phobias (mostly late teenage years or early twenties) (Marks and Gelder 1966). Typically, the first episode occurs while the person, more often a woman (see below), is waiting for public transport or shopping in a crowded store. Suddenly she becomes extremely anxious without knowing why, feels faint, and experiences palpitations. She rushes away from the place and goes home or to hospital, where she recovers rapidly. When she enters the same or similar surroundings, she becomes anxious again and makes another hurried escape. This sequence recurs over the next weeks and months; the panic attacks are experienced in more and more places, and a habit of avoidance follows. It is unusual to discover any serious immediate stress that could account for the first panic attack, though some patients describe a background of serious problems (e.g. worry about a sick child); in a few cases the symptoms begin soon after a physical illness or childbirth.

While many patients associate the onset of agoraphobic symptoms with a panic attack, some describe an onset without such an attack. In one study, two-thirds of 260 new cases of agoraphobia reported an onset without a panic attack (Eaton and Keyl 1990). This finding is relevant to the theory that agoraphobia develops as a consequence of panic disorder. It has been suggested that the methods of interviewing in community surveys underestimate the frequency of initial panic attacks; the use of more detailed interviews seems to support this opinion (Horwath *et al.* 1993).

As the condition progresses, agoraphobic patients become increasingly dependent on the spouse or other relatives for help with activities, such as shopping, that provoke anxiety. The consequent demands on the spouse often lead to arguments, but serious marital problems are no more common among agoraphobics than among other people of similar social background (Buglass *et al.* 1977).

Diagnostic conventions

Some, but not all, patients with agoraphobia have panic attacks, which may be situational or spontaneous, and many of these patients meet criteria for panic disorder. In ICD-10, the latter group are diagnosed as agoraphobia. In DSM-IV, cases with panic attacks are diagnosed as panic disorder with agoraphobia, whereas those without them are classified as agoraphobia without a history of panic attacks. The main difference between the criteria for DSM diagnosis of agoraphobia without panic and the criteria for the ICD diagnosis of agoraphobia, is the requirement for definitive anxiety symptoms in the latter (see Table 9.5). The criteria for the diagnosis of panic disorder in DSM-IV are considered on p. 238.

Table 9.5 Abbreviated diagnostic criteria for agoraphobia in ICD–10 and agoraphobia without panic in DSM-IV*

ICD–10	DSM-IV
Marked, consistent fear in, or avoidance of at least two situations from crowds, public places, travelling alone, travel away from home	• Anxiety in situations in which escape may be difficult, or help unavailable were there a panic attack, e.g. outside the home, crowds, travel, bridges • These situations are avoided, or endured with distress
At least one symptom of autonomic arousal plus one other anxiety symptom in the feared situation on at least one occasion since the onset	Criteria for panic disorder never met
Significant distress caused by the avoidance, or the anxiety, recognized as excessive or unreasonable	
Symptoms restricted to, or predominate in, the feared situations or contemplation thereof	
Not the result of another disorder, nor to cultural beliefs	Not accounted for by another disorder

* The criteria have been abbreviated and paraphrased, and the order has been changed to facilitate comparison of the two systems of classification.

Differential diagnosis

Social phobia

Some patients with agoraphobia feel anxious in social situations, and some social phobics avoid crowded buses and shops where they feel under scrutiny. Detailed enquiry into the present pattern of avoidance and into the order in which the two sets of symptoms developed will indicate the correct diagnosis.

Generalized anxiety disorder

Some patients with generalized anxiety disorder complain of anxiety in public places, but they are also anxious in many other situations not characteristic of agoraphobia. However, when the agoraphobia is severe, anxiety may develop in so many situations that the condition resembles generalized anxiety disorder. In these cases, the history of development of the disorder will usually point to the correct diagnosis.

Depressive disorder

Agoraphobic symptoms can occur in a depressive disorder, and many agoraphobic patients have depressive symptoms. However, a thorough history will show which set of symptoms developed first. Sometimes a depressive disorder develops in a person with long-standing agoraphobia; it is important to identify these cases and treat the depressive disorder (see below).

Paranoid disorders

Occasionally a patient with paranoid delusions (arising in the early stages of schizophrenia or in a delusional disorder) avoids going out and meeting people in shops and other places. The true diagnosis will usually be revealed by thorough mental state examination which will generally uncover the delusions of persecution or of reference.

Epidemiology

In a study using DSM-IIIR criteria, the 1-year prevalence of agoraphobia without panic disorder was estimated as 1.7% in men and 3.8% in women (Kessler *et al.* 1994) and the lifetime prevalence about 6–10% (Weissman and Merikangas 1986).

Aetiology

Theories of the aetiology of agoraphobia have to explain why the initial anxiety attacks occur, and why attacks spread and recur persistently. The two problems will be considered in turn.

Theories of onset

Agoraphobia begins with anxiety in a public place, generally, but not always, as a panic attack. There are three explanations for the initial anxiety.

- The *cognitive hypothesis* proposes that the anxiety attack develops because the person is unreasonably afraid of some aspect of the situation or of certain physical symptoms experienced by chance in the situation (see below under panic disorder p. 239). Although such fears are expressed by patients with established agoraphobia, it is not known whether they predated the disorder or are a consequence of it.

- *The biological theory* proposes that the initial anxiety attack results from chance environmental stimuli acting on a person who is constitutionally disposed to respond with anxiety. There is some evidence for a genetic component to this predisposition (Kendler *et al.* 1992a). The theory is considered further under panic disorder on p. 239.

- *The psychoanalytic theory* proposes, essentially, that the initial anxiety is caused by unconscious mental conflicts related to unacceptable sexual or aggressive impulses which are triggered indirectly by the original situation. Although widely held in the past, this theory has not been supported by independent evidence.

Theories of spread and maintenance

Learning theories Conditioning could account for the association of anxiety with more and more situations, and avoidance learning could account for the subsequent avoidance of these situations. Although this explanation is plausible and in keeping with observations of learning in animals, there is no direct evidence to support it.

Personality Agoraphobic patients are often described as dependent, and prone to avoid rather than confront problems. This dependency could have arisen from overprotection in childhood, which is reported more often by agoraphobics than by controls. However, despite such retrospective reports, it is not certain that the dependency was present before the onset of the agoraphobia. Furthermore, Buglass *et al.* (1977) found no difference between agoraphobics and controls in the history of separation anxiety or of other indices of dependency.

Causes in the family Agoraphobia could be maintained by family problems. However, in a well-controlled study, Buglass *et al.* (1977) found no evidence that agoraphobics had more family problems than controls. Clinical observation suggests that symptoms are sometimes prolonged by overprotective attitudes of other family members, but this feature is not found in all cases.

Mitral valve prolapse Kantor *et al.* (1980) reported that 44% of agoraphobic women had prolapse of the mitral valves. However, this finding has not been confirmed in subsequent studies.

Prognosis

Although brief cases may be seen in general practice, agoraphobia lasting for 1 year changes little in the next 5 years (Marks 1969). Brief episodes of depressive symptoms often occur in the course of chronic agoraphobia, and clinical experience suggests that patients are more likely to seek help during these episodes.

Treatment

Psychological treatment

Exposure treatment Exposure with anxiety management (see p. 740) produces better long-term results than exposure alone, with substantial and often lasting changes in avoidance behaviour as well as a reduction in phobic anxiety and panic attacks (Cohen *et al.* 1984). Despite these gains, most patients continue to experience mild anxiety in the situations in which symptoms were originally most severe (Mathews *et al.* 1981). The prognosis for this kind of treatment seems to be better in patients with good marital relationships before treatment (Monteiro *et al.* 1985) and worse in those experiencing chronic life stress (Wade *et al.* 1993).

Cognitive–behaviour therapy Studies of cognitive–behaviour therapy have used DSM criteria which make it difficult to determine the separate effects on panic disorder and agoraphobia. The trials (reviewed with panic disorder on pp. 240–1) indicate that, in the short term, cognitive therapy is about as effective as medication for this mixed group, and probably more effective in the longer term.

Medication

The drug treatment of agoraphobia resembles that for panic disorder except that medication is usually combined with repeated practice in re-entering situations that are feared and avoided. Since most studies of drug treatment use DSM diagnostic criteria, they contain both agoraphobic and panic disorder patients, and it is often difficult to judge the separate response of the two disorders. Also, some form of exposure is usually encouraged when drugs are prescribed and it is not possible to be certain of the separate effects of this exposure. The following brief account should be read in conjunction with the discussion of medication for panic disorder on p. 240.

Anxiolytic drugs These may be used for a specific, short-term purpose such as helping the patient to undertake an important engagement before other treatment has taken effect. Anxiolytic drugs should not be prescribed for more than a few weeks because of the risk of dependence (see p. 657). In some countries, though not in the UK, the high potency benzodiazepine, alprazolam, is used to treat agoraphobia with frequent panic attacks (in DSM-IV terms, panic disorder with agoraphobia). This treatment is discussed further under panic disorder (p. 240). Most studies of alprazolam have included patients with panic disorder as well as patients with agoraphobia with panic. An exception is the trial by Marks *et al.* (1993a, 1993b), in which all patients had agoraphobia; these authors found that the short-term benefit with alprazolam was about half that obtained with exposure treatment, and that relapse after treatment was more frequent with alprazolam. However, the methodology of the study has been criticized.

Antidepressant drugs These may be used to treat a concurrent depressive disorder; they also have a therapeutic effect in agoraphobic patients who are not depressed but have frequent panic attacks (Zitrin *et al.* 1983). Imipramine has been tested most thoroughly, but similar effects have been reported with clomipramine (Modigh *et al.* 1992; Gentil *et al.* 1993). The starting dose of imipramine should be very low (see p. 240) and increased gradually to reach a high final dose. If no response is obtained at lower levels, doses of up to 225 mg/day may be used provided that the patient is free from cardiac or other physical disease (see p. 240). A high rate of relapse has been reported when imipramine is stopped (Zitrin *et al.* 1983). The use of imipramine for this purpose is discussed further under panic disorder (see p. 240).

Selective serotonin re-uptake inhibitors (SSRIs) Fluvoxamine, paroxetine, sertraline, and fluoxetine have been shown to be effective in mixed groups of patients with panic disorder and panic disorder with agoraphobia (see p. 240). One meta-analysis suggested that SSRIs are superior to imipramine and alprazolam for these patients (Boyer 1995).

Monoamine oxidase inhibitors (MAIOs) One of the earliest reports of drug treatment for agoraphobia concerned the MAIOs (Sargant and Dally 1962), but they are now used infrequently because they interact with some drugs and foodstuffs (see pp. 687–8). As with imipramine, the relapse rate is high when MAIOs are stopped (Tyrer and Steinberg 1975), even after many months of treatment.

Management

In early cases, patients should be strongly encouraged to return to the situations that they are avoiding. The treatment of choice for established cases is a combination of exposure to phobic situations with training in coping with panic attacks Cognitive therapy for panic attacks may reduce relapse. There is often a waiting list for cognitive therapy, and in the meantime clinicians should supervise exposure treatment. Several self-help manuals have been published which reduce the time that therapists need to spend with patients (see, for example, Mathews *et al.* 1981; Andrews *et al.* 1994).

Medication may be offered as an alternative, or as an adjunct to behavioural treatment, especially when panic attacks are frequent and/or severe. However, medication needs to be accompanied by repeated self-exposure to previously feared and avoided situations, even if formal behaviour therapy is not carried out. In the UK, an antidepressant is usually chosen – either imipramine or more recently an SSRI – but in other countries alprazolam is a frequent choice. It is not certain how long medication should be maintained but on the analogy of depressive disorder, antidepressants are often prescribed for 9 months to a year. Any medication should be discontinued gradually, and alprazolam should be reduced particularly slowly.

Patients who have relapsed after drug treatment can be offered behaviour therapy, though no controlled evaluation has been carried out specifically to show that it is effective with such patients.

Most patients improve but few lose the symptoms completely following treatment. Relapse is common, and patients should be encouraged to seek further help at an early stage should relapse occur.

Panic disorder

Although the diagnosis of panic disorder was not used until 1980 when it was introduced in DSM-III, similar cases have been described under a variety of names for more than a century. The central feature is the occurrence of panic attacks, i.e. sudden attacks of anxiety in which physical symptoms predominate and are accompanied by fear of a serious consequence such as a heart attack. In the past, these symptoms have been variously referred to as irritable heart, Da Costa's syndrome, neurocirculatory asthenia, disorderly action of the heart, and effort syndrome. These early terms assumed that patients were correct in fearing a disorder of cardiac function. Some later authors suggested psychological causes, but it was not until the Second World War (when interest in the condition revived) that Wood (1941) showed convincingly that the condition was a form of anxiety disorder. From then until 1980 patients with panic attacks were classified as having either generalized or phobic anxiety disorders. In 1980, the authors of DSM-III introduced the new diagnostic category, panic disorder, which included patients whose panic attacks occurred with or without generalized anxiety, but excluded those whose panic attacks appeared in the course of agoraphobia. In DSM-IV, all patients with frequent panic attacks are classified as having panic disorder whether or not they have agoraphobia. (Agoraphobia without panic attacks has a separate rubric – see p. 234.) The category panic disorder did not appear in ICD-9. It was included in ICD-10, but it is not applied to patients who have marked agoraphobic anxiety and avoidance (a point of difference from DSM-IV).

Clinical features

The symptoms of a panic attack are listed in Table 9.6. Not every patient has all these symptoms. For the diagnosis of panic disorder, DSM-IV requires at least four of the symptoms in at least one attack of panic. Important features of panic attacks are that anxiety builds up quickly, the response is severe, and there is fear of a catastrophic outcome. Some patients with panic disorder hyperventilate, and this adds to their symptoms.

Hyperventilation is breathing in a rapid and shallow way with a resultant fall in the concentration of carbon dioxide in the blood. The resulting hypocapnia may cause dizziness, tinnitus, headache, a feeling of weakness, faintness, numbness

Table 9.6 Symptoms of a panic attack (from DSM-IV)

Shortness of breath and smothering sensations

Choking

Palpitations and accelerated heart rate

Chest discomfort or pain

Sweating

Dizziness, unsteady feelings or faintness

Nausea or abdominal distress

Depersonalization or derealization

Numbness or tingling sensations

Flushes or chills

Trembling or shaking

Fear of dying

Fears of going crazy or doing something uncontrolled

and tingling in the hands, feet, and face, carpopedal spasms, and precordial discomfort. There is also a paradoxical feeling of breathlessness, which may prolong the condition if the patient concludes from this feeling that he should breathe even more vigorously. When a patient has unexplained bodily symptoms, the possibility of persistent hyperventilation should always be borne in mind. The diagnosis can usually be made by watching the pattern of breathing. If there is doubt, blood gas analysis should decide the matter in acute cases though the findings may be normal in chronic cases (Hibbert 1984b).

Diagnostic criteria

In DSM-IV the diagnosis of panic disorder is made when panic attacks occur unexpectedly (i.e. not in response to a known phobic stimulus), and when more than four attacks have occurred in 4 weeks or one attack has been followed by 4 weeks of persistent fear of another attack. The criteria in ICD-10 are similar except that those concerned with course are rather less precise: the attacks must have been recurrent and not consistently associated with a phobic situation or object, or with marked exertion or exposure to dangerous or life-threatening situations.

Differential diagnosis

Panic attacks occur in generalized anxiety disorders, phobic anxiety disorders (most often agoraphobia), depressive disorders, and acute organic disorder. In DSM-IV, panic disorder can be diagnosed when these disorders are present; in the UK it is more usual to regard the panic attacks as part of the other disorder and to diagnose only what seems to be the primary disorder.

Epidemiology

Using DSM-IIIR criteria, the 1-year prevalence of panic disorder in the general population is about 13 per 1000 in men and about 32 per 1000 in women (Kessler *et al.* 1994). However, these cases include panic disorder with agoraphobia and about half of those in the general population who meet criteria for panic disorder also meet criteria for agoraphobia. In most studies, that the prevalence in women is about twice that in men has been confirmed in other studies. For panic attacks that are too mild or too infrequent to meet criteria for panic disorder, the 6-month prevalence has been estimated as 30 per 1000 (Von Korff *et al.* 1985) and the lifetime prevalence as about 56 per 1000 (Katerndahl 1993). No sharp cut-off was found for panic attacks meeting or not meeting the criteria for panic disorders; instead there seemed to be a continuous variation.

Aetiology

Panic disorder is familial (Crowe *et al.* 1983; Maier at al. 1993a; Mendelwicz *et al.* 1993). Rates in monozygotic twins are higher than in dizygotic twins, indicating that the family aggregation is due to genetic factors (Skre *et al.* 1993; Kendler *et al.* 1993e). However, in Kendler *et al.*'s study the inherited vulnerability was between only 30 and 40%. The mode of inheritance is not known. There are two main hypotheses about the origin of panic

disorder. The first proposes a biochemical abnormality, and the other a cognitive abnormality.

Biological causes

The *biochemical hypothesis* is based on three sets of observations. First, chemical agents such as sodium lactate (Pitts and McClure 1967) and yohimbine (Charney *et al.* 1984) can induce panic attacks more readily in patients with panic disorder than in healthy people. Second, panic attacks are reduced by certain drugs. Third, the genetic findings, noted above, could be mediated through biochemical mechanisms. The multitude of chemical agents that provoke panic attacks in panic disorder patients make it difficult to identify a single common mechanism. Other agents that have this effect include the benzodiazepine receptor antagonist flumazenil, cholecystokinin, and the 5-hydroxtryptamine (5-HT) receptor agonist mCCP (Bradwejn *et al.* 1991; Nutt and Lawson 1992). Suggestions about the causal mechanisms include abnormalities in the presynaptic α-adrenoceptors that normally restrain the activity of presynaptic neurons in brain areas concerned with the control of anxiety, and an abnormality of benzodiazepine or 5-HT receptor function.

The effects of drugs suggest that 5-HT mechanisms are important in panic disorder. Imipramine affects both 5-HT and noradrenergic systems. Clomipramine and fluvoxamine (which mainly affect 5-HT transmission) are effective antipanic drugs, but maprotiline, a selective noradrenergic uptake blocker, is not (Den Boer and Westerberg 1988). Clomipramine appears to be more potent than imipramine as an antipanic agent. It is possible that very high doses of imipramine are needed to suppress panic attacks because this compound is a relatively weak 5-HT uptake blocker. (See Ballenger 2000 for a review of the biological theories concerning the aetiology of panic disorder.)

Psychological causes

The *cognitive hypothesis* is based on the observation that fears about serious physical or mental illness are more frequent among patients with panic attacks than among anxious patients without panic attacks (Hibbert 1984a). It has been proposed that there is a spiral of anxiety in panic disorder as the physical symptoms of anxiety activate fears of illness and thereby generate more anxiety (Clark 1986). These observations have led to a cognitive treatment for panic disorder (see below).

Hyperventilation as a cause

A subsidiary hypothesis proposes that hyperventilation is a cause of panic disorder. Whilst there is no doubt that voluntary overbreathing can produce a panic attack (Hibbert 1984b), it has not been shown that panic disorder is caused by involuntary hyperventilation. Panic is also provoked by the inhalation of carbon dioxide more readily in panic disorder patients than in controls, and it has been proposed that panic disorder patients are unusually sensitive to feelings of suffocation, and respond with panic anxiety. (Klein 1993).

Course and prognosis

Follow-up studies have generally included patients with panic attacks and agoraphobia as well as patients with panic disorder alone. Earlier studies used categories such as effort syndrome. Early studies of effort syndrome found that most patients still had symptoms 20 years later, though most had a good social outcome (e.g. Wheeler *et al.* 1950). Studies of panic disorder also reveal a prolonged course with fluctuating anxiety and depression (Roy-Byrne and Cowley 1995). Mortality rates from unnatural causes and, among men, from cardiovascular disorders have been found to be higher than average (Coryell *et al.* 1982).

Treatment

Apart from supportive measures and attention to any causative personal or social problems, treatment is with drugs or cognitive therapy.

Benzodiazepines

Benzodiazepines control panic attacks when given in high doses. Alprazolam, a high-potency benzodiazepine, can be given in such doses without marked sedation, although it is probably no more effective in reducing panic attacks than an equivalent dose of diazepam (Dunner *et al.* 1986). The effectiveness of alprazolam over placebo has been shown in many controlled trials (see Ballenger 2000). Benzodiazepines should be withdrawn very gradually to avoid withdrawal symptoms (see p. 657). However, even when drugs are reduced over 30 days, about a third report significant withdrawal symptoms (Cross-National Collaborative Panic Study 1992).

Imipramine and clomipramine

Imipramine, a tricyclic antidepressant drug, also controls panic attacks (Klein 1964). The first effect of the drug is often to produce an unpleasant feeling of apprehension, sleeplessness, and palpitations. For this reason the initial dose should be small, for example 10 mg/day for 3 days, increasing by 10 mg every 3 days to 50 mg/day, and then by 25 mg/week to 150 mg/day. If symptoms are not controlled at this dose, further increments of 25 mg may be given to physically fit patients up to a maximum of 175–225 mg/day. Before high doses are given, an ECG should be obtained if there is any doubt about cardiac function. Full dosage is continued for 3–6 months. A relapse rate of up to 30% has been reported after stopping imipramine (Zitrin *et al.* 1978), but the rate may be less if imipramine is continued in reduced dosage for a further few months (Mavissakalian and Perel 1992).

Clomipramine appears to be at least as effective as imipramine (Cassano *et al.* 1998).

Specific serotonin re-uptake inhibitors (SSRIs)

Fluvoxamine has a therapeutic effect comparable to imipramine (Bakish *et al.* 1996). Other SSRIs with a similar effect in panic disorder include paroxetine (Ochberg *et al.* 1995) and sertraline (see Ballenger 2000).

Cognitive therapy

Cognitive therapy reduces the fears of the physical effects of anxiety, which are thought to underlie the disorder. Common fears are that palpitations indicate an impending heart attack, or that dizziness indicates impending loss of consciousness. The relevant symptoms are induced by voluntary means – usually hyperventilation or exercise – and the therapist explains that the symptoms of a panic attack have an equally benign origin so that the patient's beliefs can be questioned. The procedure is described further on p. 741. Controlled studies have shown that cognitive therapy is at least as effective as imipramine for panic disorder (Clark *et al.* 1994; Barlow *et al.* 2000). In both trials, patients treated with imipramine were more likely to relapse after the end of treatment than were those treated with cognitive–behaviour therapy.

Management

As cognitive therapy and medication appear to have comparable effects, the choice of treatment depends on the patient's preference, whether cognitive therapy is readily available, and the considerations of cost (cognitive therapy is more costly but may have more lasting effects). If medication is chosen, SSRIs may be preferred to tricyclics because they have fewer side-effects, although the evidence for their effectiveness is less complete. Alprazolam is widely used in some countries, but seldom in the UK, where a cautious approach is taken to the risk of dependency.

If panic disorder is accompanied by agoraphobic avoidance, exposure treatment should be added to the drug or cognitive–behavioural treatment (see the treatment of agoraphobia, p. 236).

Transcultural variations of anxiety disorder

In several cultures the presenting symptoms of anxiety disorder are more often somatic than mental. Leff (1981) has pointed out that this difference parallels the different vocabulary that is available for describing anxiety in the corresponding languages. Thus there is no word for anxiety in a number of African, Oriental, and American Indian languages; instead, a phrase denoting bodily experience is used. For example in Yoruba, an African language, the phrase is 'the heart is not at rest'.

Several conditions have been described that may be transcultural variants of anxiety disorders, though their exact relation to these disorders is uncertain.

Koro may be an extreme variant of anxiety disorder. It occurs amongst men in Asia, more commonly among the Chinese; the Cantonese people call it *suk-yeong*, which means shrinking of the penis. There are episodes of acute anxiety, lasting from 30 minutes to a day or two, in which the person complains of palpitations, sweating, pericardial discomfort, and trembling. At the same time he is convinced that the penis will retract into the abdomen and that when this process is complete he will die. Most episodes occur at night, sometimes after sexual activity. To prevent the feared outcome, patients may tie the penis to an object, or ask another person to hold the organ. This belief parallels the conviction held by patients during a panic attack that the heart is damaged and they will die. Epidemics of koro have been described among people made anxious by social stressors and superstitious ideas (Tseng *et al.* 1988). See Yap (1965) for a more detailed account.

Variants of social phobia have been described in the east, originally among Japanese people where it is known as *taijin-kyofu-sho* or phobia of interpersonal relations. There is an intense anxiety in social situations and an intense conviction bordering on the delusional that the person is being thought of unfavourably by others. Other symptoms include fears of producing body odours, dysmorphophobia, and aversion to eye contact (Tseng *et al.* 1992).

Mixed anxiety and depressive disorder

As explained on p. 221, anxiety and depressive symptoms often occur together. The overlap is greatest when the symptoms are mild (52% in the study of psychiatric patients by Hiller *et al.* 1989) and least when they are severe enough for a diagnosis of psychiatric disorder (29% in the study by Hiller *et al.*). Similar findings were obtained in a community epidemiological study of people meeting diagnostic criteria for anxiety disorder;

28% also met criteria for minor depression and a further 21% met criteria for major depression (Angst and Dobler-Mikola 1985). Similar rates of co-morbidity have also been reported with panic disorder, agoraphobia, and major depression (Clayton 1990).

When the anxiety and depressive symptoms are not severe enough for a diagnosis, the condition may be referred to as a minor affective disorder (these conditions are considered in Chapter 8). ICD-10 contains a category for mixed anxiety and depressive disorders. This category is for cases in which anxiety and depressive symptoms are both present, but neither set of symptoms, considered separately, is severe enough to make a diagnosis of depressive disorder or anxiety disorder. When minor anxiety and depressive symptoms are related to a change in life circumstances, adjustment disorder is diagnosed. The remaining group of persistent mixed disorder is seen commonly in general practice. The category of mixed anxiety-depressive disorders is not included in the main classification of DSM-IV, though it is included among the list of categories provided for further study.

There are three reasons why anxiety and depression may occur together:

- They may have the same predisposing causes. Brown *et al.* (1993) found that childhood adversity is associated with both anxiety and depressive disorders in adult life.
- Some stressful events combine elements of loss (which is known to be associated with depression) and danger (which is associated with anxiety).
- Persistent anxiety can lead to secondary depression. Follow-up studies have shown that onsets of depression among people with persistent anxiety are more common than onsets of anxiety among people with persistent depression.

The *prognosis* of mixed anxiety and depressive disorders is not clearly established.

Treatment is generally with a tricyclic antidepressant, which has anxiolytic as well as antidepressant effects (Rickels *et al.* 1974; Davidson *et al.* 1980; Johnstone *et al.* 1980). MAOIs are used sometimes as a second-line treatment, but care must be taken to avoid side-effects or interactions (see pp. 687–8). SSRIs may lead to an initial increase of anxiety.

Obsessive–compulsive disorder

The concise description of obsessive–compulsive disorder, contained in ICD-9, still applies:

The outstanding symptom is a feeling of subjective compulsion – which must be resisted – to carry out some action, to dwell on an idea, to recall an experience, or ruminate on an abstract topic. Unwanted thoughts, which include the insistency of words or ideas, ruminations or trains of thought, are perceived by the patient to be inappropriate or nonsensical. The obsessional urge or idea is recognized as alien to the personality but as coming from within the self. Obsessional actions may be quasi ritual performances designed to relieve anxiety, e.g. washing the hands to deal with contamination. Attempts to dispel the unwelcome thoughts or urges may lead to a severe inner struggle, with intense anxiety.

Clinical picture

Obsessive–compulsive disorders are characterized by obsessional thinking, compulsive behaviour, and varying degrees of anxiety, depression, and depersonalization. Obsessional and compulsive symptoms are described on pp. 19–21. They are listed in Table 9.7, but the reader may find it helpful to be reminded of the main features.

Obsessional thoughts These are words, ideas, and beliefs, recognized by the patient as his own, that intrude forcibly into his mind. They are usually unpleasant, and attempts are made to exclude them. It is the combination of an inner sense of compulsion and of efforts at resistance that characterize obsessional symptoms, but the effort of resistance is the more variable of the two. Obsessional thoughts may take the form of single words, phrases, or rhymes; they are usually unpleasant or shocking to the patient, and may be obscene or blasphemous. Obsessional images are vividly imag-

Table 9.7 Principal features of obsessive–compulsive disorder
Obsessional symptoms
Thoughts
Ruminations
Impulses
'Phobias'
Compulsive rituals
Abnormal slowness
Anxiety
Depression
Depersonalization

ined scenes, often of a violent or disgusting kind, involving abnormal sexual practices, for example.

Obsessional ruminations These are internal debates in which arguments for and against even the simplest everyday actions are reviewed endlessly. Some obsessional doubts concern actions that may not have been completed adequately, such as turning off a gas tap or securing a door; other doubts concern actions that might have harmed other people, for example, that driving a car past a cyclist might have caused him to fall off his bicycle. Sometimes doubts are related to religious convictions or observances ('scruples') – a phenomenon well known to those who hear confession.

Obsessional impulses These are urges to perform acts, usually of a violent or embarrassing kind, for example leaping in front of a car, injuring a child, or shouting blasphemies in church.

Obsessional rituals These include both mental activities, such as counting repeatedly in a special way or repeating a certain form of words, and repeated but senseless behaviours, such as washing the hands 20 or more times a day. Some of these have an understandable connection with obsessional thoughts

that precede them, for example, repeated hand-washing and thoughts of contamination. Other rituals have no such connection, for example, routines concerned with laying out clothes in a complicated way before dressing. Some patients feel compelled to repeat such actions a certain number of times; if this cannot be achieved, they have to start the whole sequence again. Patients are invariably aware that their rituals are illogical and usually try to hide them. Some fear that their symptoms are a sign of incipient madness and are greatly helped by reassurance that this is not so.

Obsessional slowness Although obsessional thoughts and rituals lead to slow performance, a few obsessional patients are afflicted by extreme slowness that is out of proportion to other symptoms (Rachman 1974).

Obsessional phobias Obsessional thoughts and compulsive rituals may worsen in certain situations; for example, obsessional thoughts about harming other people often increase in a kitchen or other place where knives are kept. When patients avoid such situations, the condition may resemble the avoidance of a phobic anxiety disorder, and may be called an obsessional phobia.

Anxiety Anxiety is a prominent component of obsessive–compulsive disorders. Some rituals are followed by a lessening of anxiety, whilst others are followed by increased anxiety (Walker and Beech 1969).

Depression Obsessional patients are often depressed. In some patients, depression is an understandable reaction to the obsessional symptoms; in others, depression seem to vary independently.

Depersonalization Some obsessional patients complain of depersonalization. The relationship between this distressing symptom and the other features of the disorder is not clear.

Relation to obsessional personality Obsessional personality is described in Chapter 7. It does not have a simple one-to-one relationship with obsessive–compulsive disorder: although obsessional personality is over-represented among patients who develop obsessive–compulsive disorder, about a third of obsessional patients have other types of personality (Lewis 1936). Moreover, people with obsessional personality are more likely to develop depressive disorders than obsessive–compulsive disorders (Pollitt 1960).

Differential diagnosis

Obsessive–compulsive disorders must be distinguished from other disorders in which obsessional symptoms occur.

Anxiety disorders

The distinction from generalized anxiety disorder, panic disorder, or phobic disorder should seldom be difficult provided that a careful history is taken and the mental state is examined thoroughly.

Depressive disorder

The course of obsessive–compulsive disorder is often punctuated by periods of depression in which the obsessional symptoms increase; when this happens the depressive disorder may be over-looked. Also, depressive disorders may present with obsessional symptoms, and it is important to make the correct diagnosis and give antidepressant treatment.

Schizophrenia

Obsessive–compulsive disorder may resemble schizophrenia, when the degree of resistance is doubtful, the content of the obsessional thoughts are peculiar, or the rituals are exceptionally odd. In such cases it is important to search for schizophrenic symptoms and to question relatives carefully about other aspects of the patient's behaviour.

'Organic' disorders

Obsessional symptoms are found occasionally in organic cerebral disorders. In the past they were observed in chronic cases of encephalitis lethargica following the epidemic in the 1920s.

Epidemiology

Estimates of 1-year prevalence vary from 1.1 to 1.8% when the Diagnostic Interview Schedule is used , and lifetime prevalence varies from about 2 to 3%. Closely similar estimates have been obtained in the USA, Germany, Puerto Rico, Taiwan, and New Zealand (Weissman *et al.* 1994). However, it has been suggested that use of the Diagnostic Interview Schedule by lay interviewers results in overdiagnosis and that the lifetime prevalence is between 1 and 2% (Nelson and Rice 1997; Stein *et al.* 1997a).

Estimates of the ratio of lifetime prevalence of women to men varies from 1.2 (in Puerto Rico) to 3.8 (in New Zealand). In clinic populations, the ratio is usually about 1.0. In community samples, 20–60% of people reported obsessions only. This is in contrast to those referred to psychiatric clinics, among whom 70–94% report both obsessions and compulsions (see Weissman *et al.* 1994).

Aetiology

Healthy people experience occasional intrusive thoughts, some of which are concerned with sexual, aggressive, and other themes similar to those of obsessional patients (Rachman and Hodgson 1980). It is the frequency, intensity, and, above all, the persistence of obsessional phenomena that have to be explained.

Genetics

Obsessive–compulsive disorders have been found in about 5–7% of the parents of patients with these disorders (Brown 1942; Rüdin 1953); although low, this rate is higher than in the general population. In the small number of twin studies, the concordance rate is greater in monozygotic than in dizygotic pairs (Rasmussen and Tsuang 1986), indicating that at least part of the familial loading is genetic.

Evidence of a brain disorder

Two kinds of evidence suggest a disorder of brain function in obsessive–compulsive disorder: associations between the condition and disease that has established effects on brain function, and evidence from studies using brain scanning.

Associations with other brain disorders Obsessional symptoms were recorded frequently among patients affected by encephalitis lethargica after the epidemic of the 1920s. Also, Gilles de la Tourette included obsessional symptoms in his original description of the disorder that now bears his name (Gilles de la Tourette 1885), and recent studies have confirmed this observation (Cummings and Frankel 1985; Robertson *et al.* 1988). In childhood, 70% of cases of Sydenham's chorea, a condition affecting the caudate nucleus, are reported to have obsessive–compulsive symptoms (Swedo *et al.* 1994).

Brain imaging studies Computerized tomography and magnetic resonance imaging have not revealed any consistent structural brain abnormality specific to patients with obsessive–compulsive disorder (Saxena *et al.* 1998). Studies with single-photon emission tomography (SPET) have shown increased uptake in the frontal lobe (Machlin *et al.* 1991; Rubin *et al.* 1992), which is reduced after treatment (Hoehn-Saric *et al.* 1991). Several studies using positron emission tomography (PET) have shown increased metabolic activity in the orbitofrontal cortex and possibly also in the caudate nucleus and anterior cingulate (Saxena *et al.* 1998). Although not wholly consistent, the findings taken together suggest abnormalities in the orbitofrontal cortex, anterior cingulate, and parts of the basal ganglia and thalamus. These findings have supported the suggestion that there may be abnormal activity in a neurological circuit involving these structures (Insel 1992). Treatment appears to reverse at least some of the abnormalities (Schwartz 1998).

Abnormal serotonergic function

The finding that obsessive–compulsive symptoms respond to drugs that affect 5-HT function suggests that 5-HT function might be abnormal in obsessive–compulsive disorder. The effect of 5-HT uptake inhibitors on obsessive–compulsive symptoms takes several weeks so the late effects are likely to be most relevant. However, the late effects are complex and it is not known which are important. In any case, the response of obsessive–compulsive symptoms to drugs that affect 5-HT function does not prove that 5-HT function is abnormal in obsessive–compulsive disorder. The situation might resemble that of parkinsonism in which anticholinergic drugs control symptoms by acting on the normal cholinergic systems of patients whose disorder is due to abnormal dopaminergic function.

The uncertainty as to whether 5-HT function is abnormal in obsessive–compulsive disorder is increased by the conflicting results of neuroendocrine tests of 5-HT function. (Barr *et al.* 1992; Hollander *et al.* 1992). Other studies have examined the relationship between response to treatment and measures of 5-HT function. One such study found that patients who responded to clomipramine had higher pretreatment CSF levels of the serotonin metabolite 5-hydroxyindoleacetic acid (5-HIAA) than did non-responders (Thoren *et al.* 1980). Other studies have examined the effect on symptoms of challenges with agents with effects specific to particular kinds of 5-HT receptors. These studies suggest that the relevant receptors could be the $5-HT_{1D}$ and $5-HT_{2C}$ subtypes (see Sasson and Yohar 1996).

Early experience

It is uncertain whether early experience plays a part in the aetiology of obsessive–compulsive disorder. Mothers with the disorder might be expected to transmit symptoms to their children by imitative learning. However, although the children of patients with obsessive–compulsive disorder have an increased risk of non-specific neurotic symptoms, they do not have more obsessional symptoms (Cowie 1961).

Psychoanalytical theories

Freud (1895a) originally suggested that obsessional symptoms result from unconscious impulses of an aggressive or sexual nature. These impulses could potentially cause extreme anxiety, but anxiety is reduced by the action of the defence mechanisms of repression and reaction formation. This idea fits with the aggressive and sexual fantasies of many obsessional patients, and with their restraints on their own aggressive and sexual impulses. Freud also proposed that obsessional symptoms occur when there is a regression to the anal stage of development as a way of avoiding impulses related to the subsequent genital and Oedipal stages. This idea reflects the obsessional patient's frequent concerns over excretory functions and dirt. Freud's ideas draw attention to aspects of the disorder other than the obvious symptoms. As an explanation of obsessive–compulsive disorder, however, they are convincing only within the framework of psychoanalytical theory.

Learning theory

Learning theory attempts to explain obsessive–compulsive disorder in terms of abnormalities in normal mechanisms of learning. It has been suggested that obsessional rituals are the equivalent of avoidance responses, but as a general explanation this idea cannot be sustained because anxiety increases rather than decreases after some rituals (Walker and Beech 1969).

Cognitive theory

Cognitive theory starts with the premise that it is not the occurrence of intrusive thoughts that has to be explained (they are experienced at times by healthy people – see above) but the obsessional patient's inability to control them. Salkovskis (1997) proposed that patients respond to the thoughts as if they were responsible for their consequences, for example, for harm to another person. This feeling of responsibility, it is suggested, leads to excessive attempts to ward off the supposed consequences by compulsive behaviours, avoidance, and seeking repeated reassurance. The theory is unproven but is useful in directing attention to aspects of the disorder other than the obsessions and compulsions. It has given rise to new approaches to treatment (see p. 247) though at the time of writing, their effectiveness has not been proved.

Prognosis

About two-thirds of cases improve to some extent by the end of a year. Of the cases lasting for more than a year, some run a fluctuating course, but others are chronic (Ravizza *et al.* 1997). Prognosis is better when there has been a precipitating event, social and occupational adjustment is good, and the symptoms are episodic. Prognosis is worse when there is a personality disorder, and onset is in childhood (see Iancu *et al.* 2000). Severe cases may be exceedingly persistent; for example, in a study of obsessional patients admitted to hospital, Kringlen (1965) found that three-quarters remained unchanged 13–20 years later, and in another study almost half had obsessive–compulsive disorders for more than 50 years (Skoog and Skoog 1999).

Treatment

In treatment, it is important to remember that some cases of obsessive–compulsive disorder run a fluctuating course with long periods of remission. Also, depressive disorder frequently accompanies obsessive–compulsive disorder, and in such cases effective treatment of the depressive disorder often leads to improvement in the obsessional symptoms. For this reason a thorough search for depressive disorder should be made in every patient presenting with obsessive–compulsive disorder.

Counselling

Treatment should begin with an explanation of the symptoms, and if necessary with reassurance that these symptoms are not an early sign of insanity (a common concern of obsessional patients). While waiting for the effects of treatment or for spontaneous improvement, supportive interviews can benefit patients by providing continuing hope. Joint interviews with the spouse are indicated where marital problems seem to be aggravating the symptoms. Obsessional patients often involve other family members in their rituals; and it may be necessary to counsel relatives and help them to adopt an appropriately firm but sympathetic attitude to the patient.

Medication

Clomipramine Clomipramine is a tricyclic antidepressant with potent 5-HT uptake blocking effects. When given in high doses (200–250 mg/day) it is more effective than placebo in reducing the obsessional symptoms of patients with obsessional-compulsive disorder (Clomipramine Collaborative Study Group 1991). Most patients tolerate the treatment, but at these high doses, anticholinergic side-effects are common and a few patients develop seizures. A clinically useful effect may not be reached until about 6 weeks after starting treatment; and further improvement may occur over the next 6 weeks. Many patients relapse in the first few weeks after the drug is stopped (Pato *et al.* 1988). Other tricyclic antidepressants that are less potent 5-HT uptake blockers do not have this therapeutic effect in obsessive–compulsive disorder (Foa *et al.* 1987).

Specific serotonin uptake inhibitors (SSRIs) SSRIs, including fluoxetine and fluvoxamine, paroxetine and sertraline, are effective in reducing obsessional symptoms (Goodman *et al.* 1989b; Jenike *et al.* 1990). These drugs appear to be as effective as clomipramine and produce fewer unpleasant side-effects (Freeman *et al.* 1994; Zohar and Judge 1996; Bisserbe *et al.* 1997). Nevertheless, only about half the treated patients improve substantially and attempts have been made to increased the response rate by adding a second drug to the SSRI. Beneficial effects have been reported from the addition of a neuroleptic (McDougle *et al.* 1990), but the value of this combined treatment is still uncertain. As with clomipramine, relapse is common in the few weeks after an SSRI has been stopped. It is possible that longer treatment might result in fewer relapses.

Anxiolytic drugs Anxiolytic drugs give some short-term symptomatic relief but should not be prescribed for more than about 3 weeks at a time. If anxiolytic treatment is needed for longer, small doses of a tricyclic antidepressant or an antipsychotic may be used.

Whichever medication is chosen, it should be combined with response prevention for any rituals.

Cognitive–behaviour therapy

Response prevention Obsessional rituals usually improve with a combination of response prevention (see p. 736) with exposure to any environmental cues that increase the symptoms. About two-thirds of patients with moderately severe rituals can be expected to improve substantially though not completely (Rachman and Hodgson 1980). When rituals respond to this treatment, the accompanying obsessional thoughts usually improve as well. Patients who do not consistently recognize that their beliefs are untrue appear to respond to behaviour therapy as well as those with more typical obsessional symptoms (Lelliot *et al.* 1988). The results seem comparable with those of treatment with clomipramine and SSRIs (Cox *et al.* 1993; van Bolkom *et al.* 1998).

Behavioural treatment is much less effective for obsessional thoughts occurring without rituals. The technique of thought stopping has been used for many years, but there is no good evidence that it has a specific effect. Indeed, Stern *et al.* (1973) found an effect which did not differ from that of thought-stopping directed to irrelevant thoughts.

Cognitive therapy Cognitive therapy seeks to reduce attempts to suppress and avoid obsessional thoughts, since these attempts have been shown to increase, rather than decrease, their frequency. Patients are helped to record the frequency of obsessional thoughts to compare the effects of suppression and distraction. Since suppression (and avoidance) are driven by the conviction that to think something is to make it happen, attempts are made to weaken this conviction by reviewing the evidence for and against it. These techniques may be combined with exposure to tape-recorded repetition of the thoughts, and by discussion of any other cognitive distortions along the general lines of cognitive therapy (see p. 733). At the time of writing, there is insufficient evidence to decide the long-term effectiveness of this treatment. (See

Salkovskis 1997 for an account of cognitive therapy for obsessive–compulsive disorder).

Dynamic psychotherapy

Exploratory and interpretative psychotherapy seldom helps obsessional patients. Indeed, some are made worse because these procedures encourage painful and unproductive rumination about the subjects discussed during treatment.

Neurosurgery

The immediate results of neurosurgery for severe obsessive–compulsive disorder is often a striking reduction in tension and distress. However, the long-term effects are uncertain, since no prospective controlled trial has been carried out. Uncontrolled assessments (Goktepe *et al.* 1975; Mitchell-Heggs *et al.* 1976; Jenike *et al.* 1991) and comparisons with retrospectively matched control groups (Tan *et al.* 1971) have been carried out but cannot answer the question. In a more recent study, Hay *et al.* (1993) reported a 10-year follow-up of 26 obsessive–compulsive patients treated with orbito-medial or cingulate lesions, or both. Of the 18 patients interviewed, eight had a second operation, two died by suicide, and about a third of the survivors improved. The frequency of second operations and the low improvement rates indicate the limitations of this treatment. If neurosurgery is considered for these patients, it should be only for the most chronic cases that have resisted intensive in-patient or day-patient treatment, including drug and behavioural methods, for at least a year. Using these criteria, the authors have not referred patients for surgical treatment.

Further reading

Gelder, M. G., López-Ibor, J. J. Jr, and Andreasen, N. C. (eds) (2000). *The new Oxford textbook of psychiatry*, Sections 4.7: Anxiety Disorders, and 4.8: Obsessional Disorders. Oxford University Press, Oxford. (Section 4.8 comprises chapters on: generalized anxiety disorders; social and specific phobias; and panic disorder and agoraphobia.)

Hollander, E. and Stein, D. J. (eds) (1997). *Obsessive compulsive disorders: diagnosis, etiology, treatment*. Marcel Dekker, New York. (A comprehensive review of the subject).

Nathan, P. E. and Gorman, J. M. (eds) (1998). *A guide to treatments that work*. Oxford University Press, New York. (See Chapters 15–18 concerned with psychosocial and pharmacological treatments for panic disorders, phobia, generalized anxiety disorders, and obsessional compulsive disorders.)

Noyes, R. and Hoehn-Saric, R. (1998). *The anxiety disorders*. Cambridge University Press, Cambridge. (A systematic review which includes a useful chapter on psychological and biological aspects of normal anxiety, as well as chapters on generalized anxiety disorder, panic disorder and agoraphobia, social phobia and specific phobia.)

10

CHAPTER 10

Somatoform and dissociative disorders

CHAPTER 10
Somatoform and dissociative disorders

This chapter is mainly concerned with physical symptoms which are thought to have a psychological cause (somatoform disorders). It also covers disorders characterized by disturbances of consciousness or identity, such as amnesia and multiple personality (dissociative disorders). Historically there has been thought to be an overlap between these disorders and in the underlying psychological mechanisms collectively referred to as dissociation.

The historical complexity is reflected in our current classifications and in continuing argument about mechanism and nosology; Box 10.1 lists a number of definitions of key terms.

The two groupings, somatoform disorder and dissociative disorder, were introduced by the authors of DSM-III as part of their wider attempt to rationalize what had previously been referred to as neuroses. They contain some of the oldest (and the most controversial) terms within psychiatric classification, together with new subcategories.

Both groupings are tentative, lacking a substantial evidence base, and are widely regarded as unsatisfactory. Even so, the passage of time and increasing clinical and research usage have given them a hardly justified weight. Despite important research, for example, on the relationship between dissociation and trauma and on the nature and treatment of unexplained symptoms, there have not been the wider advances in the evidence base that would enable fundamental reclassification.

Our current approaches to the disorders described in this chapter can best be understood by considering two nineteenth century terms, both of which are considered more fully later in the chapter, *dissociation* and *conversion*.

Dissociation was first used to describe an alleged psychological mechanism responsible for a wide variety of disturbances of consciousness that were believed to have been precipitated by trauma. Although attracting great attention at the time, all interest was lost until the second half of the twentieth century with renewed interest in alleged multiple personalities and in the psychological consequences of trauma (see Shorter 1992).

Conversion is a term introduced by Freud to describe the alleged conversion of psychiatric distress into physical symptoms, which he saw as underlying the historically controversial syndrome of hysteria.

Box 10.1 Some definitions

Somatoform disorders
Introduced in DSM-III for a group of disorders characterized by physical symptoms that are not explained by organic factors. Hence also somatoform *symptoms*.

Somatization
Variably defined process or processes whereby physical symptoms without adequate organic explanation are experienced and result in consultation. Hence somatization *symptoms*.

Dissociation
A mechanism whereby psychological processes relating to consciousness are split or fragmented. Also dissociative symptoms and a personality trait.

Conversion
Introduced by Freud for the conversion of distress into physical symptoms and which he proposed as the fundamental mechanism in hysteria. Used now as a diagnostic category to replace hysteria.

Classification

In an attempt to overcome continuing controversy and confusion, the authors of DSM-III attempted to create a more rational classification into dissociative and somatoform disorders (which included conversion disorder). However the inclusion of the two old words of dissociation and conversion (and their use in rather different ways in DSM and ICD) has perpetuated the confusion.

DSM-IV has entirely separate sections for dissociative disorders and somatoform disorders. ICD-10 includes somatoform disorder and dissociative (conversion) disorder as two major categories within the wider chapter of *neurotic, stress-related, and somatoform disorders*.

The principal difference between the classifications is that whereas in ICD-10 conversion disorder is included with dissociative disorders, DSM-IV states that

conversion disorder is placed in the 'somatoform disorders' section emphasizing the importance of considering neurological or other general medical conditions in the differential diagnosis.

This unusual classificatory principle further complicates a largely speculative category. This chapter follows DSM-IV for convenience.

This chapter should be read in conjunction with sections in other chapters:

- *Dissociation* is also referred to in the account of acute stress disorders and post-traumatic stress disorder (p. 192).
- Chapter 16 on psychiatry and medicine includes a wider discussion of *unexplained physical symptoms* and a section on Factitious Disorder.

Somatoform disorder

The following section should be read in conjunction with the section on unexplained physical symptoms in Chapter 16, which provides a wider perspective of the characteristics of symptoms, their epidemiology, aetiology, and treatment. This section is concerned only with the restricted and arbitrary subgroups classified within the somatoform disorder rubrics.

Somatoform disorders were included as a provisional new category in DSM-III and this remains true of both DSM-IV and ICD. Unfortunately, both classifications have been interpreted as suggesting much greater validity than originally intended. The defining feature is 'physical symptoms suggesting a physical disorder for which there are no demonstrable organic findings on known physiological mechanisms, and for which there is strong evidence, or a strong presumption, that the symptoms are linked to psychological factors or conflicts'. This is a 'dualist' explanation, which sees mind and body aetiologies as mutually exclusive alternatives. There are a number of problems in the overall concept of somatoform disorders:

- There is a lack of any clear operational definition for the overall category.
- Some types of somatoform disorder (especially severe hypochondriasis and somatization disorder) are so enduring that they might more appropriately be classified as personality disorder.
- Criteria have little meaning for cultures that do not share the Western presumption of the separation of body and mind. They instead see physical and psychological factors as contributing to the onset and course of not only 'unexplained' physical symptoms but of all illness.
- Many subjects whose symptoms satisfy criteria for somatoform disorders also report psychological symptoms of anxiety or depressive disorders. Co-morbidity, with two psychiatric diagnoses, is very common for this whole group of patients.

Classification in DSM-IV and ICD-10

There are substantial differences between ICD and DSM in the nosology of the subcategories (see Table 10.1). *Neurasthenia* is included in ICD-10

Table 10.1 Categories of somatoform disorders in ICD–10 and DSM-IV

ICD–10	DSM-IV
Somatization disorder	Somatization disorder
Undifferentiated somatoform disorder	Undifferentiated somatoform disorder
Hypochondriacal disorder	Hypochondriasis
Somatoform autonomic dysfunction	*No category*
Persistent pain disorder	Pain disorder associated with psychological factors (and a general medical condition)
Other somatoform disorders	Somatoform disorders not otherwise specified
No category	Body dysmorphic disorder
No category	Conversion disorder
Neurasthenia	*No category*

but is not used in any section of DSM-IV; *conversion disorder* is a somatoform disorder in DSM-IV but not in ICD.

Both classifications include relatively precise categories (for example, *somatization disorder* and *hypochondriasis*) and several very vaguely defined non-specific categories. It is accepted that there are major problems in both classifications:

◆ The specific categories lack reliable and valid definitions. The clinical descriptions are largely derived from hospital-based experience and are not readily applicable to the large number of people with unexplained symptoms in the community and primary care. Further problems are that diagnostic criteria are based on a mixture of principles – aetiology, symptom count, consultation, response to medical treatment.

◆ The non-specific categories include *undifferentiated somatoform disorder, somatoform autonomic*

dysfunction (ICD-10 only), and *other somatoform disorders*. Although the latter groupings have attracted much less clinical and research attention, they are by far the commonest forms of somatoform disorder in all epidemiological studies. So broad and vague are the criteria that it is possible to use them for almost all persistent unexplained physical symptoms.

◆ The differences between DSM-IV and ICD-10 mean that epidemiological research has found large discrepancies in prevalences both for overall somatoform disorder and of the subcategories (see Simon 2000).

The problems encountered in Western countries with somatoform disorders, which are described above, together with the lack of any useful meaning for cultures that do not accept the mind/body separation which underlies thir definition, means that great caution is necessary in using this category. It is important to recall that somatoform disorder remains a provisional grouping for statistical purposes rather than an evidence-based classification which has implications for clinical care.

At present we lack the knowledge for total revision in this section. There is little advantage in making trivial changes to laboriously developed but fundamentally unsatisfactory schemata. It is more realistic to encourage a critical view of the somatoform concepts that will enable some changes in terminology and definition and major improvements in DSM-IV text. At the same time, there is a need for a separate practical classification for use in everyday practice by both specialists and non-specialists. This might be multidimensional in terms of clinical syndromes, duration, number of symptoms, cognitions, and associated psychiatric disorder, such as anxiety and depression (see Mayou *et al.* 1995). Somatoform terminology should be avoided or used with tact in talking to patients and in making referrals.

Conversion disorder

Conversion disorder is the term used by DSM to replace hysteria and is the equivalent of Dissociative (Conversion) Disorder in ICD-10. It refers to a condition which has a long and controversial history and an uncertain status in modern psychiatry.

The history of hysteria

Descriptions of hysteria were included in ancient Greek medical texts. At that time the disorder was thought to result from abnormalities of position or function of the uterus, a view that persisted until the seventeenth century. Gradually, the idea of a disorder of the brain became accepted and, by the nineteenth century, the importance of predisposing constitutional and organic causes of this brain disorder were recognized, and it was also accepted that strong emotion was the usual provoking cause.

The studies of hysteria by Charcot, a French neurologist who worked at the Salpêtrière Hospital in Paris, were particularly influential in the late nineteenth century. He believed that hysteria was caused by a functional disorder of the brain which caused symptoms, and which also rendered patients susceptible to hypnosis so that new symptoms could be produced by suggestion. However, Charcot later became more interested in the probability of a psychological cause as a result of clinical studies by his pupil, Pierre Janet, who proposed that the disorder in hysteria was a tendency to dissociate (see also p. 263), i.e. to lose the normal integration between various parts of mental functioning, together with a restriction of personal awareness so that the person became unaware of certain aspects of psychological functioning that would otherwise be within his awareness. For a review of Janet's contribution see van der Kolk and van der Hart (1989).

Highly influential contributions in thinking about hysteria were made by Freud. He visited Charcot in the winter of 1895–96 and was impressed by demonstrations of the susceptibility of patients to hypnosis, and of the power of suggestion to hypnotized patients (Sulloway 1979). On his return to Vienna, Freud and his colleague Breuer studied patients with hysteria and reported their findings in a paper 'On the psychical mechanisms of hysterical phenomena' (Freud 1893). In a subsequent monograph *Studies on hysteria* (1893–5), Breuer and Freud suggested that hysteria was caused by emotionally charged ideas, usually sexual, which had become lodged in the unconscious of the patient at some previous time, and which were excluded from conscious awareness by a process which the authors called repression. They summarized this idea in the phrase 'hysterics suffer mainly from reminiscences'. Freud adopted the word 'conversion' to refer to a process whereby psychological distress was converted into physical symptoms.

Freud later concluded that his original formulations were wrong and based on fabricated stories by suggestible patients. He thereafter wrote no more on this subject. There was relatively little interest from other psychodynamic theorists and hysteria largely lost its interest. Indeed, it was seen as a declining problem in developed Western countries. Hysteria became even less popular as a diagnosis because of the pejorative associations and because of concern that it might represent misdiagnosis of organic disease. This latter view was put most vigorously by Slater (1965) who reported in a 7-year follow-up study of 85 patients that 30 had definite organic disease and 34 had definite other psychiatric disorder (see p. 263). Other writers on hysteria had very different views and emphasized the behavioural and social aspects and made comparisons with the occurrence of similar phenomena in other cultures, especially trance and possession states.

For a more complete account of the history of hysteria see Breuer and Freud (1893–5), Veith (1965), and Shorter (1992).

Clinical features

In DSM-IV conversion disorder is divided into four subtypes:

- *with motor symptom or deficit* This subtype includes such symptoms as impaired coordination or balance, paralysis or localized weakness, difficulty swallowing or 'lump in throat', aphonia, and urinary retention.

♦ *with sensory symptom or deficit* This subtype includes such symptoms as loss of touch or pain sensation, double vision, blindness, deafness, and hallucinations.

♦ *with seizures or convulsions* This subtype includes seizures or convulsions with voluntary motor or sensory components.

♦ *with mixed presentation* This subtype is used if symptoms of more than one category are evident.

Conversion symptoms do not normally reflect understandable physiological or pathological mechanisms. They are also highly suggestible and may vary considerably in response to the comments of other people, especially doctors. Symptoms may be 'reinforced' by measures such as providing a wheelchair for the patient who has difficulty walking. In addition, people with conversion disorders may show *la belle indifference* (a term used by nineteenth century French writers to denote a relative lack of concern about the nature and implications of the symptoms), but this is not an invariable feature.

It is often said that sufferers derive *secondary gain* from their symptoms; that is to say external benefits or avoidance of unwanted responsibilities (the term 'primary gain' refers to the relief allegedly obtained by the conversion of distress into physical symptoms). It is frequently impossible to identify such gains and, in any case, benefits of being ill may be observed in many psychiatric and physical disorders.

Epidemiology

The prevalence of conversion disorder in the general population is difficult to determine. However, there is no reason to accept a widely held view that hysteria is now uncommon in Western countries; it is more likely that it is the making of the diagnosis that has declined. Several recent studies have suggested that conversion disorder remains frequent in medical settings; for example, a British primary care study identified 0.5 cases per 1000 patients but concluded that there were good reasons to believe that the true prevalence was many time greater (Singh and Lee 1997).

Aetiology

The aetiology is unclear and there has been little systematic research:

♦ *Psychodynamic theories* have been poorly developed since Freud's original formulation, which he had abandoned by the early 1900s. They continue to make use of the concept of conversion of distress into physical symptoms having symbolic meaning.

♦ *Cultural explanations* It has been increasingly apparent that phenomena classed as psychiatric disorder in Western countries may, in other settings, be seen as possession states, many of which are culturally accepted (see Trance and possession disorders, p. 267).

♦ *Social factors* Social and behavioural factors appear to be major determinants of the onset and development of conversion symptoms.

♦ *Central neuropsychological and neurophysiological mechanisms* Research using functional neuroimaging and biological techniques has suggested symptoms are associated with patterns of localized abnormalities of cerebral functions (Spence 1999).

See Halligan *et al.* (2001) for reviews of neuropsychological mechanisms and other aspects of prevalence and aetiology.

Prognosis

Most patients with dissociative and conversion disorders of recent onset who are seen in general practice or hospital emergency departments recover quickly. However, those cases lasting longer than a year are likely to persist for many years. In his widely cited follow-up study, Slater (1965) described the development of major physical and psychiatric disorder in a high proportion of subjects. This finding is now seen as a reflection of the highly atypical nature of his sample of neurologically undiagnosed patients referred to a national tertiary referral neurological hospital. A more recent follow-up of much more precisely diagnosed patients attending the same hospital found a very low incidence of physical or psychiatric diagnoses which explained these patients' symptoms or disability (Crimlisk *et al.* 1998).

Treatment

For *acute conversion disorders* seen in primary care or hospital emergency departments, treatment by reassurance and suggestion is usually appropriate, together with immediate efforts to resolve any stressful circumstances that provoked the reaction (Box 10.2). The doctor's manner should be sympathetic and positive and provide a face-saving opportunity for rapid return to normal physical functioning. It is important to be aware that the condition is deserving of medical assessment, that it is a common problem, and the outcome can confidentally expected to be excellent. At the same time, it is necessary to indicate that the personal difficulties that have been identified may be contributing to the clinical picture and that they deserve assessment and treatment in their own right.

Box 10.2 Treatment of acute conversion disorder
◆ Medical and psychiatric history from patient and informants
◆ Full examination and appropriate investigation to exclude physical causes
◆ Sympathetic but positive reassurance that the patient is suffering from an acute temporary condition and does not have a disabling medical disorder
◆ Discussion of the expected rapid recovery
◆ Avoidance of reinforcement of disability or symptoms
◆ Offer continuing assessment and treatment of related psychiatric or social problems

---

Where symptoms have persisted for more than a few weeks, more elaborate treatment is required. The general approach is to focus on the elimination of factors that are reinforcing the symptoms and on the encouragement of normal behaviour. It should be explained to the patient that he has a disability (as in remembering, or moving his arm), which is not caused by serious physical disease but is made worse by psychological factors. Patients should then be told that if they try hard to regain control, they will succeed. If necessary, they can be offered help in doing this, for example, by physiotherapy.

Attention is then directed away from the symptoms and towards problems that have provoked the disorder. Staff should show concern to help the patient, and this is best done by encouraging self-help. It is important not to make undue concessions to patients' disabilities; for example, a patient who cannot walk should not be provided with a wheelchair, and a patient who has collapsed on the floor should be encouraged to get up unaided. This requires a supportive and sympathetic manner directed towards helping the patient to help himself rather than being in any way uncaring or even punitive. To achieve these ends, there must be a clear plan so that all members of staff adopt a consistent approach to the patient.

Medication has no part to play in the treatment of dissociative and conversion disorders. However, when conversion symptoms are secondary to a depressive or anxiety disorder treatment of the primary condition usually leads to an improvement of the secondary symptoms. Specific methods of behaviour therapy appear to be of little value but it is possible that cognitive methods can be helpful.

It is essential that measures to treat conversion and other symptoms are accompanied by an attempt to identify and treat underlying personal and social difficulties. Brief and focused psychological treatments are helpful, but it is essential to keep in mind that, as Freud and Breuer learned, it is often dangerous to attempt more intensive therapy as it may result in transference reactions which are difficult to manage and in false reports of dramatic previous experiences.

Those who do not improve should be reviewed thoroughly for undiscovered physical illness. All patients, whether improved or not, should be followed carefully for long enough to exclude any organic disease that might not have been detected.

Epidemic hysteria

Occasionally, dissociative (or conversion) disorder spreads within a group of people as an 'epidemic'. This spread happens most often in closed groups of young women, for example, in a girls' school, a nurses' home, or a convent. Usually anxiety has been heightened among the members of the group by some threat to the community, such as the possibility of being involved in an epidemic of actual and serious physical disease present in the neighbourhood. In many cases the anxiety may be more persistent than dissociative/conversion mechanisms. Typically, the epidemic starts in one person who is highly suggestible, histrionic, and a focus of attention in the group. This first case may result from a general apprehension about the threat of physical illness, or from a specific concern about an acquaintance who has contracted the illness. Gradually, other cases appear, first in the most suggestible and then, as anxiety mounts, among those with less predisposition. The symptoms are variable, but fainting and dizziness are common. Outbreaks among schoolchildren have been commonly reported. Some writers believe that the 'dancing manias' of the Middle Ages may have been hysterical epidemics in people aroused by religious fervour (see Wessely 1987).

Somatization disorder

The essential feature of somatization disorder is multiple somatic complaints of long duration, beginning before the age of 30. A group of psychiatrists in St Louis (Perley and Guze 1962) originally described a syndrome of chronic multiple somatic complaints with no identified organic cause, which they regarded as a form of hysteria and named it *Briquet's syndrome* after a nineteenth-century French physician who wrote a monograph on hysteria. In fact, Briquet did not describe the syndrome to which his name was given and the symptoms do not accord with usual concepts of hysteria. A similar syndrome was introduced in DSM-III and named somatization disorder. The circumstances of the description of the syndrome and the fact that it refers to a group of people whom doctors find particularly difficult to treat has resulted in the alleged syndrome attracting undue attention and being seen as having a validity that has not been confirmed by research.

In DSM-IIIR, diagnostic criteria were highly restrictive, so that many patients with chronic multiple physical complaints were excluded as insufficiently severe and had to be allocated to the residual category of *undifferentiated somatoform disorder*. In DSM-IV, the criteria for diagnosis have been made somewhat less restrictive and require four pain symptoms, two gastrointestinal symptoms, one sexual symptom, and one pseudo-neurological symptom, all of which are not fully explained by a medical condition. The ICD-10 criteria require at least six symptoms relating to at least two organ systems from among a list of fourteen predefined symptoms distributed in four groups – gastrointestinal, cardiovascular, neurogenital, and skin or pain symptoms.

Epidemiology

The reports of prevalence of somatization disorder depend on the assessment methods used. Community surveys have reported prevalences of less than 1% and primary care findings have usually been between 1 and 2%. The disorder is twice as common in women than in men. There is substantial co-morbidity with other defined psychiatric disorders, such as major depression. Diagnosis is considerably less stable over time than suggested in the original descriptions of the syndrome. See Simon (2000) and Fink (2000) for reviews.

Aetiology

The St Louis group proposed a familial association between somatization disorder in females and sociopathy and alcoholism in their male relatives. They also concluded that follow-up studies and family studies show somatization disorder to be a single stable syndrome. Their views have not been confirmed. The chronicity essential for the diagnosis of somatization disorder has led to the suggestion that it may often best be conceived as a personality disorder. Aetiology is discussed further in the section on unexplained medical symptoms in Chapter 16.

Treatment

Somatization disorder is difficult to treat. Continuing care by one doctor using only the minimum of essential investigations can reduce the patients' use of health services and may improve their functional state (Smith *et al.* 1986; G. R. Smith 1995). Psychiatric assessment can help to clarify a complicated history, to negotiate a simplified pattern of care, and to agree the aims of treatment with the patient, the family, and the responsible physician. The aim of treatment is often to limit further progression rather than to cure. See Fink (2000) for a review.

Undifferentiated somatoform disorder

This is a residual category of unexplained physical symptoms, lasting at least 6 months, which are below the threshold for a diagnosis of somatization disorder. It has a substantially higher prevalence. Since data fail to support any clear boundary based on the number of distribution of unexplained symptoms as required for somatization disorder, there have been numerous suggestions for less restrictive somatization symptoms (for example, Kroenke *et al.* 1997; Escobar *et al.* 1998). As also discussed in Chapter 16, none of the syndromes based on counting numbers of unexplained symptoms has a satisfactory evidence base and none is helpful in planning treatment.

Hypochondriasis

The term hypochondriasis is one of the oldest medical terms, originally used to describe disorders believed to be due to disease of the organs situated in the hypochondrium. Since then, the term has been used in many ways. It is now defined by DSM-IV and ICD-10 in terms of disease conviction and disease phobia. DSM-IV describes the condition as a

preoccupation with a fear or belief of having a serious disease based on the individual's interpretation of physical signs of sensations as evidence of physical illness. Appropriate physical evaluation does not support the diagnosis of any physical disorder than can account for the physical signs or sensations or for the individual's unrealistic interpretation of them. The fear of having, or belief that one has a disease, persists despite medical reassurance.

The criteria go on to exclude patients with panic disorder or delusions, and requires that symptoms have been present for at least 6 months. There is continuing argument about the status of transient hypochondriasis, a possible hypochondriacal personality disorder, and inclusion of illness phobias.

Epidemiology

Estimates of prevalence have been hindered by the absence of proven standardized assessments. Whilst some primary care surveys have estimated a prevalence of around 5%, the WHO multicentre primary care survey (Gureje *et al.* 1997) found a prevalence of only 0.8%. Using a less restrictive definition, the prevalence was 2.2%. This later definition omitted 'persistent refusal to accept medical reassurance' but retained the triad of illness worry, associated distress, and medical help-seeking. Co-morbidity with depression and anxiety disorders is frequent. See Simon (2000) for a review of epidemiology.

Prognosis

The course has not been well described but a 4–5-year follow-up by Barsky *et al.* (1998) shows that the condition is often persistent.

Aetiology

The cause is unknown; recent cognitive formulations have emphasized the faulty appraisal of bodily sensations in leading to false beliefs and to maintaining psychological reactions and behaviours. There is a marked similarity to panic disorder in which there are misinterpretations of autonomic symptoms (Salkovskis and Clark 1993). Wider issues of the aetiology of unexplained symptoms are discussed in Chapter 16.

Treatment

Treatment of hypochondriasis follows the general principles outlined on p. 468. Since the disorder is often chronic or recurrent, management is difficult. Repeated reassurance is unhelpful but measures to control investigations, to correct misattributions, and to encourage constructive ways of coping with symptoms can be helpful. Trials have shown that benefit can result from intensive cognitive–behavioural treatment. Clark *et al.* (1998), in a randomized controlled trial, compared cognitive therapy, an alternative equally credible treatment – behavioural stress management – and a waiting list control, and showed the effectiveness of cognitive therapy as a specific treatment. Both treatments were effective. Cognitive therapy was more effective for hypochondriasis but there was no difference between the treatments for mood disturbance. See Noyes (2000) for a general review of hypochondriasis.

Body dysmorphic disorder

Body dysmorphic disorder is the DSM term for a subgroup of the broader but ill-defined clinical syndrome of *dysmorphophobia*, which was first described by Morselli (1886) as 'a subjective description of ugliness and physical defect which the patient feels is noticeable to others'.

The typical patient with dysmorphophobia is convinced that some part of his body is too large, too small, or misshapen. To other people the appearance is normal, or there is a trivial abnormality. In the latter case, it may be difficult to decide whether the preoccupation is disproportionate. The common complaints are about the nose, ears, mouth, breasts, buttocks, and penis, but any part of the body may be involved. The patient

may be constantly preoccupied with and tormented by his mistaken belief. It seems to him that other people notice and talk about his supposed deformity. He may blame all his other difficulties on it: if only his nose were a better shape, he would be more successful in his work, social life, and sexual relationships. Time-consuming behaviours which aim to re-examine, improve, or hide the perceived defect are frequent. Social impairment is considerable. There is substantial co-morbidity, especially with major depression and social phobia.

The severe cases described in the psychiatric literature are infrequent, but less severe forms of dysmorphophobia are more common, especially in plastic surgery and dermatology. Some patients with this syndrome meet diagnostic criteria for other disorders. Thus Hay (1970) studied 12 men and five women with the condition, and found that 11 had severe personality disorder, five had schizophrenia, and one had a depressive illness. In these patients the preoccupation is usually delusional.

There have been no prospective studies. The condition usually begins in adolescence and is chronic, with some fluctuation over time. It is probable that there is some improvement over many years.

The term *body dysmorphic disorder* was introduced in DSM-III to denote dysmorphophobia that is not better accounted for by another psychiatric disorder. The preoccupation with the imagined defect in appearance is usually an overvalued idea, but individuals 'can receive an additional diagnosis of Delusional Disorder, Somatic type'. The separate validity of this syndrome has not yet been established; there are overlaps with delusional disorder, hypochondriasis, and obsessive–compulsive disorder. ICD-10 classifies it as a subgroup of hypochondriasis. Its features are as described above.

Assessment

The assessment should include questioning about the nature of the preoccupations with appearance and of the ways in which this has interfered with personal and social life. Diagnosis can be difficult because some sufferers keep the nature of their symptoms secret because of their embarrassment and this may result in misdiagnosis as social phobia, panic, or obsessive–compulsive disorder.

Treatment

When dysmorphophobia is secondary to a psychiatric disorder such as schizophrenia or major depression, the latter should be treated in the usual way. The treatment of body dysmorphic disorder is often difficult. It is essential to establish a working relationship in which the psychiatrist is seen as understanding of the severity of the problems and willing to provide help. Since many patients will be requesting surgery, it is important to explain the lack of success of this approach and suggest that there are other effective treatments. Some patients are helped by such reassurance and by continued support, but many are not. Counselling and practical help should be provided for any occupational, social, or sexual difficulties that accompany the condition.

Cosmetic surgery is often successful for patients who have clear reasons for requesting an operation, whether there is a definite deformity or the reasons are connected with fashion or vanity. However, surgery is usually contraindicated for those who have body dysmorphic disorder. A small proportion of such patients remain very dissatisfied after operations. Selection for surgery therefore requires careful assessment of the patient's expectations; in general, those who do not have realistic views of the possible benefits of surgery have a poor prognosis. This assessment is difficult, and collaboration between plastic surgeons, psychiatrists, and psychologists is valuable.

There is evidence of beneficial effects from antidepressant [especially selective serotonin re-uptake inhibitor (SSRI)] medication, especially in patients with prominent depressive symptoms. Whatever specific treatment is offered, it is essential that patients feel that their views have been listened to sympathetically. Unintended rebuffs by surgeons or psychiatrists can exacerbate the difficulties of management. See Phillips (1996, 2000) for reviews of dysmorphophobia.

Somatoform disorder not otherwise specified

This residual diagnostic category is used for a wide range of somatoform symptoms that do not meet the criteria for the specific somatoform categories discussed so far or for adjustment disorder with physical complaints.

Pain disorder

This term (persistent somatoform disorder in ICD-10) denotes patients with chronic pain that is not caused by any physical or specific psychiatric disorder. DSM-IV states that the essential feature of this disorder is pain that is the predominant focus of the clinical presentation and is of sufficient severity to cause distress or impairment of functioning, and that either no organic pathology or pathophysiological mechanism has been found to account for the pain, or, when there is related organic pathology, the pain or resulting social or occupational impairment is grossly in excess of what would be expected from the physical findings. The DSM-IV diagnostic requirements are:

- pain is the predominant focus of presentations;
- significant distress or impairment of function;
- psychological factors have an important role in onset, severity, exacerbation, or maintenance.

Epidemiology

Pain is widely reported in surveys of the general population. Most people report that the pain is transient, but a minority describe persistent or recurrent pain leading to disability (Von Korff *et al.* 1988; Gureje *et al.* 1998). Pain is the most common symptom among people who consult doctors. Acute pain usually has an organic cause, such as trauma surgery or cancer. In general practice, pain is a common presenting symptom of emotional problems. In psychiatric practice, it has been reported that pain is experienced by about one-fifth of in-patients and over half of out-patients. Psychological factors affect the subjective response to pain.

Pain is particularly associated with depression, anxiety, panic, and somatoform disorders. Conversely, patients with multiple pain are especially likely to suffer from psychiatric disorder (Gureje *et al.* 1998).

Aetiology

Chronic pain occurs in many conditions, including neurological or musculoskeletal disorders. It often has both physical and psychological causes. Psychiatric disorder is common. Some patients (with or without physical pathology) have a depressive disorder but it is often difficult to make DSM or ICD diagnoses. In the past, it was suggested that a 'pain-prone disorder' existed, which was a variant of depressive disorder. There is little evidence to support this idea (Von Korff and Simon 1996). It is more likely that in these cases the pain arises from personal and social factors, and that beliefs about pain are important in maintaining it (Turk 1999; Linton 2000). Chronic pain may impose great burdens on the patient's family; conversely, the attitude of family members and other care givers can influence the perception of pain, its course, and the response to treatment.

Assessment

The *assessment* of a patient complaining of pain of unknown cause should include:

- ◆ appropriate examination for, and a thorough investigation of, possible physical causes. When the results of this investigation are negative, it should be remembered that pain may be the first symptoms of a physical illness that cannot be detected at an early stage;
- ◆ a full description of the pain and the circumstances in which it occurs;
- ◆ any symptoms suggestive of a depressive or other psychiatric disorder;
- ◆ pain behaviours – verbal and non-verbal behaviours including the presentation of symptoms, requests for medication and responses to pain;

- ◆ beliefs about the causes of pain and of its implications.

Treatment

The *treatment of pain* associated with a psychiatric disorder is the treatment of the primary condition. Skill is required to maintain a working relationship with patients unwilling to accept a psychological basis for their pain. Any associated physical disorder should be treated and adequate analgesics provided.

The management of chronic pain should be individually planned, comprehensive, and involve the patient's family. Any physical cause must be treated. Psychological care is directed to two issues:

- ◆ whether there is an associated mental disorder. This assessment should be made on positive findings and not solely because no specific organic cause has been identified. If depressive illness is present it should be treated vigorously. Antidepressant medication may also be effective in patients with chronic pain in the absence of evidence of a depressive disorder (O'Malley *et al* 1999).
- ◆ whether the pain or any associated behaviours can be modified by using psychological techniques.

Behavioural treatments are useful. However, many patients with chronic pain lack the motivation needed to make full use of these methods. In some cases such treatment aims to reduce social reinforcement of maladaptive behaviour, and to encourage the patient to seek ways to overcome disability. See Morley *et al.* (1999) for a review.

Pharmacological and behavioural therapies may be combined for some patients. Multidisciplinary pain clinics provide expertise in and resources for a range of treatments. Although many patients are unwilling to accept such treatment and others are considered unsuitable, the evidence is that they are cost-effective for participants. See Benjamin (2000) for a review of pain disorder and chronic pain.

Some specific pain syndromes

Complaints of many specific kinds of pain are common in the population (Von Korff *et al.* 1988). This section is concerned with headache, facial pain, back pain, and pelvic pain. Certain other specific pain syndromes are discussed later in Chapter 16, including non-cardiac chest pain (see p. 491), abdominal pain (see p. 472), phantom limb pain (see p. 487), and fibromyalgia (see p. 473).

Headache

Patients with chronic or recurrent headache may be referred to psychiatrists. There are many physical causes of headache, notably migraine which affects about one in ten of the population at some time of their life. Many patients attending neurological clinics have headaches for which no physical cause can be found. The commonest is 'tension' headache, which is usually described as a dull generalized feeling of pressure or tightness extending around the head. It is frequently of short duration and is relieved by analgesia or a good night's sleep, but may occasionally be constant and unremitting. Some patients describe depressive symptoms and others describe anxiety in relation to obvious life stresses. Psychological factors seem to contribute to aetiology, but there is no evidence that the headaches result from increased muscle tension, and vascular mechanisms are more likely to be involved.

Most patients with headaches for which no physical cause can be found can be reassured by an explanation of the results of investigations. Some patients with persisting headaches, whether or not they have psychiatric symptoms, respond to antidepressants, or cognitive behavioural methods, or psychotherapy.

See Hopkins (1992) for a general review and Blanchard (1992) for a review of psychological treatment.

Facial pain

Facial pain has many physical causes; there are at least two forms in which psychological variables appear to be important. The more common is temporomandibular dysfunction (Costen's syndrome or facial arthralgia). There is a dull ache around the temporomandibular joint, and the condition usually presents to dentists. 'Atypical' facial pain is a deeper aching or throbbing pain which is more likely to present to neurologists. Patients with either of these symptoms are often reluctant to see a psychiatrist, but several trials suggest that antidepressants can relieve symptoms even when there is no evidence of a depressive disorder. In some cases, cognitive–behavioural methods are effective (see Feinmann 1999) for a review.

Back pain

Back pain is the second leading cause for visits to primary-care doctors and a major cause of disability. Most acute pain is transient, but in about a fifth of patients it persists for more than 6 months. Psychological and behavioural problems at the onset predict a poor outcome (Linton 2000). Treatment includes the provision of accurate information about the cause and outcome of the condition, limited use of analgesics, and a graded increase in activity. Von Korff *et al.* (1994) showed that, in primary care, systematic advice about self-care led to a functional outcome as good as that with analgesia and bed rest, cost less, and was more satisfactory to patients.

Chronic pelvic pain

Pelvic pain is one of the most common symptoms reported by women attending gynaecology clinics. The pain often persists despite negative investigations, and psychological factors appear to be significant causes of the pain and the disability. Cognitive–behavioural interventions may be effective in some cases (Glover and Pearce 1995).

Dissociative disorders

The essential feature of dissociative disorders is a disruption of the usually integrated functions of consciousness, memory, identity or perception of the environment. Disturbance may be sudden or gradual, transient or chronic. (DSM-IV).

The word dissociation can be traced back to the late nineteenth century and particularly to the work of the French philosopher and psychiatrist, Pierre Janet (1859–1947). As a young man he studied patients with hysteria and was invited by Charcot to continue his work at the Salpêtrière in Paris. He used the term 'désagregation psychologique' (subsequently loosely translated into English as dissociation) and undertook many meticulous clinical studies of sensory perception and mental integration, information processing, reactions to trauma, and the role of psychotherapy. He reported his findings in many papers and several books (see van der Kolk and van der Hart 1989). Whilst Janet himself was influenced by wide nineteenth-century interest in hypnosis, suggestibility, and other states of altered consciousness, he was a major influence on Freud and Breuer's early work on hysteria which saw symptoms as resulting from an inability to cope with the emotional consequences of severe trauma (see Shorter 1992 for an historical review). However, with the development of psychoanalysis, interest in the concept of dissociation declined.

In the 1970s the clinical problems presented by Vietnam veterans, and the increasing public concern about the consequences of physical and sexual abuse and of major disasters, resulted in much greater clinical interest in dissociative symptoms and to the inclusion of a new classification within DSM-III. Dissociative symptoms were said to include subjective numbing and detachment, reduced awareness of surroundings (feeling dazed), fragmentation or loss of memory, derealization, and depersonalization. Interest was fostered by the development of a number of screening instruments which suggested that dissociative symptoms were common. Although these instruments are widely used, they differ considerably in their content and

reflect an underlying uncertainty about the meaning of the term dissociation. This has been used to cover:

◆ a psychological mechanism

◆ a personality trait: a habitual tendency to dissociate

◆ an acute response to trauma

◆ persistent symptoms following trauma.

While this chapter describes dissociative *disorders*, much of the very large research clinical interest has concentrated on the immediate, the medium-term, and the very long-term consequences of various types of trauma – childhood abuse, major disasters, and individual trauma. Dissociative mechanisms and symptoms appear common in these situations, although it remains unclear to what extent they are fundamental features. See sections on acute stress disorder, and post-traumatic stress disorder in Chapter 8. For reviews of dissociation and trauma see Putnam (1991) and Spiegel (1991).

Dissociative disorders in clinical psychiatry

Dissociative experiences are a part of normal experiences, both in relation to highly stressful or traumatic experience, and in a variety of trance, possession or other states which may be considered as normal, even admired, in many parts of the world

Table 10.2 shows the DSM-IV classification of dissociative disorders and ICD-10 dissociative (conversion) disorders which are a subsection of the neurotic, stress-related and somatoform disorders chapter.

There is a marked discrepancy in the psychiatric literature between claims by those with a specialist interest that dissociative disorders are frequent in psychiatric populations and even in the general population (Coons 1998) and a widespread view amongst clinicians that both the whole category and its subcategories lack a convincing evidence-base (see Merskey 2000). These differing views are evident in widely varying figures for prevalence,

Table 10.2 DSM-IV classification of dissociative disorder and their ICD–10 equivalents

DSM-IV	ICD–10
Dissociative disorder	*F44 Dissociative (conversion) disorder*
Dissociative amnesia	Dissociative amnesia
Dissociative fugue	Dissociative fugue
Dissociative identity disorder	Multiple personality disorder
Depersonalization disorder	(classified in F. 48.1)
Dissociative disorder not otherwise specified	Dissociative (conversion) disorder not otherwise specified
	Dissociative stupor
	Trance and possession disorders
	Ganser's syndrome

Note: ICD–10 also includes categories of sensory and motor disturbance which DSM-IV classifies within Somatoform Disorders in a subcategory of Conversion Disorder.

ranging from extreme rarity to 50% of psychiatric inpatients.

Dissociative amnesia

The essential feature is an inability to recall important personal memories, usually of a stressful nature, that are too extensive to be explained by normal forgetfulness. As well as occurring alone, amnesia may occur during the course of other dissociative disorders and in post-traumatic stress disorder, acute stress disorder, and in somatization disorder. The diagnosis is only made when these other conditions are not present.

Dissociative amnesia must be distinguished from amnesia having a medical cause. It has been described in two forms:

◆ circumscribed amnesia for a single recent traumatic event;

◆ inability to recall long periods of childhood.

Amongst patients who present in this way, some have concurrent organic disease.

Deliberate amnesia can be extremely difficult to distinguish from genuine amnesia. See Coons (1998) for a review.

Dissociative fugue

Dissociative fugue is extremely rare in clinical practice. In a dissociative fugue, patients not only lose their memory but also wander away from their usual surroundings. When found they usually deny all memory of their whereabouts during the period of wandering, and may also deny knowledge of personal identity. There have been a number of accounts of dramatic case histories (see Hacking 1998). The disorder must be distinguished from organic disorder, for example, epilepsy and substance intoxication.

Dissociative identity disorder

In this disorder (known in ICD-10 as multiple personality disorder) there are sudden alternations between two patterns of behaviour, each of which is forgotten by the patient when the other is present (see Box 10.3). Each pattern of behaviour is a complex and integrated scheme of emotional responses, attitudes, memories, and social behaviour, and the behaviour usually contrasts strikingly with the patient's normal state. In some cases there is more than one additional behaviour pattern or

Box 10.3 **DSM-IV diagnostic criteria for dissociative identity disorder**

A The presence of two or more distinct identities or personality states (each with its own relatively enduring pattern of perceiving, relating to, and thinking about, the environment and self).

B At least two of these identities or personality states recurrently take control of the person's behaviour.

C Inability to recall important personal information that is too extensive to be explained by ordinary forgetfulness.

D The disturbance is not due to the direct physiological effects of a substance (e.g. blackouts or chaotic behaviour during alcohol intoxication) or a general medical condition (e.g. complex partial seizures).

Note In children, the symptoms are not attributable to imaginary playmates or other fantasy play.

'personality'. The condition is rare, but has been observed more frequently at some times than at others, reflecting the fluctuating interest of doctors at that time. Thus, striking examples of this disorder were described since the end of the nineteenth century which have attracted very considerable lay and literary attention. In the last 40 years there has been a dramatic increase in the number of reported cases, especially in the USA. Epidemiological studies report prevalences which vary widely from being common, especially in psychiatric populations, to being rare.

Patients often meet the criteria for other diagnoses, especially schizophrenia, personality disorder, and alcohol or drug abuse; they also have symptoms of anxiety and depression. DSM-IV criteria do not allow any clear distinction from trance and possession disorders (included in ICD-10 but in a appendix to DSM-IV). The relationship between multiple personality disorder and these other conditions would be illuminated by long-term follow-up studies, but no systematic studies of this kind have been reported.

Two issues have dominated the discussion of aetiology:

◆ *The role of severe trauma* Clinical experience and research have repeatedly emphasized that most patients describe severe childhood physical or sexual abuse. It is argued that dissociation is used as a means of psychological defence and that, over time, it has permanent consequences.

◆ *Iatrogenic factors* It has often been alleged that the wide publicity given to people of suggestible personality, combined with the credulity and enthusiasm of therapists, and frequently with the use of hypnosis, has been responsible for at least a proportion of those subject to extensive psychiatric scrutiny. See Coons (1998) and Putnam and Loewenstein (2000) for reviews; for a sceptical opinion, see Merskey (2000).

Depersonalization disorder

Depersonalization disorder is characterized by an unpleasant state of disturbed perception in which external objects or parts of the body are experienced as changed in their quality, unreal, remote, or automatized. The patient is aware of the subjective nature of this experience. The symptom of depersonalization is quite common as a minor feature of other syndromes, but depersonalization disorder is quite rare.

There is insufficient evidence about the aetiology of depersonalization disorder to be certain whether it is related to the dissociative disorders. Depersonalization disorder is classified as a dissociative disorder in DSM-IV (though has a separate place in ICD-10). For this reason and even though depersonalization is associated also with anxiety and obsessional disorders (see p. 243), we have chosen to describe the disorder here.

Clinical picture

Patients describe feelings of being unreal and experiencing an unreal quality to perceptions. They say that their emotions are dulled and that their actions feel mechanical. Paradoxically, they complain that this lack of feeling is extremely unpleasant. Insight is retained into the subjective nature of their experiences. These symptoms may be intense, and accompanied by *déjà vu* and by changes in the experience of passage of time. Some patients complain of sensory distortions affecting a single part of the body (usually the head, the nose, or a limb), which may be described as feeling as if made of cotton wool.

Two-thirds of the patients are women. The onset is often in adolescence or early adult life, with the condition starting before the age of 30 in about half the cases (Shorvon *et al.* 1946). The symptoms usually begin suddenly, sometimes when the person feels aroused but sometimes in the course of relaxation after intense physical exercise (Shorvon *et al.* 1946). Once established, the disorder often persists for years, though with periods of partial or complete remission.

Differential diagnosis

Before diagnosing depersonalization disorder, any primary disorder must be excluded, especially temporal lobe epilepsy, schizophrenia, depressive disorder, obsessional disorder, conversion or dissociative disorder, and generalized and phobic anxiety disorders. Severe and persistent depersonalization is experienced by some people with schizoid personality disorder. Most patients who present with depersonalization will be found to have one of these other disorders. The primary syndrome is rare. Ackner (1954a, 1954b) stated that all cases could be allocated to organic, depressive, anxiety, or hysterical syndromes, or to schizoid personality disorder.

Aetiology

The causes of a primary depersonalization disorder are not known. Apart from the possible association with schizoid personality disorder, no definite constitutional factors have been identified. Lader (1969) suggested that the symptoms represent a restriction of sensory input that serves to reduce intolerably high levels of anxiety. In keeping with this suggestion, a third of survivors of near fatal accidents report transient depersonalization (Noyes and Kletti 1977). Since some cases begin when the patient is tired and relaxed, this mechanism, if it exists, cannot be invariable. Also these ideas fail to explain why the condition persists as depersonalization disorder in a small minority of people

Prognosis

Secondary cases have the prognosis of the primary condition. The rare primary depersonalization disorder has not been followed systematically; clinical experience indicates that cases lasting longer than a year have a poor long-term outcome.

Treatment

When depersonalization is secondary to another disorder, treatment should be directed to the primary condition. In the rare primary depersonalization disorder, anxiolytic drugs may give short-term relief but they should not be prescribed for long periods because of the risk of dependency. Other drugs are generally ineffective, although one report suggests that SSRIs may be effective in some patients with depersonalization. (Hollander *et al.* 1990). Cognitive–behavioural treatments and dynamic psychotherapy are not effective. Supportive interviews may help the patient to function more normally despite the symptoms, and any stressors should be reduced if possible. As in other untreatable conditions, it is important to resist the temptation to give ineffective treatments in order to appear to be helping the patient; it is better to give adequate time for supportive care that enables the patient to live as normal a life as possible. See de Pauw (2000) for a review.

Other dissociative syndromes in ICD-10 (not specifically listed in DSM-IV)

Dissociative stupor

In dissociative stupor, patients show the characteristic features of stupor. They are motionless and mute, and they do not respond to stimulation, but they are aware of their surroundings. Dissociative stupor is rare. It is essential to exclude other possible conditions, namely schizophrenia, depressive disorder, mania, and organic brain diseases (see p. 418).

Ganser's syndrome

Ganser's syndrome is a very rare condition with four features: giving 'approximate answers' to questions designed to test intellectual functions, psychogenic physical symptoms, hallucinations, and apparent clouding of consciousness. The syndrome was first described among prisoners (Ganser 1898) but is not confined to them. The term 'approximate answers' denotes answers (to simple questions) that are plainly wrong but are clearly related to the correct answer in a way that suggests that the latter is known. For example, when asked to add two and two a patient might answer five. The obvious advantage to be gained from illness, coupled with the approximate answers, often suggests a crude form of malingering. However, the condition is maintained so consistently that unconscious mental mechanisms are generally thought to play a part. It is important to exclude an organic brain disease or schizophrenia; the former should be considered particularly carefully when muddled thinking and visual hallucinations are part of the clinical picture.

Trance and possession disorder

Trance and possession disorder is included in dissociative (conversion) disorder in ICD-10. DSM-IV lists it in Appendix B (Criteria Sets and Axes provided for further study) as *Dissociative Trance Disorder*. Trance and possession states are characterized by a temporary loss of the sense of personal identity and of full awareness of the person's surroundings. DSM-IV defines the condition as

an involuntary state of trance not accepted by the person's culture as a normal part of a collective cultural or religious practice and that causes clinically significant distress or functional impairment.

Some cases resemble multiple personality disorder, with the person acting as if taken over by another personality for a brief period. When the condition is induced by religious ritual, the person may feel taken over by a deity or spirit. The focus of attention is narrowed to a few aspects of the immediate environment, for example, to the priest carrying out a religious ceremony. The affected person may repeatedly perform the same movements, or adopt postures, or repeat utterances.

Such states are induced temporarily in willing participants in religious or other ceremonies. In these circumstances these states are not recorded as disorders.

Cultural syndromes

Certain patterns of unusual behaviour are found in particular cultures, which may reflect psychological mechanisms of dissociation. They may be variants of dissociative disorders even though they may have more than one cause. Some cases of so-called *'Culture Bound Syndromes'* may be classified under this heading. However this term should now be avoided in that it was applied to non-Western cultures without awareness of equivalent syndromes in Western cultures such as eating disorders, chronic fatigue and 'sick building syndrome'. Examples include the following:

- *Latah*, which is found among women in Malaya, is characterized by echolalia, echopraxia, and other kinds of abnormally compliant behaviour. The condition usually begins after a frightening experience.

- *Amok* has been described among men in Indonesia and Malaya (Van Loon 1927). It begins with a period of brooding, which is followed by violent behaviour and sometimes dangerous use of weapons. Amnesia is usually reported afterwards. It is unlikely that all patients with this pattern of behaviour are suffering from a dissociative disorder; the others may be suffering from mania, schizophrenia, or a postepileptic state.

- *Arctic hysteria* is seen among the Eskimo, more often in the women. The affected person tears off her clothing, screams and cries, runs about wildly, and may endanger her life by exposure to cold. Sometimes the behaviour is violent. The relationship of this syndrome to dissociative disorder is not firmly established, and there may be more than one cause.

Recovered memories and false-memory syndrome

In the 1980s there were increasingly frequent reports of people 'recovering apparent "memories"' of previously unknown sexual abuse. It was alleged that the memories had been repressed and dissociated. In the course of much controversy the term 'false-memory syndrome' was used by proponents of the alternative view that the recovered memories were false and created during treatment and resulted in substantial disruption of personal and social relationships. There is now a large literature and continuing argument, but little acceptable evidence. There is a high probability that most recovered memories are false. See Brandon *et al.* (1998) and Brewin (2000) for reviews. See also pp. 25, 36 and 212.

Factitious dissociative identity disorder

There is wide agreement, even among those who believe that dissociative identity disorder is common, that both factitious and malingered presentations are common (see Coons 1998).

Further reading

Gelder, M. G., López-Ibor Jr, J. J. and Andreasen, N. C. (eds) (2000). *New Oxford Textbook of* Psychiatry. Oxford University Press.
(see chapters 4.6.3; 4.9; 5.2)

Mayou, R., Bass, C., Sharpe, M. (eds) (1995). *Treatment of Functional Somatic Symptoms.* Oxford University Press. (Reviews of nature and treatment of various types of unexplained symptoms, together with review chapters by the editors)

Manu, P. (ed.) (1998). *Functional Somatic Syndromes.* Cambridge University Press.
(Edited review of common functional syndromes)

CHAPTER 11

Mood disorders

Mood disorders

Introduction

The *mood disorders* are so called because one of their main features is abnormality of mood. Nowadays the term is usually restricted to disorders in which this mood is depression or elation, but in the past some authors have included states of anxiety as well (Lewis 1956). In this book, anxiety disorders are described in Chapter 9.

It is part of normal experience to feel unhappy at times of adversity. The symptom of depressed mood is a component of many psychiatric syndromes and is also commonly found in certain physical diseases, for example, in infections such as hepatitis and some neurological disorders. In this chapter we are concerned neither with normal feelings of unhappiness nor with depressed mood as a symptom of other disorders, but with the syndromes known as *depressive disorders*.

The central features of these syndromes are:

◆ depressed mood
◆ negative thinking
◆ lack of enjoyment
◆ reduced energy
◆ slowness.

Of these, depressed mood is usually, but not invariably, the most prominent symptom.

Similar considerations apply to *states of elation*. A degree of elated mood is part of normal experience at times of good fortune. Elation can also occur as a symptom in several psychiatric syndromes, though it is less widely encountered than depressed mood. In this chapter we are concerned with a syndrome in which the central features are:

◆ overactivity
◆ elevated or irritable mood
◆ self-important ideas.

This syndrome is called *mania*. Some diagnostic classifications distinguish a less severe form of mania, *hypomania* (see below). As the dividing line between mania and hypomania is arbitrary, this book uses only the term mania whilst indicating the severity of the disorder by adding mild, moderate, or severe.

Clinical features

Depressive syndromes

The clinical presentations of depressive syndromes are varied and they can be subdivided in a number of different ways. In the following account, disorders are grouped by their *severity*. The account begins with a description of the clinical features of an episode of depression of *moderate severity*. Certain important clinical variants of these and more severe disorders are then described. Finally, the special features of the *less severe* depressive disorders are outlined. What constitutes an 'episode' of clinical depression is inevitably a somewhat arbitrary concept. The symptoms listed for the diagnosis of 'depressive episode' in the ICD-10 classification and the various levels of severity are shown in Table 11.1. Table 11.2 shows the criteria for 'major depressive episode' in DSM-IV.

Moderate depressive episode

In a moderate episode of depression, the central features are *low mood, lack of enjoyment, negative*

Table 11.1 Symptoms needed to meet criteria for 'depressive episode' in ICD–10

A Depressed mood

Loss of interest and enjoyment

Reduced energy and decreased activity

B Reduced concentration

Reduced self-esteem and confidence

Ideas of guilt and unworthiness

Pessimistic thoughts

Ideas of self-harm

Disturbed sleep

Diminished appetite

Mild depressive episode: at least 2 of A and at least 2 of B

Moderate depressive episode: at least 2 of A and at least 3 of B

Severe depressive episode: all 3 of A and at least 4 of B

Severity of symptoms and degree of functional impairment also guide classification

Table 11.2 Criteria for major depressive episode – DSM-IV

A Five (or more) of the following symptoms have been present during the same 2-week period and represent a change from previous functioning; at least one of the symptoms is either (1) depressed mood or (2) loss of interest or pleasure

(1) depressed mood most of the day, nearly every day, as indicated by either subjective report (e.g. feels sad or empty) or observation made by others (e.g. appears tearful)

(2) markedly diminished interest or pleasure in all, or almost all, activities most of the day, nearly every day (as indicated by either subjective account or observation made by others)

(3) significant weight loss when not dieting or weight gain (e.g. a change of more than 5% of body weight in a month), or decrease or increase in appetite nearly every day

(4) insomnia or hypersomnia nearly every day

(5) psychomotor agitation or retardation nearly every day (observable by others, nor merely subjective feelings of restlessness or being slowed down)

(6) fatigue or loss of energy nearly every day

(7) feelings of worthlessness or excessive or inappropriate guilt (which may be delusional) nearly every day (not merely self-reproach or guilt about being sick)

(8) diminished ability to think or concentrate, or indecisiveness, nearly every day (either by subjective account or as observed by others)

(9) recurrent thoughts of death (not just fear of dying), recurrent suicidal ideation without a specific plan, or a suicide attempt or a specific plan for committing suicide

thinking, and *reduced energy*, all of which lead to decreased *social and occupational functioning*.

Appearance

The patient's *appearance* is characteristic. *Dress and grooming* may be neglected. The facial features are characterized by a turning downwards of the corners of the mouth and by vertical furrowing of the centre of the brow. The rate of blinking may be reduced. The shoulders are bent and the head is inclined forwards so that the direction of gaze is downwards. Gestural movements are reduced. It is important to note that some patients maintain a smiling exterior despite deep feelings of depression.

Mood

The mood of the patient is one of *misery*. This mood does not improve substantially in circumstances where ordinary feelings of sadness would be alleviated, for example, in pleasant company or after hearing good news. Moreover, the mood is often experienced as different from *ordinary sadness*. Patients sometimes speak of a black cloud pervading all mental activities. Some patients can conceal this mood change from other people, at least for short periods. Some try to hide their low mood during clinical interviews, making it more difficult for the doctor to detect. The mood is often worse first thing in the morning when the patient awakes, improving a little as the day wears on. This is called *diurnal variation of mood.*

Depressive cognitions

Negative thoughts ('depressive cognitions') are important symptoms which can be divided into three groups:

◆ worthlessness

◆ pessimism

◆ guilt.

In feeling *worthless*, the patient thinks that he is failing in everything that he does and that other people see him as a failure; he no longer feels confident, and discounts any success as a chance happening for which he can take no credit. *Pessimistic thoughts* concern future prospects. The patient expects the worst. He foresees failure in his work, the ruin of his finances, misfortune for his family, and an inevitable deterioration in his health. These ideas of *hopelessness* are often accompanied by the thought that life is no longer worth living and that death would come as a welcome release. These gloomy preoccupations may progress to thoughts of, and plans for, *suicide*. It is important to ask about these ideas in every case (the assessment of suicidal risk is considered further in Chapter 17).

Feelings of *guilt* often take the form of unreasonable self-blame about minor matters; for example, a patient may feel guilty about past trivial acts of dishonesty or letting someone down. Usually these events have not been in the patient's thoughts for years but, when he becomes depressed, they flood

back into his memory, accompanied by intense feelings. Preoccupations of this kind strongly suggest depressive disorder. Some patients have similar feelings of guilt but do not attach them to any particular event. Other memories are focused on unhappy events; the patient remembers occasions when he was sad, when he failed, or when his fortunes were at a low ebb. These gloomy memories become increasingly frequent as the depression deepens. The patient blames himself for his misery and incapacity and attributes it to personal failing and moral weakness (a view not uncommonly held by the wider public).

Goal-directed behaviour

Lack of interest and enjoyment (also known as *anhedonia*) is frequent though not always complained of spontaneously. The patient shows no enthusiasm for activities and hobbies that he would normally enjoy. He feels no zest for living and no pleasure in everyday things. He often withdraws from *social encounters*. Reduced energy is characteristic (though sometimes associated with a degree of physical restlessness that can mislead the observer). The patient feels lethargic, finds everything an effort, and leaves tasks unfinished. For example, a normally house-proud woman may leave the beds unmade and dirty plates on the table. Work outside the home becomes increasingly difficult. Understandably, many patients attribute this lack of energy to physical illness.

Psychomotor changes

Psychomotor retardation is frequent (though, as described later, some patients are *agitated* rather than slowed up). In more severe depression, the retarded patient walks and acts slowly. Slowing of thought is reflected in the patient's speech; there is a long delay before questions are answered, and pauses in conversation may be so long that they would be intolerable to a non-depressed person. *Agitation* is a state of restlessness that is experienced by the patient as inability to relax and is seen by an observer as restless activity. When it is mild, the patient is seen to be plucking at his fingers and making restless movements of his legs; when it is severe, he cannot sit for long but paces up and down.

Anxiety is frequent though not invariable in moderate depression. (As described later, it is particularly common in some less severe depressive disorders.) Another common symptom is *irritability*, which is the tendency to respond with undue annoyance to minor demands and frustrations.

Biological symptoms

A group of symptoms often called *biological* is important. These biological symptoms *include sleep disturbance, diurnal variation of mood, loss of appetite, loss of weight, constipation, loss of libido*, and, among women, *amenorrhoea*. These symptoms are particularly common in severe depression and are frequent but not invariable in depressive disorders of moderate degree. (They are less usual in mild depressive disorders.) Some of these symptoms require further comment.

Sleep disturbance in depressive disorders is of several kinds. Most characteristic is *early morning waking*, but delay in falling asleep and waking during the night also occur. Early morning waking occurs 2 or 3 hours before the patient's usual time; he does not fall asleep again, but lies awake feeling unrefreshed and often restless and agitated. He thinks about the coming day with pessimism, broods about past failures, and ponders gloomily about the future. It is this combination of *early waking with depressive thinking* that is important in diagnosis. It should be noted that some depressed patients sleep excessively rather than wake early, but they still report waking unrefreshed.

Weight loss in depressive disorders often seems greater than can be accounted for merely by the patient's reported lack of appetite. In some patients the disturbances of eating and weight are towards excess – they eat more and gain weight. Usually it seems that eating brings temporary relief to their distressing feelings.

Complaints about *physical symptoms* are common in depressive disorders. They take many forms, but complaints of constipation, fatigue, and aching discomfort anywhere in the body are particularly common. Complaints about any pre-existing physical disorder usually increase and *hypochondriacal preoccupations* are common.

Other features

Several other psychiatric symptoms may occur as part of a depressive disorder, and occasionally one of them dominates the clinical picture. They include *depersonalization*, *obsessional symptoms*, *panic attacks*, and *dissociative symptoms* such as fugue or loss of function of a limb. Complaints of *poor memory* are also common; depressed patients commonly show deficits on a wide range of neuropsychological tasks, but impairments in the retrieval and recognition of recently learned material may be particularly prominent (see Elliott 1998). Sometimes the impairment of memory in a depressed patient is so severe that the clinical presentation resembles that of dementia. This presentation, which is particularly common in the elderly, is sometimes called depressive *pseudodementia* (see p. 629).

Severe depression and psychotic depression

As depressive disorders become more severe, all the features described above occur with greater intensity. There is complete loss of function in social and occupational spheres. The patient's inattention to basic hygiene and nutrition may give rise to fears for his well-being. In addition, certain distinctive features may occur in the form of delusions and hallucinations; the disorder is then sometimes called *psychotic depression*.

The delusions of severe depressive disorders are concerned with the same themes as the non-delusional thinking of moderate depressive disorders. Therefore they are termed *mood congruent*. These themes are worthlessness, guilt, ill-health, and, more rarely, poverty. Such delusions have been described in Chapter 1, but a few examples may be helpful at this point. The patient with a *delusion of guilt* may believe that some dishonest act, such as a minor concealment in making a tax return, will be discovered and that he will be punished severely and humiliated. He is likely to believe that such punishment is deserved. A patient with *hypochondriacal delusions* may be convinced that he has cancer or venereal disease. A patient with a *delusion of impoverishment* may wrongly believe that he has lost all his money in a business venture.

Persecutory delusions also occur. The patient may believe that other people are discussing him in a derogatory way or are about to take revenge on him. When persecutory delusions are part of a depressive syndrome, typically the patient accepts the supposed persecution as something that he has brought upon himself. In his view, he is ultimately to blame. Some depressed patients experience delusions and hallucinations that are not clearly related to themes of depression ('mood-incongruent'). Their presence appears to worsen the prognosis of the illness.

Particularly severe depressive delusions are found in *Cotard's syndrome*, which was described by a French psychiatrist (Cotard 1882). The characteristic feature is an extreme kind of nihilistic delusion. The nihilism is extreme. For example, some patients may complain that their bowels have been destroyed so that they will never pass faeces again. Others may assert that they are penniless and without any prospect of having money again. Still others may be convinced that their whole family has ceased to exist and that they themselves are dead. Although the extreme nature of these symptoms is striking, such cases do not appear to differ in important ways from other severe depressive disorders.

Other clinical variants of moderate and severe depression

Agitated depression

This term is applied to depressive disorders in which *agitation* is prominent. As already noted, agitation occurs in many severe depressive disorders, but in agitated depression it is particularly severe. Agitated depression is seen more commonly among the middle-aged and elderly than among younger patients. However, there is no reason to suppose that agitated depression differs in other important ways from the other depressive disorders.

Retarded depression

This name is sometimes applied to depressive disorders in which psychomotor retardation is especially prominent. There is no evidence that they represent a separate syndrome, though retardation does predict a good response to electroconvulsive therapy (ECT). If the term is used, it should be in a purely descriptive sense. In its most severe form, retarded depression shades into *depressive stupor.*

Depressive stupor

In severe depressive disorder, slowing of movement and poverty of speech may become so extreme that the patient is motionless and mute. Such depressive stupor is rarely seen now that active treatment is available. Therefore the description by Kraepelin (1921, p. 80) is of particular interest:

The patients lie mute in bed, give no answer of any sort, at most withdraw themselves timidly from approaches, but often do not defend themselves from pinpricks . . . . They sit helpless before their food, perhaps, however, they let themselves be spoon-fed without making any difficulty. . . .

Kraepelin commented that recall of the events taking place during stupor was sometimes impaired when the patient recovered. Nowadays, the general view is that on recovery patients are able to recall nearly all the events taking place during the period of stupor. It is possible that in some of Kraepelin's cases there was clouding of consciousness (possibly related to inadequate fluid intake, which is common in these patients). Patients in states of depressive stupor may exhibit catatonic motor disturbances (see p. 332).

Atypical depression

The term *atypical depression* is generally applied to disorders of moderate clinical severity. The meaning of the term has varied over the years but currently it is applied to disorders characterized by:

♦ variably depressed mood with *mood reactivity* to positive events;

♦ *overeating and oversleeping*;

♦ *extreme fatigue* and heaviness in the limbs (*leaden paralysis*);

♦ pronounced *anxiety*.

Many patients with these clinical symptoms have a lifelong tendency to react in an exaggerated way to perceived or real rejection (*rejection sensitivity*). The importance of recognizing atypical depression is that, because of their interpersonal sensitivity, patients with this disorder can be hard to manage and may be regarded as having 'difficult' personalities rather than depressive disorder. Also, atypical depression seems to be associated with a poor response to tricyclic antidepressant treatment but a better response to monoamine oxidase inhibitors (MAOIs) and perhaps to selective serotonin re-uptake inhibitors (SSRIs) (Davidson 1992).

Brief recurrent depression

Some individuals experience recurrent depressive episodes of short duration, typically 2–7 days. These episodes recur with some frequency, about once a month on average. There is no apparent link with the menstrual cycle in female sufferers. Whilst the depressive episodes are short, they are as severe as the more enduring depressive disorders. Hence they are associated with much personal distress and social and occupational impairment. The risk of a manic episode is low. Therefore it seems unlikely that this disorder is a manifestation of the rapid cycling form of bipolar disorder (Angst 1992) (see below).

Mild depressive disorders

It might be expected that *mild depressive disorders* would present with symptoms similar to those of the depressive disorders described already, but with less intensity. To some extent this is so, but in mild depressive disorder there are frequently *additional symptoms* that are less prominent in severe disorders. These symptoms have been characterized in the past as 'neurotic', and they include *anxiety, phobias,*

obsessional symptoms, and, less often, *dissociative symptoms*. In terms of classification, both DSM-IV and ICD-10 have categories of *mild depression* where criteria for a depressive episode are met but the depressive symptoms are fewer and less severe (see Table 11.1).

Apart from the 'neurotic' symptoms found in some cases, mild depressive disorders are characterized by the expected symptoms of *low mood, lack of energy and interest*, and *irritability*. There is *sleep disturbance*, but not the early morning waking that is so characteristic of more severe depressive disorders. Instead, there is more often difficulty in falling asleep and periods of waking during the night, usually followed by a period of sleep at the end of the night. *'Biological' features* (poor appetite, weight loss, and low libido) are not usually found. Although mood may vary during the day, it is usually worse in the evening than in the morning. The patient may not be obviously dejected in his appearance or slowed in his movement. Delusions and hallucinations are not present.

In their mildest forms, these cases shade into the minor affective disorders considered below. As described later, they pose considerable problems of classification. Many of these mild depressive disorders are brief, starting at a time of personal misfortune and subsiding when fortunes have changed or a new adjustment has been achieved. However, some cases persist for months or years, causing considerable suffering, even though the symptoms do not increase. These chronic depressive states are called *dysthymia*. The term *cyclothymic disorder* refers to a persistent instability of mood in which there are numerous periods of mild elation or mild depression. It is seen as a milder variant of bipolar disorder. It is not unusual for episodes of more severe mood disorder to supervene in patients who experience dysthymia or cyclothymia.

Minor affective disorders

We have already seen that anxiety and depressive symptoms often occur together. Indeed, earlier writers (see Lewis 1956) considered that anxiety and depressive disorders could not be separated clearly even in patients admitted to hospital with severe disorders. Although most psychiatrists now accept that the distinction can usually be made among the more severe forms presenting in psychiatric practice, the distinction is less easy to make in the *milder forms* presenting in primary care.

Classification

As psychiatrists work increasingly with general practitioners, the importance of minor anxiety-depressive disorders has been recognized but without any agreement about classification.

ICD10 includes a category of 'mixed anxiety and depressive disorder' which can be applied when neither anxiety symptoms nor depressive symptoms are severe enough to meet criteria for an anxiety disorder or a depressive disorder, and when the symptoms do not have the close association with stressful events or significant life changes required for a diagnosis of acute stress reaction or adjustment disorder.

According to ICD-10, patients with this presentation are seen frequently in primary care and there are many others in the general population who are not seen by doctors. In ICD-10 this diagnosis appears amongst anxiety disorders, although some psychiatrists consider that the condition is more closely related to the mood disorders, a view that is reflected in the alternative term *minor affective disorder*.

In DSM-IV, no comparable diagnosis appears in the classification. The appendix to the classification contains two provisional diagnoses that might be used for these cases: *mixed anxiety and depressive disorder* and *minor depressive disorder*. It is stated that there is insufficient factual information to justify the inclusion of either in the classification. Although little is known about these conditions or about their relationship to other disorders, patients present to doctors with this group of symptoms. A suitable category is needed even if it is not possible to write strict criteria for diagnosis.

Clinical picture

One of the best descriptions of minor affective disorder has been given by Goldberg *et al.* (1976)

who studied 88 patients from a general practice in Philadelphia. The most frequent symptoms were:

- fatigue
- anxiety
- depression
- irritability
- poor concentration
- insomnia
- somatic symptoms and bodily preoccupation.

A very similar range of symptoms was found was found in the National Psychiatric Morbidity Household Survey (Jenkins *et al.* 1997) which surveyed the frequency of 'neurotic' symptomatology in a community sample (Figure 11.1).

Patients with minor affective disorders commonly present to medical practitioners with prominent somatic symptoms. The reason for this is uncertain; some symptoms are autonomic features of anxiety, and it is possible that patients expect somatic complaints to be received more sympathetically than emotional problems (see Chapter 16). Whatever the reasons, the observation is not new (see, for example, the lengthy descriptions of physical symptoms of neurosis in Déjerine and Gauckler (1913). Another point of clinical relevance is that minor affective disorders can be prolonged and in some cases cause incapacitating difficulties in personal and occupational function. Thus the term 'minor' may not capture the serious consequences of the disorder for an individual (see Freeman 1998).

Mania

As already mentioned, the central features of the syndrome of mania are *elevation of mood*, *increased activity*, and *self-important ideas*.

Mood

When the mood is elevated, the patient seems cheerful and optimistic, and he may have a quality described by earlier writers as *infectious gaiety*. However, other patients are irritable rather than euphoric, and this irritability can easily turn to

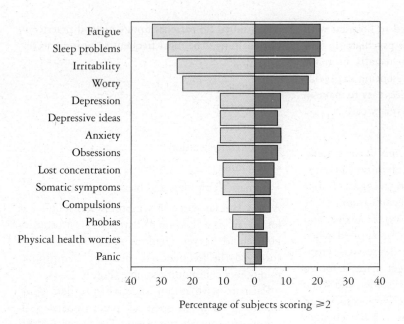

Figure 11.1 Scores for neurotic symptoms on the on the revised clinical interview schedule (CIS-R) of a randomly selected sample of 10 000 adults in the National Survey of Psychiatric Morbidity. All symptoms are commoner in women (light hatch) than men (darker hatch). The commonest symptom is 'fatigue' reported by 27% of subjects. (From Jenkins *et al.* 1997)

anger. The mood often varies during the day, though not with the regular rhythm characteristic of many severe depressive disorders. In patients who are elated, not uncommonly, high spirits are interrupted by brief episodes of *depression.*

Appearance and behaviour

The patient's appearance often reflects his prevailing mood. Clothes may be brightly coloured and ill-assorted. When the condition is more severe, the patient's appearance is often *untidy and dishevelled.* Manic patients are overactive. Sometimes their persistent overactivity leads to *physical exhaustion.* Manic patients start many activities but leave them unfinished as new ones catch their fancy. Appetite is increased and food may be eaten greedily with little attention to conventional manners. Sexual desires are increased and behaviour may be uninhibited. Women may neglect precautions against pregnancy, a point calling for particular attention when a patient is of childbearing age. Sleep is often reduced. Patients wake early, feeling lively and energetic; often they get up and busy themselves noisily, to the surprise of other people.

Speech and thought

Speech of manic patients is often *rapid and copious* as thoughts crowd into their minds in quick succession. When the disorder is more severe, there is *flight of ideas* (see p. 12) with such rapid changes that it is difficult to follow the train of thought. However, the links are usually understandable if the speech can be recorded and reviewed. This is in contrast to thought disorder in schizophrenia where changes in the flow of thought may not be comprehensible even on reflection.

Expansive ideas are common. Patients believe that their ideas are original, their opinions important, and their work of outstanding quality. Many patients become *extravagant,* spending more than they can afford on expensive cars or jewellery. Others make reckless decisions to give up good jobs, or embark on plans for hare-brained and risky business ventures.

Sometimes these expansive themes are accompanied by *grandiose delusions.* Some patients may believe that they are religious prophets or destined to advise statesmen about great issues. At times there are *delusions of persecution,* with patients believing that people are conspiring against them because of their special importance. Delusions of reference and passivity feelings also occur. Schneiderian first-rank symptoms (see Chapter 12, Table 12.3) have been reported in about 10–20% of manic patients. Neither the delusions nor the first-rank symptoms last long – most disappear or change in content within days.

Perceptual disturbances

Hallucinations also occur. They are usually consistent with the mood, taking the form of voices speaking to the patient about his special powers or, occasionally, of visions with a religious content.

Other features

Insight is invariably impaired in more severe manic states. Patients see no reason why their grandiose plans should be restrained or their extravagant expenditure curtailed. They seldom think of themselves as ill or in need of treatment.

Most patients can exert some control over their symptoms for a short time, and many do so when the question of treatment is being assessed. For this reason it is important to obtain a history from an *informant* whenever possible. Henry Maudsley (1879, p. 398) expressed the problem well:

Just as it is with a person who is not too far gone in intoxication, so it is with a person who is not too far gone in acute mania; he may on occasion pull his scattered ideas together by an effort of will, stop his irrational doings and for a short time talk with an appearance of calmness and reasonableness that may well raise false hopes in inexperienced people.

Mixed affective states

Depressive and manic symptoms sometimes occur at the same time. Patients who are overactive and over-talkative may be having profoundly depressive thoughts. In other patients, mania and depression follow each other in a sequence of rapid changes; for example, a manic patient may become intensely depressed for a few hours and then return quickly to his manic state. These changes were mentioned in early descriptions of mania by Griesinger (1867), and have been re-emphasized in recent years because they seem to predict a better response to certain mood stabilizers such as valproate.

Manic stupor

In this unusual disorder, patients are *mute and immobile*. Their facial expression suggests elation and on recovery they describe having experienced a rapid succession of thoughts typical of mania. The condition is rarely seen now that active treatment is available for mania. Hence an earlier description by Kraepelin (1921, p. 106) is of interest:

The patients are usually quite inaccessible, do not trouble themselves about their surroundings, give no answer, or at most speak in a low voice . . . smile without recognizable cause, lie perfectly quiet in bed or tidy about at their clothes and bedclothes, decorate themselves in an extraordinary way, all this without any sign of outward excitement.

On recovery, patients can remember the events that occurred during their period of stupor. The condition may begin from a state of manic excitement, but at times it is a stage in the transition between depressive stupor and mania.

Transcultural factors and clinical factors

Mania appears to be present in all cultures. In some non-Western countries, for example Nigeria, patients in hospital usually have features of mania and seldom of depression. Symptoms of mania seem to be similar in Nigerian and European patients, although reports of *auditory hallucinations* are more frequent in Nigerians (Mankanjuola 1982).

The presentation of *milder depressive disorders* seems to be influenced by culture. In developing countries, the presenting complaints are somatic in most patients. In China, many patients with mixed somatic and psychological symptoms receive a diagnosis of neurasthenia. However, in a detailed assessment, over 80% of these patients were given diagnoses of major depression (Kleinman 1986). Kim and Kim (1999) noted that depressed

Korean patients reported prominent symptoms of low mood and guilt relative to Chinese patients who experienced more somatic complaints.

Classification of depressive disorders

There is no general agreement about the best method of classifying depressive disorders. A number of approaches have been tried:

- based on presumed aetiology (*reactive* versus *endogenous*);
- based on symptomatic picture (*melancholic* versus *neurotic*);
- based on course (*unipolar* versus *bipolar*).

Classification by presumed aetiology

This reactive-endogenous classification was based on the view that depressive disorders could be divided into two kinds; in one the symptoms were caused by factors within the individual, and were independent of outside factors (*endogenous depression*), whereas in the other, the symptoms were a response to external stressors (*reactive depression*). This distinction has been recognized to be unsatisfactory for many years. For example, Lewis (1983) wrote:

every illness is a product of two factors – of the environment working on the organism – whether the constitutional factor is the determining influence or the environmental one . . . is never a question to be dealt with as either/or.

Nowadays most psychiatrists agree that it is pointless to try to allocate depressive syndromes exclusively to endogenous or reactive categories in terms of aetiology; in seeking to understand the development of depression in individual cases, the relative contributions of a variety of aetiological factors must be considered. Neither ICD-10 nor DSM-IV contains categories of reactive or endogenous depression.

Symptomatic picture

The reactive-endogenous classification of depressive disorders carried a further complication. Many supporters of this classification maintained that the two aetiological categories were associated with *characteristic patterns of symptoms*. Thus *endogenous disorders* were said to be characterized by loss of appetite, weight loss, constipation, reduced libido, amenorrhoea, and early morning waking (the *'biological' symptoms* mentioned on p. 274). *Reactive disorders* were said to be characterized by a pattern of anxiety, irritability, and phobias (*neurotic symptoms*). It has been suggested that while the reactive-endogenous distinction might not be valid in terms of *aetiology*, the differences in *symptom profile* might nevertheless represent two separable kinds of depressive disorder (see Parker 2000).

As already explained, this differential symptom profile tends to correlate with the *severity* of the depression. This raises two possibilities:

- The distinction between mild, moderate, and severe depression is one of degree with various clinical forms lying on a continuum of severity.
- There are at least two distinct kinds of depression, one with frequent *biological features* (now called *melancholic depression*), the other with predominantly *neurotic features* (*neurotic depression*).

There have been a number of studies that have attempted to distinguish between these possibilities using multivariate analysis of symptom clusters. The results have been contradictory. In a series of papers, Roth and his colleagues in Newcastle held that two separate syndromes could be distinguished (Kiloh and Garside 1963; Carney *et al.* 1965). However, Kendell (1968) did not confirm this distinction, but found evidence for a unimodal distribution of cases.

More recently, work on this neurotic/melancholic distinction has used a predominantly clinical sign-based typology to separate the two depressive subtypes. For example, the presence of signs of psychomotor retardation correlates highly with the presence of the clinical diagnosis of melancholia and when the sign-based typology is applied to groups of depressed patients, a bimodal distribution can be obtained (Parker *et al.* 1995b). However, it is still possible that this separation represents degree of severity rather than two pathophysiologically distinct disorders.

Melancholic or somatic depression

Current views are that the term *neurotic depression* is probably not useful because it covers several different disorders including, for example, mild depressive episodes, atypical depressions, and dysthymia. However, the clinical syndrome of *melancholic depression* (major depression with *melancholia* in DSM-IV, or depressive episode with *somatic symptoms* in ICD-10) (Table 11.3) as defined by symptom profile appears to have a number of validating characteristics that distinguish it from depressions lacking these features:

♦ better response to somatic treatments (for example, antidepressant medication and ECT);

♦ poorer response to placebo drug treatment;

♦ more evidence of neurobiological abnormalities (decreased latency to rapid eye movement sleep, impaired growth hormone response to clonidine).

As mentioned above, it is possible that these characteristics simply reflect a greater severity of somatic or melancholic endogenous depressions; nevertheless, the predictions for treatment response can be clinically useful.

Classification by course

Unipolar and bipolar disorders

Mood disorders are characteristically *recurrent* and Kraepelin was guided by the course of illness when he brought mania and depression together as a single entity. He found that the course was essentially the same whether the disorder was manic or depressive, and so he put the two together in a single category of *manic-depressive psychosis*.

Table 11.3 Clinical features of melancholic and somatic depression

Melancholic features (DSM-IV)

Loss of interest or pleasure in usual activities*

Lack of reactivity to pleasurable stimuli*

plus at least three of the following:

Distinct quality of mood (unlike normal sadness)

Morning worsening of mood*

Early morning waking*

Psychomotor agitation or retardation*

Significant anorexia or weight loss*

Excessive guilt

Marked loss of libido* (ICD–10 only)

* Somatic symptoms of depression in ICD–10 (at least four required for diagnosis).

This view was widely accepted until 1962 when Leonhard *et al.* suggested a division into three groups:

♦ patients who had had a depressive disorder only (*unipolar depression*);

♦ those who had had mania only (*unipolar mania*);

♦ those who had had both depressive disorder and mania (*bipolar*).

Nowadays, it is the usual practice not to use the term unipolar mania, but to include all cases of mania in the bipolar group on the grounds that nearly all patients who have mania eventually experience a depressive disorder.

In support of the distinction between unipolar and bipolar disorders, Leonhard *et al.* (1962) described differences in heredity between the groups, which have been confirmed by later studies (see p. 287). However, it is agreed that the two groups do not generally differ in their symptoms when depressed. There must be some overlap between the two groups, because a patient classified as having unipolar depression at one time may have a manic disorder later. In other words, the unipolar group inevitably contains some bipolar cases that have not yet declared themselves. Despite this limitation, the division into unipolar and bipolar cases is a useful classification because it has some implications for treatment (see p. 323).

Seasonal affective disorder

Some patients repeatedly develop a depressive disorder at the same time of year, usually the *autumn or winter*. In some cases the timing reflects extra demands placed on the person at a particular season of the year, either in his work or in other aspects of his life. In other cases there is no such cause and it has been suggested that seasonal affective disorder is related in some way to the changes in the seasons, for example, to the length of daylight. Although these seasonal affective disorders are characterized mainly by the time at which they occur, some symptoms are said to occur more often than in other mood disorders. These symptoms are:

- hypersomnia
- increased appetite with craving for carbohydrate.

The most common pattern is onset in autumn or winter, and recovery in spring or summer. This is also called 'winter depression'. Some patients show evidence of hypomania or mania in the summer, suggesting that they have a seasonal bipolar illness. This pattern has led to the suggestion that shortening of daylight is important in the pathophysiology of winter depression and treatment methods include exposure to bright artificial light during hours of darkness. For a review, see Rodin and Thompson (1997). (The use of bright light treatment is reviewed on p. 714.)

Rapid cycling disorders

Some bipolar disorders recur regularly with intervals of only weeks or months between episodes. In the nineteenth century these regularly recurring disorders were designated folie circulaire (circular insanity) by the French psychiatrist Falret (1854). At present, the frequent recurrence of mood disturbance in bipolar patients is usually called *rapid cycling disorder*. These recurrent episodes may be depressive, manic, or mixed. The main features are that recurrence is frequent (conventionally, at least four distinct episodes a year) and that episodes are separated by a period of remission or a switch to an episode of opposite polarity. A number of clinical features of rapid cycling disorder are important in management and prevention:

- they occur more frequently in women;
- concomitant hypothyroidism is common;
- they can be triggered by antidepressant drug treatment;
- lithium treatment is relatively ineffective.

For a review of the clinical features of rapid cycling see Kilzieh and Akiskal (1999).

Classification in ICD and DSM

The main categories in the sections on mood disorders in DSM-IV and the ICD-10 are shown in Tables 11.4 and 11.5. Broad similarities are evident, together with some differences. The first similarity is that both systems contain categories for *single episodes* of mood disorder as well as categories for *recurrent episodes*. The second is that both recognize mild but persistent mood disturbances in which there is either a repeated alternation of high and low mood (*cyclothymia*) or a sustained depression of mood (*dysthymia*). In neither case are the mood disturbances sufficiently severe to meet criteria for a hypomanic or depressive episode. In DSM-IV, mood disorders judged to be secondary to a medical condition are included as a subcategory of mood disorders, whereas in ICD-10 these conditions are classified as mood disorders under 'Organic mental disorders'.

Bipolar disorder

Both classifications delineate hypomania from mania on grounds of severity which include both

Table 11.4 Classification of bipolar disorder	
ICD–10	DSM-IV
Manic episode	*Hypomanic episode*
Hypomania	*Manic episode*
Mania	Mild
Mania with psychosis	Moderate
	Severe
	Severe with psychosis
Bipolar affective disorder	*Bipolar I and bipolar II disorders*
Currently hypomanic	Current (or most recent episode)
Currently manic	Hypomanic
Currently depressed	Manic*
Currently mixed	Depressed
In remission	Mixed*
Cyclothymia	*Cyclothymic disorder*

*Excludes bipolar II.

Table 11.5 Classification of depressive disorders	
ICD–10	DSM-IV
Depressive episode	*Major depressive episode*
Mild	Mild
Moderate	Moderate
Severe	Severe
Severe with psychosis	Severe with psychosis
Other depressive episodes	
Atypical depression	
Recurrent depressive disorders	*Major depressive disorder recurrent*
Currently mild	
Currently moderate	
Currently severe	
Currently severe with psychosis	
In remission	
Persistent mood disorders	*Dysthymic disorder*
Cyclothymia	
Dysthymia	
Other mood disorders	*Depressive disorders not otherwise specified*
Recurrent brief depression	Recurrent brief depression

symptomatic features and degree of social incapacity. A manic episode can be further subdivided according to severity and whether or not psychotic symptoms are present. In DSM-IV, the presence of a single episode of hypomania or mania is sufficient to meet criteria for bipolar affective disorder. In ICD-10, however, at least two episodes of mood disturbance are needed for this diagnosis. DSM-IV also separates bipolar disorder into

- bipolar I (in which *mania* has occurred on least one occasion);
- bipolar II (where *hypomania* has occurred but mania has not).

The diagnosis of bipolar II disorder is intended to indicate the importance of detecting mild hypomanic episodes in patients who might otherwise be diagnosed as having recurrent major depression. The presence of such episodes may have implica-

tions for treatment response. In DSM-IV, if a hypomanic or manic episode appears to have been precipitated by a *somatic treatment*, for example, antidepressant drug therapy, it is not counted towards the diagnosis of bipolar I or bipolar II disorder.

Depressive disorders

Both ICD-10 and DSM-IV classify depressive episodes on the basis of *severity* and whether or not *psychotic features* are present. It is also possible to specify whether the depressive episode has melancholic (DSM-IV) or somatic (ICD-10) features. In DSM-IV, an episode of major depression with appropriate clinical symptomatology (see above) can be specified as atypical depression. In ICD-10, atypical depression is classified separately under 'Other depressive episodes'. Both ICD-10 and DSM-IV allow the diagnosis of recurrent brief depression, but under slightly different headings (Table 11.5).

Classification and description in everyday practice

Although neither DSM-IV nor ICD-10 is entirely satisfactory, it seems unlikely that further rearrangement of descriptive categories will be better. The solution will come only when we have a better understanding of aetiology. Meanwhile, either ICD or DSM-IV should be used for statistical returns. For most clinical purposes, it is better to describe disorders systematically than to classify them. This can be done for every case by referring to the severity, the type of episode, distinguishing symptomatic features, and the course of the disorder, together with an evaluation of the relative importance of known aetiological factors (Table 11.6). It has become conventional to record all cases with a manic episode as bipolar, even if there has been no depressive disorder, on the grounds that:

- most manic patients develop a depressive disorder eventually; and
- in several important ways manic patients resemble patients who have had both types of episode.

This convention is followed in this textbook.

Differential diagnosis

Depressive disorder

Depressive disorders have to be distinguished from:

- normal sadness
- anxiety disorders
- schizophrenia
- organic brain syndromes.

As already explained on p. 271, the distinction from *normal sadness* is made on the presence of other symptoms of the syndrome of depressive disorder. Depressive disorders also have rates of *co-morbidity* with a wide range of other disorders, for example, anxiety disorders, eating disorders, substance misuse, and personality disorder. In all these cases, it is important to recognize and treat the depressive disorder.

Table 11.6 A systematic scheme for the clinical description of mood disorders	
The episode	
Severity	Mild, moderate, or severe
Type	Depressive, manic, mixed
Special features	With melancholic symptoms
	With neurotic symptoms
	With psychotic symptoms
	With agitation
	With retardation or stupor
The course	Unipolar or bipolar
Aetiological factors	Family history of mood disorder
	Personal history of mood disorder
	Childhood experiences
	Personality
	Social support
	Life events

Anxiety and other neurotic disorders

Mild depressive disorders are sometimes difficult to distinguish from anxiety disorders. Accurate diagnosis depends on assessment of the relative severity of anxiety and depressive symptoms, and on the order in which they appeared. Similar problems arise when there are prominent phobic or obsessional symptoms, or when there are *dissociative* symptoms with or without histrionic behaviour. In all these cases, the clinician may fail to identify the depressive symptoms and so prescribe the wrong treatment.

Schizophrenia

The differential diagnosis from *schizophrenia* depends on a careful search for the characteristic features of this condition (see Chapter 12). Difficult diagnostic problems may arise when the patient has *depressive psychosis*, but here again the distinction can usually be made on careful examination of the mental state and on the order in which symptoms appeared. Information about the past psychiatric history may also be useful. Particular difficulties also arise when symptoms characteristic of depressive disorder and of schizophrenia are found in equal measure in the same patient; these so-called schizoaffective disorders are discussed on p. 343.

Dementia and other organic conditions

In middle and late life, depressive disorders are sometimes difficult to distinguish from *dementia* because some patients with depressive symptoms complain of considerable difficulty in remembering. In fact, patients with severe depression can perform very badly on tests of cognitive function and distinction between the two conditions purely in terms of the nature of the cognitive impairment may not be possible. Here the presence of depressive symptoms is the key to diagnosis, which should be confirmed with improvement of the memory disorder as normal mood is restored.

Numerous other general medication conditions can present with depressive features (see p. 478). The key to diagnosis is a careful history and physical examination, supplemented by special investigations where appropriate.

Mania

Manic disorders have to be distinguished from:

- schizophrenia
- organic brain disease involving the frontal lobes (including brain tumour and HIV infection)
- states of brief excitement induced by amphetamines and other illicit drugs.

Schizophrenia

The diagnosis from schizophrenia can be most difficult. Auditory hallucinations and delusions, including some that are characteristic of schizophrenia such as delusions of reference, can occur in manic disorders. However, these symptoms usually change quickly in content, and seldom outlast the phase of overactivity. When there is a more or less equal mixture of features of the two syndromes, the term schizoaffective (sometimes schizomanic) is often used. This term is discussed further in Chapter 12.

Organic brain disorder and drug misuse

An organic brain lesion should always be considered, especially in middle-aged or older patients with expansive behaviour and no past history of affective disorder. In the absence of gross mood disorder, extreme social disinhibition (for example urinating in public) strongly suggests *frontal lobe pathology*. In such cases appropriate neurological investigation is essential. In younger adults infection with HIV or head injury may lead to the manifestation of mania.

The distinction between mania and excited behaviour due to *drug misuse* depends on the history and an examination of the urine for drugs before treatment with psychotropic drugs is started. Drug-induced states usually subside quickly once the patient is in hospital (see Chapter 18). It should be remembered, however, that a significant proportion of patients with bipolar disorder misuse alcohol and other drugs.

The epidemiology of mood disorders

It is difficult to determine the prevalence of depressive disorder, partly because different investigators have used different diagnostic definitions. More recent investigations have used structured diagnostic interviews linked to standardized diagnostic criteria such as the Diagnostic Interview Schedule (DIS), the Composite International Diagnostic Interview (CIDI) and the Schedule for Clinical assessment in Neuropsychiatry (SCAN) which incorporates the 10th edition of the Present State Examination (PSE) (p. 65).

Bipolar disorder

Bipolar cases are probably identified most reliably. More recent community surveys in industrialized countries (Weissman *et al.* 1996; Kessler *et al.* 1997) have suggested that:

- the lifetime risk for bipolar disorder lies between 0.3 and 1.5%;
- the 6-month prevalence of bipolar disorder is not much less than the lifetime prevalence, indicating the chronic nature of the disorder;
- the prevalence in men and women is the same;
- the mean age of onset is about 21 years of age;
- bipolar disorder is highly co-morbid with other disorders, particularly anxiety disorders and substance misuse.

Major depression

Defining the boundaries of depressive episodes in community surveys presents difficulties. However, if the DSM-IV criteria for major depression are applied, recent surveys suggest that:

- the 6-month prevalence of major depression in the community is between 2 and 5%;
- the lifetime rates in different studies show much variability (from 4 to 30%). The true figure probably lies between 10 and 20%;
- the mean age of onset is about 27 years;
- rates of major depression are about twice as great in women as men, across different cultures;
- there may be increased rates of depression in people born since 1945;
- rates of depression are higher in the unemployed and divorced;
- major depression has a high co-morbidity with other disorders, particularly anxiety disorders and substance misuse.

The reasons for *increased rates among women* are uncertain. The increase could be due in part to a greater readiness in women to admit depressive symptoms, but such selective reporting is unlikely to be the whole explanation. It is possible that some depressed men misuse alcohol and are diagnosed as suffering from alcohol-related disorders rather than depression with the consequence that the true number of depressive disorders is underestimated. Again, misdiagnosis of this kind is unlikely to account for the whole of the difference. The role of gender-related neurobiological differences in susceptibility to depression requires further investigation.

Whilst it used to be thought that the risk of depressive disorders increased with age, recent surveys suggest that major depression is most prevalent in the 18–44 age group. A number of studies have suggested that people born since 1945 in industrialized countries have both a higher lifetime risk of major depression and an earlier age of onset. These studies have mainly been retrospective and it is possible that the apparent increased rate of depression in young people is because older people forget (or are less willing to reveal) that they have been depressed. A recent prospective study supports this viewpoint (see Paykel 2000 for a discussion of this issue). For a review of the epidemiology of mood disorders, see Joyce (2000).

Dysthymia and recurrent brief depression

The lifetime risk for for *dysthymia* is about 3% (Kessler *et al.* 1994). Because of the chronic nature of the disorder, the 6-month prevalence is only a little less. Rates of dysthymia are increased in *women* and the *divorced*. There is less epidemiological information about *recurrent brief depression* but in the Zurich prospective study the 6-month prevalence for recurrent brief depression was about 5%, very similar to the rate found for major depression (Angst 1992).

Minor affective disorders

Estimates of the frequency *of minor affective disorders* show wide variations because the different studies have not defined cases in the same way. However, these disorders are probably the most prevalent psychiatric disorder in the community. For example, in the National Psychiatric Morbidity Household Survey, the overall 1-week prevalence of *neurotic disorder* was 16% (12.3% in males and 19.5% in females). Nearly half this group met ICD-10 criteria for *mixed anxiety depression* (Jenkins *et al.* 1997). There are also recent epidemiological studies of minor depression (as defined in DSM-IV). In a systematic review of community studies of people aged over 55, the prevalence of minor depression was 9.8%. A remarkably similar rate (9.9%) was identified in a group of adolescents and young adults (Kessler and Walters 1998; Beekman *et al.* 1999).

The aetiology of mood disorders

There have been many different approaches to the aetiology of mood disorders. In this section, consideration is first given to the role of *genetic* *factors* and of *childhood experience* in laying down a predisposition to mood disorders in adult life. Next, an account is given of *stressors* that may *provoke* mood disorders. This is followed by a review of *psychological* and *biochemical* factors through which predisposing factors and stressors might lead to episodes of mood disorder. In most of these topics, investigators have paid more attention to depressive disorders than to mania. More space is given to aetiology in this chapter than in most others in this book; the purpose is to show how several different kinds of enquiry can be used to throw light on the same clinical problem.

Genetic causes

Family and twin studies

Bipolar versus unipolar disorder

Familial aggregation The risk of mood disorders is increased in first-degree relatives of both bipolar and unipolar probands with the risk being about *twice as great* in relatives of bipolar patients (Table 11.7). Relatives of bipolar probands have increased risks of *unipolar depression* and *schizoaffective disorder*

Table 11.7 Epidemiology of bipolar and unipolar disorder (major depression)

	Bipolar disorder	Unipolar disorder
Lifetime risk	About 1%	10–20%
Sex ratio (M:F)	1:1	1:2
First-degree relatives:		
lifetime risk for bipolar disorder	About 10%	About 2%
lifetime risk for unipolar disorder	20–30%	20–30%
Average age of onset	21 years	27 years

as well as *bipolar disorder*. By contrast, relatives of patients with *unipolar depression* do not have increased rates of bipolar disorder or schizoaffective disorder.

Twin studies Twin studies suggest that the aggregation of mood disorders in families is due to genetic factors with the concordance rate for both bipolar and unipolar disorder being higher in monozygotic than dizygotic twins. For example, the concordance rate for mood disorder in the monozygotic co-twin of a proband with bipolar disorder is between 60 and 70%, but for dizygotic twins the rate is only about 20% (see Sanders et al. 1999). The concordance rate in unipolar depression is also greater in monozygotic twins (46%) than dizygotic twins (20%) (McGuffin et al. 1996). Overall, the genetic influence seems greater in bipolar disorder than in unipolar disorder.

Genetic evidence on classification of mood disorders
Genetic studies also throw light on the aetiological relationship between different subtypes of mood disorder. In addition, they permit assessment of how mood disorders may be related to other kinds of psychiatric illness. Much of the information in this field comes from the studies of Kendler and colleagues (1992c) who have established the population-based Virginia Twin Register to investigate the genetic epidemiology of a range of psychiatric disorders (see also Kendler 1996, 1997; Karkowski and Kendler 1997).

Some of the findings of this work are:

♦ Similar genetic influences are involved in the liability to bipolar and unipolar depression, which appear to lie on a continuum of severity rather than being aetiologically distinct.

♦ DSM-IV melancholic depression delineates a valid *clinical subtype* in terms of greater illness severity and higher familial liability than non-melancholic depression but does not appear to be a genetically distinct subtype.

♦ The liability to major depression and generalized anxiety disorder involves similar genes but different environmental risk factors.

♦ The effect of the environment on liability to depression involves experiences specific to an individual rather than shared (family) experiences.

Mode of inheritance

The familial segregation of mood disorders does not fit a simple Mendelian pattern. In addition, despite the female preponderance of depression, it does not appear as if the genetic contribution or mode of inheritance show gender-related differences. It seems likely that mood disorders result from the combined action of several genes of modest, or even small effect, so called *polygenic* inheritance (Sanders *et al.* 1999).

Molecular genetics

Linkage studies
Molecular linkage studies of mood disorders have not thus far been particularly revealing, perhaps because the genes involved are of small effect or because of genetic heterogeneity. Positive findings have emerged but have often proved difficult to replicate. More recent investigations of *bipolar disorder* have revealed a number of significant linkages involving chromosomes 4, 12, and 18 (see Owen *et al.* 2000). Replication of these findings is required.

Association studies
The monoamine theory of depression suggest that allelic variation in genes coding for monoamine synthesis or metabolism or specific receptors may contribute to the risk of mood disorders. There have been numerous association studies of such *candidate genes*, though thus far results have not been compelling (Craddock and Jones 1999; Frisch *et al.* 1999). The gene coding for the *serotonin transporter* has a number of allelic variants, one of which, in the promotor region, influences the expression of transporter sites. There is some evidence that variation in this gene is associated with mood disorders broadly defined, and also with the trait of neuroticism, a risk factor for major depression (Furlong *et al.* 1998, Owen *et al.* 2000) see p. 130. There is also some

evidence for an association between bipolar disorder and polymorphisms in the gene coding for the *A form of monoamine oxidase*, though again there are some negative studies (see Preisig *et al.* 2000).

Personality

Kraepelin (1921) suggested that people with *cyclothymic personality* (i.e. those with repeated and sustained mood swings) were more prone to develop manic-depressive disorder. Nowadays this personality type is classified as a mood disorder (cyclothymic disorder), and is seen as a mild form of bipolar disorder.

Unfortunately, most reported investigations of personality in depressed patients are of little value because measurements were made when the patients were depressed. Assessments of patients who are currently depressed may not accurately reflect the premorbid personality. Clinical experience suggests that the most relevant personality features are *perfectionist traits* and *anxiety*. Presumably these features are important because they influence the way in which people respond to stressful life events. *Neuroticism* as assessed by the Eysenck Personality Questionnaire also predisposes to major depression. The mechanism is not clear. Neuroticism is associated with lower levels of social support and low self-esteem, but also may have genes in common with major depression (see Roberts and Kendler 1999).

Early environment

Parental deprivation

Psychoanalysts have suggested that childhood deprivation of maternal affection through separation or loss predisposes to depressive disorders in adult life. Overall, however, epidemiological studies do not suggest that loss of a parent by death in childhood increases the risk of depressive disorder in adult life. By contrast, there is more support for the proposal that depressive disorder in later life is associated with *parental separation*; the main factor here appears to be *parental discord* (Tennant 1988).

Relationships with parents

It is clear that gross disruption of parent-child relationships, as occurs, for example, in *physical and sexual abuse*, is a risk factor for several kinds of adult psychiatric disorder, including major depression (Brown and Harris 1993). It is less certain whether more subtle differences in *parental style* may also predispose to depression. One problem is the difficulty of determining retrospectively what kind of relationship a patient may have had with his parents in childhood. The patient's recollection of the relationship may be distorted by many factors, including the depressive disorder itself. However, it appears that both *non-caring* and *overprotective parenting* styles are associated with non-melancholic depression in adult life. The mechanism of this association requires further study (Parker *et al.* 1995a).

Precipitating factors

Recent life events

Depression

Methodological considerations It is an everyday clinical observation that depressive disorders often follow *stressful events*. However, several other possibilities must be discounted before it can be concluded that stressful events cause the depressive disorders that succeed them. First, the association might be *coincidental*. Second, the association might be *non-specific*; there might be as many stressful events in the weeks preceding other kinds of illness. Third, it might be *spurious*; the patient might have regarded the events as stressful only in retrospect when seeking an explanation for his illness, or he might have experienced them as stressful only because he was already depressed at the time.

Research workers have tried to overcome each of these methodological difficulties. The first two problems – whether the events are coincidental or whether any association is non-specific – require the use of control groups suitably chosen from the general population and from people with other illnesses. The third problem – whether the association is spurious – requires two other approaches. The first approach is to separate events that are undoubtedly independent of illness (such as losing a job because a whole factory closes) from events that may have been secondary to the illness (such as losing a job when no one else is dismissed). The second approach is to assign a rating to each event according to the consensus view of healthy people about its stressful qualities.

Findings These methods have shown that:

- there is a sixfold excess of life events in the months before the onset of depressive disorder;
- an excess of similar events has also been shown to precede suicide attempts, and the onset of anxiety disorders and schizophrenia;
- generally, 'loss' events are associated with depression and 'threat' events with anxiety;
- life events are important antecedents of all forms of depression but appear relatively less important in established melancholic-type disorders.

Much of this work has been carried out by Brown and colleagues who have continued to refine the description of the nature of life events that trigger depression. Recent studies suggest that events that lead to feelings of *entrapment and humiliation* may be particularly relevant (Brown *et al.* 1995). It is also important to note that *genetic factors* may also be involved in the liability of an individual to experience life events. Thus certain individuals seem more prone to select *risky environments* and genetic factors also play a role in how life events are *perceived* by a particular individual (Kendler *et al.* 1999).

Mania

It is less certain whether *mania* is provoked by life events. In the past, mania was thought to arise entirely from *endogenous* causes. However, clinical experience suggests that a proportion of cases are precipitated, sometimes by events that might have been expected to induce depression, for example, *bereavement*. It is possible that the impact of life events may be more important early in the course of a recurrent manic-depressive illness because once the illness is established environmental precipitants become less important. It also appears that life events may have more effect on patients with a *later age of onset*, perhaps because their genetic loading is relatively less (Paykel and Cooper 1992; McPherson *et al.* 1993).

Vulnerability factors and life difficulties

It is a common clinical impression that the events immediately preceding a depressive disorder act as a 'last straw' for a person who has been subjected to a long period of adverse circumstances such as an unhappy marriage, problems at work, or unsatisfactory housing. Brown and Harris (1978) divided predisposing events into two kinds. The first are *prolonged stressful circumstances* which can themselves cause depression as well as adding to the effects of short-term life events. Brown and Harris gave the name *long-term difficulties* to these circumstances.

The second kind of predisposing circumstance does not itself cause depression problems; instead, it acts only by increasing the effects of short-term life events. This kind of circumstance is known as a *vulnerability factor*. In practice, the distinction between the two kinds of circumstance is not clear cut. Thus, long continued marital problems (a long-term difficulty) are likely to be associated with a lack of a confiding relationship, and the latter has been identified by Brown as a vulnerability factor.

Overall, the studies suggest that the following are vulnerability factors that increase the risk that life events will trigger a depressive episode:

- having the care of young children;
- not working outside the home;
- having no one to confide in.

Generally, there is good evidence that *poor social support*, measured as lack of intimacy or social integration, is associated with an increased risk of depression (Paykel and Cooper 1992). The mechanism of this association is not clear and is open to different interpretations. First, it may be that a lack of opportunities to confide makes people more vulnerable. Second, it may indicate that depressed people have a distorted perception of the degree of intimacy that they achieved before becoming depressed. Third, some other factor, presumably an abnormality in personality, may result in both difficulty confiding in others and vulnerability to depression.

The effects of physical illness

All medical illnesses and their treatment can act as *non-specific stressors* which may lead to mood disorders in predisposed subjects. Sometimes, however, medical conditions are believed to play a more direct role in causing the mood disorder; examples of such medical conditions are brain disease, certain infections, including HIV, and endocrine disorders. The resulting mood disorders are known as organic mood disorders; they are discussed fully in Chapter 16.

Inevitably, the above distinction is arbitrary. For example, major depression occurs in about half of patients with *Cushing's disease* (see p. 489); since not all patients with Cushing's disease suffer from depressive disorder, it follows that variables other than raised plasma cortisol levels are involved. However, organic mood disorders can give clues to aetiology. For example, depressive disorders in Cushing's disease remit after cortisol levels are restored to normal; this finding had led to the proposal that increased cortisol secretion may play a role in the pathophysiology of major depression (see p. 298). It is also worth noting here that the *puerperium* (although not an illness) is associated with an increased risk of mood disorders (see p. 501).

Psychological approaches to aetiology

These theories are concerned with the *psychological mechanisms* by which recent and remote life experiences can lead to depressive disorders. Much of the literature on this subject fails to distinguish adequately between the symptom of depression and the syndrome of depressive disorder. The main approaches to the problem are derived from the ideas of psychoanalysis, and cognitive–behavioural theories.

Psychoanalytical theory

The psychoanalytical theory of depression began with a paper by Abraham in 1911, and was developed by Freud in 1917 in a paper called 'Mourning and melancholia'. Freud drew attention to the resemblance between the *phenomena of mourning and symptoms of depressive disorders*, and suggested that their causes might be similar.

It is important to note that Freud did not suppose that all severe depressive disorders necessarily had the same cause. Thus he commented that some disorders 'suggest somatic rather than psychogenic affections' and indicated that his ideas were to be applied only to those 'whose psychogenic nature was indisputable' (Freud 1917, p. 243). Freud suggested that, just as mourning results from loss by death, so melancholia results from *loss of other kinds*. Since it was apparent that not every depressed patient had suffered an actual loss, it was necessary to postulate a loss of 'some abstraction' or internal representation, or in Freud's terms the loss of an 'object'.

Freud pointed out that depressed patients often appear critical of themselves, and he proposed that this self-accusation was really a disguised accusation of someone else for whom the patient 'felt affection'. In other words, depression was thought to occur when feelings of love and hostility were present at the same time (*ambivalence*). When a loved 'object' is lost, the patient feels despair; at the same time any hostile feelings attached to this 'object' are redirected against the patient himself as self-reproach.

Freud also put forward predisposing factors. He proposed that the depressed patient regresses to an earlier stage of development, the oral stage, at which sadistic feelings are powerful, and that problems at this stage somehow predispose to depression in later life. Klein (1934) developed this idea by suggesting that at this early stage of development, the infant gradually acquires confidence that, when his mother leaves him, she will return even when he has been angry. This proposed stage of learning was called the 'depressive position'. Klein suggested that, if this stage is not passed through successfully, the child will be more likely to develop depression when faced with loss in adult life.

Further important modifications of Freud's theory were made by Bibring (1953) and Jacobson (1953). They suggested that *loss of self-esteem* is of central importance in depressive disorders. They also proposed that self-esteem depends not only on experiences at the oral stage, but also on failures at later stages of development. However, although low self esteem is part of a depressive disorder, there is no clear evidence that it is more common among people who subsequently develop depressive disorders than among those who do not.

Psychoanalytical theory explains mania as a defence against depression; this is not a convincing explanation of most cases. For a review of the psychoanalytical literature on depression, see Mendelson (1992).

Cognitive theories

Depressed patients characteristically have *negative thoughts*. Beck (1967) proposed that these depressive cognitions consist of *automatic thoughts* that reveal negative views of the *self*, the *world*, and the *future* (the depressed patient usually reviews the past in a similar vein). These automatic thoughts appear to be sustained by illogical ways of thinking (which Beck called *cognitive distortions*). These include:

♦ *arbitrary inference* (drawing a conclusion when there is no evidence for it and even some against it);

♦ *selective abstraction* (focusing on a detail and ignoring more important features of a situation);

♦ *overgeneralization* (drawing a general conclusion on the basis of a single incident);

♦ *personalization* (relating external events to oneself in an unwarranted way).

Whilst most psychiatrists regarded these cognitions as secondary to a primary disturbance of mood, Beck suggested that another set of cognitions precede depression and predispose to it. These cognitions are *dysfunctional beliefs* such as 'If I am not perfectly successful then I am a nobody'. These beliefs are thought to affect the way a person responds to stress and adversity. For example, a failure at work is more likely to provoke depression in a person who holds the belief described above. Others have shown that, when depressed, people are more likely to remember unhappy events (Clark and Teasdale 1982). This selective recall adds to the person's depression, making it more difficult to reverse.

One of the major problems for the cognitive model is that whilst dysfunctional attitudes and

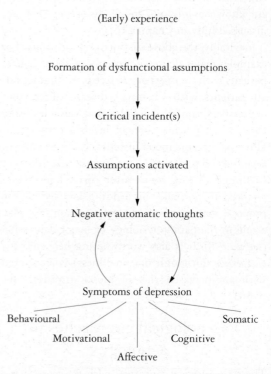

Figure 11.2 Cognitive model of how latent dysfunctional assumptions (laid down by early experience) are activated by critical incidents leading to vicious cycle of negative thinking and depressed mood. (From Fennell 1993)

beliefs, as well as negatively biased information processing, are easy to demonstrate when patients are depressed, these phenomena usually remit on clinical recovery (Peselow *et al.* 1990). Beck has suggested that dysfunctional beliefs may be present but difficult to demonstrate ('latent') until activated by a relevant stressor or by a minor change of mood (within the normal range). In this model a minor (normal) lowering of mood can activate all the concepts and constructs associated with clinical depression. An interactive cycle of low mood and negative thinking will result (see Haaga and Beck 1992 and Figure 11.2).

Recent developments of cognitive theories include the idea that mood-related biases in cognitive processing reflect changes in the *mental models* we all use to make sense of our experiences (Teasdale *et al.* 1998). Because depression is associated with its own particular mental model, when people are depressed, they inhabit a different cognitive and emotional world. Whilst this intriguing idea is not easy to test, it is in keeping with how depressed patients describe their experiences when recovered.

Neurobiological approaches to aetiology

Whatever their aetiology, the clinical manifestations of depressive disorders must ultimately be mediated through changes in brain neurochemistry and functional connectivity. Biochemical investigations in depressed patients have focused on the *monoamine neurotransmitters* because monoamine pathways appear to play an important role in the actions of effective antidepressant drugs (see below). Of course, the actions of antidepressant drugs may not reverse the cause of depression but may merely change the expression of symptoms. However, another reason for studying monoamines is that they play an important role in mediating *adaptive responses to stressful events*, and depressive disorders can be viewed as a failure of these adaptive responses.

A major problem in assessing neurobiological studies in depression is the lack of reproducibility of many of the abnormal findings reported by different laboratories. To some extent this may reflect clinical and biochemical heterogeneity in depressive disorders. However, another important point is that previous *antidepressant drug treatment* almost invariably alters the biochemical processes that have been investigated in depressed patients. Hence it is difficult to be certain that observed effects are due to the disorder rather than to the residual effects of previous drug therapy. For this reason, recent studies have aimed to investigate depressed patients who have been *unmedicated* for long periods of time.

The monoamine hypothesis

The *monoamine hypothesis* suggests that depressive disorder is due to an abnormality in a monoamine neurotransmitter system at one or more sites in the brain. In its early form, the hypothesis suggested a changed provision of the monoamine; more recent elaborations postulate alterations in receptors as well as in the concentrations or the turnover of the amines. Three monoamine transmitters have been implicated: *serotonin (5-hydroxytryptamine, 5-HT)*, *noradrenaline*, and *dopamine*. The latter two neurotransmitters are called *catecholamines*.

The hypothesis has been tested by observing three kinds of phenomenon:

- the metabolism of neurotransmitters in patients with mood disorders;
- the effects of selective drugs on measurable indices of the function of monoamine systems (usually neuroendocrine indices);
- the pharmacological properties shared by antidepressant drugs.

The biochemical effects of antidepressant drugs are considered in Chapter 21. The present chapter will consider the evidence for abnormalities in monoamine neurotransmitters in untreated depressed patients (Box 11.1). Much less work of this kind has been carried out in mania. Therefore the present discussion will be largely restricted to depressive disorders, although the dopamine hypothesis of mania will also be outlined.

Box 11.1 Abnormalities in monoamine neurotransmission in depression

5-HT

Decreased plasma tryptophan

Blunted 5-HT neuroendocrine responses

Decreased brain 5-HT$_{1A}$ receptor binding (PET)

Decreased brain serotonin transporter binding (SPET)

Clinical relapse after tryptophan depletion

Noradrenaline

Blunted noradrenaline-mediated growth hormone release

Clinical relapse after AMPT

Dopamine

Decreased homovanillic acid (HVA) levels in CSF

Increased dopamine D$_2$ receptor binding (PET/SPET)

Clinical relapse after AMPT

5-HT function

Plasma trypytophan The synthesis of 5-HT in the brain depends on the availability of its precursor amino acid, L-*tryptophan*. *Plasma tryptophan levels* are decreased in untreated depressed patients, particularly in those with melancholic depression. Studies in healthy subjects have shown that weight loss through dieting can lower plasma tryptophan, and this factor appears to explain some, but not all, of the reduction in plasma tryptophan seen in depression. Decreases in plasma tryptophan may contribute to the impairments seen in brain 5-HT function in depressed patients but are probably not an important causal factor (Anderson *et al.* 1990).

Studies of cerebrospinal fluid Indirect evidence about 5-HT function in the brains of depressed patients has been sought by examining cerebrospinal fluid (CSF). Numerous studies have been carried out, but overall the data do not suggest that drug-free patients with major depression have a consistent

reduction in CSF concentrations *of 5-hydroxyindoleacetic acid (5-HIAA)*, the main *metabolite* of 5-HT formed in the brain. However, there is more consistent evidence that depressed patients who have made suicide attempts have *low CSF 5-HIAA levels*.

This finding is not restricted to patients with depression. It has also been reported in, for example, patients with schizophrenia and personality disorder who have histories of aggressive behaviour directed towards themselves or other people. It has been proposed that low levels of CSF 5-HIAA, whilst not related specifically to depression, may be associated with a tendency of individuals to respond in an *impulsive and hostile way* to life difficulties (Brown and Linnoila 1990).

Studies of post-mortem brain Measurements of 5-HT and 5-HIAA have been made in the brains of depressed patients who have died, usually by suicide. Although this is a more direct test of the monoamine hypothesis, the results are difficult to interpret for two reasons. First, the observed changes may have taken place after death. Second, the changes may have been caused before death but by factors other than the depressive disorder, for example, by anoxia or by drugs used in treatment or taken to commit suicide. Overall there is little consistent evidence that depressed patients dying from natural causes or suicide have lowered brain concentrations of 5-HT or 5-HIAA (Horton 1992).

The observation that patients dying by suicide do not have consistently lowered brain levels of 5-HIAA is at variance with the observation that CSF 5-HIAA levels are lower in patients who have made suicide attempts. This may be because levels of 5-HIAA in the brainstem and CSF do not correlate reliably with each other. Another possibility is that decreased 5-HIAA levels may be found, particularly in patients whose suicidal behaviour is of an impulsive or violent nature (Brown and Linnoila 1990). Hence, if all kinds of suicidal behaviour are classed together, an abnormality in brain 5-HIAA in a subgroup could be obscured.

Multiple 5-HT receptors have been described in mammalian brain. There have been a number of reports that the density of brain $5-HT_2$ receptors in certain cortical regions is increased in patients dying by suicide, particularly if violent means were used. However, there are some negative studies (Horton 1992).

Neurochemical brain imaging studies Recent developments in brain imaging with selective labelled ligands has allowed assessment of certain brain 5-HT receptor subtypes *in vivo*. In contrast to the post-mortem studies in suicide victims, the density of $5-HT_2$ *receptor binding* tends, if anything, to be decreased in unmedicated depressed patients. There is also evidence of a widespread modest *decrease in $5-HT_{1A}$ receptor binding* throughout cortical and subcortical regions (Sargent *et al.* 2000). Finally, there are reductions *in brainstem 5-HT uptake sites* in depressed subjects, consistent with a decrease in the density of 5-HT cell bodies (Malison *et al.* 1998).

Neuroendocrine tests The functional activity of 5-HT systems in the brain has been assessed by giving a substance that stimulates 5-HT function and by measuring an endocrine response that is controlled by 5-HT pathways – usually the release of *prolactin*, *growth hormone*, or *cortisol*. Neuroendocrine challenge tests have the advantage that they measure an aspect of brain 5-HT *function*. However, the 5-HT synapses involved presumably reside in the *hypothalamus*, which means that important changes in 5-HT pathways in other brain regions could be missed. A number of drugs have been used to increase brain 5-HT function for the purposes of neuroendocrine challenge.

Studies in unmedicated depressed patients have shown consistent evidence that 5-HT-mediated endocrine responses are blunted in depressed patients. In most studies, these abnormalities remit upon clinical recovery, suggesting that the impairment in brain 5-HT neuroendocrine function is reversible and correlates with the presence of the depressed state. The mechanism underlying this impairment is not known; one interesting suggestion is that impaired brain 5-HT function in depression may be a consequence of *cortisol hypersecretion* (for a review see Smith and Cowen 1997).

Tryptophan depletion While the findings outlined above provide strong evidence that aspects of brain 5-HT neurotransmission are abnormal in depression, they do not reveal whether these changes are central to *pathophysiology* or might instead represent some form of *epiphenomenon*. To assess this, it is necessary to study the psychological consequences of lowering brain 5-HT function in healthy subjects and those at risk of mood disorder.

As mentioned above, the synthesis of brain 5-HT is dependent on the brain availability of its amino acid precursor, L-tryptophan. It is possible to produce a transient lowering of plasma tryptophan and brain 5-HT function over a few hours by administering a mixture of amino acids that lacks tryptophan. This procedure is called *tryptophan depletion*. Tryptophan depletion in subjects with no personal or family history of mood disorder has little measurable effect on mood and certainly does not produce significant clinical depressive symptomatology. By contrast, unmedicated euthymic patients with a personal history of mood disorder undergo a *rapid but temporary depressive relapse* when exposed to tryptophan depletion (K. A. Smith *et al.* 1997). The following conclusions can be drawn:

- Low brain 5-HT function is not *sufficient* to cause depression because tryptophan depletion fails to alter mood in those not vulnerable to mood disorder.

- In people *vulnerable to mood disorder*, lowering brain 5-HT function results in clinical depressive symptomatology.

- Low brain 5-HT function interacts with *other vulnerability factors* to cause depressive disorders in at-risk individuals.

The nature of these other vulnerability factors remain conjectural. It is possible that the 5-HT pathways of vulnerable individuals react abnormally to precursor deficit (Smith *et al.* 2000). Alternatively, there may be pre-existing deficits in central mood-regulating circuitry which are 'revealed' in the presence of low brain 5-HT states (Smith *et al.* 1999).

Noradrenaline function

Metabolism and receptors There is no consistent evidence that *brain or CSF concentrations of noradrenaline* or its major metabolite *3-methoxy–4-hydroxy-phenyleth-ylene glycol (MHPG)* are altered in depressed patients (see Anand and Charney 2000). As with 5-HT receptors, noradrenaline receptors in the brain can be divided into a number of subclasses. There is some evidence that depressed patients dying of natural causes and those who commit suicide have lowered α_1-*adrenoceptor binding* in some brain regions, though different studies have implicated different brain regions (Horton 1992).

Neuroendocrine tests Increasing brain noradrenaline function elevates plasma concentrations of *adreno-corticotropic hormone (ACTH)*, *cortisol*, and *growth hormone*. There is fairly consistent evidence that the growth hormone response to both the noradrena-line re-uptake inhibitor *desipramine* and the nora-drenaline receptor agonist *clonidine* is blunted in patients with melancholic depression (Checkley 1992). Clonidine acts directly on postsynaptic α_2-adrenoceptors in the hypothalamus to increase plasma growth hormone, and therefore the blunted response in depressed patients suggests a decreased responsivity of these postsynaptic α_2-adrenoceptors or of mechanisms linked to them.

Other biochemical and behavioural responses to clonidine, including changes in plasma MHPG and sedation, are not altered in depressed patients, suggesting that any deficit in α_2-adrenoceptor function is fairly localized, probably to the hypo-thalamus. Impaired growth hormone responses to clonidine appear to persist in recovered depressed patients, suggesting that this may be a trait abnor-mality (Checkley 1992).

Catecholamine depletion It is possible to lower the syn-thesis of catecholamines by inhibiting the *enzyme tyrosine hydroxylase*, which catalyses the conversion

of the amino acid, tyrosine to L-DOPA, a precursor of both noradrenaline and dopamine. The drug used to achieve this effect *is α-methyl-para-tyrosine (AMPT)*. In healthy subjects, AMPT produces sedation but not significant depressive symptoms. As with tryptophan depletion, however, when administered to recovered depressed patients off drug treatment, it causes a *striking clinical relapse in depressive symptomatology* (Berman *et al.* 1999). This could be mediated either by diminished dopamine or noradrenaline function, or by combined inhibi-tion of both these neurotransmitters.

These findings suggest that subjects at risk of mood disorder are *vulnerable to decreases in both 5-HT and catecholamine neurotransmission*. This is consis-tent with the clinical evidence that drugs acting selectively on noradrenaline or 5-HT pathways are effective antidepressant treatments.

Dopamine function

Depression The function of dopamine in depression has been less studied than that of 5-HT or nora-drenaline but there are a number of reasons for thinking that dopamine neurons may be involved in the pathophysiology of the depressed state:

- Dopamine neurons in the mesolimbic system play a key role in incentive behaviour and reward, processes that are disrupted in depres-sion, particularly melancholic states.
- Antidepressant treatments in animals increase the expression of dopamine receptors in part of the mesolimbic system called the *nucleus accum-bens*.

There are some pieces of evidence that suggest that dopamine function may be abnormal in depression:

- CSF levels of the dopamine metabolite homovanillic acid (HVA) are consistently low in depressed patients.
- Some brain imaging studies in depressed patients have found increased binding of dopamine D_2/D_3 receptors in striatal regions; this has been attributed to lowered presynaptic release of dopamine (see Verhoeff, 1999).

These findings, taken with the effect of AMPT to cause relapse in recovered depression, suggest that impaired dopamine function may play a role in the manifestation of the depressive syndrome and in the effects of antidepressant drug treatment.

Mania An influential hypothesis links excessive dopamine activity to the pathophysiology of schizophrenia (see p. 356). It has also been proposed that *manic states* may be attributable to dopamine overactivity (Silverstone and Cookson 1982). Studies of dopamine metabolism and function have provided little direct evidence for this suggestion, but mania can be provoked by dopamine agonists such as bromocriptine, and the euphoriant and arousing effects of psychostimulants such as amphetamine and cocaine are well known (Jacobs and Silverstone 1986). Finally, dopamine receptor antagonist drugs such as haloperidol are useful in the treatment of mania.

A recent study in recovered bipolar patients showed that they had a greater psychological response to intravenous amphetamine but no greater release of presynaptic dopamine as measured by the technique of raclopride displacement (see p. 132). This suggests that there may be a heightened responsivity to increased dopamine neurotransmission in patients at risk of mania but this is unlikely to be due to increased presynaptic dopamine release (Anand *et al.* 2000).

Monoamines and depression

There is now good evidence that unmedicated depressed patients have abnormalities in various aspects of monoamine function. However, these abnormalities vary in extent from case to case, and the changes are not large and are not sufficiently sensitive to be diagnostic.

The most convincing studies that show a key role for monoamines in the pathophysiology of depression are the 5-HT and catecholamine depletion paradigms. It is now established that in vulnerable individuals, lowering of 5-HT and noradrenaline and dopamine function is sufficient to cause clinical depression. Two major questions emerge from this work:

- What mechanisms produce low monoamine function in depressed patients?
- What are the other factors that make those at risk of depression psychologically vulnerable to manipulations of monoamine function?

Both these questions might be addressed by improving our understanding of the actions of monoamines at a cellular level. There is now increasing knowledge of the effects of monoamines on *second messenger production and intracellular signalling*. For example, recent animal experimental studies have shown that stimulating the cyclic AMP system leads to changes in expression of specific target genes including those involved in the elaboration of neurotropins such as *brain-derived neurotropic factor (BDNF)*. These neurotropins are necessary for the function and survival of CNS neurons.

BDNF expression in experimental animals is decreased by stress and enhanced by antidepressant medication. This has given rise to the hypothesis that stress-induced precipitation of mood disorders and the therapeutic effect of monoamine potentiating treatments are mediated via changes in intracellular mechanisms responsible for the production of neurotropins (see Duman *et al.* 1997). This suggestion also could account for how environmental adversity can give rise to changes in neuronal survival and perhaps thereby in the anatomy on brain structures important in mood regulation (see below).

Endocrine abnormalities

Abnormalities in endocrine function may be important in aetiology for three reasons:

- Some disorders of endocrine function are followed by depressive disorders more often than would be expected by chance, suggesting a causative relationship.
- Endocrine abnormalities found in depressive disorder indicate that there may be a disorder of the hypothalamic centres controlling the endocrine system.
- Hormones modulate the activity of monoamine neurotransmitters and could play a part in

producing some of the changes in monoamine function found in depressed patients.

Endocrine pathology and depression

About half of patients with *Cushing's syndrome* suffer from major depression, which usually remits when the cortisol hypersecretion is corrected (Checkley 1992). Depression also occurs in *Addison's disease*, *hypothyroidism*, and *hyperparathyroidism*.

Endocrine changes may account for depressive disorders occurring *premenstrually*, during the *menopause*, and after *childbirth*. These clinical associations are discussed further in Chapter 16.

Hypothalamic-pituitary-adrenal (HPA) axis

Much research effort has been concerned with abnormalities in the control of cortisol in depressive disorders. In about half of patients whose depressive disorder is at least moderately severe, *plasma cortisol secretion is increased* throughout the 24-hour cycle.

In studying depressed patients, much use has been made of the *dexamethasone suppression test*, which suppresses cortisol levels via inhibition of *ACTH* release at pituitary level. About 50% of depressed in-patients do not show the normal suppression of cortisol secretion induced by giving a 1 mg dose of the synthetic corticosteroid dexamethasone. However, not all cortisol hypersecretors are dexamethasone resistant.

Dexamethasone non-suppression is more common in depressed patients with *melancholia*, but it has not been reliably linked with any more specific psychopathological feature (Holsboer 1992). However, abnormalities in the dexamethasone suppression test are not confined to mood disorders; they have also been reported in mania, chronic schizophrenia, and dementia. This lack of diagnostic specificity diminished early hopes that dexamethasone non-suppression could be used as a diagnostic marker of melancholic depression. Nevertheless, dexamethasone non-suppression does predict a poorer response to placebo treatment in drug trials and a high risk of relapse in apparently recovered depressed patients (Ribeiro *et al.* 1993).

The cause of cortisol hypersecretion in depressed patients is not clearly established. There seem to be abnormalities at various points in the HPA axis, including:

- increased cortisol response of the adrenal gland to ACTH;
- increased number of ACTH secretory episodes;
- blunted ACTH response to pharmacological challenge with corticotropin-releasing hormone (CRH).

It has been suggested that, taken together, abnormalities in cortisol regulation in depression can best be explained by *hypersecretion of CRH* in the hypothalamus with a resultant increase in ACTH and cortisol release. Also, ACTH is a trophic hormone that can increase the responsiveness of the adrenal gland; as a consequence more cortisol will be secreted when the adrenal is stimulated. The blunted ACTH response to CRH challenge is proposed to result from a downregulation of CRH receptors as a consequence of increased endogenous CRH release. (see Holsoboer 1992).

In general, HPA axis changes in depressed patients have been regarded as *state abnormalities*, that is, they remit when the patient recovers. There is some evidence, however, that subtle changes in HPA axis function may persist in recovered depressed subjects. This suggests that some vulnerable individuals may have fairly enduring abnormalities is HPA axis regulation (Modell *et al.* 1998). Interestingly, in experimental animals, early adverse experiences produce long-standing changes in HPA axis regulation, indicating a possible neurobiological mechanism whereby childhood trauma could be translated into increased vulnerability to mood disorder. Recent studies confirm that adults who were abused as children have heightened HPA axis responses to stress (Heim *et al.* 2000).

CRH and depression In addition to its effects on cortisol secretion, CRH may play a more direct role in the aetiology of depression. It is well established that *CRH has a neurotransmitter role* in limbic regions of the brain where it is involved in regulating biochemical and behavioural responses to stress. Administration of CRH to animals produces changes in neuroendocrine regulation, sleep, and appetite that parallel those found in depressed patients. Furthermore, CRF levels may be increased in the CSF of depressed patients. Therefore it is possible that *hypersecretion of CRH* could be involved in the pathophysiology of the depressed state and non-peptide antagonists of CRH receptors may have value as antidepressant agents (see Heim and Nemeroff 2000).

Cortisol, monoamine function, and neuronal toxicity Recent work has shown that corticosteroids regulate the genomic expression and function of a number of monoamine receptors in the brain. For example, it has been shown that corticosteroids can decrease the *expression of post-synaptic 5-HT$_{1A}$ receptors in the hippocampus*; this finding has led to the suggestion that excessive cortisol secretion may precipitate depressive states through decreasing 5-HT neurotransmission. Experimental studies of animals have also linked excessive cortisol secretion to *damage to neurons in the hippocampus*. Subsequently, it has been suggested that chronic cortisol hypersecretion could be associated with the cognitive impairment which may be a particular feature of chronic depression (for reviews of this area see McAllister-Williams *et al.* 1998; Brown *et al.* 1999).

Thyroid function

Circulating plasma levels of free thyroxine appear to be normal in depressed patients, but levels of *free tri-iodothyronine* may be decreased. About a third of depressed in-patients have a *blunted thyrotropin-stimulating hormone* (TSH) response to intravenous thyrotropin-releasing hormone (TRH); this abnormality is not specific to depression, as it is also found in alcoholism and panic disorder (Checkley 1992). Like CRH, TRH has a role in brain neurotransmission and is found in brain neurons co-localized with classical monoamine neurotransmitters such as 5-HT. Therefore,

it is possible that the abnormalities in thyroid function found in depressed patients may be associated with changes in central TRH regulation.

Melatonin

The nocturnal secretion of the pineal hormone melatonin in depression has been studied with two main aims:

♦ as a measure of β-adrenergic function at post-synaptic pineal β-adrenoceptors;

♦ as a marker of circadian rhythm.

Although there are some studies suggesting that melatonin secretion is decreased in drug-free depressed patients, one well-controlled investigation found normal levels and so this finding remains in doubt (Thompson *et al.* 1988).

There is no evidence for a *phase shift of melatonin secretion in depressed patients*. In general, despite the obvious circadian changes in mood in depressed patients and the disruption of the sleep-wake cycle, there is little evidence from endocrine studies that depressed patients have a disturbance in the regulation of circadian rhythm.

Depression and the immune system

There is growing evidence that patients with depression manifest a variety of disturbances of *immune function*. Older studies found decreases in the cellular immune responses of lymphocytes in depressed patients (Herbert and Cohen 1993) but more recent work has produced evidence of immune activation with increases particularly in the release of certain *cytokines* (Box 11.2). Cytokines are known to provoke HPA axis activity and it is

---

Box 11.2 Immune changes in depression

Lowered proliferative responses of lymphocytes to mitogens

Lowered natural killer cell activity

Increases in positive acute phase proteins

Increases in cytokine levels (e.g. IL–1, IL–6)

therefore possible that changes in immune regulation may play a part in HPA axis dysfunction in depression. It is also possible that the changes seen are secondary to other depressive features, for example, lowered food intake and diminished self-care. However, the fact that medical administration of some cytokines (for example, interferon and tumour necrosis factor) can cause significant depressive symptoms argues that in some situations, changes in immune function may have a more direct role in provoking mood disorders (for a review see Griffiths *et al.* 2000).

Sleep changes in depression

Disturbed sleep is characteristic of depression. Recordings of the sleep EEG (polysomnogram) have shown a number of abnormalities in *sleep architecture* in patients with major depression:

- impaired sleep continuity and duration;
- decreased deep sleep (stages 3 and 4);
- decreased latency to the onset of rapid eye movement (REM) sleep;
- increase in the proportion of REM sleep in the early part of the night.

Decreased REM sleep latency is of interest in relation to aetiology because there is some evidence that it may persist in recovered depressed patients and indicate a vulnerability to relapse. A further link between REM sleep and depression is that many (but not all) effective antidepressant drugs decrease REM sleep time and the latency to its onset. In addition, both total *sleep deprivation* and selective REM sleep deprivation can produce a temporary alleviation of mood in depressed patients (for a review see Sharpley and Cowen 1995).

The neurochemical mechanism that links changes in REM sleep and mood is not known. The abnormalities in REM sleep in depressed patients could be attributable to excessive sensitivity of *muscarinic cholinergic receptors* (Mendelson 1991).

Brain imaging in mood disorder

Structural brain imaging

Changes in brain volume Computerized tomography (CT) and magnetic resonance imaging (MRI) have found a number of abnormalities in patients with major depression, particularly in those with more *severe and chronic disorders* (see Steffens and Krishnan 1998). The most consistent findings are:

- enlarged lateral ventricles;
- volume loss in frontal and temporal lobes;
- decreased hippocampal volume;
- decreased volume of basal ganglia structures.

Another finding that has aroused particular interest is a decrease in grey matter volume of *subgenual prefrontal cortex*, because this abnormality has been linked to lowered prefrontal perfusion in PET investigations and reduced glial cell numbers in post-mortem studies (Drevets *et al.* 1998). Changes in this brain area could represent a long-term vulnerability factor for the development of mood disorders. Another possibility is that repeated stress and depression might themselves alter brain structure. We have already noted hypotheses that link chronic cortisol hypersecretion with hippocampal atrophy and cognitive impairment. Such effects could be mediated via changes in levels of neurotropic factors such as BDNF (see above). A general theme from imaging studies is that patients with structural abnormalities are *less likely to respond to treatment*.

White and grey matter hyperintensities Hyperintense MRI *signals* can be detected in a number of regions in both normal ageing and patients with major depression. The usual sites are in the deep white matter and subcortical grey matter. In major depression, increased deep white matter hyperintensities are associated with:

- late onset of depressive disorder;
- greater illness severity and poorer treatment response;
- apathy, psychomotor slowness, and retardation;
- presence of vascular risk factors.

It has been proposed that major depression with these clinical and radiological features is more likely to be of vascular origin (Steffens and Krishnan 1998).

There are also reports that white and grey matter hyperintensities can be found in both old and young patients with bipolar disorder. However, the findings are not consistent and the significance of these abnormalities is not clear at present.

Cerebral blood flow and metabolism

Cerebral blood flow can be measured in a number of ways with, for example, single-photon emission tomography (SPET) or positron emission tomography (PET); the latter can also measure cerebral metabolism. Cerebral blood flow and metabolism are normally highly correlated (see Chapter 5).

Numerous studies have examined both cerebral metabolism and blood flow in groups of depressed patients. The findings have often been contradictory, and there are many methodological factors such as patient selection, drug status, and imaging techniques that may account for the discrepant findings. Nevertheless, there is some consensus that depressed patients have evidence of altered cerebral blood flow and metabolism in the following regions:

- prefrontal cortex
- anterior cingulate cortex
- amygdala and thalamus
- caudate nucleus.

Taken together, the abnormalities in functional brain imaging in depression support a circuitry model in which mood disorders are associated with *abnormal interactions between several brain regions* rather than a major abnormality in a single structure. The circuits implicated involve regions of the frontal and temporal lobe as well as related areas of basal ganglia and thalamus (Drevets 1998). Some tentative correlations between these brain regions and clinical depressive features are shown in Box 11.3.

> **Box 11.3 Some neuropsychological correlates of altered central perfusion in depressed patients**
>
> Dorsolateral and dorsomedial prefrontal cortex
> - Cognitive dysfunction (particularly executive dysfunction) and cognitive slowness
>
> Orbital and lateral prefrontal cortex
> - Abnormal emotional processing
> - Perseverative thinking
>
> Anterior cingulate
> - Impaired attentional processes
> - Abnormal emotional processing
>
> Amygdala
> - Abnormal emotional processing
>
> Basal ganglia
> - Impaired incentive behaviour
> - Psychomotor disturbances

Neuropsychological changes in mood disorder

Depression

Patients with depression show poor performance on several measures of neuropsychological function. Impairment is typically seen over a wide range of neuropsychological domains including attention, learning, memory, and executive function. There is disagreement as to whether these defects are best regarded as global and diffuse or whether there may be some selectivity to the changes seen. However, some have suggested that deficits in executive function may be particularly prominent in depression, which would be consistent with abnormalities seen in prefrontal perfusion in imaging studies (see Elliott 1998).

Most of the cognitive impairments resolve as the depression remits, but less striking defects have been detected in euthymic depressed patients. These may be particularly apparent in elderly patients where they appear to be independent of the age of onset of the depressive disorder (Dahabra *et al.* 1998).

Bipolar disorder

Patients with acute manic illness also perform poorly on a wide range of cognitive tasks, including sustained attention, learning and memory, and executive function (see Martnez-Aran 2000). It is possible that the defect in executive function persists in euthymic subjects (Ferrier *et al.* 1999a).

Conclusions

Predisposition

The predisposition to develop mania and severe depressive disorders has *important genetic determinants*. The level at which genetic factors operate is not known. It could be via effects on the regulation of monoamine neurotransmitters or through more remote factors such as temperament and the liability to experience life events. Adverse early experience such as *parental discord* or *abuse of various kinds* may also play a part in shaping features of personality which in turn determine whether, in adult life, certain events are experienced as stressful. In addition, early experiences could programme the HPA axis to respond to stress in a way that might predispose to the development of mood disorder.

Precipitating causes

The precipitating causes are stressful life events and certain kinds of physical illness. Some progress has been made in discovering the types of event that provoke depression and in quantifying their stressful qualities. Such studies show that *loss* can be an important precipitant, but not the only one. The effects of particular events may be modified by a number of background factors that may make a person more vulnerable, for example, caring for several small children without help and being socially isolated. As noted in the preceding paragraph, the impact of potentially stressful events also depends on personality factors and probably on genetic inheritance.

Two kinds of mechanism have been proposed to explain how precipitating events lead to the phenomena observed in depressive disorders. The first mechanism is *psychological* and the second is *neurobiological*. The two sets of mechanism are not mutually exclusive, for they may represent different levels of organization of the same pathological process. The psychological studies are at an early stage. Abnormalities have been shown in the thinking of depressed patients and they may play a part in perpetuating depressive disorder. However, there is no convincing evidence that they induce it.

Various biochemical theories can be used to explain how life stress and difficulty could be translated into the *neurochemical changes* that characterize depressive disorders. Monoamine neurotransmitters are involved in regulating responses to stress and in modifying behaviours known to be altered in mood disorders. It seems likely that both external events and a genetic predisposition bring about the changes in brain monoamine function that are seen in depressed patients. In predisposed subjects, reduction in monoamine neurotransmission can bring about clinical symptomatology. Depressive states are associated with altered cerebral activity, particularly in frontal cortex. In some patients, particularly those with a poor prognosis, there is evidence for underlying *neuropathological changes*, which probably act as a further predisposing factor (for a simplified model see Figure 11.3).

Recent studies have used sophisticated statistical techniques in an attempt to derive quantitative estimates of the roles of different risk factors in the development of depressive disorders. For example, from a prospective study of 680 female twin pairs, Kendler *et al.* (1993a) calculated that about half the liability to major depression was attributable to four main factors (in order of relative importance):

- recent stressful life events;
- genetic factors;
- previous history of major depression;
- neuroticism (as measured on the Eysenck scale).

These factors interact with each other. For example, whereas about 60% of the effect of genetic factors

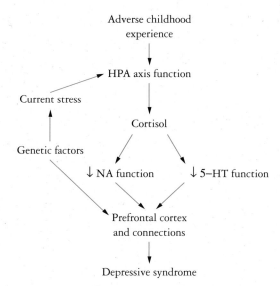

Figure 6.1 Simplified neurobiological model of the aetiology of depression. Adverse childhood experience has long-term effects on HPA axis function which is further modified by stressful life events (the susceptibility to which is partly influenced by genetic factors). An abnormal cortisol response decreases noradrenaline (NA) and 5-hydroxytryptamine (5-HT) function, leading to clinical depression in the presence of pre-existing (genetic and developmental) abnormalities of prefrontal cortical circuitry.

was directly on the risk of developing depression, the remaining 40% appeared to be expressed through increased liability to experience stressful life events and to have a high neuroticism score. By contrast, ratings of parental warmth had no direct effect on the liability to major depression, but influenced other factors of aetiological importance such as level of recent difficulties and social support.

Major depression is a disorder with important genetic, environmental, and interpersonal determinants. These factors do not interact in a simple additive manner but modify each other in direct and indirect ways. Whilst this formulation precludes the use of simple models to explain the aetiology of major depression, it does correspond more closely to clinical experience. In addition, it suggests that a number of different kinds of inter-

vention could be useful in decreasing the liability of individuals to develop mood disorders.

Course and prognosis

In considering course and prognosis it is necessary to deal with *bipolar and unipolar* disorders separately. It should be remembered, however, that any sample of patients with unipolar depression will contain a proportion of patients whose bipolar illness has not yet declared itself. It has been estimated that about 10% of patients presenting with a depressive disorder will eventually have a manic illness. Such patients are more likely to have a family history of mania or to show brief, mild manic mood swings during antidepressant treatment. From recent hospital and population-based studies, the following general conclusions can be derived (see Angst 2000).

Bipolar disorders

◆ The age of onset of bipolar disorder is typically about 21 years in hospital studies but earlier (about 17 years) in community surveys. Late-onset bipolar disorder is rare and may be precipitated by organic brain disease.

◆ The average length of a manic episode (treated or untreated) is about 6 months.

◆ At least 90% of patients with mania experience further episodes of mood disturbance.

◆ Over a 25 year follow-up, on average bipolar patients experience about 10 further episodes of mood disturbance.

◆ The interval between episodes becomes progressively shorter with both age and the number of episodes.

◆ Nearly all bipolar patients recover from acute episodes but the long-term prognosis is rather poor. For example, less than 20% of bipolar patients achieve a period of 5 years of clinical stability with good social and occupational performance. Patients with bipolar II disorder have a somewhat better outcome, whilst rapid cycling has a worse prognosis.

Unipolar depressive disorders

- The age of onset of unipolar disorders varies widely; it is generally agreed to be later than for bipolar cases. There is a fairly uniform incidence of onset of cases throughout the life span but the relative contribution of different aetiological factors probably differs between early- and late-onset cases.

- The average length of a depressive episode is about 6 months but about 25% of patients have episodes of more than a year and about 10–20% develop a chronic unremitting course.

- About 80% of patients with major depression will experience further episodes.

- Over a 25-year follow-up, on average, patients with unipolar depression experience about five further episodes.

- As with bipolar patients, the interval between episodes becomes progressively shorter.

- A high proportion (about one-third) of depressed patients do not achieve complete symptom remission between episodes.

- The longer-term prognosis of depression may be a little better in some ways than that of bipolar disorder but is still modest. For example, only about 25% of patients with unipolar depression achieve a period of 5 years of clinical stability with good social and occupational performance.

Dysthymia

Dysthymia is by definition a chronic disorder and, in the absence of effective treatment, sufferers will commonly describe depressive symptoms of many years' duration. Community studies show a low spontaneous recovery rate. Over the life span, some patients with dysthymia develop major depression (so-called *double depression*) whilst some patients originally presenting with major depression subside into dysthymia. The development of mania is rare.

Minor affective disorder

Most information is available for *minor depression* which shows a recurrence rate similar to that of major depression. Patients who meet criteria for minor depression at one point in follow-up may then subsequently be diagnosed as suffering from major depression and vice versa. Thus, similarly to dysthymia, minor depression is likely to be a *risk factor* for major depression and may also be a *residual state* following remission of major depression. Overall, the longitudinal data suggest that major and minor depression and dysthymia are not distinct conditions but are part of *spectrum of depressive disorders* (see Akiskal 2000; Angst 2000).

Mortality of mood disorders

Mortality is significantly increased in patients with mood disorders, largely, though not exclusively from *suicide.* The standardized mortality ratio in mood disorders is about twice that found in the general population. Apart from suicide, excess deaths are due to accidents, cardiovascular disease, and co-morbid substance misuse.

Rates of suicide are substantially increased in mood disorders and are at least 12 times greater than those of the general population (Harris and Barraclough, 1997). The risk varies with diagnostic subcategory but is greatest for major depression (Box 11.4). Longer-term follow-up for patients with depression have given differing rates of lifetime risk of suicide. In those with severe illnesses who have been treated as in-patients the risk may be as high as 15%. However, in community samples the risk is less (see Bostwick and Ponkretz 2001). The proportion of patients who die by suicide in mood disorders lessens as the period of follow-up increases, presumably because mortality from natural causes becomes more significant. Using a statistical modelling technique to take this effect into account, Inskip *et al.* (1998) concluded that the lifetime risk of suicide in mood disorder is about 4%. This is substantially less than that derived from other studies and requires further verification.

Box 11.4 Standardized mortality ratios for some depressive disorders	
Major depression	20.35
Bipolar disorder	15.05
Dysthymia	12.12

Harris and Barraclough (1997)

Prognostic factors

The best predictor of the future course is the history of *previous episodes*. Not surprisingly, the risk of recurrence is much greater in those with several previous episodes. An *early age of onset* is also a risk factor as is *incomplete symptomatic remission*. Other factors that predict a greater risk of future episodes are:

◆ bipolar disorder

◆ poor social support

◆ poor physical health

◆ co-morbid substance misuse

◆ co-morbid personality disorder

◆ high trait neuroticism.

The various risk factors, particularly previous pattern of recurrence, and extent of current remission have important implications for the use of longer-term maintenance treatments (see below). In many patients, depression is best conceptualized as a chronic relapsing disorder which needs an integrated long-term treatment approach (see Angst 2000).

The acute treatment of depression

This section is concerned with the *efficacy of various forms of treatment* in the acute management of depression. Details of treatment with drugs and ECT are given in Chapter 21, which should be consulted before reading this section. Advice on the selection of treatments and the day-to-day care of patients is given in the section on management.

Antidepressant drugs

Antidepressant drugs are effective in the acute treatment of depression. The largest effects relative to placebo are seen in patients with major depression whose symptoms are of at least *moderate severity*. Short-term response rates in controlled trials are about 60% for patients on active treatment and about 30% for those on placebo [number needed to treat (NNT) = 3–4] (see Anderson *et al.* 2000). In terms of efficacy there is little to choose between the various antidepressants, although some are better in certain defined situations (see below).

Similar clinical response rates are seen in *dysthymia* where again several classes of antidepressant drugs including tricyclics and SSRIs have shown therapeutic efficacy. A meta-analysis by de Lima *et al.* (1999) showed a response rate with active of treatment of 55%, compared with 30% on placebo (NNT = 3.9).

The value of antidepressant drugs in milder depressive disorders such as minor depression and mixed anxiety-depression is not established. It is generally believed that tricyclics are relatively ineffective in these disorders but whether this applies to SSRIs is not clear.

Tricyclic antidepressants

Tricyclic antidepressants have been extensively compared with placebo in both in-patients and out-patients with major depression. In all but the most severely depressed patients, tricyclic antidepressants are clearly more effective than placebo (Ball and Kiloh 1959; Morris and Beck 1974). There is little evidence that tricyclic antidepressant drugs differ from one another in clinical efficacy, but they do differ in side-effect profile (see Chapter 21). *Lofepramine* is relatively safe in overdose. Among the other classes of antidepressant drug, none is more effective than the tricyclics, although individual patients may show a preferential response to other compounds (see below).

Response in clinical subgroups

Tricyclics are appear to be less effective in the following groups of patients:

- depressive psychosis (as a sole treatment);
- milder depressive states with Hamilton Depression Scores less than about 14;
- patients with atypical depression.

Monoamine oxidase inhibitors (MAOIs)

The efficacy of *monoamine oxidase inhibitors (MAOIs)* in the treatment of major depression (particularly with melancholic features) has been a matter of controversy. However, placebo-controlled trials have shown that MAOIs are effective antidepressants and equal in therapeutic activity to tricyclic antidepressants for moderate-to-severe depressive disorders.

MAOIs are liable to produce dangerous reactions with other drugs and some foods; therefore, they are not recommended as first-line antidepressant drugs. However, controlled trials have shown that in the following situations MAOIs carry an advantage over tricyclic antidepressants:

- atypical depression;
- anergic bipolar depression (characterized by fatigue, retardation, increased appetite, and sleep);
- depression resistant to tricyclics and SSRIs.

The reversible type-A MAOI *moclobemide* has the advantage of not requiring adherence to a low-tyramine diet. However, it can still produce hazardous interactions with other drugs (see p. 690). Controlled trials have shown that moclobemide is more effective than placebo in the treatment of uncomplicated major depression but it may be a little less effective than tricyclics (Anderson 1999). It is doubtful whether moclobemide is as effective as conventional MAOIs for atypical and tricyclic-resistant depression.

Combination of MAOIs and tricyclic antidepressants

It has been reported that, in cases resistant to treatment with a tricyclic or MAOI, a combination of the two drugs is more effective than either drug given alone in corresponding dosage. This claim has not been proved; indeed, two clinical trials have

failed to confirm it (see Chalmers and Cowen 1990). However, it can be argued that neither trial was concerned with patients known to be resistant to single drugs (the patient group to whom combined treatment is most often given).

Selective serotonin re-uptake inhibitors (SSRIs) and serotonin and noradrenaline re-uptake inhibitors

Selective serotonin re-uptake inhibitors (SSRIs) have undergone extensive trials both against placebo and comparator antidepressants. There is good evidence that they are as effective as tricyclics in the broad range of depressed patients, although they may be less effective in hospitalized depressed patients (Anderson 2000). Venlafaxine also appears a little more effective than SSRIs in patients with severer depressive states. SSRIs are more effective than tricyclics (with the exception of clomipramine) in the treatment of *co-morbid depression and obsessional-compulsive disorder* (see Anderson *et al.* 2000).

Tolerance relative to tricyclics

In short-term clinical trials, compared to tricyclics SSRIs are associated with lower drop-out rates due to side-effects, but the differences are modest (relative risk of drop-out due to side-effects is 0.73, NNT = 33). However, the differences in favour of SSRIs increase in routine clinical situations, particularly when length of treatment exceeds a few weeks (see Anderson *et al.* 2000). Clearly, relative safety in overdose gives SSRIs an advantage in certain clinical situations.

Other antidepressants

A wide variety of other antidepressant drugs is now available (see Chapter 21). All have established efficacy relative to placebo. The main differences between the various preparations are in side-effect profile. Apart from reboxetine, anticholinergic-type side-effects are uncommon. Trazodone and mirtazapine are sedating. Nefazodone is relatively non-sedating, but unlike SSRIs, does not cause sexual dysfunction or sleep disruption. All are safer than tricyclics in overdose (Table 11.8).

Lithium

Lithium as a sole treatment

This section is concerned only with lithium as a treatment for depressive disorders. The use of lithium in the *treatment of mania* and in the *maintenance treatment of mood disorders* is considered later. Placebo-controlled trials suggest that lithium has antidepressant efficacy in bipolar depression (see Goodwin and Jamison 1990) but its effects in unipolar depression are modest.

Lithium in combination with antidepressants

Despite its limited utility as a sole drug treatment for depression, lithium can produce useful therapeutic effects when added to antidepressant medication in treatment-resistant patients (*lithium augmentation*). In a meta-analysis, Bauer and Dopfmer (1999) found about 50% of depressed patients responded to lithium augmentation of their antidepressant regimen, compared with about 20% of patients given placebo (NNT = 3.7).

Whilst some studies have reported a rapid amelioration of the depressed state within as little as 48 hours after the addition of lithium, the more usual pattern of response is a gradual resolution of symptoms over 2–3 weeks. Unipolar depressed patients seem to respond as well as bipolar patients and thus far there are no reliable clinical or biochemical predictors that identify depressed patients likely to respond to lithium augmentation. The effects of lithium augmentation do not seem to be restricted to any specific class of antidepressants.

Anticonvulsants

Anticonvulsants such as carbamazepine, valproate, and lamotrigine are useful in the management of bipolar disorder and in these circumstances can prevent episodes of major depression. There is little evidence that these drugs have acute antidepressant efficacy but lamotrigine has been shown to produce antidepressant effects in a placebo-controlled trial in bipolar depressed patients (Calabrese *et al.* 1999)

Electroconvulsive therapy

This treatment is described in Chapter 21, where its unwanted effects are also considered. The present section is concerned with evidence about

Table 11.8 Clinical characteristics of some antidepressant drugs

	Anticholinergic	Sedating	Weight gain	Sexual dysfunction	Toxicity and overdose
Amitriptyline	+++	+++	+++	+	+++
Lofepramine	+	+	0	+	0
SSRIs	0	0	0	+++	0*
Venlafaxine	0	0	0	+++	+
Nefazodone	0	+	0	0	0
Trazodone	0	+++	+	0	+
Reboxetine	+	0	0	++	0
Mirtazapine	0	+++	+++	0	0

0, none; +, mild; ++, moderate; +++, marked.

* Citalopram may be somewhat more toxic than other SSRIs.

the therapeutic effects of ECT for depressive disorders.

Comparison with simulated ECT

Six double-blind controlled trials have compared the efficacy of ECT and simulated ECT (anaesthesia with electrode application but no passage of current) in patients with major depression. Five of these studies found ECT to be more effective than the simulation. In the study which did not find the full procedure more effective, unilateral low-dose ECT was used, a procedure which is thought on other grounds to be relatively ineffective. The overall response rate is about 70% for ECT and 40% for simulated treatment (see review by Paykel 1989).

Comparison with other treatments

Several studies have compared depressed in-patients receiving ECT with those receiving antidepressant drugs. In nine comparisons with tricyclic antidepressants, ECT was therapeutically more effective in six studies and equally effective in the remaining three. In five comparisons with MAOIs, ECT was superior in each trial. These data suggest that in severely depressed in-patients ECT is probably superior to antidepressant drug treatment, at least in the short term (Paykel 1989).

Indications for ECT

Clinicians generally agree that the therapeutic effects of ECT are greatest in severe depressive disorders, especially those with *marked weight loss, early morning waking, retardation*, and *delusions*. From the trials comparing full ECT with simulated ECT, it appears that delusions and (less strongly) retardation are the features that distinguish patients who respond to full ECT from those who respond to placebo (Brandon *et al.* 1984; Clinical Research Centre 1984).

Other studies have established that patients with *depressive psychosis* respond better to ECT than to tricyclic antidepressants or antipsychotic drugs given alone (Kocsis *et al.* 1990). However, combined treatment with tricyclic antidepressants and *antipsychotic drugs* may be about as effective as ECT (Spiker *et al.* 1985), although no direct comparisons have been made. Another point of practical importance is that ECT may often prove effective in depressed patients who have not responded to full trials of medication, whether or not psychotic features are present (Sackheim *et al.* 1990).

Psychotherapy

All depressed patients, whatever other treatment they may be receiving, need psychotherapy in a general sense, which provides education, reassurance, and encouragement. These measures (so-called 'clinical management') can provide some symptomatic relief and can also ensure that pessimistic patients comply with specific treatments. Education and reassurance should also be given to the *patient's partner*, other close family members, and other people involved in care.

The psychological treatments used for depressive disorders can be divided as follows:

- supportive psychotherapy
- cognitive therapy
- interpersonal psychotherapy
- marital therapy
- dynamic psychotherapy.

These psychotherapies can be employed as alternatives to antidepressant medication or as adjuncts. Psychotherapies have been less well evaluated than antidepressant medication in major depression but, in general, *the more structured treatments* have a better success rate. In a meta-analysis of 29 studies (Depression Guideline Panel 1993) response rates were as follows:

- individual cognitive therapy, 50%
- interpersonal psychotherapy, 53%
- brief dynamic therapies (mainly group), 35%
- waiting-list control, 30%.

Supportive psychotherapy

Supportive psychotherapy goes beyond clinical management in focusing on the identification and resolution of current life difficulties, and in using the patient's strengths and available coping resources. A development of this approach is problem solving, in which the therapist and patient identify the main problems of concern and devise feasible step-by-step ways of tackling them. In a randomized controlled trial Mynors-Wallis *et al.* (1995) found that problem-solving treatment was as effective as amitriptyline and more effective than placebo in depressed patients in primary care.

Cognitive therapy

For depressive disorder, the essential aim of *cognitive therapy* is to help patients to modify their ways of thinking about life situations and depressive symptoms (see p. 732 for further information). There have been numerous studies of cognitive therapy in major depression and for unipolar depressive disorders of moderate severity, clinical trials indicate that the results of cognitive therapy are superior to waiting-list controls and equivalent to pharmacotherapy (Depression Giudeline Panel 1993). It has been suggested that cognitive therapy is less effective than medication in more severely depressed patients, particularly those with *melancholic illness*, but this has been disputed (DeRubies *et al.* 1999; Thase and Friedman 1999).

It has also been claimed that patients who received cognitive therapy for depression experience lower relapse rates than those treated with antidepressant medication (see, for example, Evans *et al.* 1992). This would represent an important advantage for cognitive therapy and prospective studies are needed. At present, interpretation of the findings has been hindered by the definition of relapse and by naturalistic methods of follow-up; for example, if patients seek less help after cognitive therapy, it does not necessarily mean that they are free of depression.

Interpersonal psychotherapy

Interpersonal therapy is a systematic and standardized treatment approach to personal relationships and life problems (see p. 732). It has been less studied than cognitive therapy in depression but seems to be effective. For example, Weissman *et al.* (1979) reported that the effects of interpersonal therapy on the symptoms of moderately severe depressive disorders were equal to those of amitriptyline and greater than those of minimal treatment. Drug treatment had more effect on sleep disturbance, appetite, and somatic complaints, whereas interpersonal therapy had more effect on depressed mood, guilt, suicidal ideas, interests, and work. However, the effects of psychotherapy were slower.

Interpersonal therapy was also studied in the National Institute of Mental Health (NIMH) multicentre psychotherapy study in which 240 out-patients with major depression were randomly allocated to one or other of four treatments given over 16 weeks (Elkin *et al.* 1989):

- interpersonal therapy
- cognitive therapy
- imipramine with clinical management (see above)
- placebo with clinical management.

Most patients had improved after 16 weeks. In the patient group as a whole there were few significant differences between the treatments, but interpersonal therapy was the most successful psychotherapy and as effective as imipramine except in the most severely depressed patients.

Marital therapy

Marital therapy can be given to depressed patients for whom marital discord appears to have contributed to causing or maintaining the depressive disorder. Indeed, in such patients marital therapy may have an advantage over cognitive therapy. There is also evidence that marital therapy is more effective than other psychotherapies or waiting-list control in *improving marital satisfaction* (O'Leary and Beach 1990; Depression Guideline Panel 1993). Overall, marital therapy is worth considering for depressed patients with significant marital discord, perhaps as an adjunct to drug treatment.

Dynamic psychotherapy

Dynamic psychotherapy has a different aim, which is to resolve underlying personal conflicts and attendant life difficulties that are believed to cause or maintain the depressive disorder. Opinions differ about its value. There have been few attempts to evaluate treatment, and they have mainly been concerned with brief dynamic psychotherapy in groups. The results for the treatment of depression suggest that dynamic psychotherapy is less effective than more structured psychotherapies such as cognitive therapy (Depression Guideline Panel 1993).

Other treatments

Sleep deprivation

Several studies suggest that, in some depressive disorders, rapid short-term changes in mood can be brought about by keeping patients *awake overnight*. Specific *REM sleep deprivation* can also alleviate depressed mood, but more slowly (see Wu and Bunney 1990). The alleviation of depressed mood after total sleep deprivation is nearly always *temporary*; it disappears after the next night's sleep or even during a daytime nap after the night of sleep deprivation. Whilst the antidepressant effect of sleep deprivation is of great theoretical interest, its brevity makes it unpractical. However, there are reports that sleep deprivation can be used to quicken the onset of effect of antidepressant drugs and also that some pharmacological manipulations can prolong the effect of sleep deprivation (see Wirz-Justice and van den Hoofdakker 1999).

Bright light treatment

Over 50% of patients with recurrent winter depression respond to *bright light treatment* (about 10,000 lux). Treatment is usually given for an hour or two in the morning but the timing of light treatment is not always critical and evening light or even midday exposure can be effective. The duration of exposure usually needs to be 1–2 hours.

Designing placebo-controlled trials of bright light for winter depression presents problems, because most patients are aware before treatment that bright light is believed to be the important therapeutic ingredient. Within this limitation, most studies have found that dim light is less effective than bright light. The usual onset of the antidepressant effect of bright light is within 2–5 days, but longer periods of treatment seem to be needed in some patients. Patients with *'atypical'* depressive features such as *overeating and oversleeping* appear to respond best. To avoid relapse, light treatment usually needs to be maintained until the usual time of natural remission, in the early spring (for a review of bright light treatment and winter depression see Rodin and Thompson 1997 and p. 714).

The acute treatment of mania

The treatment of mania presents a formidable clinical challenge calling for great clinical management skills from the psychiatric team. Drug treatment plays a pivotal role in the management of mania and has the aim of reducing physical and mental overactivity, improving features of psychosis, and preventing deterioration in health due to exhaustion, sleep deprivation, and poor fluid intake. It is worth noting that before the advent of modern drug treatment the mortality of mania in hospital setting was over 20%; nearly half these patients died from exhaustion (Derby 1933).

Medication

Antipsychotic drugs

Typical antipsychotic drugs

Several randomized controlled trials have shown efficacy of *chlorpromazine* and *haloperidol* in manic symptoms, whether or not patients have clear psychotic features. However, the use of typical antipsychotic drugs has limitations; manic patients often receive high doses and may be particularly susceptible to extrapyramidal side-effects. In addition, antipsychotic drugs do not protect against the depressive downswings that can follow resolution of a manic illness. Particularly in the USA, *mood stabilizers* such as lithium and valproate are now advocated as the primary pharmacological treatment of acute mania. However, audit of drug prescription shows that antipsychotic drugs are, in fact, prescribed to the majority of hospitalized manic patients in the USA (Chou *et al.* 1996).

Atypical antipsychotic drugs

Because of their improved tolerability profile, atypical antipsychotic agents such as *risperidone* and *olanzapine* are being increasingly used in mania. In a randomized controlled trial, Tohen *et al.* (1999) found that the response to olanzapine in manic patients (48%) was significantly greater than that to placebo (24%). There have been no placebo-controlled trials of risperidone in mania yet published, but in a randomized study, Segal *et al.* (1998) found that risperidone (6 mg) and haloperidol (10 mg) were equivalent in acute antimanic effect to lithium. There also are case reports that *clozapine* can be of value in patients with intractable manic symptoms (see McElroy *et al.* 1996).

Mood stabilizers

Lithium

Five placebo-controlled trials have shown that lithium is effective in the acute treatment of mania. Early studies gave high improvement rates (see Goodwin and Jamison 1990); however, the most recent investigation (Bowden *et al.* 1994) found a response rate of 49% for lithium and 25% for placebo. Lithium is at least as effective as antipsychotic medication but its onset of action is slower (American Psychiatric Association 1994b; Bowden 1996).

There is little evidence from the controlled studies that patients receiving combined treatment with lithium and antipsychotic drugs have a better short-term outcome than patients receiving either drug alone (Chou 1991). Prominent depressive symptoms and psychotic features predict a poorer response to lithium alone, as does a rapid cycling disorder.

Carbamazepine

Assessment of the efficacy of *carbamazepine* in acute mania is limited by problems in study design. These include small numbers, the use of adjunctive medications, and mixed diagnostic groupings (see Chou 1991). In general, carbamazepine appears equivalent in efficacy to antipsychotic drugs, although a slight inferiority to lithium cannot be excluded (American Psychiatric Association 1994b).

Clinical studies suggest that carbamazepine may be useful for manic patients who have not been helped by lithium, including those with dysphoric symptoms and rapid-cycling disorders. In some patients, the combination of lithium and carbamazepine may be effective when neither drug alone has proved beneficial.

Valproate

Several randomized controlled trials have shown that *valproate* possesses antimanic activity greater than placebo and equivalent to lithium. For example, in the study of Bowden *et al.* (1994), the response rate of manic patients to valproate (48%) was the same as that of lithium (49%) and significantly greater than placebo (25%). In this study, valproate was more effective than lithium in patients with dysphoric symptoms and rapid-cycling disorders.

An advantage possessed by valproate is that the time of onset of its activity is faster than other mood stabilizers (Bowden 1996). For example, with 'valproate loading' (20 mg/kg/day) the onset of manic effect can be as early as within 1–4 days. This is probably because the tolerability of valproate allows rapid dose escalation whilst lithium and carbamazepine must be introduced more gradually. Studies have suggested that an antimanic response to valproate is more likely to occur with plasma levels above 50 μg/ml (see Hirschfeld *et al.* 1999).

Other mood stabilizers

Studies of *lamotrigine* and *gabapentin* in mania are less well developed, although there are positive reports from case series of manic patients for both drugs. A recent small randomized trial in manic patients showed no difference in efficacy between lithium and lamotrigine (Ichim *et al.* 2000).

Benzodiazepines

Benzodiazepines are useful *adjuncts* in the treatment of mania because they can rapidly diminish overactivity, and restore sleep. Benzodiazepines have been used as a sole therapy in the treatment of mania but this carries a risk of disinhibition. Their most useful role is an adjunct to mood stabilizers because the latter drugs can take several days to become effective. Benzodiazepines can also be given in combination with antipsychotic drugs because this lowers the doses of antipsychotic drug needed to calm agitated and overactive patients. The usual benzodiazepines employed are the high-potency agents, lorazepam and clonazepam. Use should be 'as needed' and for as short a time as possible to minimize the risk of tolerance and dependence (see Chou 1991).

Electroconvulsive therapy

ECT has been widely used to treat mania, although there are only two recent prospective controlled trials. In one, bilateral ECT was found to be superior to lithium (Small *et al.* 1988). In another study, unilateral and bilateral ECT were compared with a combination of lithium and haloperidol in patients who had not responded to antipsychotic drugs alone. The response rate of these patients to ECT (13 of 22) was greater than that to combined drug treatment (none of five). The efficacy of unilateral and bilateral ECT did not differ (Mukherjee *et al.* 1988).

Retrospective investigations have shown ECT to be effective in acute mania, with the overall response rate being about 80%. Many of the patients had been unresponsive to medication (Mukherjee *et al.* 1994). In clinical practice, there is a tendency to give ECT to patients unresponsive to drug treatment, or to patients with a manic illness of life-threatening proportions due to extreme overactivity and physical exhaustion. ECT is often given at shorter intervals in the treatment of mania than in the treatment of depression, but there is no evidence that this regimen is necessary or speeds treatment response. It is unclear whether bilateral electrode placement is better than unilateral placement in manic patients (for a review see Mukherjee *et al.* 1994).

The longer-term treatment of mood disorders

Follow-up studies have shown that mood disorders often recur and, untreated, have a rather poor long-term prognosis. For this reason there is now increasing emphasis on *long-term management*.

Prevention of relapse and recurrence

Strictly, the word *relapse* refers to the worsening of symptoms after an initial improvement during the treatment of a single episode of mood disorder, whilst *recurrence* refers to a new episode after a period of complete recovery. Treatment to prevent relapse should be called *continuation treatment*, and treatment to prevent recurrence should be called *prophylactic or maintenance treatment*. In practice, however, it is not always easy to maintain the distinction between these two kinds of treatment because a therapy may be given at first to prevent relapse and then may be used to prevent recurrence.

Drug treatment of unipolar depression

Continuation treatment

It is now well established that stopping anti-depressants soon after treatment response is associated with a high risk of *relapse*. About *a third* of patients withdrawn from medication relapse over the next year with the majority of the relapses occurring in the first 6 months. Placebo-controlled studies of the role of continuation therapy have reached the following conclusions (see Anderson *et al.* 2000):

- continuing antidepressant treatment for 6 months past the point of remission halves the relapse rate;

- treatment should be at the originally effective dose of medication if possible;

◆ in patients at low risk of further episodes, continuation of antidepressant treatment longer than 6 months confers little extra benefit except in the elderly where 12 months continuation therapy is more appropriate;

◆ in patients at higher risk of relapse, longer-term maintenance antidepressant treatment should be considered.

Maintenance treatment

Controlled studies involving patients with recurrent depression (usually defined as at least three episodes over the last 5 years) have shown that maintenance antidepressant treatment can substantially reduce relapse rates. For example, in a 3-year study of 128 patients, Frank *et al.* (1990) found a relapse rate of 22% in patients taking imipramine compared with 78% in patients treated with placebo. In this latter study, patients were maintained on the same dose of imipramine as they had received during their acute illness. During longer-term treatment, it is common practice to lower the dose of tricyclic antidepressant to a 'maintenance' level, but this may lessen prophylactic efficacy (Frank *et al.* 1993). There are also data to support maintenance using a range of newer antidepressants, which may be better tolerated over the longer term that full-dose tricyclic treatment (Edwards 1999).

Lithium carbonate is also effective in the prevention of recurrent unipolar depression. A meta-analysis of eight small studies found that lithium was more effective than placebo and about equivalent to antidepressants in preventing recurrence (Souza and Goodwin 1991). Lithium may be the preferred treatment for patients who have shown any sign of elevated mood because (unlike antidepressant drugs) it also prevents mania (see below).

Drug treatment of bipolar disorder

Continuation treatment

The role of continuation treatment in bipolar disorder following an episode of mania has been less studied. However, it a common clinical experience that too rapid a reduction in doses of drug treatment can lead to the sudden recrudescence of an apparently treated manic disorder. Since the average length of a manic episode is about 6 months, it seems prudent to continue some form of medication for at least this period. Patients who have been severely ill will often be taking a mood stabilizer and an antipsychotic agent. Because of the adverse effects of antipsychotic drugs, it will often be appropriate slowly to withdraw this form of treatment first.

Maintenance treatment

Lithium There is substantial evidence for the efficacy of *lithium* in the maintenance treatment of recurrent mood disturbances in patients with bipolar disorders. *About 50%* of such patients respond well to lithium, whilst the rest show either a partial response or no response (Goodwin and Jamison 1990). It has been argued more recently that the prophylactic effect of lithium in the earlier controlled studies was exaggerated because the use of placebo-controlled crossover designs resulted in sudden lithium withdrawal and manic rebound (see p. 700). This would falsely inflate the incidence of recurrence off lithium treatment. However, even allowing for this effect, lithium is an effective prophylactic agent (for an account of this controversy, see Moncrieff and Goodwin 1995).

In bipolar patients, lithium seems to be equally effective in preventing recurrences of depression and recurrences of mania. The following predict a relatively poorer response to lithium maintenance treatment:

◆ rapid-cycling disorders or chronic depression;

◆ mixed affective states;

◆ alcohol and drug misuse;

◆ mood-incongruent psychotic features.

There is also evidence that use of lithium in patients with recurrent mood disorders is associated with a *significant reduction in mortality from suicide*. This effect is most often seen in dedicated lithium clinics and the mechanism and specificity of the association requires further study. Nevertheless, it is clinically important that the carefully supervised use of lithium is associated with a lowered risk of suicidal behaviour. This effect is not necessarily shared by other mood stabilizers (Thies-Flechtner *et al.* 1996; Tondo *et al.* 1998).

Carbamazepine Although the number of patients studied in randomized controlled studies is relatively few, *carbamazepine* appears to be about as effective as lithium in the prophylaxis of bipolar disorder (Post 1991). Therefore, carbamazepine can be considered in patients who are intolerant of lithium. In addition, patients who respond poorly to lithium, particularly those with rapid-cycling disorders, may benefit from carbamazepine given either alone or in combination with lithium.

On the results of both controlled and uncontrolled trials, Post (1991) estimated that about 65% of bipolar patients show a good response to carbamazepine, or to *lithium and carbamazepine* given in combination. It is not clear from the literature what proportion of these patients had not responded to lithium before receiving carbamazepine. Also, in studies of lithium-resistant patients, carbamazepine is often added to lithium; it is then difficult to determine whether the therapeutic effect is caused by carbamazepine alone, or by lithium and carbamazepine together.

Whilst these results with carbamazepine are promising, it is worth noting that a group of 24 treatment-resistant patients initially showed a good response to carbamazepine, but about half reported the *re-emergence of mood swings* after 2 years of continuous treatment (Post *et al.* 1990). This finding suggests that in some patients tolerance to the mood-stabilizing properties of carbamazepine may attenuate the therapeutic effect.

Valproate Valproate is increasingly used in the treatment of acute mania and therefore evidence of its longer-term maintenance effects is needed. Bowden *et al.* (2000) randomized 372 patients to 1-year maintenance treatment with valproate, lithium, and placebo. There were no significant differences between the three treatments on the primary outcome measure of time to recurrence, but patients on valproate had better outcomes on a number of secondary measures including lower depression scores and lower rates of discontinuation.

There are numerous case series indicating that valproate may have useful prophylactic effects in patients with refractory bipolar illness, even when there has been a poor response to lithium and carbamazepine. In these studies valproate has often been combined with lithium or other mood stabilizers (see Frye *et al.* 2000).

There are also case series documenting improvement of maintenance treatment when lamotrigine or gabapentin have been added to unsuccessful mood-stabilizing regimens. Controlled trials of these treatments are awaited (see Nassir-Ghaemi and Gaughan 2000).

Antipsychotic drugs In clinical practice, patients with bipolar disorder are sometimes maintained on *antipsychotic drugs*. It is usually wise to minimize this form of treatment where possible because antipsychotic drugs do not protect against depression and may be more liable to cause tardive dyskinesia in bipolar patients. Whether newer antipsychotic drugs such as risperidone and olanzapine will find a place in the maintenance treatment of bipolar illness remains to be seen.

Psychotherapy

Cognitive therapy

Unipolar depression

As noted above, there is some evidence that cognitive therapy given during an acute phase of depression decreases the risk of subsequent relapse and recurrence. There is also growing interest in the use of continuation and maintenance treatment with cognitive therapy, particularly in patients who have *residual depressive symptomatology* and are thereby at increased risk of relapse. For example, Paykel *et al.* (1999) studied 158 patients who experienced significant residual symptoms after treatment of an episode of major depression. All patients received clinical management and continuation treatment with antidepressant medication and half also received 16 sessions of cognitive therapy. Over the next 16 months, the relapse rate in the patients receiving cognitive therapy was 29%, compared with 47% in the group who received clinical management only.

Bipolar disorder

Psychotherapy has been less studied in bipolar patients but cognitive techniques may be valuable in helping patients accept their illness and the need for medical treatment (Jamison and Goodwin, 1990). A randomized study showed that education about early signs of relapse, reduced rates of manic illness in bipolar patients over 18 months by 30% (Perry *et al.*, 1999).

Interpersonal therapy

In patients with recurrent depressive episodes, *interpersonal therapy* given once monthly delayed, but did not prevent, depressive relapse compared with standard clinical management. In the same study, interpersonal therapy was less effective than imipramine maintenance treatment and the combination of psychotherapy and imipramine was no better than imipramine alone (Frank *et al.* 1990). However, a more recent study in elderly depressed patients found that a combination of nortriptyline and interpersonal therapy was superior to nortriptyline and clinical management in preventing depressive relapse over 3 years (Reynolds *et al.* 1999) (Box 11.5).

The assessment of depressive disorders

The steps in assessment are:

- to decide whether the diagnosis is depressive disorder;
- to judge the severity of the disorder, including the risk of suicide;
- to form an opinion about the causes;
- to assess the patient's social resources;
- to gauge the effect of the disorder on other people.

Box 11.5 Effect of nortriptyline and interpersonal therapy (IPT) on relapse rate over 3 years in depressed patients aged 60 years and over

Treatment	n	Relapse rate (95% CI)
Nortriptyline + IPT	22	20% (4–36)
Nortriptyline	24	43% (25–61)
IPT and placebo	21	64% (45–83)
Placebo	29	90% (79–100)

Diagnosis depends on thorough *history taking* and examination of the *physical and mental state*. It has been discussed earlier in this chapter. Particular care should be taken not to overlook a depressive disorder in the patient who does not complain spontaneously of being depressed ('masked depression'). It is equally important not to diagnose a depressive disorder simply on the grounds of prominent depressive symptoms; the latter could be part of another disorder, for example, a general medical condition. It should also be remembered that certain drugs both legal and illegal can induce depression (see p. 479 and Chapter 18).

The *history of previous mood disturbance* is important in assessment. Some patients will have had recurrent episodes of mood disorder. A history of these episodes often provides clues to the probable course of the current disorder and its response to treatment. It is particularly important to ask about possible previous episodes of *mania*, even if mild and short-lived. If there is a history of mania, the mood disorder is bipolar. Interviews with relatives and close friends may help to establish whether such episodes have occurred.

The *severity* of the disorder is judged from the symptoms. Considerable severity is indicated by 'biological' symptoms, hallucinations, and delusions, particularly the latter two. It is also important to assess how the depressive disorder has reduced the patient's capacity to work or to engage

in family life and social activities. In this assessment, the duration and course of the condition
should be taken into account as well as the severity
of the present symptoms. Not only does the length
of history affect prognosis, but it also gives an indication of the patient's capacity to tolerate further
distress. A long-continued disorder, even if not
severe, can bring the patient to the point of desper-
ation. The *risk of suicide* must be judged in every
case (the methods of assessment are described on
p. 515).

Aetiology is assessed next, with reference to
precipitating, predisposing, and maintaining
factors. No attempt need be made to allocate the
syndrome to an exclusively 'endogenous' or 'reactive' category; instead, the importance of all relevant risk factors should be evaluated in every case.

Provoking causes may be psychological and social
(the 'life events' discussed earlier in this chapter),
or they may be physical illness and its treatment.
In assessing such cases, it is good practice to
enquire routinely into the patient's work, finances,
family life, social activities, general living conditions, and physical health. Problems in these areas
may be recent and acute, or may take the form of
chronic background difficulties such as prolonged
marital tension, problems with children, and financial hardship.

The patient's *social resources* are considered next.
Enquires should cover family, friends, and work. A
loving family can help to support a patient through
a period of depressive disorder by providing
company, encouraging him when he has lost confidence, and guiding him into suitable activities. For
some patients, work is a valuable social resource,
providing distraction and comradeship. For others
it is a source of stress. A careful assessment is
needed in each case.

The *effects of the disorder on other people* must be
considered carefully. The most obvious problems
arise when a severely depressed patient is the
mother of young children who depend on her. This
clinical observation has been confirmed in objective studies which have demonstrated that depressive disorder in either parent is associated with

emotional disorder in the children (Cooper and
Murray 1998). It is important to consider whether
the patient could endanger other people by
remaining at work, for example, as a bus driver.
When there are *depressive delusions*, it is necessary to
consider what would happen if the patient were to
act on them. For example, severely depressed
mothers may occasionally kill their children
because they believe them doomed to suffer if they
remain alive.

The management of depressive disorders

This section starts with the management of a
patient with a depressive disorder of moderate or
greater severity. The first question is whether the
patient requires *in-patient or day-patient care*. The
answer depends on the *severity of the disorder* and the
quality of the patient's *social resources*. In judging
severity, particular attention should be paid to the
risk of suicide (or any risk to the life or welfare of
family members, particularly dependent children)
and to any failure to eat or drink that might
endanger the patient's life. Provided that these
risks are absent, most patients with a supportive
family can be treated at home, even when severely
depressed. Patients who live alone, or whose families cannot care for them during the day, may need
in-patient or day-patient care, unless intensive
community treatment is available.

If the patient is to remain out of hospital, the
next question is whether he should continue to
work. If the disorder is mild, work can provide a
valuable distraction from depressive thoughts and
a source of companionship. When the disorder is
more severe, retardation, poor concentration, and
lack of drive are likely to impair performance at
work, and such failure may add to the patient's feelings of hopelessness. In severe disorders, there may
be dangers to other people if the patient remains at
his job.

The need for *antidepressant drug treatment* should
be considered next. This treatment is indicated for

most patients with a *major depressive syndrome* of at least moderate severity, and particularly those with *melancholic symptoms*. Other indications include a family history or personal history of depression, particularly if there has been a clear response to drug treatment. *Dysthymia* is also an indication for antidepressant medication but the role of antidepressants in *minor affective disorders* is not established.

Choice of antidepressant drug

Several kinds of antidepressant drug treatment are available, and the choice should be made according to the needs of the individual patient, with particular consideration of likely side-effects. These are fully described in Chapter 21. *Tricyclic antidepressants* may be the first choice for patients with severe depression, and particularly for depressed in-patients. For severely ill patients unable to tolerate tricyclics or where there are medical contraindications or a high risk of deliberate overdose, *venlafaxine* is a suitable alternative.

Newer antidepressants such as *SSRIs* should be used for most other depressed patients because of their ease of dosing, lack of toxicity in overdose, and better tolerability, particularly in the medium and longer term. SSRIs (or clomipramine) should be used when a depressive disorder occurs in the context of an obsessional disorder (see p. 247). Finally, *trazodone* or *mirtazapine* may be considered if patients need sedation but anticholinergic effects are contraindicated or there is a risk of deliberate overdose.

The dosage of these drugs, the precautions to be observed in using them, and the instructions to be given to patients are described in Chapter 21. Here it is necessary only to emphasize again the importance of explaining to the patient that, although side-effects will appear quickly, the therapeutic effect is likely to be delayed for 2 weeks, with maximum improvement occurring over 6–12 weeks. During this time patients should be seen regularly to provide suitable clinical management (see above); those with more severe disorders may

need to be seen every 2 or 3 days, and other patients once a week. It is important to make sure that the drugs are taken in the prescribed dose. Patients should be warned about the effects of *taking alcohol*. They should be advised about *driving,* particularly that they should not drive while experiencing sedative side-effects or any other effects that might impair their performance in an emergency.

The use of ECT

ECT will seldom be part of the first-line treatment of depression and will usually be considered only for patients already admitted to hospital. The only indication for ECT as a first measure is the need to bring about improvement as rapidly as possible. In practice this applies to two main groups of patients: those who refuse to drink enough fluid to maintain an adequate output of urine (including the rare cases of depressive stupor), and those who present a highly dangerous suicidal risk.

Occasionally, ECT is indicated for a patient who is suffering such extreme distress that the most rapid form of treatment is deemed justifiable. Such cases are rare. It should be remembered that, with the exception of patients who are unresponsive to antidepressant drugs, the effects of ECT differ from those of antidepressant drugs in greater rapidity of action rather than in the final therapeutic result. In patients with *depressive psychosis*, ECT is considerably more effective than a tricyclic antidepressant given alone, but probably about the same therapeutic effect can be achieved, albeit more slowly, if a combination of an antidepressant drug and an antipsychotic drug is used.

Activity

The need for *suitable activity* should be considered for every patient. Depressed patients give up activities and withdraw from other people. In this way they become deprived of social stimulation and rewarding experiences, and their original feelings of depression are increased. It is important to make sure that the patient is occupied adequately, though he should not be pushed into activities where he is likely to fail because of slowness or poor concentration. Hence there is a fairly narrow range of activity that is appropriate for the individual depressed patient, and the range changes as the illness runs its course. If the patient remains at home, it is important to discuss with relatives how much he should be encouraged to do each day. If he is in hospital, the question should be decided by the clinical team. Relatives may also need to be helped to accept the disorder as an illness and to avoid criticizing the patient.

Psychotherapy

The kind of appropriate psychological treatment should also be decided in every case. As noted earlier, all depressed patients require support, encouragement, and a thorough explanation that they are suffering from illness and not moral failure. Similar counselling of partners and other family members is often useful.

The use of one of the more specific psychotherapies discussed earlier should also be considered. These treatments can be used as the sole therapy for patients with mild-to-moderate depression without melancholic features, particularly when the patient prefers not to take drug therapy (Depression Guideline Panel 1993). The kind of psychotherapy used depends largely on the availability of a suitably trained therapist and the preference of the patient. The more structured therapies (such as interpersonal therapy and cognitive therapy) have greater efficacy in the treatment of depression. The therapeutic response to antidepressant drugs is usually quicker than that to psychotherapy.

In general, there is little evidence that *combining specific psychotherapy with medication* adds much to the effect of the latter in resolving an acute depressive episode (Depression Guideline Panel 1993). In individual patients, however, it often seems worthwhile tackling psychosocial problems that make an important contribution to the depression. In particular, *marital therapy* can be a helpful addition in depressed patients with marital problems.

If the depressive disorder is severe, too much discussion of problems at an early stage is likely to increase the patient's feeling of hopelessness. Therapy directed to self-examination is particularly likely to make the disorder worse. During intervals between acute episodes, such therapy may be given to patients who have recurrent depressive disorders largely caused by their ways of reacting to life events.

Resistant depression

If a depressive disorder does not respond within a reasonable time to a chosen combination of antidepressant drugs, graded activity, and psychological treatment, the plan should be reviewed. The first step is to check again that the patient has been *taking medication* as prescribed. If not, the reasons should be sought. The patient may be convinced that no treatment can help, or may find the side-effects unpleasant. The diagnosis should also be reviewed carefully, and a check made that important stressful life events or continuing difficulties have not been overlooked.

If this enquiry reveals nothing, antidepressants should be continued at increased dose if possible. With certain tricyclic antidepressants, particularly in doses greater than 150 mg daily, it may be worth checking plasma concentrations (see p. 678). If it becomes clear that the patient is not improving, a number of further steps can be taken (Table 11.9).

Change in antidepressant drug treatment

If a patient cannot tolerate a full dose of an antidepressant of one class, for example, a tricyclic antidepressant, it is worthwhile trying another kind of drug that may be better tolerated such as an SSRI or venlafaxine. Some patients do not respond to one class of antidepressant despite an adequate trial, but improve if switched to an antidepressant of a different class. Overall, about 50% of depressed patients who do not respond to a primary antidepressant improve when another antidepressant is substituted (Depression Guideline Panel 1993).

Table 11.9 Some pharmacological treatments for resistant depression

Increase antidepressant to maximum tolerated dose; measure tricyclic antidepressant levels; if patient has depressive psychosis add an antipsychotic drug; try different class of antidepressant drug, including venlafaxine

Add lithium to antidepressant drug treatment

Add tri-iodothyronine to tricyclic antidepressant treatment

MAOIs (can be usefully combined with lithium)

ECT

Usually such 'switch' studies are open in design and cannot take account of spontaneous improvement. However, there is evidence from controlled investigations that both venlafaxine and the MAOI, tranylcypromine are effective in patients resistant to other antidepressant medications (Nolen *et al.* 1988; Poirier and Boyer 1999). Nevertheless, in view of the food and drug interactions with MAOIs, it is unusual to use them early in drug-resistant depression unless a patient has clear-cut features of atypical depression (see above) or has responded well to them in the past.

Augmentation of antidepressant drug treatment

In switching antidepressant preparations, a problem is that withdrawal of the first compound may not be straightforward. Patients may have gained some small benefit from the treatment, for example, improved sleep or reduced tension, and this benefit may be lost. Also, if the first medication is stopped quickly, withdrawal symptoms may result (see Chapter 21); however, if the dose is reduced gradually, the changeover in medication may be protracted and may not be easily tolerated by a depressed and despairing patient.

For this reason, in patients unresponsive to first-line medication it may be more appropriate to add a second compound to the antidepressant – so-called '*augmentation therapy*'. A disadvantage of augmentation therapy is the increased risk of adverse effects through drug interaction.

Lithium augmentation

We have already seen that data from randomized trials indicates that lithium can be effective in the treatment of resistant depression. Provided that there are no contraindications (see p. 700), the addition of lithium to antidepressant drug treatment is usually safe and well tolerated. About half of depressed patients will show a useful response over 1–3 weeks. Lithium can be added to any primary antidepressant medication with good effect, although combination with SSRIs and venlafaxine should be used with caution because of the risk of *5-HT neurotoxicity* (see p. 688). In augmentation treatment, the aim should be to obtain the same lithium level as that used for prophylactic purposes (0.5–0.8 mmol/l) and the dosage schedule is the same.

Tri-iodothyronine

Among patients who have not responded to tricyclic antidepressants, some improve promptly when tri-iodothyronine (20–50 μg) is added. This improvement is unlikely to be a pharmacokinetic effect because it is not accompanied by a change in plasma concentrations of the antidepressant drug. There seems to be no relationship between thyroid status and the efficacy of this combination. In a study of depressed out-patients who had not responded to imipramine, the addition of tri-iodothyronine (37.5 μg) was as effective as the addition of lithium and both were superior to the addition of placebo (Joffe *et al.* 1993).

A meta-analysis of tri-iodothyronine augmentation gave mixed results. When all evaluable studies were incorporated, patients treated with tri-iodothyronine augmentation were twice as likely to respond as controls (OR = 2.09, NNT = 4.3). However, when only randomized trials were considered, the therapeutic effects of tri-iodothyronine were substantially less and not statistically significant (OR = 1.53, NNT = 12.5) (Aronson *et al.* 1996).

In general, the combination of tri-iodothyronine and tricyclics appears safe, but it should be used with caution in patients with cardiovascular disease. There are no controlled trials of tri-iodothyronine addition in patients receiving newer antidepressants, but in clinical practice the combination is sometimes used.

MAOI combinations

In patients who do not respond to the augmentation strategies described above, the use of an *MAOI* may be considered. At this stage patients often receive lithium as part of their treatment; if the lithium is well tolerated, it should be continued with the MAOI because evidence from open studies indicates that this combined treatment can be effective in refractory depressed states (Price *et al.* 1985). MAOIs must not be given with clomipramine, SSRIs, or venlafaxine, but can be added cautiously to some tricyclic antidepressants (the method of addition is explained on p. 689).

It is not established whether MAOIs and tricyclic antidepressants can potentiate one another in resistant depression (see above). However, this combination can help to prevent MAOI-induced sleep disturbance, although there is an increased risk of weight gain and postural hypotension (see Chalmers and Cowen 1990). Of the MAOIs available, tranylcypromine is often used for the more severely depressed patients, but it has been implicated more often than phenelzine and isocarboxazid in food and drug interactions. The reversible type-A selective MAOI, *moclobemide*, is the safest of the MAOIs from the point of view of food and drug interaction (Dingemanse 1993), but it has not been studied systematically in resistant depression.

Pindolol

Pindolol is a β-adrenoceptor antagonist which also binds to 5-HT$_{1A}$ receptors. Animal studies indicate that 5-HT$_{1A}$ autoreceptor antagonists can potentiate the ability of SSRIs to facilitate 5-HT neurotransmission. From this it has been suggested that pindolol addition to SSRIs might speed the *onset of antidepressant effect* and perhaps be of value in *treatment-resistant depression*. Both these matters are currently controversial. The best-designed controlled trial of pindolol addition in SSRI-unresponsive patients showed no antidepressant effect (Perez *et al.* 1999). However, brain imaging studies suggests that the dose of pindolol employed (7.5 mg daily) may have been insufficient to provide adequate blockade of human 5-HT$_{1A}$ receptors (Rabiner *et al.* 2000).

Olanzapine

The atypical antipsychotic agent, olanzapine, has modest antidepressant properties in patients with schizophrenia. In a small, randomized controlled trial, the addition of olanzapine to ineffective fluoxetine treatment produced a significantly greater antidepressant effect than placebo addition or olanzapine as a sole treatment. The mechanism of this potentiation requires further study but it is possible that in the presence of fluoxetine, the 5-HT$_2$ receptor antagonist properties of olanzapine might facilitate dopamine release in mesolimbic regions. Further studies on the efficacy of atypical antipsychotic agents in resistant depression are needed.

The use of ECT in resistant depression

If severe depression persists, ECT should be considered. ECT is often beneficial to patients who have not responded to antidepressant drugs, and it is probably more effective than drugs in the most severe depressions, particularly when psychotic features are present. Nevertheless, naturalistic studies suggest that the response rate in depressed patients *resistant to medication* (about 50%) is lower than that expected in patients who are not medication resistant (about 80%) (Prudic *et al.* 1990).

It is important to note that, among patients who have not responded to full-dose antidepressant medication, the relapse rate in the year after ECT may be as high as 50%. This may be because patients are often continued on the same antidepressant medication to which they previously failed to respond (Sackheim *et al.* 1990). In these circumstances it seems reasonable to use an antidepressant of a different class or lithium for continuation treatment after ECT, but there is currently no evidence that this procedure lowers the relapse rate.

Other measures

Continuing support is required for patients who do not respond to treatment. Lack of improvement increases the pessimism experienced by the depressed patient. Hence it is important to give reassurance that depressive disorders have a good chance of recovering eventually, whether or not treatment speeds recovery. Meanwhile, if the patient is not too depressed, any problems that have contributed to his depressed state should be discussed further. Techniques derived from cognitive therapy can be used to help the patient to limit distorted thinking and judgement. In resistant cases, it is particularly important to watch carefully for suicidal intentions.

Prevention of relapse and recurrence

Drug treatment

Continuation therapy

After recovery, the patient should be followed up for several months by the psychiatric team or general practitioner. If the recovery appears to have been brought about by an antidepressant drug, the drug should usually be continued for about 6 months and then gradually withdrawn over several weeks. If residual symptoms are still present, it is safer not to withdraw medication. At follow-up interviews, a careful watch should be kept for *signs of discontinuation reactions* or *relapse*.

Relatives should be warned that relapse may occur, and they should be asked to report any signs of it.

Maintenance treatment

Major depression is often recurrent, and long-term maintenance treatment may need to be considered. The risk factors for recurrence have been noted above (p. 305). In addition, the clinician will need to take into account other individual factors:

- the likely impact of a recurrence on the patient's life;
- the previous response to drug treatment;
- the patient's view of long-term drug treatment.

It is estimated that, among patients who have had three episodes of major depression, the chance of another episode is 90% (National Institute of Mental Health 1985). The usual recommendation is that maintenance drug treatment should be considered if a patient has had two episodes of depression in a 5-year period, particularly if there is a family history of recurrent major depression, bipolar disorder, or onset at an early age (Prien 1992).

Choice of medication

In most patients, the choice of antidepressant will be derived from their response in the acute or continuation phase of treatment. In this case, the same medication can be continued, if possible at the same dose. As noted earlier, newer antidepressant drugs are better tolerated in the longer term and may be preferred for maintenance treatment. If a change needs to be made because of adverse effects (for example, sexual dysfunction with SSRIs), an alternative choice should be determined by side-effect profile.

Lithium is also effective for long-term maintenance of recurrent depression. Its adverse effect profile and the need for plasma monitoring means that it will not be a first choice for most patients but its use should be considered if there is any history of manic episodes, even where these have been mild and transient. In addition, lithium will sometimes be effective in patients who do not respond to maintenance treatment with antidepressants.

Other measures

If a depressive disorder was related to self-imposed stressors, such as overwork or complicated social relationships, the patient should be encouraged to change to a lifestyle that is less likely to lead to further illness. These readjustments may be helped by psychotherapy, which may be individual, marital, or group therapy. As noted above, cognitive therapy appears to be helpful in lowering the risk of relapse in patients with residual depressive symptomatology. Whether this effect extends to patients with other risk factors for frequent recurrence is not known.

The assessment of mania

In the assessment of mania, the steps are the same as those for depressive disorders, as outlined above:

♦ decide the diagnosis;

♦ assess the severity of the disorder;

♦ form an opinion about the causes;

♦ assess the patient's social resources;

♦ judge the effects on other people.

Diagnosis depends on a *careful history and examination*. Whenever possible, the history should be taken from relatives as well as from the patient because the latter may not recognize the extent of his abnormal behaviour. Differential diagnosis has been discussed earlier in this chapter. It is always important to remember that mildly disinhibited behaviour can result from frontal lobe lesions (such as tumours) as well as from mania. There should be a routine urine screen for illegal substances.

Severity is judged next. For this purpose, it is essential to interview an informant as well as the patient. Manic patients may exert some self-control during an interview with a doctor, and may then behave in a disinhibited and grandiose way immediately afterwards. At an early stage of mania, the doctor can easily be misled and may lose the opportunity to persuade the patient to enter hospital before causing himself long-term difficulties, for example, ill-judged decisions or unjustified extravagance.

Where possible, it is important to identify any life events that may have provoked the onset of manic illness. Some manic episodes follow physical illness, treatment by drugs (especially steroids or antidepressants), or operations. *Sleep deprivation* may trigger mania in some susceptible individuals.

The patient's resources and the effect of the illness on other people are assessed in the ways described above for depressive disorders. Even for the most supportive family, it is extremely difficult to care for a manic patient at home for more than a few days unless the disorder is exceptionally mild. The patient's responsibilities in the care of dependent children or at work should always be considered carefully.

The management of manic patients

Acute episodes

The first decision is whether to *admit the patient to hospital*. In all but the mildest cases, admission is nearly always advisable to protect the patient from the consequences of his own behaviour. If the disorder is not too severe, the patient will usually agree to enter hospital after some persuasion. When the disorder is more severe, compulsory admission is likely to be needed.

Clinical management

Development of a *therapeutic alliance* with the manic patient is an important goal of treatment although lack of insight and anger at involuntary detention can make this a testing and time-consuming process. It is best to use an understanding, yet firm, approach which minimizes confrontation. For example, it is often possible to avoid an argument by taking advantage of the manic patient's easy distractibility; instead of refusing his demands, it is better to delay until his attention turns to another topic that he can be encouraged to pursue. In hospital, nursing staff play a pivotal role in this kind of management where they attempt to provide manic patients with a low-stimulus and safe environment which limits confrontations and ill-judged sexual liaisons.

Supportive, reality-orientated psychotherapy is an important part of treatment and may need to be extended to partners and family who often will have suffered great strain through the manic episode. *Educational sessions* are important when patients are more settled. Patients may need much practical help to limit financial, legal, and occupational repercussions of the illness.

Medication

Medication plays an important role in the acute management of mania. However, all current drug treatments have limitations in terms of efficacy and tolerability. As noted above, there are differences in practice between different centres and different countries. In the USA, for example, initial treatment with mood stabilizers is encouraged with the aim of limiting antipsychotic medication as much as possible (although the use of antipsychotic agents remains common) (see American Psychiatric Assocation 1994b). In the UK, antipsychotic drugs are generally used as primary agents in acute mania, with mood stabilizers being reserved for longer-term prophylaxis or where the initial response to antipsychotic drugs is unsatisfactory. From this latter viewpoint, the drug management can summarized as follows:

- begin treatment with modest doses of haloperidol (risperidone and olanzapine are alternatives);
- where needed, use adjunctive high-potency benzodiazepines (for example, lorazepam or clonazepam) to prevent the need for high-dose antipsychotic therapy and to ensure satisfactory sleep;
- add a mood stabilizer if the response to this treatment is unsatisfactory (use lithium for 'classical' mania and valproate for mania with atypical features (see above)) or where lithium is contraindicated.

If it is decided to use a mood stabilizer as the initial treatment, the choice lies between lithium and valproate. Valproate is somewhat easier to use and has a faster onset of action. As before, benzodiazepines can be used as an adjunct to reduce overactivity and permit sleep, whilst antipsychotic agents can be reserved for patients unresponsive to these measures.

Progress of a manic episode can be judged not only by the *mental state* and *general behaviour*, but also by the *pattern of sleep* and the regaining of any weight lost during the illness. As progress continues, antipsychotic drug treatment is reduced gradually. It is important not to discontinue the drug too soon; otherwise, there may be a relapse and a return of all the original problems of management.

As explained already (p. 312), *ECT* was used to treat mania before antipsychotic drugs were introduced, but evidence about its effectiveness is still limited. It is appropriate to consider the treatment for the unusual patients who do not respond to drug treatment even when given at maximum doses. In such cases, clinical experience suggests that ECT may often be followed by a significant reduction in symptoms sufficient to allow treatment to be continued with drugs. ECT may also be helpful for *mixed affective states* in which depressive symptoms are prominent.

Whatever treatment is adopted, a careful watch should be kept for symptoms of *depressive disorder*. It should be remembered that transient but profound depressive mood change, accompanied by depressive ideas, is common among manic patients. The clinical picture may also change rapidly to a sustained depressive disorder. If either change happens, the patient may develop suicidal ideas. A sustained change to a depressive syndrome is likely to require antidepressant drug treatment unless the disorder is mild.

Treatment of bipolar depression

Depressive episodes are common in bipolar illness. Treatment of depression in the context of a bipolar disorder can be problematic because standard antidepressant treatments carry a number of disadvantages:

- apparent lower efficacy than in unipolar depression;
- risk of inducing mania;
- risk of inducing rapid cycling.

There is general agreement that the best current treatment of bipolar depression is *lithium*. Lithium is a useful antidepressant in bipolar patients and does not cause mania. On the other hand, it is ineffective in a significant proportion of cases and many bipolar patients become depressed despite taking lithium. In these circumstances, the use of antidepressants is common and SSRIs are a usual choice because they are probably less likely than tricyclics to induce mania or rapid cycling.

Conventional MAOIs are useful in anergic bipolar depression, which is characterized by lethargy and hypersomnia, but the role of moclobemide in this situation is uncertain. There is also interest in possible antidepressant properties of the mood stabilizer *lamotrogine* in bipolar patients. When treating a bipolar depressed patients with an antidepressant, it is prudent to combine the antidepressant with a mood stabilizer because this may lower the risk of mania (for a review see Compton and Nemeroff 2000).

Prevention of relapse and recurrence

Continuation treatment

Since the untreated duration of a manic episode can be several months (see above), some form of *continuation treatment,* as in the management of depression, is advisable for at least 6 months. As a guide, treatment should not be withdrawn finally until patients have been asymptomatic for at least 8 weeks. Withdrawal of lithium should be particularly cautious (for example, by not more than about 100 mg a week) because sudden discontination can lead to 'rebound' mania (Faedda *et al.* 1993).

Maintenance treatment

Medication

We have already seen that the majority of patients with bipolar disorder will experience recurrence, suffering both depressive and manic episodes, though the pattern in individual patients is variable. For patients who have had two or more episodes of illness in less than 5 years, particularly where the illnesses have proved personally disruptive or hazardous, longer-term maintenance treatment should be considered. This will usually involve long-term treatment with a mood stabilizer.

In the UK, lithium is still regarded as the first choice of mood stabilizer, although in the USA valproate is the most popular because of its better tolerability. However, the evidence for its long-term prophylactic efficacy is less complete. In addition, there is evidence that the supervised use of lithium is associated with a decreased risk of suicidal behaviour in bipolar illness.

The practical aspects of using lithium to prevent further episodes are discussed on p. 700. There are two aspects of maintenance that require emphasis. First, patients should be seen and plasma lithium and renal and thyroid function assessed at regular intervals. Second, some patients stop lithium of their own accord because they fear that the drug may have harmful long-term effects or because it makes them feel 'flat'. The risk of stopping lithium suddenly is that it may well lead to relapse. Therefore, patients should be advised to discontinue lithium slowly under supervision.

With carefully supervised follow-up, the chances of relapse can be reduced substantially by maintenance treatment, though lesser degrees of mood change often continue. These mood changes can often be treated successfully with adjunctive antidepressant or antipsychotic drug treatment (Peselow *et al.* 1994). Maintenance antipsychotic treatment should be used as little as possible because of the risk of movement disorders. However, antipsychotic drugs still have a limited place in patients with frequent recurrence who do not benefit from or adhere to mood-stabilizing drugs (Cookson 1998). It is possible that the role of maintenance antipsychotic treatment will grow with the advent of atypical antipsychotic drugs. In the USA, clozapine is sometimes used for the treatment of intractable bipolar illness.

For patients who do not show a good response to lithium, alternative mood-stabilizing drugs can be used. It is possible to use combinations of mood stabilizers, although the risk of adverse reactions is increased.

Rapid-cycling disorder Some patients with bipolar disorder develop rapid-cycling mood disorder (see p. 282). Sometimes this disorder is apparently provoked by antidepressant treatment, in which case the best plan is to try to withdraw the antidepressant drug. Valproate and carbamazepine may have a useful role in the treatment of rapid cycling; for resistant cases, thyroid hormone has been advocated (see Kilzieh and Akiskal 1999).

Psychosocial approaches

Bipolar disorder is often a life-long, disruptive illness which carries a substantial morbidity (Scott 1995). There are several areas of psychosocial function where problems may arise:

- adjustment to diagnosis and need for lifestyle limitations;
- interpersonal and marital difficulties;
- occupational problems;
- misuse of both illegal and legal substances;
- problems relating to compliance with medication.

There are relatively few formal studies of specific psychotherapy, but Jamison (1992) has stressed that cognitive and educational techniques are an important part of a collaborative management plan. The issues that should be addressed include:

- education of patients and families about the symptoms, course and treatment of bipolar illness;
- advice about lifestyle (regular social and sleep routines, avoidance of illicit drugs);
- identification and avoidance of triggers for relapse (for example, sleep deprivation, substance misuse);

- identification of early subjective signs of relapse (for example, feeling driven, sleeping badly) with contingency plans for action;
- education (compliance therapy) about the importance of medication. Sensitivity to side-effects and active measures to reduce them.

Although there are some useful drug therapies for bipolar illness, the effectiveness of treatment in clinical practice is often disappointing. The use of the psychosocial measures outlined above should enhance the overall effectiveness of treatment plans but randomized trials are needed to confirm this proposal.

Further reading

Goodwin, F. K. and Jamison, K. R. (1990). *Manic Depressive Illness*. Oxford University Press, Oxford. Comprehensive overview of clinical and scientific basis of bipolar illness.

Jamison, K. R. (1997) *An unquiet mind*. Picador, London. A superb autobiographical account of the experience of bipolar illness and its treatment

Kraepelin, E. (1921). Manic-depressive insanity and paranoia (transl. R. M. Barclay), pp.1–164. Churchill Livingstone, Edinburgh. [Reprinted in 1976 by Arno Press, New York] (The classical account. See especially the description of untreated mania – seldom seen today.)

Lewis, A. J. (1934). Melancholia: a clinical survey of depressive states. *Journal of Mental Science* **80**, 277–378. [Reprinted in Lewis, A. J. (1967). *Inquiries in Psychiatry*, pp. 30–117. Routledge and Kegan Paul, London]. (This landmark study contains a detailed account of the clinical picture of depressive disorder.)

Schizophrenia and schizophrenia-like disorders

CHAPTER 12

Schizophrenia and schizophrenia-like disorders

Of all the major psychiatric syndromes, schizophrenia is much the most difficult to define and describe. The main reason for this difficulty is that, over the past 100 years, many widely divergent concepts of schizophrenia have been held in different countries and by different psychiatrists. Radical differences of opinion persist to the present day. If these conflicting ideas are to be made intelligible, it is useful to start with a simple comparison between two basic concepts – *acute schizophrenia* and *chronic schizophrenia*. Such a comparison can pave the way for a description of the many varieties of clinical picture encountered in clinical practice, and for discussion of the main theories and arguments about schizophrenia.

Accordingly, after a brief section on epidemiology, the features of 'typical' acute and chronic syndromes are described. The reader should bear in mind that these will be idealized descriptions, but it is useful to oversimplify at first before introducing controversial issues.

Essentially, the predominant clinical features in acute schizophrenia are *delusions, hallucinations*, and *interference with thinking* (Table 12.1). Features of this kind are often called 'positive' symptoms. Some patients recover from the acute illness, whilst others progress to the chronic syndrome. By contrast, the main features of chronic schizophrenia are *apathy*, *lack of drive*, *slowness*, and *social withdrawal* (Table 12.2). These features are often called 'negative' symptoms. Once the chronic syndrome is established, few patients recover completely.

Most of the disagreements about the diagnosis of schizophrenia are concerned with the acute syndrome. The criteria for diagnosis are concerned with both the pattern of symptoms and the course of the disorder. There are disagreements about both the range of symptoms that are required and the length of time that these symptoms should have been present in order to make the diagnosis. This point is illustrated later in the chapter when the criteria for diagnosis in DSM-IV and ICD-10 are discussed.

Epidemiology

Schizophrenia is a disorder with a *low incidence but a relatively high prevalence*. Estimates of the incidence and prevalence of schizophrenia depend on the criteria for diagnosis and the population surveyed (problems of diagnosis are discussed on

Table 12.1 **The most frequent symptoms of acute schizophrenia**

Symptom	Frequency (%)
Lack of insight	97
Auditory hallucinations	74
Ideas of reference	70
Suspiciousness	66
Flatness of affect	66
Voices speaking to the patient	65
Delusional mood	64
Delusions of persecution	64
Thought alienation	2
Thoughts spoken aloud	50

Source: World Health Organization (1973).

Table 12.2 Behavioural characteristics of chronic schizophrenic patients in rank order of frequency

Characteristic	Frequency (%)
Social withdrawal	74
Underactivity	56
Lack of conversation	54
Few leisure interests	50
Slowness	48
Overactivity	41
Odd ideas	34
Depression	34
Odd behaviour	34
Neglect of appearance	30
Odd postures and movements	25
Threats or violence	25
Poor mealtime behaviour	13
Socially embarrassing behaviour	8
Sexually unusual behaviour	8
Suicidal attempts	4
Incontinence	4

Source: Creer and Wing (1975).

p. 335). The annual incidence using current diagnostic criteria is probably between 0.17 and 0.54 per 1000 population using a broad definition of schizophrenia. For more restrictive diagnoses such as DSM-IV or ICD-10, the incidence is about two to three times lower (see Jablensky 2000b). The onset of schizophrenia characteristically occurs between the ages of 15 and 45. While schizophrenia occurs equally in men and women, the mean age of onset is about 5 years earlier in men.

The prevalence of schizophrenia is probably about 1.4–4.6 per thousand population at risk (Jablensky 2000b) and is similar in different countries. For example, the British National Psychiatric Morbidity Survey found an annual prevalence of 'functional psychosis' of 4 per 1000 (Jenkins *et al.* 1998). There are, however, exceptions to this general uniformity of rates with high rates being reported in certain isolated communities in Sweden and Finland and in the *Afro-Carribean population* in the UK (see section on aetiology). By contrast, a consistently low prevalence of about 1.2 per 1000 has been reported among the Hutterites and the Anabaptist sect in the USA (Nimgaonkar *et al.* 2000). These reported differences in prevalence may have more than one cause. First, they may reflect differences in diagnostic criteria. Second, they may be affected by differences in migration. For example, people predisposed to schizophrenia may stay in the remote north of Sweden because they are more able to tolerate extreme isolation, whilst those predisposed to schizophrenia may leave a Hutterite community because they are less able to tolerate a close-knit society. Finally, there may be differences between populations in their genetic susceptibility to schizophrenia.

Some recent studies have suggested that the incidence of schizophrenia, as measured by the diagnosis rate in first admissions to hospital, may be falling in industrialized countries. For example, Eagles and Whalley (1985) reported a 40% fall in first admission rates for schizophrenia in Scotland between 1969 and 1978. This observation has been supported by some, but not all, subsequent investigations (Jablensky 2000b). Whether the observed decline represents a true fall in the inception rate for schizophrenia remains an open question; for example, Kendell *et al.* (1993) found that in Scotland, at least, the apparent decline may be attributable to changing diagnostic criteria and inaccurate recording of true first admissions.

Epidemiological studies of the demographic and social correlates of schizophrenia are considered later under aetiology.

Clinical features

The acute sydrome

Some of the main clinical features are illustrated by a short description of a patient. A previously healthy 20-year-old male student had been behaving in an increasingly odd way. At times he appeared angry and told his friends that he was being persecuted; at other times he was seen to be laughing to himself for no apparent reason. For several months he had seemed increasingly preoccupied with his own thoughts. His academic work had deteriorated. When interviewed, he was restless and awkward. He described hearing voices commenting on his actions and abusing him. He said that he believed that the police had conspired with his university teachers to harm his brain with poisonous gases and take away his thoughts. He also believed that other people could read his thoughts.

This case history illustrates the following common features of acute schizophrenia: prominent *persecutory ideas* with accompanying *hallucinations*, gradual *social withdrawal* and *impaired performance at work*, and the odd idea that other people can *read one's thoughts*. In describing the features of schizophrenia here, it is assumed that the reader has read the descriptions of symptoms and signs in Chapter 1. Reference will be made to that chapter in the following account.

In appearance and behaviour some patients with acute schizophrenia are entirely normal. Others seem changed and different, although not always in a way that would immediately point to psychosis. They may be preoccupied with their health, their appearance, religion, or other intense interests. Social withdrawal may occur. Some patients smile or laugh without obvious reason. Some appear to be constantly perplexed. Some are restless and noisy, or show sudden and unexpected changes of behaviour. Others retire from company, spending a long time in their rooms, perhaps lying immobile on the bed apparently preoccupied in thought.

The speech often reflects an underlying thought disorder. In the early stages, there is vagueness in the patient's talk that makes it difficult to grasp his meaning. Some patients have difficulty in dealing with abstract ideas (a phenomenon called concrete thinking). Other patients become preoccupied with vague pseudoscientific or mystical ideas.

When the disturbance is more severe, two characteristic kinds of abnormality may occur. Disorders of the *stream of thought* include *pressure of thought*, *poverty of thought*, and *thought blocking*, which are described on p. 12. Thought withdrawal (the conviction that one's thoughts have been taken away) is sometimes classified as a disorder of the stream of thought, but it is more usefully considered as a form of delusion (see p. 18).

Disorders of the *form of thought* are reflected in the *loosening of association* between expressed ideas. This may be detected in illogical thinking (for example, 'knight's move' p. 13) or talking past the point (*Vorbeireden*). In the severest form of loosening, the structure and coherence of thinking is lost, so that utterances are jumbled (word salad or verbigeration). Some patients use ordinary words or phrases in unusual ways (metonyms or paraphrases), and a few coin new words (neologisms).

Abnormalities of mood are common and are of three main kinds. First, there may be sustained abnormalities of mood such as anxiety, depression, irritability, or euphoria. Second, there may be *blunting of affect*, sometimes known as flattening of affect. Essentially this is sustained emotional indifference or diminution of emotional response. Third, there is *incongruity of affect*. Here the expressed mood is not in keeping with the situation or with the patient's own feelings. For example, a patient may laugh when told about a bereavement. Incongruity of affect is usually observed as a sign, and it can be difficult to distinguish from social gaucherie. Occasionally patients are able to describe this experience, which can resolve diagnostic doubt. Without such a description, although the abnormality of incongruity of affect is said to be highly characteristic of schizophrenia, different interviewers tend to disagree about its presence.

Auditory hallucinations are among the most frequent symptoms. They may take the form of noises, music, single words, brief phrases, or whole conversations. They may be unobtrusive or so severe as to cause great distress. Some voices seem to give commands to the patient. Some patients hear their own thoughts apparently spoken out loud either as they think them (*Gedankenlautwerden*) or immediately afterwards (*écho de la pensée*). Some voices seem to discuss the patient in the third person. Others comment on his actions. As described later, these last three symptoms can have particular diagnostic value.

Visual hallucinations are less frequent and usually occur with other kinds of hallucination. Tactile, olfactory, gustatory, and somatic hallucinations are reported by some patients. They are often interpreted in a delusional way; for example, hallucinatory sensations in the lower abdomen are attributed to unwanted sexual interference by a persecutor.

Delusions are characteristic. *Primary delusions* (see p. 15) are infrequent and are difficult to identify with certainty. Delusions may originate against a background of so-called *primary delusional mood* (*Wahnstimmung*, see p. 15). *Persecutory delusions* are common, but are not specific to schizophrenia. Less common but of greater diagnostic value are *delusions of reference and of control*, and delusions about the *possession of thought*. The latter are delusions that thoughts are being inserted into or withdrawn from one's mind, or 'broadcast' to other people (see p. 18).

In acute schizophrenia, orientation is usually normal. However, it is now recognized that patients with schizophrenia have *generalized deficits in cognitive function*, including learning, memory, perception, and motor skills, and that these are present from the early stages of the illness (see David 2000). Executive function that involves planning and the integration of different cognitive abilities is particularly compromised. *Insight* is usually impaired. Most patients do not accept that their experiences result from illness, but usually ascribe them to the malevolent actions of other people. This lack of insight is often accompanied by unwillingness to accept treatment.

Patients with schizophrenia do not necessarily experience all these symptoms. The clinical picture is variable, as described later in this chapter. At this stage the reader is referred to Table 12.1, which lists the most frequent symptoms found in one large survey.

The chronic syndrome

In contrast with the 'positive' symptoms of the acute syndrome, the chronic syndrome is characterized by thought disorder and the 'negative' symptoms of underactivity, lack of drive, social withdrawal, and emotional apathy. The syndrome can be illustrated by a brief example. A middle-aged man lives in a group home and attends a sheltered workshop. He spends most of his time alone. He is usually dishevelled and unshaven, and cares for himself only when encouraged to do so by others. His social behaviour seems odd and stilted. His speech is slow, and its content is vague and incoherent. He shows few signs of emotion. For several years this clinical picture has changed little except for brief periods of acute symptoms which are usually related to upsets in the ordered life of the hostel.

This description illustrates several of the negative features of what is sometimes called schizophrenic defect state. The most striking feature is diminished *volition*, that is, a lack of drive and initiative. Left to himself, the patient may be inactive for long periods, or may engage in aimless and repeated activity. He withdraws from social encounters and his behaviour may deteriorate in ways that embarrass other people. A few patients neglect themselves to the point of incontinence.

A variety of motor disturbances occur, but most are uncommon. They are outlined here because they are the only symptoms of schizophrenia not described in Chapter 1.

Disorders of motor activity are often called *catatonic*. In the past, a separate syndrome of catatonia was recognized, but nowadays the symptoms more often occur individually than as a distinct syndrome. *Stupor and excitement* are the most striking catatonic symptoms. A patient in stupor is immobile, mute, and unresponsive, although fully conscious. Stupor may change (sometimes quickly) to a state of uncontrolled motor activity and excitement.

Occasionally, schizophrenic patients show a disorder of muscle tone called *waxy flexibility* (or flexibilitas cerea). The patient allows himself to be placed in an awkward posture, which he then maintains apparently without distress for much longer than most people could achieve without severe discomfort. This phenomenon is also called *catalepsy* (a term that is also used to describe similar phenomena in patients who have been hypnotized). Some patients themselves take up odd and uncomfortable postures and maintain them for long periods. At times these postures have obvious symbolic significance (for example crucifixion). Occasionally a patient lies for a long period with his head raised a little above the pillow (the so-called psychological pillow). Healthy people would experience extreme discomfort if they tried to do the same.

Various disorders of movement occur in schizophrenia. A *stereotypy* is a repeated movement that does not appear to be goal directed. It is more complex than a tic. The movement may be repeated in a regular sequence, for example rocking forwards and backwards or rotating the trunk. A *mannerism* is a normal goal-directed movement that appears to have social significance but is odd in appearance, stilted, and out of context, for example, a repeated hand movement resembling a military salute. It is often difficult to decide whether an abnormal movement is a stereotypy or a mannerism, but the distinction is of no diagnostic importance.

Ambitendence is a special form of ambivalence in which a patient begins to make a movement but, before completing it, starts the opposite movement, for example, putting the hand back and forth to an object but without reaching it. Some patients, on the point of entering a room, repeatedly walk backwards and forwards across the threshold. *Mitgehen* is moving a limb in response to slight pressure on it, despite being told to resist the pressure (the last point is important). Mitgehen is often associated with forced grasping, which is repeated grasping (despite instructions to the contrary) at the interviewer's outstretched hand. In automatic obedience the patient obeys every command, though he has first been told not to do so. These disorders were described in more detail by Hamilton (1984) whose account is still unrivalled.

Social behaviour may deteriorate. Self-care may be poor and, particularly in women, the style of dress and presentation may be careful but somewhat inappropriate. Some patients collect and hoard objects, so that their surroundings become cluttered and dirty. Others break social conventions by talking intimately to strangers or shouting obscenities in public.

Speech is often abnormal, showing evidence of thought disorder of the kinds found in the acute syndrome described above. *Affect is* generally blunted; when emotion is shown, it is often incongruous. *Hallucinations* are common, again in any of the forms occurring in the acute syndrome. *Delusions* are often systematized. In chronic schizophrenia, delusions may be held with little emotional response. For example, patients may be convinced that they are being persecuted but show neither fear nor anger. Delusions may also be 'encapsulated' from the rest of the patient's beliefs. Thus, although a patient may be convinced that his private sexual fantasies and practices are widely discussed by strangers, his remaining beliefs may be normal and his working and social life well preserved.

The symptoms and signs are combined in many ways so that the clinical picture is variable. The reader is referred to Table 12.2, which shows the range and frequency of the symptoms and behavioural abnormalities found in one survey of patients with chronic schizophrenia .

Variations of the clinical picture

As anticipated in the introduction to this chapter, so far an account has been given of the typical features of acute and chronic syndromes. Such an account makes description easier, but it is an over-simplification. Two points need to be stressed. First, different features may predominate within a syndrome; for example, in the acute syndrome one patient may have predominantly paranoid delusions, and another mainly thought disorder. Second, some patients have features of both the acute and the chronic syndromes. For example, it is not unusual to see patients with acute schizophrenia who also have negative symptoms in addition to delusions and hallucinations. Clinicians have attempted to identify various clinical subtypes, and these will be described later in the chapter.

Depressive symptoms in schizophrenia

It has been recognized since the time of Kraepelin that *depressive symptoms* commonly occur in schizophrenia, in both the acute and chronic stages. More recently these clinical observations have been confirmed using standardized methods of assessment. It is not uncommon for patients to experience depressive symptoms some time before more florid symptoms of schizophrenia become apparent. In addition, following resolution of psychotic symptoms, about a quarter of patients exhibit persistent and significant depression, which may respond to antidepressant drug treatment.

There are several reasons why depressive symptoms may be associated with schizophrenia:

♦ *Depression may be a side-effect of antipsychotic medication*. This is not the only explanation since depressive symptoms can occur in the absence of antipsychotic drug therapy, for example before the diagnosis of schizophrenia has been made (see above). However, the dopamine receptor antagonist properties of antipsychotic medication might plausibly cause loss of motivation and anhedonia.

♦ In the post-psychotic phase, *depressive symptoms may be a response to recovery of insight* into the nature of the illness and the problems to be faced. Again, this may happen at times, but it does not provide a convincing general explanation.

♦ *Depression may be an integral part of schizophrenia.* This view is supported by the observation that about 50% of patients with acute schizophrenia experience significant depressive symptomatology which improves as the psychosis remits.

It is important that depressive symptoms should not be confused with *motor side-effects of medication* or *negative symptoms*. For a review of the relationship between depression and schizophrenia see Mulholland and Cooper (2000).

Water intoxication in schizophrenia

A few chronic schizophrenic patients drink excessive amounts of water, thus developing a state of *water intoxication* characterized by polyuria and hyponatraemia. When this condition is severe, it may give rise to seizures, coma, visceral and cerebral oedema, and sometimes death. The reasons for this behaviour cannot be explained by the patients and has not been uncovered by investigation. The possible mechanisms include a response to a delusional belief, changes in the secretion of antidiuretic hormone, or abnormalities in the hypothalamic centre that regulates thirst and fluid intake (see Merceir-Guidez and Loas 1998). Treatment involves fluid restriction, but in more severe cases diuretics or urea may be needed.

Factors modifying the clinical features

The amount of *social stimulation* has a considerable effect on the clinical picture. Understimulation increases 'negative' symptoms such as poverty of speech, social withdrawal, apathy, and lack of drive. Overstimulation precipitates 'positive' symptoms such as hallucinations, delusions, and restlessness. Modern treatment is designed to avoid understimulation, and as a result 'negative' features are less frequent than in the past.

The social background of the patient may affect the content of some symptoms. For example, religious delusions are less common now than a century ago. Age also seems to modify the clinical features of schizophrenia. In adolescents and young adults, the clinical features often include thought disorder, mood disturbance, passivity phenomena, thought insertion, and withdrawal. With increasing age paranoid symptomatology is more common, with more organized delusions (Hafner *et al.* 1993).

Low intelligence also affects the clinical features. Patients with learning disability usually present with a less complex clinical picture, sometimes referred to as pfropfschizophrenie (described in Chapter 25, p. 871).

Diagnosis

The development of ideas about schizophrenia

Some of the diagnostic problems encountered today can be understood better with some knowledge of the historical developments of ideas about schizophrenia.

In the nineteenth century, one view was that all serious mental disorders were expressions of a single entity which Griesinger called *Einheitpsychose* (unitary psychosis). The alternative view, which was put forward by Morel in France, was that mental disorders could be separated and classified. Morel searched for specific entities, and argued for a classification based on cause, symptoms, and outcome (Morel 1860). In 1852 he gave the name *démence précoce* to a disorder which he described as starting in adolescence and leading first to withdrawal, odd mannerisms, and self-neglect, and eventually to intellectual deterioration. Not long

after, Kahlbaum (1863) described the syndrome of *catatonia*, and Hecker (1871) wrote an account of a condition he called *hebephrenia* (an English translation has been published by Sedler 1985).

Emil Kraepelin (1855–1926) derived his ideas from study of the course of the disorder as well as the symptoms. His observations led him to argue against the idea of a single psychosis, and to propose a division into *dementia praecox* and *manic-depressive psychosis*. This grouping brought together as subclasses of dementia praecox the previously separate entities of hebephrenia and catatonia. Kraepelin's description of dementia praecox appeared for the first time in 1893, in the fourth edition of his textbook, and the account was expanded in subsequent editions (see Kraepelin 1897 for a translation of the description in the fifth edition).

Kraepelin described the illness as occurring in clear consciousness and consisting of

a series of states, the common characteristic of which is a peculiar destruction of the internal connections of the psychic personality. The effects of this injury predominate in the *emotional* and *volitional* spheres of mental life. (Kraepelin 1919)

He originally divided dementia praecox into three subtypes (catatonic, hebephrenic, and paranoid) and later added a fourth (simple). Kraepelin separated the condition he named *paraphrenia* from dementia praecox on the grounds that it started in middle life and seemed to be free from the changes in emotion and volition found in dementia praecox. It is commonly held that Kraepelin regarded dementia praecox as invariably progressing to chronic deterioration. However, he reported that, in his series of cases, 13% recovered completely (though some relapsed later) and 17% were ultimately able to live and work without difficulty.

Eugen Bleuler (1857–1959) was the Director of Burghlozli Clinic and Professor of Psychiatry in Zurich. He based his work on that of Kraepelin, and in his own book wrote 'the whole idea of dementia praecox originates with Kraepelin' (Bleuler 1911). He also acknowledged the help of his younger colleague, Carl Gustav Jung, in trying to apply some of Freud's ideas to dementia praecox. Compared with Kraepelin, Bleuler was concerned less with prognosis and more with the mechanisms of symptom formation. Bleuler proposed the name *schizophrenia* to denote a *'splitting' of psychic functions*, which he thought to be of central importance.

Bleuler believed in a distinction between *fundamental* and *accessory symptoms*. Fundamental symptoms included disturbances of associations, changes in emotional reactions, and autism (withdrawal from reality into an inner world of fantasy). It is interesting that, in Bleuler's view, some of the most frequent and striking symptoms were accessory (secondary), for example, hallucinations, delusions, catatonia, and abnormal behaviours. Bleuler was interested in the psychological study of his cases, but did not deny the possibility of a neuropathological cause for schizophrenia. Compared with Kraepelin, Bleuler took a more optimistic view of the outcome, but still held that one should not 'speak of cure but of far reaching improvement'. He also wrote:

as yet I have never released a schizophrenic in whom I could not still see distinct signs of the disease, indeed there are very few in whom one would have to search for such signs. (Bleuler 1911)

Since Bleuler was preoccupied more with psychopathological mechanisms than with symptoms themselves, his approach to diagnosis was less precise than that of Kraepelin.

Kurt Schneider (1887–1967) tried to make the diagnosis more reliable by identifying a group of symptoms characteristic of schizophrenia, but rarely found in other disorders. Unlike Bleuler's fundamental symptoms, Schneider's symptoms were not supposed to have any central psychopathological role. Thus Schneider (1959) wrote:

Among the many abnormal modes of experience that occur in schizophrenia, there are some which we put in the first rank of importance, not because we think of them as basic disturbances, but because they have this special value in helping us to determine the diagnosis of schizophrenia. When any one of these modes of experience is undeniably present and no basic somatic illness

can be found, we may make the diagnosis of schizophrenia . . . Symptoms of first rank importance do not always have to be present for a diagnosis to be made.

The last point is important. Schneider's first-rank symptoms are listed in Table 12.3. Some of these symptoms are included in the diagnostic criteria for schizophrenia used in DSM-IV and ICD-10 (see pp. 339–342).

Several German psychiatrists tried to define subgroupings within schizophrenia. Karl Kleist, a pupil of the neurologist Wernicke, looked for associations between brain pathology and different subtypes of psychotic illness. He accepted Kraepelin's main diagnostic framework but used careful clinical observation in an attempt to distinguish various subdivisions within schizophrenia and other atypical disorders. His attempt to match these subtypes to specific kinds of brain pathology was ingenious but not successful (Kleist 1928).

Leonhard continued this approach of careful clinical observation, but did not pursue Kleist's interest in cerebral pathology. He published a complicated classification which distinguishes schizophrenia from the *'cycloid' psychoses*, which are a group of non-affective psychoses of good outcome (Leonhard 1957). Cycloid psychoses are described later in this chapter. Leonhard also divided schizophrenia into two groups. The first

Table 12.3 Schneider's symptoms of the first rank
Hearing thoughts spoken aloud
Third-person hallucinations
Hallucinations in the form of a commentary
Somatic hallucinations
Thought withdrawal or insertion
Thought broadcasting
Delusional perception
Feelings or actions experienced as made or influenced by external agents

group is characterized by a progressive course, and is divided into catatonias, hebephrenias, and paraphrenias. Leonhard gave this group a name which is often translated as *systematic*. The second group, called *non-systematic*, is divided into *affect-laden paraphrenia*, *schizophasia*, and *periodic catatonia*. Affect-laden paraphrenia is characterized by paranoid delusions and the expression of strong emotion about their content. In schizophasia, speech is grossly disordered and difficult to understand. Periodic catatonia is a condition with regular remissions; during an episode, akinetic symptoms are sometimes interrupted by hyperkinetic symptoms.

Scandinavian psychiatrists have been influenced by Jaspers' distinction between process schizophrenia and reactive psychoses. In the late 1930s, Langfeldt, using follow-up data on patients in Oslo, proposed a distinction between true schizophrenia, which had a poor prognosis, and *schizophreniform states*, which had a good prognosis (Langfeldt 1961). True schizophrenia was defined narrowly and was essentially similar to Kraepelin's dementia praecox. It was characterized by emotional blunting, lack of initiative, paranoid symptoms, and primary delusions. Schizophreniform states were described as often precipitated by stress and frequently accompanied by confusional and affective symptoms. Langfeldt's proposed distinction between cases with good and bad prognosis has been influential but, as explained later, other psychiatrists have not found that his criteria predict prognosis accurately (see p. 363). According to modern diagnostic criteria, most of Langfeldt's cases of schizophreniform psychosis would, in fact, be classified as mood disorders (Bergen *et al.* 1990). In DSM-IV the term schizophreniform disorder is used in a different way to define a disorder that meets the diagnostic criteria schizophrenia but whose duration is less than the 6 months required.

In Denmark and Norway, cases of psychosis arising after stressful events have received much attention. The terms *reactive psychosis* or *psychogenic psychosis* are commonly applied to conditions which appear to be precipitated by stress, are to some extent understandable in their symptoms, and have a good prognosis (see Pitta and Blay 1997). In current diagnostic schemes such disorders would be classified as *brief psychotic disorder* or *schizophreniform disorder* (see p. 343).

International differences in diagnostic practice

By the 1960s there were wide divergences in the criteria for the diagnosis of schizophrenia. In the UK and continental Europe, psychiatrists generally employed Schneider's approach, using first rank symptoms to identify a narrowly delineated group of cases. In the USA, however, interest in psychodynamic processes led to diagnosis on the basis of mental mechanisms and to the inclusion of a much wider group of cases.

First admission rates for schizophrenia were much higher in the USA than in the UK. This discrepancy prompted two major cross-national studies of diagnostic practice. The US-UK Diagnostic Project (Cooper *et al.* 1972) showed that the diagnostic concept of schizophrenia was much wider in New York than in the UK. In New York the concept included cases that were diagnosed as depressive illness, mania, or personality disorder in the UK.

The International Pilot Study of Schizophrenia (IPSS) was concerned with the diagnosis of schizophrenia in nine countries (World Health Organization 1973). The main finding was that similar criteria were adopted in seven of the nine countries: Colombia, Czechoslovakia, Denmark, India, Nigeria, Taiwan, and the UK. Broader criteria were used in the USA and the former USSR. Despite these differences, it was found that when standard diagnostic techniques were used, a core of cases with similar features could be identified in all the countries. In France, schizophrenia is not defined in Kraepelian terms. It is regarded as a chronic disorder with an onset before the age of 30. The diagnosis is made largely on symptoms, especially the fundamental symptoms proposed by Bleuler. The term *bouffée délirante* is used for a sudden-onset syndrome of good prognosis (Pichot 1984; Ferrey and Zebdi 1999).

Reasons for diagnostic inconsistencies

To agree about the diagnosis of schizophrenia, clinicians must first agree about the symptoms that make up the syndrome, about the criteria for deciding whether these symptoms are present, and about the length of time that these features must last before the diagnosis can be made. The criteria for diagnosing the various symptoms of schizophrenia were discussed in Chapter 1. Here we consider the other two issues.

The narrower the range of symptoms that are accepted as diagnostic of schizophrenia, the more reliable is the diagnosis. However, a narrow definition may exclude cases that are aetiologically related; this problem cannot be settled until we know more about the causes of schizophrenia. An example of a well-known narrow definition is that requiring the presence of Schneider's first-rank symptoms (Table 12.3). The use of this criterion leads to high reliability in diagnosis but not to effective prediction of outcome. In addition, whilst genetic factors are known to play a part in the aetiology of schizophrenia, Schneider's first-rank symptoms delineate a syndrome with no apparent heritability (McGuffin *et al.* 1984). It is also now clear that first-rank symptoms can occur in cases that otherwise meet generally agreed diagnostic criteria for mania. Both ICD-10 and DSM-IV use wider definitions of schizophrenia, including other symptoms as well as Schneider's first-rank symptoms.

There is disagreement about the *duration of symptoms* required before schizophrenia can be diagnosed. ICD-10 requires 1 month, and DSM-IV requires 6 months. Both periods are arbitrary. The longer time is more likely to identify patients with a poor prognosis, but the importance of prognosis in defining schizophrenia is not yet clear.

Standardized diagnosis

An important example of a standardized diagnostic system is CATEGO, a computer program designed to process data from a standard interview known as the *Present State Examination* (Wing *et al.* 1974). The program incorporates diagnostic rules, which give a series of standard diagnoses. The narrowest syndrome (S+) is diagnosed mainly on the symptoms of thought intrusion, broadcast, or withdrawal, delusions of control, and voices discussing the patient in the third person or commenting on his actions.

The Feighner criteria (Feighner *et al.* 1972) were developed in St Louis to identify patients with a poor prognosis. They include symptomatic criteria that are less precise than those in CATEGO, and a criterion of 6 months' continuous illness. They also require the exclusion of cases meeting diagnostic criteria for mood disorder, drug misuse, or alcohol dependence. The criteria are reliable but restrictive, leaving many cases without a diagnosis. Patients with a poor prognosis are identified well (probably because of the criterion of 6 months' continuous illness). These criteria have been widely used in research.

The Research Diagnostic Criteria (RDC) were developed from those of Feighner by Spitzer *et al.* (1978). The main difference is in the length of history required before the diagnosis of schizophrenia can be made: 2 weeks, instead of 6 months in the Feighner criteria. A structured interview, the Schedule of Affective Disorders and Schizophrenia (SADS), has been developed for use with RDC. Both the Feighner criteria and the RDC influenced the development of DSM-III and DSM-IV (see below).

Schizophrenia secondary to other medical conditions

If the symptoms of schizophrenia occur apparently as a result of some identifiable disease of the central nervous system, the condition is generally referred to as a *psychotic disorder secondary to a general medical condition* (DSM-IV) or an *organic delusional disorder*

(ICD-10). These conditions are sometimes known as 'symptomatic schizophrenia'. Certain disorders that can produce a secondary schizophrenic syndrome are discussed elsewhere in this book. They include temporal lobe epilepsy (complex partial seizures) (p. 436), encephalitis (p. 426), substance misuse of some kinds (p. 573), and alcohol misuse (p. 547). In addition, schizophrenia-like syndromes can occur post partum (see p. 500) and in the post-operative period (p. 486).

Classification in DSM-IV and ICD-10

The classification of schizophrenia and schizophrenia-like disorders is summarized in Table 12.4.

Table 12.4 Classification of schizophrenia and schizophrenia-like disorders in ICD–10 and DSM-IV*

ICD–10	DSM-IV
Schizophrenia	*Schizophrenia*
Paranoid	Paranoid
Hebephrenic	Disorganized
Catatonic	Catatonic
Undifferentiated	Undifferentiated
Residual	Residual
Simple schizophrenia	
Post-schizophrenic depression	
Other schizophrenia	
Unspecified schizophrenia	
Schizotypal disorder	
Schizoaffective disorder	*Schizoaffective disorder*
Persistent delusional disorders	*Delusional disorder*
Delusional disorder	
Other persistent delusional disorders	
Acute and transient psychotic disorders	*Brief psychotic disorder*
Acute polymorphic psychotic disorder	*Schizophreniform disorder*
Schizophrenia-like psychotic disorder	
Other acute psychotic disorder	
Induced delusional disorder	*Shared psychotic disorder*
Other non-organic psychotic disorders	
Unspecified non-organic psychosis	*Psychotic disorder not otherwise specified*

* The order of categories in the two systems has been changed slightly to show their comparable features more clearly.

Both classifications distinguish schizophrenic illness, though in DSM-IV more emphasis is placed on *course and functional impairment*, whereas in ICD-10 *Schneider's first-rank signs* are given more weight. Both classifications separate out disorders with especially prominent mood disturbance (*schizoaffective disorders*), and also identify illnesses that meet symptomatic criteria for schizophrenia but have a brief duration of symptomatology (*brief psychotic disorder* and *schizophreniform disorder* in DSM-IV and *acute and transient psychotic disturbance* in ICD-10). In addition, both DSM-IV and ICD-10 distinguish illnesses that centre around relatively enduring non-bizarre delusions without other features of schizophrenia (*delusional disorder*).

DSM-IV

In this classification schizophrenia is defined in terms of the symptoms in the *acute phase* and also of the *course*, for which the requirement is continuous signs of disturbance for at least 6 months. The acute symptoms can include delusions, hallucinations, disorganized speech or behaviour, and negative symptoms. At least two of these symptoms must have been present for a period of one month (unless successful treatment has occurred). Where subjects have major disturbances of mood occurring concurrently with the acute-phase symptoms, a diagnosis of a *schizoaffective disorder* or *mood disorder with psychotic features* should be made (Table 12.5) (see below).

A further criterion for the diagnosis of schizophrenia in DSM-IV is that the patient must have exhibited deficiencies in their expected level of *occupational or social functioning* since the onset of the disorder. As noted above, for the diagnosis to be made there must have been at least 6 months of continuous disturbance; this can include prodromal and residual periods when acute-phase symptoms, as described above, are not evident. Patients whose symptom duration does not meet this criterion 6-month period will be classified as suffering from a *schizophreniform disorder* or a *brief psychotic disorder* (see below).

In DSM-IV, schizophrenic disorders are divided into a number of subtypes, defined by the predominant symptomatology at the time of evaluation (Table 12.4) (see below). In addition, after at least 1 year has elapsed since the onset of active phase symptoms, DSM-IV allows the schizophrenic disorder to be classified by longitudinal course. This classification takes into account the pattern of illness so that remissions and their quality and the presence of relapse can be coded.

In DSM-IV, schizophrenia is distinguished from two other major categories: *delusional disorder* (discussed in Chapter 13) and the mixed group of *psychotic disorders not elsewhere classified*.

ICD-10

The ICD-10 definition of schizophrenia places more reliance than DSM-IV on *first-rank symptoms*, and requires a duration of illness of only 1 month, with prodromal symptoms being excluded (Table 12.6) There are several clinical subtypes of schizophrenia; these differ most obviously from DSM-IV in the inclusion of categories of simple schizophrenia and post-schizophrenic depression. The ICD-10 category of hebephrenic schizophrenia corresponds to the DSM-IV category of schizophrenia, disorganized type. Like DSM-IV, cases in which symptoms of schizophrenia are accompanied by prominent mood disturbances are classified as schizoaffective disorders.

Certain kinds of personality disorder such as schizotypal personality (p. 349) are genetically associated with schizophrenia. ICD-10 includes *schizotypal disorder* among schizophrenic disorders, whereas in DSM-IV, this condition is classified as a personality disorder. Schizotypal disorder is associated with social isolation and restriction of affect; in addition there are perceptual distortions with disorders of thinking and speech and striking eccentricity or oddness of behaviour.

Similarly to DSM-IV, ICD-10 classifies delusional disorders separately from schizophrenia (see Chapter 13). In addition, a group of acute and transient psychotic disorders are recognized that have an acute onset and complete recovery within 2–3 months (see below).

Table 12.5 Criteria for schizophrenia in DSM-IV

A *Characteristic symptoms of the active phase*

Two (or more) of the following, each present for a significant portion of time during a 1-month period (or less if successfully treated):

(1) Delusions

(2) Hallucinations

(3) Disorganized speech (e.g. frequent derailment or incoherence)

(4) Grossly disorganized or catatonic behaviour

(5) Negative symptoms, i.e. affective flattening, alogia, or avolition

B *Social/occupational dysfunction*

For a significant portion of the time since the onset of the disturbance, one or more major areas of functioning such as work, interpersonal relations, or self-care are markedly below the level achieved prior to the onset (or when the onset is in childhood or adolescence, failure to achieve expected level of interpersonal, academic, or occupational achievement)

C *Duration*

Continuous signs of the disturbance persist for at least 6 months. This 6-month period must include at least 1 month of symptoms (or less if successfully treated) that meet criterion A (i.e. active-phase symptoms) and may include

periods of prodromal or residual symptoms, the signs of the disturbance may be manifested by only negative symptoms or two or more symptoms listed in criterion A present in an attenuated form (e.g. odd beliefs, unusual perceptual experiences)

D *Schizoaffective and mood disorder exclusion*

Schizoaffective disorder and mood disorder with psychotic features have been ruled out because either (1) no major depressive, manic, or mixed episodes have occurred concurrently with the active-phase symptoms, or (2) if mood episodes have occurred during active-phase symptoms, their total duration has been brief relative to the duration of the active and residual periods

E *Substance/general medical condition exclusion*

The disturbance is not due to the direct physiological effects of a substance (e.g. a drug of abuse, a medication) or a general medical condition

F *Relationship to a pervasive developmental disorder*

If there is a history of autistic disorder or another pervasive development disorder, the additional diagnosis of schizophrenia is made only if prominent delusions or hallucinations are also present for at least 1 month (or less if successfully treated)

Table 12.6 Symptomatic criteria for schizophrenia in ICD–10

The normal requirement for a diagnosis of schizophrenia is that a minimum of one very clear symptom (and usually two or more if less clear-cut) belonging to any one of the groups listed as (a)–(d) below, or symptoms from at least two of the groups referred to as (e)–(h), should have been clearly present for most of the time *during a period of 1 month or more*.

(a) Thought echo, thought insertion or withdrawal, and thought broadcasting

(b) Delusions of control, influence, or passivity, clearly referred to body or limb movements or specific thoughts, actions, or sensations; delusional perception

(c) Hallucinatory voices giving a running commentary on the patient's behaviour, or discussing the patient among themselves, or other types of hallucinatory voices coming from some part of the body

(d) Persistent delusions of other kinds that are culturally inappropriate and completely impossible

(e) Persistent hallucinations in any modality, when accompanied either by fleeting or half formed delusions without clear affective content, or by persistent overvalued ideas, or when occurring every day for weeks or months on end

(f) Breaks or interpolations in the train of thought, resulting in incoherence or irrelevant speech, or neologisms

(g) Catatonic behaviour, such as excitement, posturing, or waxy flexibility, negativism, mutism, and stupor

(h) 'Negative' symptoms such as marked apathy, paucity of speech, and blunting or incongruity of emotional responses, usually resulting in social withdrawal and lowering of social performance; it must be clear that these are not due to depression or to neuroleptic medication

(i) A significant and consistent change in the overall quality of some aspects of personal behaviour, manifest as loss of interest, aimlessness, idleness, a self-absorbed attitude, and social withdrawal

Subtypes of schizophrenia

The variety of the symptoms and course of schizophrenia has led to several attempts to define subgroups. This section is concerned only with the traditional subgroups of hebephrenic, catatonic, paranoid, and simple schizophrenia.

Patients with *hebephrenic schizophrenia* (disorganized type in DSM-IV) often appear silly and childish in their behaviour. Affective symptoms and thought disorder are prominent. Delusions are common and not highly organized. Hallucinations also are common, and are not elaborate.

Catatonic schizophrenia is characterized by motor symptoms of the kind described on p. 322 and by changes in activity varying between excitement and stupor. Hallucinations, delusions, and affective symptoms occur but are usually less obvious. In paranoid schizophrenia, the clinical picture is dominated by well-organized paranoid delusions. Thought processes and mood are relatively spared, and the patient may appear normal until his abnormal beliefs are uncovered.

Simple schizophrenia is characterized by the insidious development of odd behaviour, social withdrawal, and declining performance at work. Since clear schizophrenic symptoms are absent, simple schizophrenia is difficult to identify reliably.

With the possible exception of *paranoid schizophrenia*, these 'subgroups' are of uncertain validity. There is some genetic evidence for separating cases with the paranoid picture but not enough to recommend doing so in everyday clinical work. Follow-up studies suggest that paranoid schizophrenia has a later and more acute onset than other subtypes of schizophrenia and tends to run a more a remittent course (Fenton and McGlashan 1991).

Catatonic symptoms are much less common now than 50 years ago, perhaps because of improvements in the social environment in which patients are treated or because of the use of more effective physical treatments. Other explanations are possible; for example, organic syndromes may have been included in some earlier series.

Schizophrenia-like disorders

Whatever definition of schizophrenia is adopted, there will be cases that resemble schizophrenia in some respects and yet do not meet the criteria for diagnosis. Schizophrenia-like disorders can be divided into four groups:

- delusional or paranoid disorders
- brief disorders
- disorders accompanied by prominent affective symptoms
- disorders without all the required symptoms for schizophrenia.

The latter three groups will be discussed below: delusional or paranoid disorders are discussed in Chapter 13.

Brief disorders

DSM-IV uses the term *brief psychotic disorder* for a syndrome characterized by at least one of the acute-phase positive symptoms shown in Table 12.4. The disorder lasts for at least 1 day but not more than 1 month, by which time full recovery has occurred. The disorder may or may not follow a stressor, but psychoses induced by the direct physiological effects of drugs or medical illness are excluded. *Schizophreniform psychosis* is a syndrome similar to schizophrenia (meeting criterion A) which has lasted more than 1 month (and so cannot be classified as brief psychotic disorder) but less than the 6 months required for a diagnosis of schizophrenia

to be made. Social and occupational dysfunction are not needed to make the diagnosis (although they may occur).

In ICD-10, more short-lived psychotic illnesses are grouped under the term acute and transient psychotic disorder. These disorders are of acute onset, and complete recovery within 2–3 months is the rule. The disorder may or may not be precipitated by a stressful life event. In the first two subtypes (*acute polymorphic psychotic disorders, with or without symptoms of schizophrenia*) hallucinations, delusions, and perceptual disturbance are obvious but change rapidly in nature and extent. There are often accompanying changes in mood and motor behaviour. The two subtypes are distinguished from each other by whether or not typical schizophrenic symptoms are also present, although if they are, the duration of the disorder must not have exceeded 1 month or schizophrenia will be diagnosed. The terms *bouffée délirante* and cycloid psychosis are given as synonyms for these categories. A third subtype, *schizophrenia-like episode*, is a non-committal term for cases meeting the symptom criteria for schizophrenia but lasting for less than a month. Such cases could turn out to be schizophrenia or acute delusional episodes, depending on the subsequent course. The fourth subtype, for cases that do not fit the other three, is called *other acute psychotic episodes*.

Disorders with prominent affective symptoms

Some patients have a more or less equal mixture of schizophrenic and affective symptoms. As mentioned earlier, such patients are classified under *schizoaffective disorder* in both DSM-IV and ICD-10.

The term schizoaffective disorder has been used in several distinct ways. It was first applied by Kasanin (1933) to a small group of young patients with severe mental disorders

characterized by a very sudden onset in a setting of marked emotional turmoil with a distortion of the outside world. The psychosis lasts a few weeks and is followed by recovery.

The definitions of schizoaffective disorder in DSM-IV and ICD-10 differ substantially from this description. For example, DSM-IV requires that

there should have been an uninterrupted period of illness during which, at some time there is either a major depressive episode, a manic episode or a mixed episode concurrent with symptoms that meet criterion A for schizophrenia.

During this continuous episode of illness, the acute-phase psychotic symptoms must have been present for at least 2 weeks in the absence of prominent mood symptoms (or the diagnosis would be a mood disorder with psychotic features). However, the episode of mood disturbance must have been present for a substantial part of the illness.

The definition of schizoaffective disorder in ICD-10 is similar. It specifies that the diagnosis

should only be made when both definite schizophrenic and definite affective symptoms are equally prominent and present simultaneously, or within a few days of each other.

ICD-10 classifies schizoaffective disorder by whether the mood disturbance is depressive, manic, or mixed. In DSM-IV schizoaffective disorder is specified either as depressive type or bipolar.

Family studies have shown that the more recent diagnostic concepts of schizoaffective disorder delineate a syndrome in which *first-degree relatives* have an increased risk of both *mood disorders* and *schizophrenia* (see below). In addition, the outcome of schizoaffective disorder may be generally rather better than that for schizophrenia, particularly where affective symptoms have been consistently prominent (Tsuang *et al.* 2000).

As noted above, it is not uncommon for patients with schizophrenia to *develop depression* as the symptoms of acute psychosis subside. This is recognized in ICD-10 as *post-schizophrenic depression* where prominent depressive symptoms have been present for at least 2 weeks while some symptoms of schizophrenia (either positive or negative) still remain. It is important to distinguish depressive symptoms in these circumstances from the side-effects of antipsychotic drug treatment or the impaired volition and affective flattening that may occur in the context of a schizophrenic disorder (see p. 334).

Disorders without all the required symptoms for schizophrenia

A difficult problem is presented by cases with symptoms which resemble those of schizophrenia but fail strict criteria for diagnosis and which endure for years. There are three groups:

- people who from an early age have *behaved oddly* and shown features seen in schizophrenia, for example, ideas of reference, persecutory beliefs, and unusual types of thinking. When long-standing, these disorders can be classified as personality disorders as in DSM-IV (*schizotypal personality disorder*, see p. 167), or with schizophrenia as in ICD-10 (*schizotypal disorder*). Because of a suggested close relationship to schizophrenia, these disorders have also been called latent schizophrenia. They are more frequent in families of patients with schizophrenia than in other families, suggesting a genetic relationship (see p. 349).

- people who develop symptoms after a period of more normal development. There is a gradual development of social withdrawal, lack of initiative, odd behaviour, and blunting of emotion. These 'negative' symptoms are not accompanied by any of the 'positive' symptoms of schizophrenia such as hallucinations and delusions. Such cases are classified as *simple schizophrenia* in ICD-10; in DSM-IV they are classified as *schizotypal personality disorder*.

- patients who have shown the full clinical picture of schizophrenia in the past but no longer have all the symptoms required to make the diagnosis. These cases are classified as *residual schizophrenia* in both DSM-IV and ICD-10.

Borderline disorders

In the USA there has been much interest in states intermediate between schizophrenia and the neuroses and personality disorders. The term *borderline states* has been applied to them, but has been used in several different ways. Current usage applies the term borderline to certain kinds of personality disorder, for example, *borderline personality* in DSM-IV and *emotionally unstable personality, borderline type* in ICD-10. The characteristics of this personality disorder are described on p. 168. Although patients with borderline personality disorder may experience transient psychotic symptoms, family studies do not suggest that this disorder is related to schizophrenia (Kendler *et al.* 1993a, 1993b, 1993c).

Some other notable terms

Schizophreniform states

As mentioned earlier, this term was applied by Langfeldt (1961) to good prognosis cases as distinct from 'true' schizophrenia. The main features of schizophreniform states were the presence of a precipitating factor, acute onset, clouding of consciousness, and depressive and hysterical features. It is unfortunate that DSM-IV uses the term schizophreniform quite differently to describe a condition identical to schizophrenia but with a course of less than 6 months.

Cycloid psychoses

Kleist introduced the term *cycloid marginal psychoses* to denote functional psychoses which were neither typically schizophrenic nor manic-depressive. Leonhard (1957) developed these ideas by describing three forms of cycloid psychosis which are distinguished by their predominant symptoms; these conditions are all bipolar and are described as having a good prognosis and leaving no chronic defect state. The first is anxiety-elation psychosis, in which the prominent symptom is a mood change. At one 'pole' anxiety is associated with ideas of reference and sometimes with hallucinations. At the other 'pole' the mood is elated, often with an ecstatic quality. The second is confusion psychosis, in which thought disorder is the prominent symptom and the clinical picture varies

between excitement and a state of underactivity with poverty of speech. The third is motility psychosis, in which the striking changes are in psychomotor activity.

A study, using the statistical technique of latent class analysis, suggested that a group of variously described disorders including *cycloid psychosis, bouffée délirante*, and *Kasanin's schizoaffective disorder* may form a cluster of *atypical psychoses* which can be distinguished on clinical grounds from ICD-10 and DSM-IV concepts of schizophrenia (McGorry *et al.* 1992).

Type I and type II schizophrenia

For many years a distinction has been made between positive and negative symptoms of schizophrenia. There is not complete agreement on the specification of negative symptoms but it is generally agreed that they include:

- poverty of speech
- blunting of affect
- lack of volition
- social withdrawal.

Crow and his colleagues (1985) described two syndromes. Type I has an acute onset, mainly positive symptoms, and good social functioning during remissions. It has a good response to antipsychotic drugs with biochemical evidence of dopamine overactivity. By contrast, type 2 is said to have an insidious onset, mainly negative symptoms, and poor outcome. It has a poor response to antipsychotic drugs without evidence of dopamine overactivity. In type 2 there is evidence of structural change in the brain (especially ventricular enlargement). (Cognitive, biochemical, and neurological aspects of schizophrenia are considered later in this chapter.) In practice, although some patients can be recognized to have type I syndrome, those with pure type II are much less common and most patients show a mixture of types I and II symptoms. In addition, structural brain abnormalities, for example, enlarged cerebral ventricles, do not correlate consistently with symptomatology or outcome (see Harrison 2000a).

Table 12.7 Cerebral and psychological correlate of three symptom clusters

Syndrome	Symptoms	Regional cerebral bloodflow correlates	Impaired psychological performance
Reality disturbance	Delusions, hallucinations	Left medial temporal lobe, cingulate cortex	Disorders of self-monitoring
Disorganization	Formal thought disorder inappropriate affect, bizarre behaviour	Anterior cingulate, right ventral frontal cortex, bilateral parietal regions	Tests of selective attention
Psychomotor poverty	Flat affect, poverty of speech, decreased spontaneous movement	Underactivity of frontal cortex	Word generation tasks, planning tests

See Liddle (2000).

Three clinical syndromes

Recent studies have proposed more complex delineations of psychopathology than that offered by the positive and negative dichotomy. For example, Liddle (1987), studying patients with chronic schizophrenia, described three overlapping clinical syndromes, each linked to a particular symptom cluster in association with patterns of neuropsychological deficit and regional cerebral blood flow (Liddle *et al.* 1992). At present the most reproducible finding seems to be the link between psychomotor poverty (negative symptoms), impaired performance on frontal lobe tasks, and decreased frontal blood flow (Table 12.7).

Gjessing's syndrome

Gjessing (1947) described a rare disorder in which catatonic symptoms recurred in phases. He also found changes in nitrogen balance, which were not always in phase with the symptoms. Gjessing believed that there were underlying changes in thyroid function and that the disorder could be treated successfully with thyroid hormone. The condition, if it exists, is exceedingly rare. It is possible that it may have been a variant of rapid cycling bipolar disorder for which some authorities currently recommend thyroid treatment (p. 282).

Differential diagnosis

Schizophrenia has to be distinguished mainly from:

♦ *organic syndromes.* There must be careful observation for *clouding of consciousness, obvious disorientation*, and other symptoms and signs that are not characteristic of schizophrenia. Some diffuse brain diseases can present a schizophrenia-like picture in the absence of neurological disorder; a rare but important example is general paralysis of the insane. Temporal lobe epilepsy (see p. 436) should also be considered.

♦ *drug-induced states (including substance misuse).* Certain medically prescribed drugs, particularly steroids and dopamine agonists, can cause florid psychotic states. Among younger patients substance misuse, particularly with psychostimulants and phencyclidine, should be considered. Urine testing for illicit drugs can be helpful in diagnosis.

♦ *mood disorder with psychotic features.* The distinction between mood disorder and schizophrenia depends on the degree and persistence of the mood disorder, the relation of any hallucinations or delusions to the prevailing mood, and the nature of the symptoms in any previous episodes. The distinction from mania in young people can be particularly difficult, and sometimes the diagnosis can be clarified only by *longer-term follow-up. A family history of mood disorder* may be a useful pointer.

◆ *personality disorder.* Differential diagnosis from personality disorder can also be difficult when insidious changes are reported in a young person. Prolonged lengthy observation for acute symptoms of psychosis may be required. Some patients with borderline personality can also exhibit psychotic symptoms. Again previous history and follow-up should help clarify the diagnosis.

Aetiology

Before reviewing evidence on the causation of schizophrenia, it may be helpful to outline the main areas of inquiry. Of the predisposing causes, *genetic factors* are most strongly supported by the evidence, but the fact that monozygotic twins may be discordant for the disorder suggests that *environmental factors* are likely to play a part as well. The nature of these environmental factors is uncertain. *Neurological damage* around the time of birth has been suggested, and so have *interpersonal* and *social influences.* The evidence for all these factors is indirect and incomplete.

There is growing evidence that schizophrenic disorders presenting in adulthood have distinguishable *childhood antecedents* characterized by *cognitive* and *social impairments.* Research on precipitating causes has been concerned mainly with *life events.* Although such precipitants seem to have a definite effect, the size of the effect is uncertain. Among perpetuating factors, *social and family influences* seem important; however, they are not considered in this section but in the later section on course and prognosis.

The neurodevelopmental hypothesis

In recent years there has been accumulating evidence that patients with schizophrenia have abnormalities in *brain structure and morphology.* In addition, neuropsychological testing provides evidence of deficits in aspects of *psychological performance,* often in association with altered *patterns of cerebral blood flow.* Some of these abnormalities have been shown to be present when patients with schizophrenia first present for treatment and they do not seem to worsen as the disease progresses. In addition, whilst neuropathological studies provide evidence of disordered cellular architecture in some cortical and subcortical brain regions, *gliosis* is not consistently present. This is taken to indicate that the pathological changes are neurodevelopmental in origin, or that if an injury of some kind occurred to the brain, it happened before the end of the second trimester *in utero* (after which time gliosis would be seen).

These findings have given rise to the *neurodevelopmental hypothesis* of schizophrenia in which the pathological changes of the disorder are laid down early in life, presumably through genetic influences, and then modified by maturational and environmental factors (see Weinberger 1995). The neurodevelopmental theory provides a useful framework in which to consider the aetiology of schizophrenia, particularly the various neurobiological changes that have been linked to the clinical disorder. A number of these changes are discussed below, followed by a consideration of how far psychological, social, and epidemiological findings in schizophrenia are consistent with the neurodevelopmental approach to aetiology (Table 12.8).

Genetics

The genetic study of schizophrenia has been directed towards four questions:

◆ Is there a genetic basis?

◆ Is there a relationship between clinical form and inheritance?

Table 12.8 Some findings compatible with the neurodevelopment hypothesis of schizophrenia

Structural brain lesions present at illness onset

Cognitive impairment present at illness onset

Cytoarchitectural disturbances without gliosis

Cognitive and social impairments in childhood

'Soft' neurological signs

Excess of winter births

♦ What is the mode of inheritance?
♦ What is the phenotype?

These four questions will be considered in turn. (Readers requiring a more detailed account are referred to Murray and Castle 2000 and Maier *et al.* 2000.)

Is there a genetic basis?

Family studies

The first systematic family study of dementia praecox was carried out in Kraepelin's department by Ernst Rudin, who showed that the rate of dementia praecox was higher among the siblings of probands than in the general population (Rudin 1916). More recent research has used better criteria for diagnosis in probands and relatives, and better ways of selecting the probands. These improved methods yield estimates of an average lifetime risk of about 5–10% among first-degree relatives of schizophrenics, compared with 0.2–0.6% among first-degree relatives of controls (Table 12.9).

To some extent, the risk depends on the *definition of the phenotype*. For example, in a prospective study of over 200 children of mothers with schizophrenia, Parnas *et al.* (1993) found not only a significant excess of schizophrenia (16.2% versus 1.9% in controls) but also an excess of *schizotypal*, *paranoid*, and *schizoid personality disorders* (21.3% versus 5%). Similar findings were reported by Kendler *et al.* (1993b, 1993c, 1993d) in a study of

first-degree relatives of patients with schizophrenia (Table 12.10).

Taken together, the family studies provide clear evidence of a *familial aetiology* but do not distinguish between the effects of genetic factors and those of the family environment. To make this distinction *twin* and *adoption* studies are required.

An additional value of family studies is to determine whether the liability to schizophrenia and mood disorders is transmitted independently, which should be the observed pattern if the two disorders are separate syndromes with differing aetiology. However, the findings from the various studies have been contradictory, with some workers arguing for separate familial transmission of mood disorders and schizophrenia, while others suggest that what is transmitted is a general vulnerability to psychotic illness (Crow 1994). The following conclusions can be drawn from the more recent studies (Kendler *et al.* 1993a, 1993b, 1993c,

Table 12.9 Approximate lifetime expectancy of developing schizophrenia for relatives of schizophrenics

Relationship	Risk (%)	
	Definite cases only	Definite and probable cases
Parents	4.4	5.5
All siblings	8.5	10.2
Siblings (one parent schizophrenic)	13.8	17.2
Children	12.3	13.9
Children (both parents schizophrenic)	36.6	46.3
Half siblings	3.2	3.5
Nephews and nieces	2.2	2.6

Adapted from Shields (1980).

1993d; Maier *et al.* 1993b; Parnas *et al.* 1993) (Table 12.10).

- The risk of schizophrenia, schizoaffective disorder, and schizotypal personality is increased in first-degree relatives of patients with schizophrenia.
- The risk of both schizophrenia and mood disorder is increased in first-degree relatives of patients with schizoaffective disorder (as defined in DSM-IIIR).
- The risk of bipolar illness is not increased in first-degree relatives of patients with schizophrenia.

Possible familial links between schizophrenia and mood disorders remain controversial (Kendler *et al.* 1993d). For example, Maier *et al.* (1993b) reported an excess of unipolar depression in first-degree relatives of patients with schizophrenia. While this observation is of interest in view of the frequent coexistence of depression and schizophrenia, it has not been reliably confirmed (Kendler *et al.* 1993d; Parnas *et al.* 1993). Another interesting finding comes from the Roscommon study carried out by Kendler *et al.* (1993a, 1993b,

1993c, 1993d) who investigated the families of patients with schizophrenia in County Roscommon, Ireland. Whilst the overall incidence of mood disorders was not increased in first-degree relatives of schizophrenic probands, if the relatives suffered a mood disorder, it was more likely to be of a psychotic type (Table 12.10). Again, other workers have not identified such an effect (Parnas *et al.* 1993).

At present, the findings from family studies suggest some familial specificity for schizophrenia and schizotypal disorder and for bipolar illness. However, schizoaffective illness, even quite narrowly defined, appears to predispose to both schizophrenia and mood disorder. Whether, as the data of Kendler *et al.* (1993d) suggest, a vulnerability to psychosis might be transmitted in families together with a vulnerability to schizophrenia remains to be determined.

Twin studies

These studies compare the concordance rates for schizophrenia in *monozygotic (MZ) and dizygotic (DZ) twins*. The methodological problems of such studies have been considered already (see p. 126).

Table 12.10 Lifetime risk of psychiatric disorder in first-degree relatives of probands with DSM-IIIR schizophrenia, schizoaffective disorder, and controls

	Diagnosis of proband		
Disorder	Schizophrenia	Schizoaffective disorder	Control
Schizophrenia	6.5%	6.7%	0.5%
Schizotypal disorder	6.9%	2.8%	1.4%
Schizoaffective disorder	2.3%	1.8%	0.7%
All affective illness	24.9%	49.7%	22.8%
Psychotic affective illness	8.3%	12.4%	2.6%
Bipolar disorder	1.2%	4.8%	1.4%

From Kendler *et al.* (1993b, 1993c, 1993d).

The first substantial twin study was carried out in Munich by Luxenberger (1928), who found concordance in 11 of his 19 MZ pairs and in none of his 13 DZ pairs. Although this finding for DZ pairs casts doubt on the selection of the sample, subsequent investigations using improved methods have led to similar results. In these studies, concordance rates in MZ pairs have varied considerably, but they have always been higher than the concordance rates in DZ pairs. Representative figures for concordance are *about 50% for MZ pairs and about 10% for DZ pairs* (McGuffin 1988). A recent analysis from the Maudsley Twin Series using current operational diagnoses gave concordance rates for ICD-10 schizophrenia of 42% in MZ twins and 1.7% in DZ twins (see Murray and Castle 2000).

It might be expected that studies of MZ twins discordant for schizophrenia would reveal some environmental factors relevant to aetiology (see below). However, it is worth noting that the risk of schizophrenia in the offspring of an unaffected twin is the same as that of an affected twin. This means that an unaffected twin has the same genetic susceptibility to developing schizophrenia as the affected twin but for some reason the susceptibility is not expressed. This lack of expression may not necessarily be linked to environmental factors; for example even identical twins may be subject to differential gene expression (see McGuffin *et al.* 1994).

Adoption studies

Heston (1966) studied 47 adults who had been born to mothers with schizophrenia and separated from them within 3 days of birth. As children they had been brought up in a variety of circumstances, though not by the mother's family. At the time of the study their mean age was 36. Heston compared them with controls who were matched for circumstances of upbringing, but whose mothers had not suffered from schizophrenia. Amongst the offspring of the affected mothers, five were diagnosed as having schizophrenia compared with none of the controls. There was also an excess of antisocial

personality and neurotic disorders among the children of the affected mothers. The age-correlated rate for schizophrenia among the index cases was comparable with that among non-adopted children with one parent with schizophrenia. In this investigation, no account was taken of the fathers.

Further evidence has come from a series of studies started in 1965 by a group of Danish and American investigators. The work has been carried out in Denmark, which has national registers of psychiatric cases and adoptions. In one major project (Kety *et al.* 1975) two groups of adoptees were identified: 33 who had schizophrenia, and a matched group who were free from schizophrenia. Rates of disorder were compared in the biological and adoptive families of the two groups of adoptees. The rate for schizophrenia was greater among the *biological relatives of the adoptees* with *schizophrenia* than among the relatives of controls, a finding which supports the genetic hypothesis. Furthermore, the rate for schizophrenia was not increased amongst couples who adopted the affected children, suggesting that environmental factors were not of substantial importance. Recent follow-up studies using a national sample of adoptees in Denmark has confirmed that biological first-degree relatives of patients with schizophrenia have an approximately tenfold increased risk of suffering from schizophrenia or a related ('spectrum') disorder (Kety *et al.* 1994) (see below).

The Danish investigators viewed schizophrenia as a spectrum of illnesses with four divisions: (1) process schizophrenia, (2) reactive schizophrenia, (3) borderline schizophrenia, and (4) schizoid states. The last three are sometimes referred to collectively as *schizophrenia spectrum disease*. The adoption study findings reported above were for process schizophrenia, but the investigators also reported an excess of schizophrenia spectrum disease in biological relatives. These data have been reanalysed using DSM-III criteria for diagnosis, and an excess of *schizophrenia*, *schizoaffective psychosis* (mainly schizophrenic type), and *schizotypal personality disorder* has been confirmed among the biological relatives of schizophrenic probands (Kendler *et al.* 1993a, 1993b, 1993c).

Adoption studies cannot rule out environmental causes in the adoptive family, but they indicate that, if there are such environmental causes, they act only on genetically predisposed children.

Is there a relationship between clinical form and inheritance?

Family and twin studies of hebephrenic and paranoid subtypes have shown that there is some tendency for these subtypes to 'breed true' in families, although this is by no means clear cut (McGuffin 1988). There is some evidence that, compared with the hebephrenic subtype, probands with paranoid schizophrenia have a lower incidence of affected first-degree relatives and also that in paranoid schizophrenia the concordance ratio between MZ and DZ twins is less than that in other subtypes. This may mean that paranoid schizophrenia is a less genetic form of schizophrenia. Another way of viewing this distinction is by means of a threshold liability model in which hebephrenic and catatonic subtypes of schizophrenia are more severe forms of the illness and carry a greater genetic loading (McGuffin 1988).

What is the mode of inheritance?

The genetic evidence does not permit definite conclusions about the mode of inheritance. There have been three main theories.

Monogenic theory (single-gene models)

As the ratios of the frequencies of schizophrenia among people with different degrees of relationship with the proband do not fit any simple *Mendelian pattern*, it is necessary to propose modifying factors, for example, a dominant gene of *variable penetrance*. Penetrance depends on the *definition of the phenotype*, and as mentioned above this can be expanded to include various other disorders including schizotypal disorder. Despite these modifications, molecular genetic linkage studies have made it unlikely that schizophrenia, broadly or narrowly defined, is associated with a single

gene of main effect (see below and Maier *et al.* 2000).

Polygenic theory

This theory proposes a *cumulative effect of several genes*. It is proposed that the liability to schizophrenia lies on a continuum in the population and is expressed when a certain threshold of susceptibility is exceeded. In the polygenic model this liability is composed of predominantly additive effects of genes at different loci, together with additional environmental effects (McGuffin 1988). This model is less precise than the monogenic theory and more difficult to test, particularly with molecular genetic linkage techniques. However, increasingly systematic scans of the human genome with polymorphic markers have identified several areas of the genome that may contain susceptibility genes, for example, on chromosomes 6 and 10. The problem in assessing the significance of these findings is the lack of reproducibility between studies (see Maier *et al.* 2000).

Genetic heterogeneity theory

Monogenic and polygenic theories assume that schizophrenia is a single disease. Heterogeneity theories explain the observed patterns of inheritance by proposing that schizophrenia is a group of disorders of different genetic make-up or perhaps with genetic and non-genetic forms. Several attempts have been made to test these hypotheses, but the results have been ambiguous and will remain so until a definite biological or genetic marker is identified.

What is the phenotype?

Identification of genetic markers is made much easier if the boundaries of the inherited phenotype can be delineated. We have already seen that first-degree relatives of patients with schizophrenia have an excess of other disorders such as *schizotypal personality*, which appear to be inherited as part of the predisposition to schizophrenia. Studies of *non-affected relatives* have identified a number of neurobiological abnormalities, which are also found in patients with schizophrenia but not in controls with no family history of schizophrenia. These include enlarged lateral ventricles, loss of cerebral asymmetry, abnormal eye tracking performance and delayed P300 event potentials. Murray and Castle (2000) suggest that these abnormalities indicate familial transmission of genes for a variety of neurobiological characteristics, each of which may increase the risk of schizophrenia in an additive way.

Molecular genetic studies

As described in Chapter 5, two main approaches have been used to investigate the molecular genetic basis of schizophrenia. First, *linkage analysis* has been applied to multiply-affected families. Recent studies have identified multiple susceptibility markers that may represent genes of small effect. However, many of these findings require replication (see DeLisi 1999). As mentioned above, it is of course possible that the clinical syndrome of schizophrenia is genetically heterogenous and different genes may underlie the disorder in different populations.

In addition, studies of *candidate genes* have explored *associations* between particular genetic polymorphisms and the disease state. One difficulty is the current lack of really convincing candidate genes because of our poor understanding of the neurobiology and neurochemistry of schizophrenia. Overall there is some evidence of an association between schizophrenia and a polymorphism within the coding region of the *5-HT$_{2A}$ receptor gene* (Williams *et al.* 1997). This is of interest given the high affinity of atypical antipsychotic drugs for the 5-HT$_{2A}$ receptor. Associations have also been reported between schizophrenia and polymorphisms of the genes for *catecholamine O-methyl transferase* and the *dopamine D$_3$ receptor*. Even if these associations are confirmed, however, their contribution to the excess risk of schizophrenia in an individual will be small (see Maier *et al.* 2000).

In view of the neurodevelopmental hypothesis of schizophrenia, genes coding for brain development will also be important candidates. For example, Crow has hypothesized that the genes predisposing

to psychosis may be those which code for brain size and lateralization. Increasing knowledge of the genetic control of neurodevelopment will facilitate investigation of these interesting ideas.

Changes in brain structure in schizophrenia

Neuropathological studies

In the past, many investigators searched for gross pathological changes in the brains of schizophrenic patients but, with a few exceptions, found none. Later *post-mortem studies*, however, have indicated that, in comparison with psychiatric and healthy controls, the brains of patients with schizophrenia are *lighter* and somewhat *smaller*. There is *enlargement of the lateral ventricles*, particularly in the anterior and temporal horns. This is associated with a reduction in the volume of *medial temporal structures* such as the hippocampus and parahippocampal gyrus. The thalamus is reduced is size (Falkai and Bogerts 1993).

More detailed *histopathological investigations* have shown evidence of *cytoarchitectural disturbances* in the hippocampus and entorhinal cortex. These subtle abnormalities, which are not consistently associated with gliosis, are likely to be due to disturbances in the late migration or in the final differentiation of neurons during brain development. The consequence could be the misplacement of neurons from their intended sites and a disruption of the normal pattern of cortical connections. However, it is important to note that these abnormalities have not been widely replicated. There are more consistent reports of *decreased neuronal size* in a number of brain regions including hippocampus, dorsolateral prefrontal cortex, and Purkinje cells in the cerebellum. In addition, the *number of cells* in dorsomedial nucleus of the thalamus is reduced. Finally, there is also reasonably consistent evidence of a reduction in *synaptic density* in hippocampus and areas of prefrontal cortex. This may particularly involve *excitatory glutamatergic connections*. (For a review see Harrison 2000a).

Structural brain imaging

Lateral ventricular enlargement in schizophrenia was first reported from studies using *air encephalography* (Haug 1962). Using *computerized tomographic (CT)* scanning, which provides a non-invasive alternative, Johnstone *et al.* (1976) found significantly larger ventricles in 17 elderly hospitalized patients with schizophrenia than in eight normal controls. Much work has followed with both CT scanning and *magnetic resonance imaging (MRI)*, which allows better detection of localized brain changes.

A recent meta-analysis of MRI studies concluded that there are reliable and significant differences in ventricular volume and medial temporal structures in schizophrenia (Wright *et al.* 2000). However, the changes are relatively modest and there is *significant overlap between patient groups and controls*. The changes in regional brain volume in patients with schizophrenia show a *unimodal distribution*, indicating that the abnormality is not confined to a subgroup of subjects. There is no clear association with *gender*. They are present at the *onset of illness*, suggesting that they are not due to treatment.

In cross-sectional studies, the structural abnormalities do not correlate with *duration of illness*, suggesting a lack of progression. However, longitudinal studies in some patients have demonstrated apparent worsening of the brain changes. This is a controversial issue but it is possible that a subgroup of patients may undergo a *continuing neurotoxic process* after illness onset (see Harrison 2000a). Finally, first-degree relatives of patients with schizophrenia tend to show changes in brain structure that are midway between those of the patients and healthy controls (Lawrie *et al.* 1999). This suggests that some of the brain abnormalities are associated with genetic predisposition to the disorder. However, patients who express the illness phenotype appear to have additional cerebral damage, perhaps due to environmental causes such as birth injury (McNeil *et al.* 2000).

Clinical neurological aspects of schizophrenia

The increasing evidence of abnormal brain morphology has restimulated interest into whether patients with schizophrenia have objective evidence of *clinical neurological signs*. Clinicians have often detected signs of minor neurological abnormalities in schizophrenic patients. Although it is possible that some of these signs resulted from coincidental neurological disease, in the majority of cases they are likely to reflect the neuropathological changes described above.

Movement disorders are common in patients with schizophrenia and have often been attributed to antipsychotic drugs. However, similar movement disorders including tardive dyskinesia can be found in patients who have never apparently received antipsychotic drug treatment. The prevalence increases with age, suggesting that ageing can interact with a schizophrenic illness to increase the risk of movement disorders. Movement disorders unrelated to antipsychotic drug treatment have been associated with an early onset of illness and more severe symptomatology (see Hollister and Cannon 1999).

In view of the changes found in the temporal lobe in schizophrenia, it is of interest to note that patients with chronic *temporal lobe seizures* have an increased risk of developing symptoms of schizophrenia (see p. 436), as do patients with Huntington's chorea (see p. 423). Interestingly, as first suggested by Flor-Henry (1969), patients with epileptic foci in the *left temporal lobe* are at higher risk of developing a schizophrenia-like illness (see Trimble 1999).

Neurophysiological changes in schizophrenia

The EEGs of patients with schizophrenia generally show increased amounts of theta activity, fast activity, and paroxysmal activity compared with those of healthy controls. The significance of these findings is unknown.

There has been long-standing interest in the *P300 response*, an evoked potential which occurs 300 ms after a subject identifies a target stimulus embedded in a series of irrelevant stimuli. Therefore this response provides a measure of auditory information processing. In patients with schizophrenia, the *amplitude of the P300 wave is reduced* and the same abnormality can be found in a proportion of first-degree relatives of schizophrenic patients, suggesting that a reduction in P300 amplitude is a genetically transmitted marker for vulnerability to schizophrenia. However, similar abnormalities can be found in other patient groups, such as those with alcohol misuse and personality disorder. This questions the specificity of P300 abnormalities for schizophrenia (see Blackwood 2000). Abnormalities in another evoked potential, *the P50 wave*, have also been reported in patients with schizophrenia, their relatives and subjects with schizotypal personality. Molecular genetic studies in families with schizophrenia have shown that deficits in the P50 wave are linked to the gene coding for a subunit of the *nicotinic cholinergic receptor*. This implies that alterations in cholinergic neurotransmission could underlie abnormalities in information processing in schizophrenia (see Cadenhead *et al.* 2000).

There is evidence that more than 50% of patients with schizophrenia have defective performance in tests of *eye tracking*. A similar abnormality affects about 25% of first-degree relatives. Eye-tracking performance involves an integrated neural network involving middle and superior temporal areas of the extrastriate cortex. Holzman (2000) has proposed that eye-tracking dysfunction is a genetically transmitted and phenotypically mild variant of schizophrenia that, in the presence of other risk factors, can lead to the development of the overt clinical illness.

Functional brain imaging in schizophrenia

As described in Chapter 5, a number of techniques, particularly positron emission tomography (PET), single-photon emission tomography (SPET), and functional magnetic resonance imaging (fMRI), have been used to assess patterns of cerebral blood flow in patients with schizophrenia. There are two general approaches that have been proved useful:

- correlation of patterns of regional cerebral blood flow with the presence of specific symptomatology;
- patterns of cerebral activation and deactivation after specific neuropsychological tasks.

The link between three domains of symptom clusters (psychomotor poverty, reality distortion, and disorganization) and regional cerebral blood flow has been described above (Table 12.7). Other studies have looked at the cerebral correlates of more specific symptomatology. For example, in an fMRI investigation, it was found that when patients listened to externally generated speech, the presence of *auditory hallucinations* was linked to reduced activity of the temporal regions that normally process external speech. This could represent competition for a common neural substrate (see David and Busatto 1999). In another study using PET, patients with *passivity phenomena* showed hyperactivation of parietal and cingulate cortex in a motor task. The latter regions are involved in attributing significance to sensory information from both internal and external sources, and it is possible that dysfunction in these brain areas could lead to internally generated motor acts being attributed to an external source (see Vogeley and Falkai 1999; Liddle 2000).

Several functional imaging studies have indicated that the activation of prefrontal cortex associated with tasks such as the Wisconsin Card Sorting Test is impaired in patients with schizophrenia. Abnormalities in activation of prefrontal cortex have also been demonstrated in response to other psychological tasks including word generation and planning tasks. Some workers have concluded that the abnormalities in prefrontal activation in schizophrenia may reflect an abnormal relationship between activity in prefrontal cortex and other cerebral sites. This is often referred to as an abnormality in *functional connectivity* (see McGuire and Frith 1996).

The clinical relevance of the changes in blood flow in prefrontal cortex were demonstrated by Berman *et al.* (1992) who studied a group of nine MZ twins, discordant for schizophrenia. These workers found that all affected twins had lower prefrontal blood flow than their unaffected co-twin during the Wisconsin Card Sort Test. Moreover, the affected twin almost invariably had reduced hippocampal volume, which correlated with the decrement in prefrontal blood flow. This study suggests that the expression of clinical schizophrenia is associated with abnormal functional connectivity of temporal and frontal lobes.

Neuropsychological abnormalities in schizophrenia

It is now well established that patients with schizophrenia have widespread cognitive deficits particularly in tasks involving learning and memory. Neuropsychological studies aim to answer two rather different questions:

◆ What is the pattern of neuropsychological defects in schizophrenia and how might this reflect abnormalities in the various brain regions that subsume these psychological functions?

◆ How might specific cognitive abnormalities account for the characteristic symptoms of schizophrenia?

Although there is evidence that patients who develop schizophrenia have lower than average scores on IQ tests before they become ill, the onset of illness is associated with a further cognitive decline. There are generalized deficits in attention, perception, motor skills, language comprehension, together with several aspects of memory and executive 'planning' function (see Bilder *et al.* 2000; David 2000). *Semantic memory* and *executive functions* appear to be disproportionately affected. This is consistent with the abnormalities found in temporal cortex and hippocampus on MRI scans and the decrease in prefrontal activation revealed by functional imaging. Cognitive impairment is more profound in patients with prominent negative symptoms. Symptom resolution does not necessarily reverse cognitive decline, which is often the limiting factor in efforts at rehabilitation. Once established it is unclear whether cognitive decline increases over and above the usual ageing process (see Mortimer 2000).

As noted above, *attention deficits* are common in patients with schizophrenia and probably contribute to many of the impairments seen in psychological performance tests. Disorders of attention have been proposed to account for some of the clinical features of schizophrenia, particularly the positive symptoms. For example, Hemsley (1993) has argued that patients with schizophrenia over-attend to irrelevant stimuli with the result that they are unable to apply past experience to organize current perceptions. The result is an ambiguous unstructured sensory input, which predisposes to formation of delusions.

Using a different model, Frith (1996) has argued that in schizophrenia there is a breakdown in the *internal representation of mental events*. For example, a failure to monitor and identify one's own willed intentions might give rise to the idea that thoughts and actions arise from external sources, resulting in delusions of control. Such formulations are difficult to test experimentally, and presumably might apply to the pathophysiology of psychotic symptoms in general rather than schizophrenia specifically.

Biochemical abnormalities in schizophrenia

Many findings of early biochemical investigations turned out to be the result of unusual diet or medication rather than of schizophrenia itself. Recent studies have usually attempted to control these extraneous variables. Several hypotheses have been suggested, but the most dominant proposal has concerned the role of dopamine.

The dopamine hypothesis

Two lines of research have converged on the neurotransmitter *dopamine*. The first concerns the effects of *amphetamine*, which, among other actions, releases dopamine at central synapses. Repeated use of amphetamine at high doses can induce a disorder similar to acute schizophrenia in some normal people. In addition, acute amphetamine administration worsens psychotic symptoms in people with schizophrenia. The second approach starts from the finding that the various antipsychotic drugs *share dopamine receptor blocking properties*.

Recent studies have demonstrated that dopamine receptors in the brain exist in multiple subtypes, which differ in their pharmacological characteristics and neuroanatomical localization. Virtually all antipsychotic drugs bind to dopamine D_2 receptors and it is this property that correlates best with their clinical potency. In addition, drugs that are highly selective D_2 receptor antagonists, such as sulpiride, are effective antipsychotic agents. The exception to this rule is *clozapine*, which during usual clinical dosing occupies fewer D_2 receptors than other antipsychotic drugs. However, clozapine has a wide spectrum of other pharmacological effects including potent $5\text{-}HT_2$ receptor antagonist action, and it has been hypothesized that this may account for its unusual therapeutic efficacy (see Stahl 1999).

Although the evidence that dopamine is central to the action of antipsychotic drugs is strong, evidence for the corollary – that dopamine neurotransmission is abnormal in schizophrenia – has been weaker. For example, while biochemical studies of post-mortem brains from schizophrenic patients show increased dopamine receptor density in various brain regions, these changes could be a consequence of previous treatment with antipsychotic drugs, which produce reliable increases in brain D_2 receptor binding when administered to experimental animals (see Harrison 2000a).

PET and SPET studies provide a way of investigating dopamine receptor binding in the brain of living, unmedicated patients by using appropriately labelled dopamine receptor ligands. The balance of evidence suggests that D_2 receptor densities are unchanged in the basal ganglia of patients with schizophrenia. This does not rule out possible abnormalities in these receptors in mesolimbic and mesocortical regions. There are also some data indicating that D_1 receptors may be decreased in patients with schizophrenia, particularly in the presence of negative symptoms (Sedvall *et al.* 2000).

As explained earlier (Chapter 5) it is possible to measure the release of dopamine *in vivo* following pharmacological challenge by measuring the displacement of a D_2 radioligand such as $[^{11}C]$raclopride. In patients with acute schizophrenia, administration of amphetamine causes a greater decrease in $[^{11}C]$raclopride binding than is seen in healthy controls; this suggests that there may be excessive presynaptic dopamine release in acute schizophrenia (Laruelle 1998). Further studies have shown that the extent of the increase in presynaptic dopamine release in acute schizophrenia correlates with the therapeutic response to treatment with D_2 receptor antagonists. However, in patients not experiencing acute psychosis, dopamine release returns to normal. Current evidence therefore suggests:

- In patients with acute psychosis, presynaptic dopamine release is increased.
- Blocking the effects of increased dopamine release with D_2 receptor antagonists attenuates psychotic symptoms.
- Increased dopamine release cannot account for the symptoms of chronic schizophrenia.

Serotonin in schizophrenia

There has been long-standing interest in the possible role of *serotonin (5-HT)* in schizophrenia because the hallucinogen, lysergic acid diethylamide, is an agonist at $5\text{-}HT_2$ receptors. More recently it has become apparent that $5\text{-}HT_2$ receptor antagonism may supplement the therapeutic effect of D_2 blockade in schizophrenia and allelic variation in the $5\text{-}HT_{2A}$ gene is a risk factor for schizophrenia (see above). Additional support for a role for 5-HT pathways in pathophysiology is the finding of *decreased expression of 5-HT$_{2A}$ receptors in prefrontal cortex* in post-mortem studies and diminished cortical 5-HT$_{2A}$ receptor binding in unmedicated subjects with schizophrenia (Ngan et al. 2000). Increases in 5-HT$_{1A}$ receptor binding has also been reported in post-mortem studies (see Harrison 2000a; Sedvall *et al.* 2000). The findings are of interest because of the role of 5-HT neurons in neurodevelopment. Also, there are well-recognized interactions between 5-HT, dopamine, and glutamate pathways (see Carlsson *et al.* 1999).

Amino acid neurotransmitters in schizophrenia

There is increasing interest in the possible role of the amino acid neurotransmitter *glutamate* in the pathogenesis of schizophrenia (Carlsson *et al.* 1999). Glutamate is the major excitatory neurotransmitter in the brain and has a well-recognized role in neurotoxicity, which could be involved in abnormal neurodevelopment in schizophrenia. Post-mortem studies in patients with schizophrenia have revealed a variety of abnormalities in glutamatergic neurotransmission, which vary in nature depending on the brain region examined. For example, in medial temporal lobe, glutamatergic markers are decreased and there is a reduced expression of non-N-methyl-D-aspartate (non-NMDA) glutamate receptors. By contrast, in frontal brain regions there is an increase in the density of certain post-synaptic glutamate receptors (see Harrison 2000a).

These complex changes are of interest in the light of the clinical effects of *phencyclidine* and *ketamine*, both of which are glutamate NMDA receptor antagonists. Like amphetamine, these drugs can produce hallucinations and delusions but, in addition, they can cause negative-like symptoms, such as blunted affect and emotional withdrawal (Krystal *et al.* 1994). *Glycine* is a modulator of NMDA neurotransmission and it may therefore be significant that glycine treatment may be of benefit in some patients resistant to conventional antipsychotic drug therapy treatment (Heresco-Levy *et al.* 1999).

Drug misuse as a cause of schizophrenia

Misuse of a number of psychoactive substances can give rise to psychotic symptoms that may resemble some of the features of schizophrenia (see Chapter 18). Sometimes drug misuse is associated with a more prolonged illness that meets criteria for schizophrenia. In these circumstances it is usually considered that substance misuse may have precipitated the disorder but has not caused it. It is not clear whether prolonged and heavy substance misuse can lead to a schizophrenic illness in someone who would not otherwise have developed the disorder.

Andreasson *et al.* (1987) followed up 45 570 Swedish conscripts for 15 years. They found that the relative risk of developing schizophrenia was 2.5 times greater in subjects who used *cannabis*, and the relative risk for heavy users was six times greater. These data have led to two interpretations: first, that cannabis misuse is indeed a risk factor for the development of schizophrenia; second, that those predisposed to develop the illness are also predisposed to misuse cannabis. Which of these explanations may be correct is uncertain. It is, however, fairly clear that continuing substance misuse can *worsen the outcome* of an established schizophrenic illness (see Lowe 1999).

Developmental factors

Intrauterine events

Whilst genetic influences are of major importance in the aetiology of schizophrenia, it seems likely that environmental factors also play a role (see above). A number of workers have suggested that factors acting before or around the time of birth may contribute to the neuropathological abnormalities found in adult patients with schizophrenia. In support of this idea, there is indirect evidence from studies of *birth complications* and *season of birth*.

As evidence of birth complications, retrospective studies of schizophrenic patients have reported more obstetric complications than do studies of normal controls. In a meta-analysis of 12 case-control studies, Geddes and Lawrie (1995) concluded that patients with schizophrenia have had an increased risk (odds ratio 1.38) of being exposed to a definite birth complication. However, more recent case-control studies (Kendell *et al.* 2000) and a prospective investigation (Done *et al.* 1991) have failed to confirm this. It has been suggested that the association between obstetric complications and schizophrenia may be confined to males, or that birth injury may correlate with other aspects of the disorder such as early age of onset. It is also possible that in children with a genetic predisposition to schizophrenia, obstetric complications may increase the risk of a clinical schizophrenic disorder and of lateral ventricular enlargement in brain imaging studies (McNeil *et al.* 2000).

Schizophrenia is more frequent among people *born in the winter* than among those born in the summer, with about an 8% excess of schizophrenic births taking place in the first 3 months of the year. Interestingly, winter birth may be more common in patients without a family history of schizophrenia. Kendell *et al.* (1993) found that the incidence of schizophrenia in those born between February and May correlated inversely with climate temperature the previous autumn, i.e. the colder the temperature around the third month of gestation, the higher was the risk of a subsequent schizophrenic illness. It has been argued that these findings suggest a seasonal environmental influence of aetiological importance, perhaps viral in origin (see below). Some studies have linked increases in the incidence of schizophrenia with *prenatal exposure to influenza*, but the data do not suggest that such an effect has an important role in aetiology (see Crow 2000).

Childhood development

Parnas *et al.* (1982) reported a study of 207 children of mothers with schizophrenia who were first assessed when they were 8–12 years old and then again, as adults, 18 years later. Thirteen had developed schizophrenia (CATEGO diagnoses), 29 had 'borderline schizophrenia', and five had died by suicide. Of the measures made on the first occasion, those predicting schizophrenia were:

- poor rapport at interview;
- socially isolated from peers;
- disciplinary problems mentioned in school reports;
- reports by the parents that the person had been passive as a baby.

More recently, Done *et al.* (1994) found that in a cohort of more than 16 000 children prospectively studied over a 16-year period, those who developed schizophrenia could be distinguished at age 11 by greater hostility towards adults and speech and reading difficulties. In a similar study, Jones *et al.* (1994) found that individuals out of a large cohort of children who eventually developed schizophrenia showed delayed milestones and speech problems, together with lower education test scores and less social play. In a study linking information from the Israeli Draft Board Registry with a Psychiatric Case Register, Davidson *et al.* (1999) found that male adolescents who eventually developed schizophrenia exhibited defects in social functioning, organizational ability, and intellectual functioning.

There is therefore reasonable evidence that people who will develop schizophrenia show in their childhood development, some signs of *cognitive dysfunction* and *poor social competence* compared with controls. However, it is not clear how specific these changes are, nor how they may be related to the subsequent development of a schizophrenic illness.

Personality factors

Several early writers, including Bleuler (1911), commented on the frequency of abnormalities of personality preceding the onset of schizophrenia. Kretschmer (1936) proposed that both personality type and schizophrenia were related to the asthenic type of body build. He suggested a continuous variation between normal personality, schizoid personality (see p. 167), and schizophrenia. He regarded schizoid personality as a partial expression of the psychological abnormalities that manifest in their full form in schizophrenia. Such ideas must be treated with caution, since it is difficult to distinguish between premorbid personality and the prodromal phase of slowly developing illness. However, current findings from family studies suggest that the schizophrenic illness may share a common diathesis with schizotypal personality and some related personality disorders (Kendler *et al.* 1993b, 1994; Parnas *et al.* 1993).

Taken together, the findings suggest that abnormal personality features are not uncommon among people who later develop schizophrenia and among their first-degree relatives. However, many people with schizophrenia have no obvious disorder of personality before the onset of the illness and only a minority of people with schizoptypal or schizoid personalities develop schizophrenia.

Gender and age of onset

As noted above, although the incidence of schizophrenia in men and women is about equal over the life span, the age of onset of schizophrenia is *earlier in men than in women*. In men the onset peaks steeply at about 20 years age, declines and is thereafter fairly constant. In women there is also a small peak of age of onset in the early twenties but the incidence rises again in the late thirties.

It has been argued that many of the neurodevelopmental abnormalities described above are more common in males with schizophrenia. For example, men with schizophrenia are more likely than females to have poor premorbid adjustment, with more frequent and severe relapses and more evidence of structural brain abnormalities. However, Eaton *et al.* (1992) found that, if the age of onset was controlled for, the gender of the patient did not predict outcome. This suggests that the key variable determining severity of the illness is, in fact, age of onset. Jablensky (2000a) concluded that there is no unequivocal evidence of consistent gender differences in the clinical symptomatology of schizophrenia.

Conclusion

The neurodevelopmental view of schizophrenia is that abnormalities in brain structure and function are present for many years before the onset of a schizophrenic illness. While the studies reviewed above provide some evidence that cognitive and social abnormalities may be present before the onset of psychosis, these changes are usually modest and many patients appear to have functioned normally or even at a high level. This raises the question as to why, in most cases, the onset of schizophrenia becomes apparent only in early adulthood. Various ideas have been proposed. For example, the frontal cortex matures relatively late in development, and in non-human primates the full behavioural effects of early frontal lesions are not apparent until maturity, with the attendant development of cerebral specialization (Gold and Weinberger 1991). Also, following puberty, predisposed individuals will be subject to effects of late myelination in frontal and limbic cortex, changing sex hormone environments, and the psychosocial stressors consequent upon development into adulthood. At the moment there is no firm evidence to favour one proposal rather than another.

Dynamic and interpersonal factors in aetiology

Psychodynamic theories

From the point of view of aetiology, psychodynamic theories of schizophrenia are now largely of historical interest. However, they do focus attention on *interpersonal aspects* of schizophrenia, which are important in view of the evidence described above suggesting that patients with schizophrenia have abnormal social development during childhood. Freud's theory of schizophrenia was stated most clearly in his 1911 analysis of the *Schreber* case and in his 1914 paper 'On narcissism: an introduction'. According to Freud, in the first stage, libido was withdrawn from external objects and attached to the ego. The result was exaggerated self-importance. Since the withdrawal of libido made the external world meaningless, the patient attempted to restore meaning by developing abnormal beliefs. Because of libidinal withdrawal, the patient could not form a transference and therefore could not be treated by psychoanalysis. Although Freud developed his general ideas considerably after 1914, he elaborated his original theory of schizophrenia but did not replace it.

Melanie Klein (1952) believed that the origins of schizophrenia were in infancy. In the 'paranoid-schizoid position' the infant was thought to deal with innate aggressive impulses by splitting both his own ego and his representation of his mother into two incompatible parts, one wholly bad and the other wholly good. Only later did the child realize that the same person could be good at one time and bad at another. Failure to pass through this stage adequately was the basis for the later development of schizophrenia.

Psychodynamic views on aetiology and treatment have been discussed by Jackson and Cawley (1992).

The family as a cause of schizophrenia

Two kinds of theory have been proposed about the family as a cause of the onset of schizophrenia: *deviant role relationships* and *disordered communication*. The different role of the family in determining the course of established schizophrenia is discussed later (p. 366).

Deviant role relationships

The concept of the *'schizophrenogenic' mother* was suggested by the analyst Fromm-Reichmann in 1948. Lidz and his colleagues (1965) used intensive psychoanalytical methods to study the families of 17 patients with schizophrenia, of whom 14 were in social classes I or II. Two types of abnormal family pattern were reported:

♦ *marital skew*, in which one parent yielded to the other's (usually the mother's) eccentricities, which dominated the family;

♦ *marital schism*, in which the parents maintained contrary views so that the child had divided

loyalties. It was suggested that these abnormalities were the cause rather than the result of the schizophrenia.

Investigations by other clinicians have not confirmed these findings Even if they were confirmed, the abnormalities in the parents could be an expression of genetic causes or secondary to the disorder in the patient. These and other speculations about the causative role of family relationships have had the unfortunate consequence of inducing unjustified guilt in parents.

Disordered family communication

Research on disordered communication in families originated from the idea of the *double bind* (Bateson *et al.* 1956). A double bind is said to occur when an instruction is given overtly, but is contradicted by a second more covert instruction. For example, a mother may overtly tell her child to come to her, whilst conveying by manner and tone of voice that she rejects him. According to Bateson, double binds leave the child able to make only ambiguous or meaningless responses, and schizophrenia develops when this process persists. The theory is ingenious but not supported by evidence.

Studies of communication in families of patients with schizophrenia have given rather conflicting results (Singer and Wynne 1965; Hirsch and Leff 1975). However, it is worth noting that an association between abnormal social communication in parents and schizophrenic illness in children may, in fact, be a consequence of a shared genetic inheritance. This is because the incidence of *schizotypal disorder* (characterized by abnormalities of thought and speech) is raised in first-degree relatives of patients with schizophrenia (Table 12.10). Interestingly, parents of children with schizophrenia are more likely to suffer from schizotypal disorder than schizophrenia, presumably because the former impairs reproductive fitness somewhat less than the latter (Kendler *et al.* 1993b, 1993c).

Social factors in aetiology

Culture

If cultural factors are important in the aetiology of schizophrenia, differences in the incidence of the disorder might be expected in countries with contrasting cultures. As already explained (p. 329), the incidence rates of schizophrenia are remarkably similar in widely different places (Jablensky 2000b), and the possible exceptional rates are in areas (northern Sweden and Slovenia) with cultures that do not differ much from others in the Western world.

Occupation and social class

Several studies have shown that schizophrenia is over-represented among people of lower social class. In Chicago, for example, Hollingshead and Redlich (1958) found both the incidence and the prevalence of schizophrenia to be *highest in the lowest socioeconomic groups*. At first, these findings were thought to be of aetiological significance, but they could be a consequence of schizophrenia. For instance Goldberg and Morrison (1963) found that people with schizophrenia were of lower social status than their fathers and that this was usually because they had changed status after the illness began. However, Castle *et al.* (1993) found that, compared with controls, patients with schizophrenia were more likely to have been *born into socially deprived households*. The authors proposed that some environmental factor of aetiological importance was more likely to affect those of lower economic status living in inner cities.

Place of residence

Faris and Dunham (1939) studied the place of residence of mentally ill people in Chicago, and found that schizophrenics were over-represented in the *disadvantaged inner-city areas*. This distribution has been confirmed in other cities and it has been suggested that unsatisfactory living conditions caused schizophrenia. However, the findings can be explained equally plausibly by the occupational and social decline described above, or by a search for social isolation by people about to develop schizophrenia.

Migration

High rates of schizophrenia have been reported among some migrants. In a study of Norwegians who had migrated to Minnesota, Ødegaard (1932) found that the inception rate for schizophrenia was twice that of Norwegians in Norway. The reasons for these high rates are not clear, but they are probably due mainly to a disproportionate migration of people who are unsettled because they are becoming mentally ill. The effects of a new environment may also play a part in provoking illness in predisposed people. Thus 'social selection' and 'social causation' may both contribute to an excess of schizophrenia among migrants (see Cheng and Chang 1999).

Recent studies in the UK have suggested a strikingly increased incidence of schizophrenia (about 6 per 1000 in *Afro-Caribbeans* (Harrison *et al.* 1988), particularly in the 'second generation' born in the UK. By contrast, rates in the Carribean are not appreciably increased. The familial nature of schizophrenia in Afro-Caribbeans living in the UK seems similar to that of the remainder of the population (Sugarman and Crawford 1994). Therefore, if the incidence of schizophrenia is indeed increased, some environmental factor is likely to be involved. Various possibilities have been put forward, including an increased risk of viral infection *in utero*, high prevalence of cannabis use, and increased social adversity through racial discrimination (see Jablensky 2000a, 2000b).

Psychosocial stresses

Social isolation

People with schizophrenia often live alone, unmarried, and with few friends. The findings reviewed above suggest the pattern of isolation may begin before the illness, sometimes in early childhood. Of course, some patients may choose to isolate themselves as a way of decreasing social stimulation. In this sense social isolation, though undesirable in a general sense, is not a straightforward stressor.

Psychosocial stresses

Life events and difficulties have often been put forward as precipitants of schizophrenia, but few satisfactory studies have been carried out. In one of the most convincing, Brown and Birley (1968) used a standardized procedure to collect information from 50 patients newly admitted with a precisely datable first onset or relapse of schizophrenia. By comparison with a control group, the rate of 'independent' events in the schizophrenics was increased in the 3 weeks before the onset of the acute symptoms. When the events (which included moving house, starting or losing a job, and domestic crises) were compared with events preceding depression, neurosis, and suicide attempts, they were found to be non-specific. As a rough guide to the size of the effect, Paykel (1978) calculated that experiencing a life event doubles the risk of developing schizophrenia over the subsequent 6 months. Other workers have confirmed these findings for both first episodes and relapse of schizophrenia (see, for example, Bebbington *et al.* 1993).

In a review of studies, Norman and Malla (1993) concluded that in patients with chronic schizophrenia, the level of symptoms over time correlated with life events; however, there was little evidence that patients with schizophrenia suffered more life events than the general population.

Conclusions

There is strong evidence that schizophrenia has important *genetic causes*, although the mode of inheritance is not known. There is increasing evidence that there are *neurodevelopmental antecedents* in some patients, as judged by the presence of childhood cognitive and social impairments, but whether neurodevelopmental abnormalities are present in all patients to some degree is not clear. Most researchers believe that schizophrenia results from an interaction of genetic predisposition and environmental factors, although some have concluded that genetic explanations will eventually prove sufficient (Crow 1994). Environmental

factors proposed as important include *infection in utero*, *obstetric injury*, and *social adversit*, but the evidence for these is currently inconsistent. There is good reason to think that *stressful life events* often provoke the disorder; however, the events appear to be non-specific and are similar to those which precede mood disorders.

Patients with a schizophrenic illness have changes in *cerebral structural and function*, particularly involving the temporal and frontal lobes. These changes are associated with a generally non-progressive neuropsychological impairment. Although neurochemical disorders are likely to accompany these changes in cerebral morphology, the key abnormalities have not yet been identified with certainty. There is however, reliable evidence of *increased dopamine release* and *abnormal expression of some 5-HT receptor subtypes* (Box 12.1). Current theories propose disorders in *functional connectivity* between temporal and frontal cortex accompanied by alterations in dopamine, serotonin, and glutamatergic neurotransmission (see Carlsson *et al.* 1999).

Box 12.1 Some neurobiological abnormalities in schizophrenia

Neuropathology

Enlarged cerebral ventricles

Decreased medial temporal structures

Decreased neuronal size in hippocampus and pre-frontal cortex

Decreased number of cells in thalamus

Biochemistry

Increased dopamine release

Decreased dopamine D_1 receptor binding

Altered 5-HT receptor expression

Altered indices of glutamate neurotransmission

Course and prognosis

It is generally agreed that the outcome of schizophrenia is worse than that of most psychiatric disorders, but there have been surprisingly few long-term follow-up studies. Fewer still have included satisfactory criteria for diagnosis, samples of adequate size, and outcome measures that distinguish between symptoms and social adjustment. It is generally accepted that there are *wide variations in outcome*. This variation can be explained in three ways:

- Schizophrenia may be a single condition with a course that is modified by extraneous factors.
- Schizophrenia may consist of separate subtypes with different prognoses.
- Good prognosis cases may not be schizophrenia but some other condition.

The second and third explanations have already been discussed; the rest of this section is concerned with the first explanation.

It is essential to distinguish between data from studies of first admissions to hospital and data from investigations that study second or subsequent admissions or give no information on this point. When successive reports are studied, it appears that prognosis may have improved since the beginning of the century. Kraepelin (1919) concluded that only 17% of his patients in Heidelberg were socially well adjusted many years later. In 1932, Mayer-Gross, from the same clinic, reported social recovery in about 30% of patients after 16 years. By 1966, Brown *et al.* reported social recovery in 56% of patients after 5 years.

An important long-term study was carried out by Manfred Bleuler (1972, 1974) who personally followed up 208 patients who had been admitted to hospital in Switzerland between 1942 and 1943. Twenty years after admission, 20% had a complete remission of symptoms and 24% were severely disturbed. Bleuler considered that these proportions had changed little since the introduction of modern treatments, although advances in drug and social treatments had substantially benefited patients whose illnesses had a fluctuating course. When social adjustment was examined, a good outcome was found in about 30% of the whole group, and in 40% of those who had originally been first admissions. When full recovery had occurred, it was usually in the first 2 years and seldom after 5 years of continuous illness.

Bleuler's diagnostic criteria were narrow, and his findings suggest that the traditional view of schizophrenia as a generally progressive and disabling condition must be reconsidered. Nevertheless, 10% of his patients suffered an illness of such severity that they required long-term sheltered care. When the illness was recurrent, each subsequent episode usually resembled the first in its clinical features.

Bleuler's conclusions are broadly supported by Ciompi's larger but less detailed study of long-term outcome in Lausanne (Ciompi 1980). The study was based on the well-kept records of 1642 patients diagnosed as having schizophrenia from the beginning of the century to 1962. The average follow-up was 37 years. A third of the patients were found to have a good or fair social outcome. Symptoms often became less severe in the later years of life.

More recent studies are in general agreement with these findings. For example, in a 3–13-year follow-up study of patients with schizophrenia discharged between 1975 and 1985, Johnstone (1991) found that almost half had a good social outcome. In a 15-year follow-up of 330 Chinese patients with first admission schizophrenia, almost one-third recovered, but about 17% remained unable to function outside the hospital (Tsoi and Wong 1991). In the USA, however, Carone *et al.* (1991) found that only about 15% of patients meeting DSM-III criteria for schizophrenia recovered after 5 years, consistent with the proposal that DSM criteria identify a group of subjects with a poorer prognosis (see below).

Mortality in schizophrenia

All studies with prolonged follow-up report an *increased mortality* in patients with schizophrenia. In a meta-analysis of 36 000 patients Harris and

Table 12.11 **Factors predicting the outcome of schizophrenia**

Good prognosis	Poor prognosis
Sudden onset	Insidious onset
Short episode	Long episode
No previous psychiatric history	Previous psychiatric history
Prominent affective symptoms	Negative symptoms
Paranoid type of illness	Enlarged lateral ventricles
	Male gender
Older age at onset	Younger age at onset
Married	Single, separated, widowed, divorced
Good psychosexual adjustment	Poor psychosexual adjustment
Good previous personality	Abnormal previous personality
Good work record	Poor work record
Good social relationships	Social isolation
Good compliance	Poor compliance

Barraclough (1998) found that risk of death from all causes was increased 1.6-fold. Almost 40% of the excess mortality was accounted for by unnatural causes, mainly *suicide*, the risk of which was *increased tenfold*. The lifetime risk of suicide in schizophrenia is usually quoted at about 10%, although longer-term follow-up suggests that the rate may be somewhat lower, perhaps about 4% (Inskip *et al.* 1998). This is probably because the highest risk of suicide in schizophrenia is soon after diagnosis and declines somewhat thereafter. Deaths due to smoking-related diseases are also substantially increased in schizophrenia.

Predictors of outcome

There have been several attempts to find satisfactory predictors of the outcome of schizophrenia. In the International Pilot Study of Schizophrenia (World Health Organization 1973) tests were made of the predictive value of several sets of criteria based on symptoms, including Langfeldt's criteria, Feighner's diagnostic criteria, and others. All these symptom criteria proved to be largely unsuccessful at predicting outcome at 2 years or 5 years. The best predictors of poor outcome appear to be the criteria used for diagnosis in DSM-III, probably because they stipulate that the syndrome should have been present for 6 months before the diagnosis can be made.

More recent studies suggest that poor outcome in schizophrenia is associated with younger age of onset, male sex, and poor premorbid functioning (Lieberman and Sobel 1993). There is also evidence that the duration of psychotic symptoms prior to antipsychotic drug treatment correlates with time to remission and level of remission, that is, the greater the delay the worse the outcome (see McGorry *et al.* 2000). Whilst reluctance to seek treatment could be associated with other predictors of poor outcome, it is also possible that early antipsychotic drug treatment may improve the prognosis for some patients. Negative symptoms that persist after resolution of positive symptoms also predict a poorer outcome (Lieberman and Sobel 1993).

Some of the predictors that have emerged from the various studies are listed in Table 12.11 and may be taken as a moderately useful guide. However, it is wise for clinicians to be cautious when asked to predict the outcome of individual cases.

So far this discussion has been concerned with factors operating before or at the onset of schizophrenia. An account will now be given of factors acting after the illness has been established.

Social environment and course

Cultural background

As noted above, international studies suggest that the incidence of schizophrenia is similar in different countries; however, the course and outcome are not similar. In a 12-year follow-up study of 90 patients in Mauritius, Murphy and Raman (1971) observed a better prognosis than that reported in the UK by Brown *et al.* (1966). More Mauritian patients were able to leave hospital and return to a normal way of life. Nearly two-thirds were classified as socially independent and symptom-free at follow-up, compared with only half the English sample.

Comparable differences were reported at 2-year follow-up in the International Pilot Study of Schizophrenia (World Health Organization 1973). Outcome was better in India, Colombia, and Nigeria than in the other centres. This finding could not be explained by any recorded differences in the initial characteristics of the patients. The possibility of selection bias remains; for example, in these three countries patients with acute illness may be more likely to be taken to hospital than patients with illness of insidious onset. However, more recent studies designed to overcome these objections also found a *more favourable course of illness in less developed countries* (see Jablensky 2000a). The major difference in outcome was that patients in developing countries were more likely to achieve a complete remission than those in developed coun-

tries, who tended to be impaired by continual residual symptoms.

Life events

As explained above, some patients experience an excess of life events in the weeks before the onset of acute symptoms of schizophrenia. This applies not only to first illnesses but also to relapses (Bebbington *et al.* 1993). In addition, patients with increased numbers of life events experience a more symptomatic course.

Social stimulation

In the 1940s and 1950s clinicians recognized that among schizophrenics living in institutions many clinical features were associated with an unstimulating environment. Soon after this, Brown and colleagues (Brown *et al.* 1966; Wing and Brown 1970) investigated patients at three mental hospitals. One was a traditional institution, another had an active rehabilitation programme, and the third had a reputation for progressive policies and short admissions. The research team devised a measure of 'poverty of the social milieu' which took into account little contact with the outside world, few personal possessions, lack of constructive occupation, and pessimistic expectations on the part of ward staff. Poverty of social milieu was found to be closely related to three aspects of the patients' clinical condition: *social withdrawal*, *blunting of affect*, and *poverty of speech*. The causal significance of these social conditions was strongly supported by a further survey of the same hospitals 4 years later. Improvements had taken place in the environment of the hospitals, and these changes were accompanied by corresponding improvements in the three aspects of the patients' clinical state.

While an understimulating hospital environment is associated with worsening of the so-called poverty syndrome, an overstimulating environment can precipitate positive symptoms and lead to relapse. Since factors in a hospital environment play an important part in determining prognosis, it seems likely that similar factors are important to patients living in the community.

Family life

Brown *et al.* (1958) found that, on discharge from hospital, patients with schizophrenia returning to their families generally had a *worse prognosis than those entering hostels*. Brown *et al.* (1962) found that relapse rates were greater in families where relatives showed 'high expressed emotion' by making critical comments, expressing hostility, and showing signs of emotional over-involvement. In such families the risk of relapse was greater if the patients were in contact with their close relatives for more than 35 hours a week. The work was confirmed and extended when Leff and Vaughn (1981) investigated the interaction between 'expressed emotion' in relatives and life events in the 3 months before relapse. The onset of illness was associated either with a high level of expressed emotion or with an independent life event.

Vaughn and Leff (1976) also suggested an association between expressed emotion in relatives and the patient's response to *antipsychotic medication*. Among patients who were spending more than 35 hours a week in contact with relatives showing high emotional expression, the relapse rate was 92% for those not taking antipsychotic medication and only 53% for those taking antipsychotic medication. Among patients taking antipsychotic drugs and spending less than 35 hours in contact with relatives showing high emotional expression, the relapse rate was as low as 15%. In this study patients had not been allocated randomly to the treatment conditions.

Further studies (Leff *et al.* 1985) strongly suggested that high emotional expression has a causal role. Twenty-four families were selected in which a schizophrenic patient had extended contact with relatives showing high emotional expression. All patients were on maintenance neuroleptic drugs. Half the families were randomly assigned to routine out-patient care. The other half took part in a programme including education about schizophrenia, relatives' groups, and family sessions for relatives and patients. The relapse rate was significantly lower in this group than in the controls at 9-month and 2-year follow-up. Apart from providing further evidence of the importance of relatives' expressed emotion in relapse, this study showed the effectiveness of combined social intervention and drug treatment.

Expressed emotion has now been widely investigated as a predictor of schizophrenic relapse. Whilst not all studies concur, overall there seems little doubt that patients living in families with high levels of expressed emotion have a two- to threefold increased risk of psychotic relapse. Similar findings have been found across cultures, although high levels of expressed emotion are more common in Western countries (Kavanagh 1992). Further evidence has accumulated that family intervention aimed at improving the knowledge and skills of relatives can lower expressed emotion levels and decrease relapse rate (Kavanagh 1992). However, in a meta-analysis of the published studies, De Jesus Mari and Streiner (1994) found that inclusion of treatment withdrawals and drop-outs (an intention to treat analysis) reduced the apparent effectiveness of family intervention to prevent relapse. This suggests that the results of family intervention may be useful in those who persist with it, while the others need an alternative approach.

Levels of expressed emotion probably depend on interactions between the patient, their symptomatology, and their relatives. Thus certain types of symptoms may be more likely to provoke high expressed emotion (see below). However, no clear relationships have emerged between the form and severity of the schizophrenic disorder and levels of expressed emotion (Kavanagh 1992), although relatives with low levels of expressed emotion are more likely than those with high levels to regard the schizophrenic disorder and associated behaviour as an illness beyond the control of the patient. Interestingly, the nature of these causal attributions, like expressed emotion, are significant predictors of relapse (Barrowclough *et al.* 1994).

Effects of schizophrenia on the family

With the increasing care of patients in the community rather than in hospital, difficulties have arisen for some families. Relatives of patients with schizophrenia describe two main groups of problems. The first group relates to *social withdrawal* patients tend not interact with other family members; they seem slow, lack conversation, have few interests, and neglect themselves. The second group relates to more obviously *disturbed and socially embarrassing behaviour* such as restlessness, odd or uninhibited social behaviour, and threats of violence. These problems are likely to play a part in the development of high levels of expressed emotion in relatives, which may in turn worsen the behaviours.

Relatives of patients with schizophrenia may often feel anxious, depressed, guilty, or bewildered. They may be understandably uncertain of how to deal with difficult and odd behaviour. Further difficulties arise from differences in opinion between family members, and more commonly from a lack of understanding and sympathy among neighbours and friends. The effects on the lives of relatives and families are often serious. Unfortunately, in the UK and other countries community services for patients with chronic schizophrenia and their relatives are often less than adequate. Improving help, advice, and services to carers of patients is a priority of the recent National Service Framework for Mental Health (Department of Health 1999a). Leff (1998) has commented:

Relatives should be respected for the caring they undertake day and night for years on end. They do not want to be considered pathogenic and suitable cases for treatment. Instead they wish to be regarded as partners in the struggle against schizophrenia.

Conclusion

Social factors play a role in the onset of schizophrenia and the level of symptomatology in established cases. The emotional involvement of relatives can affect the risk of relapse, and it is possible that the lower degree of expressed emotion typically found in families in developing countries could play a part in the improved prognosis of schizophrenia in these cultures. In terms of the general environment in which patients live, too

much stimulation appears to precipitate relapse into positive symptoms, whilst understimulation leads to worsening of negative symptoms.

Treatment

The treatment of schizophrenia is concerned with both the acute illness and chronic disability. In general, the best results are obtained by *combining drug and social treatments*, whereas methods aimed at providing psychodynamic insight are unhelpful.

This section is concerned with evidence from clinical trials about the efficacy of various forms of treatment. A later section on management deals with the use of these treatments in everyday clinical practice. The pharmacological aspects of antipsychotic drugs and their use are discussed in Chapter 21. The organization of community care and care planning is discussed in Chapter 23.

Antipsychotic drugs

Treatment of acute schizophrenia

The effectiveness of *antipsychotic medication* in the treatment of acute schizophrenia has been established by several well-controlled double-blind studies. For example, the National Institute of Mental Health collaborative project (Cole *et al.* 1964) compared chlorpromazine, fluphenazine, and thioridazine with placebo. Three-quarters of the patients receiving antipsychotic treatment for 6 weeks improved, whatever the drug, whilst half of those receiving placebo worsened. In a meta-analysis, Thornley *et al.* (1997) reviewed 42 randomized studies of chlorpromazine. Relative to placebo, chlorpromazine was more likely to lead to global clinical improvement at 8 weeks (55% versus 37%, NNT = 6). In addition, treatment with chlorpromazine was associated with lower relapse rates over the following 2 years (40% versus 71%, NNT = 4). The most common adverse effects were weight gain (41%), and sedation (28%). The incidence of Parkinsonian side-effects was fairly low (12%) but chlorpromazine is less liable to produce this adverse effect than higher-potency antipsychotic drugs such as haloperidol.

Drug treatment has most effect on the positive symptoms of schizophrenia, such as hallucinations and delusions, and least effect on the negative symptoms. The sedative and calming action may be immediate, but the antipsychotic effect develops more slowly, sometimes taking up to several weeks to be clearly apparent.

Differences between antipsychotic drugs

Studies have failed to show differences in efficacy between the various *typical* antipsychotic drugs. *Clozapine*, however, does have a significantly greater efficacy than conventional agents in both treatment-responsive and treatment-resistant schizo-

phrenia (Wahlbeck *et al.* 1999) (Figure 12.1). Whether other atypical agents are more effective than conventional drugs is still a matter of debate. Both *olanzapine* and *risperidone* have proved superior to haloperidol in some studies, with greater efficacy against both positive and negative symptoms; however, the clinical relevance of these differences has been disputed (NHS Centre For Reviews and Dissemination 1999).

The adverse-effect profiles of both typical and atypical agents does vary and for many patients this is the best basis on which to choose a suitable agent (p. 661). In general, atypical agents produce fewer *extrapyramidal movement disorders* than typical antipsychotics, although low doses of typical agents may, in fact, be well tolerated. Recent studies suggest that, for many patients, modest doses of

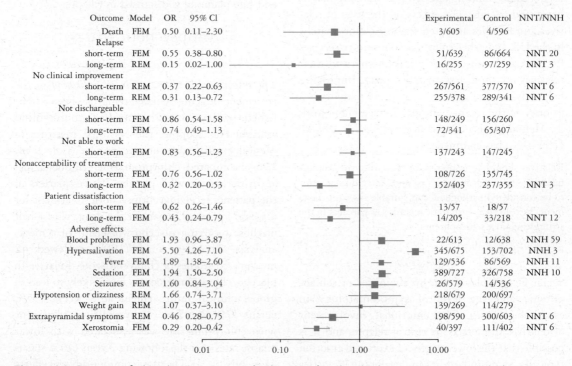

Outcome	Model	OR	95% CI	Experimental	Control	NNT/NNH
Death	FEM	0.50	0.11–2.30	3/605	4/596	
Relapse						
short-term	FEM	0.55	0.38–0.80	51/639	86/664	NNT 20
long-term	REM	0.15	0.02–1.00	16/255	97/259	NNT 3
No clinical improvement						
short-term	REM	0.37	0.22–0.63	267/561	377/570	NNT 6
long-term	REM	0.31	0.13–0.72	255/378	289/341	NNT 6
Not dischargeable						
short-term	FEM	0.86	0.54–1.58	148/249	156/260	
long-term	FEM	0.74	0.49–1.13	72/341	65/307	
Not able to work						
short-term	FEM	0.83	0.56–1.23	137/243	147/245	
Nonacceptability of treatment						
short-term	FEM	0.76	0.56–1.02	108/726	135/745	
long-term	REM	0.32	0.20–0.53	152/403	237/355	NNT 3
Patient dissatisfaction						
short-term	FEM	0.62	0.26–1.46	13/57	18/57	
long-term	FEM	0.43	0.24–0.79	14/205	33/218	NNT 12
Adverse effects						
Blood problems	FEM	1.93	0.96–3.87	22/613	12/638	NNH 59
Hypersalivation	FEM	5.50	4.26–7.10	345/675	153/702	NNH 3
Fever	FEM	1.89	1.38–2.60	129/536	86/569	NNH 11
Sedation	FEM	1.94	1.50–2.50	389/727	326/758	NNH 10
Seizures	FEM	1.60	0.84–3.04	26/579	14/536	
Hypotension or dizziness	REM	1.66	0.74–3.71	218/679	200/697	
Weight gain	REM	1.07	0.37–3.10	139/269	114/279	
Extrapyramidal symptoms	REM	0.46	0.28–0.75	198/590	300/603	NNT 6
Xerostomia	FEM	0.29	0.20–0.42	40/397	111/402	NNT 6

0.01   0.10   1.00   10.00

Figure 12.1 Outcomes of schizophrenic patients randomly assigned to short- or long-term treatment with clozapine (experimental) or conventional neuroleptics (control) in 30 trials. OR, odds ratio; CI, confidence interval; NNT, number needed to treat; NNH, number needed to harm; FEM, fixed effects model; REM, random effects model. Columns with headings Experimental and Control refer to numbers of subjects. See Chapter 5 for explanation of terms.

antipsychotic drugs (for example 5–10 mg halo-peridol) are as effective as higher doses and have significantly less risk of side-effects such as movement disorders and hyperprolactinaemia (Kapur *et al.* 1999). If rapid sedation is required, it is usually preferable to combine the antipsychotic drug with a *benzodiazepine* (Taylor *et al.* 1999).

Treatment after the acute phase

Since the original demonstration by Pasmanick *et al.* (1964), many controlled trials have shown the effectiveness of continued oral and depot antipsychotic therapy in *preventing relapse*. It has also become clear that some patients with chronic schizophrenia do not respond even to long-term medication, and that other patients remain well without drugs. Unfortunately, there has been no success in predicting which patients benefit from longer-term drug treatment. Since long-continued antipsychotic medication may lead to problematic side-effects including substantial weight gain, sexual dysfunction, and irreversible dyskinesias, it is important to know how long such treatment needs to be given. There is still no clear answer to this question, but chlorpromazine was still more effective than placebo in preventing relapse over 2–5 years of treatment (55% versus 83%, NNT = 4) (Thornley *et al.* 1997). The general consensus is that even long periods of remission produced by antipsychotic medication do not protect patients from relapse once medication is withdrawn (see Cunningham Owens and Johnstone 2000).

There is a widespread clinical impression that *depot injections* are more successful than continued oral medication in preventing relapses of schizophrenia and this view is supported by much investigation (Davis *et al.* 1993). This is presumably due to improved compliance. Studies of intermittent treatment, where antipsychotic drugs are given at the first sign of relapse, have shown it to be less effective than continuous prophylaxis (Jolley *et al.* 1990).

Antidepressants and mood stabilizers

As already explained, symptoms of depression occur commonly in the syndrome of schizophrenia (p. 334). Since it is not easy to distinguish between depressive symptoms and the various negative symptoms of schizophrenia, it is difficult to assess the effects of *antidepressant medication* in chronic schizophrenia. As yet, there have been few satisfactory clinical trials.

Siris *et al.* (1987) carried out a placebo-controlled trial of imipramine in schizophrenic patients receiving maintenance fluphenazine in whom a depressive episode became apparent following resolution of the psychotic symptoms. Imipramine was significantly better than placebo in these patients, improving depressed mood but not altering psychotic symptoms. A more recent study by the same group confirmed the beneficial effect of imipramine in post-psychotic depression and also suggested some benefit on negative symptoms (Siris *et al.* 1991). In patients where depressive symptoms coexist with an active psychosis, antidepressant drugs do not seem to be helpful and in fact there is some evidence that they may worsen psychotic symptoms (Plasky 1991). Newer antidepressants such as selective serotonin re-uptake inhibitors (SSRIs) are now used to treat depressive symptoms in schizophrenia but have not been rigorously evaluated (Kirli and Caliskan 1998).

The value of *lithium* in treating schizophrenia is uncertain. Occasional beneficial effects could be due to the treatment of patients with schizoaffective disorder. There is some evidence that lithium has a therapeutic action in this diagnostic group. In two small trials, Brockington *et al.* (1978) found that chlorpromazine was more effective than lithium for patients who satisfied criteria for both depressive disorder and schizophrenia. However, lithium and chlorpromazine were equally effective for patients with mania and schizophrenia. In the Northwick Park Functional Psychosis study, lithium decreased elevated mood, whatever the diagnosis of the patient, but had no significant effect on positive or negative symptoms (Johnstone *et al.* 1988).

Prophylactic studies of other mood stabilizers such as carbamazepine and sodium valproate often include patients with diagnoses of schizoaffective disorder. The current evidence suggests that patients with more prominent manic symptoms are likely to be helped by these drugs (see Chapter 21).

Electroconvulsive therapy

In the treatment of schizophrenia, the traditional indications for ECT are catatonic stupor and severe depressive symptoms accompanying schizophrenia. The effects of ECT are often rapid and striking in both these conditions. Nowadays, ECT is seldom used for other presentations of schizophrenia, although there is some evidence that it is rapidly effective in acute episodes (Taylor and Fleminger 1980). ECT is occasionally used in patients whose positive symptoms have not responded to adequate antipsychotic drug treatment, but its effectiveness for this indication has not been formally evaluated.

Psychosocial approaches

The development of community-based services has led to increasing emphasis on psychosocial interventions in the treatment of schizophrenia. These interventions are of several different kinds but share similar purposes (see Mueser and Bond 2000) (Box 12.2):

- enhancement of interpersonal and social functioning;
- promotion of independent living in the community;

Box 12.2 **Psychosocial treatment approach in schizophrenia**

Assertive community treatment

Family intervention

Social skills training and illness self-management

Cognitive behaviour therapy

- attenuation of symptom severity and associated co-morbidity (for example, substance misuse);
- improvement in personal illness management.

Dynamic psychotherapy

In the past, *individual dynamic psychotherapy* was used quite commonly for schizophrenia, though much more in the USA than in the UK. Evidence from clinical trials is scanty, but it does not support the use of this kind of psychological treatment. An investigation by May (1968) found that psychotherapy had little benefit, but the treatment was short and provided by relatively inexperienced psychiatrists. Apart from the lack of convincing evidence that intensive individual psychotherapy is effective in schizophrenia, there may be some danger that the treatment will cause overstimulation and consequent relapse (see Malmberg and Fenton 2000).

Group therapy

Many kinds of group therapy have been used to treat schizophrenia. When the results have been compared with routine hospital treatment, the general finding in the better-controlled evaluations has been that group therapy is of little benefit in the acute stage of the disorder. There may be a place for *supportive groups* for patients who are re-settling after the resolution of an acute illness.

Family therapy

As noted above, schizophrenia places a considerable burden on patients' families and *family therapy* of various kinds is often employed at various stages of treatment. The most systematically evaluated family intervention is that designed to decrease expressed emotion in family members. The procedure is usually combined with education about the illness and its consequences, together with practical advice on management. The controlled studies reviewed above (see p. 366) suggest that these interventions are beneficial in preventing relapse, although their utility in routine clinical practice is uncertain (see Pharoah *et al.* 2000). A recent meta-analysis of controlled trials confirmed

Box 12.3 Elements in family intervention in schizophrenia

Box 12.3 Elements in family intervention in schizophrenia

Education about schizophrenia
Improving communication
Lowering expressed emotion
Expanding social networks
Adjusting expectations
Reducing hours of daily contact

Source: Leff (1998)

that such interventions may lower rates of hospitalization (NNT to prevent relapse = 6.5) and improve medication compliance. However, the studies showed a wide range of outcome with more recent investigations showing less effect (Pharoah *et al.* 2000). Leff (1998) has reviewed the key ingredients of family therapy in schizophrenia (Box 12.3).

Social skills training and illness self-management

Social skills training uses a variety of approaches to teach complex interpersonal skills, including behavioural rehearsal, feedback and *in vivo* training. Skills training may be combined with illness self-management in which patients learn to adjust their own medication and organize their lives to minimize troublesome symptomatology. The results of these interventions are generally positive but concerns remain about whether the gains are maintained when treatment ends and whether benefit is restricted to patients who have a good prognosis (see Mueser and Bond 2000).

Cognitive behaviour therapy

The use of *cognitive behaviour therapy* in schizophrenia is based on the rationale that positive psychotic symptoms are amenable to structured reasoning and behavioural modification. With delusional beliefs, for example, individual ideas are traced back to their origin and alternative explanations are explored. However, direct confrontation is avoided. Similarly, it may be possible to modify a patient's beliefs about the omnipotence, identity, and purpose of auditory hallucinations, with a resulting decrease in the distress that accompanies the experience and, perhaps, in its frequency. A recent controlled trial found that cognitive behaviour therapy combined with medication was more effective than supportive counselling in decreasing positive symptoms of schizophrenia (Tarrier *et al.* 1998). Another study found that both cognitive behaviour therapy and a less specific 'befriending' intervention led to significant reductions in both positive and negative symptoms over 9 months of treatment but that gains were more enduring in the cognitive therapy group 9 months after treatment had ended (Sensky *et al.* 2000). How far these beneficial effects could be obtained in routine clinical settings is an important question.

Interaction of maintenance drug treatment and psychosocial treatment

The psychosocial treatments mentioned above are usually given in conjunction with antipsychotic medication. Successful psychosocial treatment often improves compliance with medication but this is not usually sufficient to explain symptomatic improvement. In the case of expressed emotion, for example, it seems likely that antipsychotic treatment is more effective if adverse psychological stress is lowered. However, it is worth noting that psychological intervention designed specifically to improve adherence to medication is also a useful treatment adjunct (Kemp *et al.* 1996).

Assessment

Assessment begins with *differential diagnosis*, which is particularly concerned with the exclusion of organic disorder (especially a drug-induced state), mood disorder, and personality disorder. In practice, the main difficulty is often to elicit all the symptoms from a withdrawn or suspicious patient. This procedure may require several psychiatric interviews as well as careful observations by nursing staff. The differential diagnosis from mood disorder can be particularly difficult and may require prolonged observation for discriminating symptoms of schizophrenia. Information from relatives or close friends will always be helpful.

While the psychiatric diagnosis is being confirmed, a *social assessment* should be carried out. This includes assessment of the patient's previous personality, work record, accommodation, and leisure pursuits, and especially the attitudes to the patient of relatives and any close friends. The doctor or social worker can proceed with this enquiry, while an evaluation of the patient's social functioning in the ward is made by nurses and occupational therapists.

Management

Success in management depends on establishing a *good relationship* with the patient so that his cooperation is enlisted. It is often difficult to establish a working relationship with patients suffering from chronic illness who are paranoid or emotionally unresponsive, but with skill and patience progress can usually be made. It is important to make plans that are realistic, especially for the more handicapped patient. Overenthusiastic schemes of rehabilitation may increase the patient's symptoms and, if he lives in the community, place unacceptable burdens on relatives. Minimizing the side-effects of medication is also important if compliance is to be facilitated. It is important that plans are acceptable to the patient's family and general practitioner.

The acute illness

Treatment in hospital is usually needed for both first episodes of schizophrenia and acute relapses, although with adequate resources home treatment is possible and may carry some advantages (Dedman 1993). However, hospital admission allows a thorough assessment and provides a secure environment for the patient. It also gives a period of relief to the family, who have often experienced considerable distress during the period of pro-dromal symptoms of the illness.

There are important advantages in a few days of observation without drugs, although some acutely disturbed patients may require immediate treatment. A drug-free period allows thorough assessment of the patient's mental state and behaviour as described above. It also shows whether mental abnormalities and disturbed behaviour are likely to improve simply with change of environment. If they do not improve, an *antipsychotic drug* should be prescribed, with the dose depending on the severity of the symptoms.

There is a wide choice of drugs (see p. 661), but the clinician should become thoroughly familiar with a few. For acutely disturbed patients, the sedating effects of modest doses of *chlorpromazine* (200–400 mg daily) are useful. An alternative approach is to use a modest dose of a high-potency agent (for example 5–10 mg *haloperidol*) with additional *benzodiazepine treatment* for a short period. This approach permits lower doses of antipsychotic drugs to be used, which is important in lessening toxicity and improving patient compliance. Potential complications such as behavioural disinhibition and benzodiazepine dependence seem to be rare if benzodiazepine treatment is co-prescribed with an antipsychotic drug and given as needed for a limited period.

Whether *atypical antipsychotic drugs* should be used initially, particularly in first episode cases, has been debated. Recent UK guidelines have recommended the use of atypical agents (National Institute of Clinical Excellence 2002). Such drugs are particularly indicated when there is a high risk of movement disorder (see McGrath and Emmerson 1999). The choice should be discussed with the patient and the family. Clinicians should be aware of new evidence as it emerges (see for example, Geddes et al. 2000, Csernansky et al. 2002). As noted above, *cognitive deficit* appears to be a fundamental part of schizophrenia. There are hints that, in contrast to typical agents, some of the atypical agents may improve cognitive performance (see Harvey and Keefe 2000). If this is confirmed, it would give such drugs a significant advantage.

Oral medication is usually given at this stage, although occasional intramuscular doses may be needed for patients who exhibit acutely disturbed behaviour and are unwilling to comply with oral treatment. If there are doubts about whether the patient is swallowing tablets, the drug can be given as syrup. An alternative is *zuclopenthixol acetate* given as a short-acting depot preparation, but this approach must be used with caution because it is not possible to titrate the dose with precision. It has been recommended that zuclopenthixol acetate should not be given to patients whose tolerance of antipsychotic drugs is undetermined (Royal College of Psychiatrists 1993).

Medication should be continued at a fairly constant level for a number of weeks because the antipsychotic effects of treatment need time to become established. Benzodiazepines may be useful for intermittent agitation, and insomnia. *Antiparkinsonian drugs* should be prescribed if parkinsonian side-effects are troublesome, but they need not be given routinely. Symptoms of excitement, restlessness, irritability, and insomnia can be expected to improve within days. Symptoms of mood disturbance, delusions, and hallucinations respond more slowly, often persisting for several weeks. Lack of improvement at this stage suggests inadequate dosage or failure to take the drugs prescribed, but a few cases resist all efforts at treatment. Once there is undoubted evidence of sustained improvement, dosage can be reduced cautiously while careful watch is kept for any return of symptoms. This reduced dose is continued then for a further period (see below).

As soon as possible it is important to explain the need for drug treatment to the patient and to obtain full consent (see p. 652). Where a patient is not judged able to make decisions of this nature, the appropriate legal safeguards under the Mental Health Act and its code of practice should be employed. It is important to involve the patient and their family as far as possible in their treatment. The use of *patient advocates* is also helpful.

During the early days of treatment, the clinical team will have taken histories from the patient, relatives, and other informants, in order to build up a picture of the patient's previous personality, premorbid adjustment, and social circumstances, and any precipitants of illness. By the time that symptomatic improvement has taken place, the team should have formulated a provisional plan for continuing care. Although it is difficult to predict the long-term prognosis at this stage, a judgement has to be made about the likely immediate outcome. The judgement is based on the degree and speed of response to treatment, the history of previous episodes, and on the factors listed in Table 12.11. The aim is to decide how much after-care patients will require, and to make realistic plans accordingly.

After-care of 'good-prognosis' patients

After a first episode of schizophrenia, patients judged to have a good immediate prognosis have two principal needs for treatment following discharge from hospital. The first is to take medication in decreasing dosage for 3–6 months. The second is to be given advice about avoiding obviously stressful events. The patient should be seen regularly as an out-patient or at home by a community nurse until a few months after medication has been stopped and symptoms have ceased. Thereafter, a cautiously optimistic prognosis can be given, but the patient and his family should be warned to seek medical help quickly if there is any suggestion of the condition returning. The patient's GP has an important role to play in this phase of treatment.

After-care of the 'poor-prognosis' patients without major social handicaps

When it is judged that further relapse is likely, continuing care will be required and this will probably include *prophylactic medication*. It may be better to give such medication by injection (for example, as fluphenazine or flupenthixol decanoate) since some patients fail to take oral medication regularly over long periods. The dosage, which should be the minimum required to suppress symptoms, can be determined by cautiously varying its size and frequency while observing the patient's clinical state. Some patients show little response to continued antipsychotic medication even in substantial doses.

Particularly where response is poor, it is worthwhile considering a trial of an *atypical agent*. *Clozapine* is the only drug with proven efficacy in treatment-resistant patients but clinical experience suggests that some patients who do not respond to typical agents can do well with safer atypicals such as *risperidone* or *olanzapine*. Failure with these agents should prompt consideration of a trial of clozapine (Stahl 1999).

Patients who respond poorly to medication will usually have a mixture of positive and negative symptoms. Generally it is worthwhile continuing modest doses of a well-tolerated antipsychotic agent because the patient's mental state may well worsen without it. The follow-up plan should include regular review of mental state and medication, social adjustment, and occupation. It may be helpful for advice to be given about stressful situations and family problems. Specific interventions may be needed to help the family understand the patient's illness, to have realistic expectations of what the patient can accomplish, and to decrease their emotional involvement where appropriate. Work of this nature can be undertaken by community psychiatric nurses, social workers, psychiatrists, and GPs working together. Leff (1998) has suggested that family interventions may be particularly appropriate in families:

- where the patient relapses despite being compliant with medication;
- where arguments can erupt into violence;
- where the police are called to restore order;
- where relatives constantly make demands on staff.

The most difficult problem in continuing management is likely to be the patient's tendency to withdraw from treatment. *Assertive community treatment* has a useful role to play in this respect (see Chapter 23) (Marshall and Lockwood 2000).

Patients with poor prognosis and significant chronic handicap

When patients have poor social adjustment and behavioural defects characteristic of chronic schizophrenia, they require more elaborate after-care. They should be identified as early as possible so that long-term plans can be made for both rehabilitation in hospital and resettlement outside hospital. Maintenance drug therapy plays an important part, but the main emphasis is on a programme of rehabilitation tailored to the needs of the individual patient. Contributions from an occupational therapist and clinical psychologist can be particularly helpful. Particular issues that require attention are:

- *living accomodation and circumstances*. Will the patient be able to live alone or will he return to live with parents or other relatives. Will a group home or hostel be needed?
- *occupational activities*. Will the patient be able to undertake some form of paid employed or voluntary work?
- *activities of everyday living*. Patients often need help to relearn basic living skills such as cooking, budgeting, shopping, housework, and personal hygiene.
- *social skills training and leisure activities*. Social skills training can benefit everyday living activities and leisure pursuits.

It can be expected that the least handicapped patients will live more or less independently. Sheltered work and accommodation are likely to be needed for the remainder. The essential requirements are a management plan that focuses on one or two aspects of behaviour disorder (for example, problems with personal hygiene) at any one time, and a consistent approach between the members of staff carrying it out.

Despite the present emphasis on treatment outside hospital, early rehabilitation in hospital has significant advantages because it allows greater consistency of approach over the whole of the patient's day. Wards organized mainly for the treatment of acute illness are often too stimulating for patients with chronic schizophrenia in need of rehabilitation. Hence it is appropriate to set aside a special area for rehabilitation.

Most handicapped patients are able to live outside hospital, albeit in sheltered provisions. A minority require long-term care in hospital. The components of a community service for these patients are described in Chapter 23. Success depends less on physical provisions than on well-trained staff who have tolerant attitudes and the capacity to obtain satisfaction from work that produces small improvements over long periods.

When a patient has persisting abnormalities of behaviour, particular attention needs to be given to the problems of his family, as noted above. Relatives may be helped by joining a voluntary group and meeting others who have learned to deal with similar problems. They also need to know that professional help will be provided whenever problems become too great. Advice is needed about the best ways of responding to abnormal behaviour, and about the expectations that they should have of the patient. Such advice is often given best by community nurses who have experience of treating chronic schizophrenic patients in hospital as well as in the community (see Gournay 2000). Social workers also have a part to play in advising and helping relatives.

Care plans

There is increasing emphasis on the use of *care plans* in the management of psychiatric disorders. While this approach is applicable to all patients, it is particularly appropriate for those with a schizophrenic illness who will often require long-term support in the community. The essential elements of a care plan are:

- systematic assessment of health and social needs;

- a treatment plan agreed by the relevant staff, the patient, and the relatives;

- the allocation of a key worker whose task is to maintain contact with patient, monitor progress, and ensure that the treatment programme is being delivered.

- regular review of the patient's progress and needs (for further discussion of care planning and the role of psychiatric services, see Chapter 23).

Early intervention

There is growing interest in the idea that *early treatment* of schizophrenia may improve the long-term prognosis (see DeQuardo 1998). This is based on a number of pieces of evidence:

- Patients with a longer duration of untreated psychosis have a worse longer-term prognosis.

- There is an increasing time of response to treatment during subsequent psychotic episodes.

- Much of the deterioration in social function takes place in the first 2 years after diagnosis.

This implies that it may be worthwhile recognizing patients with psychosis as early as possible so that effective treatment can be instituted. Also, psychosocial interventions at this time should be particularly aimed at maintaining interpersonal skills and social function. In the future it may be possible to target relevant psychosocial interventions at people at high risk of schizophrenia (for example, children of parents with schizophrenia), before development of overt psychosis. Preliminary findings have suggested that such an approach could be worthwhile (Falloon *et al.* 1996).

Substance misuse and management

Many patients with schizophrenia also *misuse psychoactive substances*, both legal and illegal. For example, the Epidemiological Catchment Area Study in the USA found that patients with schizophrenia had a four- to fivefold increased risk of substance misuse The reasons for this are likely to be complex but include:

◆ exposure to socioeconomic factors associated with substance misuse in the general population;

◆ relief of personal distress, induced by psychiatric symptoms and perhaps antipsychotic drug treatment;

◆ increased genetic susceptibility (see McEvoy 2000).

Patients who misuse substances are likely to have a *worse course symptomatically* and be more difficult to engage in treatment. Also, substance misuse is associated with increased risks of *homelessness*, *violent behaviour*, and *poor general health*.

Patients with substance misuse and schizophrenia (so-called 'dual-diagnosis' patients) may not be adequately served by standard psychiatric services. Recent studies suggest that benefit can be obtained with comprehensive out-patient and assertive community programmes that address both substance misuse and psychotic illness in an integrated way (Drake *et al.* 1998). Key features appear to be assertive outreach, case management, and a staged, motivational approach to the substance misuse disorder (see McEvoy 2000).

The violent patient

Overactivity and disturbances of behaviour are common in schizophrenia, and although major violence towards others is not common, it certainly does occur. For example, Humphreys *et al.* (1992) found that, in a group of 253 patients with a first schizophrenic episode, 52 behaved in a way threatening to the lives of others. In about half the patients, the behaviour was directly attributable to psychotic symptoms, usually delusions. As noted above, substance misuse increases the risk of violence (see Citrome and Volavka 2000).

General management for the potentially violent patient is the same as that for any other patient with schizophrenia, although a compulsory order is more likely to be required. Whilst medication is often needed to bring disturbed behaviour under immediate control, much can be done by providing a calm, reassuring, and consistent environment in which provocation is avoided. A special ward area with an adequate number of experienced staff is much better than the use of heavy medication. Threats of violence should be taken seriously, especially if there is a history of such behaviour in the past, whether or not the patient was ill at the time. The danger usually resolves as acute symptoms are brought under control, but a few patients pose a continuing threat. The management of violence is considered further in Chapter 26.

Suicide and schizophrenia

We have already seen that suicide is not infrequent in schizophrenia, and in the early stages of illness about one patient in ten dies by suicide. In schizophrenia as in other psychiatric disorders general risk factors such as male gender, social isolation, unemployment, and a previous episode of suicidal behaviour are important. Other risk factors include:

◆ depression and hopelessness

◆ frequent exacerbations

◆ good premorbid functioning

◆ early in the course of the disorder

◆ during hospitalization or shortly after discharge.

Patients with pronounced negative symptoms are less likely to make suicide attempts. Whilst suicide may be associated with active positive symptoms such as delusions of control or auditory hallucinations, more often suicide occurs in those with previously high educational attainment in a relatively non-psychotic stage of their illness. Such patients often have depressive symptoms in the context of high premorbid expectations of themselves and a negative appraisal of the way their illness had damaged their future prospects.

Lowering the risk of suicide in schizophrenia means being aware of the *relevant risk factors* and *treating depressive symptomatology* as vigorously as possible with pharmacological and psychoscial interventions. Interestingly, clozapine treatment may reduce suicide risk in schizophrenia but the mechanism of this effect requires further study (Meltzer and Okayli 1995). For a review of the risk factors for suicide in schizophrenia see De Hert and Peuskens (2000).

Further reading

Bleuler, E. (1911). Dementia praecox or the group of schizophrenias (English edition 1950). International University Press, New York. (see especially the sections concerned with the concept of schizophrenia, basic and accessory symptoms, and sub-types.)

Kraepelin, E. (1919). *Dementia praecox and paraphrenia*. Churchill Livingstone, Edinburgh.

Kraepelin, E. (1986). Dementia praecox. *Psychiatrie*, 5th edn, pp. 426–41. Translated in Cutting, J. and Shepherd, M. (eds), *The clinical roots of schizophrenia concept*. Cambridge University Press, Cambridge. (The classical description of the syndrome.)

Reveley, M. A. and Deakin, J. F. W. (2000). *The psychopharmacology of schizophrenia*. Oxford University Press, New York. Contemporary approach to the psychopharmacology and biochemistry of schizophrenia.

CHAPTER 13

Paranoid symptoms and paranoid syndromes

Paranoid symptoms and paranoid syndromes

Introduction

The term *paranoid* can be applied to *symptoms*, *syndromes*, or *personality types*. Paranoid symptoms are *overvalued ideas* or *delusional beliefs* which are most commonly persecutory but not always so. Paranoid syndromes are those syndromes in which paranoid symptoms form a prominent part of a characteristic *constellation of symptoms*, such as pathological jealousy or erotomania (described later). Paranoid personalities are those personalities in which there is excessive *self-reference and undue sensitiveness* to real or imaginary humiliations and rebuffs, often combined with self-importance, combativeness, and aggressiveness. The term paranoid is *descriptive* and not diagnostic. If we recognize a symptom or syndrome as paranoid, this is not making a diagnosis, but it is a preliminary to doing so. In this respect it is like recognizing stupor or depersonalization.

Paranoid syndromes present considerable problems of classification and diagnosis. The reasons for this can be understood by dividing them into two groups. In the first group, paranoid symptoms occur as part of a *primary mental illness* such as schizophrenia, mood disorder, or an organic mental disorder. In the second group, paranoid symptoms occur but no other primary disorder can be detected – the paranoid symptoms appear to have arisen independently.

In this book, following the DSM-IV and ICD-10 classifications, the term *delusional disorders* is applied to this second group. It is this second group that has given rise to difficulties and confusion over classification and diagnosis. For example, there has been much argument as to whether these conditions are an alternative form of schizophrenia, or a stage in the evolution of schizophrenia, or a quite separate entity. It is because these problems arise frequently in clinical practice that a whole chapter is devoted to them.

This chapter begins with definitions of the commonest paranoid symptoms and then reviews the causes of such symptoms. Next comes a short account of paranoid personality. This is followed by discussion of primary psychiatric disorders such as organic mental states, mood disorders, and schizophrenia, with which paranoid features are frequently associated. These primary disorders are dealt with elsewhere in the book, but the focus here is on differentiating them from *delusional disorders*. These disorders are then reviewed, with particular reference to paranoia and paraphrenia. The latter terms are considered against their historical background. Next, an account is given of a number of distinctive paranoid symptoms and syndromes, some of which are fairly common and some exceedingly rare. This chapter finishes with a description of the assessment and treatment of patients with paranoid features.

Paranoid symptoms

In the introduction it was pointed out that the commonest paranoid delusions are *persecutory*. The term paranoid is also applied to the less common delusions of grandeur and jealousy, and sometimes to delusions concerning love, litigation, or religion. It may seem puzzling that such varied delusions should be grouped together. The reason is that the central abnormality implied by the term paranoid is a morbid distortion of beliefs or attitudes concerning *relationships between oneself and other people*. If someone believes falsely or on inadequate grounds that he is being victimized, or exalted, or deceived, or loved by a famous person, then in each case he is construing the relationship between himself and other people in a morbidly distorted way.

The varieties of paranoid symptom are discussed in Chapter 1, but the main ones are outlined here for convenience. The following definitions are derived from those in the glossary to the Present State Examination (PSE) (Wing *et al.* 1974).

Ideas of reference

Ideas of reference are held by people who are unduly self-conscious. The subject cannot help feeling that people take notice of him in buses, restaurants, or other public places, and that they observe things about him that he would prefer not to be seen. He realizes that this feeling originates within himself and that he is no more noticed than other people, but all the same he cannot help the feeling, quite out of proportion to any possible cause.

Delusions of reference

Delusions of reference consist of a further elaboration of simple ideas of self-reference, and the person does not recognize that the ideas are false. The whole neighbourhood may seem to be gossiping about the subject, far beyond the bounds of possibility, or he may see references to himself on the television or in newspapers. The subject may hear someone on the radio say something connected with some topic that he has just been thinking about, or he may seem to be followed, his movements observed, and what he says tape-recorded.

Delusions of persecution

When a person has *delusions of persecution* he believes that someone, or some organization, or some force or power is trying to harm him in some way, to damage his reputation, to cause him bodily injury, to drive him mad, or to bring about his death. The symptom may take many forms, ranging from the direct belief that people are hunting him down to

complex and bizarre plots with every kind of science fiction elaboration.

Delusions of grandeur

The glossary of the PSE proposes that *delusions of grandeur* should be divided into

- delusions of grandiose ability
- delusions of grandiose identity.

The subject with delusions of *grandiose ability* thinks that he is chosen by some power, or by destiny, for a special mission or purpose because of his unusual talents. He thinks that he is able to read people's thoughts or that he is particularly good at helping them, that he is much cleverer than anyone else, or that he has invented machines, composed music, or solved mathematical problems beyond most people's comprehension. The subject with delusions of *grandiose identity* believes that he is famous, rich, titled, or related to prominent people. He may believe that he is a changeling and that his real parents are royalty.

Causes of paranoid symptoms

When paranoid symptoms occur in association with a primary organic illness, a mood disorder, or schizophrenic illness, the main aetiological factors are those determining this primary illness. The question still arises as to why some people develop paranoid symptoms, whilst others do not. It has usually been answered in terms of *premorbid personality* and of factors causing *social isolation*.

Premorbid personality

Many writers, including Kraepelin, have held that paranoid symptoms are most likely to occur in patients with premorbid personalities of a *paranoid type* (see next section). Kretschmer (1927) also believed that paranoid disorders were more likely in people with predisposed or sensitive personalities. In such people a precipitating event could induce what Kretschmer called *sensitive delusions of reference* (*sensitive Beziehungswahn*), occurring as an understandable psychological reaction. Modern studies of so-called *late-onset paraphrenia* have supported these views (see Chapter 20, p. 632). Thus Kay and Roth (1961) found paranoid or hypersensitive personalities in over half of their group of 99 subjects with late-onset paraphrenia.

Freud (1911) proposed that, in predisposed people, paranoid symptoms could arise through the defence mechanisms of *denial and projection*. He held that a person does not consciously admit his own inadequacy and self-distrust, but projects them on to the outside world. Freud also held that paranoid symptoms could arise when denial and projection were being used as defences against *unconscious homosexual tendencies*. These ideas were derived from his study of *Daniel Schreber*, the presiding judge of the Dresden appeal court (Freud 1911). Freud never met Schreber, but read the latter's autobiographical account of his paranoid illness (now generally accepted to be paranoid schizophrenia), together with a report by Weber, the physician in charge.

Freud held that Schreber could not consciously admit his homosexuality, and so the idea 'I love him' was dealt with by denial and changed by a reaction formation to 'I hate him'; this was further changed by projection into 'it is not I who hate him, but he who hates me', and this in turn became transformed to 'I am persecuted by him'. Freud believed that all paranoid delusions could be represented as contradictions of the idea 'I (a man) love him (a man)'. He went so far as to argue that *delusions of jealousy* could be explained in terms of unconscious homosexuality; the jealous husband was unconsciously attracted to the man whom he accused his wife of loving. In this case the formulation was 'it is not I who love him; it is she who loves him'. At one time these ideas were widely taken up, but nowadays they gain little acceptance. They are not supported by clinical experience.

Social isolation

Apart from premorbid disposition, *social isolation* may also lead to the emergence of paranoid symptoms. As mentioned later in this chapter, prisoners in solitary confinement, refugees, and migrants may be prone to paranoid symptoms

and syndromes, although the evidence on this is conflicting.

Social isolation can also be produced by *deafness*. In 1915, Kraepelin pointed out that chronic deafness could lead to paranoid attitudes. Houston and Royse (1954) found an association between deafness and paranoid schizophrenia, whilst Kay and Roth (1961) found hearing impairment in 40% of patients with late-onset paraphrenia. However, it should be remembered that the great majority of deaf people do not become paranoid.

Paranoid personality disorder

The concept of personality disorder was discussed in Chapter 7, and *paranoid personality disorder* was briefly described there. It is characterized by:

◆ extensive sensitivity to setbacks and rebuffs;

◆ suspiciousness;

◆ a tendency to misconstrue the actions of others as hostile or contemptuous;

◆ a combative and inappropriate sense of personal rights.

It is implied in the DSM-IV and ICD-10 definitions that paranoid personality embraces a wide range of types. At one extreme is the excessively sensitive youth who shrinks from social encounters and thinks that everyone disapproves of him. At the other is the assertive and challenging man who flares up at the least provocation. Many grades lie between these two extremes.

Because of the implications for treatment, it is important to distinguish these paranoid personalities from the paranoid syndromes to be described later. The distinction can be very difficult to make. Sometimes one shades into the other in the course of a single life history, as appears to have happened to the philosopher, *Jean Jaques Rousseau* and the dictator, *Joseph Stalin* (Hachinski 1999). The basis for making the distinction is that in paranoid personalities there are no delusions but only dominant, often overvalued ideas, and no hallucinations. Separating paranoid ideas from delusions calls for considerable skill. The criteria for doing so are given in Chapter 1 (p. 13). Family studies suggest that paranoid personality disorder is related genetically to *schizophrenia* and *delusional disorder* (see below).

Primary psychiatric disorders with paranoid symptoms

It was mentioned in the introduction to this chapter that paranoid symptoms occur in association with *primary mental disorders*. This association occurs commonly in clinical practice. As the primary disorders are described at length in other chapters, they are mentioned only briefly here.

Cognitive mental disorders (delirium and dementia)

Paranoid symptoms are common in *delirium*. Impaired grasp of what is going on around the patient may give rise to apprehension and misinterpretation, and so to suspicion. Delusions may then emerge which are usually transient and disorganized; they may lead to disturbed behaviour, such as querulousness or aggression. Examples are drug-induced states. Similarly, paranoid delusions may occur in dementia arising from any cause, including trauma, degenerations, infections, metabolic, and endocrine disorders (see Chapter 20). In clinical practice it is important to remember that in elderly patients with dementia, paranoid delusions may appear before any intellectual deterioration is detectable.

Mood disorders

Paranoid delusions not uncommonly occur in patients with *severe depressive disorders*. The latter are often characterized by guilt and retardation, and by biological features such as loss of appetite and weight, sleep disturbance, and reduced sex drive. These disorders are more common in middle or later life. In depressive disorder, the patient typically accepts the supposed activities of the persecutors as *justified* by his own guilt or wickedness, but in schizophrenia he often resents them bitterly.

It is sometimes difficult to determine whether the paranoid features are secondary to depressive disorder, or whether depressed mood is secondary to paranoid symptoms arising from another cause. Primary depressive disorder is likely if the mood changes have occurred earlier and are of greater intensity than the paranoid features. Previous psychiatric history and family history may also be useful pointers.

The distinction may have some importance from the point of view of prognosis, because patients with a primary mood disorder will usually have a better long-term outcome. Furthermore, if depressive disorder is primary, patients will probably need antidepressant medication or ECT, in addition to treatment with antipsychotic drugs (see Chapter 11).

Paranoid delusions also occur in *manic patients*. Often the delusions are *grandiose* rather than persecutory – the patient claims to be extremely wealthy or of exalted rank or importance.

Paranoid schizophrenia

Paranoid schizophrenia has been described in Chapter 12. In contrast with the hebephrenic and catatonic forms of schizophrenia, the paranoid form usually begins later in life – in the thirties rather than in the twenties. The dominant feature of paranoid schizophrenia is delusions that are relatively stable over time. The delusions are frequently of persecution, but may also be of jealousy, exalted birth, Messianic mission, or bodily change. They may be accompanied by hallucinatory voices which sometimes, but not invariably, have a persecutory or grandiose content.

It is important to consider the differential diagnosis of paranoid schizophrenia from other paranoid conditions. The criteria for the diagnosis of schizophrenia in DSM-IV and ICD-10 were described on p. 339. In cases of doubt, the diagnosis of schizophrenia rather than delusional disorder is suggested if the paranoid delusions are *particularly odd* in content (often referred to by psychiatrists as *bizarre delusions*). For example, a middle-aged woman became convinced that a

Cabinet Minister was taking a special interest in her and was promoting her well-being. She believed that he was the pilot of an aeroplane that flew over her house shortly after noon each day. Therefore she waited in her garden each day and threw a large red beachball into the sky when the plane flew over. She maintained that the pilot always acknowledged this action by 'waggling the wings' of the plane.

When the delusions are less extreme than this, a judgement as to how bizarre they are must be arbitrary. DSM-IV defines non-bizarre delusions as involving situations that could conceivably occur in real life, for example, being followed, poisoned, or loved at a distance.

There are two other diagnostic points. First, in schizophrenia delusions are most likely to be *fragmented* and *multiple*, rather than systematized and unitary. Second, patients with paranoid schizophrenia often have *auditory hallucinations* that seem to be totally *unrelated to their delusions*, whereas patients with paranoid conditions other than schizophrenia frequently have no auditory hallucinations, or else fleeting hallucinations that are related in content to their delusional ideas.

Schizophrenia-like syndromes

Paranoid syndromes are also common in several *schizophrenia-like syndromes* discussed in Chapter 12 (and listed in Table 12.4). These include the DSM-IV categories of brief psychotic disorders and schizophreniform disorder, and the ICD-10 categories grouped under the heading acute and transient psychotic disorders.

Delusional disorders (paranoid psychoses)

DSM-IV uses *delusional disorder* for a disorder with persistent, non-bizarre delusion that is not due to any other mental disorder. ICD-10 has a rather similar category of *persistent delusional disorders*.

Historical background: paranoia and paraphrenia

The terms *paranoia* and *paraphrenia* have played a prominent part in psychiatric thought. Much can be learned from reviewing the conceptual difficulties associated with them. For this reason, their history will be traced in some detail, starting with paranoia.

The term *paranoia*, from which the modern adjective paranoid is derived, has a long and chequered history. It has probably given rise to more controversy and confusion of thought than any other term used in psychiatry. A comprehensive review of the large literature, which is mostly German, and from the period before the 1970s has been provided by Lewis (1970).

The term paranoia came into prominence in the last quarter of the nineteenth century, but its origins are much older. The word paranoia is derived from the Greek *para* (beside) and *nous* (mind). It was used in ancient Greek literature to mean 'out of mind', i.e. of unsound mind or insane. This broad usage was revived in the eighteenth century.

However, in the mid-nineteenth century German psychiatrists became interested in conditions that were particularly characterized by delusions of persecution and grandeur. The German term *Verrucktheit* was often applied to these conditions, but eventually was superseded by *paranoia*. There were many different conceptions of these disorders. The main issues can be summarized as follows:

- Did these conditions constitute a primary disorder, or were they secondary to a mood disorder or other disorder?

- Did they persist unchanged for many years, or were they a stage in an illness which later manifested deterioration of intellect and personality?

- Did they sometimes occur in the absence of hallucinations, or were hallucinations an invariable accompaniment?

- Were there forms with good prognosis?

Kahlbaum raised these issues as early as 1863, when he classified paranoia as an independent or primary delusional condition, which would remain unchanged over the years. Kraepelin had a strong influence on the conceptual history of paranoia, although he was never comfortable with the term, and his views changed strikingly over the years . In 1896 he used the term only for incurable, chronic, and systematized delusions without severe personality disorder. In the sixth edition of his textbook he wrote:

The delusions in dementia praecox are extremely fantastic, changing beyond all reason, with an absence of system and a failure to harmonize them with events of their past life; while in paranoia the delusions are largely confined to morbid interpretations of real events, are woven together into a coherent whole, gradually becoming extended to include even events of recent date, and contradictions and objects are apprehended and explained. (Kraepelin 1904, p. 199)

In later descriptions Kraepelin (1919) used the distinction made by Jaspers (1913) between personality development and disease process. He proposed paranoia as an example of the former, in contrast to the disease process of dementia praecox. In his final account, Kraepelin (1919) developed these ideas by distinguishing between *dementia praecox*, *paranoia*, and a third paranoid psychosis, *paraphrenia*. He suggested that:

- *Dementia praecox* had an early onset and a poor outcome ending in mental deterioration, and was fundamentally a disturbance of affect and volition.

- *Paranoia* was restricted to patients with the late onset of completely systematized delusions and a prolonged course usually without recovery but not inevitably deteriorating. An important point was that the patients did not have hallucinations.

- *Paraphrenia* was somewhat intermediary, in that the patient had unremitting systematized delusions but did not progress to dementia. The main difference from paranoia was that the patient with paraphrenia had hallucinations.

Bleuler's concept of the paranoid form of dementia praecox (which he later called paranoid schizophrenia) was broader than that of Kraepelin (Bleuler 1906, 1911). Thus Bleuler did not regard paraphrenia as a separate condition, but as part of dementia praecox. However, he accepted Kraepelin's view of paranoia as a separate entity, although he differed from Kraepelin in maintaining that hallucinations could occur in many cases.

Bleuler was particularly interested in the psychological development of paranoia; at the same time he left open the question of whether paranoia had a somatic pathology.

From this time, two main views were prominent in the history of paranoia. The first theme was that paranoia was distinct from schizophrenia and mainly *psychogenic* in origin. The second theme was that paranoia was *part of schizophrenia*.

Some celebrated studies of individual cases appeared to support the first theme – the psychogenic origins of paranoid delusions. For example, Gaupp (1914) made an intensive study of the diaries and mental state of the mass murderer Wagner who murdered his wife, four children, and eight other people as part of a careful plan to revenge himself on his supposed enemies. Gaupp concluded that Wagner suffered from paranoia in the sense described by Kraepelin, as discussed above. At the same time, he believed that Wagner's first recognizable delusions developed as a psychogenic reaction.

The most detailed argument for psychogenesis was put forward by Kretschmer (1927) in his monograph 'Der Sensitive Beziehungswahn'. Kretschmer believed that paranoia should not be regarded as a disease, but as a psychogenic reaction occurring in people with particularly sensitive personalities. However, many of Kretschmer's cases would nowadays be classified as suffering from schizophrenia.

In 1931, Kolle put forward evidence for the second view, that paranoia is part of schizophrenia. He analysed a series of 66 patients with so-called paranoia, including those diagnosed by Kraepelin in his Munich clinic. For several reasons, both symptomatic and genetic, Kolle came to the conclusion that so-called paranoia was really a mild form of schizophrenia.

Considerably less has been written about *paraphrenia*. However, it is interesting that Mayer (1921), following up Kraepelin's series of 78 paraphrenic patients, found that 50 of them had developed schizophrenia. He found no difference in original clinical presentation between those who developed schizophrenia and those who did not. Since then paraphrenia has increasingly been regarded as late-onset schizophrenia or schizophrenia-like disorder of good prognosis. Kay and Roth (1961) used the term *late paraphrenia* to denote paranoid conditions in the elderly that were not due to primary organic or affective illnesses. These authors found that a large majority of their 99 patients had the characteristic features of schizophrenia (see Chapter 12). Modern classifications do not use separate categories for early- and late-onset schizophrenia.

Modern usage: DSM-IV and ICD-10

In DSM-IV, *delusional disorder* replaces the traditional category of paranoia. The criteria require *non-bizarre delusions* of at least 1 month's duration and that auditory or visual hallucinations, if present, are not prominent. However, *olfactory* and *tactile* hallucinations may be present as part of the delusional disorder (for example, a patient may experience itching associated with a delusion of infestation) (Table 13.1).

In DSM-IV, there are five specific subtypes of delusional disorder and two other categories:

- persecutory
- jealous
- erotomanic
- somatic
- grandiose
- mixed (more than one type and no one theme predominates)
- unspecified.

Table 13.1 DSM-IV criteria for delusional disorder

A Non-bizarre delusions (i.e. involving situations that occur in real life, such as being followed, poisoned, infected, loved at a distance, or deceived by spouse or lover, or having a disease) of at least 1 month's duration

B Criterion A for schizophrenia has never been met. *Note:* Tactile and olfactory hallucinations may be present in delusional disorder if they are related to the delusional theme

C Apart from the impact of the delusion(s) or its ramifications, functioning is not markedly impaired and behaviour is not obviously odd or bizarre

D If mood episodes have occurred concurrently with delusions, their total duration has been brief relative to the duration of the delusional periods

E The disturbance is not due to the direct physiological effects of a substance (e.g. a drug of abuse, a medication) or a general medical condition

---

The somatic form covers the disorder sometimes referred to as *monosymptomatic hypochondriacal psychosis*. Delusional disorder appears to be rare, to occur predominantly in mid-life, and to have a prolonged course.

ICD-10 gives a similar definition for the principal category of persistent delusion disorders, of which delusional disorder is the main diagnosis. However, the symptoms must have been present for at least 3 months rather than the 1 month required in DSM-IV and the subtypes are not specified. In addition the delusions are not required to be 'non-bizarre.'

The essence of the modern concept of delusional disorder is that of a permanent and unshakeable delusional system developing insidiously in a person in middle or late life. This delusional system is encapsulated, and there is no impairment of other mental functions. The patient can often go on working, and his social life may sometimes be maintained fairly well. In clinical practice, cases conforming strictly to the definitions are rare. The term paraphrenia does not appear in DSM-IV or ICD-10.

Epidemiology of delusional disorder

Delusional disorder is regarded as being an uncommon illness. In a community survey of over 5000 people aged 65 and over, Copeland *et al.* (1998) found a prevalence for DSM-IIIR schizophrenia of 0.12% and delusional disorder 0.04%. In a retrospective study of over 10 000 outpatients, Hsiao *et al.* (1999) diagnosed 86 (0.83%) as meeting DSM-IV criteria for delusional disorder (Box 13.1). The disorder was a little more common in women than men and the mean age of onset of symptoms was 42 years. Significant depressive symptoms were present in about a third of subjects. About 5% of psychiatric inpatients with a diagnosis of functional psychosis met criteria for delusional disorder (Kendler and Walsh 1995).

Box 13.1 Subtypes of delusional disorder in 86 Chinese out-patients

Persecutory – 61

Mixed – 12

Jealous – 7

Somatic – 2

Erotomanic – 1

Grandiose – 1

Unspecified – 2

Hsiao *et al.* (1999)

Aetiology of delusional disorder

To understand the aetiology of delusional disorder, it is important to establish its relationship with schizophrenia and paranoid personality disorder.

This question has been addressed by family studies and comparative studies of neurobiological abnormalities.

Family studies

Paranoid personality disorder, *delusional disorder*, and *schizophrenia* have been the subject of family studies designed to clarify the possible relationships between these disorders. The findings of the various investigations have been somewhat contradictory, but recent studies have found that the incidence of paranoid personality disorder is increased in first-degree relatives of patients with schizophrenia, although not to the same extent as schizotypal personality (Kendler *et al.* 1993b, 1993c). First-degree relatives of patients with delusional disorder also have an increased incidence of paranoid personality disorder, perhaps more so than first-degree relatives of patients with schizophrenia (Kendler *et al.* 1985a, 1985b).

The familial relationship of delusional disorder to schizophrenia is less clear. At present it appears that, while the risk of delusional disorder is increased in first-degree relatives of patients with schizophrenia, relatives of patients with delusional disorder do not have an increased risk of schizophrenia or schizotypal personality (Kendler and Walsh 1995). This familial association pattern has been called *asymmetric co-aggregation* and may be due to a number of factors:

◆ differences in the incidence rates of the two disorders in the general population;

◆ differences in diagnostic error rate between probands and relatives (probands are usually subject to more intensive assessment);

◆ a higher genetic loading for severe illness in those who come to medical attention (and are therefore assessed as probands).

There does seem to be a familial association between *alcoholism* and delusional disorder (Kendler and Walsh 1995) which could explain the association between delusional jealousy and alcohol misuse.

Neurobiological studies

Structural MRI studies have revealed that patients with delusional disorder have changes in cerebral ventricles similar to those of patients with schizophrenia (Howard *et al.* 1995). The two groups also show similar abnormalities in tasks of eye tracking. Other eye-tracking abnormalities in delusional patients may relate more to depressed mood, suggesting heterogeneity in the neurobiology of delusional disorder (Campana *et al.* 1998). There are inconsistent reports that delusional disorder may be associated with polymorphisms in the gene for the dopamine D_4 receptor (see Zenner *et al.* 1998).

Special paranoid conditions

Certain paranoid conditions are recognizable by their distinctive features. They can be divided into two groups:

- those with *special symptoms*
- those occurring in *special situations*.

The special symptoms include *jealous*, *erotic*, and *querulant* delusions, and also the delusions associated with the names of *Capgras* and *Fregoli*. The special situations include intimate relationships (*folie à deux*), also known as *induced delusional disorder* (ICD-10) or *shared psychotic disorder* (DSM-IV), as well as *migration* and *imprisonment psychoses*. Many of these symptoms have been of particular interest to French psychiatrists (Pichot 1982, 1984). None, apart from 'shared psychotic disorder' or 'induced delusional disorder', is recognized as a separate category in DSM-IV or ICD-10.

Among the conditions with special symptoms, *pathological jealousy* will be described first and in the greatest detail because of its importance in clinical practice. It is probably the most common, and is often *dangerous*.

Pathological jealousy

In *pathological (or morbid) jealousy*, the essential feature is an abnormal belief that the marital partner is being *unfaithful*. The condition is called pathological because the belief, which may be a *delusion* or an *overvalued idea*, is held on inadequate grounds and is unaffected by rational argument. Pathological jealousy has been reviewed in a classic paper by Shepherd (1961) and by Mullen and Maack (1985). Various other names have been used for pathological jealousy, including sexual jealousy, erotic jealousy, morbid jealousy, psychotic jealousy, and the Othello syndrome.

The belief is often accompanied by strong emotions and characteristic behaviour, but these do not in themselves constitute pathological jealousy. A man who finds his wife in bed with a lover may experience extreme jealousy and may behave in an uncontrolled way, but this should not be called pathological jealousy. *The term should be used only when the jealousy is based on unsound evidence and reasoning.*

The main sources of information about pathological jealousy are the surveys carried out by Shepherd (1961), Langfeldt (1961), Vaukhonen (1968), and Mullen and Maack (1985). Shepherd examined the hospital case notes of 81 patients in London and Langfeldt did the same for 66 patients in Norway. Vaukhonen made an interview study of 55 patients in Finland; Mullen and Mack examined the hospital case notes of 138 patients.

The frequency of pathological jealousy in the general population is unknown, although jealous feelings are ubiquitous (Mullen and Martin 1994). Pathological jealousy is not uncommon in psychiatric practice (Table 13.2), and most full-time clinicians probably see one or two cases a year. They merit careful attention, not only because of the great distress that they cause within marriages and families, but also because they may be *highly dangerous*.

It is likely that pathological jealousy is more common in men than in women. For example, the surveys noted above found that about two men are affected for every woman. However, the precise sex ratio may depend on the particular group studied and in particular whether the jealousy is secondary to another disorder. For example, in a retrospective

Table 13.2 Disorders associated with pathological jealousy
Schizophrenia
Mood disorder
Organic disorder
Substance misuse (including alcohol)
Personality disorder

survey of psychiatric in-patients, Soyka *et al.* (1991) found that amongst patients with paranoid schizophrenia more females than males had delusions of jealousy, whilst amongst patients with alcoholic psychosis more men developed delusional jealousy (even allowing for the fact that more men than women were affected with alcoholic psychosis).

Clinical features

As indicated above, the main feature is an *abnormal belief in the partner's infidelity*. This may be accompanied by other abnormal beliefs, for example, that the partner is plotting against the patient, trying to poison him, taking away his sexual capacities, or infecting him with venereal disease. The *mood* of the pathologically jealous patient may vary with the underlying disorder, but often it is a mixture of misery, apprehension, irritability, and anger.

The *behaviour* of the patient is often characteristic. Commonly there is intensive seeking for evidence of the partner's infidelity, for example, by searching in diaries and correspondence, and by examining bedlinen and underwear for signs of sexual secretions. The patient may follow the partner about, or engage a private detective to spy on the partner. Typically the jealous person cross-questions the partner incessantly. This may lead to violent quarrelling and paroxysms of rage in the patient. Sometimes the partner becomes exasperated and worn out, and is finally goaded into making a false confession. If this happens, the jealousy is inflamed rather than assuaged.

An interesting feature is that the jealous person often has no idea as to who the supposed lover may be, or what kind of person he or she may be. Moreover, he may avoid taking steps that could produce unequivocal proof one way or the other.

The behaviour of patients with pathological jealousy may be strikingly abnormal. A successful city businessman carried a briefcase that contained not only his financial documents but also a machete for use against any lover who might be detected. A carpenter installed an elaborate system of mirrors in his house so that he could watch his wife from another room. A third patient avoided waiting alongside another car at traffic lights, in case his wife in the passenger seat might surreptitiously make an assignation with the other driver.

Aetiology

In the above surveys, pathological jealousy was found to be associated with a range of *primary disorders*. The frequencies varied, depending on the population studied and the diagnostic scheme used. For example, *paranoid schizophrenia* (or paranoia or paraphrenia) was reported in 17–44% of patients, depressive disorder in 3–16%, *neurosis* and *personality disorder* in 38–57%, *alcoholism* in 5–7%, and *organic disorders* in 6–20%. Primary organic causes include misuse of exogenous substances such as amphetamine and cocaine, but more commonly a wide range of brain disorders including infections, neoplasms, metabolic and endocrine disorders, and degenerative conditions (see Tsai *et al.* 1997).

The role of *personality* in the genesis of pathological jealousy should be stressed. It is often found that the patient has a pervasive sense of his own inadequacy, together with *low self-esteem*. There is a discrepancy between his ambitions and his attainments. Such a personality is particularly vulnerable to anything that may threaten this sense of inadequacy, such as loss of status or advancing age. In the face of such threats the person may project the blame onto others, and this may take the form of jealous accusations of infidelity. As mentioned earlier, Freud believed that unconscious homosexual urges played a part in all jealousy, particularly the delusional kind. He held that this could occur when such urges were dealt with by repression, denial, and reaction formation. However, clinical studies do not support an association between homosexuality and pathological jealousy.

Many writers have held that pathological jealousy may be induced by the onset of *erectile difficulties* in men or *sexual dysfunction* in women. In their surveys, Langfeldt and Shepherd found little or no evidence of such associations. However, Vaukhonen reported sexual difficulties in over half the men and women in his series, but his sample was drawn partly from a marriage guidance clinic.

Prognosis

The *prognosis* depends on a number of factors, including the nature of any underlying psychiatric disorder and the patient's *premorbid personality*. There is little statistical evidence on prognosis. When Langfeldt followed up 27 of his patients after 17 years, he found that over half of them still had persistent or recurrent jealousy. This confirms a general clinical impression that the prognosis is often poor.

Risk of violence

Although there is no direct statistical evidence of the risks of violence, there is no doubt that people with pathological jealousy can be highly dangerous (A. J. Silva *et al.* 1998). In Shepherd's (1961) series of 81 patients with pathological jealousy, three had shown homicidal tendencies. In addition to homicide, the risk of physical injury inflicted by jealous patients is undoubtedly considerable. In Mullen and Maack's (1985) series, few of the 138 patients had received criminal convictions, but a quarter had threatened to kill or injure their partner, and 56% of men and 43% of women had been violent to or threatened the supposed rival. There is also be a risk of *suicide*, particularly when an accused partner finally decides to end the relationship.

Assessment

The assessment of a patient with pathological jealousy should be particularly thorough. Full psychiatric assessment of the patient is essential and the partner should be seen alone at first, and with the patient afterwards.

The partner may give a much more detailed account of the patient's morbid beliefs and actions than can be elicited from the patient. The doctor should try to find out tactfully how firmly the patient believes in the partner's infidelity, how much resentment he feels, and whether he has contemplated any vengeful action. What factors provoke outbursts of resentment, accusation, and cross-questioning? How does the partner respond to such outbursts by the patient? How does the patient respond in turn to the partner's behaviour? Has there been any violence so far? If so, how was it inflicted? Has there been any serious injury?

In addition to these enquiries, the doctor should take a detailed *marital and sexual history* from both partners. It is also important to diagnose any underlying psychiatric disorder, as this will have implications for treatment.

Treatment

The treatment of pathological jealousy is often difficult, because the jealous person may regard it as obtrusive and may show little compliance. Adequate treatment of any associated disorder such as schizophrenia or a mood disorder is a first requisite. If alcohol or other substance misuse is present, specific treatment will be needed. In other cases the pathological jealousy may be the symptom of a delusional disorder, or an overvalued idea in a patient with low self-esteem and personality difficulties.

When the jealousy seems to be *delusional* in nature, a careful trial of an antipsychotic drug is worthwhile, though results are often disappointing. When the jealousy is an overvalued idea, treatment with *selective serotonin re-uptake inhibitors* (SSRIs) may be useful (Stein *et al.* 1994); however, no randomized trials have yet been reported. As noted above, even when depressive disorder is not the primary diagnosis, it frequently complicates pathological jealousy and may worsen it. Treatment with an antidepressant drug may help in these circumstances.

Psychotherapy may be given to patients where the jealousy appears to arise from personality problems. One aim is to reduce tensions by allowing the patient (and partner) to ventilate feelings. Behavioural methods include encouraging the partner to produce behaviour that reduces jealousy, for example, by refusal to argue, depending on the individual case. A study of *cognitive therapy*, in which patients were encouraged to identify faulty assumptions and taught strategies of emotional control, gave superior results relative to a waiting list control group (Dolan and Bishay 1996).

If there is no response to out-patient treatment or if the risk of violence is high, in-patient care may be necessary. Not uncommonly, however, the patient appears to improve as an in-patient, only to relapse on discharge.

If there appears to be a *risk of violence*, the doctor should warn the partner. In some cases the safest procedure is to advise separation. It is not uncommon for feelings of pathological jealousy to wane once a relationship has ended. Sometimes, however, the problem re-emerges if the patient enters a new relationship.

Erotic delusions (De Clérambault's syndrome)

De Clérambault (1921, see also 1987) proposed that a distinction should be made between paranoid delusions and *delusions of passion*. The latter differed in their pathogenesis and in being accompanied by excitement. They had a sense of purpose:

patients in this category whether they display *erotomania*, *litigious behaviour*, or *morbid jealousy* all have a precise aim in view from the onset of the illness, which brings the will into play from the beginning. This constitutes a distinguishing feature of the illness.

This distinction is of historical interest only, as it is not made nowadays. However, the syndrome of *erotomania* is still known as De Clérambault's

syndrome. It is a rare disorder. Although erotomania is usually a disorder of women, Taylor *et al.* (1983) have reported four cases in a series of 112 men charged with violent offences.

In erotomania, the subject, usually a single woman, believes that an exalted person is in love with her. The supposed lover is usually inaccessible, as he is already married, or famous as an entertainer or public figure. According to De Clérambault, the infatuated woman believes that it is the supposed lover who first fell in love with her, and that he is more in love than she. She derives satisfaction and pride from this belief. She is convinced that the supposed lover cannot be a happy or complete person without her.

The patient often believes that the supposed lover is unable to reveal his love for various reasons that he has withheld from her, and that he has difficulties in approaching her, has indirect conversations with her, and has to behave in a paradoxical and contradictory way. The woman may be a considerable nuisance to the supposed lover, who may complain to the police and the courts. Sometimes the patient's delusion remains unshakeable, and she invents explanations for the other person's paradoxical behaviour. She may be extremely tenacious and impervious to reality. Other patients turn from a delusion of love to a delusion of persecution. They become abusive and make public complaints about the supposed lover. This was described by De Clérambault as two phases – hope followed by resentment.

Many patients with erotic delusions are suffering from *paranoid schizophrenia*. Sometimes there is insufficient evidence to make a final diagnosis at the time, and they can be classified as delusional disorder erotomanic type in DSM-IV.

'Stalking'

A proportion of 'stalkers' appear to suffer from *erotomania*, which is why the topic is mentioned briefly here. There is no clear consensus about the definition of stalking. Most formulations contain the following elements (Meloy 1998):

- a pattern of intrusive behaviour;
- the intrusive behaviour is associated with implicit or explicit threats;
- the person being stalked experiences fear and distress.

Stalkers typically follow their victim around and loiter outside their house or place of work. Unwanted communications by telephone, letter, graffiti, and, more recently, e-mail, are very common. Behaviour can then become more threatening with hoax advertisements or orders for services, scandalous rumour mongering, damage to the victim's property, threats of violence, and actual assault.

Stalkers compose a *heterogenous* group with differing underlying psychopathologies. Some suffer from *erotomania*, occasionally as a primary disorder but also secondary to other illnesses such as schizophrenia or a mood disorder. Patients with *delusions of jealousy* can also stalk their victims (Silva *et al.* 2000). More commonly stalkers suffer from *personality disorder*, predominantly with borderline, narcissistic, and sociopathic traits. They have often had a relationship with their victim that may have been quite superficial; in other cases, however, a serious relationship has cooled. A previous history of *domestic violence* in the relationship puts the victim at particularly high risk of assault and injury (Walker and Meloy 1998). Whether or not victims suffer actual assault, they invariably experience severe psychological stress, which can lead to anxiety and mood disorders and post-traumatic stress disorder. (For a review of stalking see Kamphuis and Emmelkamp 2000 or Mullen *et al.* 2000; see also Chapter 26.)

Somatic delusional disorder

People with *somatic delusional disorder* believe that they suffer from a physical illness or a physical deformity. As noted above, this term also covers *monosymptomatic hypochondriacal psychosis* where there is a single delusional belief about health or body function. Somatic delusional disorder needs to be distinguished from the hypochondriacal delusions that can occur in severe depression and schizophrenia. Treatment with antipsychotic drugs, particularly pimozide, has been advocated but therapeutic effects may be limited (Munro and Mok 1995).

Some patients with *body dysmorphobic disorder* (see p. 259) can hold beliefs about defects in appearance with delusional intensity. In fact, there appears to be much overlap clinically between delusional and non-delusional forms of body dysmorphobic disorder, suggesting they differ mainly in severity. For both delusional and non-delusional forms, treatment with selective serotonin inhibitors may be useful, perhaps more so than antipsychotic drugs (see Thomson 1998).

Querulant delusions and reformist delusions

Querulant delusions were the subject of a special study by Krafft-Ebing (1888). Patients with this kind of delusion indulge in a series of complaints and claims lodged against the authorities. Closely related to querulant patients are *paranoid litigants* who undertake a succession of lawsuits; they become involved in numerous court hearings, in which they may become passionately angry and make threats against the magistrates. Baruk (1959) described 'reformist delusions', which are centred on religious, philosophical, or political themes. People with these delusions constantly criticize society and sometimes embark on elaborate courses of action. Their behaviour may be violent, particularly when the delusions are political. Some political assassins fall within this group. It is extremely important that this diagnosis is made on clear *psychiatric grounds* rather than *political grounds* (Bloch and Chodoff 1981).

Capgras delusion

Although there had been previous case reports, the condition now known as *Capgras syndrome* was well described by Capgras and Reboul-Lachauz in 1923. They called it *l'illusion des sosies (illusion of doubles)*. Strictly speaking, it is not a syndrome but a symptom, and it is better termed the delusion (rather than illusion) of doubles.

The patient believes that a person closely related to him has been replaced by a double. He accepts that the misidentified person has a great resemblance to the familiar person, but still believes that they are different people. It is a rare condition, seen more often in women than men. A history of *depersonalization*, *derealization*, or *déjà vu* is not unusual . The misidentified person is usually the patient's partner or another relative. It is important to note that some patients with Capgras syndrome may *behave dangerously* by attacking the presumed doubles.

Capgras syndrome is traditionally linked with schizophrenia but it is now recognized that up to half the cases may be associated with organic brain disease of various kinds including dementia, head injury, and vascular disease. The right hemisphere, which has a recognized role in facial processing, may be preferentially affected (see Edelstyn and Oyebode 1999). Research on the process of facial recognition has revealed two dissociable neural systems, one of which generates semantic and biographical information about the observed face whilst the other produces an affective response. It is possible that a disconnection between these two systems could account for the delusional misidentification of Capgras syndrome (see Breen *et al.* 2000).

Fregoli delusion

This is usually referred to as the *Fregoli syndrome*, and derives its name from an actor called Fregoli who had remarkable skill in changing his facial appearance. The condition is even rarer than the Capgras delusion. It was originally described by Courbon and Fail in 1927. The patient identifies a familiar person (usually someone whom he believes to be his persecutor) in various other people he encounters. He maintains that, although there is no physical resemblance between the familiar person and the others, nevertheless they are psychologically identical. This symptom is usually associated with schizophrenia, although as with the Capgras syndrome, underlying organic

brain disease may also be a factor (Portwich and Barocka 1998).

Paranoid conditions occurring in special situations

Induced delusional disorder (folie à deux)

An *induced delusional disorder* is a paranoid delusional system which appears to have developed in a person as a result of a close relationship with another person who already has an established and similar delusional system. The delusions are nearly always persecutory. These cases are classified as *shared psychotic disorder* in DSM-IV, and as *induced delusional disorder (folie à deux)* in ICD-10. The frequency of induced psychosis is not known, but it is low. Sometimes more than two people are involved, but this is exceedingly rare.

Over 90% or more of reported cases are members of the same family but the condition has occasionally been described in two people who are not family relations. Usually there is a dominant partner with fixed delusions who appears to induce similar delusions in a dependent or suggestible partner, sometimes after initial resistance. Generally the two have lived together for a long time in close intimacy, often in isolation from the outside world. The partner in whom the psychosis is induced may also suffer premorbidly from dementia, depression, or learning difficulties. Once established, the condition runs a chronic course.

It is usually necessary to advise separation of the affected people. This separation may lead to resolution of the delusional state in the recipient. The induced should be treated along the lines for other paranoid disorders. Induced delusional disorder is reviewed by Enoch and Trethowan (1979) and Silveira and Seeman (1995).

Migration psychoses

It might be expected that people migrating to foreign countries would be likely to develop paranoid symptoms because their appearance, speech, and behaviour attract attention. Ødegaard (1932) found that rates for schizophrenia (including paranoid schizophrenia) were twice as high amongst Norwegian-born immigrants to the USA as amongst the general population of Norway. However, the explanation of the finding appeared to be not so much that emigration was a pathogenic experience as that people vulnerable to the development of schizophrenia were more likely to emigrate. This finding has been confirmed in a more recent study (Mortensen *et al.* 1997).

Recent studies suggest that the relationship between migration and mental illness is not straightforward and some groups can expect an improvement in their mental health (see Cheng and Chang 1999). However, in the UK, there is an increase in the risk of psychosis in the *children* of Afro-Caribbean immigrants to the UK but not in the immigrants themselves. This suggests that an *environmental factor* may be responsible for the increase in schizophrenia in the second generation.

Prison psychosis

The evidence about imprisonment is conflicting. The work of Birnbaum (1908) suggests that isolation in prison, and especially *solitary confinement*, may lead to paranoid disorders that clear up when the prisoners are allowed to mix with others. Eitinger (1960) reported that paranoid states were not uncommon in prisoners of war. However, Faergeman (1963) concluded that such developments were rare even amongst the inmates of concentration camps. The strong association between prison and psychotic illness in modern states is probably accounted for in large part by the incarceration of mentally ill people and substance misuse (Gunn 2000) (see Chapter 26 for a review of psychiatric disorders in prisons).

Cultural psychoses

In some developing countries there is a high incidence of transient and acute psychotic states, in which paranoid symptoms commonly occur. Some of these acute states may be due to organic causes such as tropical infections. Because of the conditions of observation, information about these disorders is incomplete.

Paranoid symptoms: assessment and diagnosis

In the assessment of paranoid symptoms there are two stages, the *recognition* of the symptoms themselves and the *diagnosis* of the underlying condition.

Sometimes it is obvious to everyone that the patient has persecutory ideas or delusions. At other times recognition of paranoid symptoms may be exceedingly difficult. The patient may be suspicious or angry. He may say very little, simply staring silently at the interviewer, or he may talk fluently and convincingly about other things, whilst steering away from delusional ideas or beliefs, or denying them completely. Considerable skill may be needed to elicit the false beliefs. The psychiatrist should be tolerant and impartial. He should present himself as a detached but interested listener who wants to understand the patient's point of view. He should show compassion and ask how he can help, but without colluding in the delusions and without giving promises that cannot be fulfilled. Tact is required to avoid any argument that may cause the patient to take offence. Despite skill and tact, experienced psychiatrists may interview a patient for a long time without detecting the morbid thoughts.

If apparently false beliefs are disclosed, before concluding that they are delusions it may be necessary to check the patient's statements against those of an informant and to ensure that the patient has had an opportunity to recognize the falsity of his beliefs. As with all apparent delusions, they must be judged against the *cultural background*, since the patient may hold a false belief that is generally held by his own group.

If paranoid delusions are detected, the next step is to diagnose the underlying psychiatric disorder.

This means looking for the diagnostic features of *organic mental disorders (including disorders of substance misuse), schizophrenia*, and *mood disorders*, which are described in other chapters. It is important to determine whether any persecutory or jealous delusions are likely to make the patient *behave dangerously* by trying to kill or injure his supposed persecutor. This calls for close study of the patient's personality and the characteristics of his delusions and any associated hallucinations. Hints or threats of homicide should be taken seriously, in the same way as for suicide.

A full risk assessment (see p. 924) is needed in these circumstances. The doctor should be prepared to ask tactfully about possible homicidal plans and preparations to enact them. In many ways the method of enquiry resembles the assessment of suicide risk: 'Have you ever thought of doing anything about it?' 'Have you made any plans?' 'What might prompt you to do it?'

Sometimes a patient with persecutory delusions does not know the identity of a supposed persecutor, but may still be dangerous. For example, an overseas visitor in his early twenties was seen in a psychiatric emergency clinic. Careful enquiry revealed that he believed that unidentified conspirators were trying to kill him, and that his life was in imminent danger. When asked if he had taken any steps to protect himself, he said that he had made a brief trip to Brussels to buy a pistol, which he was now carrying. When asked what he might do with the gun, he said that he was waiting until the voices told him to shoot someone.

The assessment of dangerousness is discussed further in Chapter 26. The most reliable guideline is that the risk of violence is greatest in patients with a history of previous violence.

The treatment of patients with paranoid symptoms

In the management of patients with paranoid symptoms, both *psychological* and *physical* measures should be considered.

Psychological management is frequently difficult. The patient may be suspicious and distrustful, and may believe that psychiatric treatment is intended to harm him. Even if he is not suspicious, he is likely to regard his delusional beliefs as justified, and to see no need for treatment. Considerable tact and skill are needed to persuade patients with paranoid symptoms to accept treatment. Sometimes this can be done by offering to help non-specific symptoms such as anxiety or insomnia. Thus a patient who believes that he is surrounded by persecutors may agree that his nerves are being strained as a result, and that this nervous strain needs treatment.

It is usually necessary at an early stage to decide whether to admit the patient for in-patient care. This may be indicated if the delusions are causing *aggressive behaviour* or there is a significant risk of such behaviour. In assessing such factors, it is usually best to consult other informants and to obtain a history of the patient's behaviour in the past. If voluntary admission is refused, compulsory admission may be justified to protect the patient or other people, although this is likely to add to the patient's resentment.

During treatment the psychiatrist should strive to maintain a good relationship. He should be dependable and should avoid provoking resentment by letting the patient down. He should show compassionate interest in the patient's beliefs, and neither condemn them nor collude with them.

Patients with paranoid delusions may be helped by psychological support, encouragement, and reassurance. Interpretative psychotherapy and group psychotherapy are unsuitable because suspiciousness and hypersensitivity may easily lead the patient to misinterpret what is being said. *Cognitive techniques* as used for the treatment of delusions in schizophrenia (p. 371) may also be worth trying if a sufficiently good therapeutic rapport exists.

Treatment by *medication* may be indicated for a primary psychiatric disorder, such as schizophrenia, mood disorder, or an organic mental state. In delusional states, with no detectable primary disorder, symptoms may be relieved by antipsychotic medication but results may be disappointing (H. Silva *et al.* 1998). The choice of drug and dosage depends on the patient's age, physical condition, degree of agitation, and response to previous medication. Some workers have suggested that *pimozide* may be the most effective antipsychotic agent for various forms of delusional disorder, particularly monosymptomatic hypochondriacal psychosis (delusional disorder, somatic type in DSM-IV) and pathological jealousy (Munro and Mok 1995); however, it is doubtful whether pimozide is more effective than other non-sedating antipsychotic drugs. Newer antipsychotic agents such as risperidone may be better tolerated (Kiraly *et al.* 1998). Finally, as noted above, *SSRIs* may be of benefit in the treatment in the delusional from of body dysmorphophobic disorder (Phillips *et al.* 1998), but whether this applies to other kinds of somatic delusional disorder is uncertain.

A common reason for failure of drug treatment is that patients do not take their medication because they suspect that it will harm them. It may then be necessary to prescribe a long-acting depot preparation such as fluphenazine decanoate if the patient can be persuaded to take it. In some patients the dosage can be reduced or stopped later without ill effects, whilst in others it must be maintained for long periods of time. This issue can be judged only by careful clinical trial and regular monitoring of mental state.

Further reading

Hirsch, S. R. and Shepherd, M. (eds) (1974). *Themes and variations in European psychiatry*. John Wright, Bristol. See following sections: E. Strömgren, Psychogenic psychoses; R. Gaupp, The scientific significance of the case of Ernst Wagner; and The illness and death of the paranoid mass murderer schoolmaster Wagner: a case history; E. Kretschmer, The sensitive delusion of reference; H. Baruk, Delusions of passion; H. Ey, P. Barnard, and C. Brisset, Acute delusional psychoses (*bouffées délirantes*).

Lewis, A. (1970). Paranoia and paranoid: a historical perspective. *Psychological Medicine* 1, 2–12. (A searching and scholarly review of the origin and development of the term paranoid and related concepts.)

McEwan, I, (1999) *Enduring love*. Fascinating novelist's account of De Clérambault's syndrome. Anchor Books, London

CHAPTER 14

Neuropsychiatry and sleep disorders

Neuropsychiatry and sleep disorders

Introduction

The term neuropsychiatry refers to psychiatric disorders which all arise from demonstrable abnormalities of brain structure and function. These frequently affect cognitive processes, but behavioural and emotional disturbances are also common and may be the sole manifestations of the brain disease. The boundaries are ill-defined; other psychiatric disorders, such as major depression and schizophrenia, have been shown to have, in part, a neurobiological basis whilst psychological factors influence or precipitate neurological syndromes, such as the paroxysmal movement disorders (Jarman *et al.* 2000).

This chapter is mainly concerned with three main categories of disorder:

- acute generalized cognitive impairment, usually referred to as *delirium*. The most important clinical feature is alteration of consciousness. There is global derangement of brain function; however, the primary cause often lies outside the brain.

- chronic generalized cognitive impairment, often used synonymously with *dementia*. The primary cause is usually within the brain, and is often degenerative. Cognitive impairment is frequently selective early in the course, becoming generalized as the process evolves.

- *specific neuropsychiatric syndromes*. These include the focal cerebral syndromes, the amnestic syndrome, and organic disorders selectively affecting perception and mood.

Later sections of the chapter describe common specific diseases, representing a broad spectrum of

neurobiological processes, which illustrate the application of these principles. General medical conditions, which may cause secondary or symptomatic cognitive impairment, are described in Chapter 18. For convenience, sleep disorders are also described in this chapter.

Classification systems

In ICD-10, the organic psychiatric disorders are termed *'organic, including symptomatic, mental disorders'*, and in DSM-IV, *'delirium, dementia, amnestic and other cognitive disorders'*. The two classifications are compared in Table 14.1. The main differences are as follows:

- The decision by the authors of DSM-IV to omit the word organic from the section title has led to rearrangement of the classification of some conditions formerly grouped under the heading organic. Thus major depression with organic aetiology is classified under mood disorders either as secondary to a general medical condition, or substance induced. As a result of these changes, DSM-IV avoids the problems within ICD-10 of the definition of the terms organic, symptomatic, and secondary (Spitzer *et al.* 1992).

- In both classifications the specific medical conditions causing cognitive disorder can be coded in addition to the latter disorder. In DSM-IV, this additional code is recorded on Axis III.

- In ICD-10, the section on organic disorder includes subcategories for mental disorders due to brain damage and dysfunction and to physical disease, and for personality and

Table 14.1 Classification of organic mental disorders

DSM-IV	ICD–10
Delirium, dementia, amnestic and other cognitive disorders	Organic, including symptomatic mental disorders
Delirium	
Delirium due to a general medical condition	Delirium, not induced by alcohol and other psychoactive drugs
Substance-induced delirium	
Substance-withdrawal delirium	
Delirium due to multiple aetiologies	
Dementia	
Dementia of Alzheimer's type with early onset	Dementia in Alzheimer's disease with early onset
Dementia of Alzheimer's type with late onset	Dementia in Alzheimer's disease with late onset
Vascular dementia	Vascular dementia
Dementia due to HIV disease	Multi-infarct dementia
Dementia due to head trauma	Subcortical vascular dementia
Dementia due to Parkinson's disease	HIV disease
Dementia due to Huntington's disease	Parkinson's disease
Dementia due to Pick's disease	Huntington's disease
Dementia due to Creutzfeldt–Jakob disease	Pick's disease
Dementia due to substance abuse	Creutzfeldt–Jakob disease
	Dementia in other diseases, classified elsewhere
Amnestic disorders	
Amnestic disorder due to general medical condition	Organic amnestic syndrome, not induced by alcohol or other psychoactive substance
Substance-induced persisting amnestic disorder	Other mental disorders due to brain damage and dysfunction and to physical disease
	Organic hallucinosis
	Organic delusional (schizophrenia-like) disorder
	Organic mood (affective) disorders
	Organic anxiety disorder
	Personality and behavioural disorders due to brain disease, damage, and dysfunction
	Organic personality disorder
	Postencephalitic syndrome
	Post-concussional syndrome

behavioural factors due to brain disease, damage, and dysfunction. In DSM-IV these conditions are not classified under delirium, dementia, and amnestic disorders, but under the relevant psychiatric disorder with the addition of a code to indicate that the disorder is secondary to a medical condition.

♦ DSM-IV includes under delirium, dementia, and amnestic disorders, a category for substance-induced delirium, substance-induced dementia, and substance-induced amnestic syndrome. In ICD-10 these conditions are recorded in the section on mental and behavioural disorders due to psychoactive substance abuse. In this book, these disorders are described in Chapter 18.

Delirium

In both DSM-IV and ICD-10, delirium is used as a general term for the acute cognitive impairment syndrome. In the past, a number of other terms such as 'confusional state' and 'acute organic syndrome' were used, but they should now be avoided. See Liptzin *et al.* (1994) for a review of terminology and classification.

Delirium is characterized by global impairment in consciousness, resulting in reduced level of alertness, attention, and perception of the environment. It occurs in 5–15% of patients in general medical or surgical wards, and a higher proportion of patients in intensive care units (Lipowski 1990). It is more common in the elderly and other individuals with diminished 'cerebral reserve', notably those with pre-existing dementia. The importance of recognizing delirium cannot be overstated as it is, if not adequately treated, associated with a high mortality.

Clinical features

The cardinal feature is disturbed consciousness with disorientation in time and place, which typically fluctuates over the course of 24 hours with nocturnal deterioration. Other features include mental slowness, distractibility, perceptual anomalies, and disorganization of the sleep-wake cycle. Symptoms and signs vary widely between patients, and in the same patient at different times of day. Lipowski (1980) distinguished two broad patterns of presentation:

♦ the patient is restless, irritable, and oversensitive to stimuli, with psychotic symptoms;

♦ psychomotor retardation and perseveration, without psychotic symptoms.

Repetitive, purposeless movements are common in both forms. Thinking is slow and muddled, but often rich in content ('dream-like'). Ideas of reference and delusions (often persecutory) are common, but usually transient and poorly elaborated. Visual perception is often distorted, with illusions, misinterpretations, and visual hallucinations, sometimes with fantastic content. Tactile and auditory hallucinations also occur. Anxiety, depression, and emotional lability are common. Patients may be frightened, or perplexed. Experiences of depersonalization and derealization are sometimes described. Attention and registration are particularly impaired, and on recovery there is usually amnesia for the period of the delirium.

Aetiology

Some of the main causes of delirium are shown in Table 14.2. The condition occurs particularly in association with increasing age, anxiety, sensory under- or overstimulation, drug dependence, and brain damage of all types. Engel and Romano (1959) showed that the severity of the clinical disturbance correlates with the degree of slowing of cerebral rhythms in the EEG. Cognitive changes resulting from major cardiac surgery have been shown to be associated with brain damage attributable to aspects of surgical and bypass procedures (Newman and Stygall 1999, Selnes and McKann 2001). See Trzepacz (1994) for a review of recent research on neuropathogenesis.

Table 14.2 Some causes of delirium

Drug intoxication and withdrawal

Alcohol, anticholinergics, anxiolytic-hypnotics, corticosteroids, anticonvulsants, digoxin, opiates, L-dopa, dopaminergic agonists, neuroleptic malignant syndrome, illicit drugs, heavy metals, herbicides (organophosphates), industrial poisons, carbon monoxide, prescription of multiple drugs

Withdrawal of alcohol, opiates, and anxiolytic sedatives

Metabolic disturbance

Uraemia, liver failure, respiratory failure, cardiac failure, disorders of electrolyte balance (especially hyponatraemia, hypercalcaemia), dehydration, severe anaemia

Endocrinopathies

Hypoglycaemia, diabetic ketoacidosis and non-ketotic hyperglycaemic coma, Cushing's syndrome, hypothyroidism, hyperthyroidism, hypopituitarism

Systemic infection

Urinary tract infection, viral exanthemata, septicaemia, endocarditis, pneumonia

Intracranial infection

Encephalitis (especially herpes simplex), meningitis, brain abscess, HIV, cerebral malaria, neurocysticercosis.

Other intacranial causes

Intracranial inflammation

Vasculitis

Head injury

Post-concussional syndrome, diffuse axonal injury, subdural haematoma

Epilepsy

Epileptic status (non-convulsive), post-ictal states

Vascular

Subarachnoid haemorrhage, venous sinus thrombosis, arterial stroke

Neoplastic

Focal space-occupying lesions, raised intracranial pressure (including acute hydrocephalus), carcinomatous or lymphomatous meningitis, paraneoplastic limbic encephalitis

Vitamin and other nutritional deficiency

Thiamine, nicotinic acid

Other

Pain, sleep deprivation, sensory deprivation and distortion (as in Intensive Treatment Units)

General principles of management

It is essential to identify and treat the underlying cause. General measures are necessary to relieve distress, control agitation, and prevent exhaustion. These include frequent explanation, reorientation, and reassurance. Frequent changes in the staff caring for the patient should be avoided if possible, and relatives and friends should visit the patient frequently. The patient should ideally be nursed in a quiet single room whilst taking care to avoid sensory deprivation which could perpetuate delirium. Relatives should be encouraged to visit regularly. At night, lighting should be sufficient to promote orientation, while not preventing sleep. See American Psychiatric Association (1999) for a review of treatment.

Drug treatment

Drug treatment of the underlying physical problem should be reviewed to ensure that it is the minimum required. Occasionally patients require medication to control distress, prevent exhaustion, and permit adequate sleep.

For agitation the drugs of choice are antipsychotics. Haloperidol is suitable, in a dose carefully titrated to achieve the desired calming without excess sedation or side-effects, generally between 3 and 15 mg/day. If necessary, the first 2–5 mg can be given intramuscularly. The utility of chlorpromazine and other phenothiazines is limited by side-effects such as hypotension, hepatotoxicity, and lowered seizure threshold. In patients with dementia with Lewy bodies and other extrapyramidal syndromes (which predispose to delirium), the use of neuroleptics is potentially dangerous, and should be avoided. If absolutely necessary, new generation, 'atypical' agents (such as risperidone, quetiapine, and olanzapine) with more selective effects on dopaminergic receptor subpopulations (see below, 'Parkinson's disease: hallucinations'), are preferable.

Short-acting benzodiazepines may be appropriate at night to promote sleep; they should be avoided during the day, because their sedative effects may worsen confusion.

All sedative drugs should be used sparingly in liver failure because of the danger of precipitating hepatic coma. See Liptzin (2000) for a review.

Dementia

Dementia is an acquired, usually progressive, impairment of intellect and personality which frequently becomes generalized, with no alteration of consciousness. Dementia may begin with focal cognitive or behavioural disturbances, but both DSM-IV and ICD-10 definitions require impairment in two or more cognitive domains (memory, language, abstract thinking and judgement, praxis, visuoperceptual skills, personality, and social conduct), sufficient to interfere with social or occupational functioning. It is increasingly recognized that cognitive impairment may initially be too mild or circumscribed to fulfil this definition. The fluctuations in alertness which characterize delirium are usually absent, unless, of course, the two coexist. Fluctuating impairment of consciousness is, however, a feature of dementia with Lewy bodies (see below). Although most cases of dementia are irreversible, a small but important group are treatable (see Table 14.3). See Growdon and Rossor (1998) and Lovestone (2000) for reviews of contemporary concepts in dementia.

Clinical features

The presenting complaint is usually of poor memory. Other features include disturbances of behaviour, personality, mood, or perception. Dementia is often exposed by a change in social circumstances or an intercurrent illness; indeed, patients with dementia are especially susceptible to superimposed delirium.

The clinical picture is much determined by the patient's premorbid personality. People with good social skills may continue to function adequately despite severe intellectual deterioration. The elderly, socially isolated, or deaf are less likely to

Table 14.3 Examples of cortical, subcortical and mixed dementias

Cortical

Alzheimer's disease

Frontotemporal dementias

Creutzfeldt-Jacob disease

Subcortical

Normal pressure hydrocephalus

Huntington's disease

Parkinson's disease

Focal thalamic and basal ganglia lesions

Multiple sclerosis

AIDS-dementia complex

Hypothyroidism

Dementia pugilistica

Mixed

Multi-infarct dementia

Dementia with Lewy bodies

Corticobasal degeneration

Neurosyphilis

bicycle), and, at least initially, general knowledge about the world at large. By contrast, words and, ultimately, the very objects to which they refer, lose their meaning for patients with semantic memory impairment (as in certain frontotemporal dementias). Two major behavioural syndromes are commonly observed, and may coexist:

- apathy, inertia, and loss of interest in work and hobbies;
- restlessness, disinhibition, distractibility, loss of empathy, and social skills.

Loss of flexibility and adaptability in new situations, with the appearance of rigid and stereotyped routines ('organic orderliness'), and, when taxed beyond restricted abilities, sudden explosions of rage or grief ('catastrophic reaction') are frequent.

Early, prominent behavioural and emotional disturbances with relative preservation of memory and general intellect are characteristic of the frontotemporal dementias. Prominent visual processing difficulties (such as finding the door or locating food with utensils) suggest dementia with Lewy bodies; similar phenomena are, however, also common in later Alzheimer's disease. Visual hallucinations are often prominent and vivid, but (unlike those in psychiatric disease or drug-induced states) typically silent and non-threatening

As dementia worsens, patients are less able to care for themselves and they neglect social conventions. Disorientation for time, and later for place and person, is common. Behaviour becomes aimless, and stereotypies and mannerisms may appear. Thinking slows and becomes impoverished in content and perseverative. False ideas, often of a persecutory kind, gain ground easily. In the later stages, thinking becomes grossly fragmented and incoherent. This is reflected in the patient's speech, with syntactical and dysnomic errors. Eventually, the patient may become mute.

Mood disturbances commonly occur during the course of most dementias. It is likely that these, in part, have a biological basis (see for example, Hirono *et al.* 2000). They include anxiety, irritability, aggression, and depression. Retained insight

compensate for failing intellectual abilities; however, their difficulties may be unrecognized or dismissed.

Forgetfulness is usually early and prominent, but may sometimes be difficult to detect in the early stages. Poor memory is not anatomically localizing: it may reflect disrupted registration (frontotemporal interactions), encoding (mesial temporal lobes), or retrieval (frontal lobes). Impaired attention and concentration are common and non-specific features. Difficulty in new learning is usually the most conspicuous feature. Memory loss is more evident for recent than for more remote material. Disturbed episodic memory (for example, in Alzheimer's disease) manifests as forgetfulness for recent day-to-day events, with relative preservation of procedural memory (for instance, riding a

in the earlier stages may give rise to considerable distress and reactive depression. Later, emotional responses become blunted, and sudden, apparently random mood changes occur.

Subcortical and cortical dementia syndromes

The term 'subcortical dementia' refers to a syndrome of slowness of thought, difficulty with complex, sequential intellectual tasks, impoverishment of affect and personality, with relative preservation of language, calculation, and learning. It contrasts with the spectrum of cortical dysfunction (including early, prominent impairments of memory, word finding, or visuospatial abilities) seen in 'cortical dementia' of Alzheimer's disease.

The concept of subcortical dementia is part of increasing awareness of the cognitive functions of subcortical pathways and nuclei, notably the thalamus and basal ganglia (see below, 'Subcortical syndromes'). A network approach to human cognitive neurology has replaced traditional views of topographical localization (Varma and Trimble 1997). At least five large-scale neurocognitive networks can be identified in the human brain (Mesulam 1998):

- a right hemisphere spatial awareness network including posterior parietal cortex and frontal eye fields;
- a left hemisphere language network including Broca's and Wernicke's areas;
- a memory-emotion network including hippocampus, amygdala and cingulate cortex;
- a working memory-executive function network including prefrontal cortex and posterior parietal cortex; and
- a face and object recognition network in temporoparietal and temporo-occipital cortex.

Subcortical structures, in particular the basal ganglia, may facilitate, via massive reciprocal connections with multiple cortical (especially frontal) areas, the synchronization of cortical activity underlying the selection and execution of an appropriate movement or sequence of thoughts (Brown and Marsden 1998).

Some causes of subcortical dementia are listed in Table 14.4. Although the distinction between the cortical and subcortical dementias is frequently blurred clinically and pathologically, the terms are useful as clinical descriptions.

Semantic dementia

Recent years have seen growing awareness of a dementia syndrome distinguished by selective, progressive loss of meaning for verbal and non-verbal material, accompanied by striking difficulty in naming, categorization and comprehension. Autobiographical memory is relatively preserved (though it may be difficult to access). When asked to demonstrate an object or action, patients typically stare at the examiner uncomprehendingly, repeating the instruction as if it had been asked in a foreign language. Associated cognitive, psychiatric or neurological signs are minimal in the early stages and the increasingly severe semantic impairment may remain circumscribed for many years; yet the implications for independent life are often devastating. There is selective, often asymmetric temporal lobe atrophy. The concept and its development have been usefully reviewed by Garrard and Hodges (2000).

Dementia or normal ageing?

The distinction between age-related cognitive change and early dementia (especially Alzheimer's disease) is a common diagnostic problem, which at present relies on clinical judgement. In normal ageing, although the speed of cognitive processing slows, the accuracy of responses is not affected, new learning can be demonstrated with repetition, and verbal abilities remain stable. In practice, doubtful cases are resolved by repeated neuropsychometric assessments over time, and if available, serial magnetic resonance imaging (MRI) to detect progressive atrophy (Fox *et al.* 1996).

Aetiology

Dementia has many causes, of which some are listed in Table 14.3. Among the elderly, degenera-

Table 14.4 Some causes of dementia

Primary degenerative

Sporadic Alzheimer's disease, dementia with Lewy bodies, Pick's disease and other frontotemporal dementias, Parkinson's disease

Genetically determined

Familial Alzheimer's disease, frontotemporal dementia linked to chromosome 17, familial prion diseases, Huntington's disease

Vascular

Multiple strokes,* focal thalamic and basal ganglia strokes, subdural haematoma*

Inflammatory and autoimmune

SLE,* systemic vasculitides* with neurological involvement, isolated vasculitis of CNS, Behçet's disease,* neurosarcoidosis,* Hashimoto's encephalopathy,* multiple sclerosis

Traumatic

Severe single head injuries, repeated head injury in boxers ('dementia pugilistica') and others

Infections and related conditions

HIV,* sporadic and new variant CJD, neurosyphilis,* post-encephalitic, Lyme disease*

Metabolic and endocrine

Sustained uraemia,* renal dialysis,* liver failure,* hypothyroidism,* hyperthyroidism ('apathetic' or masked), chronic hypoglycaemia,* Cushing's syndrome,* hypopituitarism,* adrenal insufficiency*

Neoplastic

Intracranial space-occupying lesions,* carcinomatous or lymphomatous meningitis, paraneoplastic 'limbic encephalitis'

Post-radiation

Acute and subacute radionecrosis, radiation thromboangiopathy, accelerated cerebral atherosclerosis, radiation leucodystrophy

Post-anoxic

Severe anaemia, post-surgical (especially cardiac bypass), carbon monoxide poisoning, cardiac arrest, chronic respiratory failure

Vitamin and other nutritional deficiency

Sustained lack of vitamin B12,* thiamine* (Wernicke-Korsakov syndrome)

Toxic

Alcohol, poisoning with heavy metals,* organic solvents, organophosphates*

Other

Normal pressure hydrocephalus*

*Therapy available.

tive and vascular disorders predominate; however (especially in younger patients), the clinician should consider a broad range of possible causes, taking particular care to exclude those which are treatable (see Table 14.4).

General principles of management

As in delirium, the cause must be identified and treated if possible. General management of any dementia begins with an assessment of the nature and degree of disability and the social resources of the patient and family.

The treatment plan aims to achieve optimal daily function, relieve distress, and provide practical help for the patient and carers. It should make clear the part to be played by all members of the multidisciplinary team, whether the patient is living in hospital or in the community. Personality change and restlessness at night cause particular difficulties for carers.

It may be necessary to make legal arrangements for the administration of the patient's financial affairs. It is essential that the patient's capacity and safety to drive be regularly re-evaluated; in practice, this means informing the Licensing Authority at the time of diagnosis in most cases. It is also useful to ask the patient's spouse if he or she feels safe as a passenger when the patient takes the wheel.

As the patient's capacity for self-care decreases, scrupulous attention must be paid to personal hygiene, safety, exercise, and, in particular, nutrition, which is frequently inadequate in demented elderly people. Incontinence of urine and faeces becomes an important determinant of the level of care the patient requires in more advanced disease.

Drug treatment

There is no curative treatment for the neurodegenerative dementias; however, effective symptomatic therapies which may improve specific capacities, such as memory (notably, acetylcholinesterase inhibitors in Alzheimer's disease), have recently become available (see p. 628).

Medications such as antipsychotics or benzodiazepines can be helpful for such symptoms as anxiety and agitation. If the patient has depressive symptoms, a trial of antidepressant medication is worthwhile, since the functional gain can be great.

As a general principle however, drugs are more likely to aggravate than to improve cognitive impairment in demented patients, and medications should be reviewed regularly to ensure that they are being used rationally. Neuroleptics should be used cautiously, if at all, and introduced slowly. Disastrous extrapyramidal reactions may be produced in dementia with Lewy bodies and in some frontotemporal dementias.

Behavioural strategies

Careful assessment of the patient's functional abilities and limitations, and setting of attainable goals is an essential part of care. A regular daily routine is desirable; however, at the same time, social isolation must be avoided. Ideally, the patient's capacities should be challenged, but not exceeded. Behavioural methods include positive reinforcement, shaping, desensitization, prompts and other practical aids to coping with forgetfulness. Difficulties in coping with unfamiliar environments and situations should be anticipated, and regular reorientation and reassurance should be offered. See Prigatano (1999) and Wilson (1999) for reviews of neurophysiological rehabilitation. See Fleminger (2000) and references in Chapter 20 for reviews of the management of dementia.

Specific neuropsychiatric syndromes

Focal cerebral syndromes

There are a number of syndromes of specific cognitive and psychiatric impairment, characterized by more or less selective derangements of cortical functions, memory, mood, or personality. In many, specific or localized brain pathology can be demonstrated. This chapter concentrates on features of particular relevance to the psychiatrist. The many forms of dysphasia, agnosia, and dyspraxia lie traditionally (if arbitrarily) within the province of the neurologist, and have been excluded; they are well described by Lishman (1998), and in standard neurology texts.

Frontal lobe

The frontal lobes have a crucial role in personality and judgement. Recent research (reviewed by Dolan 1999) has demonstrated that they have an intricate physiology with reciprocal connections to other cortical and subcortical regions. The patient with a frontal lobe syndrome may present with a variety of clinical syndromes, which are probably associated with different anatomical localizations. He may:

- be disinhibited, overfamiliar, tactless, and garrulous, make fatuous jokes and puns ('Witzelsucht'), commit errors of judgement and sexual indiscretions, and disregard the feelings of others;
- appear inert (abulic) and apathetic, with a paucity of spontaneous speech, movement, and emotional expressions;
- engage in obsessive, ritualistic behaviours with perseveration of thought and gesture.

See Lishman (1998) and Garrard and Hodges (2000).

Measures of formal intelligence are generally unimpaired in frontal lobe disease; however, there may be difficulties in abstract reasoning ('How are glass and ice different?') and cognitive estimates are typically inaccurate but precise ('364 miles from London to New York'). Concentration and attention are reduced. Insight is often markedly impaired. Verbal fluency, assessed using word generation by letter (for example, number of words beginning with 's' in one minute) and category (for example, number of animals), is reduced and unusual (low-frequency) examples may be volunteered. The patient has difficulty switching between tasks (perseveration), carrying out sequenced movements, and understanding rules.

Utilization behaviour (for example, donning several pairs of spectacles) may be evident.

Posterior extension of a dominant frontal lobe lesion may involve Broca's area and produce an expressive (non-fluent) dysphasia. Encroachment on the motor cortex or deep projections may result in a contralateral hemiparesis. Other signs may include ipsilateral optic atrophy or anosmia, a grasp or other primitive reflexes and, if the process is bilateral or in the midline, incontinence of urine. See Gustafson (2000) for a review of psychiatric manifestations of frontal lobe tumours.

Parietal lobe

Lesions of the parietal lobe may cause various neuropsychological disturbances which are easily mistaken for hysteria. Involvement of the non-dominant parietal lobe characteristically gives rise to visuospatial difficulties, with neglect of contra-lateral space, constructional and dressing apraxias. Lesions of the dominant lobe may be associated with receptive dysphasia, limb apraxia, body image disorders, right-left disorientation, dyscalculia, finger agnosia and agraphia in various combinations. Other signs may include contralateral cortical sensory loss, with sensory inattention, astereognosis and agraphaesthesia, and (with more extensive lesions) a contralateral hemiparesis or homonymous inferior quadrantanopia.

Persistent denial of neurological deficit (anosognosia) is not uncommon, especially with non-dominant parietal lesions. In extreme cases, the patient may deny that paretic limbs belong to him. This should be distinguished from denial due to a psychological unwillingness to recognize disability and its consequences.

Temporal lobe

The temporolimbic syndromes (see Trimble 1997) are characterized by complex and wide-ranging neuropsychiatric clinical pictures. There may be personality change resembling that of frontal lobe lesions, but more often accompanied by specific cognitive deficits and neurological signs. Temporal lobe lesions are sometimes associated with a schizophrenia-like psychosis. Right medial temporal atrophy has been associated with paranoid delusions in Alzheimer's disease (Geroldi *et al.* 2000). The florid behavioural disturbances which characterize the frontotemporal dementias (see p. 420) may implicate the mesial temporal-limbic structures and their frontotemporal connections.

Unilateral temporal lobe lesions may produce lateralizing memory deficits, broadly speaking, verbal on the left, non-verbal on the right (in nearly all right-handed people and most left-handers, too). Pathology involving the dominant temporal lobe may declare itself in a semantic impairment, fluent dysphasia, and receptive language difficulties.

Occipital lobe

Occipital lobe lesions may cause disturbances of visual processing which are easily misinterpreted as benign of psychological origin. Such phenomena occasionally accompany migraine or occipital lobe seizures, in the absence of structural pathology. Complex visual hallucinations may occur with lesions involving visual association areas, sometimes referred to a hemianopic field. These include multiple visual images (polyopia), persistent after-traces of the features of an image (visual perseveration or palinopia), and distortions of the visual scene (metamorphopsia). Lesions which impinge anteriorly on the parietal or temporal lobes may produce visual disorientation (inability to localize objects in space under visual guidance) with asimultagnosia (difficulty perceiving the visual scene as a unity), or prosopagnosia (inability to recognize familiar faces), respectively. In patients with suspected occipital lobe pathology, the visual fields should be mapped using perimetry, and neuropsychological tests performed to delineate visual agnosias and other higher-order derangements of visual processing.

Corpus callosum

Corpus callosum lesions (classically, the 'butterfly glioma') typically extend laterally into both hemispheres. They then produce a picture of severe and rapid intellectual deterioration, with localized neurological signs varying with the degree of extension into the frontal or occipital lobes or the diencephalon. In isolated callosal lesions (for example, post-surgical), specialized neuropsychological testing may expose a 'disconnection syndrome', reflecting disruption of interhemispheric communication. These unique patients raise intriguing questions concerning the mechanisms which normally bind the two hemispheres together to generate a consistent, unitary sense of the self (see Gazzaniga 2000). The rare syndrome of *Marchiafava and Bignami* is associated with callosal degeneration in those with severe alcohol dependence.

Subcortical syndromes

As indicated earlier, the role of thalamus, basal ganglia and other subcortical structures in large-scale, distributed neural networks is increasingly emphasized in accounts of a wide range of cognitive (notably executive, language, and memory) functions, behaviours, and affective states (see Varma and Trimble 1997). It is likely that subcortical structures have a specific functional role within these networks, as well as exerting a more diffuse, activating or facilitatory influence over the cortical mantle.

Thalamus and basal ganglia

A variety of cognitive and psychiatric consequences have been described following lesions of subcortical grey matter structures. These include memory, language, and mood disturbance.

Rostral brainstem

Behavioural disturbances frequently accompany lesions of the rostral brainstem (see Varma and Trimble 1997). The most characteristic features are an amnestic syndrome (see below), hypersomnia, and the syndrome of 'akinetic mutism' ('vigilant coma').

Disorders of memory

Classification and neuroanatomy of memory functions

Clinical, neuropsychological, and brain imaging studies (both structural and functional) support the existence of multiple memory systems in the human brain. The classification of memory functions has been clearly outlined by Hodges (1994) and is discussed on p. 23 in Chapter 1. It is, for convenience, also described here. These functions may all be affected more or less selectively by brain lesions. The most basic division lies between *implicit (procedural)* and *explicit (declarative) memory*. The former includes a range of phenomena not usually subject to conscious analysis, such as motor skills, conditioned behaviours, and repetition priming. The latter comprises consciously accessed material, which may be subject to short-term or long-term storage.

The short-term store underpins working memory (for example, when dialling an unfamiliar telephone number). Distinct anatomical substrates for short-term storage of verbal and visuospatial information, both controlled by a central executive, have been proposed. In neuropsychological terms, short-term refers to *immediate recall*. By contrast, the concept of 'short-term' memory as sometimes applied by clinicians to *recall over minutes and days*, does not correspond to an anatomical substrate.

The long-term store is often further subclassified into *episodic* (autobiographical events) and *semantic* (knowledge of the world) functions.

Specific types of memories, such as faces and topographical information, may engage dedicated subsystems. Episodic memory has both anterograde (new learning) and retrograde (recall of past events) components. It appears to be mediated by a network of cortical and subcortical structures, which includes the hippocampus, parahippocampal and entorrhinal cortices, amygdala, mammillary bodies, fornix, cingulate, thalamus, and frontobasal cortex, whereas semantic memory may be subserved by a partly independent network overlapping the language areas of the left hemisphere.

Table 14.5 Some important causes of amnesia
Transient
Transient global amnesia
Transient epileptic amnesia
Head injury
Alcoholic blackouts
Post-electroconvulsive therapy
Post-traumatic stress disorder
Psychogenic fugue
Amnesia for criminal offence
Persistent
Amnestic syndrome
Herpes encephalitis
Vascular disorder
Head injury

Broadly speaking, verbal memories are mediated by the left (dominant) hemisphere and non-verbal by the right; however, interhemispheric cooperation is likely to be extensive under normal circumstances.

Table 14.5 lists important causes of memory disorder.

Amnestic syndrome

Amnestic disorder is defined by DSM-IV as a specific impairment of episodic memory, manifesting as inability to learn new information (anterograde amnesia) and to recall past events (retrograde amnesia), in the absence of evidence for generalized intellectual dysfunction, accompanied by 'significant impairment in social or occupational functioning' and evidence of a general medical condition 'aetiologically related to the memory impairment'. The syndrome classically results from lesions in the medial thalamus, adjacent midline structures, or hippocampi.

A syndrome of severe memory impairment accompanied by confabulation and irritability was first described by the Russian neuropsychiatrist, Korsakov, in 1889. The term 'Korsakov's syndrome' has been used to denote both a clinical picture and a pathological entity. The alternative *Wernicke-Korsakov syndrome* was proposed by Victor *et al.* (1971), because the chronic amnestic syndrome often follows an acute neurological syndrome (described by Wernicke in 1881) comprising impaired consciousness and disorientation, episodic memory impairment, truncal ataxia, pupillary abnormalities, ophthalmoplegia, nystagmus, and a peripheral neuropathy. Historically, bilateral temporal lobe resection has also produced the amnestic syndrome.

The information processing defect in the amnestic syndrome is likely to involve the encoding of new material, consolidation of this material into long-term storage, and subsequent retrieval, to a variable degree dependent on the precise anatomy of the causative lesion (Hodges 1994).

Clinical features

The cardinal sign is a profound deficit of episodic memory. Wernicke-Korsakov syndrome and the syndrome of 'diencephalic amnesia' after bilateral medial thalamic lesions comprise a similar, striking clinical picture: disorientation for time, loss of autobiographical information (often extending back for many years), confabulation, and severe anterograde amnesia for verbal and visual material. Events are recalled immediately after they occur, but forgotten a few minutes later. Thus digit span, testing the short-term memory store, is typically normal. New learning is grossly defective, but retrograde memory is variably preserved and shows a temporal gradient. Gaps in memory may be filled by confabulation: the patient is often highly suggestible, and may give a vivid and detailed but wholly fictitious account of recent activities. *Confabulation* is widely believed to be a specific symptom of the amnestic syndrome. It is more correctly seen as a sign of delirium and of frontal lobe disease. Other cognitive functions are

relatively well preserved, although some emotional blunting and inertia are often observed, suggesting disruption of frontotemporal or frontosubcortical connections.

Aetiology and pathology

Chronic alcohol abuse associated with thiamine deficiency is the most frequent cause of the Wernicke-Korsakov syndrome. The differential diagnosis of amnesia is outlined in Table 14.5. Post-mortem findings in this condition typically include petechial haemorrhages with astrocytic degeneration in the mammillary bodies, the region of the third ventricle, the periaqueductal grey matter, pons, and medial dorsal thalamic nuclei.

Investigation and management

Alertness to the possibility of the amnestic syndrome is essential; the patient may not fit the stereotype of chronic alcohol misuse, and this is a potentially reversible condition. Useful findings from investigations include a reduced red cell transketolase level, which is a marker of thiamine deficiency, and an abnormal increased MRI signal in midline structures. Management involves administration of parenteral thiamine (before giving glucose-containing solutions, which will otherwise exacerbate the deficiency), rehydration, general nutritional support, and frequently, treatment of supervening alcohol withdrawal. Thiamine should be given without delay wherever there is even suspicion of deficiency and without awaiting investigations. Progressive amnesia suggests a slowly expanding structural lesion, such as a midbrain tumour.

Course and prognosis

In the series of Victor *et al.* (1971) comprising 245 patients with Wernicke-Korsakov syndrome, 96% presented with Wernicke's encephalopathy. Mortality was 17% in the acute stage, and 84% of survivors developed a typical amnestic syndrome. There was no improvement in half, complete recovery in a quarter, and partial recovery in the remainder. Favourable prognostic factors were a short history before diagnosis and prompt commencement of thiamine replacement.

The prognosis is poor in cases of amnestic syndrome due to encephalitis and other causes of irreversible bilateral hippocampal or diencephalic damage; however, other aetiologies (such as head injury) have a relatively favourable outlook.

Transient global amnesia

This syndrome is important in the differential diagnosis of episodic neurological and psychiatric disturbance (see Table 14.6). It occurs in middle or late life. The clinical picture is of sudden onset of isolated anterograde amnesia in a clear sensorium generally lasting less than 24 hours. Functional imaging studies during transient global amnesia have demonstrated localized transient hypo- or hyperperfusion consistent with dysfunction of circuits mediating episodic memory.

The patient appears bewildered, and requires repeated reorientation, only to ask the same questions moments later; however, there is no disturbance of alertness and (in contrast to psychogenic fugue) personal identity is retained. Procedural memory is spared (for example, the patient may carry on driving competently during the episode). Apart from the memory disturbance, the neurological examination is entirely normal.

Complete recovery, with amnesia for the period of the episode, is usual and recurrence is rare. However, investigation is always indicated since the condition may be exactly mimicked by a temporal lobe tumour. Other causes of the amnestic syndrome (see above and Table 14.5) must also be excluded. Patients with transient global amnesia often present as emergencies to general practitioners and casualty departments; the syndrome is not infrequently misdiagnosed as a dissociative fugue. See Kopelman (2000) and Berrios and Hodges (2000) for reviews of memory disorders.

Secondary psychiatric syndromes

A variety of psychological symptoms, including changes in personality, perception, and mood, may result from brain dysfunction due to cerebral or systemic disease. Causes for some of these syndromes are listed in Table 14.7. The phenomenological features are generally identical to those in

---

Table 14.6 Differential diagnosis of paroxysmal neurological and psychiatric symptoms

Organic

Vasovagal syncope

Cardiogenic syncope (Stokes-Adams attacks)

Reflex syncope (cough, micturition, deglutition)

Transient ischaemic attacks

Migraine

Epilepsy (simple partial, complex partial, absence, generalized tonic-clonic, myoclonic, atonic)

Hypoglycaemia, other metabolic encephalopathies, phaeochromocytoma

Transient global amnesia

Narcolepsy, cataplexy, somnambulism, REM sleep behaviour disorder, periodic leg movements of sleep

Episodic ataxias

Paroxysmal choreoathetoses

Spasticity with flexor spasms

Myoclonus (brainstem, spinal, peripheral)

Tonic spasms of multiple sclerosis

Treatment-related complications in Parkinson's disease

Drug abuse (covert)

Psychiatric

Panic attacks and hyperventilation

Dissociative disorder

Schizophrenia

Bipolar affective disorder

Aggressive outburst in personality disorder

Temper tantrums (children)

Breath-holding spells (children)

Table 14.7 Some causes of symptomatic or secondary psychiatric syndromes

Syndrome	Causes
Psychosis	Temporal lobe disorder, Huntington's disease, focal basal ganglia lesions, endocrinopathies
Mood disorder	Alzheimer's disease, stroke (multiple syndromes), head trauma, Parkinson's disease (including effects of medical and surgical therapy), multiple sclerosis, Huntington's disease, CJD, paraneoplastic limbic encephalitis, endocrinopathies, metabolic disorders (especially hypercalcaemia), neurosyphilis
Delusional disorder	Alzheimer's disease, dementia with Lewy bodies, metabolic disorder, thalamic lesions, neurosyphilis
Organic hallucinosis (especially visual)	Dementia with Lewy bodies, Parkinson's disease (especially with dopaminergic agonists), Alzheimer's disease, occipital lobe lesions, temporal and occipital epilepsy, CJD, paraneoplastic limbic encephalitis, migraine
Personality disorder	Frontotemporal dementias, frontal lesions, Huntington's disease, focal basal ganglia lesions, neurosyphilis, CJD, paraneoplastic limbic encephalitis
Obsessive–compulsive behaviours	Frontotemporal dementias, temporal lobe epilepsy, encephalitis lethargica, other basal ganglia disorders, Rett syndrome
Self-mutilation	Lesch-Nyhan syndrome

primary psychiatric illness. Clues to specific neural circuitry underpinning emotional experiences and behaviour are evident in the accounts of consequences of certain focal brain lesions.

Awareness of possible physical causes of psychiatric disorders is reflected in recent diagnostic classification schemes (Spitzer *et al.* 1992). Since these syndromes are phenomenologically indistinguishable from primary psychiatric illness, diagnosis of a secondary syndrome depends on associated features. In ICD-10, the following clinical guidelines are suggested as supporting an aetiology secondary to a physical condition:

- evidence of cerebral disease, damage or dysfunction, or of systematic physical disease, known to be associated with one of the listed syndromes;
- temporal relationship (weeks or a few months) between the development of the underlying disease and the onset of the mental syndrome;

- recovery from the mental disorder following removal or improvement of the underlying presumed cause;
- absence of evidence suggesting an alternative cause of the mental syndrome

Assessment of the patient with suspected cognitive impairment

Any suspicion of cognitive impairment should lead to detailed questioning about intellectual function and neurological symptoms. It is particularly important to interview other informants separately. The mode of onset and progression of symptoms should be determined in detail. A thorough physical examination is essential.

Initial investigations

With every patient a judgement needs to be made concerning the extent of investigation required to allow accurate diagnosis, and to identify reversible processes. A basic initial battery includes:

- full blood count and differential; erythrocyte sedimentation rate;
- biochemistry including serum calcium, renal, liver and thyroid function tests, serum B12 and folate;
- serology for syphilis;
- a chest radiograph;
- brain imaging (CT or MRI) and an EEG.

Care is needed in interpreting the significance of the results; for example, a low serum B12 is common in the elderly, but it is rarely the sole cause of cognitive decline.

Further investigations

The clinical picture should dictate which (if any) further investigations are required. Neuropsychometry may be valuable in defining the psychological profile more precisely (see below). HIV testing is not routine, but in the presence of specific risk factors or other indications it should be considered and discussed with the patient. Vasculitic, autoimmune, neoplastic, and toxicological screens, and in younger patients, copper studies and white cell enzymes, may be indicated, as may genetic testing in familial dementias.

Neuroimaging

Computerized tomography (CT) has a key role as a first line imaging modality in the diagnosis of both focal and diffuse cerebral pathology. Magnetic resonance imaging (MRI) is superior to CT in detecting white matter disease (especially in vascular dementia), and, using thin slice T1-weighted images, focal (especially temporal lobe) atrophy. It also has an emerging role in serial assessment of progressive regional atrophy for diagnosis and prognosis.

Electroencephalography

EEG can indicate diffuse cortical dysfunction (useful, for example, in distinguishing Alzheimer's disease from the frontotemporal dementias, in which the EEG is typically normal), and is essential in detecting non-convulsive seizure activity, which may present as psychosis.

Cerebrospinal fluid (CSF) examination

If an infectious or inflammatory process is suspected, CSF examination is mandatory, provided there are no contraindications. Features may include a raised cell count (pleocytosis), raised protein, low CSF:serum glucose ratio, or unmatched oligoclonal bands (indicating local synthesis of immunoglobulin in the central nervous system). Polymerase chain reaction (PCR) can be used to amplify and detect viral and other infective DNA. Cytological examination may reveal atypical or malignant cells in neoplastic conditions. Elevated levels of brain-specific proteins such as 14–3–3, S–100 and tau may be detectable in certain neurodegenerative disorders.

Specialized investigations

Functional brain imaging techniques, such as single photon emission computed tomography (SPECT), positron emission tomography (PET) and functional magnetic resonance imaging (fMRI) may occasionally be useful. These techniques provide information about regional cerebral blood flow or metabolism, and may assist in the diagnosis of dementia and certain other disorders. Interpretation is difficult, and the availability of such techniques is likely to remain limited.

In exceptional cases, brain biopsy (usually right frontal lobe) may be indicated to exclude a potentially treatable (especially, inflammatory) process, if the diagnosis cannot be made by less invasive means. This carries an approximately 1% combined risk of significant morbidity or mortality, and should always be a carefully weighed decision.

Neuropsychometry

Neuropsychometric tests depend on (among many other factors) the patient's cooperation, and should be administered and interpreted by an experienced examiner. Discrimination between organic and functional disorders is sometimes difficult. Psychometry is of particular value in monitoring changes in psychological functioning over time, and in assessing patterns of disability as a basis for planning rehabilitation. Some of the more frequently used tests are outlined below (for further information, see Hodges 1994).

Wechsler Adult Intelligence Scale (WAIS)

This is a well-standardized test providing a profile of verbal and non-verbal abilities. It is most useful for screening; however, analysis of subscores can provide useful diagnostic information. The WAIS is best interpreted together with a measure of premorbid attainment, such as the National Adult Reading Test (NART).

Perceptual functions, especially spatial relationships

This kind of test is exemplified by the Benton Revised Visual Retention Test, which requires the patient to study and reproduce ten designs.

New learning as a test of memory

There are many new word learning tasks, for example, the Walton-Black Modified Word Learning Test and the Paired Associated Learning Test, both of which give a useful quantitative estimate of memory impairment.

Specific tests

Examples of specific tests are the Wisconsin Card Sorting Test for frontal lobe damage, and the Token Test for receptive language disturbance.

Standardized mental state schedules

There are numerous mental state schedules, ranging in complexity from the ten-item Hodkinson Mental Test to lengthy research instruments. Two of the most commonly used brief schedules are the Mini-Mental State Examination (MMSE) (see p. 68) and the Hodkinson Mental Test. An example of a longer research procedure is the Cambridge Cognitive Examination (CAMCOG), which is part of a standardized assessment schedule (CAMDEX) designed specifically for the use with elderly people with the diagnosis of dementia. Such instruments are convenient to administer, but have a number of shortcomings, including insensitivity to circumscribed cognitive deficits and frontal executive dysfunction. They are perhaps most useful in detecting progression over serial assessments (Hodges 1994).

Aspects of differential diagnosis

Organic or functional?

It is sometimes difficult to distinguish between organic and functional cognitive symptoms. An organic disorder may be misdiagnosed as functional if the patient has personality features (for example, depressive or paranoid) which distort the clinical presentation. This applies to diseases in which behavioural and emotional disturbances are integral to the disease process (such as the frontotemporal dementias), as well as disorders in which prominent mood symptoms may be a manifestation of retained insight. The opposite error is also frequent, for example, misdiagnosing dementia in a depressed patient whose presenting complaint is poor memory. Either type of error has serious implications if a reversible process is missed.

Despite advances in brain imaging and other investigative techniques, the essential requirements remain a complete history (including information from a reliable informant), and a thorough physical and cognitive examination. The mode of onset of the symptoms is of particular importance. Personal and cultural information should be gathered to build up an accurate picture of premorbid functioning and to set the present illness in context.

If psychiatric symptoms cannot be understood psychologically, enquiry should always be directed to a possible primary cognitive disorder. Conversion or dissociative disorder should never be diagnosed until all possible organic causes have been excluded *and* a psychological causation established, even in patients with a history of psychiatric illness. Brain diseases frequently present with symptoms that resemble those of a conversion, dissociative or mood disorder, and should be considered in any patient with an unexplained episode of disturbed behaviour. Certain symptoms should always arouse suspicion of an organic process, for example, isolated visual hallucinations, or complaints which would be distinctly unusual in a functional disorder, such as ataxia, incontinence, or micrographia. Important signs may be evident during the examination (for example, certain frontal phenomena, such as utilization behaviour and perseveration, which almost never accompany psychiatric illness).

'Pseudodementia'

Although non-convulsive status epilepticus may produce an 'epileptic pseudodementia' (see below), the term is chiefly reserved for primary psychiatric illness (especially depression and conversion disorder) and factitious disorders. Pseudodementia is most common in elderly depressed patients (see p. 629). The patient complains of poor memory and concentration, and neurovegetative symptoms may be elicited. There may be a personal or family history of psychiatric illness. 'Don't know' responses and poor involvement with neuropsychological tests are characteristic. It must be kept in mind that depression is a common feature early in the course of some organic disorders, notably Alzheimer's disease.

In distinguishing pseudodementia from true dementia, it is necessary to establish which symptoms developed first, since in the former other psychological symptoms generally precede the apparent intellectual decline.

Dissociative cognitive impairment is generally distinguished by its relatively abrupt onset, the presence of an identifiable emotional precipitant, lack of progression, and inconsistencies on formal testing, with performance far inferior to that expected from daily life performance; the patient who, having found his way to clinic unaccompanied, is quite unable to recall test material probably has a pseudodementia. In contrast to patients with organic memory impairment, those with dissociative or conversion disorders may fail to recall the most emotionally salient material. In factitious dementia, a source of secondary gain may be apparent. The possibility of an elaborated, underlying organic impairment should always be considered, and in practice, the distinction between organic and psychiatric disorder may be difficult. Clinical reassessment over time is the key to resolving this dilemma.

Acute or chronic?

The time course of evolution of the illness is critical, but may be difficult to establish, usually because a clear history is lacking. The testimony of family and friends is usually decisive. Delirium may be superimposed on a long-standing dementia; it may obscure the underlying diagnosis, or alternatively draw attention to the background impairment. The most helpful clinical clues to an acute syndrome are impairment of consciousness, perceptual abnormalities, disturbed attention, poor sleep, and thinking that is disorganized but rich in content. Although a fluctuating course is characteristic of delirium, it is also a central feature of some forms of dementia, notably dementia with Lewy bodies.

Diagnosis of stupor

'Stupor' is sometimes used to describe a state of immobility (or sometimes hyperactivity) and diminished engagement with the environment from which the sufferer can be briefly roused by vigorous stimulation. However, a precise description of the patient's capacities is preferable. The main psychiatric causes are severe depression, schizophrenia, and, rarely, hysteria and mania. Some organic causes are listed in Table 14.8. The common pathway in these disorders is impaired function of the anatomical network subserving alertness, especially the ascending reticular formation in the brainstem, and its projections to

Table 14.8 Differential diagnosis of organic stupor
Focal brain lesions
Diffuse brain lesions
Metabolic disturbances
Drugs
Prescription
Recreational
Toxic exposures

midbrain, thalami, and forebrain. Diagnosis can usually be made on the history and examination. The possible role of drugs (recreational and prescribed) should not be overlooked. An EEG (to demonstrate slowing of cerebral rhythms) and CT or MRI (to reveal structural brain lesions) may be helpful in distinguishing between organic and psychogenic causes. See Lishman (1998) for a review.

Identifying a cause

The history and findings on physical and neuropsychological examination should be reviewed in terms of one of the recognized patterns of cognitive dysfunction. The central questions are 'Where in the brain does the process reside?' and 'What is its nature?' The answers depend on an accurate picture of duration, mode of onset, and pattern of evolution of the symptoms. Specific enquiry should be made about any history of head injuries, fits, alcohol or drug abuse, and recent physical illness. Dietary deficiency should be considered if the patient is elderly, of low intelligence, or alcoholic. A searching family history is important, recognizing that this may be incomplete or concealed. It is essential to enquire about symptoms of raised intracranial pressure (headaches, vomiting, and visual disturbance), as well as those suggesting a focal lesion in the brain.

Physical examination must be systematic and thorough since signs may not be conspicuous.

Appropriate investigations should then be guided by the differential diagnostic formulation.

Important neuropsychiatric disorders

Primary neurodegenerative dementias

The most common causes of dementia are degenerative diseases of the central nervous system presenting in middle or late life, sometimes called *primary dementias*. Recent developments in genetics and biochemistry have transformed understanding of a large and varied group of disorders, which are clinically, pathologically, and biochemically distinct. For example, Alzheimer's disease itself is not a single entity in terms of its molecular biology, though a characteristic histopathological final common pathway is involved. It is important that the diagnosis is as accurate as possible, since this aids prognosis and, ultimately, the design of specific therapies will depend on this. However, experience shows that at present the correlation of the clinical picture with pathological findings is imperfect.

Common sporadic disorders, such Alzheimer's and Parkinson's disease, together with rarer entities such as the frontotemporal dementias, MND-dementia-parkinsonism syndromes, 'Pick's disease', and the prion disease (see below) can all be understood in terms of a common model of neurodegeneration. Specific populations of neurons in these diseases may be implicated by their biochemistry, synaptic connections, and unidentified factors which render them vulnerable to environmental insults. Genomic and environmental factors interact to produce abnormal structural proteins, enzymes, and mitochondria. A disturbance in the functioning of any one of these may disrupt the other elements, with complex consequences for both the mechanical and metabolic integrity of the cell. Abnormal proteins may accumulate as a result, in the form of insoluble cytoskeletal inclusions which in turn interact with unidentified susceptibility factors, leading to cell death.

Alzheimer's disease

See Chapter 20.

Dementia with Lewy bodies

See Chapter 20.

Frontotemporal dementias

Background and clinical syndromes

The group of frontotemporal dementias (FTD) is the second most common form of primary dementia before old age and they are also evident in 3–10% of patients with late life dementia who come to post mortem. Many of this group have a clinical syndrome comprising early, prominent behavioural disturbances (disinhibition, apathy, obsessionality, hyperorality, development of a 'sweet tooth'), cognitive impairment (executive dysfunction, mutism, relatively preserved memory) and motor signs (deltoid fasciculations, extrapyramidal syndrome without resting tremor, or corticospinal involvement). Language disturbances are frequent, and verbal fluency is typically reduced. Because behavioural changes often occur early, while there is still sparing of general intellect, patients with frontotemporal dementias not infrequently present to the psychiatrist.

There are a variety of distinctive clinical syndromes, with overlapping pathological features. These include the *focal cortical atrophies* first described by Mesulam (primary progressive aphasia, primary progressive apraxia, progressive prosopagnosia), *Pick's disease, familial progressive subcortical gliosis*, and also subtypes associated with amyotrophic lateral sclerosis and parkinsonism. Three cognitive profiles – apathetic, ritualistic, and disinhibited – may correlate with the distribution of atrophy within the frontal lobes.

FTD is hereditary in a small proportion of cases and in a number of these, autosomal dominant inheritance linked to the *tau* gene on chromosome 17q21 (see below) has been established in the families. The mean age of onset in these families ranges from 40 to 65 years, but is typically in the fifth decade, with average duration of 7–10 years.

Pathology and pathophysiology

There is selective frontal and anterior temporal atrophy; hemispheric involvement may be asymmetric. Microscopic examination reveals neuropil loss, neuropil vacuolation of superficial layers of cerebral cortex, and variable gliosis of grey and white matter, most severe in frontal and temporal cortices and substantia nigra. The hippocampi are relatively preserved, and Alzheimer-type changes are absent. Neuronal loss and gliosis in the amygdala are often pronounced. Intraneuronal inclusions, with variable histochemical characteristics, are frequent and may hold an important clue to the pathogenesis of neurodegeneration in these conditions.

Functional imaging evidence supports the concept that behavioural disturbances in these (and other dementing) illnesses are mirrored by hypoactivity in frontotemporal networks, especially within the left hemisphere (Hirono *et al.* 2000).

Pick's disease

The term Pick's disease has become a source of considerable unresolved nosological confusion (Garrard and Hodges 2000). It is used both as a *clinical description*, synonymously with frontotemporal dementia and, more strictly, as a *pathological entity* characterized by circumscribed, asymmetric 'knife-blade' frontotemporal atrophy, and histologically by ballooned cells, astrocytic gliosis, and intraneuronal argyrophilic inclusions (Pick bodies) containing the proteins tau and ubiquitin.

The role of tau

Microtubule-associated proteins (MAPs) are a diverse group of cytoskeletal proteins which interact with other subcellular components. Tau is a MAP, localized to the axonal segment of peripheral and central neurons, which can organize microtubules into bundles. Aberrant forms of tau which have lost their affinity for microtubules and collect as insoluble aggregates, are present in neurofibrillary tangles and paired helical filaments in Alzheimer's disease and in a range of other neurodegenerative diseases. A mutation in the *tau* gene has been identified in a large proportion of families with a FTD phenotype linked to chromosome17, although alternative loci have been implicated in others. The study of affected families has greatly enhanced our appreciation of tau function in health and disease, and the more general role played by cytoskeletal proteins in neurological illness (see Delacourte and Buée 2000; Wolozin and Behl 2000). Disruption of tau microtubule binding may cause cell death directly, by promoting microtubule degeneration, or indirectly, via the accumulation of filaments and tangles 'choking' cell metabolism. A single copy of the *tau* gene is present in the human genome on chromosome 17q21, consisting of 15 exons of which 11 encode the major tau isoforms in the brain. The primary RNA transcript undergoes complex, regulated alternative splicing to encode the different protein isoforms, which can be detected on Western immunoblots of normal brain. Western blots reveal abnormal tau 'fingerprints' in various neuro-degenerative disorders ('tau-opathies') including Alzheimer's disease, Steele-Richardson disease, corticobasal degeneration, and Pick's disease.

Assessment

Diagnosis is based on clinical and neuropsychological assessment, together with brain imaging (MRI if available), which can demonstrate selective, often asymmetric atrophy of frontal and temporal regions. Left anterior temporal atrophy is much more frequently observed than right, for unknown reasons. Measurement of the pattern of cytoskeletal proteins in cerebrospinal fluid may aid in distinguishing FTD from Alzheimer's disease; however, this remains largely a research tool. Genetic testing is appropriate in familial forms, in consultation with a clinical genetics service.

Treatment

There is no specific therapy. Cholinesterase inhibitors may worsen behavioural disturbances and should be avoided. Good carer support is particularly important, as the consequences of the disintegration of personality in these diseases can be very distressing. Obsessional behaviours are common; practical support and the use of

distractions may ease the burden of continual supervision. Antidepressant medication is helpful if depressive symptoms are prominent. As in dementia with Lewy bodies, neuroleptics must be used with great caution, since they may exacerbate an associated extrapyramidal syndrome. See Gustafson (2000) for a review of Pick's disease and frontal lobe dementias.

Parkinson's disease

Pathophysiological mechanisms

Dementia and psychiatric disturbances are features of several diseases traditionally classified as extrapyramidal disorders: idiopathic Parkinson's disease, and other related syndromes. All produce rigidity, slowness, and impoverishment of voluntary movement, hence their designation as akinetic-rigid syndromes. All share a pathology based on the accumulation of abnormal neuronal inclusions, and dysfunction within neurotransmitter projection systems, especially those utilizing dopamine. There is primary dysfunction in frontosubcortical circuits, with a 'subcortical' clinical dementia. This account focuses on *idiopathic Parkinson's disease.*

Idiopathic Parkinson's disease is among the most common illnesses of the elderly world-wide, with an overall prevalence of approximately 1 per 1000. It results primarily from degeneration of the basal ganglia nigrostriatal pathway, the pathological hallmarks being neuronal loss and gliosis within the zona compacta of the substantia nigra and the presence of intracytoplasmic eosinophilic Lewy bodies containing the protein α-synuclein within surviving neurons in substantia nigra, brainstem nuclei, and neocortex. Neuronal loss occurs in all these areas, and the pathological demarcation from diffuse Lewy body disease (see p. 625) is ill-defined. Functionally, the fundamental defect is depletion of dopaminergic projection systems.

Clinical features

The cardinal neurological features of idiopathic Parkinson's disease are tremor at rest, rigidity, and

Table 14.9 Neuropsychiatric manifestations in idiopathic Parkinson's disease
Delirium, stupor (especially drugs, intercurrent infection)
Cognitive decline (subcortical dementia)
Depression, mania
Hallucinations (chiefly visual), illusions of presence
Delusions, psychosis
Sleep attacks, REM sleep behaviour disorder
Sexual disorders

bradykinesia. The main psychological consequences are cognitive impairment and depression (see Table 14.9).

Dementia

Estimates of the prevalence of dementia in Parkinson's disease vary widely, probably because different populations have been studied and diagnostic criteria have varied. Recent estimates using DSM-IIIR criteria are in the range 11–15% (Biggins *et al.* 1992). In a controlled longitudinal study the incidence was 19% in 54 months, higher than in the general population (Biggins *et al.* 1992). Cognitive impairment correlates with the severity of the movement disorder and disease duration of the disease.

The cognitive impairment may result from a number of mechanisms (Varma and Trimble 1997). A subcortical pattern of dementia with predominant frontal-executive impairment is most frequent (Gibb 1989; Ring 1993) but some patients have symptoms of Alzheimer-type. See Mindham (2000) for a review.

Depression

The association of Parkinson's disease with depression is well established with a prevalence of approximately 40%. It is most common in the early and in the very advanced stages of the disease. The mechanism is uncertain; depression correlates poorly with degree of disability and disease duration, and may be related to frontal lobe abnormalities and disturbed dopaminorgic mechanisms (Duffy and Coffey 1997). Antidepressants must be used with care, to avoid exacerbation of cognitive impairment or induction of delirium or organic hallucinosis (see below). Selective serotonin re-uptake blockers and newer generation agents, with less anticholinergic activity, may be preferable to tricyclics. Electroconvulsive therapy should be considered in patients with refractory symptoms.

Anxiety

Anxiety is common and usually associated with depression. Panic may occur in advanced Parkinson's disease, especially in the weaning-off phase of medication. Management may be difficult, as attempts to intensify dopaminergic therapy may lead to psychiatric side-effects.

Psychotic symptoms

Psychotic symptoms occur at some stage in 20% of patients. Visual hallucinations in clear consciousness occur in 30% (Fenelon *et al.* 2000) and are associated with increasing age, disease duration and severity, depression, cognitive impairment, reduced visual acuity, and sleep-wake cycle disruption. Delusions are less frequent and are usually paranoid in content. Antiparkinson drugs have been implicated as causes; whenever possible these should be reduced. When this results in unacceptable worsening of the physical symptoms, antipsychotic medication is necessary. Newer drugs, such as clozapine, are preferable.

Other neuropsychiatric manifestations

Excessive somnolence, a disordered sleep-wake cycle, sleep attacks, and REM sleep behaviour disorder are more common in Parkinson's disease (Arnulf *et al.* 2000). Drugs, especially dopaminergic agents such as pramipexole and ropinirole, have been linked to sleep attacks which may cause accidents when driving, and patients must be warned that they should not drive if they experience any such episodes.

Neuropsychiatric manifestations in Parkinson's disease are summarized in Table 14.9.

See Marsh (2000) for a review.

Huntington's disease

This disease has a worldwide distribution, with estimated prevalence 4–7 per 100 000 (Oliver 1970). Onset is typically in middle life, with relentless progression of cognitive and behavioural decline in most cases. The tell-tale choreiform movements may be subtle, taking the form of excessive, purposeless 'fidgeting' which the patient may attempt to disguise.

The disease may present to the psychiatrist, since these patients commonly become depressed early in the course while insight is retained, and later often become withdrawn, 'eccentric', and socially isolated. The onset may be difficult to determine, as patients may disguise symptoms or there may have been long-standing personality and behavioural problems arising from an upbringing disturbed by the effects of the disease in a parent. A high rate of bipolar disorder has also been reported (Peyser and Folstein 1993). The clinical features of depression are similar to those of major depression, and both biological and reactive components probably contribute (Dufy and Coffey 1997). Paranoid symptoms are common and schizophrenia may occur more frequently than in the general population. Cognitive impairment with subcortical features is usual in the later stages, but its severity and progress vary widely. Distractibility is characteristic, with reduced ability to regulate attention and psychomotor speed (Rothlind et al. 1993), and apathy later in the course. A gaze apraxia and inability to sustain tongue protrusion ('serpentine tongue') are typically found. The pathological changes mainly affect the frontal lobes and the caudate nucleus. Neuronal loss, which is most marked in the frontal lobes, is accompanied by gliosis; polyglutamine nuclear inclusions are present.

Huntington's disease is inherited in autosomal dominant fashion, penetrance is complete, and new mutations are very rare; most apparently sporadic cases reflect an incomplete family history or lack of knowledge of true paternity. The gene on chromosome 4p encodes a protein, huntingtin, of unknown function. The pathogenic mechanism by which the mutation causes disease remains unknown. Decreased concentrations of the neuro-inhibitory transmitter gamma-aminobutyric acid (GABA) in the caudate nucleus, and increased dopaminorgic activity, have been described.

Diagnostic and predictive genetic testing for the causative mutation, an expanded DNA 'triplet repeat' coding for glutamine (Huntington's Disease Collaborative Research Group 1993), is now widely available. Because of the devastating implications for sufferer and descendants, expert genetic counselling is required before and after mutation analysis.

There is no specific therapy; dopaminergic blockade may occasionally be required to suppress severe chorea if it is producing exhaustion or limiting mobility. Antidepressants are useful for major depressive symptoms.

See Rosenblatt and Leroi (2000) and Folstein (2000) for reviews of the psychiatric aspects of Huntingdon's disease.

Cerebrovascular syndromes

Vascular dementia

See Chapter 20.

Stroke

Cognitive deficits

The nature and degree of cognitive impairment depend crucially on the site and size of the vascular event. A particular pattern of cognitive impairment (for example, dysphasia) may result from strokes in diverse locations; conversely, a single strategically located stroke (for example, in the dominant middle cerebral artery territory) may impair multiple cognitive domains. Deficits of higher cortical function such as dysphasia, anosognosia, and dyspraxia may handicap the patient to a degree that is often underestimated. Successive strokes may lead to the stepwise accumulation of deficits: vascular dementia (see p. 625). If small perforating vessels are predominantly affected, the presentation may take the form of a diffuse, sub-cortical dementia (so-called 'Binswanger's disease'), without any history of a symptomatic acute stroke

Personality change

Irritability, apathy, lability of mood, and occasion-ally aggressiveness may occur. Inflexibility in coping with problems is common and may be seen in extreme form as a *catastrophic reaction*. Such changes are probably due more to associated wide-spread arteriosclerotic vascular disease than to a single stroke; they may continue to worsen even though the focal signs of a stroke are improving. When a person has had a stroke, the family is likely to complain mainly of the subsequent personality change. Impersistence, a physical sign of frontal lobe damage, is commonly misinterpreted as perversity and uncooperativeness.

Mood disorder

Depressed mood is common after stroke (House *et al.* 1991) and may contribute to the apparent intellectual impairment or impede rehabilitation. Estimates of prevalence range from 12 to 64%. Undoubtedly its development is influenced by the premorbid psychological and social factors demon-strated for all mood disorder (Sharpe *et al.* 1994). There has been much controversy about the suggestion that the risk of depression is deter-mined by the location of the lesion (see Starkstein and Robinson 1993). A systematic review has not supported this hypothesis (Carson *et al.* 2000).

Treatment of depression depends in part on active rehabilitation. A trial of an antidepressant is usually indicated, but the drug should be given cautiously as side-effects are frequent in these patients.

Post-stroke *anxiety* and (less commonly) *mania* may also have an organic basis; however, there are no consistent anatomical associations. The variable neuroanatomical substrate of post-stroke mood disorders may reflect disruption of distributed neural networks and neurotransmitter projection

systems mediating emotion (Duffy and Coffey 1997). Patients who have suffered strokes have a significantly increased risk of suicide (Stenager *et al.* 1998).

Emotionalism

Abnormal emotionalism (pathological affect) sometimes develops after stroke (House *et al.* 1989). Odd mixtures of spontaneous laughter and crying may occur, the emotional display frequently at odds with the patient's mood. Both tricyclic and SSRI antidepressants are helpful, perhaps by compensating for serotonergic dysfunction.

Subdural haematoma

Subdural haematoma is not uncommon after falls in elderly patients, and especially those associated with alcoholism. A history of head trauma is commonly lacking. Acute haematomas may cause coma or fluctuating impairment of consciousness, and are often associated with hemiparesis and oculomotor signs. The psychiatrist is more likely to see the chronic syndromes, in which patients present with headache, poor concentration, vague physical complaints, and fluctuating conscious-ness, but often few localizing neurological signs. It is particularly important to consider this possi-bility as a cause for accelerated deterioration in patients with a neurodegenerative dementia. Treatment is by surgical evacuation, which may reverse the symptoms.

Prion diseases

The prion diseases are a group of neurodegenerative conditions, characterized by diffuse spongiosis, neuronal loss, gliosis and amyloid deposition, which can be transferred between individuals, hence their designation as *transmissible spongiform encephalopathies*. Human prion diseases occur in sporadic, acquired (often iatrogenic), and inherited forms. Creutzfeldt–Jakob disease (CJD) is the most common and important, with an approximate inci-dence of one case per million in populations world-wide. Sporadic disease accounts for approximately 90% of cases. Kuru, described in the Fore linguistic group of New Guinea highlanders, was transmitted by ritual cannibalism; the disease has largely disappeared since this practice was abolished in the 1950s, although occasional new cases may suggest a very long presymptomatic phase. The inherited prion diseases include familial CJD, fatal familial insomnia, Gerstmann– Sträussler–Scheinker syndrome, and atypical Alzheimer-like illnesses. All have autosomal dominant inheritance.

Sporadic CJD affects both sexes equally and typically between 60–65 years. It is usually heralded by cognitive decline (often memory impairment), which may be accompanied by prominent behavioural abnormalities or personality change, prompting initial referral to a psychiatrist. Visual symptoms, extrapyramidal, pyramidal, and cerebellar signs, and involuntary movements are all frequent. Seizures are frequent later in the course. There is usually a relentless progression to death, often within 6 months, but occasional patients have a more protracted illness (up to several years).

The name 'prion' denotes proteinaceous infectious particles. Deposits in the brain of the abnormal fibrillar prion glycoprotein, PrP, can be detected using special stains. The prion protein is encoded by a gene on chromosome 20, designated *PRNP*. Different PrP conformations and glycosylation patterns give rise to various strains, which show species specificity. The paradigm disorder is scrapie, a disease of sheep and goats, in which experimental transfer between animals was first demonstrated in 1938. Analogues of scrapie exist in a number of other species, including cattle, mink, and cats.

Prion diseases share a unique pathogenetic mechanism, based on the aggregation in affected brains of a conformational isomer (PrP^{Sc}) of the native prion protein, PrP^C. Sporadic disease is assumed to result from rare spontaneous conversions of PrP^C to PrP^{Sc}, whereas the inherited prion diseases arise from mutations in the *PRNP* gene. The PrP^{Sc} isomer accumulates as amyloid fibrils (molecularly distinct from the β amyloid of Alzheimer's disease), due to its relative insolubility, resistance to digestion by proteases, and propensity to self-aggregate. The mechanisms by which this accumulation leads to cell death remain unclear. CJD has been transmitted to experimental animals, and there are approximately 200 well-documented iatrogenic cases in which the disease has been transmitted to humans by neurosurgical procedures, dural and corneal grafts, and pooled donor pituitary extract prior to the advent of recombinant human growth hormone. Susceptibility to acquired and sporadic disease is determined by a common polymorphism (valine or methionine) at residue 129 of the PrP gene, heterozygotes being relatively protected against development of disease.

Variant Creutzfeldt–Jakob disease

Intense interest in the human prion diseases has resulted from the description of variant Creutzfeldt–Jakob disease (vCJD), first identified in the UK in 1996. This is linked with bovine spongiform encephalopathy (BSE), epidemic in Britain at that time. A number of lines of evidence indicate that BSE and vCJD are caused by the same prion strain. The full public health implications are still uncertain. By analogy with other prion diseases, it is probable that new cases of vCJD will continue to appear for some years to come. All patients so far have been homozygous for methionine at codon 129 of the PrP gene (compared with 37% of controls and 80% of patients with sporadic CJD), and no mutation has been identified. See Collinge (2000) for a review of prion diseases.

Other intracranial infections

Many intracranial infections cause cognitive impairment, and effective treatment is available for the majority. HIV infection is considered in Chapter 16. Unusual infections should always be considered as a cause of otherwise unexplained cognitive and psychiatric symptoms.

Neurosyphilis

Neurosyphilis, a manifestation of the tertiary stage of infection, is now rare in Western countries; however, increasing numbers of cases have been reported in association with HIV. An asymptomatic (latent) stage precedes clinical disease with variable latency. Of every 12 patients with symptomatic neurosyphilis, approximately five have general paresis, four have meningovascular syphilis, and three have tabes dorsalis. Parenchymal syphilis or 'general paralysis of the insane' (GPI) is of most interest to psychiatry, since discovery of its cause was an important landmark in the history of the subject, stimulating a search for organic causes of other psychiatric syndromes. See Hare (1959) for a historical review.

Encephalitis

Encephalitis may occur with primary (generally viral) infection of the brain parenchyma, or as a complication of bacterial meningitis, septicaemia, or a brain abscess (cerebritis). A great many viral causes have been identified, of which *herpes simplex* is the most common and important in the UK. Effective treatment (intravenous acyclovir) is available. The sequelae of the untreated disease may be devastating. In the acute stage, headache, vomiting, and impaired consciousness are usual, and seizures are common. Presentation may be with delirium. The psychiatrist may be involved in initial diagnosis but is more likely to see chronic complications which may include prolonged anxiety and depression, a profound amnestic syndrome, personality change, or temporal lobe epilepsy.

Other significant encephalitides in adults include those produced by arthropod-borne viruses (including Japanese B and Murray Valley) and (especially in the immunocompromised) varicella zoster, which, in addition, rarely causes an angiitis with focal neurological signs.

Encephalitis lethargica (Von Economo's)

A small outbreak of encephalitis lethargica was first reported in 1917 by Von Economo at the Vienna Psychiatric Clinic (Von Economo 1929). The condition attained epidemic proportions in the 1920s. By the 1930s, it had largely disappeared, although rare sporadic cases do still occur. It probably represents a common pathological response to a variety of (presumably viral) agents. Parkinsonism is a disabling complication; another is personality change with antisocial behaviour. Some patients develop a clinical state resembling schizophrenia. Sacks (1973) has given a vivid description of such cases, and the striking but temporary 'awakening' brought about in some by L-dopa.

Brain tumours

Many brain tumours cause psychological symptoms at some stage in their course, and a significant proportion present with such symptoms. Psychiatrists are likely to see patients with slow-growing tumours in 'silent' (especially frontal) areas which produce psychological effects, but few neurological signs, for example, subfrontal meningioma or butterfly glioma of the corpus callosum. The nature of psychological symptoms is influenced by the global effects of raised intracranial pressure, in addition to tumour location. The rate of tumour growth is also important; rapidly expanding tumours with raised intracranial pressure can present as delirium, whereas less aggressive tumours are more likely to cause chronic cognitive deficits. Focal lesions give rise to a variety of specific neuropsychiatric syndromes; those near the frontal poles typically manifest initially as a subtle personality change. The possibility of such an aetiology justifies brain imaging in patients with a first presentation of atypical cognitive or affective symptoms. See Ron (1989) for a review.

Cancer

The cognitive complications of *cancer* are classified in Table 14.10.

Table 14.10 Some causes of cognitive decline in patients with cancer

Mass effects
Primary and metastatic brain tumours

Haemorrhagic change (especially melanoma, renal cell carcinoma, choriocarcinoma)

Diffuse infiltration
Gliomatosis cerebri

Carcinomatous and lymphomatous meningitis

En plaque meningioma

Paraneoplastic limbic encephalitis

Metabolic derangements
Hypercalcaemia

Hyponatraemia

Acidosis

Hypoglycaemia

Radiotherapy
Acute and subacute radionecrosis

Radiation thromboangiopathy

Accelerated cerebral atherosclerosis

Radiation leucodystrophy

Second malignancies (especially glioma, meningioma)

Chemotherapy
Metabolic encephalopathies

Opportunistic infections secondary to immunosuppression (herpes zoster, progressive multifocal leucoencephalopathy)

Multiple sclerosis

Multiple sclerosis is the most common cause of chronic neurological disability in young adults in developed countries, and commonly imposes a heavy burden on families and carers in its later stages. Its consequences for work and relationships may be profound. The disease may be difficult to diagnose early in the course, and physical symptoms are sometimes misinterpreted as psychiatric. Psychological symptoms are rarely the presenting feature but two-thirds of patients will experience such symptoms at some stage, and in a third of cases they are severe enough to meet the criteria for major depression. Euphoria occurs in approximately 10%, usually in those with the most severe cognitive impairment, and accompanied by other frontal signs. Fatigue is also a prominent symptom; it may be physically or emotionally based. Emotional lability is frequent. There is a sevenfold increase in the risk of suicide (Stenager *et al.* 1992).

Depression is more common in multiple sclerosis than in other disabling illnesses, with a lifetime risk of the order of 50% (Ron and Logsdail 1989). It does not appear to be closely related to the severity of the clinical syndrome or the site of lesions; nevertheless, biological factors may play a role. Standard antidepressant medication is usually effective.

Cognitive impairment may be an early manifestation of the illness, and occasionally a rapidly progressive dementia occurs. In most cases, however, intellectual deterioration is less severe and progresses slowly. Older males with primary progressive multiple sclerosis are the subgroup most likely to present with dementia. Cognitive impairment is present in 40% of patients from community samples; it is common late in the disease (approximately 50–60% of clinic attenders). It correlates with total lesion load and degree of callosal atrophy on MRI (Varma and Trimble 1997) and probably reflects axonal loss rather than demyelination per se. In the early stages, well-practised verbal skills are often preserved despite deficits in problem solving, abstraction, memory, and learning. See Ron (2000) for a review of psychiatric aspects of multiple sclerosis.

Normal pressure hydrocephalus

In this variety of hydrocephalus, there may be block to cerebrospinal fluid flow within the ventricular system due to non-tumoral aqueduct stenosis, or in the subarachnoid space; however, the precise pathogenesis of the clinical syndrome remains obscure.

Ventricular pressure is generally normal or low (though episodes of raised pressure may occur). The characteristic clinical triad comprises an early, striking 'gait apraxia' (a broad-based, small-stepped gait with difficulty in initiation) on which supervene a progressive frontal subcortical syndrome with bradyphrenia and, later, urinary incontinence. Ventricular enlargement out of proportion to the degree of cortical atrophy, often with periventricular signal change, is the hallmark finding on brain imaging. The prevalence is uncertain, ranging from 0 to 6% of cases of late-life dementia in published series. The condition is more common in the elderly, but sometimes occurs in middle life. Often, no cause for the obstruction can be discovered although there may be a history of subarachnoid haemorrhage, head injury, or meningitis. It is most important to differentiate this condition from the degenerative dementias, or depression with mental slowness. Cases with a short history and prominent gait disturbance with relative sparing of intellect may be amenable to a neurosurgical shunt procedure to improve the circulation of cerebrospinal fluid; however, the outcome is variable and difficult to predict. The presence of hippocampal atrophy on imaging suggests associated Alzheimer's disease and predicts a poor response to shunting.

Head injury

Most head injuries do not have serious long-term consequences. The psychiatrist is likely to see two main groups of patients who have suffered a head injury:

- a small number of patients with serious, permanent cognitive sequelae;
- a larger group with emotional symptoms and personality change.

The latter, though less conspicuous, are often disabling. Improved care of severe injuries has led to increasing numbers of young, otherwise physically fit people surviving with severe, chronic neurological and psychiatric disability. See National Institutes of Health Consensus Development Panel (1999) for a review.

Concussive head injury disrupts cholinergic transmission in animals and a similar mechanism may be relevant in dementia pugilistica and other forms of head injury in humans. There is a well-established association between head trauma and subsequent development of Alzheimer's disease (Guo *et al.* 2000), the risk correlating with the severity of the injury. Formation of amyloid precursor protein may be induced by neuronal stress, and a substantial proportion of those surviving severe head injury have diffuse plaques containing βA4 protein; a similar observation has been made in dementia pugilistica (see below). The factors governing susceptibility remain unknown; however, apolipoprotein E (APOE) ε 4 may play a role (Jordan 2000).

Acute psychological effects

Impairment of consciousness occurs after all but the mildest closed injuries, but is less common after penetrating injuries. On recovery of consciousness, defects of memory are usually apparent. Even apparently 'minor' head injuries can cause brain damage acutely (Kushner 1998). Diffuse shear caused by rotational forces (Kelly 2000) may give rise to both structural and metabolic axonal damage.

After severe injury there is often a prolonged phase of delirium, with disordered behaviour, anxiety, and mood disturbance. The duration of post-traumatic amnesia correlates closely with neurological complications, persistent deficits in memory, psychiatric disability, generalized intellectual impairment, and personality change. Conversely, the period of retrograde amnesia is not a good predictor of outcome.

Chronic psychological effects

Both primary and secondary damage (the effects of brain swelling and raised intracranial pressure) determine the neurological and cognitive deficits. Long-term outcome is also importantly influenced by premorbid personality traits, occupational attainment, availability of social supports, and compensation issues. Post-traumatic epilepsy may be a further significant complicating factor in more serious injuries. The risk of suicide is increased after head injury.

Post-concussional syndrome

After head injury, many patients describe a group of symptoms known as the post-concussional syndrome. The main features are anxiety, depression, and irritability, accompanied by headache, dizziness, fatigue, poor concentration, and insomnia. The duration and severity of these symptoms are highly variable. Since this syndrome often occurs after mild head injury, it has been suggested that it is psychologically based. It is probable (Lishman 1988) that 'there is . . . an interplay of factors in the genesis of post-concussional syndrome with an intertwining of organic and nonorganic contributions' (see also Jacobson 1995). Most cases do, however, eventually resolve without specific medical intervention.

Lasting cognitive impairment

Although head injuries accompanied only by transient loss of consciousness can cause diffuse brain damage and cognitive impairment, injuries followed by post-traumatic amnesia of more than 24 hours are more likely to give rise to persisting cognitive impairment, which is proportional to their severity. In penetrating injuries, there may be focal cognitive deficits, but some evidence of more widespread impairment is usually found. Lishman (1968) found that the amount of tissue destruction was related both to intellectual impairment and to 'organic' psychological symptoms such as apathy, euphoria, poor judgement, and disinhibition 1–5 years later. Cognitive impairment was particularly associated with parietal and temporal damage (especially left-sided).

Personality change

Personality change is common after severe injuries, particularly if there is frontal lobe damage, when there may be irritability, apathy, loss of spontaneity and drive, disinhibition and occasionally reduced control of aggressive impulses. Management is difficult, demanding heavy social support and, in some cases, prolonged neuro-rehabilitation.

Emotional disorder

Depression and anxiety are very common after brain damage. Persistent depression and anxiety occur in about a quarter of cases, a frequency similar to that in other serious physical disorders. Antidepressant medication is often useful. Organic mania has also been reported (Jorge *et al.* 1993).

Schizophrenia-like syndromes

Delusions are not uncommon after recovery from prolonged unconsciousness. It is difficult to draw firm conclusions about the incidence of schizophrenia-like syndromes after head injury; however, Davison and Bagley (1969) concluded that this was well above chance. The pathogenesis is uncertain. See Fann (1997) for a review of the psychiatric consequences of head injury. See Wrightson and Gronwall (1999) for a guide to management of mild head injury.

Boxing and head injury

For many years, the significance of 'punch-drunk' states in boxers has been disputed. The numerous published reports of 'punch-drunk' syndrome (dementia pugilistica) typically lack adequate controls. In a study of a random sample of 224 retired professional boxers (Roberts 1969), 37 had a characteristic syndrome related to the cumulative extent of head injuries over the course of a career.

The syndrome typically develops and progresses after retirement from the ring, and appears to interact with the effects of age. The principal early features are executive dysfunction, bradyphrenia, mild dysarthria and incoordination, followed by parkinsonism, spasticity, and ataxia. The fully developed syndrome may comprise cerebellar, pyramidal, and extrapyramidal features, mixed cortical and subcortical cognitive deficits, and a variety of behavioural manifestations.

Radiological findings are typically non-specific; however, diffuse cerebral atrophy and a cavum septum pellucidum may be evident. At post-mortem examination, there is loss of neurons in cortex and substantia nigra with widespread neurofibrillary tangles (Corsellis *et al.* 1973), and scarring of cerebellar folia with Purkinje cell drop-out. Diffuse neuritic plaques containing βA4 amyloid protein, believed to be a key precursor to Alzheimer's disease, are present.

Concussive head injury disrupts cholinergic transmission in animals, and a similar mechanism may be relevant in dementia pugilistica and other forms of head injury in humans (Jordan 2000).

There is a well established association between head trauma and subsequent development of Alzheimer's disease (Guo *et al* 2000), the risk correlating with the severity of the injury. Formation of amyloid precursor protein may be induced by neuronal stress, and a substantial proportion of those surviving severe head injury have diffuse plaques containing βA4 protein; a similar observation has been made in dementia pugilistica. The factors governing susceptibility remain unknown, however APOE ε 4 may play a role (Jordan 2000).

Treatment

Long-term treatment plans should be made as early as possible after head injury. Prospective studies demonstrate that early assessment of the extent of neurological signs provides a useful guide to the likely pattern of long-term physical disability. Neuropsychiatric problems should be assessed and their impact anticipated, and a comprehensive social assessment is crucial. The clinical psychologist can sometimes contribute behavioural and cognitive techniques (see Wilson 2000). Practical support is needed for family and carers. Issues of compensation and litigation should be settled as quickly as possible. See National Institutes of Health Consensus Development Panel (1999) for a review of the management of head injury and Fleminger (2000) for a review of the neuropsychiatry of head injury.

Dystonias

Focal dystonias are uncontrolled muscle spasms leading to involuntary movements of the eyelids, face, neck, jaw, shoulders, larynx, hands, and, rarely, other part of the body. They are uncommon but disabling.

The *aetiology* is uncertain. In the past, dystonias were regarded as conversion phenomena; now there is evidence that they are idiopathic or drug-induced neurological disorders, and that psychogenic cases are rare. However, psychiatric factors may exacerbate symptoms and disability.

Clinical types include blepharospasm, torticollis, writer's cramp, and laryngeal dystonia. The most effective treatment is the injection of botulinum toxin directly into the affected muscles.

Psychiatric symptoms secondary to the physical disorder can usually be treated with antidepressants or behavioural therapy.

Occupational dystonia

Muscular problems are common amongst musicians and may threaten to end their careers. There are many causes, including overuse injury, pressure on peripheral nerves, and focal dystonias. These problems should be assessed by a physician with experience in this special field. Performance anxiety is also frequent, and may impair or prevent performance. β-Blockers alleviate this symptom and are used by many musicians, sometimes without medical supervision. Anxiety management is effective in some cases. Other occupations and activities also have their characteristic afflictions, for example 'auctioneer's jaw' and 'golfer's hip'. See Frucht (1999) for a review.

Tics

Tics are purposeless, stereotyped, and repetitive jerking movements occurring most commonly in the face and neck. They are much more common in childhood than in adult life, though a few cases begin at ages of up to 40 years. The peak of onset is about 7 years, and the onset is often at a time of emotional disturbance. They are especially common in boys. Most sufferers have just one kind of abnormal movement, but a few people have more than one (multiple tics). Like almost all involuntary movements, tics are worsened by anxiety. They can be controlled briefly by voluntary effort, but this results in an increasing unpleasant feeling of tension. Many tics occurring in childhood last only a few weeks; others last longer but 80–90% of cases improve within 5 years. A few cases become chronic. The subject of tics has been reviewed by Lees (1988).

Gilles de la Tourette syndrome

This condition was described first by Itard in 1825 and subsequently by Gilles de la Tourette in 1885. The main clinical features are *multiple tics* beginning before the age of 16, together with *vocal tics* (grunting, snarling, and similar ejaculations). About a third of the people affected show *coprolalia* (involuntary uttering of obscenities), but few of these are children. Between 10 and 40% show *echolalia* or *echopraxia*. There may be stereotyped movements such as jumping and dancing. The tics are often preceded by *premonitory sensations*. Associated features include overactivity, difficulties in learning, emotional disturbances, and social problems.

Obsessive–compulsive symptoms occur frequently in patients with the Gilles de la Tourette syndrome, and more often among the families of these patients than in the general population. Attention-deficit hyperactivity disorder has also been reported to be more frequent in these patients than in the general population.

The reported *prevalence* of the condition varies according to the criteria for diagnosis and method of enquiry. A generally accepted figure is about 0.5 per 1000 population. The disorder is three to four times more common in males than in females and about ten times more prevalent in children and adolescents than in adults.

The *aetiology* of the Gilles de la Tourette syndrome is uncertain. A *neurochemical disorder* has been suggested, possibly of dopamine function since dopamine-blocking drugs produce improvements. Post-mortem studies suggest decreased 5-hydroxytryptamine and glutamate in several areas of the basic ganglia.

Family genetic studies, including segregation analysis studies, strongly suggest a *genetic basis for the disorder*. The concordance rate in monozygotic twins is reported to be 53% compared with 8% for dizygotic twins. Multiple tics without vocal tics are more frequent in the families of probands with Gilles de la Tourette syndrome than in the general population, suggesting that the two conditions are related.

Treatment

Mild cases may not require specific treatment. Many treatments have been tried. Haloperidol appears to be the most effective, but the side-effects can be troublesome. Treatment of co-morbid psychiatric disorder, such as obsessive–compulsive disorder and attention-deficit hyperactivity disorder, may be clinically more important than treatment of the core features of the syndrome. Selective serotonin re-uptake inhibitors (SSRIs) have been reported to control the obsessional symptoms of the patients as they do in obsessive–compulsive disorder (see p. 247). There is not enough follow-up information to indicate the prognosis, but clinical experience suggests that although two-thirds of patients can expect improvement or lasting remission in early adult life, the outcome is frequently poor. Coprolalia disappears in one-third of patients, but the tics and obsessive–compulsive symptoms may be lifelong. For reviews of the syndrome see Robertson (2000) and Ron (2000).

Carbon monoxide poisoning

Carbon monoxide poisoning usually arises from deliberate self-harm by car exhaust fumes. After poisoning, the course is variable. Milder cases recover over days or weeks. Recovery of consciousness is often followed by an organic psychiatric syndrome; this clears up, leaving an amnestic syndrome which in turn gradually improves. Extrapyramidal and other neurological signs occur at an early stage and then resolve. In more severe cases there is a characteristic period of partial recovery, followed by relapse with a return of an acute organic syndrome and extrapyramidal symptoms. Occasionally, death occurs at this stage. Some patients are left with permanent extrapyramidal symptoms or become demented.

The frequency of these complications is uncertain. Shillito *et al.* (1936) surveyed 21 000 cases of carbon monoxide poisoning in New York City and found few lasting problems. By contrast, Smith and Brandon (1973) made a detailed study of 206 cases from a defined area. They followed-up 74 patients for an average of 3 years: eight patients had sustained gross neurological damage; eight patients had died; of those alive at follow-up, eight had improved, 21 had shown personality deterioration, and 27 reported memory impairment. See Ernst and Zibrak (1998) for a review of all aspects of carbon monoxide poisoning.

Epilepsy

Epilepsy may be defined as tendency to recurrent seizures, a seizure consisting of a paroxysmal electrical discharge in the brain and its clinical sequelae. It is crucial to distinguish the tendency to recurrent seizures, which defines epilepsy, from isolated seizures which may be provoked by drugs, sleep deprivation, hypoglycaemia, intercurrent illnesses, syncope (especially if the person is held upright), or other factors. The psychiatrist is likely to meet four kinds of problem in relation to epilepsy:

- differential diagnosis of episodic disturbances of behaviour (particularly 'atypical' attacks, aggressive behaviour, and sleep problems);
- the treatment of the psychiatric and social complications of epilepsy;
- the treatment of epilepsy itself;
- the psychological side-effects of anticonvulsant drugs.

Types of seizures

The International League Against Epilepsy proposed a classification of seizures (Gastaut 1969), which has since been revised (Dreifuss *et al.* 1981). A simplified outline is shown in Table 14.11. The principal distinction is between *partial* (focal onset) and *generalized* seizures. Since partial seizures may

Table 14.11 **Classification of seizures**
Partial seizures or seizures beginning focally
Simple motor or sensory (without impaired consciousness)
Complex partial (with impaired consciousness)
Partial seizures with secondary generalization
Generalized seizures without focal onset
Tonic-clonic
Myoclonic
Atonic
Absence
Unclassified

become generalized, an accurate description of the onset is essential. It is also necessary to distinguish between types of epilepsy and types of seizure. Traditional terms such as 'petit mal' and 'grand mal' are ambiguous, and are best avoided. It should be remembered that an 'aura' is in fact a partial seizure; most so-called 'absences' are actually complex partial seizures (often of temporal lobe origin), implying a focal rather than generalized disturbance, as in true absences.

A brief clinical description of the more common seizure types follows.

Simple partial seizures

The content depends upon the site of the focus. They include Jacksonian motor seizures and a variety of sensory seizures in which the phenomena are relatively unformed. Awareness is not impaired, unless secondary generalization occurs. Focal neurological or cognitive dysfunction may persist for a variable period following the seizure.

Complex partial seizures

These are characterized by altered awareness of self and environment. Consciousness is retained, unless secondary generalization occurs. Patients often have great difficulty in describing their experiences. The seizures arise most commonly in the

Table 14.12 Clinical features of complex partial seizures

Domain	Features
Consciousness	Altered
Autonomic and visceral	'Epigastric aura', dizziness, flushing, tachycardia, and other bodily sensations
Perceptual	Distorted perceptions, *déjà vu*, *jamais vu*, visual, auditory, olfactory, gustatory, somatic hallucinations
Cognitive	Disturbances of speech, thought, and memory, derealization, depersonalization
Affective	Fear and anxiety; occasionally, euphoric or ecstatic states
Psychomotor	Automatisms, grimacing and other bodily movements; repetitive or more complex stereotyped behaviours

temporal lobe. However 'temporal lobe epilepsy' should not be used synonymously with complex partial seizure. Those originating in the frontal lobe are particularly likely to be misdiagnosed as functional, since they are frequently accompanied by bizarre posturing and other semi-purposeful, complex motor behaviours. Complex partial seizures of temporal lobe origin are often heralded by an *aura*, which may take the form of olfactory, gustatory, auditory, visual, or somatic hallucinations. Particularly common is the 'epigastric aura', a sensation of churning in the stomach which rises toward the neck. The patient may also experience odd disturbances of thought or emotion, including an intense sense of familarity (*déjà vu*) or unfamiliarity (*jamais vu*), depersonalization or derealization, or, rarely, vivid hallucinations of past experiences ('experiential phenomena'). The clinical features of complex partial seizures are summarized in Table 14.12. The sequence of events in the seizure tends to be stereotyped in the individual

patient, an important diagnostic aid. The whole ictal phase usually lasts up to 1–2 minutes. During this period, the subject appears out of touch with the surroundings, and may show automatisms or dystonic posturing of a limb. After recovery, only the aura may be recalled. Non-convulsive status epilepticus may take the form of a prolonged single seizure, or a rapid succession of brief seizures. In such cases, a protracted period of automatic behaviour may be mistaken for a dissociative fugue or other psychiatric disorder.

Absences

The *true* absence attack starts suddenly, without an aura, lasts for seconds, and ends abruptly. Loss of awareness is a cardinal feature. There are no post-ictal abnormalities, and simple automatisms (such as eyelid fluttering) often accompany the attack. For purposes of diagnosis and treatment, it is essential to distinguish between typical absence seizures and complex partial seizures. The latter last longer, recovery occurs more slowly, there may be complex automatisms during the episode, and the patient may subsequently recall an aura. An EEG will often aid the distinction.

Generalized tonic-clonic seizures

This is the familiar epileptic convulsion with a sudden onset, tonic and clonic phases, and a succeeding period of variable duration (up to many hours) in which the patient is unrousable, sleeping, confused, or disorientated. Incontinence, tongue-biting, or other injuries may occur. Generalized tonic-clonic seizures may be initiated by a partial seizure, implying localized brain disease, often overlooked. This is an issue of fundamental importance, since primary and secondary generalized seizures have quite different significance and management.

Myoclonic, atonic, and other seizure types

There are several types of seizures with predominantly motor symptoms, including myoclonic jerks and drop attacks with loss of postural tone. They are unlikely to present to the psychiatrist.

Epidemiology

Population surveys show that epilepsy is usually of short duration and only becomes a chronic and potentially handicapping condition in about a fifth of subjects. This means that regular attenders at specialist clinics are a minority of all those with epilepsy who are especially likely to suffer from medical and social complications related to epilepsy. In the UK, general practice data indicate the prevalence of epilepsy is at least 4–6 per 1000. The inception rate is highest in early childhood, and there are further peaks in adolescence and over the age of 65. Childhood epilepsies are more often associated with significant cognitive impairment. The high prevalence in prison populations is discussed on p. 905.

Aetiology

Age at onset is an important clue to aetiology. For example, in the newborn, birth injury, congenital malformations, metabolic disorders, and infections are common causes. Many cases of childhood-onset epilepsy are genetically determined. In adults, identifiable causes include cerebrovascular disease, brain tumours, head injury, and neurodegenerative disorders. Patterns of alcohol and other drug use should always be established, particularly in young adults. Although advances in neuroimaging increasingly permit identification of structural anomalies, no specific cause is found in up to three-quarters of patients with epilepsy.

Seizure threshold may be lowered by drug therapy, including neuroleptics and tricyclic antidepressants. Sudden withdrawal of substantial doses of any drug with anticonvulsant properties, most commonly diazepam and alcohol, is likely to precipitate seizures and not infrequently, status epilepticus.

Making the diagnosis

Epilepsy is essentially a clinical diagnosis which depends upon detailed accounts of the attacks given by witnesses as well as by the patient. The background history, physical examination, and special investigations are directed to establishing aetiology. The extent of investigation is guided by the initial findings, the type of attack, and the patient's age. Only an outline can be given here; for a full account the reader is referred to textbooks, for instance Hopkins *et al.* (1995). An EEG can confirm but cannot exclude the diagnosis of epilepsy. It is more useful in determining the type of epilepsy and site of origin. The standard recording may be supplemented by sleep recording, ambulatory monitoring, and split-screen video (telemetry) techniques.

Epilepsy is often erroneously diagnosed as the cause of paroxysmal neurological and psychiatric symptoms, and it is important to keep in mind the extensive differential diagnosis (see Table 14.6). A clear description of the circumstances surrounding the episode and the mode of onset is fundamental. The most important differential diagnosis of generalized seizures are vasovagal syncope (commonly associated with involuntary movements, a fact not always appreciated) and cardiac arrhythmias. Hyperventilation (of which the patient is often unaware) and panic attacks frequently produce symptoms similar to complex partial seizures, and may lead to actual loss of consciousness if prolonged. Sudden changes in motor activity, affect, and cognition can occur in schizophrenia.

Factors that together suggest a seizure include abrupt onset, a stereotyped course lasting many seconds to a few minutes, tongue-biting, urinary incontinence, cyanosis, sustaining injury during the attack, and prolonged post-ictal drowsiness or confusion; however, none alone is necessary or sufficient to make the diagnosis. Epilepsy is often considered in the diagnosis of aggressive outbursts; however, true ictal aggression is very rare. Some forms of frontal lobe epilepsy are particularly likely to be misdiagnosed as psychogenic. If the diagnosis remains uncertain, and attacks are frequent, close observation in hospital, including video recording and EEG telemetry and ambulatory monitoring, may be worthwhile.

Non-epileptic attacks ('pseudoseizures') and dissociative states can be very difficult to distinguish; indeed, up to 50% of patients referred to epilepsy services have non-epileptic attacks exclusively or in combination (Brown and Trimble 2000). A detailed description and careful history of the background of the attacks are crucial. Features that suggest non-epileptic episodes include identifiable psychosocial precipitants, a past history of physical or sexual abuse, a personal or family history of psychopathology, an unusual or variable pattern of attacks, occurrence only in public or while alone, and absence of autonomic signs or change in colour during 'generalized' attacks. The patient may be suggestible, or betray other evidence of retained awareness during the episode. Complex, purposeful behaviour is more often seen in dissociative states. Ambulatory EEG may be helpful; however, some types of seizure may not be reflected in the surface EEG and conversely, EEG abnormalities occur in perhaps 3% of healthy individuals. Post-ictal serum prolactin is useful in a minority of cases but should not be relied upon to make the distinction. See Fenton (1986), Lowman and Richardson (1987) and Brown and Trimble (2000) for reviews of the distinction between epilepsy and psychiatric disorder.

Social aspects of epilepsy

The consequences for quality of life correlate with the severity of the seizure disorder and the presence of structural brain pathology. The social implications and stigma attached to a diagnosis of epilepsy can be far-reaching. In counselling patients and their families, it is important to be sensitive to these issues and to allay groundless fears and misconceptions. Restrictions on driving are a major burden for many patients, whose livelihood may be at stake. To obtain a British driving licence, the patient must have had at least 1 year with no seizures while awake, whether or not he is still taking antiepileptic drugs. Those who suffer seizures only while asleep may hold a licence if this pattern has been stable for at least 3 years.

Table 14.13 Associations between epilepsy and psychological disturbance

Psychiatric and cognitive disorders associated with the underlying cause

Behavioural disturbances associated with seizures

    Pre-ictal: prodromal states and mood disturbance

    Ictal: complex partial seizures (affective disturbances, hallucinations, experiential phenomena, automatisms); absence seizures (altered awareness, automatisms)

    Post-ictal: impaired consciousness; delirium; psychosis; Todd's paresis (hemiparesis, dysphasia, other focal signs)

Epileptic pseudodementia (non-convulsive status)

Inter-ictal disorders

    Cognitive

    Personality change

    Sexual behaviour

    Depression and emotional disorder

    Suicide and deliberate self-harm

    Crime and other antisocial behaviour

    Psychoses

Psychiatric consequences of epilepsy

There are a number of ways in which epilepsy predisposes to psychiatric and cognitive disturbances (see Table 14.13).

Psychiatric and cognitive disorders associated with the underlying cause

The underlying cause of epilepsy may contribute to intellectual impairment or personality problems, especially if there is extensive brain damage, or give rise to the focal cerebral syndromes (see p. 409) if localized.

Behavioural and cognitive disturbances associated with seizures

Increasing tension, irritability, and depression are sometimes apparent as prodromata for several days before a seizure. Transient confusional states, hallucinations, affective disturbances, automatisms, and other abnormal behaviours may occur during seizures (especially complex partial) and after seizures (usually those involving generalized convulsions, and complex partial seizures). Less commonly, an abnormal mental state may be the only sign of non-convulsive (complex partial or absence) status epilepticus, and the diagnosis is easily overlooked. The syndrome of 'epileptic pseudodementia' is gaining increasing recognition as a cause of reversible cognitive decline. Waxing and waning memory impairment is characteristic, and discrete episodes may be apparent, 'transient epileptic amnesia' (distinguished from transient global amnesia by the tendency to recurrence and association with overt seizures in most cases). Prolonged post-ictal memory impairment may cause confusion with Alzheimer's disease, and EEG telemetry may be required to make the diagnosis.

Psychoses may occur as an ictal phenomenon. Clues to this possibility include sudden onset and termination of psychiatric disturbance, a relative lack of first-rank symptoms, and amnesia for the period of the disturbance. Crimes committed during epileptic automatisms are extremely rare, an important medico-legal finding (see p. 905).

Inter-ictal disorders

Aside from the phenomenology of seizures themselves, there are several less direct associations between epilepsy and psychiatric disturbance.

Cognitive function

In the nineteenth century, it was widely held, based on experience with institutionalized populations, that epilepsy was associated with an inevitable decline in intellectual functioning; however, it is now established that relatively few people with epilepsy show cognitive changes. When these do occur, they are likely to reflect brain damage, unrecognized non-convulsive seizures, or the effects of antiepileptic drugs. A few epileptic patients show a progressive decline in cognitive function. In such cases, careful investigation is required to exclude an underlying progressive neurological disorder; this is a particular concern in paediatric practice.

Personality

The historical concept of an 'epileptic personality', characterized by egocentricity, irritability, religiosity, quarrelsomeness, and 'sticky' thought processes, has been discarded. Community surveys indicate that only a minority have serious personality difficulties and these probably reflect the adverse consequences of brain damage on education, employment, and social life rather than a specific association with epilepsy (Trimble 1997). It has been suggested that personality defects are associated with mesial temporal lobe lesions.

Depression and other emotional disorders

Depression and certain other emotional disorders are more common in people with epilepsy than in the general population. The incidence of bipolar affective disorder is not increased. Depression is most common in those with adverse social factors, but may be rooted in biological (temporolimbic) processes. Suicide is four times, and deliberate self-harm six times, more frequent among people with epilepsy than among the general population (see p. 905).

Inter-ictal psychoses

The nature and prevalence of inter-ictal schizophrenia has long been controversial. An important study by Slater *et al.* (1963) concluded that some patients with 'temporal lobe epilepsy' developed a psychosis that resembled schizophrenia; however, affective and religious overtones are typically more prominent. It is difficult to obtain epidemiological evidence free from selection bias and based on precise diagnostic criteria. Nevertheless, it is likely that a schizophrenia-like psychosis is more common among patients with foci in the temporal lobes than in those with primary generalized seizures (Krishnamoorthy and Trimble 1999). Other possible associations include onset in adolescence, left hemisphere lesions, abnormal neurological signs, and left-handedness. No firm biological explanation has emerged.

Treatment

The drug treatment of epilepsy is undertaken by neurologists. Here, discussion will be restricted to some key points. The importance of distinguishing between peri-ictal and inter-ictal psychiatric disorders when planning treatment deserves emphasis. For peri-ictal psychiatric disorders, treatment is aimed at control of the seizures. Treatment of inter-ictal psychiatric disorders is similar to those in non-epileptic patients, though it should be re-membered that many antidepressants and other psychotropic drugs may increase seizure frequency. Conversely, anticonvulsant drugs can cause a variety of cognitive and psychiatric symptoms. Newer generation agents, especially vigabatrin and topiramate, can give rise to a psychotic or major affective disorder. Vigabatrin leads to visual field loss (probably a retinopathy) in an uncertain proportion of patients, which may not be reversible (Johnson *et al* 2000): regular ophthalmological assessment with perimetry is therefore mandatory if this agent is to be used. Topiramate frequently produces marked cognitive impairment, particularly affecting language (in some cases, verbal IQ falls by more than 20 points), which is reversible on stopping the drug. See Toone (2000) for a review of the psychiatric aspects of epilepsy.

Sleep disorders

Psychiatrists may be asked to see patients whose main problem is either difficulty in sleeping or, less often, excessive sleep. Such problems are important:

Table 14.14 Sleep disorders mistaken for psychological disorder or behaviour problems/hallucinations

Excessive daytime sleepiness
    Laziness and disinterest
    Misbehaviour
    Opting out
Automatic behaviour
    Misbehaviour
    Laziness
    Dissociative states
Parasomnias
    Panic attacks
    Sleep disorders causing violence in sleep

- as primary sleep disorders;
- as causes of psychological symptoms;
- as features of *mental illness*;
- because they may be mistaken for psychological disorder (Table 14.14).

Many patients who sleep badly complain of tiredness during the day and mood disturbance. Although prolonged sleep deprivation leads to some impairment of intellectual performance and disturbance of mood, loss of sleep on occasional nights is usually of little significance. However, it is of importance in those whose responsibilities or activities require maximum alertness. The daytime symptoms of people who sleep badly are probably related more to the cause of their insomnia (often a depressive disorder or anxiety disorder) than to insomnia itself.

Classification

Table 14.15 shows the DSM-IV classification of sleep disorders, which is compatible with the considerably more elaborate International Classification of Sleep Disorders. Classifiction in ICD-10 is rather different, with sleep disorders occurring in three different parts of the classification.

Table 14.15 **Classification of primary sleep disorders in DSM-IV**

Dyssomnias

    Primary insomnia

    Primary hypersomnia

    Narcolepsy

    Breathing-related sleep disorder

    Circadian rhythm sleep disorder

    Dyssomnia not otherwise specified

Parasomnias

    Nightmare disorder (dream anxiety disorder)

    Sleep terror disorder

    Sleep-walking disorder

    Parasomnia not otherwise specified

Sleep disorder related to another mental disorder

    Insomnia

    Hypersomnia

Other sleep disorders

    Secondary sleep disorder due to a general medical condition

    Substance-induced sleep disorder

Box 14.1 **Assessment of sleep disturbance (see Stores 2000)**

Screening questions

    Do you sleep well enough and long enough?

    Are your very sleepy during the day?

    Is your sleep disturbed at night?

Sleep history

    Detailed history of the sleep complaint

    Pattern of occurrence, factors making sleep better or worse

    Consequences for mood, everyday life, family

    Past and present treatment

    Typical 24-hour sleep/wake schedule

    Sleep diary

    Systematic 2 week or longer record

History from bed partner

    Investigation

    Video recording

    Wrist scintigraphy (monitoring body movement)

    Polysomnography (EEG, EMG)

Epidemiology

Sleep disorders are frequent in the general population. There is a wide range of variation in estimates of the prevalence of insomnia depending on the definition and on the population studied. Up to 30% of adults complain of insomnia, a third as a chronic problem. Excessive sleepiness occurs in 5% of adults, and possibly 15% of adolescents and 14% of the adult population suffer some form of chronic sleep-wake disorder.

In the Epidemiologic Catchment Area Study (Ford and Kamerow 1989), 10.2% of the community sample reported insomnia and 3.2% reported hypersomnia. Forty per cent of those who suffered insomnia and 46.5% of those with hypersomnia had a psychiatric disorder compared with 16.4% of those with no sleep complaints. Groups at special risk of persistent sleep problems include young children, adolescents, the physically ill, those with learning disability, and those with dementia.

Assessment

Assessment requires a full psychiatric and medical history, together with detailed enquiries about the sleep complaint (Box 14.1). In several cases specialist investigation is necessary (see Stores 2000).

Insomnia

Transient insomnia occurs at times of stress or as 'jet lag'; short-term insomnia is often associated with personal problems, for example, illness or bereavement. Insomnia in clinical practice is usually secondary to other disorders, notably painful physical conditions, depressive disorders, and anxiety disorders, and is often clinically overlooked (Berlin 1984). Insomnia also occurs with excessive use of alcohol or caffeine, and in dementia. Sleep may be disturbed for several weeks after stopping heavy drinking. Sleep problems are also common in association with any medical illness that results in significant pain or discomfort or is associated with metabolic disturbances. They may also be provoked by prescribed drugs.

In about 15% of cases of insomnia, no cause can be found (*primary insomnia*). People vary in the amount of sleep they require, and some of those who complain of insomnia may be having enough sleep without realizing it.

Assessment

Usually the diagnosis of insomnia can be based on the account given by the patient. EEG recordings made in a sleep laboratory or at home are occasionally helpful when there is continuing doubt about the extent and nature of the insomnia. These observations often show that, despite the patient's complaint, sleeping time is within the normal range.

Treatment

If insomnia is secondary to another condition, the latter should be treated together with general measures to promote good sleep (Box 14.2) and avoidance of the disruptions to sleep and short-term hypnotics. In primary insomnia it is useful to encourage regular habits and exercise, and discourage overindulgence in tobacco, caffeine, and alcohol.

Although it may sometimes be justifiable to give a hypnotic for a few nights, demands for prolonged medication should be resisted. This is because withdrawal of hypnotics may lead to insomnia that is as distressing as the original sleep disturbance. Continuation of hypnotics may be associated with impaired performance during the day, tolerance to the sedative effects, and dependency. The use of hypnotic drugs is described further on p. 659.

> **Box 14.2 Principles of sleep education (hygiene)**
>
> *Sleep environment*
> > Familiar and comfortable
> > Dark
> > Quiet
>
> *Encourage*
> > Bedtime routines
> > Consistent bedtime and waking up time
> > Going to bed only when tired
> > Thinking about problems *before* going to bed
> > Regular exercise
>
> *Avoid*
> > Overexcitement before going to bed
> > Late evening exercise
> > Caffeine-containing drinks late in the day
> > Excessive alcohol and smoking
> > Excessive daytime sleep
> > Large late meals
> > Too much time in bed lying awake

Psychological treatments, especially cognitive behavioural treatments, have been shown to be effective in numerous controlled trials; strategies include behavioural procedures such as stimulus control and sleep restriction, and cognitive interventions such as paradoxical intervention and thought restructuring.

See Espie (2000) for a review.

Excessive daytime sleepiness

Excessive daytime sleepiness is common (with a reported prevalence between 3 and 5%) and underdiagnosed. Many cases are secondary to loss of night-time sleep. Table 14.16 shows the principal causes.

Idiopathic hypersomnia

In this uncommon condition patients complain that they are unable to wake completely until

> ### Table 14.16 Causes of excessive daytime sleepiness
>
> **Insufficient night-time sleep**
>
> Unsatisfactory irregular sleep routines or circumstances
>
> Circadian rhythm sleep disorders
>
> Frequent parasomnias
>
> Chronic physical illness
>
> Psychiatric disorders
>
> **Pathological sleep**
>
> Obstructive sleep apnoea
>
> Narcolepsy
>
> Other central nervous system disease
>
> Drug effects
>
> Kleine–Levin syndrome
>
> Depressive illness

several hours after getting up. During this time they feel confused and possibly disorientated ('sleep drunkenness'). They usually report prolonged and deep night-time sleep. Almost half have periods of daytime automatic behaviour, the aetiology of which is obscure. Most patients respond well to small doses of central nervous system stimulant drugs.

Narcolepsy

Narcolepsy usually begins between the ages of 10 and 20 years, though it may start earlier. Onset is rare after middle age. Narcolepsy is more frequent among males. Cataplexy (sudden temporary episodes of paralysis with loss of muscle tone) occurs in most cases, but sleep paralysis and hypnagogic hallucinations occur in only a quarter of patients.

Many aetiological theories have been advanced but none is convincing. There is a family history of narcolepsy in about a third of patients, and in occasional families the disorder appears to be trans-

mitted as an autosomal dominant. These findings, together with a high incidence of HLA concordance, imply a major genetic predisposition.

Psychiatric aspects of narcolepsy

Strong emotions sometimes precipitate cataplexy but apparently not narcolepsy. Patients with narcolepsy often have secondary emotional and social difficulties, and their difficulties are increased by other people's lack of understanding. Schizophrenia-like mental disorders have been reported to occur more frequently in patients with narcolepsy than in the general population.

Treatment

Patients need considerable help in adjusting to a disabling chronic illness They should be encouraged to follow a regular routine with planned short periods of sleep during the day. If stressful events seem to provoke attacks, efforts should be made to avoid them. Regular dosage with a stimulant drug has some effect in reducing narcoleptic attack but little effect on cataplexy. These drugs have to be given in high doses that lead to side-effects and problems of dependency. Tricyclic and SSRI antidepressants do not affect the sleep disorder but may reduce the frequency of cataplexy.

Breathing-related sleep disorder

This syndrome consists of daytime drowsiness together with periodic respiration and excessive snoring at night. It is usually associated with upper airways obstruction. The prevalence is about 4% in the male population. The typical patient is a middle-aged overweight man who snores loudly. Treatment consists of relieving the cause of the respiratory obstruction and encouraging weight loss. Continuous positive pressure ventilation using a face mask is often effective. Compliance with advice is often poor.

See Billard (2000) for a review of excessive sleepiness.

The Kleine–Levin syndrome

This very rare secondary sleep disorder consists of episodes of somnolence and increased appetite, often lasting for days or weeks and with long intervals of normality between them. Although the combination of appetite disorder and sleep disturbance suggests a hypothalamic disorder, there is no convincing evidence about the aetiology.

Circadian rhythm sleep disorder (sleep-wake schedule disorders)

There are several forms of circadian sleep disorder of which jet lag is the most familiar. Shift-work type is a common and increasing problem whose consequences are widely underestimated. Fatigue and transient difficulties in sleeping accompany regular changes of shift, or the irregular alternation of night work and days off may lead to chronic problems of poor sleep, fatigue, impaired concentration, and an increased liability to accidents as well as adverse effects on family life.

Parasomnias (dream anxiety disorder)

Nightmares

A nightmare is an awakening from REM sleep to full consciousness with detailed dream recall. Children experience nightmares with a peak frequency around the ages of 5 or 6 years. Nightmares may be stimulated by frightening experiences during the day, and frequent nightmares usually occur during a period of anxiety. Other causes include post-traumatic stress disorder, fever, psychotropic drugs, and alcohol detoxification.

Night terror disorder

Night terrors are much less common than nightmares. They are sometimes familial. The condition begins in childhood and usually ends there, but occasionally persists into adult life. A few hours after going to sleep, the child, whilst in stage 3–4 non-REM sleep, sits up and appears terrified. He may scream and usually appears confused. There are marked increases in heart and respiratory rates.

After a few minutes the child slowly settles and returns to normal calm sleep. There is little or no dream recall. A regular bedtime routine and improved sleep hygiene have been shown to be helpful. Benzodiazepines and imipramine have been shown to be effective in preventing night terrors, but their prolonged use should be avoided.

Sleep-walking disorder

Sleep-walking is an automatism occurring during deep non-REM sleep, usually in the early part of the night. It is most common between the ages of 5 and 12 years, and 15% of children in this age group walk in their sleep at least once. Occasionally, the disorder persists into adult life. Sleep-walking may be familial. Most children do not actually walk, but sit up and make repetitive movements. Some walk around, usually with their eyes open, in a mechanical manner but avoiding familiar objects. They do not respond to questions and are very difficult to wake. They can usually be led back to bed. Most episodes last for a few seconds or minutes, but rarely as long as an hour.

As sleep-walkers can occasionally harm themselves, they need to be protected from injury. Doors and windows should be locked and dangerous objects removed. Adults with severe problems should be given advice about safety, avoidance of sleep deprivation, and any other circumstances that might make them excessively sleepy (for example, drinking alcohol before going to bed). See Schenck and Mahowald (2000) for a review of parasomnias.

Further reading

Gelder, M. G., López-Ibor, J. J., Andreasen, N. C. (eds) (2001) 4.1 Delirium, dementia, amnesic and other cognitive disorders; 4.14 Sleep – wake disorder; 5.3.2 & 5.3.3 Epilepsy – Psychiatric aspects of neurological disease. *New Oxford textbook of psychiatry*. Oxford University Press

Lishman, W. A. (1998). *Organic Psychiatry*. Blackwells, Oxford.
(The standard textbook on Neuropsychiatry – an essential reference work)

15

CHAPTER 15

Eating disorders

Eating disorders

Until the late 1970s, eating disorders were believed to be uncommon. Following the description of bulimia nervosa, they have increasingly been seen as conspicuous and disabling. It remains uncertain whether the rapid rise in presentation and diagnosis reflects a true increase (Van Hoeken *et al.* 1998). Many are still clinically unrecognized and it is estimated that general practitioners recognize only 12% of bulimia nervosa and 45% of anorexia nervosa.

Anorexia nervosa and bulimia nervosa appear to be subgroups of a wider range of eating disorders which include those that may be incomplete expressions of the two main diagnoses, as well as others that appear qualitatively different. These atypical disorders are classified within DSM-IV as Eating Disorders Not Otherwise Specified (EDNOS). The relationship between these disorders is shown in Figure 15.1.

Anorexia nervosa

Although there were many previous case histories, anorexia nervosa was named in 1868 by the English physician William Gull, who emphasized the psychological causes of the condition, the need to restore weight, and the role of the family. The other key description at this time was by Charles Lasegue in Paris (see Palmer 2000). The main features are very low body weight (defined as being 15% below the standard weight or body mass index, BMI, below 17.5), an extreme concern about weight and shape characterized by an intense fear of gaining weight and becoming fat, a strong desire to be thin and, in women, amenorrhoea (see Box 15.1 for DSM-IV criteria).

Most patients are young women (see epidemiology, below). The condition usually begins in adolescence, although childhood-onset and older-onset cases are encountered. It generally begins with ordinary efforts at dieting, which then get out of control. The central psychological features are the characteristic overvalued ideas about body shape and weight. The patient may have a distorted image of her body, believing herself to be too fat even when severely underweight. This belief explains why most patients do not want to be helped to gain weight.

The pursuit of thinness may take several forms. Patients generally eat little and set themselves very low daily calorie limits (often between 600 and 1000 kcal). Some try to achieve weight loss by inducing vomiting, excessive exercising, and misusing laxatives. Patients are often preoccupied with thoughts of food, and sometimes enjoy cooking elaborate meals for other people. Some patients with anorexia nervosa admit to stealing

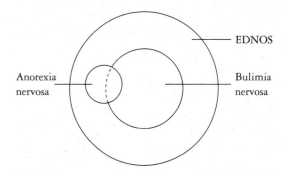

Figure 15.1 Venn diagram illustrating the relationship between the diagnoses of anorexia nervosa, bulimia nervosa, and eating disorder not otherwise specified (EDNOS). (Reproduced with permission from Fairburn and Wilson 1993).

food, either by shoplifting or in other ways. A subgroup of the patients have repeated episodes of binge eating (uncontrollable overeating). This behaviour becomes more frequent with chronicity and increasing age. During binges, the patients typically eat foods that are usually avoided. After overeating they feel bloated and may induce vomiting. Binges are followed by remorse and intensified efforts to lose weight. If other people encourage them to eat, patients are often resentful; they may hide food or vomit secretly as soon as the meal is over. In DSM-IV, anorexia nervosa with binge eating and purging (self-induced vomiting or the misuse of laxatives or diuretics) is recognized as a distinct type, differing from the restricting type.

Amenorrhoea is one of several physical abnormalities that have traditionally been incorporated in diagnostic criteria. It occurs early in the development of the condition, and in about a fifth of cases it precedes obvious weight loss, although careful history taking generally reveals that these patients had already started dieting. Some cases first come to medical attention with amenorrhoea rather than disordered eating.

Depressive, anxiety and obsessional symptoms, lability of mood, and social withdrawal are all common. In women and men lack of sexual interest is usual.

Physical consequences

A number of important symptoms and signs of anorexia nervosa are secondary to starvation, including sensitivity to cold, slow gastric emptying, constipation, low blood pressure, bradycardia, and hypothermia. Investigations may show leucopenia and abnormalities of water regulation. Vomiting and abuse of laxatives may lead to a variety of electrolyte disturbances, the most serious being hypokalaemia. Rarely, these abnormalities may cause epileptic seizures or death from cardiac arrhythmia. Hormonal abnormalities also occur: growth hormone levels are raised, plasma cortisol is increased and its normal diurnal variation lost, and levels of gonadotrophin are reduced. Thyroxine and thyrotropin-stimulating hormone are usually normal, but tri-iodothyronine (T3) may be reduced (Sharp and Freeman 1993). These hormonal abnormalities and the accompanying amenorrhoea are now thought to be secondary to the restricted eating and weight loss.

Hypothalamic dysfunction

In anorexia nervosa there is profound disturbance of weight regulation. In some cases amenorrhoea apparently begins before significant weight loss.

This combination has suggested a primary disorder of hypothalamic function, since it can occur with structural lesions of the hypothalamus. However, post-mortem studies have not revealed any regular occurrence of hypothalamic lesions in anorexia nervosa. The balance of evidence now suggests that endocrine and metabolic abnormalities are secondary to low weight and disturbed eating habits (see Russell 2000).

Epidemiology

Estimates of incidence based on case registers in the UK and the USA range from 0.37 to 4.06 per 100, 000 population per year. These are likely to be underestimates. Reported incidence rates have increased recently, but these changes may reflect greater awareness of the condition as well as some real increase of incidence (Van Hoeken *et al.* 1998). It is difficult to determine the true prevalence of anorexia nervosa because many people with the condition deny their symptoms. Surveys have suggested prevalence rates of up to 0.5% among schoolgirls and female university students. Many more young women have amenorrhoea and weight loss less than that required for the diagnosis of anorexia nervosa. Amongst anorexic patients seen in clinical practice only 5–10% are male. The condition is more common in the upper than the lower social classes, and is reported to be rare in non-Western countries or in the non-white population of Western countries (see Van Hoeken *et al.* 1998).

Genetics

Among the female siblings of patients with established anorexia nervosa, 6–10% suffer from the condition compared with the 1–2% found in the general population of the same age. This increase might be due to family environment or to genetic influences. There is evidence of a greater concordance in monozygotic than in dizygotic twins, suggesting genetic influences. Family genetic studies show an association between eating disorders and affective disorders. It seems probable that this is not due to a single, shared, aetiological factor for the two groups of disorders (see Lilenfeld and Kay 1998).

Social factors

Surveys show that most schoolgirls and female college students diet at one time or another. However, there is evidence that those who develop anorexia nervosa (or bulimia nervosa) come from family and social backgrounds which are likely to promote concerns about eating, shape, and weight (Fairburn *et al.* 1999). There are raised rates of family dieting and concerns about shape and weight and raised rates of overt eating disorders.

Individual psychological causes

Bruch (1974) was one of the first writers to discuss the psychological antecedents to anorexia nervosa. She suggested that these patients are engaged in 'a struggle for control, for a sense of identity and effectiveness with the relentless pursuit of thinness as a final step in this effort'. These clinical observations are supported by epidemiological studies, which implicate low self-esteem, undue compliance, and extreme perfectionism in the aetiology of the disorder. Crisp (1977) proposed that, whilst anorexia nervosa is at one level a 'weight phobia', the consequent changes in body shape and menstruation can be regarded as a regression to childhood and an escape from the emotional problems of adolescence. Certainly the timing of onset of the disorder suggests that developmental issues are important. It has been suggested that the premorbid personality traits of these people equips them particularly poorly for the demands of adolescence, an idea now demonstrated epidemiologically in case-control designs (Fairburn *et al.* 1999). In addition, clinical experience suggests that traits of low self-esteem, perfectionism, and undue compliance commonly precede the disorder (Vitousek and Manke 1994).

Causes within the family

Disturbed relationships are often found in the families of patients with anorexia nervosa, and some authors have suggested that they have an important causal role. Minuchin *et al.* (1978) held that a specific pattern of relationships could be identified, consisting of 'enmeshment, over protectiveness, rigidity and lack of conflict resolution'. They also suggested that the development of anorexia nervosa in the patient served to prevent dissent within the family. From a study of 56 families in which one member had anorexia nervosa, Kalucy *et al.* (1977) concluded that the other family members had an unusual interest in food and physical appearance, and that the families were unusually close knit to an extent that might impede the patient's adolescent development. Neither these studies nor others in the literature have shown convincingly that such patterns of behaviour differ significantly from the patterns in families of normal adolescents. On the other hand, there is a raised rate of parental problems preceding the onset of the disorder (Fairburn *et al.* 1999).

Course and prognosis

In its early stages, anorexia nervosa often runs a fluctuating course with exacerbations and periods of partial remission. Full recovery is not uncommon in cases with a short history. The long-term prognosis is difficult to judge because most published series are based on selected cases or are incomplete in their follow-up. Outcome is very variable. Although weight and menstrual functioning usually improve, eating habits often remain abnormal and some patients develop bulimia nervosa. It does not evolve into other forms of psychiatric disorder.

Long-term outcome studies show that, although the disorder may run a chronic course, recovery can occur even after many years. Reported mortality rates from long-term follow-up studies of severe cases are high at around 15%; this represents a sixfold increase in the standardized mortality rate. It is believed that the mortality rate is lower in more representative samples, falling with improved methods of treatment. About a fifth of patients make a full recovery, and another fifth

remain severely ill; the remainder show some degree of chronic or fluctuating disturbance.

The main factors predictive of outcome are the length of illness at presentation and age of onset; disorders with a short history and starting at a younger age are associated with a better prognosis (see Palmer 2000).

Assessment

Most patients with anorexia nervosa are reluctant to see a psychiatrist, and so it is important to try to establish a good relationship. This means listening to the patient's views, explaining treatment alternatives, and being willing to contemplate compromises. A thorough history should be taken of the development of the disorder, the present pattern of eating and weight control, and the patient's ideas about body weight (see Boxes 15.2 and 15.3). In the mental state examination, particular attention should be given to depressive symptoms. More than one interview may be needed to obtain this information and gain the patient's confidence. The parents or other informants should be interviewed whenever possible. It is essential to perform a physical examination, with particular attention to the degree of emaciation, cardiovascular status, and signs of vitamin deficiency. Other wasting disorders, such as malabsorption, endocrine disorder, or cancer, should be excluded. Electrolytes should be measured if there is any possibility that the patient has been inducing vomiting or abusing purgatives.

Evidence about treatment

There is a lack of good evidence about treatment and management. In part, this reflects the rarity of the disorder, but it also reflects the wide range in severity and the difficulty of evaluating complex interventions. Although there have been several well-conducted trials, there have been too few to establish a reliable evidence base. This means that current views about treatment depend upon clinical experience and opinion.

Box 15.2 **Assessment of eating issues: some topics to be included**

What is a typical day's eating? To what degree is the patient attempting restraint?

Is there a pattern? Does it vary? Is eating ritualized?

Does she avoid particular foods? And if so why?

Does she restrict fluids?

What is the patient's experience of hunger or of any urge to eat?

Does she binge? Are these objectively large binges? Does she feel out of control?

Are the binges planned? How do they begin? How do they end? How often?

Does she make herself vomit? If so how? Does she vomit blood? Does she wash out with copious fluids afterwards?

Does she take laxatives, diuretics, emetics, appetite suppressants? With what effects?

Does she chew and spit? Does she fast for a day to more?

Can she eat in front of others?

Does she exercise? Is this to 'burn off calories'?

(Reproduced with permission from Palmer, B. (ed.) (2000). *Helping people with eating disorders. A clinical guide to assessment and treatment.* John Wiley, Chichester)

Box 15.3 **Assessment of psychological issues: some topics to be included**

What does the patient feel about her body and her weight?

If she is restraining her eating, what is her motivation?

Does she feel fat? Does she dislike her body? If so, in what way?

Does she have a distorted body image? If so, in what way?

What does she feel would happen if she did not control her weight or eating?

Does she fear loss of control? Is she able to say what she means by this?

Does she feel guilt or self-disgust? If so, what leads her to feel this?

Does anything about her disorder lead her to feel good?

If she binges, what are her feelings before, during, and after bingeing?

What has she told others about her eating disorder – if anything?

How does she think about her disorder? What does she make of it?

(Reproduced with permission from Palmer, B. (ed.) (2000) *Helping people with eating disorders. A clinical guide to assessment and treatment.* John Wiley, Chichester)

Management

Starting treatment

Success largely depends on establishing a good relationship with the patient. It should be made clear that achieving an adequate weight is essential in order to reverse the physical and psychological effects of starvation. It is important to agree a definite dietary plan but not to become involved in wrangles about it. At the same time, it should be emphasized that weight control is only one aspect of the problem, and help should be offered with the accompanying psychological problems (see Palmer 2000).

Educating the patient and family about the disorder and its treatment is important. Admission to hospital is indicated if:

- the patient's weight is dangerously low;
- weight loss is rapid;
- there is severe depression;
- out-patient care has failed.

Less serious cases may be treated as day patients or out-patients. The former follows the general principles described for in-patient care in the next section.

Restoring weight

Weight restoration is normally accomplished on an out-patient basis but if the patient is admitted it should be on the understanding that she will stay in hospital until her agreed target weight has been reached and maintained and there is detailed discussion of the treatment plan. The target usually has to be a compromise between a healthy weight (a BMI above 20) and the patient's idea of what her weight should be. A balanced diet of about 3000 kcal is provided as three or four meals a day, with supplementary snacks. Successful treatment depends on good nursing care, with clear aims and firmness, and understanding. In the past, strict behavioural regimens were used. However, it appears that these had no advantage and often appeared punitive. A more informal but clear and predictable approach appears more effective and acceptable. Eating must be supervised by a nurse, who has two important roles: to reassure the patient that she can eat without the risk of losing control over her weight and to be firm about agreed targets, and to ensure that the patient does not induce vomiting or take purgatives. It is reasonable to aim for a weight gain of between 0.5 and 1.0 kg each week. Weight restoration usually takes between 8 and 12 weeks.

Some patients demand to leave hospital before their treatment is finished, but with patience the staff can usually persuade them to stay.

Rarely, the patient's weight loss is so severe as to pose an immediate threat to life. If such a patient cannot be persuaded to enter hospital, compulsory admission is necessary (see Box 15.4).

The role of psychotherapy

Many forms of psychotherapy have been tried. It is generally agreed that intensive psychoanalytical methods are not helpful. Clinical experience suggests that there is some value in simple supportive measures directed to improving personal relationships and increasing the patient's sense of personal effectiveness.

In recent years, family therapy has been advocated for younger patients. The results of a con-

---

Box 15.4 Compulsory treatment

Laws about compulsory treatment require evidence of mental illness to enable involuntary treatment. Their application to anorexia nervosa is controversial. Is anorexia a mental illness in the legal sense? Is successful treatment possible without consent?

In practice, compulsory treatment is used rarely and as a last resort when the patient is in physical danger. In these circumstances it may save the patient's live and gain the time to establish long-term voluntary treatment.

Compulsory treatment has many disadvantages, including losing the possibility of the patient ever cooperating with any reasonable treatment plan.

---

trolled evaluation suggest that there may be benefits with younger patients but do not support the general use of family therapy (Russell *et al.* 1987). If this treatment is used, it should be for selected cases in which family problems seem particularly relevant and the family members are willing to participate. Cognitive–behaviour therapy has also been used with the aim of modifying abnormal cognitions about shape, weight, and eating, but it has to be formally evaluated. Many patients and families find self-help groups valuable. For guidelines on treatment see Bell *et al.* (2000). For reviews of anorexia nervosa see Palmer (2000) and Russell (2000).

Bulimia nervosa

The term bulimia refers to episodes of uncontrolled excessive eating, sometimes called 'binges'. As mentioned above, the symptom of bulimia occurs in some cases of anorexia nervosa. The syndrome of bulimia nervosa was first described by Russell (1979) in a highly influential paper in which he named the condition and described the key clinical features in 30 patients seen between 1972 and 1978. Thereafter the syndrome 'bulimia' was included in DSM-III and it very soon became

Recurrent episodes of binge eating. An episode of binge eating is characterized by both of the following:

◆ eating, in a discrete period of time (e.g. within any 2-hour period) an amount of food that is definitely larger than most people would eat during a similar period of time and similar circumstances;

◆ a sense of lack of control over eating during the episode (e.g. a feeling that one cannot stop eating or control what or how much one is eating).

Recurrent inappropriate compensatory behaviour in order to prevent weight gain, such as self-induced vomiting; misuse of laxatives, diuretics, enemas, or other medication; fasting; or excessive exercise.

The binge eating and inappropriate compensatory behaviour both occur, on average, at least twice a week for 3 months.

The disturbance does not occur exclusively during episodes of anorexia nervosa.

Types
Purging type During the current episode of bulimia nervosa the person has regularly engaged in self-induced vomiting or the misuse of laxatives, diuretics, or enemas.

Non-purging type During the current episode of bulimia nervosa, the person has used other inappropriate compensatory behaviours, such as fasting or excessive exercise, but has not regularly engaged in self-induced vomiting or the misuse of laxatives, diuretics, or enemas.

evident that bulima nervosa was common in the general population (see Fairburn 2000 for a review).

Although the syndrome was described by Russell as an 'ominous variant' of anorexia nervosa, only a quarter have a history of preceding anorexia nervosa. The central features are an irresistible urge to overeat, extreme measures to control body weight, and overvalued ideas concerning shape and weight of the type seen in anorexia nervosa. Two subtypes are recognized in DSM-IV (see Box 15.5), the purging type characterized by the use of self-induced vomiting, laxatives, and diuretics to prevent weight gain, and the non-purging type in which 'purging' symptoms do not occur regularly but the person uses other behaviours to avoid weight gain, such as fasting and excessive exercise. Patients with bulimia nervosa are usually of normal weight; patients who are substantially underweight usually qualify for a diagnosis of anorexia nervosa, which takes precedence. Most patients are female and they often have normal menses.

Patients have a profound loss of control over eating. Episodes of bulimia may be precipitated by stress or by the breaking of self-imposed dietary rules, or may occasionally be planned. In the episodes large amounts of food are consumed, on average over 2000 kcal per episode; for example, a loaf of bread, a whole pot of jam, a cake, and biscuits. This voracious eating usually takes place alone. At first it brings relief from tension, but relief is soon followed by guilt and disgust. The patient may then induce vomiting or take laxatives. There may be many episodes of bulimia and purging each day.

Depressive symptoms are more prominent than in anorexia nervosa, and are probably secondary to the eating disorder. A high proportion of patients meet criteria for major depression. The symptoms usually remit as the eating disorder improves. A few patients appear to suffer from a depressive disorder requiring antidepressant drugs.

Physical consequences

Repeated vomiting leads to several complications. Potassium depletion is particularly serious, resulting in weakness, cardiac arrhythmia, and renal damage. Rarely, urinary infections, tetany, and epileptic fits may occur. The teeth become pitted by the acid gastric contents in a way that dentists can recognize as characteristic.

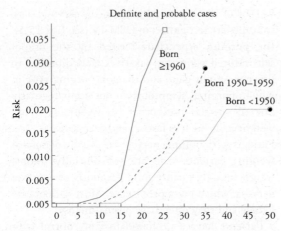

Definite and probable cases

Figure 15.2 Lifetime cumulative risk of bulimia nervosa amongst different birth cohorts of female twins. (Reproduced with permission from Kendler *et al.* 1991)

Epidemiology

The prevalence of bulimia nervosa is around 1% among women aged between 16 and 40 years (Van Hoeken *et al.* 1998). It is uncommon among men. Bulimia nervosa has only been identified in developed countries. The dramatic increase in presentation and diagnosis (see Figure 15.2) suggests that there has been a real increase in recent years, especially in young women aged between 15 and 24. However, there is still a lack of totally convincing evidence that there has been a real increase rather than increased awareness leading to greater numbers presenting and to improved recognition by doctors.

Development of the disorder

Bulimia nervosa usually has an onset in late adolescence (i.e. several years later than anorexia nervosa). It usually follows a period of concern about shape and weight and a quarter of patients have a history of a previous episode of anorexia nervosa. It commonly follows a period of dietary restriction which, after a variable length of time, but usually within 3 years, breaks down with increasingly frequent episodes of overeating. As the overeating becomes more frequent, the body weight returns to

a more normal level. At some stage self-induced vomiting and laxative misuse are adopted to compensate for the overeating. However, this may result in even less control of eating.

Aetiology

Bulimia nervosa appears to be the result of exposure to general risk factors of psychiatric disorder and of risk factors for dieting. General factors include a family history of psychiatric disorder, especially depression, and a range of adverse childhood experiences. It used to be thought that sexual abuse was especially common but the evidence now suggests the rate is no higher than amongst those who develop other types of psychiatric disorder. Other predisposing factors include perfectionism and low self-esteem. The role of genetic factors remains unclear with contradictory evidence. It remains possible that there is an inherited abnormality in the regulation of weight and eating habits (see Lilenfeld and Kaye 1998). Once established, the continuing concerns about body shape and weight, together with the vicious cycle of overeating and weight control by vomiting or purging, maintain the disorder.

Course and prognosis

This is uncertain since there have been few long-term studies. The course and outcome in those who do not present for treatment is unknown. Those who do present tend to do so after a prolonged duration, indicating that among this subgroup the disorder is already chronic. It is probable that abnormal eating habits persist for many years, but that they vary in severity. The overall outcome is very variable. The evidence to date suggests that cases of clinical severity tend to run a chronic course. The findings of treatment studies indicate that the outcome is considerably better than suggested by original descriptive accounts. Even so, even with cognitive behavioural therapy, only about half the patients make a full recovery. At 10-year follow-up, about 10% meet diagnostic criteria for bulimia nervosa and a further 15% have an atypical eating disorder. There is no evidence that bulimia nervosa is associated with the onset of any other psychiatric disorder. In contrast with anorexia nervosa, the mortality rate is not raised. The disorder tends to improve during pregnancy but subsequent relapse is common. No convincing predictors of course or outcome have been identified.

It is also probable that severe bulimia nervosa in mothers of young children may have considerable consequences for maternal care. It is also apparent that disturbed eating habits and attitudes among mothers are associated with feeding disorders among children (Stein *et al.* 1995).

Evidence about treatment effectiveness

There is a substantial evidence base, especially for psychological treatments. This has principally been concerned with cognitive–behavioural therapy but other psychological treatments, such as interpersonal therapy, have also been shown to be effective, as have some drug and 'self-help' treatments.

The most extensively studied psychological treatment is a manual-based, cognitive–behaviour therapy which helps patients regain control over their eating (see Fairburn 2000). This out-patient treatment uses procedures that aim to normalize eating habits and cognitive techniques designed to modify the excessive concerns about shape and weight. Patients attend as out-patients, keep records of their food intake and episodes of vomiting, and attempt to identify and modify any environment stimuli, thoughts, or emotional changes that regularly precede the urge to overeat. There is good evidence that up to two-thirds of patients treated in this way achieve substantial and lasting change. Cognitive behavioural therapy is acceptable to most patients, with a drop-out rate of about 15%, half that seen with antidepressant drugs. The effects are well maintained, with low relapse rates. Apart from benefits for the main features of eating and weight control, mood improves and social functioning and self-esteem improve. No consistent predictors have been identified. See

Fairburn (2000) for a review of cognitive–behavioural methods.

There is evidence that *interpersonal therapy*, which is a short-term focal psychotherapy, is equally effective but much slower to act. A recent multicentre trial (Agras *et al.* 2000) compared cognitive–behavioural and interpersonal therapy; cognitive–behavioural therapy achieved improvements significantly more rapidly than interpersonal therapy. The authors concluded that cognitive–behavioural therapy should be considered the preferred psychotherapeutic treatment for bulimia nervosa.

There is also evidence from several studies that cognitive–behavioural *self-help* treatment with minimal specialist supervision may be effective in milder cases (see, for example, Fairburn and Carter 1997). Treatment with antidepressant drugs results in a reduction in the frequency of binge eating but frequently the benefits do not last. Whilst there is no doubt that psychological treatments are more effective than drug therapy, drug treatments may be particularly useful where skilled therapists are not available, as an additional therapy for depressive symptoms and where psychological treatment has failed.

Management

The management of bulimia nervosa is easier than that of anorexia nervosa because the patient is more likely to wish to recover and a good working relationship can often be established. Also, there is no need for weight restoration. It is necessary to assess the patient's physical state and to identify the few cases that might benefit from treatment with antidepressant drugs. It is unusual to need drug treatment for depression but antidepressants are widely used in the USA for their antibulimic effect. Out-patient treatment is posible in the great majority of cases, and admission to hospital is indicated only if there are severe depressive symptoms or physical complications, or if out-patient treatment has failed. See Palmer (2000) for a review.

As with many common disorders, a 'stepped-care' approach appears to be the best way of providing appropriate care to large numbers of people with varying degrees of severity of disorder. Four main steps have been described (see Fairburn 2000):

◆ *Step one* Identify the small minority (less than 5%) who require specialist treatment because of severe depression, physical complications requiring in-patient or day-patient care, or severe substance abuse requiring treatment in its own right.

◆ *Step two* Guided cognitive–behavioural self-help as appropriate using a self-help book and with the guidance of a non-specialist facilitator. Treatment usually takes about 4 months and requires eight to ten meetings with the facilitator. Such treatment is appropriate for primary care and appears to lead to good progress in a third to half of patients.

◆ *Step three* Patients who do not show benefit within around 6 weeks of step two require full cognitive–behavioural therapy. In a minority of cases it is worthwhile adding an antidepressant drug.

◆ *Step four* Patients who do not improve with cognitive–behavioural therapy require comprehensive specialist reassessment. In some cases, measures to provide better cognitive therapy or an antidepressant drug may be useful. It is important to review the initial treatment with the patient with the aim of agreeing a treatment approach that is more acceptable and in which compliance is likely to improve.

See Fairburn (2000) and Palmer (2000) for reviews of bulimia nervosa.

Eating disorder not otherwise specified (atypical eating disorders)

These DSM-IV and ICD categories are for disorders of eating that do not meet the criteria for anorexia nervosa or bulimia nervosa, but are of clinical severity. They are frequent, and are diagnosed in at least a third of referrals.

A subgroup within EDNOS is recognized in DSM-IV as 'requiring further study'. It has been named *binge-eating disorder*; its definition and validity remain elusive and uncertain (see Palmer 2000). It is characterized by recurrent bulimic episodes in the absence of the other diagnostic features of bulimia nervosa. It appears to be associated with exposure to risk factors for psychiatric disorder in general and for obesity. Compared with bulimia nervosa, the risk factors are weaker (Fairburn *et al.* 1998). Treatment is similar in principle to that of cases that meet the criteria for diagnosis of anorexia nervosa or bulimia nervosa.

Obesity

Obesity is a medical condition characterized by excess body fat. It is diagnosed when the BMI (weight in kg/height in m^2) exceeds 30%. Almost 20% of the adults in the UK meet this criteria and this figure is rising. Obesity is associated with an increased mortality, and severe obesity (BMI greater than 40) is associated with a 12-fold increase of risk in those aged 25–35 years. It has been estimated that in the USA, 300 000 deaths each year can be attributed to obesity, making it a public health problem second only to smoking as a potentially preventative cause of death (see Stunkard and Wadden 2000 and Devlin *et al.* 2000 for reviews).

Aetiology

Most obesity is attributable to genetic factors exacerbated by social factors that encourage overeating. Psychological causes do not seem to be of great importance in most cases, but psychiatrists are sometimes asked to see obese people whose excessive eating seems to be determined by emotional factors.

Psychological consequences

Although there have been many reports of emotional disturbance amongst the obese, numerous careful studies have shown little difference in psychopathology as compared with non-obese people in the general population. Concern appears to be most common between teenage and young women of upper and middle socioeconomic status who are likely to live in social circumstances in which prejudice and discrimination are most common.

One form of psychopathology that is specific to obesity is a distortion of body image, feeling grotesque, and a belief that others feel contempt. This disorder, which is associated with self-consciousness and social limitations, occurs only in the minority of obese people who have been obese since childhood and also have low self-esteem. See Stunkard and Waddon (2000).

Another form of psychopathology is that underlying so-called 'binge-eating disorder' (see p. 454). This is increasingly prevalent with increasing body weight and described by between 10 and 20% of people entering obesity treatment programmes.

Course

Obesity is a chronic, indeed lifelong, problem. Obese children and adolescents are unlikely to grow out of their obesity unless treated. Most untreated adults continue to gain weight at the rate of approximately 1 kg per year.

Treatment

It is now widely accepted that the goal of treatment should be one of reduction by as little as 5–15% rather than unrealistically attempting to attain an ideal weight which is unlikely to be achieved or maintained. Such more modest goals may have medical benefits and also improve mood and body image. They are also appropriate to attaining long-term weight management. The main treatment options (see Devlin *et al.* 2000) are:

♦ *behavioural weight control.* There is consistent evidence that although this approach is effective in the short term, weight is then gradually re-gained. It is therefore usually seen as an initial phase of a longer-term approach to care. Behavioural approaches appear to be considerably more effective in children.

♦ *diet.* This is also disappointing in that weight is usually slowly regained after successful short-term weight loss. It is important that programmes concentrate on achieving long-term changes in dietary content and habits accompanied by increased physical activity.

♦ *physical activity.* Physical activity is an important element both in achieving initial weight loss but also, especially, in maintaining loss.

♦ *pharmacological treatments.* These are usually more effective than behavioural treatment in achieving weight loss and maintaining a stable weight in the medium term. Long-term follow-up suggests that gradual re-gain of weight occurs in many patients. Weight is quickly re-gained when medication is discontinued. It is probable that newer medications will achieve a more substantial place in the short-term and maintenance therapy of obesity.

The long-term results of all kinds of treatment are disappointing, whether supervised by a doctor or not (G. T. Wilson 1993; Devlin *et al.* 2000). Group therapy and self-help groups produce short-term benefit but do not improve long-term results. The same is true for appetite-suppressing drugs and behavioural methods. The results with children are somewhat more encouraging (Epstein *et al.* 1994), although there is concern that treatment *may* encourage the later development of bulimia nervosa (Wilson 1994).

Surgical treatment

Surgical treatment is probably indicated for very severe obesity (BMI >40). The most common form is gastric restriction. As the risks of this form of surgery are significant in severely overweight patients, it should be offered only when other treatments have failed. Jaw wiring is sometimes recommended as a means of losing substantial amounts of weight, but weight may be re-gained when the wires are removed (see Devlin *et al.* 2000; Stunkard and Wadden 2000).

Early treatment

The lack of effective treatments in adult life highlights the need for a greater emphasis on environmental change and public policy to achieve primary prevention. It is also important to intervene early with children because of their high risk of lifelong obesity. While it is likely that there will be some improvements in treatments with adults, we need to ensure that aims for weight loss are reasonable and achievable (which may not always be acceptable to obese subjects) and that efforts are made to improve self-esteem and quality of everyday life, whatever the person's weight.

Management

Most treatment is provided in primary care and medical clinics. Psychiatrists need to be aware of the standard treatments for obesity, including the role of self-help and commercial programmes. Whilst the effectiveness of the latter remains unclear, the dependence of Weight Watchers and some other programmes on sound principles of nutrition and activity mean that they are probably helpful to those with moderate degrees of obesity and health risk.

Mildly overweight people need nothing more than advice about diet and exercise. Although there has been concern that dieting may be associated with adverse physiological and psychological effects, it would seem that these are not of clinical significance for moderate changes in eating and exercise (French and Jeffery 1994). It is important to be aware that aiming at an 'ideal' weight is unrealistic and even inappropriate. Severely overweight people require assessment and treatment in specialized clinics. For a review of obesity see Stunkard and Wadden (2000) and Devlin *et al.* (2000).

Psychogenic vomiting

Psychogenic vomiting is chronic and episodic vomiting without an organic cause which commonly occurs after meals and in the absence of nausea. It should be distinguished from the more common syndrome of bulimia nervosa, in which self-induced vomiting follows episodes of binge eating (uncontrolled overeating). Psychogenic vomiting appears to be more common in women than in men and usually presents in early or middle adult life. It is reported that both psychotherapeutic and behavioural treatments can be helpful.

Further reading

Fairburn, C. G. (2000). Bulimia nervosa. In *The new Oxford textbook of psychiatry* (eds M. G. Gelder, J. J López-Ibor Jr, and N. C. Andreasen), Chapter 4.10.2. Oxford University Press, Oxford.

Palmer, B. (2000). *Helping people with eating disorders. A clinical guide to assessment and treatment.* John Wiley, Chichester.

Stunkard, A. and Wadden, T. A. (2000). Obesity. In *The new Oxford textbook of psychiatry* (eds M. G. Gelder, J. J López-Ibor Jr, and N. C. Andreasen), Chapter 4.10.3. Oxford University Press, Oxford.

CHAPTER 16

Psychiatry and medicine

Psychiatry and medicine

Introduction

This chapter is concerned with the frequent occurrence together of psychiatric disorder and physical illness in patients presenting in primary care or in general hospital practice. It also covers psychological symptoms that are not severe enough to satisfy diagnostic criteria but may also cause considerable morbidity and lead to an increased use of medical services. It is important that psychological problems should not be missed:

♦ Severe conditions are likely to need specific psychiatric treatment; simpler measures may alleviate mild disorders.

♦ Psychiatric disorder in patients with chronic medical conditions is associated with markedly worse quality of everyday life.

♦ They are a frequent cause of poor compliance with medical treatment and of inappropriate use of medical services.

♦ They may be associated with behaviours and lifestyles (such as smoking, excessive alcohol, and physical inactivity) that predispose to or exacerbate medical illness.

When treatment is needed for the psychiatric disorder, it is usually provided as part of overall medical care by the practitioner who is treating the physical illness. However, the more severe disorders are likely to require treatment by psychiatrists or psychologist.

Epidemiology

In the general population physical illness and physical symptoms are associated with an increase of psychiatric disorder (Wells *et al.* 1988; Kroenke and Price 1993). The WHO collaborative study of patients presenting to *primary care* in 14 countries showed a strong association between somatic symptoms and psychiatric morbidity in all the centres, despite their different cultural approaches to illness and its care. Moderate and severe physical disorder was associated with psychiatric disorder, whilst there was a linear relationship between number of medically unexplained symptoms (i.e. symptoms in which no adequate pathological cause was evident) and psychiatric disorder. Medically unexplained symptoms were more common than those with a physical explanation. Medically and non-medically explained somatic symptoms often occurred together (see Kisely and Goldberg 1996; Simon *et al.* 1996; Kisely *et al.* 1997; G. Simon 2000).

Numerous studies have found associations between physical and psychiatric disorders among *general hospital in-patients, out-patients and emergency department attenders.* For example, surveys in medical wards have shown that over a quarter of in-patients have a psychiatric disorder. The frequency and nature of these disorders depend on the age and sex of the patients and the nature of the specialty of the ward. For example, affective and adjustment disorders are more common in the elderly, and drinking problems in younger men. Psychological problems are frequent among patients attending emergency clinics, as well as gynaecological and medical out-patient clinics. Organic mental disorders are frequent in geriatric wards, and drinking problems in liver units.

Non-specialist management

Recognition

There is much evidence that primary-care practitioners often fail to recognize psychiatric disorder in patients with physical illness (Goldberg and Huxley 1980). Similarly, psychiatric disorder in patients in medical and surgical wards often goes undetected. Subsequent studies have confirmed that many affective and organic disorders and most drinking problems are not detected among patients in general hospitals. Recognition of psychological problems depends upon awareness of their clinical importance and willingness to ask general screening questions together with further probes as necessary. Screening instruments for psychological problems may have a role provided that staff have the skill to interpret and use findings.

Most psychological care of the physically ill is provided by doctors other than psychiatrists and their clinical teams, either in primary care or in the general medical services. It is therefore important that medical, nursing, and other professional staff have the knowledge and skills to provide appropriate care themselves and to identify patients who need specialist treatment. They also need to be aware that, in all populations, use of alternative or complementary therapies is very considerable (Diehl and Eisenberg 2000). Cross-cultural studies have emphasized widely differing practice and attitudes towards the use of traditional remedies.

Discussion, advice, and information, willingness to enquire about the patient's beliefs and worries, talking to relatives, and a willingness to spend more time on the minority of patients with greater needs is all part of general medical care. Nurses and other members of the clinical team can have an essential role, but the specialized problems discussed in this chapter may require referral to psychiatric or clinical psychology services.

> #### Box 16.1 Association between psychological factors and physical illness
>
> Psychological factors affecting the onset and course of physical illness.
>
> Psychological factors and unexplained physical symptoms (see also Chapter 10)
>
> Psychiatric consequences of physical illness:
>
> - dementia, delirium, and other cognitive disorders (see also Chapter 14)
> - side-effects of drugs
> - stress-related, anxiety, and mood disorders (see also Chapters 8, 9, and 11).
>
> Psychiatric and physical disorder occurring together by chance.
>
> Psychiatric problems with physical complications:
>
> - suicide and deliberate self-harm (Chapter 17)
> - alcohol and other substance abuse (Chapter 18)
> - eating disorders (Chapter 15)

The organization of this chapter

This chapter covers most of the association between psychological factors and physical illness shown in Box 16.1. However, it should be read in conjunction with other chapters, especially those on dissociative and somatoform disorders, neuropsychiatry, and suicide and attempted suicide. In particular, the discussion of medically unexplained symptoms is divided between the main account in this chapter and the section on DSM and ICD classifications of somatoform disorders in Chapter 10.

Psychiatric and physical disorders occurring together by chance

Psychiatric and physical disorders often arise independently of one another and then interact. Psychiatric disorder may affect the patient's response to physical symptoms and increase the problems of medical management. For example, an eating disorder may greatly complicate the treatment of diabetes; depression is a risk factor for increased mortality and morbidity following myocardial infarction (see p. 491). Anxiety and depression are also risk factors for non-compliance with medical treatment (DiMatteo *et al.* 2000).

On the other hand, physical illness may lead to deterioration of psychiatric disorder. The presence of a physical illness has been shown to be an adverse risk factor for minor affective disorder in primary care and for anxiety and depressive disorder. Occasionally the onset of a major medical problem is associated with considerable improvement in chronic psychiatric difficulties.

Psychological factors affecting the onset and course of physical illness

Historical background

Throughout the twentieth century there was very considerable interest in the role of psychological factors as *causes* of major physical disorders – *psychosomatic medicine*. Advances in medical knowledge, together with a sceptical view of psychodynamic theory and of the methodological inadequacies of the older evidence have resulted in a much more cautious and critical view of the ways in which psychological and social factors may interact with other risk factors in the onset an course of medical illness.

A number of psychodynamic theorists, mainly working in North America but strongly influenced by Freud and his followers, developed the original concepts of psychosomatic illnesses. The term initially referred to a belief that psychological variables could be direct causes via psychophysiological mechanisms of a physical disorder (it continues to be used, but in a much broader sense, for all the ways in which psychological and physical factors interact in the medically ill). In the 1930s, there were two particularly well-known theoretical approaches. Flanders Dunbar, the founder of the American Psychosomatic Society, suggested that personality types might be associated with particular illness; Franz Alexander, a Chicago-based analyst who wrote the best known major book (see Alexander 1950) proposed that psychological conflict was important in a number of specifically psychosomatic physical conditions, which included ischaemic heart disease, ulcerative colitis, and hypertension. The original theories and evidence are no longer credible. This is in large part because of the very substantial advances in the methodology of psychiatric research in recent years. However, a continuing influence of older views is still evident in some of the more precisely formulated current theories.

One more recent theoretical example is the suggestion by Nemiah and Sifneos (1970) that *alexithymia* (i.e. inability to recognize and describe feelings, difficulty in discriminating between emotional states and bodily sensations, and inability to fantasize) is important in the onset, course, and presentation of physical illness. Although these characteristics are recognizable in clinical practice, there is no agreed way of defining them for research. They have not been shown to constitute a valid syndrome, to be specifically associated with physical disorder, or to have significance in treatment. Nonetheless, the concept remains widely popular. See Salminen *et al.* (1995) for a review.

Current research

Over the last 30 years there have been major advances in several research disciplines (see Steptoe and Wardle 1994 for a useful annotated collection of some of the most important papers).

Current research is concerned as much with the effects of psychosocial variables on the *course* of physical illness as with *onset*.

- *Social factors* A wide range of research has considered the influence of unemployment, job strain, and issues arising from social relationships, such as isolation and social support. Increasingly, sophisticated individual and population studies have begun to define the significance of unpleasant circumstances and the ways in which they interact with a person's personal and social resources. For example, social isolation has been shown to be an independent risk factor for mortality amongst survivors of myocardial infarction.

- *Stressful events* There has been considerable research on the role of stressful life events (see p. 121). This originally used the Schedule of Recent Experience (Holmes and Rahe 1967) or modifications of it; recent work has used more recent and elaborate instruments. The role of life events is likely to be as a precipitant rather than a 'formative' cause.

- *Personality* Current research is still concerned with the ways in which personality traits may be risk factors for the onset or for the course of major illness. For example, it now seems probable that the personality trait of hostility contributes to the development and course of ischaemic heart disease (see p. 491). Similarly, there appears to be a growing body of evidence that psychological and behavioural variables affect the course of various types of cancer.

- *Psychiatric disorder* Depression may have a direct effect on, as well as being an important determinant of, compliance with medical care. For example, there is substantial evidence that depressed mood is a major risk factor for mortality following myocardial infarction (Frasure-Smith *et al.* 1995).

- *Lifestyle and health-related behaviours* Behavioural risk factors are increasingly seen as having an important role in many conditions; a common example is smoking and diet and ischaemic heart disease. Understanding of the role of lifestyle in the aetiology of many major diseases in both the developed and developing world has very large implications for public health and medical interventions, which can be expected to have a large impact on mortality or morbidity.

- *Mechanisms* Other work has dealt with the mechanisms through which emotions could induce physical changes. For example, in a pioneering study, Wolf and Wolff (1947) studied a patient with a gastric fistula and found that emotional changes were accompanied by characteristic changes in the colour, motility, and secretory activity of the stomach mucosa. More recent research has focused on neuroendocrine and immunological mechanisms that may mediate the effects of psychological factors on physical processes (for example, see McEwan *et al.* 1997).

As a result of research and clinical experience in all these areas, the traditional concept of separate psychosomatic illnesses of predominantly psychological aetiology has been abandoned. It has been replaced by a general acceptance that psychological and behavioural factors interact with pathological processes in the development and course of physical disorders and that they also have substantial effects on consultation and compliance with treatment.

Implications for clinical practice

Whilst current evidence is patchy, and there are missing links in proposed causal relationships, there is now a substantial body of research – psychological, physiological, and pathological – to suggest that psychological factors are amongst the determinants on the onset and course of a number of common physical disorders. There are public health implications in reducing lifestyle risk factors within whole populations and also for reducing the large inequalities of need and resource allocation within poor populations. At the level of the individual patient it is possible to propose effective interventions for use alongside physical interventions. These include:

- psychological and behavioural procedures to modify lifestyle risks, for example in those at risk of ischaemic heart disease;

- treatment of depression and other psychiatric disorders that have been shown to affect the course of several illnesses;

◆ individual or group psychosocial treatments designed to increase survival in those with established illness, for example, group therapy for people with metastatic cancer (Spiegel and Barlow 2000).

Classification

Classifications have taken some account of new knowledge. Thus, DSM-IV has a rubric for *psychological factors affecting physical conditions* in one of four ways:

◆ influencing the course of the medical condition;

◆ interfering with its treatment;

◆ constituting additional health risks;

◆ precipitating or exacerbating the physical condition.

When using this rubric, one or more of six factors may be specified as affecting the medical disorder: a mental disorder; psychological symptoms; personality traits or coping style; maladaptive health behaviours; stress-related physiological responses; or other unspecified factors. Unfortunately, the description is so broad that it could be applied to most medical disorders and the category has not been used consistently or extensively.

Psychological factors contributing to medically unexplained symptoms

Non-specific physical symptoms which do not have any adequate organic explanation are extremely frequent in the general population and in all medical settings (see Mayou *et al.* 1995; Simon 2000). Most are transient but a minority are persistent and disabling and lead to frequent consultation. Medically unexplained symptoms are also due to factitious disorder and malingering. (Box 16.2). This chapter deals with general issues of the characteristics, aetiology, and treatment of such symptoms. Somatoform disorders are described in Chapter 10. However, many people who present to doctors with unexplained symptoms do not suffer

---

> **Box 16.2 Clinical problems associated with medically unexplained symptoms**
>
> Minor transient symptoms
> Persistent symptoms and syndromes, often associated with psychiatric disorder
> Factitious disorder
> 'Factitious disorder by proxy'
> Malingering

---

from somatoform or other psychiatric disorder. Even so, psychological and social factors may be of considerable importance in the aetiology of the presenting symptoms and psychological and psychiatric treatments often have a major role.

Terminology

All cultures seem to recognize categories of non-specific symptoms in which there is no major sinister organic cause and most have descriptive terms for them. Many terms have been used, including psychiatric terms, such as hysteria and hypochondriasis, and more general terms, such as functional symptoms, somatization, somatoform symptoms, as well as pejorative non-psychiatric terms, such as 'functional overlay' (to describe the symptoms), and the 'worried well' or 'heartsink patient' (to describe the people who complain of them).

◆ *Somatization* is the most widely used general term. It was introduced at the beginning of the twentieth century by Stekl, a German psycho-analyst, and implied the expression of emotional distress as bodily symptoms. More recently, somatization has become a popular general term, both as a process and as a category. Some current definitions are very broad, covering both the *perception* of bodily sensations and *consultation*. Most definitions implicitly contain Stekl's original idea that physical symptoms are an alternative expression of emotional distress, for example 'a tendency to experience and communicate psychological distress in the form of somatic symptoms and to seek medical help for them' (Lipowski 1988). Current research suggests that the level of distress and the severity and number of physical symptoms are positively related rather than alternatives. Narrower definitions reject Stekl's view and use criteria that require physical symptoms to be accompanied by anxiety or affective disorder satisfying standard criteria. Because of the lack of an agreed definition and the aetiological assumptions that it conveys, we believe that somatization is an unsatisfactory term.

♦ *Somatoform* is a term used originally in DSM-III to describe a new category of disorders which included traditional psychiatric disorders such as hysteria and hypochondriasis, together with newly proposed categories, such as somatization disorder (see p. 257).

♦ *Functional somatic symptoms* is a term frequently used for physical problems in which disturbance of function is more conspicuous than evidence of pathological processes. The wider use of the word functional (as opposed to organic) in psychiatry has been much criticized and this is a disadvantage in applying it to this subgroup of clinical problems.

♦ A different and much broader descriptive approach has been to refer to *medically unexplained symptoms*. This has advantages of describing a clinical problem without assumptions of aetiology but is unsatisfactory in that it wrongly implies that there is in fact no medical explanation.

Epidemiology of medically unexplained symptoms

The many reports of symptoms and syndromes in the general population and in primary care all show that unexplained symptoms are very common and that they are more frequent in women than in men. Although most are seen by patients as trivial and are self-limiting, a sizeable minority are associated with time off work, consulting doctors or taking medication, and distress (Kroenke and Price 1993; von Korff *et al.* 1998). A WHO multicentre primary care study of psychiatric disorder presenting in attenders at centres in the less developed countries reported more somatic symptoms than individuals attending centres in developed countries (see Simon 2000). The preponderance of unexplained symptoms among women appeared to be entirely due to their increased experience of psychiatric disorder (Piccinelli and Simon 1997). The more detailed findings for different types of somatoform disorder are discussed in Chapter 10.

Aetiology

The Western *dualist* view of aetiology as being *either* physical *or* psychological, which underlies current concepts of somatoform disorder, has resulted in great problems in psychiatric and lay understanding, classification, and treatment of unexplained symptoms. It has, for instance, resulted in the polarized argument about the causes of chronic fatigue syndrome which has resulted in the totally rejection of any contribution by psychological factors by proponents of particular physical aetiologies. It has also caused bewilderment in other cultures that do not share a dualist approach to illness and where the large group of symptoms without specific known cause do not result in any major classification problem. An alternative view, for which there is compelling evidence, is that the aetiology of unexplained medical symptoms involves the interaction of physiological, pathological, and psychological variables.

The majority of 'unexplained' symptoms arise from a primary bodily sensation or concern (Table 16.1) which is then attributed or interpreted as being of sinister significance. Concern and anxiety result in focusing on the subjective symptoms and physiological, behavioural, and emotional consequences, which then exacerbate and maintain the original perception. For example, awareness of abnormal heart rate at a time of excitement or anxiety may precipitate panic (see p. 240) but also worry about heart disease, and lead to restriction of

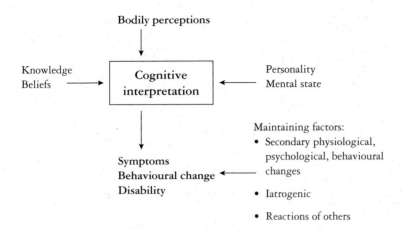

Figure 16.1
Aetiology of medically
unexplained symptoms.

Table 16.1 Some causes of bodily sensations

Major pathology

Minor pathology

Physiological processes

  Sinus tachycardia and benign minor arrhythmias

  Effects of fatigue

  Hangover

  Effects of overeating

  Effects of prolonged inactivity

  Autonomic effects of anxiety

  Lack of sleep

daily activities and repeated consultation to seek investigation and reassurance. It may often be that physiological or minor pathological causes are prominent at the onset of a clinical problems but, as time goes by, symptoms are largely maintained by anxiety and other psychological and behavioural factors (Figure 16.1).

There is considerable evidence on the ways in which psychological processes affect the interpretation of physical symptoms, whatever the underlying major or minor pathology or to physiological processes. Cognitive behavioural formulations emphasize the central significance of anxiety about illness (Salkovskis and Clark 1993) and the reinforcing effects of physiological, cognitive, affective, and behavioural consequences. See Mayou *et al.* (1995) for a review of aetiology.

The *interpretation* of bodily sensations is affected by several sets of factors:

- *previous illness and treatment experience* (Table 16.2) Adult patients with unexplained symptoms report a variety of adversities in childhood, for example, poor parenting and various forms of abuse. There is also evidence that a high proportion of children with unexplained symptoms come from families where there are potential 'models' for their symptoms and complaining. Much of this evidence is retrospective but in a prospective cohort study, Hotopf *et al.* (2000) showed a clear association between experience of illness in parents during childhood and subsequent physical symptoms during adult life.

- *illness beliefs* (attribution and cognitions) Illness amongst family and friends and media publicity influenced presentation, characteristics and understanding of symptoms (Table 16.2).

- *social circumstances* In addition to the cross-cultural differences in the reported experience and presentation of unexplained symptoms,

Table 16.2 Illness experience which may affect interpretation of bodily sensations and concern
Childhood illness
Family illness and consultation in childhood
Childhood consultation and school absence
Physical illness in adult life
Experience and satisfaction with medical consultation
Illness in family and friends
Publicity in television, newspapers, etc.
Knowledge of illness and its treatment

medically unexplained symptoms are associated with poor socioeconomic circumstances and acute or chronic adversity.

♦ *personality and mental state* Many of those who present with more disabling unexplained symptoms have a predisposition to concern about bodily health which is evident in frequent consultation. They are also difficult to reassure.

Once symptoms have developed they may be *maintained* by:

♦ behavioural, psychological, and emotional consequences which reinforce the underlying perceptions and interpretation;

♦ peripheral and central neurobiological mechanisms associated with chronic anxiety;

♦ the reactions of others; particularly important are misconceptions arising from medical advice which is not accompanied by an explanation, or by ambiguous or contradictory advice. Doctors' uncertainty about how to manage symptoms which are upsetting to patients but for which they can find no specific organic cause means that they have difficulty in giving information and treatment advice which is adequate for the patient's concerns about a serious physical cause.

The association with psychiatric disorder

The majority of medically unexplained symptoms in the general population are not associated with psychiatric disorder, but those that are persistent or multiple are more likely to be associated. The psychiatric disorder is frequently anxiety or mood disorder and this is true for all cultures. Both small local studies and major international collaborative research indicate that association is strongest for those who have the greatest number of unexplained symptoms (Simon *et al.* 1996; Kisely *et al.* 1997). Research suggests three overlapping types of psychiatric association: anxiety and depression, worry about illness (which may be referred to as health anxiety or as hypochondriasis) and pre-occupation with multiple physical symptoms (Kirmayer and Robbins 1991).

Associations between longer-established categories of psychiatric disorder are discussed below and elsewhere in this book and somatoform disorders are considered in Chapter 10.

Classification of unexplained symptoms

Classification of those with persistent and disabling medically unexplained symptoms has been considered from two rather separate perspectives. The medical view of *descriptive syndromes* covers patterns of symptoms, some of which are of considerable antiquity, such as irritable bowel and fibromyalgia. Many incorporate assumptions about aetiology and there is little evidence for their validity; there are striking cross-cultural differences, for instance, low blood pressure syndrome in Germany, *mal de foie* in France, and myalgic encephalomyelitis (ME) in the UK. An increasing number of syndromes have been introduced by lay groups to describe their own predicaments and the apparent lack of success of conventional medicine. Although these syndromes are seen as entities by doctors who treat them, they appear to overlap and be strongly affected by cultural differences in presentation and treatment (Wessely *et al.* 1999).

A few have now received *operational diagnostic criteria*, which have proved valuable in planning treatment, for example, the criteria for chronic fatigue (see below).

The alternative applicable approach from psychiatry has been to attempt to identify psychiatric syndromes. These include both the standard categories of *anxiety and depressive disorders* and the new concept, first introduced in DSM-III, of *somatoform disorder* (Chapter 10). DSM-III also introduced the further new category of *factitious disorder* for self-inflicted physical problems (see below).

Classification in clinical practice

The following chapters of this book describe syndromes that have proved to have some operational value despite the acknowledged lack of validity. Anxiety and depression are considered fully elsewhere. In everyday clinical practice, it is rarely necessary (or helpful) to use somatoform categories, but the recognition of anxiety and depression is important because it has therapeutic implications. It is probably most useful to be able to provide brief descriptions of the clinical problem which can be a basis for formulating treatment:

◆ acute or chronic;

◆ number of symptoms;

◆ the pattern of symptoms (i.e. clinical syndromes such as fatigue);

◆ any association with anxiety, depression, or other specific psychiatric disorder;

◆ the patient's beliefs about cause.

Evidence about treatment

The evidence base for specific treatments remains limited. High-quality trials have mainly been concerned with drug treatments and with cognitive–behavioural psychological treatment. Examples are cited in the following sections of this chapter and in Chapter 10.

Antidepressant medication has been shown to have a limited role in a range of syndromes including facial pain and irritable bowel, and this is especially so for patients with marked depressive symptoms. Cognitive–behavioural treatments are effective in hypochondriasis and in the treatment of presenting problems such as non-cardiac chest pain, irritable bowel, and chronic fatigue.

The wider principles of specialist and non-specialist treatment described in this chapter are largely based on clinical experience. See Mayou *et al.* (1995) and Manu (1998) for reviews.

Management

Assessment

The treatment of medically unexplained symptoms presents two general requirements. The first is to ensure that all those involved in care have a consistent approach. The second is to make sure that patients understand that, although their symptoms are not due to physical illness, their complaints are accepted as real and are taken seriously. To these ends physicians should explain clearly the purpose and results of all investigations, and the likely value of psychological assessment and referral. The psychiatrist should be aware of the results of physical investigations, and the explanation and advice given to the patient by other clinicians (see Table 16.3).

Table 16.3 General principles of assessment of 'unexplained' symptoms

Consider psychological factors from outset

Appropriate physical investigation to exclude physical cause

Clarify psychological and physical complaints

Clarify previous personality and concerns about physical illness

Understand patient's beliefs and expectations

Identify depression or other psychiatric disorder

Identify psychosocial problems

Many patients are reluctant to accept that their somatic symptoms may have psychological causes and that referral to a psychiatrist may be appropriate. Hence the clinician should adopt a tactful and sensitive approach. As noted above, it is important to discover the patient's views about the causes of his symptoms and to discuss them seriously. The patient should be made aware that the doctor believes his symptoms to be real. Physicians and psychiatrists should liaise closely to ensure consistency. The usual scheme of history taking and assessment should be followed. Special attention should be directed to eliciting the patient's beliefs about the symptoms and to describing the behavioural consequences, and to the relatives' reactions. It is important to obtain information from other informants as well as from the patient.

When a patient has unexplained physical symptoms, a psychiatric diagnosis should be made only on positive grounds. It should not be assumed that such symptoms are of psychological origin merely because they occur in relation to stressful events. Such events are common and may coincide with physical disease which, while not yet identifiable, is far enough advanced to produce symptoms. For the diagnosis of psychiatric disorder, the same strict criteria should be used for the physically ill as for the physically healthy.

Treatment

Symptoms that are persistent or recurrent despite reassurance are generally difficult to treat. Continuing symptoms without any specific medical explanation are likely to confirm and maintain worries about serious illness and those worries may be further exacerbated by secondary anxiety and behavioural consequences. Effective treatment should meet the patient's needs and also those of the family. A multicausal view of aetiology leads to conclusions about treatment and avoids psychiatric diagnoses that may be unacceptable to the patient.

The general principles of treatment (Table 16.4) are similar for all forms of unexplained symptoms, single or multiple, but individual treatment plans

Taable 16.4 **General principles of treatment of medically 'unexplained' symptoms**
Emphasize symptoms are real and familiar and that medical care is appropriate
Provide physical treatment for any associated established disease and co-ordinate physical and other care
Offer explanation and discuss
Allow patients and families to ask questions
Discuss the role of psychological factors in all medical care
Treat any primary psychiatric disorder
Agree a treatment plan

must take account of psychiatric diagnoses of anxiety or depression and the particular type of physical symptoms. The specific treatment of particular forms of somatoform disorders are described in Chapter 10. Sections below describe the treatment of chronic fatigue and some other common clinical syndromes. The therapist needs to be familiar with the clinical characteristics of common syndromes and be able to provide an appropriate combination of treatment methods. For example, the management of physical deconditioning is central to the treatment of chronic fatigue, whereas antidepressant medication has a major role in the treatment of atypical facial pain.

Many patients with somatic complaints seek repeated investigation and reassurance. Once all medically necessary investigations have been carried out, the patient should be told clearly that no further investigation is required. This information should be given with a combination of authority and willingness to discuss the investigations and their results. After this explanation, the aim should be to combine psychological management with treatment of any associated physical disorder.

It is important to avoid arguments about the causes of the symptoms. Many patients who do not fully accept psychological causes for their symptoms are, nevertheless, willing to accept that psychological factors may influence their perception of these symptoms. Such patients may accept guidance on learning to live more positively with their symptoms. Explanation and reassurance are usually effective in cases of recent onset. In chronic cases, however, reassurance is seldom helpful; sometimes repeated reassurance may even encourage increased complaining and seeking of more and more frequent reassurance (Salkovskis and Warwick 1986).

Specific treatments should be based on a formulation of the individual's difficulties. They include antidepressant medication for an underlying mood disorder and specific behavioural techniques such as anxiety management, graded practice, and cognitive therapy to modify beliefs about the origin and significance of symptoms.

Much can be achieved by good non-specialist care in primary care or by hospital physicians (Table 16.5), but chronic and recurrent problems may need specialist psychiatric and psychological treatment (Table 16.6). There is good evidence for the effectiveness of a range of treatments in specialist care, but there is much less evidence about simple, routine measures. Outlook for simpler syndromes of relatively recent onset is

Table 16.5 **Treatments suitable for non-specialist care**
Discussion and explanation of aetiology
Treatment of any minor underlying physical problem
Anxiety management (including tapes and handouts)
Advice on diary monitoring and graded return to full activities
Specific self-help programmes (e.g. chronic fatigue, irritable bowel)
Involvement of relatives and explanation of the treatment

Table 16.6 **Specialist treatments**
Psychotropic medication
Antidepressants
Anxiolytics
Cognitive-behavioural therapy
Interpretative psychotherapy: individual and group
Specific psychiatric treatment for associated psychiatric and social problems
Programme to coordinate and control all medical care

good but the prognosis for very prolonged chronic, multiple, or recurrent syndromes (for example, somatization disorder) is much less good. In these circumstances the control of medical care and the prevention of further iatrogenic disability may be more realistic than cure.

Chronic fatigue

Many terms, including post-viral fatigue syndrome, neurasthenia, and lay terms such as myalgic encephalomyelitis (ME), have been used to describe a disabling syndrome of chronic fatigue. Since there are many causes and in individual cases the aetiology is often uncertain, the descriptive term chronic fatigue syndrome is preferred. The main complaints are excessive and disabling fatigue at rest and prolonged exhaustion after minor physical and mental exertion, though other symptoms such as muscle pain and poor concentration are typically present. Operational criteria for diagnosis (Fukuda *et al.* 1994) require that the illness has lasted for at least 6 months and that other causes of fatigue have been excluded.

Clinical features

A central symptom is fatigue. Other common symptoms include muscular pains, poor concentration and those listed in Table 16.7. Other common characteristics are beliefs that the illness is purely physical, that the symptoms should indicate that it is important to avoid activity, marked and erratic variations in the extent of activity from day to day, frustration, depression, and loss of physical fitness.

Chronic fatigue syndrome has a long history. In the nineteenth century the symptoms were diagnosed as neurasthenia. In ICD-10 the syndrome can still be coded as *neurasthenia* (a diagnosis that is used widely in several countries including China (Lee 1994). There is considerable overlap between the operational definition of chronic fatigue and a number of other psychiatric symptoms, most notably depression, anxiety, and various somatoform disorders. Even so, the operational definition does have current clinical justification in assessment and treatment.

Epidemiology

Surveys of the general population indicate that persistent fatigue is experienced by about a quarter of the population at any one time. It is a common complaint amongst people attending in primary-care and out-patient clinics, but a small proportion of people who complain of excessive fatigue meet the criteria for chronic fatigue syndrome. Methodological problems make it difficult to determine prevalence but best estimates are between 0.3 and 1% of the general population.

The symptom of chronic fatigue is common in patients with other functional somatic syndromes, such as chronic pain, fibromyalgia, and irritable bowel. It is unlikely that these are truly separate entities; they appear to represent different presentations of multiple medically unexplained symptoms (Wessely *et al.* 1999).

Aetiology

The causes of chronic fatigue are controversial. Most research is of poor quality and discussion is made difficult by the activities of pressure groups convinced that the cause is entirely physical without any psychological component.

Suggested factors include:

♦ *physical causes* There is no convincing evidence for a general physical cause of the chronic fatigue syndrome. Many have been suggested,

---

Table 16.7 Case definition of chronic fatigue syndrome

Inclusion criteria

Clinically evaluated, medically unexplained fatigue of at least 6 months duration that is:

♦ of new onset (not life long)

♦ not result of ongoing exertion

♦ not substantially alleviated by rest

♦ a substantial reduction in previous level of activities

The occurrence of 4 or more of the following symptoms:

♦ subjective memory impairment

♦ sore throat

♦ tender lymph nodes

♦ muscle pain

♦ joint pain

♦ headache

♦ unrefreshing sleep

♦ post-exertional malaise lasting more than 24 hours

Exclusion criteria

Active, unresolved or suspected disease

Psychotic, melancholic or bipolar depression (but not uncomplicated major depression

Psychotic disorders

Dementia

Anorexia or bulimia nervosa

Alcohol or other substance misuse

Severe obesity

From Sharpe, M. and Wessely, S. (2000). Chronic fatigue syndrome. In *The new Oxford textbook of psychiatry* (eds M. G. Gelder, J. J. López-Ibor Jr, and N. C. Andreasen). Oxford University Press, Oxford. Reproduced by permission of Oxford University Press.

including chronic infection, immune dysfunction, a muscle disorder, neuroendocrine dysfunction, and ill-defined neurological disorders.

◆ *psychological factors* are important and there is evidence relating to attribution, perceptual processes, coping behaviours, and difficulties in communication.

◆ *physical activity* Inactivity leads to physical deconditioning which increases fatigues and discomfort. Patients characteristically alternate between relative overactivity, which results in tiredness and muscular discomfort, and periods of prolonged rest.

Although research into aetiology has been hindered by poor methodology, there is now evidence to support an interactive scheme of predisposing, precipitating, and perpetuating factors (Table 16.8). Probable *predisposing* factors include a past history of major depressive disorder and perhaps personality characteristics such as perfectionism. The *precipitation* by viral infection and life stresses appears to be important. *Perpetuating factors* may include neuroendocrine dysfunction, emotional disorder, physical disease attributions, and coping by avoidance. Chronic personal and social difficulties and media misinformation are also significant influences. See Sharpe and Wessely

(2000) and Wessely *et al.* (1998) for reviews of aetiology.

Course and prognosis

Clinical experience and systematic studies agree in suggesting a poor outcome with continuing long-term ill-health. However, it must be remembered that the majority of studies relate to patients referred to specialist centres and to patients with long histories prior to referral. Also, most refer to course before the introduction of the modern treatments reviewed below.

Evidence about treatment

Many treatments have been suggested but very few are of proven efficacy. Clinical experience suggests they do have a role, especially if there are marked depressive symptoms. There have been several randomized controlled trials of cognitive–behavioural therapy which have shown its advantage of standard medical care and relaxation therapy. For example, Sharpe *et al.* (1996) compared intensive rehabilitative cognitive–behavioural therapy with standard medical care. The superiority of cognitive–behavioural therapy was evident in improvement in disability and in subjective ratings of fatigue and depression. It was notable that disability improved only slowly and continued

Table 16.8 **Possible causal factors in chronic fatigue syndrome**			
	Predisposing	**Precipitating**	**Perpetuating**
Biological	Genetic	Virus	HPA axis disturbance
	Previous depression		Inactivity
Psychological	Personality (perfectionism)	Response to stress	Disease attribution
			Avoidant coping style
Social	?	Stresses	Life conflicts
			Iatrogenic factors

From Sharpe, M. and Wessely, S. (2000). Chronic fatigue syndrome. In *The new Oxford textbook of psychiatry* (eds M. G. Gelder, J. J. López-

during the follow-up period. Three-quarters of those in the intervention group returned to normal daily functioning, compared with only a quarter of those in the standard medical care condition.

Management

Assessment

Assessment should exclude any treatable organic or psychiatric cause of chronic fatigue. There should be a detailed description of the course of the symptoms and their consequences for the patient. It is important to enquire carefully about depressive symptoms, especially as patients may not at first reveal them. Although extensive physical investigations are unlikely to be rewarding, the psychiatrist can usefully collaborate with a physician when assessing these patients. The formulation should refer to the relevant factors summarized in Table 16.8. Sharpe and Wessely (2000) outline five basic steps essential to care:

◆ acknowledge the reality of the patient's symptoms and the disability associated with them;

◆ provide appropriate information about the nature of the syndrome to both the patient and their family, whilst avoiding unproductive argument about aetiology;

◆ treat identifiable depression and anxiety;

◆ encourage return to normal functioning by overcoming avoidance and regaining the capacity for physical activity;

◆ provide help with occupational and practical problems.

Drug treatment

When there is a definite depressive disorder, antidepressant drugs should be prescribed in usual doses. Clinical experience suggests selective serotonin re-uptake inhibitor (SSRI) drugs are best tolerated. Antidepressant drugs are also useful in reducing anxiety, improving sleep, and reducing pain.

Psychological (cognitive–behavioural) treatment

This includes education about the condition, correcting misconceptions about cause, and treatment.

Specific treatment includes *cognitive strategies* to correct misconceptions about the nature of the condition and excessive concern about activity, together with *behavioural strategies* to encourage a gradual increase in activity. In recent controlled trials, cognitive–behavioural treatment has been shown to be superior to standard care. Any other associated personal or social difficulties should be discussed using a problem-solving approach.

It is appropriate to explain that there is no evidence that the condition is due to chronic viral infection, even though the syndrome may be precipitated by an acute infection or other minor physical disorder. The role of psychological factors in perpetuating the disorder should be explained, and the doctor should emphasize that the syndrome is a real and disabling problem that is deserving of medical care. Arguments about the role of physical factors should be avoided; instead the effectiveness of graded activities in reducing the fatigue should be explained together with advice about the importance of avoiding bouts of strenuous exertion. See Wessely *et al.* (1998) and Sharpe and Wessely (2000) for reviews of chronic fatigue.

Irritable bowel syndrome

The irritable bowel syndrome is abdominal pain or discomfort, with or without an alteration of bowel habits, persisting for longer than 3 months in the absence of any demonstrable organic disease. The condition is common in gastroenterology clinics, and also amongst people who have not consulted a doctor. It is uncertain whether the condition is related to a disorder of intestinal motility, dietary fibre deficiency, or other physical factors. Research has proved little evidence of an association with life events, social factors, or psychiatric symptoms. However, psychological and social factors make it more likely that patients with these symptoms will seek treatment. These factors are associated with greater disability and may make management more difficult. Psychiatric disorder is common among clinic attenders, particularly those who fail to respond to treatment.

Patients with mild symptoms usually respond to education, reassurance about the disorder, dietary modification, and, when required, antimotility agents. More severe and chronic symptoms may be helped by specific psychological treatments. There is evidence that psychotherapy, behavioural methods, and antidepressants are effective with some patients (see Guthrie *et al.* 1991; Drossman 1998; Creed 1999; Blanchard 2001).

Fibromyalgia

The term fibromyalgia refers to a syndrome of generalized muscle aching, tenderness, stiffness, and fatigue, often accompanied by poor sleep. Women are affected more than men, and the condition is more common in middle age. The most important sign is the presence of multiple tender points. There is a marked overlap with chronic fatigue syndrome (Wessely *et al.* 1998).

The aetiology is uncertain. There may be physical causes, but the common association of the condition with other functional somatic symptoms suggests that psychological factors may play a part. (see McBeth and Silman 1999; Wessely and Hotopf 1999; see also Box 16.3). Controlled trials have shown that behavioural intervention is effective in preventing acute musculoskeletal pain from becoming chronic. There is no specific physical treatment, but the patient may be helped by the general psychological measures described above for the management of medically unexplained symptoms

Factitious disorder

This term was introduced in DSM-III to refer to self-inflicted signs and symptoms. DSM-IV defines factitious disorder as the 'intentional production or feigning of physical or psychological symptoms which can be attributed to a need to assume the sick role'. The category is divided further into cases with psychological symptoms only, those with physical symptoms only, and those with both. The classification in ICD-10 is similar. Factitious disorder differs from malingering (see p. 475) in that it does not bring any external reward such as

---

> **Box 16.3 Some other 'unexplained' symptoms**
>
> Facial pain
> Back pain
> Non-cardiac chest pain
> Palpitation
> Vertigo
> Non-ulcer dyspepsia
> Environmental allergy
> Forearm pain (repetitive strain injury)
> Gulf War syndrome

---

financial compensation. The term Munchausen syndrome is sometimes used to denote a small but striking subgroup of patients with the condition which is seen mainly in emergency departments and has a poor prognosis (see p, 475).

The prevalence of factitious disorder is not known with certainty, but it accounts for about 1% of referrals to consultation liaison services. Clinical features are very diverse, with both physical and psychological presentations. Factitious disorders usually begin before the age of 30 and there is often a history of an unexpectedly large number of childhood consultations with high rates of previous substance abuse, mood disorder, and personality disorder. Over half the reported patients in the major studies have worked in medically related occupations.

In the absence of large studies and with the knowledge that many patients' histories are substantially untrue, there is little good evidence about aetiology. Frequently reported themes include: parental abuse or neglect, early experiences of chronic illness or hospital care, and previous alleged medical mismanagement.

Course is variable but usually chronic. Few accept treatment, but others appear to improve during generally supportive medical care. In a proportion of cases there is evidence of other disturbed behaviours, such as child abuse and (for those working in health professions) harm to patients.

Management

Assessment

The suspicion of a factitious cause for physical symptoms should lead to a careful review of the available information, including the history given by informants as well as that provided by the patient. A psychiatrist may be able to assist in this assessment, and in cases of doubt further specialist physical investigation may be needed (Wallach 1994). Additional evidence may be obtained by careful observation of the patient, but the ethical and legal aspects of any decision to make covert observations should be considered.

Treatment

Once the diagnosis seems likely, the senior doctor should explain to the patient the findings and their implications. This should be done in a way that conveys an understanding of the patient's distress and enables a full discussion of the possible reasons for the behaviour. There are two main approaches:

♦ *Confrontation with evidence of the diagnosis* This is easier and more appropriate if there is clear evidence as to fabrication. The approach should be non-punitive and supportive, stressing the need for continuing care and suggesting what is available.

♦ *Non-confrontational* This approach is concerned with face-saving procedures to involve the patient in constructive treatment without the need to admit, and be confronted with, the original behaviours.

Although some patients admit their behaviour, others persistently deny that the symptoms are self-inflicted. In the latter cases, management should be directed to any associated psychological and social difficulties, and other appropriate care provided with the patient clearly aware of the doctors' views about aetiology. Patients with factitious disorder often cause difficulties on medical and surgical wards and in other medical settings. Staff anger on discovery of the deception may make continuing management the more difficult. A psychiatrist can help staff members by allowing them to discuss their feelings, the nature of the patient's behaviour, and the severity of the underlying psychological problems. Discussion and agreement between all the involved staff can be very helpful in enabling a treatment plan which will carefully define future medical care and offer appropriate help to the patient and family.

When factitious disorder is diagnosed in a health-care worker, the psychiatrist should consider whether the patient's continuing in clinical work would pose risks to patients, especially children, who may be harmed by interference in their treatment. Highly publicized cases of serious physical harm have rightly aroused considerable concern. It is essential for all those concerned in management to consider the issues carefully and seek expert medico-legal advice.

It is often helpful for staff discussion to include the ethical and legal issues summarized in Box 16.4. It may be sensible to obtain expert advice on breaching confidentiality in cases where it is thought there is a serious risk to others. Many experienced physicians feel it is unethical to search patients' belongings without having initially told the patient that factitious disorder is being considered and requesting permission to search belongings. This ethical problem does not arise in relation to discoveries (for instance, needles or syringes) made during the course of routine treatment. See Bass and Gill (2000) for a review of factitious disorder.

Box 16.4 Ethical and legal issues in factitious disorder

Confidentiality
♦ Disclosure to other parties (e.g. employers)
♦ Circulation of registers or 'blacklists'
Invasion of privacy
♦ Searching patients' belongings
♦ Videotaping
Involuntary treatment

'Munchausen syndrome'

Asher (1951) suggested the term Munchausen syndrome for the patient who is

admitted to hospital with apparent acute illness supported by a plausible or dramatic history. Usually his story is largely made up of falsehoods; he is found to have attended and deceived an astounding number of hospitals; and he nearly always discharged himself against advice after quarrelling violently with both doctors and nurses. A large number of scars is particularly characteristic of this condition.

This type of factitious disorder occurs mainly in early adult life and among men, and is usually encountered in dramatic manner in emergency departments. There is gross lying (pseudologia fantastica), which includes the giving of false names and invented medical histories. They may obstruct efforts to obtain information about themselves and may interfere with diagnostic investigations. They invariably discharge themselves prematurely. When further information is obtained, it often reveals many recurrent previous simulated illnesses. The aetiology and long-term outcome are unknown.

Factitious disorder by proxy

In 1977, Meadow described a form of child abuse in which parents (or other carers) give false accounts of symptoms in their children and may fake signs of illness (Meadow 1985). They seek repeated medical investigations and needless treatment for the children. Despite the name, it is *not* a factitious disorder as defined in DSM-IV.

The signs reported most commonly are neurological signs, bleeding, and rashes. Some children collude in the production of the symptoms and signs. The perpetrators usually have severe personality disorders and may themselves suffer from factitious disorder. Hazards for the children include disruption of education and social development. The prognosis is probably poor for both children and perpetrators, and there is a significant mortality. Some children may progress to the adult factitious disorder (Bools *et al.* 1993). Occasional

cases of murder of children by professional carers have been described as an extreme form of this disorder; some of these people also had factitious disorder.

Malingering

Malingering is the fraudulent simulation or exaggeration of symptoms. In DSM-IV it is said to differ from factitious disorder in that the production of symptoms is motivated by external incentives, whereas in factitious disorder there are no external incentives but a psychological need for the sick role. This distinction as well as the distinction from somatoform disorder can be difficult.

Malingering occurs most often among prisoners, the military, and people seeking compensation for accidents. Numerous types of clinical picture have been described:

- malingered psychosis, seen in those wishing to obtain admission to hospital for shelter, previously psychotic patients whose discharge is imminent or in criminal defendants trying to avoid standing trial or influence sentencing;

- 'Ganser's syndrome', a syndrome of so-called 'approximate answers' which is described on p. 267;

- malingered or exaggerated post-traumatic stress disorder;

- malingered cognitive deficit;

- malingered physical disease and disability.

Before malingering is diagnosed, there should always be a full medical examination. DSM-IV suggests that malingering should be strongly suspected if the following are observed:

- marked discrepancy between the person's claimed stress or disability and the objective findings;

- lack of cooperation during the diagnostic evaluation and treatment;

- the presence of antisocial personality disorder; and

- the medicolegal context.

When the diagnosis is certain, the patient should be informed tactfully. He should be encouraged to deal more appropriately with any problems that led to the symptoms, and in appropriate cases offered a face-saving way to give up the symptoms. It is always necessary to remember that people who are known to malinger also suffer genuine physical illness.

Surveillance by video or other means is used by lawyers or insurers, although seldom by clinicians for ethical reasons. Psychological tests and a number of specialist instruments have been suggested as aids in diagnosis. Careful and cautious interpretation is appropriate within consideration of the whole clinical picture. See Bass and Gill (2000) for a review.

Psychological and psychiatric consequences of physical illness

The most conspicuous feature of the emotional response of most people to serious physical illness is their resilience. Although distress is common, only in a minority is it severe enough to be classified as a psychiatric disorder. The general features of emotional reactions to stress have been described in Chapter 8, together with accounts of psychological defence mechanisms, coping responses, and the concepts of illness behaviour and sick role. Delirium, dementia, and cognitive disorders associated with specific medical conditions are discussed in Chapter 14. This section is concerned with emotional disorders consequent upon physical illness.

The usual emotional response to acute illness is anxiety, but as illness progresses, depressive symptoms become more prominent. The defence mechanisms of *denial* (see p. 188) and its partial form *minimization* are frequent, and may result in an unwillingness to accept the diagnosis or its implications. Such denial is usually short-lived but, if prolonged, may lead to poor compliance with treatment. In more chronic illness, depression is usually more prominent than anxiety, although fluctua-

tions in the course and treatment of events may evoke further periods of anxiety.

Psychiatric disorder

Psychiatric disorder is present in up to 30% of patients with serious acute, recurrent, or progressive physical illness. However, there are difficulties in the use of standard criteria for the diagnosis of psychiatric disorder in the physically ill; this is especially true of depression. Physical illness may cause symptoms such as fatigue and poor sleep, which are among the criteria of psychiatric disorder. Although modifications to the criteria have been suggested to make them more appropriate for patients with physical as well as psychiatric disorder, none is wholly satisfactory.

Although *adjustment disorders*, *anxiety*, and *depression* are the commonest psychiatric consequences, physical illness may precipitate many types of psychiatric disorder (Table 16.9). There is also a raised rate of suicide in the physically ill as compared with the general population, specific

Table 16.9 Psychiatric disorder in the physically ill

Adjustment disorder

Major depression

Anxiety disorder:

    Generalized anxiety disorder

    Panic disorder

    Phobic disorder

    Acute stress disorder

    Post-traumatic stress disorder

Somatoform disorder

Substance misuse

Eating disorder

Sleep disorder

Factitious disorder

Sexual disorders

associations being reported for cancer, multiple sclerosis, and a number of other conditions. See Harris and Barraclough (1995) for a review of suicide, Mayou and Sharpe (1995) for a review of the epidemiology of psychiatric disorder in association with physical illness.

Other psychologically determined consequences

Physical morbidity and mortality

It has been shown that psychosocial variables have direct effects on the course of physical disorder, for example, ischaemic heart disease (Frasure-Smith *et al.* 1995) and cancer (Spiegel and Classen 1999).

Quality of everyday life

Patients vary in their capacity to adjust to physical illness; most manage well but a few develop social handicaps out of proportion to the severity of the illness. A few patients use physical illness as a reason to avoid responsibilities, for others illness is an opportunity to reconsider their way of life and improve its quality. Sexual function is often affected by physical illnesses and treatments (Table 16.10).

Effects on the family

Physical illness may place a considerable burden on the family. Although family ties may be strengthened when a member becomes ill, others may experience considerable distress or develop psychiatric disorder. These effects may result in increased use of medical services by other family members. Children are affected as well as adults; some have to assist in caring for a parent.

Effects on compliance and on the use of medical resources

Marital state, beliefs, and other psychological variables are amongst the most important determinants of patient consultation and attitudes to the use of medical care (for example see DiMatteo *et al.* 2000). Psychoeducational interventions have a substantial place in improving outcome and cost-effectiveness.

Table 16.10 Some medical conditions associated with impaired sexual function

Endocrine disorder
   Diabetes
   Hypogonadism
   Hypopituitarism
Cardiovascular disorders
   Myocardial infarction
   Vascular disease
Respiratory failure
Chronic renal failure
Neurological disorders
   Spinal cord damage
   Damage to higher centres
Pelvic surgery
Disabling arthritis
Medication
   Anticholinergic drugs
   Hormones
   Psychotropic drugs (phenothiazines, antidepressants)
   Antihypertensive drugs
   Diuretics
   L-Dopa
   Indomethacin

Determinants of psychiatric consequences of physical illness

The prevalence and nature of psychiatric disorder is determined by factors relating to the physical illness and its treatment on one hand, and to the patient's personality and circumstances on the other (Table 16.11).

The physical disease as a cause of

    Symptomatic psychiatric disorder

    Threat to normal life

    Disability

    Pain

Nature of the treatment

    Side-effects

    Mutilation

    Demands for self-care

Factors in the patient

    Psychological vulnerability

    Social circumstances

    Other life stresses

Reactions of others

    Family

    Employers

    Doctors

The physical illness and its treatment

Certain types of physical illness are particularly likely to provoke serious psychiatric consequences. These include life-threatening acute illnesses and recurrent progressive conditions. Psychiatric disorder is more common in chronic illness when there are distressing symptoms such as severe pain, persistent vomiting, and severe breathlessness; self-care is demanding when there is severe disability. Physical illness is likely to have more serious psychological consequences when its effects are particularly significant to the patient's life, for example, arthritis of the hands of a pianist.

Psychiatric disorder directly caused by physical illness

In addition to delirium and dementia, a number of other psychiatric disorders are directly caused by physical illnesses, for example acute infection, endocrine disorders, and some forms of malignancy (see p. 494).

Psychological symptoms induced directly by physical illness

Some of the many psychological symptoms that can be caused directly by physical illness are shown in Table 16.12. Because all the symptoms listed in this table are commonly encountered in psychiatric practice, the psychiatrist should be on the lookout for undetected physical illness in any patient presenting with such symptoms. Occasionally they are presenting features before physical symptoms have become conspicuous.

Table 16.12 **Some organic causes of common psychiatric symptoms**

Depression
Carcinoma, infections, neurological disorders including dementias, diabetes, thyroid disorder, Addison's disease, systemic lupus erythematosus

Anxiety
Hyperthyroidism, hyperventilation, phaeochromocytoma, hypoglycaemia, neurological disorders, drug withdrawal

Fatigue
Anaemia, sleep disorders, chronic infection, diabetes, hypothyroidism, Addison's disease, carcinoma, Cushing's syndrome, radiotherapy

Weakness
Myasthenia gravis, McArdle's disease and primary muscle disorder, peripheral neuropathy, other neurological disorders

Episodes of epilepsy
Hypoglycaemia, phaeochromocytoma, porphyria, early dementia, toxic states, transient global amnesia

Headache
Migraine, giant-cell arteritis, space-occupying lesions

Loss of weight
Carcinoma, diabetes, tuberculosis, hyperthyroidism, malabsorption

Treatments causing physical symptoms

Table 16.13 lists some commonly used therapeutic drugs that may produce psychiatric symptoms as side-effects. Whenever psychological symptoms are found in a medical or surgical patient, the possibility should be considered that they have been induced by medication. Other treatments associated with psychiatric disorder include radiotherapy, cancer chemotherapy, and mutilating operations such as mastectomy.

Individual psychological factors and beliefs

Patients who have histories of previous psychological problems in relation to stress, and those who have suffered other adverse life events or are in difficult social circumstances, are at greater risk of both acute and persistent psychiatric distress associated with physical illness.

Illness perceptions

The ways in which people perceive their illness and medical care determines the subjective experience of the symptoms, distress, and behaviour (see Petrie and Weinmann 1997; Weinmann and Petrie 2000). Illness meanings include: threat, loss and failure, feelings of stigma, and feeling isolated.

Coping

There is considerable variation in coping behaviours, active or passive. They are most constructively directed to seeking appropriate information and finding ways of overcoming or minimizing the effects of symptoms and limitations.

The reaction of others

The reactions of family, friends, employers, and doctors may affect the psychological impact of

---

Table 16.13 Some drugs with psychological side-effects

Drug	Side-effect
Antiparkinsonian agents	
Anticholinergic drugs (benzhexol, benztropine, procyclidine)	Disorientation, agitation, confusion, visual hallucinations
L-Dopa	Acute organic syndrome, depression, psychotic symptoms
Antihypertensive drugs	
Methyldopa	Tiredness, weakness, depression
Calcium-channel blockers	
Clonidine	
Sympathetic blockers	Impotence, mild depression
Digitalis	Disorientation, confusion, and mood disturbance
Diuretics	Weakness, apathy, and depression (due to electrolyte depletion)
Analgesics	
Salicylamide	Confusion, agitation, amnesia
Phenacetin	Dementia with chronic abuse
Antituberculous therapy	
Isoniazid	Acute organic syndrome and mania
Cycloserine	Confusion, schizophrenia-like syndrome
Steroids	

physical illness. They may reduce the consequences by their support, reassurance, and other help, or they may increase it by their excessive caution, contradictory advice, or lack of sympathy.

Prevention

Good, well organized care for the physical illness is fundamental in minimizing the psychological and psychiatric consequences. Additional help should be focused on patients suffering illnesses or undergoing treatments which are known to be associated with psychiatric disorder, and on patients who are psychologically vulnerable.

Evidence on treatment

There have been relatively few randomized controlled trials of drug or psychological treatments for those with physical illness and many of these are methodologically inadequate. There is relatively good evidence of the effectiveness of both tricyclic and SSRI antidepressants. Cognitive– behavioural and other psychological interventions have been widely used in clinical practice but there have been rather few adequate clinicial trials. In the absence of high-quality evidence it is reasonable to assume that the treatments shown to be effective in those who are not physically ill would also be effective in those with a medical disorder.

Management

Assessment

Assessment is similar to that for psychiatric disorder in other circumstances, except that the doctor needs to be well informed about the nature and prognosis of the physical illness. Doctors should be aware that certain symptoms, such as tiredness and malaise, may be features of both physical and psychiatric disorders. It is important to distinguish anxiety and depressive disorders from normal emotional responses to physical illness and its treatment. This distinction is based partly on clinical experience of the reactions of other patients with similar illness, and partly on eliciting

symptoms that seldom occur in normal distress (such as hopelessness, guilt, loss of interest, and severe insomnia). Assessment of sexual problems should take account of the known association between medical conditions and treatments and impaired sexual function (Table 16.10).

The initial diagnostic assessment should also be considered as an important part of treatment (Price 2000). This includes simple measures to understand the patient's beliefs and worries, explanation of the diagnosis and its implications, and clear and informative communication with others who will be involved in care. Advice on ways of coping with the effects of treatment is always helpful. Written booklets and audio or video tapes are useful in providing information about the effects of the disorder, but patients and families also need to be able to ask questions and discuss their individual concerns.

Treatment

Although emotional distress is inevitable in physical illness, it can be reduced by emotional support, appropriate reassurance, advice, information, and practical help. It is essential to reduce the patient's fears and uncertainty by clear explanation of the illness and its treatment and the opportunity to allow patients to express their worries and fears. The patient must be involved in decision making and, wherever possible, the family should have an opportunity to discuss plans and the ways in which they can help. Psychiatric disorder is treated with the methods appropriate for the same disorder occurring in a physically healthy person.

Successful treatment of chronic illness depends on clearly formulated plans agreed with patients. These should include sympathetic support, information and advice, collaborative use of medical, social, voluntary, and other services, active regular follow-up, a behavioural approach to activity and self-care, and the involvement of families and carers. A minority require specialist psychiatric and psychological treatments (see Vonkorff *et al.*, 1997).

Drug therapy

Hypnotic and anxiolytic drugs are valuable for short periods when distress is severe, for example, during treatment in hospital. The indications for antidepressants are probably the same as those for patients who are not physically ill, but there have been too few satisfactory trials to be certain about the precise indications for the drug treatment of depression in medically ill patients. The side-effects and interactions of psychotropic drugs should be considered before prescribing for patients who are physically ill.

Cognitive and behavioural methods

Much medical advice is behavioural. Specific specialist interventions have varied aims, for example, to prevent side-effects of treatment, increase medication compliance, reduce disproportionate disability, and to modify lifestyle risk factors. Many of the psychological treatments used in everyday clinical practice are poorly planned and lack an evidence base. However, more clearly defined cognitive–behavioural methods are increasingly available and popular (see Abel and Rouleau 2000; Kroenke and Swindle 2000; Yates and Bowers 2000).

Consultation and liaison psychiatry

Psychiatric services for general hospitals are widely referred to as consultation-liaison services. The two components of this term refer to two separate ways of conducting psychiatric work in a general hospital.

In *consultation work*, the psychiatrist is available to give opinions on patients referred by physicians and surgeons. In *liaison work* the psychiatrist is a member of a medical or surgical team, and offers advice about any patient to whose care he feels able to contribute. The liaison psychiatrist also assists other staff to deal with day-to-day psychological problems encountered in their work, including the problems of patients whom he does not interview himself. One of the aims of liaison is to increase the skills of other staff in assessment and management of psychological problems; by contrast, the consultation approach implicitly assumes that the other staff possess these skills.

In practice, most consultation liaison psychiatrists work in a way that combines elements of the two approaches. Either approach requires close personal professional contact between the psychiatrist and the physician.

General hospital consultation and liaison units vary in their size and organization. Some are staffed entirely by psychiatrists, and others by a team of psychiatrists, nurses, social workers, and clinical psychologists. In some countries, clinical psychologists provide a separate 'behavioural medicine' service. Some liaison services have in-patient beds for patients who are both medically ill and psychiatrically disturbed. In a few North American general hospitals with large consultation-liaison services, up to 5% of all admissions are referred to psychiatrists. In the UK and many other countries, a smaller proportion of in-patients are referred, most being emergencies including deliberate self-harm (see Chapter 17).

Most of the literature on consultation-liaison psychiatry has focused on referral of in-patients. By contrast, the majority of the workload in most established units relates to those who have not been admitted – emergency department attenders, and out-patients. The future of consultation-liaison is increasingly seen as lying in the provision of specialist psychiatric and psychological expertise, to attenders with medically unexplained symptoms and collaborative management of patients with psychiatric difficulties associated with chronic physical illness. This requires the administrative and clinical skills to work with hospital clinical teams and with primary care. For further information about consultation and liaison psychiatry see Stoudemire *et al.* (2000).

The psychiatric consultation

The consultation has two parts: assessment of the patient and communication with the doctor making the referral. Assessment is not essentially different from that of any other patient referred for a psychiatric opinion but it is necessary to take into account the patient's physical state and willingness to see a psychiatrist.

The referral

On receiving the request for a consultation, the psychiatrist should make sure that the referring doctor has discussed the psychiatric referral with the patient. Before interviewing the patient, the psychiatrist reads the relevant medical notes and asks the nursing staff about the patient's mental state and behaviour. The psychiatrist finds out what treatment the patient is receiving, and if necessary consults a reference book about the side-effects of any drugs.

The assessment interview

At the start of the interview the psychiatrist makes clear to the patient the purpose of the consultation. It may be necessary to discuss the patient's anxieties about seeing a psychiatrist and to explain how the interview may contribute to the treatment plan. Next, an appropriately detailed history is obtained and the mental state examined. Usually the physical state is already recorded in the notes, but occasionally it will be necessary to extend the examination of the nervous system. It is essential for the psychiatrist to have a full understanding of the patient's physical condition. At this stage it may be necessary to ask further questions of the ward staff or social worker, to interview relatives, or to telephone the family doctor and enquire about the patient's social background and any previous psychiatric disorder.

Clinical notes

The psychiatrist should keep separate full notes of the examination of the patient and of interviews with informants. His entry in the medical notes should differ from conventional psychiatric case notes. The entry should be brief and free of jargon, and should contain only essential background information. It should omit confidential information as far as possible and should concentrate on practical issues, including answering the questions

raised by the referring doctor. When an opinion is entered in the medical notes, the principles are similar to those adopted in writing to the primary care practitioner (see p. 64). It is important to make clear the nature of any immediate treatment that is recommended, and who is to carry it out. If the assessment is provisional until other informants have been interviewed, the psychiatrist should state when the final opinion will be given.

Discussion with the referrer

It is often appropriate to discuss the proposed plan of management with the consultant, ward doctor, or nurse in charge before writing a final opinion. In this way the psychiatrist can make sure that recommendations are feasible and acceptable, and that answers have been given to the relevant questions about the patient. The note should be signed legibly, and should tell the ward staff where the psychiatrist or a deputy can be found should further help be required.

Management

Recommendations about treatment are similar to those for a similar psychiatric disorder in a physically well patient. When psychiatric drugs are prescribed, attention should be paid to the possible effects of the patient's physical state on their metabolism and excretion, and to any possible interactions with other drugs prescribed for the physical illness. A realistic assessment should be made of the amount of supervision available on a medical or surgical ward, for example, for a depressed patient with suicidal ideas. No undue demands should be made, but with support from a psychiatrist the nursing staff can manage most brief psychiatric disorders that arise in a general hospital.

Continuing care

It is often difficult to ensure that psychiatric recommendations made during in-patient stay are acted upon and continued following discharge. It is sensible for the psychiatrist to give information directly to primary care and, on occasion, either to continue to see the patient as an out-patient or to refer to a community-based psychiatric team.

Some practical emergency problems

The successful management of a psychiatric emergency depends strongly on the initial clinical interview. The aims are to establish a good relationship with the patient, elicit information from the patient and other informants, and observe the patient's behaviour and mental state. A calm, yet firm, sympathetic approach often enables the doctor to understand the patient's worries and to deal with them in a way that makes it possible to agree about a solution. Although the pressures on the doctor in an emergency often make it difficult to follow this systematic approach, time can be saved and mistakes avoided if the assessment is as complete as the circumstances permit, and a calm and deliberate approach is adopted.

The anxious patient

The physical symptoms of panic are a frequent reason for emergency presentations. The patient can be talked through the episodes of panic, and *hyperventilation* responds to rebreathing into a paper bag. There may occasionally be an indication for a small dosage of a benzodiazepine. Explanation and review in primary care helps to identify underlying causes.

Anxiety may also be a complicating factor. Attending as an emergency can be an upsetting or bewildering experience and can be made worse by the response of uncomprehending staff. It is very often possible to relieve distress by an understanding manner and by explaining what is happening. Again, a small dosage of a benzodiazepine or hypnotic may be useful.

The angry patient

It can be very upsetting to doctors when a patient or relative is angry, but it is essential to keep calm, avoid doing or saying anything that may make the situation worse, and to be careful about physical safety (see below). The doctor should be honest and willing to give straightforward information. The doctor should try to understand what the patient wants and to find out why he is angry. Sometimes it may be helpful to comment on the patient's anger and to ask directly why he is so upset. It may be appropriate for a doctor to admit to feeling upset by any accusations that are being made, but it is never sensible to show anger or to be unduly submissive in manner. It may be necessary to apologize if it is appropriate (for example, if the patient has been kept waiting).

The aggressive or violent patient

If the patient is actually or potentially violent, it is essential to arrange for adequate but unobtrusive help to be available. If restraint cannot be avoided, it should be accomplished quickly by an adequate number of people using the minimum of force. Staff should always avoid attempting single-handed restraint. Physical contact (including physical examination) should not be attempted unless the purpose has been clearly understood by and agreed with the patient. Extreme caution is, of course, required with a patient thought to possess any kind of offensive weapon.

Emergency drug treatment of disturbed or violent patients

Diazepam (5–10 mg) may be useful for a patient who is frightened. For a more disturbed patient, rapid calming is best achieved with 2–5 mg haloperidol injected intramuscularly and repeated, if necessary, up to a usual maximum of 30 mg in 24 hours depending upon the patient's body size and physical condition. When distress and agitation are particularly severe, it may be helpful to combine haloperidol with a benzodiazepine. When the patient is calm, haloperidol may be continued in smaller doses, usually three to four times a day and preferably by mouth, using a syrup if the patient will not swallow tablets. The dosage depends on the patient's weight and on the initial response to the drug. Careful observations by nurses of the physical state and behaviour are necessary during this treatment. Extrapyramidal side-effects may require treatment with an anti-parkinsonian drug (see p. 674).

Problems in consent to treatment

The general principles relating to consent to treatment are discussed in Chapter 3. Psychiatrists are sometimes asked to give urgent advice about patients who are refusing to accept medical treatment. Patients may be unwilling to accept their doctors' advice for many reasons. Commonly it is because they are frightened or angry, or do not understand what is happening; occasionally the cause is a mental illness that interferes with the patient's ability to make an informed decision.

It has to be accepted that some patients will refuse treatment even after a full and rational discussion of the reasons for carrying it out, and, of course, it is a right of a conscious mentally compe-

---

Box 16.5 Medico-legal and ethical issues: patients who refuse to accept advice about emergency treatment

◆ *In life-threatening emergencies* where it is not possible to obtain the patient's consent (impaired consciousness, evidence of psychiatric disorder which cannot be immediately assessed), opinions should be obtained from medical and nursing colleagues, and, if possible, from the patient's relatives. Detailed records should be kept of the reasons for the decision. It is essential for all doctors to know the law about these matters in the country in which they are practising.

◆ If a patient has a *mental disorder that impairs the ability to give informed consent*, it may be appropriate to use legal powers of compulsory assessment and treatment of the mental disorder. The powers for compulsory treatment of a mental disorder do not give the doctor a right to treat concurrent physical illness against the patient's wishes. Successful compulsory treatment of the psychiatric disorder may result in the patient giving informed consent for the treatment of the physical illness.

---

tent adult to do so. However, in many countries (including the UK), it is accepted that the doctor in charge of the patient does have the right to give immediate treatment in life-threatening emergencies when he cannot obtain the patient's consent. Box 16.5 summarizes medico-legal issues. See Strain *et al.* (2000) for a review of ethical issues in the care of the medically ill. See Boland *et al.* (2000) for a review of the management of psychiatric syndromes in intensive care units.

Psychiatric aspects of medical procedures and conditions

Genetic counselling

The prevalence of genetic disease is between 4 and 5% of the population. Major single-gene diseases include cystic fibrosis and Duchenne muscular dystrophy, as well as sickle cell anaemia, which is common in some ethnic groups. Conditions with polygenic multifactorial inheritance are more common; they include coronary artery disease, hypertension, and diabetes. At present, genetic counselling is mainly concerned with the first group of conditions, although increasing knowledge of the genetics of polygenic conditions will increase the scope of counselling in the future. Genetic counselling is based on the results of two distinct approaches to detection:

◆ *genetic testing* for those who are known to be at high risk, such as close relatives of those who have inherited disorders;

◆ *genetic screening* of populations.

Genetic counselling about the *reproductive* risks of hereditary disease is mainly given to couples contemplating marriage or planning or expecting a child. The scope of counselling is growing rapidly because of increasing understanding of genetic mechanisms, improved methods for identifying carriers and for making prenatal diagnoses, and the prospects of gene therapy. It includes providing information about risks, helping family members to cope with worries caused by the diagnosis, and enabling them to take informed decisions about family planning. *Predictive* screening, which gives people information about their own chances of developing a disease, is increasingly frequent. This includes presymptomatic tests for conditions such as Huntingdon's disease and predispositional tests for risk factors. The latter indicate an increased risk, but not a certainty, of developing a disease – for example, genetic tests for hereditary breast and ovarian cancer. Predispositional testing will become the main type of genetic test in the near future, as genes predisposing to common conditions such as cancer, Alzheimer's disease, heart disease, and diabetes are discovered. Uptake rates for genetic tests depend on whether there are effective ways of treating or preventing the condition and also on how the test is offered.

Those who find that they have a genetic risk that predisposes themselves or a possible child to disease are more distressed than those whose test results are negative, although it is uncommon for this distress to be of psychiatric severity. Indeed, some people receiving positive test results have found relief as the uncertainty about their genetic status has been removed. Somewhat surprisingly, some people receiving negative test results experience difficulties in adjustment. Inevitably relationships amongst siblings, parents, and offspring may be complicated by the outcome of genetic testing. Box 16.6 summarizes the implications for good practice. See Marteau and Croyle (1998) for a review of psychological responses to genetic testing.

Genetic counselling is usually provided by the staff of genetic clinics, but there is also a need for counselling by primary-care doctors and specialists other than geneticists. Genetic counselling needs to be guided by a clear understanding of ethical issues, which affect both individuals and wider society (Box 16.7). It is often difficult to weigh the benefits of genetic testing for the individual and for other family members. As genetic testing increases, more guidance will be required about the best ways of dealing with the psychosocial impact of the results.

Box 16.6 Best practice in genetic counselling

In the light of current evidence, best practice for the conduct of genetic testing (presymptomatic, predispositional, and prenatal) includes the following points:

- The written protocol for the conduct of the testing programme should include how the laboratory tests are to be conducted and how communication with patients is to be managed.

- Before they decide whether to undergo a test, clear and simple information should be presented to those eligible for testing. Such information should include the advantages and disadvantages of testing, as well as the meaning of any possible test result.

- The initial offer of a test should be separated in time (a day or more) from the taking of a biological sample.

- Test results should be explained and support offered to all those tested and their relatives.

- The effectiveness of a testing programme in achieving good understanding as well as facilitating behaviours that reduce risk, without high levels of emotional distress or false reassurance, needs to be assessed, not assumed.

Box 16.7 Genetic counselling: ethical and legal issues

- Confidentiality
- Consent
- Storage and use of genetic information
- Testing children: It is generally believed that it is wise to delay testing until an age at which individuals can make their own decisions.
- Implications for life insurance

Counselling involves giving information about the results of tests and dealing with problems arising from these results. It should be non-directive, allowing those counselled to make decisions for themselves after receiving complete and up-to-date information. Counselling may be concerned with anxiety while awaiting the results of prenatal tests, distress before and after termination of pregnancy for medical reasons, distress about being a disease carrier, and worry about children at risk of an inherited disorder.

The nature of the information that should be given varies with the type of genetic risk. Usually, counselling is an opportunity to allay anxiety and to reassure, but occasionally it is necessary to help a couple to confront distressing facts and make difficult decisions. Successful counselling requires an awareness of the couple's circumstances, knowledge of the likely psychological and personal consequences of information about genetic risks, and, in appropriate cases, an understanding of the ethical and other aspects of termination of pregnancy. Receiving information about risk can be very distressing, especially for parents who have experienced a previous abnormal pregnancy.

After giving information about the risk of an inherited disorder, the counsellor should discuss alternative actions with the couple. These actions include effective contraception (which may include sterilization) and, where this is possible, prenatal diagnosis with the opportunity for termination. Counselling is more effective in imparting knowledge than in changing behaviour, and many couples choose to accept that their future children will be at high risk. See Svenson and Folstein (2000) for a review of the psychological aspects of testing for genetic disorders.

Screening for disease

Presymptomatic screening for disease is becoming widely established. Examples include prenatal screening for fetal abnormalities, and screening for breast and cervical cancers and for hypertension. The success of any programme depends in part upon psychological factors, which determine whether people attend for screening and whether those who attend are distressed by the experience. Participation in many screening programmes is low, and there have been few studies of ways of increasing uptake.

Screening can relieve long-standing worries about health. Most people cope well with the findings, but a few of those screened suffer marked distress. When the result of screening is negative, patients should be reassured. However, negative findings do not always allay anxiety, and screening may increase fears about health. These problems are greater in those recalled for further assessment. Although a positive finding on screening is distressing, so is the discovery of disease when symptoms or signs have developed. Psychiatrists can contribute to screening programmes by assisting in staff training, by helping in the production of information for patients, and by assessing and treating the most distressed patients. See Shaw *et al.* (1999) and Rimes and Salkovskis (2000) for reviews.

Psychiatric aspects of surgical treatment

Preoperative mental state and outcome

It is a matter of everyday observation that patients about to undergo surgery are often anxious. There is a linear relationship between anxiety before and after surgery. Most research shows, as would be expected, that those who show more general ability to cope with stress suffer fewer postoperative problems. Many, but not all, studies of psychological preparation for surgery have shown that intervention can reduce postoperative distress and problems, especially if it includes cognitive coping techniques rather than mere information. Psychiatrists may be asked to provide a preoperative assessment. Common reasons include:

- clarification of the role of emotional factors in the patient's physical complaints;
- uncertainty about the patient's cognitive state and capacity to provide informed consent;

- help in the management of current psychiatric problems;
- help in predicting the patient's response to surgery and ability to comply with continuing treatment requirements.

Psychiatric problems in the postoperative period

Delirium

Delirium is common after major surgery, especially in the elderly. The development of postoperative delirium also depends on the type of surgery, the type of anaesthetic, postoperative physical complications, and medication. Delirium is associated with increased mortality and longer stay in hospital. Distressing pain, poor sleep and poor compliance are all frequent problems which can normally be managed as part of routine postoperative care.

Pain

Patients who are given greater control over the timing of analgesia experience less pain and make less use of analgesia. Psychiatrists are sometimes asked to advise on the management of patients with unusually severe postoperative pain. Useful interventions include advice on the flexible use of analgesia, anxiety management, and resolution of any disagreements between the patient and staff.

Long-term psychological problems after surgery

Long-term psychological problems may follow surgery. Adjustment problems are particularly common after mastectomy and laryngectomy, and after surgery that has not led to the expected benefit. A psychiatrist may be able to help with these problems of adjustment, especially when the surgery is part of the management of a relapsing, chronic, or progressive disorder. It may be helpful to provide further information, to allow the expression of feelings, and to encourage problem solving. A minority of patients require specific psychological treatment or antidepressant medication. See Rodin and Abbey (2000) and Stoddard *et al.* (2000) for reviews.

Plastic surgery

People with physical deformities often suffer teasing, embarrassment, and distress, which may markedly restrict the lives of both adults and children. When patients are psychiatrically healthy, reconstructive plastic surgery usually gives good results. Even when there is no major objective defect, cosmetic surgery to the nose, face, breast, or other parts of the body is usually successful. Nevertheless, it is appropriate to carry out psychological assessment before plastic surgery because the outcome is likely to be poor in patients who have unrealistic expectations, a history of dissatisfaction with previous surgery, or delusions about their appearance. See Sarwer *et al.* (1998) for a review.

Limb amputation

Limb amputation has different psychological consequences for young and for elderly people. Young adult amputees, such as those losing a leg in military action or a road accident, characteristically show denial at first, and later experience depression and phantom limb pains, which resolve slowly. The outcome for children and adolescents seems similar. Older subjects usually undergo amputation after prolonged medical and surgical problems associated with vascular disease. Such patients do not commonly report severe distress immediately after the operation, but they often develop phantom limb pain. Some have difficulty with the prosthesis and show a degree of functional incapacity disproportionate to the physical state.

Organ transplantation

Technical advances in surgery and intensive care, and particularly the introduction of the immunosuppressant drug cyclosporin, have led to a rapid increase in availability of organ transplantation procedures, although these are limited by a shortage of donor organs. As procedures become routine, medical and psychiatric complications have diminished and are in many ways comparable to reactions to other major medical procedures. However, the nature of the surgery and the need for intensive continuing medical assessment and treatment are associated with considerable neuropsychiatric and other psychiatric consequences.

Selection for transplantation is stressful, particularly for seriously ill patients awaiting vital organ transplants as compared with kidney transplants for which continuing dialysis is available as an alternative treatment. Whilst psychological assessment is often said to have a role in selection for surgery, there are probably few psychological contraindications, most of which relate to inability to cope with demanding long-term medical care. Psychiatric assessment is more useful in planning support during the stressful time of waiting for surgery and during convalescence.

Transplantation is associated with the same psychiatric and emotional consequences described above for other major treatments. The nature of the surgery, the immunosuppressive drug regimen, and the social and family consequences all mean that delirium, anxiety, and depression are common. In addition to the general consequences of organ transplantation, there are issues specific to each type of organ transplant; for example, liver transplantation has the highest rate of pre- and postoperation neuropsychiatric complications.

The frequency and seriousness of psychiatric problems is such that specific psychiatric liaison should be available both to train and support staff and to advise on management of individual patients. See Trzepacz and DiMartini (2000) and House (2000) for reviews of transplantation.

Diabetes and endocrine disorders

Diabetes mellitus

Diabetes is a chronic condition requiring prolonged medical supervision and informed self-care, and many physicians emphasize the psychological aspect of treatment.

Psychological factors and diabetic control

Psychological factors are highly important in the course of established diabetes because they influence its control, and it is now generally accepted that good control of blood glucose is the single most important factor in preventing long-term complications. Psychological factors can impair control in two ways. First, stressful experiences can lead directly to endocrine changes. Second, many diabetics show poor self-care and poor compliance with medical advice, especially at times of stress, and this is an important cause of 'brittle' diabetes.

Problems of being diabetic

For the diabetic person, psychological and social problems may be caused by restrictions of diet and activity, the need for self-care, and the possibility of serious physical complications such as vascular disease and impaired vision. Although most diabetic patients adapt well to the limitations of their illness, an important minority of those with insulin-dependent and non-insulin-dependent diabetes have difficulties. Compliance with blood testing, diet, and insulin use is frequently unsatisfactory and as a result glycaemic control is often less than optimal. These problems are particularly prominent in adolescence.

Psychiatric problems include depression and anxiety. The prevalence of eating disorders amongst adolescent and young adult diabetic women may be slightly greater than in the non-diabetic population. When the two are combined, treatment is more difficult. Insulin misuse to promote weight loss is frequent among young women with diabetes. Psychological and social problems are especially common in diabetics with severe medical complications such as loss of sight, renal failure, and vascular disease.

Sexual problems are common among diabetics. Two kinds of impotence occur in diabetic men. The first is psychogenic impotence of the kind found in other chronic debilitating diseases. The second kind, which is more common in diabetes, may predate other features of the disease. It is thought to be associated with pelvic autonomic neuropathy, although vascular and endocrine factors may also contribute.

Pregnancy is a difficult time for diabetic women,

since there may be problems in the control of diabetes and increased risks of miscarriage and fetal malformations.

Organic psychiatric syndromes in diabetic patients

Evidence of acute cognitive impairment occurs in the prodromal stage of diabetic (hyperglycaemic) coma. It may present as an episode of disturbed behaviour, which may begin either abruptly or insidiously. Other prodromal physical symptoms include thirst, headaches, abdominal pain, nausea, and vomiting. The pulse is rapid and blood pressure is low. Dehydration is marked and acetone may be smelt on the breath

Mild dementia is not uncommon among those with chronic diabetes. It may be caused by recurrent attacks of hypoglycaemia or by cerebral arteriosclerosis. Dementia may develop in patients with associated cerebrovascular disease.

Psychiatric management

Medical treatment can be usefully supplemented with certain forms of specialist psychological intervention. The latter includes the treatment of depressive disorder, blood glucose awareness training to improve the ability to recognize and act on fluctuations in blood glucose concentrations, behavioural methods to improve self-care and relieve associated psychological and social problems, weight management programmes, and psychological and pharmacological treatment of sexual dysfunction. Tricyclic antidepressants may

---

Box 16.8 Endocrine disorders

Hyperthyroidism (thyrotoxicosis)

Presentation with psychiatric symptoms is common – anxiety, irritability, emotional lability, difficulty in concentrating. These, together with hyperactivity, fatigue and tremor, may make differential diagnosis from anxiety disorder difficult. Treatment of thyroid dysfunction usually results in improvement of the psychiatric symptoms. See p. 299 for relevance to aetiology of affective disorder.

Hypothyroidism (myxoedema)

Cognitive impairment is usual and other psychiatric disorders are common. Affective disorder may be rapid cycling form (see p. 282). Replacement therapy may reverse the psychiatric features but neuropsychiatric problems may be permanent. See Dugbartey (1998).

Hyperadrenalism (Cushing's syndrome)

Emotional disorder occurs in a high proportion of cases. Depressive symptoms are the most common but paranoid symptoms also occur, especially in those with the most severe physical illness. The severity of depressive symptoms is not closely related to plasma cortisol concentrations and premorbid personality and stressful life events appeared to predispose to affective disorder (see p. 298 for relevance of aetiology of affective disorder). Psychological symptoms usually improve quickly when the medical condition is controlled. See W. F. Kelly (1996) and Sonino and Fava (1998).

Steroid therapy

Affective symptoms, especially euphoria or mild mania, are frequent. Less common are paranoid symptoms. Severity of the mental disorder is not closely associated with dosage. Symptoms usually improve when the dosage is reduced but severe depressive mental disorder may require specific treatment. Lithium prophylactic should be considered for patients who need to continue steroid treatment after an affective disorder has been bought under control. Withdrawal of cortisol steroids may cause lethargy, weakness, and joint pain.

Anabolic steroids

Anabolic – androgenic – steroids are very widely used by athletes. Mood disturbances and increased aggression have been reported. See Wroblewska (1997).

be helpful in relieving the pain of neuropathy. See Jacobson (1996) for a review of psychological care of patients with insulin-dependent diabetes.

Other endocrine disorders

Many endocrine disorders, and most conspicuously thyroid dysfunction, have been associated with psychiatric complications. Box 16.8 summarizes some of the more common associations. See Kornstein *et al.* (2000) for a review of the psychiatric aspects of endocrine disorder.

Cardiac disorders

For many years, it has been assumed that emotional disorder predisposes to ischaemic heart disease and Dunbar (1954) described a 'coronary personality'. Such ideas are difficult to test because only prospective studies can separate psychological factors present before the heart disease from the psychological effects of being ill. Recent research has concentrated on several groups of possible risk factors including chronic emotional disturbance, social and economic disadvantage, overwork or other chronic stress, and the type A behaviour pattern. The most intensively investigated of these factors is the type A behaviour pattern, which is defined as hostility, excessive competitive drive, ambitiousness, a chronic sense of urgency, and a preoccupation with deadlines (Friedman and Rosenman 1959). Although type A behaviour has been widely accepted to be an independent risk factor for ischaemic heart disease, recent evidence has cast doubt on this conclusion. A systematic review (Hemingway and Marmot 1999) suggests the following conclusions:

- In prospective cohort studies, a possible primary aetiological role has been shown for type A: hostility, depression and anxiety, psychosocial work characteristics and lack of social support.

- In populations of patients with established coronary heart disease, prospective studies show a prognostic role for depression and anxiety, psychosocial work characteristics, and

lack of social support. There is no evidence of a prognostic role for type A or hostility.

- Stressful life events can precipitate acute ischaemic syndromes.

Primary and secondary prevention have largely concentrated on changing lifestyle risk factors such as smoking, diet, and lack of physical activity. Attempts have also been made to alter type A behaviour (Friedman *et al.* 1986). The positive findings need replication and there are unanswered questions about the mechanisms and interpretation of the findings.

More recent research has concentrated on the findings that depression (Frasure-Smith *et al.* 1995), anxiety, and social isolation are important risk factors for the outcome of coronary artery disease (see Frasure-Smith and Lespérance 2000; Januzzi *et al.* 2000). As a result, considerable current research is concerned with evaluating interventions to treat depression and to reduce social isolation.

Angina

Angina is often precipitated by emotions such as anxiety, anger, and excitement. It can be a frightening symptom, and some patients become overcautious despite reassurance and encouragement to resume normal activities. Angina may be accompanied by atypical chest pain and breathlessness caused by anxiety or hyperventilation. There is often little relationship between objectively measured exercise tolerance and the patient's complaints of chest pain and limitation of activity. Patients with silent ischaemia on exercise testing appear to be less sensitive to pain and other bodily sensations than those with angina. Surgical and medical treatment together with regular and appropriate exercise can be highly effective. Individually planned programmes of information and training in self-help skills can produce increased confidence, a reduced frequency of symptoms, and less disability (see Lewin 1999). It has been claimed that an intensive programme designed to change lifestyle can result in regression of coronary atherosclerosis (Ornish *et al.* 1990), but this finding requires confirmation.

Myocardial infarction

Patients often respond to the early symptoms of myocardial infarction with denial, and consequently delay seeking treatment. In the first few days in hospital acute organic mental disorders and anxiety symptoms are common. Emotional distress may be an important cause of arrhythmias and sudden death. Mood disorder is associated with an increase of subsequent mortality (Frasure-Smith *et al.* 1995).

Survivors of cardiac arrest may suffer cognitive impairment. When such impairment is mild, it often manifests later as personality change or behavioural symptoms which may be attributed wrongly to an emotional reaction to the illness.

When patients return home from hospital, they commonly report non-specific symptoms such as fatigue, insomnia, and poor concentration, as well as excessive concern about somatic symptoms and an unnecessarily cautious attitude to exertion. Most patients overcome these problems and return to a fully active life. A few continue with emotional distress and social disability out of proportion to their physical state, often accompanied by atypical somatic symptoms. Such problems are more common in patients with long-standing psychiatric or social problems, overprotective families, and myocardial infarction with a complicated course.

Attempts have been made to reduce these psychological problems by using various forms of rehabilitation, in which the most important component seems to be early mobilization. Other components include exercise training, education, and group therapy. Exercise training has been used widely but does not seem to be particularly effective in reducing psychological problems. A self-help programme including anxiety management and behavioural advice has been reported to lead to an improved return to full activities (Lewin *et al.* 1992). It is important to treat the small minority of patients with persistent depression or with other emotional or social problems (Lespérance and Frasure-Smith 2000). Major depression should be treated with an antidepressant drug that is not cardiotoxic, such as an SSRI (see Seiner and Mallya 1999).

Non-cardiac chest pain

During the American Civil War, Da Costa (1871) described a condition which he called 'irritable heart'. This syndrome consisted of a conviction that the heart was diseased, together with palpitations, breathlessness, fatigue, and inframammary pain. This combination has also been named 'disorderly action of the heart', 'effort syndrome', and 'neuro-circulatory asthenia'. The symptoms were originally thought to indicate a functional disorder of the heart.

Non-cardiac chest pain, in the absence of heart disease and often associated with complaints of breathlessness and palpitations, is very common among patients in primary care and in cardiac out-patient clinics. Most patients with the symptoms are reassured by a thorough assessment, but a significant minority continue to complain of physical and psychological symptoms and to limit their everyday activities. Follow-up studies of patients with chest pain and normal coronary angiograms have consistently found subsequent mortality and cardiac morbidity to be little greater than expectation, but persistent disability to be common.

Many causes have been suggested for atypical cardiac symptoms including pain originating in the chest wall, oesophageal reflex and spasm, microvascular angina, mitral valve prolapse, and psychiatric disorder. In most patients chest pain appears to be due to minor non-cardiac physical causes or to hyperventilation, together with anxiety, which are then misconstrued as heart disease. The aetiology is as described for medically unexplained symptoms (see p. 464). The most common psychiatric concomitant is panic disorder; less common are depressive disorder and hypochondriasis.

Management should follow the general principles described on p. 468 with a particular emphasis on the treatment of hyperventilation, graded increase in activity, and discussion of beliefs about the course of the pain. Cognitive–behavioural treatments are effective in the management of anxiety and hyperventilation (Mayou *et al.* 1998). Depressive disorder should be treated with antidepressant medication. See Chambers *et al.* (1999) for a review.

Sensory disorders

Sensory disorders of deafness and blindness cause difficulties for doctors as well as for sufferers. It is essential to make special efforts in communication and to do so in a way that ensures the patient is not made to feel a burden on the clinician.

The onset of sensory loss leads to fear, frustration, and grief for patients and for relatives. These are often made worse by lack of sympathy and understanding from other people. Although many people adjust in the long term, a large minority suffer continuing anxiety and depression with a wide range of personal and social difficulties.

In the majority of cases where the sensory loss is gradual it is possible to promote measures that will provide information and practical techniques and also enable the patient and family to begin the processes of grief and adjustment. Contacts with voluntary organizations of sufferers and their relatives are often very helpful. Those responsible for medical care need to encourage the use of rehabilitation and voluntary and other services, and be ready to refer those who do not make progress to specialist services. See Fitzgerald and Parkes (1998) for a review.

Deafness

Deafness may develop before speech is learned (prelingual deafness) or afterwards. Profound early deafness interferes with speech and language development, and with emotional development. When patients with this condition leave school at age 16, they are on average 8 years behind children with normal hearing. Prelingually deaf adults often keep together in their own social groups and communicate by sign language. They appear to develop behaviour problems and social maladjustment more often than emotional disorder. For the management of such problems, special knowledge of the practical problems of deafness is required.

Deafness of later onset has less severe effects than those just described. However, the acute onset of profound deafness can be extremely distressing, whilst milder restriction of hearing may cause depression and considerable social disability.

Kraepelin was the first to suggest that deafness is an important factor in the development of persecutory delusions. Current evidence supports an association between deafness and paranoid disorders in the elderly (see p. 633). See Hindley and Kitson (1999) for a review.

Tinnitus

Tinnitus is very common, but few patients seek treatment and most are able to live a normal life. Persistent tinnitus may be associated with low mood. Some patients are helped by devices that mask tinnitus with a more acceptable sound. Antidepressant medication may improve mood and reduce the intensity of the tinnitus. Cognitive and behavioural methods may enable people to accept their tinnitus and to minimize their social handicaps.

Blindness

Although it imposes many difficulties, blindness in early life need not lead to abnormal psychological development in childhood (Graham and Rutter 1968; Ammerman *et al.* 1986) or to unsuccessful later development. In previously sighted people, the later onset of blindness causes considerable distress. Initial denial and subsequent depression are common, as are prolonged difficulties in adjustment. See Fitzgerald and Parkes (1998).

Infections

Viral encephalitis is often accompanied by psychiatric symptoms. In addition, some infectious diseases, for example hepatitis A, influenza, and brucellosis, are frequently followed by periods of depression. Psychological factors may affect the course of recovery from an acute infection (Hotopf *et al.*, 1996). In one early study, psychological tests were completed by 600 people who subsequently developed Asian influenza. Delayed recovery from the influenza was no more common among people whose initial illness had been severe, but it was more frequent among those who had obtained more abnormal scores on the psychological tests before the illness (Imboden *et al.* 1961). Recent findings of research on viral illness in general practice and infectious mononucleosis have reported similar conclusions (see White *et al.*, 1998). The role of infection as a cause of chronic fatigue syndrome is discussed on p. 470.

HIV infection

HIV infection is common. The brain is affected at an early stage and the disease has a chronic progressive course associated with a wide range of psychiatric consequences. The nature of the physical symptoms, their relentless progressive course, and the reactions of other people all explain why emotional distress is common in patients with HIV infection. A further reason is that some of the groups at high risk for HIV (for example, those with haemophilia and drug abusers) may have other psychological problems. Neuropsychiatric disorders also occur in people with HIV infection. Even so, many patients with AIDS manage to lead relatively normal lives for substantial periods. Men with AIDS and haemophilia do not appear to have psychological problems greater than those of other AIDS patients.

Fears of infection and reaction to testing

Although surveys suggest that worry about having AIDS is not uncommon in the general population, severe concern is infrequent. Although HIV antibody testing is worrying for most of those who undergo it, the distress is usually short-lived whatever the outcome of the test. People who have persistent and unjustified worries about having AIDS require psychiatric help of the kind appropriate for other illness fears (see p. 468).

Psychiatric problems include adjustment disorder, depressive disorder, and anxiety disorder. These disorders may occur at any stage of the disease, but are particularly frequent at the time of diagnosis. People with previous psychological problems, long-standing social difficulties, or lack of social support are especially vulnerable.

Suicide and deliberate self-harm may occur in people who are concerned about the possibility of HIV infection as well as in people with proven disease. Among the latter, the risk is greater in those with advanced symptoms. However, it is not certain how much greater is the risk of suicide and deliberate self-harm in AIDS patients than in the general population. Effects on the family may be considerable, as they may be with any serious medical disorder. These effects are particularly significant where the partner and especially the children also suffer from the infection.

In general, women have a similar psychiatric morbidity to men but they are especially concerned about the effects on childbearing.

Neuropsychiatric disorders are common, both secondary to the complications of immune suppression and as direct effects of HIV on the brain. HIV-associated dementia (AIDS-dementia complex), HIV encephalopathy and subacute encephalitis occur late in the illness in around a third of patients. There is usually an insidious onset with progression to profound dementia. Minor cognitive disorders are frequent. HIV infection can also result in neurological symptoms and dementia in those who do not have AIDS. Several acute and subacute organic syndromes have been described, of which the most frequent is subacute encephalitis. Delirium may occur when there is an opportunistic infection or cerebral malignancy. See Maj (2000) for a review of dementia associated with HIV infection.

Social consequences are considerable both because of the public fears of the condition and stigma; they are much greater than for other major neuropsychiatric conditions. Cultural differences in acceptance or rejection and in the availability of family and other support are major determinants of quality of life.

Problems in relation to illicit drug use are considered on p. 562. The disorganized way of life of some drug users and their personal and social problems make the treatment of HIV difficult.

Treatment

Psychiatrists should be involved in planning services for AIDS patients; they may provide counselling and specialist treatment for neuropsychiatric and other psychiatric complications. It is not yet known what scale of long-term care-scale facilities may be required for AIDS patients who develop dementia.

Ethical and legal issues

The public fear and stigma of AIDS and the dangers of transmission of HIV have led to considerable debate about ethical and legal aspects of the infection:

♦ the importance of maintaining confidentiality;

♦ disclosure to third parties at risk of infection;

♦ disclosure to insurers and to employers;

♦ protection of the public from any risk of transmission from HIV-infected health-care workers.

Psychiatrists confronted by any of these issues should seek local legal or other informed advice.

See Bialer *et al.* (2000) and Grant and Atkinson (2000) for reviews of the psychiatric aspects of HIV infection.

Cancer

Psychological factors in aetiology and prognosis

It is not surprising that cancer patients have emotional reactions to the disease. Some writers have suggested the opposite relationship, namely that psychological factors, including depression, personality traits, the suppression of anger, and stressful life events, may play a part in the aetiology of cancer. Overall, much of the evidence for this idea is not convincing, partly because the research on which it is based has severe limitations of methodology, including reliance on retrospective accounts and on subjective or non-standardized methods of assessment. There is more convincing evidence of the role of these factors on the course and outcome of cancer. For example, studies of group therapy (Spiegel and Barlow 2000) have led to the claim that this treatment improves prognosis. Research with animals has indicated that the rate of tumour growth may be increased in animals exposed to stressful situations that are only partially under their control. This finding suggested the possibility that endocrine or immunological mechanisms may mediate the effects of emotion on the prognosis of malignancy. See Spiegel and Kato (1996) and Spiegel and Classen (1999) for reviews of the effects of psychological treatment on prognosis.

It has been suggested that depressive symptoms may be a precursor of cancer in various sites. The issue remains unproved, and it is unlikely that with one possible exception, *carcinoma of the pancreas*, any association is of practical significance.

Psychological consequences of cancer

The psychological consequences of cancer are similar to those of any serious physical illness:

♦ Some patients *delay seeking medical help* because they fear or deny symptoms (Ramirez *et al.* 1999).

♦ *The diagnosis of cancer* may cause shock, anger, and disbelief, as well as anxiety and depression. The most common associated psychiatric disorder is adjustment disorder (Van't Spijker *et al.* 1997). The risk of suicide is increased in the early stages (Harris and Barraclough 1995). Depressed mood is particularly likely at the time of diagnosis and following relapse but is usually transient.

♦ *Longer-term consequences* Major depression occurs throughout the course of cancer affecting 10–20% of patients and appears to be more frequent in those suffering pain. However, patients with cancer are no more depressed than other physically ill patients, and the majority do not experience long-term distress unless the disorder progresses or unless they are particularly vulnerable to stress (Holland 1998).

♦ Both the *progression* and the *recurrence* of cancer are often associated with increased psychiatric disturbance, which may result from a worsening of physical symptoms such as pain and nausea, from fear of dying, or from the development of an organic psychiatric syndrome.

♦ *Delirium and dementia* may arise from brain metastases, which originate most often from carcinoma of the lung, but also from tumours of the breast and alimentary tract, and from melanomas. Occasionally, brain metastases produce psychiatric symptoms before the primary lesion is discovered.

♦ *Neuropsychiatric problems (paraneoplastic syndromes)* are sometimes induced by certain kinds of cancer in the absence of metastases, notably by carcinoma of the lung, ovary, breast, stomach and Hodgkin's lymphoma. The aetiology is thought to be an autoimmune response to the tumour.

Treatment for cancer may cause psychological disorder. Emotional distress is particularly common after mastectomy and other mutilating surgery. *Radiotherapy* causes nausea, fatigue, and emotional distress. *Chemotherapy* often causes malaise and nausea, and anxiety about chemotherapy may cause anticipatory nausea before the treatment. The latter may be helped by behavioural treatments in addition to antiemetic medication.

Family and other close relatives of cancer patients may experience psychological problems, which may persist even if the cancer is cured. Nevertheless, many patients and relatives make a good adjustment to cancer. The extent of their adjustment depends partly on the information they receive.

Psychological treatment

In the past doctors have been reluctant to tell patients that the diagnosis is cancer, but most patients prefer to know the diagnosis and how it will affect their lives. The quality of communication is often unsatisfactory and when this happens there may be consequences for psychological adjustment. The problem is particularly difficult when the patient is a child; even then it is generally better to explain the diagnosis in terms appropriate to the child's stage of development.

Depression (see Newport and Nemeroff 1998) and anxiety disorders should be recognized early and treated according to standard psychiatric procedures. Various other specific psychiatric interventions for patients with cancer have been evaluated, including counselling and social support groups (Fawzy *et al.* 1995). Recent studies of support groups (Fawzy and Fawzy 1998; Spiegel and Classen 1999) and of cognitive–behavioural treatments (Moorey and Greer 1989) have shown benefits to survival time associated with effects on and immune function (see Baum and Anderson 2001).

Although the psychological problems of patients with cancer can often be alleviated, many are undetected. One possibility is to provide educational programmes, counselling, or group therapy for all cancer patients whether or not they report problems. However, it seems more appropriate to select suitable patients, particularly as there is some evidence that counselling may increase distress in some vulnerable patients who have denied their anxieties. The patients most likely to need psychological treatment include those with a history of previous psychiatric disorder or poor adjustment to other problems and those who lack a supportive family

Childhood cancer

Childhood cancer presents special problems. The child often reacts to the illness and its treatment with behaviour problems. Many parents react at first with shock and disbelief, taking months to accept the full implications of the diagnosis. About one mother in five develops an anxiety or depressive disorder during the first 2 years of treatment of childhood leukaemia, and other family members may be affected. In the early stages of the illness parents are usually helped by advice about practical matters, and later by discussions of their feelings, which often include guilt. Adult survivors of cancer in childhood or adolescence appear to be at risk of social difficulties. See Rouhani and Holland (2000) and Roth *et al.* (2000) for reviews and Holland (1998) for reviews of all aspects of psycho-oncology.

Accidents

Psychiatric factors as causes

Personality and psychiatric illness are among the important causes of accidents in the home, at work, and on the roads. In childhood, psychiatric reasons for 'accident proneness' include overactivity and conduct disorders. Among young adults, alcohol, drug abuse, and mood disorders are important. In the elderly, organic mental disorders are important causes (McDonald and Davey 1996).

Psychiatric consequences

A wide range of psychiatric consequences are commonly described. They include adjustment disorder, anxiety disorders, and depression, as well as post-traumatic stress disorder (see p. 194). Avoidance is frequent and may be severe enough to be diagnosed as phobic anxiety disorder. Cognitive disorders may complicate head injury (see p. 428). There are also more specific psychiatric and social consequences related to the type of trauma.

Types of accident

Criminal assault is frequent and can have severe and persistent consequences for victims (Acierno *et al.* 1997; Kilpatrick *et al.* 1997; Resnick *et al.* 1997). Victims' problems are discussed further on p. 916.

Road traffic accidents are the leading cause of death in people aged under 40 and are a major cause of physical morbidity. As well as the abuse of alcohol and drugs, psychiatric factors in the causation of road accidents include severe psychiatric disorder, suicidal and risk-taking behaviour, and the side-effects of prescribed psychotropic drugs.

Psychiatric problems following a road accident include those consequent upon injury to the brain, acute stress disorder, anxiety and depression, post-traumatic stress disorder, and phobias of travel. Though some of these conditions are transient, many persist and give rise to considerable disability. Most of those affected do not seem to have been psychologically vulnerable before the accident (see Hickling and Blanchard 1999). Chronic psychiatric complications are mainly predicted by factors relating to the accident threat, initial distress and dissociation, and by maintaining psychological variables.

Occupational injury

The psychiatric consequences of occupational injury resemble those of other accidents. It is often alleged that hopes of compensation or other benefits are important in maintaining the symptoms and disability (see the discussion of compensation neurosis below). Although people who suffer occupational injury seem to have more time off work than those suffering similar injuries unrelated to work, deliberate exaggeration or simulation are rare.

Spinal cord injury

Around a quarter of patients admitted to a spinal injury unit suffer from psychiatric problems requiring treatment. Depression is common in the period immediately after a spinal cord injury, but recent follow-up studies have generally found that most patients are not psychologically disturbed a year after the injury. Nevertheless, suicide appears to be more common among these patients than in the general population. Depressive disorder is related to social isolation and unemployment, rather than to the degree of medical impairment (Radnitz *et al.* 1996).

Burns

Psychological and social problems may contribute to the causation of burns in both children and adults. In children, burns are associated with over-activity and mental retardation, and also with child abuse and neglect. In adults, burns are associated with alcohol and drug abuse, deliberate self-harm, and dementia. Severe burns and their protracted treatment may cause severe psychological problems. Hamburg *et al.* (1953) described three stages:

◆ *Stage 1* lasts days or weeks; denial is common. The most frequent psychiatric disorders are organic syndromes. At this stage the relatives often need considerable help.

◆ *Stage 2* is prolonged and painful; here denial recedes and emotional disorders are more common. Patients need to be helped to withstand pain, to express their feelings, and gradually accept disfigurement.

◆ In *stage 3* the patient leaves hospital and has to make further adjustments to deformity or physical disability and the reaction of other people to his appearance.

Recent reports have confirmed early case reports that post-traumatic disorder is a common complication of severe burn injury.

Persistent anxiety and depression occurs in more than a third of those suffering severe burns. It is generally agreed that the outcome is worse in patients with burns affecting the appearance of the face. Such patients are likely to withdraw permanently from social activities. These patients need considerable support from the staff of the burns unit, but only a minority require referral to a psychiatrist. See Bernstein (2000) for a review.

'Compensation neurosis'

The term compensation neurosis (or accident neurosis) refers to psychologically determined physical or mental symptoms occurring when there is an unsettled claim for compensation. From his experience as a neurologist, Miller (1961) claimed a psychological basis for persistent physical disability after occupational injuries and road accidents. He emphasized the role of the compensation claim in prolonging symptoms and suggested that settlement was followed by recovery. More recent evidence has failed to substantiate this extreme view, though it remains prevalent in medico-legal practice.

In fact many accident victims do not claim compensation, and few become involved in prolonged litigation. For example, amongst patients with mild head injuries, several studies have found that few people with prolonged psychological consequences were engaged in court proceedings or hoped for compensation. However, it does appear that time off work and disability are affected by the type of accident, social factors, and the prospect of compensation, social security, or other benefits. It has usually been assumed that settlement of a compensation claim is followed by improvement. This assumption is not supported by follow-up studies (Mendelson 1995). See Malt (2000) for a review of the psychiatric aspects of accidents, burns, and other trauma.

Psychiatric aspects of obstetrics and gynaecology

Pregnancy

Psychiatric disorder is more common in the first and third trimesters of pregnancy than in the second. In the first trimester unwanted pregnancies are associated with anxiety and depression. In the third trimester there may be fears about the impending delivery or doubts about the normality of the fetus. Psychiatric symptoms in pregnancy are more common in women with a history of previous psychiatric disorder and probably also in those with serious medical problems affecting the course of pregnancy, such as diabetes. Although minor affective symptoms are common in pregnancy, serious psychiatric disorders are probably less common than in non-pregnant women of the same age.

Some *women who had chronic psychological problems before being pregnant* report improvement in these problems during pregnancy whilst others require extra psychiatric care. The latter are often late or poor attenders at antenatal care, thus increasing the risk of obstetric and psychiatric problems. Misuse of alcohol, opiates, and other substances should be strongly discouraged in pregnancy, especially in the first trimester when the risk to the fetus is greatest (see p. 652). Eating disorders do not appear to be precipitated by pregnancy, and bulimic symptoms often improve.

Geat care must be taken in the use of psychotropic drugs during pregnancy because of the risk of fetal malformations, impaired growth, and prenatal problems (see Box 16.9). Pharmacokinetics may be altered. Benzodiazepines should be avoided throughout the pregnancy and during breast-feeding because of the danger of depressed respiration and withdrawal symptoms in the neonate. Lithium should be stopped if possible throughout the first trimester of pregnancy but can be restarted later if there are pressing reasons; it should be stopped again at the onset of labour.

Box 16.9 Use of psychotropic medicine in pregnancy and during breast-feeding

Pregnancy

Avoid all medication if possible. Use only if expected benefit to the mother is greater than the possibility of risk to the fetus.

Antidepressants No evidence that tricyclics or SSRIs cause fetal abnormality, but use only where there are very clear indications and in minimal dosage.

Lithium Risk of teratogenicity and of toxic effects on fetus in late pregnancy. Risks reduced by careful monitoring of levels. Ideally should be avoided in period of conception and early pregnancy, but possible careful re-prescription in final trimester. Unplanned pregnancy during long-term therapy: discuss with parents, consider termination, careful screening for malformations. Omit perinatally.

Antipsychotics Continue in minimal dose if major clinical indications.

Breast-feeding

Care with all medications

Antidepressants Evidence not clear but no definite contraindications. Avoid if possible. Need for careful consideration of risks and benefits with parents

Lithium Evidence uncertain. Breast-feeding cannot be recommended with confidence.

Antipsychotic drugs Risk probably small, but avoid if possible.

Mothers taking lithium should not breast-feed. It is preferable to avoid using tricyclic antidepressants or neuroleptics during pregnancy unless there are compelling clinical indications. See Chapter 21 for further information on drug treatment.

Hyperemesis gravidarum

About half of all pregnant women experience nausea and vomiting in the first trimester. Some authors have suggested that these symptoms, as well as the severe condition of hyperemesis gravidarum, are primarily of psychological aetiology. However, there is no reason to doubt that physical factors are of primary importance, although psychological factors may substantially influence the severity and course of the symptoms.

Pseudocyesis

Pseudocyesis is a rare condition in which a woman believes that she is pregnant when she is not, and develops amenorrhoea, abdominal distension, and other changes similar to those of early pregnancy. The condition is more common in younger women. Pseudocyesis usually resolves quickly once diagnosed, but some patients persist in believing that they are pregnant. Recurrence is common. The condition may be associated with psychiatric disorder.

Couvade syndrome

In this syndrome, the husband of the pregnant woman reports that he is himself experiencing some of the symptoms of pregnancy. This condition may occur in the early months of the woman's pregnancy, when the man complains usually of nausea and morning sickness and often of toothache. These complaints generally resolve after a few weeks.

Unwanted pregnancy

In the past, psychiatrists in the UK were often asked to see pregnant women who were seeking a therapeutic abortion on the grounds of mental illness. The provisions of current legislation in many countries now make it generally more appropriate for decisions to be made by the family doctor and the gynaecologist, without involving a psychiatrist. The situation and role of the psychiatrist is different in other jurisdictions. However, psychiatric opinions are still sought at times, not only about the grounds for termination of pregnancy but also for an assessment of the likely psychological effects of termination in a particular patient. Most of the evidence suggests that the psychological consequences of abortion are usually mild and transient, but that they are greater for mothers who have cultural or religious beliefs against abortion (see Major *et al.* 2000).

Spontaneous abortion

Approximately 20% of diagnosed pregnancies do not progress beyond 20 weeks, mainly because of fetal defects. Friedman and Gath (1989) interviewed women 4 weeks after spontaneous abortion and found that half were psychiatric cases of depression (a rate four times higher than in the general population of women). Many women showed features typical of grief. Depressive symptoms were most frequent in women with a history of previous spontaneous abortion. Although the majority improve with time (Janssen *et al.* 1996), the extent of morbidity indicates the importance of recognition of the needs of those who suffer miscarriage.

Therapeutic abortion

Iles and Gath (1993) compared a group of women who had a termination of pregnancy for medical reasons with a group who suffered a spontaneous abortion. In both groups psychiatric morbidity was high at 1 month. At follow-up there were significant improvements in psychiatric symptoms, guilt, and interpersonal and sexual adjustments. Adverse psychiatric and social consequences were rare. However, there is a need for sympathetic routine care and the recognition of the extra treatment needs of a minority. See p. 484 for a discussion of genetic counselling.

Antenatal death

Antenatal death (stillbirth) causes an acute bereavement reaction, increased long-term psychiatric problems, and concern about future pregnancy. In the past, such problems were ignored and stillbirth was seen as a trivial and routine event. Parents need to be helped to mourn and should be encouraged to see and hold the baby, to name it, and to have a proper funeral. The next pregnancy may be a particularly worrying time.

Caesarian section

Caesarian section is extremely frequent and is becoming more frequent in Western countries; it has been said to have adverse psychological consequences for parents and infants. Much of the research has failed to separate the effects of surgery from other adverse material factors. However, it would seem sensible to pay particular attention to parental support and to initial bonding.

See Brockington (1998) and Brockington (2000) for reviews of the psychiatric aspects of pregnancy.

Post-partum mental disorders

These disorders can be divided into maternity blues, puerperal psychosis, and chronic depressive disorders of moderate severity.

Minor mood disturbance – 'maternity blues'

Amongst women delivered of a normal child, between half and two-thirds experience brief episodes of irritability, lability of mood, and episodes of crying. Lability of mood is particularly characteristic, taking the form of rapid alternations between euphoria and misery. The symptoms reach their peak on the third or fourth day post partum. Patients often speak of being 'confused', but tests of cognitive function are normal. Although frequently tearful, patients may not be feeling depressed at the time but tense and irritable.

'Maternity blues' is more frequent among primigravida. The condition is not related to complications at delivery or to the use of anaesthesia. 'Blues' patients have often experienced anxiety and depressive symptoms in the last trimester of pregnancy; they are also more likely to give a history of premenstrual tension, fears of labour, and poor social adjustment.

Both the frequency of the emotional changes and their timing suggest that maternity blues may be related to readjustment in hormones after delivery. Oestrogens and progesterone both increase greatly during late pregnancy and fall precipitously after childbirth. Changes also occur in adrenal steroids, but they are complicated by associated changes in corticosteroid-binding globulin. However, there is no convincing evidence that these changes lead to the emotional symptoms, and at present the cause of maternity blues is unknown. No treatment is required because the condition resolves spontaneously in a few days.

Post-partum psychosis

In the nineteenth century, puerperal and lactational psychoses were thought to be specific entities distinct from other mental illnesses (Esquirol 1845). Later psychiatrists such as Bleuler and Kraepelin regarded the puerperal psychoses as no different from other mental illnesses. This latter view is widely held today on the grounds that puerperal psychoses generally resemble other psychoses in their clinical picture.

The incidence of post-partum (puerperal) psychoses has been estimated in terms of admission rates to psychiatric hospital (Pugh *et al.* 1963; Kendell *et al.* 1987). The reported rates vary, but a representative figure is one admission per 500 births. This incidence is substantially above the expected rate for non-puerperal women of the same age. Puerperal psychoses are more frequent in primiparous women, those who have suffered previous major psychiatric illness, those with a family history of mental illness, and probably in unmarried mothers. There is no clear relationship between psychosis and obstetric factors. The onset of puerperal psychosis is usually within the first 1–2 weeks after delivery, but rarely in the first 2 days. Puerperal illnesses are especially common in

developing countries and the excess may be cases with an organic aetiology.

The early onset of puerperal psychoses has led to speculation that they might be caused by hormonal changes such as those discussed above in relation to the blues syndrome. There is no evidence that hormonal changes in women with puerperal psychoses differ from those in other women in the early puerperium. Hence if endocrine factors do play a part, they probably act only as precipitating factors in predisposed women. Some research has implicated a supersensitivity of dopamine receptors in the pathophysiology of puerperal psychoses, perhaps precipitated by oestrogen withdrawal (Wieck *et al.* 1991). In depressive disorders stress appears a less important factor than in depression at other times.

Clinical features

Three types of clinical picture are observed: delirium, affective, and schizophreniform. Delirium was common in the past, but is now much less frequent since the incidence of puer-peral sepsis was reduced by antibiotics. Nowadays affective syndromes predominate; either bipolar disorder or schizoaffective disorder. Schizophrenia-like illnesses presenting for the first time are rare. The clinical features of these syndromes are generally regarded as being much the same as those of corresponding non-puerperal syndromes. Insomnia and overactivity are often early features. Perplexity and confusion are frequent.

Management

In the *assessment* of patients with post-partum psychosis, it is essential to ascertain the mother's ideas concerning the baby. Severely depressed patients may have delusional ideas that the child is malformed or otherwise imperfect. These false ideas may lead to attempts to kill the child to spare it from future suffering. Schizophrenic patients may also have delusional beliefs about the child; for example, they may be convinced that the child is abnormal or evil. Again, such beliefs may point to the risk of an attempt to kill the child. Patients with depression or schizophrenia may also make suicide attempts.

Treatment is given according to the clinical syndrome, as described in other chapters. Admission to hospital is normally required. For in-patient care it has been argued that there should be special mother and baby units to minimize adverse effects on maternal bonding. However, it is very difficult to supervise safe care and the presence of the baby may complicate treatment. The benefits of such units for outcome have not been established in controlled trials. All contact between mother and baby should initially be supervised by nursing staff and thereafter reviewed in the light of clinical progress.

Electroconvulsive therapy (ECT) is often the best treatment for patients with depressive or manic disorders of marked or moderate severity, because it is rapidly effective and enables the mother to resume the care of her baby quickly. For less urgent depressive disorders, antidepressant medication may be tried first. If the patient has predominantly schizophrenia-like symptoms, an antipsychotic drug may be prescribed; if definite improvement does not occur within a short period, ECT should be considered, especially if the onset was acute.

Most patients recover fully from a puerperal psychosis, but some of those with a schizophrenic disorder remain chronically ill. After subsequent childbirth the recurrence rate for depressive illness in the puerperium is approximately 20–30%. According to Protheroe (1969), at least half of women who have suffered a puerperal depressive illness will later suffer a depressive illness that is not puerperal. See Chapter 11 for a discussion of bipolar illness.

All mothers who have suffered post-partum psychosis should be considered for special psychiatric review during any further pregnancies so that post-partum problems can be treated rapidly and effectively.

Postnatal depression of mild or moderate severity

Less severe depressive disorders are much more common than the puerperal psychoses, occurring in 10% of women in the early weeks post partum. Tiredness, irritability, and anxiety are often more prominent than depressive mood change, and there may be prominent phobic symptoms. Most patients recover after 2–6 months.

Clinical observation suggests that these disorders are often precipitated in vulnerable mothers by the psychological adjustment required after childbirth, as well as by the loss of sleep and hard work involved in the care of the baby. There is little evidence of a biological basis. The main risk factors are a previous history of depression (especially when accompanied by obstetric complications) and indications of social adversity.

The only large-scale study of the predictive value of antenatal factors produced an index of only modest clinical usefulness; it is likely that its value could be improved by the inclusion of perinatal factors. There has been much argument as to whether the prevalence of depression is raised post partum. In a controlled study, Cooper *et al.* (1988) examined 483 pregnant women 6 weeks before the expected date of delivery, and re-examined them 3, 6, and 12 months after childbirth. At all stages of assessment, the point prevalence of psychiatric disorder was no higher than in a matched sample of women from the general population. However, it did seem that the inception rate was raised in the first 3 months compared with the subsequent 9 months. There was no evidence that the postnatal psychiatric disorder differed either diagnostically or in duration from psychiatric disorders arising at other times.

Those providing care to mother and baby need to be alert to the possibility of depression. In treatment, psychological and social measures are usually as important as antidepressant drugs. Despite the medical and other care given to women after childbirth, many post-partum depressions are undetected or, if detected, untreated. Most women can be treated effectively in primary care by brief, supportive, or problem-solving treatments together with practical support. A small proportion may benefit from antidepressant medication and others may require referral to specialist psychiatric services.

There is evidence that postnatal depression adversely affects the *mother–infant relationship* and the cognitive and emotional development of the infant (Stein *et al.* 1991). Evidence on the consequences in early childhood is less clear. See Murray and Cooper (1997) for a review.

See Cooper and Murray (1998) for a review of postnatal depression. See Brockington (1998, 2000) for reviews of all aspects of post-partum psychological complications. See Viguera and Cohen (2000) for a review of psychopharmacology during pregnancy and the post-partum period.

Psychiatric aspects of gynaecology

Premenstrual syndrome

This term denotes a group of distressing psychological and physical symptoms starting a few days before and ending shortly after the onset of a menstrual period. The psychological symptoms include anxiety, irritability, food cravings, and depression; the physical symptoms include breast tenderness, abdominal discomfort, and a feeling of distension. Premenstrual syndrome is not included in current classifications of psychiatric disorder, although premenstrual dysphoric disorder is listed as a condition for future study in DSM-IV. The syndrome should be distinguished from the much more frequent occurrence of similar symptoms that are not strictly premenstrual in timing.

The estimated frequency of the premenstrual syndrome in the general population varies widely from 30 to 80% of women of reproductive age. There are several reasons for this wide variation in reported rates. First, there is a problem of definition. Mild and brief symptoms are frequent premenstrually, and it is difficult to decide when they should be classified as premenstrual syndrome. Second, information about symptoms is often collected retrospectively by asking women to recall earlier menstrual periods, and this is an unreliable way of establishing the time relations. Third, the description of premenstrual symptoms may vary according to whether or not the woman knows that the enquiry is concerned specifically with the premenstrual syndrome.

The aetiology is uncertain. Physical explanations have been based on ovarian hormones (excess oestrogen, lack of progesterone), pituitary hormones, and disturbed fluid and electrolyte balance. None of these theories has been proved. Various psychological explanations have been based on possible associations of the syndrome with neuroticism or with individual or public attitudes towards menstruation.

The syndrome has been widely treated with progesterone, and also with oral contraceptives, bromocriptine, diuretics, and psychotropic drugs. There is no convincing evidence that any of these is effective, and treatment trials suggest a high placebo response (up to 65%). Psychological support and encouragement may be as helpful as medication. There have been encouraging reports of the effectiveness of SSRI antidepressants during the vulnerable period and of a cognitive behavioural treatment. See Blake *et al.* (1995) for a review of the syndrome and its psychological treatment.

The menopause

In addition to the physical symptoms of flushing, sweating, and vaginal dryness, menopausal women often complain of headache, dizziness, and depression. It is not certain whether depressive symptoms are more common in menopausal women than in non-menopausal women. Nevertheless, amongst patients who consult general practitioners because of emotional symptoms, a disproportionately large number of women are in the middle-age group that spans the menopausal years.

Depressive and anxiety-related symptoms at the time of the menopause could have several causes. Hormonal changes have often been suggested, notably deficiency of oestrogen. In some countries, notably the USA, oestrogen has been used to treat emotional symptoms in women of menopausal age, but the results of trials of treatment with oestrogens have been disappointing (see Pearce *et al.* 1995). Psychiatric symptoms at this time of life could equally well reflect changes in the woman's role as her children leave home, her relationship with her husband alters, and her own parents become ill or die. It seems best to treat depressed menopausal women with methods that have been shown to be effective for depressive disorder at any other time of life

Hysterectomy

Several retrospective studies have indicated an increased frequency of depressive disorder after hysterectomy. A prospective investigation using standardized methods showed that patients who are free from psychiatric symptoms before hysterectomy seldom develop them afterwards. Some patients with psychiatric symptoms before hysterectomy lose them afterwards, but others continue to have symptoms after the operation (Gath *et al.* 1982a, 1982b). It is likely that these latter persisting cases (those with symptoms before and after surgery) are identified in the retrospective studies, and lead to the erroneous conclusion that hysterectomy causes depressive disorder. This finding provides a general warning about inferring the effects of treatment from the results of retrospective investigations.

Sterilization

Considerations similar to those for hysterectomy apply to these procedures. Retrospective studies have suggested that sterilization leads to psychiatric disorder, sexual dysfunction, and frequent regrets after the operation. However, prospective enquiry has shown that the operation does not lead to significant psychiatric disorder; sexual relationships are more likely to improve than worsen, and definite regrets are reported by fewer than one patient in 20.

See Robinson (2000) and Brockington (2000) for reviews of the psychological aspects of gynaecology.

Further reading

Gelder, M. G., López-Ibor, J. J. Jr, and Andreasen, N.C. (eds) (2000). *The new Oxford textbook of psychiatry.* Oxford University Press. (See Section 5 on Psychiatry and Medicine by various authors.)

Guthrie, F. and Creed, F. (eds) (1996). *Liaison psychiatry.* Gaskell, London.

Rundell, J. R. and Wise, M. G. (eds) (1999). *Essentials of consultation liaison psychiatry.* American Psychiatric Press, Washington, DC. (A short reference work. Short account of basic clinical issues.)

Stoudemire, A., Fogel, B. S., and Greenbury, D. (eds) (2000). *Psychiatric care of the medical patient,* 2nd edn. Oxford University Press, New York. (A comprehensive reference book.)

CHAPTER 17

Suicide and deliberate self-harm

Suicide and deliberate self-harm

Suicide is among the ten leading causes of death in most countries around the world for which information is available. In the UK it is the third most important contributor to life years lost after coronary heart disease and cancer. Treatment of those who are at risk and management of the aftermath is an issue for all doctors. Over the last two decades several countries have reported a considerable increase in the number of young men who kill themselves. This increase has been one of the factors that have led to a series of national and international initiatives to promote the prevention of suicide and to reverse this trend (World Health Organization 1998; Department of Health 1999c).

For every suicide it is estimated that that more than 30 non-fatal episodes of self-harm occur. Depression, substance misuse, and other mental health problems are more common in people who deliberately harm themselves and the rate of suicide in the year following an episodes of deliberate self-harm is 100 times that of the general population. The rate of suicide is also raised in the period following discharge from in-patient psychiatric care. For these reasons psychiatrists need to be well informed about the nature of suicidal behaviour and strategies aimed at its prevention. For reviews of all aspects of suicide and deliberate self-harm see Hawton and van Heeringen (2000).

Suicide

The act of suicide

Suicide has been defined as an act with a fatal outcome, that is deliberately initiated and performed by the person in the knowledge or expectation of its fatal outcome. People who take their lives do so in several different ways. In England and Wales, self-poisoning using car exhaust fumes has become the most commonly used method for suicide by men, accounting for a third of all deaths (Charlton et al. 1992, Charlton et al. 1993). Hanging (28%) and overdose (15%) are also frequently used. By contrast, in the USA, gunshot and other violent methods are frequent. In women, drug overdose accounts for almost 50% of suicides in England and Wales. Hanging, drowning, and jumping account for most of the remaining deaths. Women use self-poisoning with car exhaust fumes far less often than men; however, it is the only method of suicide in women where rates are increasing.

Most completed suicides have been planned. Precautions against discovery are often taken, for example, choosing a lonely place or a time when no one is expected. However, in most cases a warning is given. In a survey in the USA, interviews were held with relatives and friends of people who had committed suicide. It was found that suicidal ideas had been expressed by more than two-thirds of the deceased and clear suicidal intent by more than a third. Often the warning had been given to more than one person. In a similar British study of people who had committed suicide, Barraclough et al. (1974) found that two-thirds had consulted their general practitioner in the previous month, and 40% had done so in the previous week. A quarter were seeing a psychiatrist, of whom half had seen the psychiatrist in the week before their suicide. More recent evidence confirms high rates of contact with mental health services in the period before suicide though rates are relatively lower among young men.

The epidemiology of suicide

Accurate statistics about suicide are difficult to obtain because information about the cause of a fatal event is not always available. For example, in England and Wales, official figures depend on the verdicts reached in coroners' courts. A verdict of suicide is only recorded by a coroner if there is clear evidence that the injury was self-inflicted and that the deceased intended to kill himself. If there is any doubt about either point, an accidental or open verdict is recorded. In England and Wales over recent years, the proportion of open verdicts to suicide verdicts has risen. Open verdicts are more often recorded when the method of self-harm is less active (e.g. drowning compared with hanging) and may be more likely to occur when the deceased is young rather than old (Neeleman and Wessely 1997). For these reasons it is accepted that official statistics underestimate the true rates of suicide. Barraclough (1973) demonstrated that amongst people whose deaths are recorded as accidental, many have recently been depressed or dependent on drugs or alcohol, thus resembling people who commit suicide. For example, in Dublin at that time, psychiatrists ascertained four times as many suicides as the coroners did and similar discrepancies have been reported elsewhere. An attempt has been made to overcome these problems by reporting 'probable suicides', which combine deaths attributed to suicide and 'open verdicts'. Caution therefore needs to be exercised when comparing rates of suicide in different time periods and different locations around the world. Despite these problems, long-standing and fairly stable differences in rates of suicide between different countries are apparent. Sainsbury and Barraclough (1968) presented indirect evidence that differences in rates of suicide among different nations are real by demonstrating that, within the USA, the rank order of suicide rates among immigrants from 11 different nations was similar to the rank order of national rates within the 11 countries of origin. Table 17.1 shows ranking of the top 10 countries by total number reported and rates of suicide. The

Table 17.1 Ranking of the top ten countries by number of suicides (estimated for the year 2000) and suicide rates (most recent year available).

Country	Number of suicides	Rate per 100 000	Ranking by suicide rate	Country	Number of suicides	Rate per 100 000	Ranking by number of suicides
China	195 000	16.1	24	Lithuania	1600	41.9	22
India	87 000	9.7	45	Estonia	600	40.1	25
Russia	52 500	41.5	3	Russia	52 500	37.6	3
USA	31 000	11.9	38	Latvia	850	33.9	23
Japan	20 000	16.8	23	Hungary	3000	32.9	16
Germany	12 500	15.8	25	Sri Lanka	5400	31.0	9
France	11 600	20.7	14	Kazakhstan	4500	28.6	13
Ukraine	11 000	22.6	11	Belarus	2800	28.0	17
Brazil	5400	3.5	71	Slovenia	600	26.6	24
Sri Lanka	5400	31.0	7	Finland	1300	24.3	21

See World Health Organization (1999). *Facts and figures about suicide*. World Health Organization, Geneva.

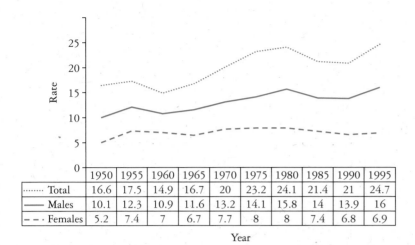

Figure 17.1 Global suicide rates (per 100 000), by gender, 1950–95 (selected countries indicated in Table 17.1). Reproduced with permission World Health Organization Figures and Facts about Suicide World Health Organization, Geneva, 1999

	1950	1955	1960	1965	1970	1975	1980	1985	1990	1995
Total	16.6	17.5	14.9	16.7	20	23.2	24.1	21.4	21	24.7
Males	10.1	12.3	10.9	11.6	13.2	14.1	15.8	14	13.9	16
Females	5.2	7.4	7	6.7	7.7	8	8	7.4	6.8	6.9

Year

official suicide rate in the UK is in the lower range of those reported in Western countries. Generally, higher rates are reported in eastern and northern European countries, and lower rates in Mediterranean countries. Reported suicide rates are very low in Islamic countries. The sex differences are less in Asian than in Western countries; methods reflect local culture with specific methods such as self-immolation or ritual disembowelment (Cantor 2000; Cheng and Lee 2000).

Changes in suicide rates

Global suicide rates have increased since 1950 (Figure 17.1). Changes within individual countries are complex. Thus, over the years since 1900, suicide rates in the UK have changed substantially at different times. Recorded rates for men and women fell during both world wars. There were also two periods when rates were unusually high. The first, 1932–33, was a time of economic depression and high unemployment; the second, between the late 1950s and the early 1960s, was not. Another unusual period was 1963–74, when rates declined in England and Wales but not in other European countries (except Greece) or in North America.

These changes mask more dramatic changes that have occurred among young men, especially in English-speaking countries (Figure 17.2). There has been little change in Asian cultures where the occurrence of suicide tends to increase with age. However, rates in one subgroup, men aged 15–24, have increased substantially. (See also Charlton *et al.* 1992)

Variations with the seasons

In England and Wales, suicide rates have been highest in spring and summer for every decade since 1921–30. A similar pattern has been found in other countries in the northern hemisphere. In the southern hemisphere, a similar rise occurs during the spring and early summer, even though these seasons are in different months of the year. The reason for these fluctuations is not known.

Demographic characteristics

Suicide is three times as common in men as in women. The highest rates of suicide in both men and women continue to be seen in the elderly (see Figure 17.2). Suicide rates are lowest among the married, and increase progressively with the never married, widowers and widows, and the divorced. Rates are higher in the unemployed compared with the employed. In terms of social class, the highest rates are seen in social class V (unskilled workers) followed by social class I (professional), in which rates are higher than in social classes II, III, and IV. Rates are particularly high in certain professions.

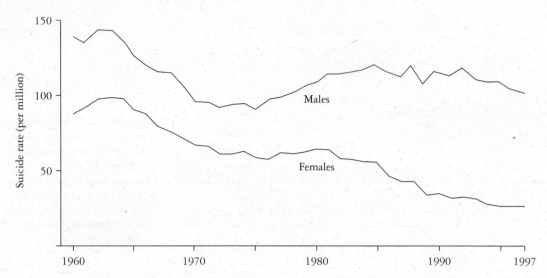

Figure 17.2 Suicide rate for all ages in England and Wales, 1960–97. Reproduced with permission from McClure G. M. G. (2000). Changes in suicide in England and Wales 1960–1997. *British Journal of Psychiatry*, **176**, 64–7.

Veterinary surgeons have three times the expected rate, and pharmacists, farmers, and medical practitioners have double the expected rate (Charlton *et al.* 1994). High rates of suicide occur in prisoners, especially amongst those on remand.

The causes of suicide

Attempts to investigate the causes of suicide face several substantial barriers. Retrospective information concerning the health and well-being of the deceased at the time of suicide cannot be directly obtained. Prospective studies of suicide are problematic because of its relative rarity. Two main strategies have been used in an attempt to overcome these barriers. First, retrospective studies have pieced together the circumstances that surrounded the suicide by examining records and interviewing those who knew the deceased prior to death. Second, studies have examined associations between social and demographic factors and rates of suicide in different populations at different times. Each approach has methodological problems. However, the first type of study, which has become known as 'psychological autopsy' study, has helped identify factors that precede suicide. The latter approach has informed our under-

standing of social circumstances that may give rise to increased rates of suicide.

Individual psychiatric and medical factors

In several studies, interviews have been held with doctors, relatives, and friends of people who have committed suicide, and detailed histories of the deceased have been compiled. The most consistent finding of these studies is that the large majority of those who die from suicide have some form of mental disorder (Table 17.2) at the time of death (Barraclough *et al.* 1974). This finding has been consistent wherever studies have been conducted (Cheng and Lee 2000).

♦ *Personality disorder* is diagnosed in a third to half of people who commit suicide (Foster *et al.* 1997).

♦ *Mood disorder* It is estimated that about 6% of those who suffer from a mood disorder will die by suicide. Depressed patients who die by suicide are more likely to have a past history of self-harm and to have been noted to experience a sense of hopelessness (Fawcett *et al.* 1990). However, they differ in that they have made

Table 17.2 **Rates (%) of mental disorders in five psychological autopsy studies on completed suicides using DSM-III or DSM-III-R criteria**	
Depressive disorders	36–90
Alcohol dependence or abuse	43–54
Drug dependence or abuse	4–45
Schizophrenic disorders	3–10
Organic mental disorders	2–7
Personality disorders	5–44

From Lonnqvist, J. K. (2000). Epidemiology and causes of suicide. In *The new Oxford textbook of psychiatry* (eds M. G. Gelder, J. J. López-Ibor Jr, and N. C. Andreasen), Chapter 4.15.1. Oxford University Press, Oxford.

more previous suicide attempts, are more often single, separated, or widowed, are older, and are more often male.

- *Alcohol misuse* Follow-up studies of patients dependent on alcohol show a continuing risk of suicide, with a lifetime risk of 7% (Inskip *et al.* 1998). Among those who are alcohol dependent, suicide is more likely when the patient is male, of older age, has a long history of drinking, past history of depression, and a history of previous suicidal attempts. It is also increased among those whose drinking has caused physical complications, marital problems, difficulties at work, or arrests for drunkenness offences.

- *Drug misuse* is relatively common, particularly in the young (Oyefeso *et al.* 1999).

- In *schizophrenia*, suicide is more likely among young men early in the course of the disorder, particularly when there have been relapses, when there are depressive symptoms, and when previous academic success has been turned to failure by the illness. The lifetime risk has been estimated at 7% (Inskip *et al.* 1998).

Other factors associated with suicide are a *past history of deliberate self-harm* (see p. 524) and *concurrent physical ill-health,* especially *epilepsy* and other *chronic medical conditions.* (See Harris and Barraclough 1995 and Stenager and Stenager 2000 for reviews.)

Social factors associated with suicide.

Comparisons of rates of suicide between and within different countries have been conducted over many years. None has been more influential than that conducted by Emile Durkheim at the end of the nineteenth century (see Durkheim 1951). Durkheim examined variations in the rate of suicide within France and between France and other European countries. He demonstrated that a range of social factors impact on rates of suicide. Rates were lower at times of war and revolution, and increased during periods of both economic prosperity and economic depression. This led him to the conclusion that social integration and social regulation were central to the rate of suicide. He suggested that where there was a lack of social integration, for instance due to lack of religious faith, 'egoistic' suicide may result. When society lacked 'collective order' because it was in the midst of major social upheaval, 'anomic' suicide may result.

More recent studies have repeatedly demonstrated that areas with *high unemployment, poverty* (Gunnel *et al.* 1995), *divorce,* and *social fragmentation* (Whitley *et al.* 1999) have higher rates of suicide. Whilst the results of such studies cannot be used as a means of examining the characteristics of individuals who kill themselves, they provide important information about factors within society that may affect the rate of suicide. *Cross-cultural evidence* indicates wide variation in the meaning of suicide and social attitudes to it which appear to be associated with differences in suicide rates.

Another social factor that seems to affect rates of suicide is *media coverage of suicide.* Suicide and attempted suicide rates have been shown to increase after the showing of fictional television programmes and films depicting suicide (Hawton *et al.* 1999). On other occasions the means of suicide and its timing seem to have been influenced by the circumstances of a suicide that attracted attention within a local community or received wide publicity in newspapers or on television (Eisenberg 1986; Gould *et al.* 1990).

Biological factors

There is a strong association between suicidal behaviour and both impulsivity and aggression. Recent research has focused on genetic and other biological mechanisms. Adoption studies suggest that genetic factors may be responsible for the concordance of suicide in some families. It is suggested the mechanism may be independent of the inheritance of specific psychiatric disorders (Roy *et al.* 2000).

Investigations of biological factors that may be important in the aetiology of suicidal behaviour present ethical and technical problems. There is evidence that under-functioning of brain seroton-ergic systems may be linked to suicidal behaviour. This may be an association with a personality trait predisposing to suicide rather than with episodes of overt psychiatric disorder. See Amsel and Mann (2000).

Psychological factors

Psychological factors implicated in suicide tend to be extrapolated from the studies of non-fatal deliberate self-harm, but it cannot be assumed that factors are the same. An exception to this is work by Beck and colleagues who followed more than 200 patients who had been hospitalized because of suicidal ideation (Beck *et al.* 1985). They demonstrated that those who scored highly on a measure of hopelessness had very high rates of suicide over the following 5–10 years. More recent work indicates a range of psychological variables that may be associated with suicidal behaviour – impulsivity, dichotomous thinking, cognitive constriction, hopelessness, problem-solving deficits, and over-generalized autobiographical memory. These may predispose the person to react impulsively (Williams and Pollock 2000).

Conclusion

The associations between suicide and the various factors mentioned above do not, of course, establish causation. Nevertheless, they point to the importance of two sets of interacting influences. Amongst medical factors, depressive disorders, alcohol misuse, and abnormal personality are particularly prominent. Amongst social factors, social isolation and poverty stand out. Recent research also suggests the need to consider biological variables, although it is not yet certain what these are.

Special groups

Suicide in patients in contact with psychiatric services

Given the strong association between mental disorder and suicide, it is no surprise that many people who kill themselves are in contact with psychiatric services. In England and Wales an attempt has been made to collect information on all patients who have committed suicide who have had contact with mental health services in the previous 12 months as part of a National Confidential Inquiry (Appleby *et al.* 1999). Early findings of this study demonstrate high rates of suicide during the course of in-patient treatment. Suicide was most likely to occur within the first week of the admission to hospital (23%) and when discharge was being planned (40%). The highest rate of suicide among out-patients was in the first week following discharge from in-patient treatment, many prior to the first out-patient appointment. Suicides were particularly likely to occur following short admissions and when patients had taken discharge against medical advice.

Most deaths among out-patients followed recent contact with psychiatric services. When asked to provide retrospective accounts of patient management prior to the suicide, mental health teams stated that for most patients the immediate risk of suicide was believed to be low (84%), and judged that in 78% of cases the death had not been preventable. When teams stated that additional measures could have reduced the risk of suicide, improved patient compliance and closer supervision were the factors most often mentioned.

Among patients treated for depression, the risk of suicide may be increased following initial treatment when psychomotor retardation decreases. However, most patients who kill themselves have probably not been taking antidepressant medication prior to their death (Isacsson *et al.* 1994). The suggestion that some antidepressants might increase the risk of suicidal behaviour is not supported by evidence from prospective studies (Leon *et al.* 1999).

'Rational' suicide

Despite the findings reviewed above, there can be no doubt that suicide is occasionally the rational act of a mentally healthy person. Moreover, mass suicides have been described among groups of people, for instance religious communities, and it is unlikely that they were all suffering from mental disorder. Nevertheless, in the clinical assessment of someone who is talking of suicide, it is a good rule to assume that his suicidal inclinations are likely to be influenced by an abnormal state of mind.

If this assumption is correct – as it usually will be – the patient's urge to suicide is likely to diminish with recovery from the abnormal mental state. Even if the assumption is wrong (i.e. if the patient is one of the few who have reached a rational decision to die), the doctor should still try to protect him from harming himself. Given more time for reflection, most people with suicidal intent change their intentions. For example, they may discover that death from a cancer need not be as painful as they believed. Hence they may change a decision that was made rationally but on false premises (see Emanuel 1994 for a review of issues relating to euthanasia) (Box 17.1).

Older people

In most countries the highest rate of suicide is in people aged over 75 years. As with suicide in younger people, depression, social isolation, and impaired physical health are important risk factors.

> **Box 17.1 Physician-assisted suicide: ethical issues**
>
> - Importance and efficacy of treating depression and symptoms in those who say they wish to die.
> - Importance of establishing working relationships and understanding the patient's and their family's views on death.
> - Need to assess patient's competence and/or review any advance directive.
> - Need to provide high quality care and support to patient and family.
> - Effective symptomatic relief may hasten death.
> - Decision not to use aggressive treatment in the terminally ill.
> - Withdrawal of life support.
>
> See Emanuel (1998)

However, older people are less likely than the young to have talked about suicide or made previous suicide attempts. In addition to active self-harm, some older adults die from deliberate self-neglect, such as refusing food or non-compliance with therapy. These 'silent suicides' are usually the result of self-starvation or non-compliance with essential medical treatment. Respecting the autonomy of competent patients is central to proper medical practice whatever age the patient is. Equally, decisions about the appropriate treatment of depression in patients should not be influenced by the patients age. See Harwood and Jacoby (2000).

Children and adolescents

Accurate estimation of suicide rates is even more difficult for children than for adults. However, suicide is known to be rare in children. In 1989, the suicide rate for children aged 5–14 years was 0.7 per 100 000 in the USA and 0.8 per 100 000 in the UK. Little is known about factors leading to suicide in childhood, except that it is associated with severe personal and social morbidity. Shaffer

(1974) reported that suicidal behaviour and depressive disorders were common among the parents and siblings, and that children who died by suicide had usually shown antisocial behaviour. Shaffer distinguished two groups of children. The first comprised children of superior intelligence who seemed to be isolated from less educated parents. Many of their mothers were mentally ill. Before death, the children had seemed depressed and withdrawn, and some had stayed away from school. The second group consisted of children who were impetuous, prone to violence, and resentful of criticism (Pfeffer 2000; Shaffer *et al.* 2000).

In several countries there is evidence of a recent marked increase in suicide by older adolescents (WHO); in some countries, including the USA, there has also been an increase among younger children. In England and Wales the only recent change in rates has been an increase in males aged 15–19 years (McClure 2000). Psychological autopsy studies shows that the majority of adolescents who kill themselves have severe psychosocial problems, approximately two-thirds have expressed suicidal intent, and half made a previous suicide attempt. See de Wilde (2000).

Ethnic groups

Rates amongst immigrants closely reflect those of their countries of origin. In the UK, there is particular concern about high rates amongst Asian women.

High-risk occupational groups

The suicide rate among *doctors* is greater than that in the general population, but similar to several other occupations. There are no consistent findings of differences between medical specialties. Many reasons have been suggested, such as the ready availability of drugs, increased rates of addiction to alcohol and drugs, the extra stresses of work, reluctance to seek treatment for depressive disorders, and the selection into the medical profession of predisposed personalities. Whatever the true reasons, it is clear that the profession could do useful preventive work within its own ranks.

Farmers also have high rates of suicide. Possible causes include the ready availability of means of self-harm (such as poisons and guns), together with stress related to work and financial difficulties (Malmberg *et al.* 1999).

In contrast to many suggestions that students are a high-risk group, suicide rates are generally close to expectations for the age group in the wider population.

Suicide pacts

In suicide pacts, two people agree that at the same time each will take his or her own life. Completed suicide pacts are uncommon. It is estimated that they are responsible for 0.28–1.00% in the USA and UK and 0.77–3.10% in Japan and India. In Far Eastern countries, those involved are usually lovers aged less than 30 years and in Western countries usually interdependent couples aged more than 50 years. Suicide pacts have to be distinguished from cases where murder is followed by suicide (especially when the first person dies but the second is revived), or where one person aids another person's suicide without intending to die himself.

The psychological causes for these pacts are not known. Usually there is a particularly close relationship between the two members of the pact. The partners in the pact are usually socially isolated and a dominant partner is important in initiating the suicide.

Mass suicide pacts are occasionally reported, for example, the deaths of 960 Jews at Masada in AD 73. More recently, 913 followers of the Peoples Temple cult died at Jamestown, Guyana in 1978 and 39 members of the Heavens Gate cult in California in 1997. They are generally initiated by charismatic leaders who may be deluded and there may be evidence of murder as well as suicide. See Nock and Marzuk (2000) for a review of suicide pacts and of suicide and violence.

Murder followed by suicide

See p. 909.

The assessment of suicidal risk

General issues

Every doctor should be able to assess the risk of suicide. The first requirement is a willingness to make tactful but direct enquiries about a patient's intentions. Asking a patient about suicidal inclinations does not make suicidal behaviour more likely. On the contrary, the patient who has already thought of suicide will feel better understood when the doctor raises the issue and this feeling may reduce the risk. For a review of general issues see Hawton (2000a, 2000b).

The second requirement is to be alert to the general factors signifying an increased risk. Even so, prediction has a low sensitivity and specificity, and it is even more difficult to distinguish between long-term risk and risk at a particular time. For example, Goldstein et al. (1991) tried to develop a statistical model to predict the occurrence of 46 suicides from amongst a group of high-risk hospital patients, but failed to identify a single patient who later committed suicide.

Assessing risk

The most obvious warning sign is a direct statement of intent. It is now well recognized, but cannot be repeated too often, that there is no truth in the idea that people who talk of suicide do not enact it. On the contrary, two-thirds of those who die by suicide have told someone of their intentions. The greatest difficulty arises with people who talk repeatedly of suicide. In time their statements may no longer be taken seriously, but may be discounted as threats intended to influence other people. However, some people who repeatedly make threats do kill themselves in the end. Just before the act, there may be a subtle change in their way of talking about dying, sometimes in the form of oblique hints instead of former more open statements.

Risk is also assessed by considering the factors that surveys have shown to be associated with suicide (see p. 510). Older patients are more at risk, as are the lonely and those suffering from chronic painful illness. Those who have previously attempted suicide are especially at risk and 30–40% of those who die by suicide have made a previous attempt. Depressive disorders are highly important, especially when there is severe mood change with insomnia, anorexia, and weight loss (Barraclough et al. 1974). Patients with marked hopelessness are also of concern.

As noted earlier, there is an increased risk of suicide with alcohol dependence, especially when associated with physical complications or severe social damage, drug dependence, epilepsy, and abnormal personality. In schizophrenia, suicide is particularly likely in young men with recurrent severe illness and intellectual deterioration.

Completing the history

When these general risk factors have been assessed, the rest of the history should be evaluated. The interview should be conducted in an unhurried and sympathetic way that allows the patient to admit any despair or self-destructive intentions. It is usually appropriate to start by asking about current problems and the patient's reaction to them. Enquiries should cover losses, both personal (such as bereavement or divorce) and financial, as well as loss of status. Information about conflict with other people and social isolation should also be elicited. Physical illness should always be asked about, particularly any painful condition in the elderly. (Some depressed suicides have unwarranted fears of some physical illness as a feature of the psychiatric disorder.)

In assessing previous personality, it should be borne in mind that the patient's self-description might be coloured by depression. Whenever possible, another informant should be interviewed. The important points include mood swings, impulsive or aggressive tendencies, and attitudes towards religion and death.

Mental state examination

The assessment of mood should be particularly thorough, and cognitive function must not be overlooked. The interviewer should then assess suicidal intent. It is usually appropriate to begin by asking whether patients think that life is too much for them, or whether they no longer want to go on. This question can lead to more direct questions about thoughts of suicide, specific plans, and actions such as saving tablets. It is important always to remember that severely depressed patients occasionally have homicidal ideas; they may believe that it would be an act of mercy to kill other people, often the spouse or a child, to spare them intolerable suffering. Such homicidal ideas should not be missed, and should always be taken extremely seriously.

The management of suicidal patients

General issues

Having assessed the suicidal risk, the clinician should make a treatment plan and try to persuade the patient to accept it. The first step is to decide whether the patient should be admitted to hospital or treated as an out-patient or day-patient. This decision depends on the intensity of the suicidal intention, the severity of any associated psychiatric illness, and the availability of social support outside hospital. If out-patient treatment is chosen, patients should be given a telephone number with which they can, at all times, obtain help if feeling worse. Frustrated attempts to find a doctor can be the last straw for a patient with suicidal inclinations.

If suicidal risk is judged to be high, in-patient care is nearly always required. An occasional exception may be made when the patient lives with reliable relatives, but only if those relatives wish to care for the patient themselves, understand their responsibilities, and are able to fulfil them. Such a decision requires an exceptionally thorough knowledge of the patient and his problems. If hospital treatment is essential but the patient refuses it, admission under a compulsory order will be necessary. Readers should consult local legislation.

Table 17.3 Care of the suicidal patient in the community

Full assessment of patient and key relatives, including review of the suicidal risk

Organization of adequate social support

Regular review

Full dosage of safe psychiatric treatments
 Choose less toxic drugs
 Small prescriptions
 Involve relatives in care of tablets

Arrange immediate access to extra help for patient and relatives

Management in the community

The management of patients identified as being at risk of suicide but not requiring admission depends upon recognition and continuing assessment of the suicidal risk together with clear plans to provide appropriate treatment and support (Table 17.3). Regular liaison between the key worker and members of the multidisciplinary psychiatric team is required. Where available, relatives should also be involved. Mutually agreed plans for treatment will often include the patient's support for taking therapeutic doses of medication. The support of the patient's GP may need to be sought in order to ensure that the quantity and toxicity of medication the patient has is limited. Both patients and carers need to know how to access emergency help at all times.

Management in hospital

The obvious first requirement is to prevent patients from harming themselves. These arrangements require adequate staffing in a safe ward environment. A clear policy (Table 17.4) should be agreed with all staff members on admission.

Consideration needs to be given to minimizing the availability of means of self-harm. This includes preventing access to open windows and other areas of buildings where jumping could lead

Table 17.4 Care of the suicidal patient in hospital

Safe ward environment

Adequate well-trained staff with good working relationship

Clear policies for assessment, review, and observation

On admission

  Assess risk

  Agree level of observation

  Remove objects which might be used as means of suicide

  Discuss plans with patient

  Agree policy for visitors (number, duration, information)

During admission

  Regular review of risk and plans

  Clear plans for level of supervision

  If patient leaves ward without notice, take immediate action

Discharge

  Plan and agree in advance

  Prescribe adequate but non-dangerous amount of drugs

  Early follow-up

to serious medical injury. It may involve limiting or preventing access to areas of a ward where self-injury would be easier to enact and removal of potentially dangerous objects such as belts and razors. Special nursing arrangements may be needed at times so that the patient is never alone.

The management policy should be reconsidered carefully at frequent intervals until the danger passes. It is particularly important that any changes in policy should be made clear when staff change between shifts. The agreement of patients should also be sought; when this is not possible, the reasons for action being taken need to be carefully explained and when necessary compulsory treatment provided under the terms of local statutory powers.

When intensive supervision is needed for more than a few days, increasing difficulties may arise. Patients under constant observation may become irritated and resentful, and may evade supervision. Staff should be aware of such problems, and treatment of any associated mental illness should not be delayed. Appropriate physical treatment should be accompanied by supportive psychotherapy. However determined the patient is to die, there is usually some small remaining wish to go on living. If doctors and nurses adopt a caring and hopeful attitude, these positive feelings can be encouraged and patients can be helped towards a more realistic and balanced view of their future. At the same time, they can be helped to see how an apparently overwhelming accumulation of problems can be dealt with one by one. The period that precedes the patient's discharge from hospital is also a time of increased risk of suicide. Clear plans for periods of leave away from the ward may need to be agreed to aid this transition. Care should be taken to make adequate arrangements for psychological and social support following discharge from hospital. The patient should be encouraged to discuss any concerns about plans for discharge; when necessary, plans should be modified to deal with the concerns.

However carefully patients are managed, occasionally a patient will die by suicide despite all the efforts of the staff. The doctor then has an important role in supporting other staff, particularly any nurses who have come to know the patient well through taking part in constant observation. Although it is essential to review every suicide carefully to determine whether any useful lessons can be learned, this process should never become a search for a scapegoat.

The relatives

When a patient has died by suicide, the relatives require not only the support that is appropriate for any bereaved person, but also help with particular difficulties such as anger, guilt, and a feeling that the suicide could have been prevented. In a study by Barraclough and Shepherd (1976), the relatives usually reported that the police conducted their enquiries in a considerate way, but nearly all found the public inquest distressing. The subsequent newspaper publicity caused further grief, reactivating the events surrounding the death and increasing any feelings of stigma. Sympathetic listening, explanation, and counselling are likely to help relatives with these difficulties. It is essential to understand that anger is often a part of grief and that it should be met by a patient willingness to listen and to give full information. See Wertheimer (1992) for a review of consequences of suicide for relatives.

Suicide prevention

In population terms, suicide is a rare event; in western Europe this approximates to between one and two deaths per every 10 000 people per year. A controlled trial that aimed to demonstrate the effect of an intervention on the number of people who commit suicide would therefore need to include many thousands of participants even if the effect of the intervention were dramatic. However, evidence from observational studies does suggest that medical interventions and public health measures (Table 17.5) may have an impact on the rate of suicide. See Lewis *et al.* (1997) and Hawton (2000b) for a review of these issues.

Medical interventions for high-risk groups

Improvements in psychiatric services might be expected to lead to earlier recognition and better treatment of the psychiatric disorders and problems associated with suicide. However, published studies have found generally disappointing effects of psychosocial and psychiatric treatments of mental disorder on suicide rates. Although the use of 'prophylactic' antidepressants in the period following an episode of depression reduces the risk of a subsequent episode of depression, reduction in suicidal behaviour has not been achieved.

Table 17.5 **Suicide prevention**
Primary
Better and more available psychiatric services
Restricting the means of suicide
Educational programmes
Restricting opportunities for imitation
Secondary
Better and more available psychiatric care
Crisis centres and 'hot lines'

Although the results of observational studies have shown that patients attending 'lithium clinics' have lower rates of suicide than matched patients who do not attend clinics, it is unclear whether or not patient factors, the general effects of attendance at clinics, or the pharmacological effects of lithium are responsible for this difference.

A further clinical approach is to target high-risk groups such as patients who have recently received in-patient psychiatric treatment, people who have recently deliberately harmed themselves (intervention aimed at reducing the incidence of suicidal behaviour in the period following deliberate self-harm are reviewed on p. 529) and high-risk occupational groups and prisoners.

Population strategies

Educating primary care physicians

The effectiveness of interventions based in primary care is equivocal. Rutz and colleagues conducted an intervention study involving all general practitioners on the Swedish island of Gotland in 1983 and 1984. The study aimed to evaluate the impact of teaching the island's GPs about the diagnosis and treatment of affective disorder. After the programme was introduced, the suicide rate dropped to an extent that was significantly different from both the long-term suicide trend on Gotland and that for Sweden as a whole. A further study found that by 1988, 3 years after the project had ended, the suicide rate had returned almost to baseline values (Rutz *et al.* 1992). The researchers concluded that the programme had been effective but that it would need to be repeated every 2 years to have long-term benefits. These findings have, so far, not been replicated.

Reducing the availability of methods of suicide

Just as professions that involve easy access to potentially lethal methods of self-harm appear to have higher rates of suicide, the ease with which the population as a whole can access lethal methods of self-harm may affect the rate of suicide in that population.

Gas detoxification In Britain, in the period 1948–50, poisoning by domestic coal gas accounted for 40% of reported suicides among men and 60% among women. Following the introduction of less toxic North Sea gas, the number using this method reduced dramatically. During this period the national rate of suicide also fell. It has been argued that the removal of coal gas was responsible for this change and this view is supported by evidence that that suicide rates are higher in places where access to firearms is less restricted.

Car exhausts The fitting of catalytic converters to motor vehicles to reduce the toxicity of car exhaust fumes might be expected to reduce suicides by this course.

Modifying drug prescription Replacing prescriptions of tricyclic antidepressants with less toxic selective serotonin re-uptake inhibitors (SSRIs) may be helpful. Recent UK government legislation that has limited the amount of paracetamol that people can buy at one time will provide an opportunity to examine the effectiveness of this measure.

Physical barriers Physical barriers on bridges, train platforms, and other popular sites, together with special precautions in hospital wards, police cells, and other areas where risk is especially high, may help to reduce suicides.

It is clear that no matter what changes are made, methods by which people can fatally harm themselves will continue to be available. However, it is equally clear that a proportion of people who attempt to kill themselves are ambivalent about their plan and restricting methods for self-harm can only decrease the likelihood that suicide occurs.

Responsible media reporting The evidence on the importance of imitation as a factor in precipitating suicide suggests the need to persuade the media to take a responsible view of the reporting and portrayal of suicide. There is some evidence that restricting media reporting of suicides may reduce the number of deaths that occur.

Crisis counselling An alternative public health approach to preventing suicide has been the development of crisis counselling services, one of the most prominent of which is the Samaritan organization founded in London in 1953 by the Reverend Chad Varah. People in despair are encouraged to contact a widely publicized telephone number. The help offered ('befriending') is provided by non-professional volunteers, all trained to listen sympathetically without attempting to take on tasks that are in the province of a doctor or social worker. There is some evidence that, amongst people who telephone the Samaritans, the suicide rate in the ensuing year is higher than in the general population (Barraclough and Shea 1970). This finding suggests that the organization has attracted an appropriate group of people, but it also raises the question of the efficacy of the help offered. Comparisons of matched towns with and without services suggest little difference in suicide rates (Jennings *et al.* 1978). Even so, whether or not they prevent suicides, the Samaritans appear to perform a useful role providing for the needs of many lonely and despairing people.

Social policy Given the repeatedly demonstrated association between unemployment and suicide, Lewis and colleagues recently argued that policies aimed at reducing rates of unemployment may be among the most effective ways of reducing the rate of suicide (Lewis *et al.* 1997). Others have argued that other factors such as increasing social isolation also need to be tackled in this way. While the means to achieve such strategies are far from clear and efforts to demonstrate their effectiveness would be complex, such calls reflect our knowledge of those factors which contribute to suicide rates and should be one part of a wider debate of the relationship between social policy and health.

Public education There have been numerous public campaigns to educate the public about mental illness and its treatment. These have included several approaches in schools, such as teaching about the facts of suicide, programmes on problem-solving and also efforts to protect children and adolescents at risk.

The value of these various approaches remains uncertain.

Deliberate self-harm

People who have deliberately harmed themselves commonly present to doctors, especially in emergency departments. They are widely seen as un-popular, troublesome, and difficult to manage. However, it is evident that many have severe personal and social difficulties and that well planned care can help them.

Before the 1950s little distinction was made between people who killed themselves and those who survived after an apparent suicidal act. Stengel (1952) identified epidemiological differences between the two groups in the UK, and proposed the term 'attempted suicide' to describe an episode of self-injury consciously aimed at self-destruction that the patient could not be sure to survive. However, subsequent studies of suicidal behaviour that investigated the motivation for such episodes demonstrated that the intention of many surviving patients had not been to kill themselves. As a result terms such as 'deliberate self-poisoning', 'parasui-cide' and 'deliberate self-harm' were used to describe episodes of intentional self-harm that may or may not have been motivated by a desire to end

life. Kreitman (1977) defined this behaviour as 'a non-fatal act in which an individual deliberately causes self-injury or ingests a substance in excess of any prescribed or generally recognized dosage'. This definition is helpful because it does not specify the extent of suicidal intent. In this chapter, the term deliberate self-harm will be used to describe such incidents.

The distinction between suicide and deliberate self-harm is not absolute. There is an important overlap. Some people who had no intention of dying succumb to the effects of an overdose. Others who intended to die are revived. Moreover, many patients were ambivalent at the time, uncertain whether they wished to die or live. It should be remembered that, among patients who have been involved in deliberate self-harm, the suicide rate in the subsequent 12 months is about a hundred times greater than in the general population. For this reason and for other reasons, deliberate self-harm should not be regarded lightly.

The act of deliberate self-harm

The drugs used in deliberate self-poisoning.

In the UK, about 90% of the cases of deliberate self-harm referred to general hospitals involve a drug overdose, and most of them present no serious threat to life. The type of drug used varies some-what with age, local prescription practices, and the availability of drugs. The most commonly used drugs are the non-opiate analgesics, such as parac-etamol and aspirin. Paracetamol is particularly dangerous because it damages the liver and may lead to the delayed death of patients who had not intended to die. It is particularly worrying that younger patients who are usually unaware of the serious risks often take this drug. Amongst all cases of deliberate self-harm, about 40% of people have taken alcohol in the 6 hours before the act (Hawton *et al.* 1989).

Methods of deliberate self-injury

Deliberate self-injury accounts for 5–15% of all deliberate self-harm presenting to general hospitals in Britain. The commonest method of self-injury is laceration, usually of the forearm or wrists; it accounts for about four-fifths of the self-injuries referred to a general hospital. (Self-laceration is discussed further below.) Other forms of self-injury are jumping from heights or in front of a train or motor vehicle, shooting, and drowning. These violent acts occur mainly among older people who intended to die (Harwood and Jacoby 2000).

Deliberate self-laceration

There are three forms of deliberate self-laceration: deep and dangerous wounds inflicted with serious suicidal intent, more often by men; self-mutilation by schizophrenic patients (often in response to hallucinatory voices); and superficial wounds that do not endanger life. Only the last group will be described here. It is estimated that the majority of people who superficially cut themselves do not present to services following the attempt. Of those who are in contact with services, the majority are young and female. Personality problems characterized by low self-esteem, impulsive or aggressive behaviour, unstable moods, difficulty in interpersonal relationships are common, as are problems of alcohol and drug misuse. There is a strong association with childhood sexual abuse. Self-injury is a common and disabling problem among those with learning disability.

Usually, increasing tension and irritability precede self-laceration, and are then relieved by it. Some patients say that the lacerations were inflicted during a state in which they felt detached from their surroundings and experienced little or no pain. The lacerations are usually multiple, and are made with glass or a razor blade on the forearms or wrists. Some patients cause other injuries as well, for example by burning with cigarettes or inflicting bruises. After the act, the patient often feels shame and disgust. Some psychiatric in-patients, especially adolescents, lacerate themselves in imitation of others on the same ward. For a review see Hawton (1990).

The epidemiology of deliberate self-harm

In the early 1960s a substantial increase in deliberate self-harm began in most Western countries. In the UK, the rates of admission to general hospitals increased about fourfold in the 10 years up to 1973. The rates continued to increase more slowly in the mid–1970s, but then fell in the late 1970s. Rates are now rising again. Current estimates of the rate of deliberate self-harm in Britain suggest a figure of about 3 per 1000 per year. This results in over 100 000 hospital admissions each year. Rates in most European countries are lower (see Kerkhof 2000).

Variations according to personal characteristics

Deliberate self-harm is more common among younger people, with the rates declining sharply in middle age (Figure 17.3). Over recent years, the proportion of men presenting following deliberate self-harm has risen. In the 1960s and 1970s a female-to-male ratio of 2:1 was common; recent studies suggest that almost as many men as women now attend hospital following an episode of deliberate self-harm. The peak age for men is older than that for women. For both sexes rates are very low under the age of 12 years. Deliberate self-harm is more prevalent in the lower social classes. There are also differences related to marital status. The highest rates for both men and women are among the divorced, and high rates are also found among teenage wives and younger single men and women.

There has been little recent change in the rates of deliberate self-harm in the elderly. The characteristics of such people seem to be rather more similar to those who kill themselves than do those of younger deliberate self-harm subjects (Harwood and Jacoby 2000).

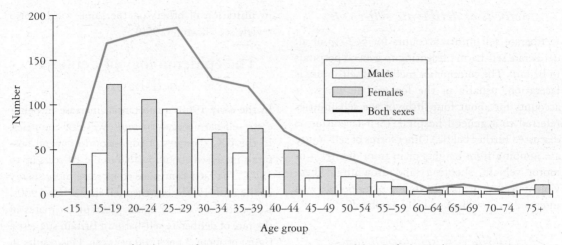

Figure 17.3 Age groups of deliberate self-harm patients presenting to hospital in Oxford, UK, by gender in 1999. Reproduced by permission of Professor K.E. Hawton, Oxford University

Variations according to place of residence

High rates are found in areas characterized by high unemployment, overcrowding, many children in care, and substantial social mobility (Gunnel *et al* 1995).

Causes of deliberate self-harm

Precipitating factors

Compared with the general population, people who deliberately harm themselves experience four times as many stressful life problems in the 6 months before the act (Paykel *et al.* 1975). The events are various, but a recent quarrel with a spouse, girlfriend, or boyfriend is particularly common. Other events include separation from or rejection by a sexual partner, the illness of a family member, recent personal physical illness, and a court appearance.

Predisposing factors

Familial and developmental factors predispose to self-harm in later life. Recent evidence suggests that familial factors may also be important in determining predisposition to acts of deliberate self-harm (Statham *et al.* 1998). There is some evidence

that early parental loss through bereavement, or a history of parental neglect or abuse, is more frequent among cases of deliberate self-harm.

There is also evidence for *personality variables*. They include poor skills in solving interpersonal problems and in planning for the future. Hopelessness and impulsiveness are the two psychological factors most often implicated in the aetiology of deliberate self-harm.

The precipitating events often occur against a *background of long-term problems concerning marriage, children, work, and health*. About two-thirds of the patients in one early study (Bancroft *et al.* 1977) had some kind of marital problem; half the men had been involved in an extramarital relationship, and a further quarter said that their wives had been unfaithful. Among the unmarried, a similar proportion has difficulties in their relationships with sexual partners. Incidents of deliberate self-harm are four times more common in women who have a past history of childhood sexual abuse when compared with women who were not abused.

Amongst men who deliberately harm themselves, the proportion who are unemployed has been increasing in recent years, and the rate of deliberate self-harm increases with length of unemployment. However, unemployment is related to other social factors associated with deliberate self-harm, such as financial difficulties, and it is difficult to determine whether unemployment is a direct cause. The association between female unemployment and attempted suicide has attracted less attention. The rates of attempted suicide are considerably higher amongst unemployed than amongst employed women, and are particularly high in women unemployed for more than a year. As with men, it is unclear whether unemployment and its consequences are a direct cause of attempted suicide, or whether women already predisposed in other ways to attempt suicides are more likely to become unemployed.

A background of poor physical health is common. This applies particularly to people with epilepsy.

Psychiatric disorder

Interviews with patients admitted to hospital following deliberate self-harm reveal high rates of depression at the time of their initial presentation. An important minority, between 5 and 15%, of patients also suffer from psychiatric disorders (Nordentoft and Rubin 1993). Few studies have followed up patients to examine the persistence of psychological symptoms and those that have attempted this have been beset by high rates of drop-out. However, a proportion of patients have enduring mental health problems and problems of alcohol and substance misuse are also more common than in the general population (Deykin and Buka 1994). Among a large series of people who deliberately harmed themselves, about half had consulted a general practitioner, psychiatrist, social worker, or another helping agency in the previous week.

Motivation and deliberate self-harm

The motives for deliberate self-harm are usually mixed and difficult to identify for certain (Table 17.6). Even if patients know their own motives, they may try to hide them from other people. For

Table 17.6 **Motives or reasons for deliberate self-harm**
To die
To escape from unbearable anguish
To get relief
To change the behaviour of others
To escape from a situation
To show desperation to others
To get back at other people/make them feel guilty
To get help

From Hawton, K. (2000). Treatment of suicide attempters and prevention of suicide and attempted suicide. In *The new Oxford textbook of psychiatry* (eds M. G. Gelder, J. J. López-Ibor Jr, and N. C. Andreasen), Chapter 4.15.4. Oxford University Press, Oxford.

example, people who have taken an overdose in frustration and anger may feel ashamed and say instead that they wished to die. Conversely, people who truly intended to kill themselves may deny it. For this reason, more emphasis should be placed on a common-sense evaluation of the patients' actions leading up to self-harm than on their subsequent accounts of their own motives.

Despite this limitation, useful information has been obtained by questioning groups of patients about their motives. Only a few say that the act was premeditated. About a quarter say that they wished to die. Some say that they are uncertain whether they wanted to die or not, others that they were leaving it to 'fate' to decide, and others that they were seeking unconsciousness as a temporary escape from their problems. Another group admit that they were trying to influence someone, for example, that they were seeking to make a relative feel guilty for having failed them in some way. This motive of influencing other people was first emphasized by Stengel and Cook (1958), who described the patients' hope of 'calling forth action from the human environment'. This behaviour has since been referred to as 'a cry for help'. Although some acts of deliberate self-harm result in increased help for the patient, others may arouse resentment, particularly if they are repeated.

The outcome of deliberate self-harm

Repetition of self-harm

Repetition rates are based on groups of patients, some of whom have received psychiatric treatment after the act. Reported rates vary between about 15 and 25% in the year after the act (Kreitman 1977). Factors associated with repetition of deliberate self-harm (Kreitman 1977; Appleby 1993) are listed in Table 17.7.

Suicide following deliberate self-harm

Among people who have intentionally harmed themselves, the risk of later suicide is much increased (Figure 17.4). For example, in the first year afterwards, the risk of suicide is about 1–2%, which is 100 times that of the general population (Kreitman 1977). An 8-year follow-up showed that, amongst patients who were previously

Table 17.7 Factors associated with risk of repetition of attempted suicide
Previous attempt(s)
Personality disorder
Alcohol or drug abuse
Previous psychiatric treatment
Unemployment
Lower social class
Criminal record
History of violence
Age 25–54 years
Single, divorced, or separated

From Hawton, K. (2000). Treatment of suicide attempters and prevention of suicide and attempted suicide. In *The new Oxford textbook of psychiatry* (eds M. G. Gelder, J. J. López-Ibor Jr, and N. C. Andreasen), Chapter 4.15.4. Oxford University Press, Oxford.

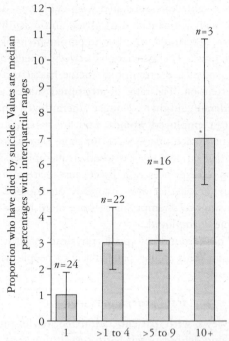

Figure 17.4 Suicide after non-fatal deliberate self-harm (DSH) according to duration of follow-up. *n* refers to number of published studies in group. Reproduced with permission Deliberate Self Harm, *Effective Health Care*, **4** (6), 1998.

admitted with deliberate self-harm, almost 3% eventually take their own lives and about twice the expected number die from natural causes (Hawton and Fagg 1988).

Among people who deliberately harm themselves, the risk of eventual suicide is greater in those with other risk factors for suicide. Thus the risk is greater among older patients who are male, depressed, or alcoholic. A non-dangerous method of self-harm does not necessarily indicate a low risk of subsequent suicide, partly because patients have little knowledge of the dangerousness of many methods. However, the risk is certainly high when violence or highly dangerous drug overdoses have been used.

In the weeks after deliberate self-harm, many patients report changes for the better. People with psychiatric symptoms often report a decrease in their intensity. Improvements may result from help provided by psychiatrists and other professionals or from improvements in relationships, attitudes, and behaviour. However, some patients fare much worse and repeatedly harm themselves within months of the first act, and some relatives are unsympathetic and even hostile.

There have been numerous attempts to construct scales to predict repetition with an accuracy that could be clinically useful. For example, Kreitman and Foster (1991) proposed a scale that allows allocation of patients to low-, moderate-, and high-risk groups. However, all instruments are of relatively low specificity, identifying no more than half of those at high risk and an even lower proportion of the numerically largest group of repeaters at moderate risk.

The results of intervention studies

Evidence that management of deliberate self-harm affects the rate of repetition of self-harm came initially from observational studies. An early study reported that the rate of repetition of deliberate self-harm among patients attending accident and emergency departments who had been assessed by a psychiatrist was half that of patients who were discharged without psychiatric assessment. A study in Oxford (Hawton *et al.* 1987) demonstrated that among women who had been admitted to hospital following deliberate self-harm, lower rates of repetition of self-harm were seen in those who had been referred for psychiatric assessment compared with those who had not been referred. No difference was seen in the rate of repetition among men.

The results of observational studies can, however, be misleading. Many factors that influence decisions about patient management are known to affect the rate of repetition of self-harm. Whilst attempts can be made to control for the potential confounding effects of these factors, the possibility that apparent effects are due to other variables that were not measured remains. The best way to reduce the impact of these other variables is to conduct an experiment and to assign large numbers of patients to different types of treatment purely on the basis of chance.

The results of experimental studies in which patients were randomly assigned to different treatments following deliberate self harm have recently been reviewed. A meta-analysis of randomized controlled trials of interventions following deliberate self-harm identified 20 trials in which repetition of deliberate self-harm was used as an outcome measure (Hawton *et al.* 1998). Trials were divided into ten different groups of treatments.

Statistically significant reductions in rates of repetition of suicidal behaviour in a subgroup with personality disorder were demonstrated for dialectical behaviour therapy compared with standard after-care. In those with a history of multiple repetition of deliberate self-harm, depot flupenthixol was shown to be superior to placebo in reducing the rate of repetition. Both these findings are based on the results of single trials and both require further evaluation. Trends towards reduction of repetition of suicidal behaviour were found for problem-solving therapy, provision of an emergency contact card, and community outreach when compared with standard after-care.

The authors of this paper conclude that 'there remains considerable uncertainty about which forms of psychosocial and physical intervention are most effective' and suggested that this was, in part, due to insufficient numbers of patients being included in studies conducted to date. Three interventions seemed promising:

♦ Although the greatest reductions in rates were found by an evaluation of the provision of *an emergency contact card*, the effectiveness of this simple intervention has since been questioned by a subsequent study that showed an increase in the rate of repetition of deliberate self-harm among those given a crisis card (M. O. Evans *et al.* 1999).

♦ Problem solving, which has been shown to be an effective treatment of depression in some settings, may also be valuable in at least a proportion of those who have harmed themselves.

◆ Dialectic behaviour therapy was introduced as a method of treatment for those with chronic repetitive self-harm and abnormal personality characteristics (Linehan *et al.* 1993). It requires intensive treatment and the benefits may not be sustained. However, it may make it possible to develop an effective intervention for people who are normally regarded as extremely difficult to treat.

Randomized controlled studies, which have included measures of outcome other than repetition of deliberate self-harm, have demonstrated reductions in contact with services, decreases in psychopathology, and improvements in social problems and social adjustment. Thus, even though there is a lack of evidence about effectiveness of interventions, there are strong reasons for believing that well-organized care has other benefits. It enables recognition and treatment of major mental disorders and also appropriate care for a range of personal and social difficulties. See Hawton (2000a) for a review.

The assessment of patients after deliberate self-harm

General aims

Assessment is concerned with three main issues: the immediate risks of suicide, the subsequent risks of further deliberate self-harm, and current medical or social problems. The assessment should be carried out in a way that encourages the patient to undertake a constructive review of his problems and of the ways in which he can deal with them himself. This encouragement of self-help is important, because many patients are unwilling to be seen again by a psychiatrist.

Usually the assessment has to be carried out in an accident and emergency department or a ward of a general hospital, in which there may be little privacy. Whenever possible, the interview should be in a side room so that it will not be overheard or interrupted. If the patient has taken an overdose, the interviewer should first make sure that the patient has recovered sufficiently to be able to give a satisfactory history. If consciousness is still impaired, the interview should be delayed. Information should also be obtained from relatives or friends, the family doctor, and any other person (such as a social worker) already attempting to help the patient. Wide enquiry is important because sometimes information from other sources may differ substantially from the account given by the patient. See Hawton (2000b) for reviews of general hospital assessment.

Specific enquiries

The interview is directed to five questions:

◆ What were the patient's intentions when he harmed himself?

◆ Does he now intend to die?

◆ What are the patient's current problems?

◆ Is there a psychiatric disorder?

◆ What helpful resources are available to this patient?

Each question will be considered in turn.

What were the patient's intentions when he harmed himself?

As mentioned already, patients sometimes misrepresent their intentions. For this reason the interviewer should reconstruct, as fully as possible, the events that led up to the act of self-harm in order to find the answers to five subsidiary questions:

◆ *Was the act planned or carried out on impulse?* The longer and more carefully the plans have been made, the greater is the risk of a fatal repetition.

◆ *Were precautions taken against being found?* The more thorough the precaution, the greater is the risk of a further fatal overdose. Of course, events do not always take place as the patient expected; for example, a spouse may arrive home earlier than usual so that the patient is discovered alive. In such circumstances it is the patient's reasonable expectations that count in predicting the future risk.

Box 17.2 Beck Suicide Intent Scale

Circumstances related to suicidal attempt

Isolation

0 Somebody present

1 Somebody nearby or in contact (as by phone)

2 No-one nearby or in contact

Timing

0 Timed so that intervention is probable

1 Timed so that intervention is not likely

2 Timed so that intervention is highly unlikely

Precautions against discovery and/or intervention

0 No precautions

1 Passive precautions as: avoiding others but doing nothing to prevent their intervention (alone in a room with unlocked door)

2 Active precaution as: locked door

Acting to gain help during/after attempt

0 Notified potential helper regarding the attempt

1 Contacted but did not specifically notify potential helper regarding the attempt

2 Did not contact or notify potential helper

Final acts in anticipation of death

0 None

1 Partial preparation or ideation

2 Definite plans made (changes in Will, giving of gifts, taking out insurance)

Degree of planning for suicide attempt

0 No preparation

1 Minimal preparation

2 Extensive preparation

Suicide note

0 Absence of note

1 Note written but torn up

2 Presence of note

Overt communication of intent before act

0 None

1 Equivocal communication

2 Unequivocal communication

Purpose of attempt

0 Mainly to change environment

1 Components of '0' and '2'

2 Mainly to remove self from environment

Self-report

Expectations regarding fatality of act

0 Patient thought that death was unlikely

1 Patient thought that death was possible but not probable

2 Patient thought that death was probable or certain

Conception of method's lethality

0 Patient did less to himself than he thought would be lethal

1 Patient wasn't sure, or did what he thought might be lethal

2 Act equalled or exceeded patient's concept of its medical lethality

'Seriousness of attempt'

0 Patient did not consider act to be a serious attempt to end his life

1 Patient was uncertain whether act was a serious attempt to end his life

2 Patient considered act to be a serious attempt to end his life

Ambivalence towards living

0 Patient did not want to die

1 Patient did not care whether he lived or died

2 Patient wanted to die

Conception of reversibility

0 Patient thought that death would be unlikely if he received medical attention

1 Patient was uncertain whether death could be averted by medical attention

2 Patient was certain of death even if he received medical attention

Degree of premeditation

0 None, impulsive

1 Suicide contemplated for 3 hours or less prior to attempt

2 Suicide contemplated for more than 3 hours prior to attempt

Reprinted with permission from Beck, A. T. *et al* (1974). *The prediction of suicide.* Charles Press, Philadelphia

♦ *Did the patient seek help?* Serious intent can be inferred if there were no attempts to obtain help after the act.

♦ *Was the method thought to be dangerous?* If drugs were used, what were they and what amount was taken? Did the patient take all the drugs available? If self-injury was used, what form did it take? (As noted above, the greater the suicidal intent the greater is the risk of a further suicide attempt.) Not only should the actual dangerousness be assessed, but also that anticipated by the patient, which may be inaccurate. For example, some people wrongly believe that paracetamol overdoses are harmless or that benzodiazepines are dangerous.

♦ *Was there a 'final act' such as writing a suicide note or making a will?* If so, the risk of a further fatal attempt is greater.

By reviewing the answers to these questions, the interviewer makes a judgement of the patient's intentions at the time of the act (Table 17.8).

Table 17.8 Factors that suggest high suicidal intent

Act carried out in isolation

Act timed so that intervention unlikely

Precautions taken to avoid discovery

Preparations made in anticipation of death (e.g. making Will, organizing insurance)

Preparations made for the act (e.g. purchasing means, saving up tablets)

Communicating intent to others beforehand

Extensive premeditation

Leaving a note

Not alerting potential helpers after the act

Admission of suicidal intent

From Hawton, K. (2000). Treatment of suicide attempters and prevention of suicide and attempted suicide. In *The new Oxford textbook of psychiatry* (eds M. G. Gelder, J. J. López-Ibor Jr, and N. C. Andreasen), Chapter 4.15.4. Oxford University Press, Oxford.

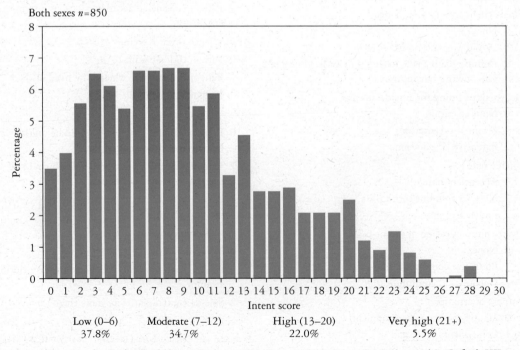

Figure 17.5 Scores on the Beck Suicide Intent Scale in 1999. From patients presenting to hospital in Oxford, UK. Reproduced by permission, Professor K.E. Hawton, Oxford University.

A similar approach has been formalized in Beck's Suicide Intent Scale (Box 17.2 and Figure 17.5; Beck *et al.* 1974) which gives a score for the degree of intent.

Does the patient now intend to die?

The interviewer should ask directly whether the patient is pleased to have recovered or wishes that he had died. If the act suggested serious suicidal intent and if the patient now denies such intent, the interviewer should try to find out by tactful questioning whether there has been a genuine change of resolve.

What are the current problems?

Many patients will have experienced a mounting series of difficulties in the weeks or months leading up to the act. Some of these difficulties may have been resolved by the time that he is interviewed; for example, a husband who planned to leave his wife may now have agreed to stay. The more serious the problems that remain, the greater is the risk of a fatal repetition. This risk is particularly strong if there are problems of loneliness or ill-health. The review of problems should be systematic and should cover the following:

- intimate relationships with the spouse or another person;
- relations with children and other relatives;
- employment, finance, and housing;
- legal problems;
- social isolation, bereavement, and other losses.

Drug and alcohol problems can be considered at this stage or when the psychiatric state is reviewed.

Is there psychiatric disorder?

It should be possible to answer this question from the history and from a brief but systematic examination of the mental state. Particular attention should be directed to depressive disorder, alcoholism, and personality disorder. Schizophrenia and dementia should also be considered, though they will found less often.

What are the patient's resources?

These include his capacity to solve his own problems, his material resources, and the help that others may provide. The best guide to patients' ability to solve future problems is their record of dealing with difficulties in the past, for example, the loss of a job or a broken relationship. The availability of help should be assessed by asking about the patients' friends and confidants, and about any support they may be receiving from their general practitioners, social workers, or voluntary agencies.

Is there a continuing risk of suicide?

The interviewer now has the information required to answer this important question. The answers to the first four questions outlined above are reviewed:

- Did the patient originally intend to die?
- Does he intend it now?
- Are the problems which provoked the act still present?
- Is he suffering from a mental disorder?

The interviewer also decides what help other people are likely to provide after the patient leaves hospital ('What are the patient's resources', above). Having reviewed the individual factors in this way, the interviewer compares the patient's characteristics with those found in groups of people who have died by suicide. These characteristics are summarized in Table 17.8.

Is there a risk of further non-fatal self-harm?

The predictive factors, which have been outlined (see p. 524), are summarized in Table 17.7. The interviewer should consider all the points in turn before making a judgement about the risk.

Is treatment required and will the patient agree to it?

If the patient is actively suicidal, the procedures are those outlined in the first part of this chapter (see p. 515). About 5–10% of deliberate self-harm patients require admission to a psychiatric unit for

- There are wide differences in national procedures, practice, and legislation.
- The patient who has harmed himself and is alert and conscious should be presumed to be competent to refuse medical advice and treatment unless there is evidence to the contrary.
- The most senior experienced doctor available should be prepared to discuss the need for treatment, the alternatives, and the patient's anxieties. It is often appropriate to involve relatives. Calm, sympathetic discussion is often effective in enabling the patient to decide to consent to treatment.
- Competence should be assessed (see p. 80), preferably by a psychiatrist.
- If the patient is competent and continues to refuse to consent, the consequences should be clearly outlined to the patient and the discussion fully recorded. The patient should be allowed to go, but encouraged to return. Where possible, an alternative plan should be agreed with the patient and, if possible, relatives or friends. If the patient is assessed as being incompetent, then the reasons should be recorded fully. Emergency treatment should proceed and a compulsory order under mental health legislation sought.

further management; most need treatment for depression, schizophrenia, or alcoholism, but a few require only a brief respite from overwhelming domestic stress. The best methods of treating the remaining patients are less certain. A quarter to a third are probably best referred to general practitioners, social workers, or others who may already be involved in their case. Many patients (up to half) may benefit from out-patient care, usually problem-oriented counselling for personal problems rather than treatment for psychiatric disorder. Many patients refuse the offer of out-patient help; their care should be discussed with the general

practitioner before they are allowed to return home. It is useful to provide an emergency telephone number enabling patients to obtain immediate advice or an urgent appointment in any further crisis.

Special groups

Mothers of young children

Mothers of young children require special consideration because of the known association between deliberate self-harm and child abuse. It is important to ask about the mother's feeling towards her children, and to enquire about their welfare. In the UK, information about the children can usually be obtained from the general practitioner, who may ask his health visitor to investigate the case.

Children and adolescents

Despite problems of case definition and identification, it appears that there has been a striking increase in the frequency of deliberate self-harm amongst children and adolescents in many parts of the developed world. Deliberate self-harm is rare but not unknown among pre-school children; it becomes increasingly common after the age of 12. It is more common amongst girls except at younger ages. The most common method is drug overdose, which is usually not dangerous, though occasionally life-threatening. The more dangerous methods of self-injury are more frequent amongst boys. Epidemics of deliberate self-harm occasionally occur amongst adolescents in psychiatric hospitals and other institutions. See de Wilde (2000).

It is difficult to determine the motivation of self-harm in young children, especially as a clear concept of death is not usually developed until around the age of 12. It is probable that only a few of the younger children have any serious suicidal intent. Possibly their motivation is more often to communicate distress, to escape from stress, or to influence other people.

Deliberate self-harm in children and adolescents is associated with histories of broken homes, family psychiatric disorder, and child abuse. It is often precipitated by social problems such as difficulties with parents, boyfriends, or schoolwork. It is also associated with mood disorder and personality disorder.

For most children and adolescents, the outcome of deliberate self-harm is relatively good, but an important minority continue to have social and psychiatric problems, and to repeat acts of deliberate self-harm. A poor outcome is associated with poor psychosocial adjustment, a history of previous deliberate self-harm, and severe family problems. There is a significant risk of suicide amongst adolescents, especially boys. When children harm themselves, it is better for them to be assessed by child psychiatrists rather than members of the adult services for deliberate self-harm. Treatment is usually directed towards the family. In the case of adolescents, treatment largely follows the general principles of management described in this chapter (see Shaffer *et al.* 2000).

The organization of services

In the UK, up until the mid–1980s, patients who presented to hospital following an episode of deliberate self-harm would receive general medical care and then be referred to psychiatric services for psychosocial assessment. However, evidence that other suitably trained staff, such as junior medical staff, nurses, and social workers, were able to carry out adequate assessments of patients following self-harm, led to a change in recommended practice. In 1984, a Department of Health circular stated that the policy of automatic referral of all patients to psychiatric services following deliberate self-harm was no longer justified (Department of Health and Social Security 1984). It recommended that other, suitably trained staff could make the initial assessment and then refer on to psychiatric services if required.

Since that time, concerns have repeatedly been expressed about the quality of psychosocial assessment of patients. In one study, the vast majority of patients appeared to have been inadequately assessed and for one in ten there was no evidence that a psychosocial assessment had been conducted (Ebbage *et al.* 1994). Such reports emphasize the need to make sure those conducting assessments

are adequately trained and supervised, and training staff has been demonstrated to improve the quality of assessment of patients (Crawford *et al.* 1998). Liaison psychiatrists are well placed to make a contribution to these tasks. At each hospital site a code of practice that details how the psychosocial assessment of patients following deliberate self-harm should be delivered should be drawn up and agreed by general medical and psychiatric services. See Hawton (2000b) for a review.

Management

All hospitals will need to have a system in place that will allow the small minority (perhaps 5–10%) who require in-patient treatment in a psychiatric unit to be identified and receive appropriate care. A larger proportion (perhaps a third) has clear mental health problems that require further treatment, usually on an out-patient basis. The management of the remaining two-thirds is less clear. This is reflected in the large variation in the proportion of patients offered follow-up from different hospitals (Kapur *et al.* 1998). The main problem is that, once they have left hospital, many patients are disinclined to take part in any treatment. For those who do agree to be seen, evidence for the effectiveness of treatment is not sufficiently well developed to make specific recommendations.

For those who are offered follow-up and attend, the main aim of treatment is to enable the patient first to resolve the difficulties that led up to the act of self-harm, and second to deal with any future crisis without resorting to further self-harm. The starting point of treatment is the list of problems compiled during the assessment procedure. Patients are encouraged to consider what steps they could take to resolve each of these problems, and to formulate a practical plan for tackling them one at a time. Throughout this discussion, the therapist tries to persuade patients to do as much as possible for themselves.

Many cases are associated with interpersonal problems. It is often helpful to interview the other person involved, first alone and then in a few joint interviews with the patient. This procedure may help to resolve problems that the couple have been unable to discuss on their own. When deliberate self-harm follows bereavement or another kind of loss, a different approach is needed. The first step should be sympathetic listening while patients express their feelings of loss. Then patients are encouraged to seek ways of gradually rebuilding their lives without the lost person. Appropriate measures will depend on the nature of the loss – whether it was through death, or the break-up of a marriage, or the end of another relationship. Again, the emphasis should be on self-help. For a review of treatment see Hawton (2000a).

Some special problems of management

Patients refusing assessment

After deliberate self-harm, some patients refuse to be interviewed, and others seek to discharge themselves before the assessment is complete. Such patients have very high rates of repetition of self-harm (Crawford and Wessely 1998). In these cases it is essential to gather as much information as possible from other sources in order to exclude serious suicidal risk of psychiatric disorder before letting the patient leave hospital. If the patient has left hospital, liaison with local community-based mental health services forms an important part of the management. Occasionally, detention under a compulsory order is appropriate.

Frequent repeaters

Some patients take overdoses repeatedly at times of stress. Often the behaviour seems intended to reduce tension or gain attention. However, when overdoses are taken repeatedly, relatives often become unsympathetic or even overtly hostile, and staff of hospital emergency departments become angry and bewildered. These patients usually have a personality disorder and many insoluble social problems, but neither counselling nor intensive psychotherapy is usually effective. It is helpful if all those involved in management agree a clear plan whereby the patient

is rewarded for constructive behaviour. An opportunity for continuing support by one person should be arranged. However, whatever help is arranged, the risk of eventual death by suicide is high.

Repeated self-cutting

The management of self-laceration presents many problems. Patients often have difficulty in expressing their feelings in words, and so formal psychotherapy may not be helpful. Simple efforts to gain the patients' confidence and increase their self-esteem are more likely to succeed. Assessment should include a behavioural analysis of the sequences of events that lead to self-cutting. This may help to formulate ways in which treatment could either interrupt the chain of events which leads to self-cutting, or replace the cutting by an alternative method of relieving methods.

Medication appears to have a limited role, although neuroleptics such as chlorpromazine or haloperidol may be valuable as a short-term measure to reduce tension. Many people who cut themselves have severe personality difficulties. Treatment should be directed towards these problems, although it may be difficult and prolonged. Admission to a psychiatric unit is occasionally necessary, and it is essential that a clear and detailed policy is agreed by those involved since self-cutting is very often difficult to manage in an in-patient unit and, indeed, may be imitated by other patients.

Further reading

Gelder, M. G., López-Ibor, J. J. Jr, and Andreasen N. C. (eds) (2000). Clinical syndromes in psychiatry. Section 4.1.5, Suicide. In *The new Oxford textbook of psychiatry*. Oxford University Press, Oxford. (The four chapters in this section review comprehensively deliberate self-harm and suicide.)

Hawton, K. E. and van Heeringen, K. (2000). *The international handbook of suicide and attempted suicide*. John Wiley, Chichester.
(Substantial and highly authoritative reviews on all aspects of suicide and attempted suicide by leading writers)

18

CHAPTER 18

The misuse of alcohol and drugs

CHAPTER 18

The misuse of alcohol and drugs

The presentation of alcohol and drug misuse is not limited to any particular psychiatric or indeed medical speciality. Alcohol and drug use may play an important part in all aspects of psychiatric practice, and is relevant for example, in the assessment of a patient with acute confusion on a medical ward, a suicidal patient in the accident and emergency department, the elderly patient whose self-care has deteriorated, the troubled adolescent, or a disturbed child who may be inhaling volatile substances.

The phrases *substance use disorder* (DSM-IV) or *disorders due to psychoactive drug use* (ICD-10) are used to refer to conditions arising from the misuse of alcohol, psychoactive drugs, and other chemicals such as volatile substances. In this chapter, problems related to alcohol will be discussed first under the general heading of alcohol use disorders; problems related to drugs and other chemicals will be discussed second under the general heading of other substance use disorders.

Classification of substance use disorders

The two classification systems, DSM-IV and ICD-10, use similar categories of substance use disorders but group them in different ways. Both schemes recognize the following disorders: intoxication, abuse (or harmful use), dependence, withdrawal states, psychotic disorders, and amnestic syndromes. These and some additional categories are shown in Table 18.1.

In both diagnostic systems the first step in classification is to specify the *substance or class of substance*

that is involved (Table 18.2); this provides the primary diagnostic category.

Although many drug users take more than one kind of drug, the diagnosis of the disorder is made on the basis of the most important substance used. Where this judgement is difficult or where use is chaotic and indiscriminate, the categories *polysubstance-related disorder* (DSM-IV) or *disorder due to multiple drug use* (ICD-10) may be employed. Then the relevant disorder listed in Table 18.1 is added to the substance misused. In this system any kind of disorder can, in principle, be attached to any drug, though in practice certain disorders do not

Table 18.1 Substance-related disorders

DSM-IV	ICD–10
Intoxication	Intoxication
Abuse	Harmful use
Dependence	Dependence syndrome
Withdrawal	Withdrawal state
Withdrawal delirium	Withdrawal state with delirium
Psychotic disorders	Psychotic disorder
Dementia	
Amnestic disorder	Amnestic syndrome
Mood disorders	Residual and late onset psychotic disorder
Anxiety disorders	Other mental and behavioural disorders
Sexual dysfunctions	
Sleep disorders	

develop with individual drugs. ICD-10 also has a specific category *residual and late-onset psychotic disorder*, which describes physiological or psychological changes that occur when a drug is taken but then persist beyond the period during which a direct effect of the substance would reasonably be expected to be operating. Such categories might include hallucinogen-induced flashbacks or alcohol-related dementia.

Definitions in DSM-IV and ICD-10

Both DSM-IV and ICD-10 provide definitions of *intoxication*. In both systems, intoxication is seen as a transient syndrome due to recent substance ingestion that produces clinically significant psychological and physical impairment. These changes disappear when the substance is eliminated from the body. The nature of the psychological changes varies with the person as well as with the drug; for example, some people intoxicated with alcohol become aggressive, but others become maudlin.

The term *abuse* in DSM-IV and *harmful use* in ICD-10 refer to maladaptive patterns of substance use that impair health in a broad sense (Table 18.3). (The widely used term *misuse* carries a similar meaning). The definition in ICD-10 is likely to depend more on the experience and judgement of the clinician and therefore may be more inclusive. Some individuals show definite evidence of substance abuse but do not meet criteria for substance dependence (Table 18.4). However, if they do, the diagnosis of dependence should be made and not that of abuse or harmful use.

The term *dependence* refers to certain physiological and psychological phenomena induced by the repeated taking of a substance; the criteria for diagnosing dependence are similar in DSM-IV and ICD-10, and include:

♦ a strong desire to take the substance;

♦ progressive neglect of alternative sources of satisfaction;

♦ the development of tolerance;

♦ a physical withdrawal state (see Table 18.4).

Tolerance is a state in which, after repeated administration, a drug produces a decreased effect, or increasing doses are required to produce the same effect. A *withdrawal state* is a group of symptoms and signs occurring when a drug is reduced in amount or withdrawn, which last for a limited time. The nature of the withdrawal state is related to the class of substance used.

Alcohol-related disorders

Terminology

In the past, the term *alcoholism* was generally used in medical writing. Although the word is still widely used in everyday language, it is unsatisfactory as a technical term because it has more than one meaning. It can be applied to habitual alcohol consumption that is deemed excessive in amount according to some arbitrary criterion. Alcoholism may also refer to damage, whether mental, physical, or social, resulting from such excessive consumption. In a more specialized sense, alcoholism may imply a specific disease entity that is supposed to require medical treatment. However, to speak of an alcoholic often has a pejorative meaning, suggesting behaviour that is morally bad.

For most purposes it is better to use three terms that relate to the classifications outlined above: *excessive consumption of alcohol*, *alcohol misuse* (the term *abuse* is used in DSM-IV but is not favoured generally because of its pejorative overtones), and *alcohol dependence*. *Excessive consumption of alcohol* refers to a daily or weekly intake of alcohol exceeding a specified amount (see below). *Alcohol misuse* describes drinking that causes mental, physical, or social harm to an individual. The term *alcohol dependence* can be used when the additional criteria for a dependence syndrome listed in Table 18.4 are met.

A fourth term that is often used is *problem drinking*, which is applied to those in whom drinking has caused an alcohol-related disorder or disability. Its meaning is essentially similar to alcohol misuse but it can also include drinkers who

Table 18.2 Classes of substances	
DSM-IV	**ICD–10***
Alcohol	Alcohol
Amphetamines	Other stimulants, including caffeine
Caffeine	
Cannabis	Cannabinoids
Cocaine	Cocaine
Hallucinogens	Hallucinogens
Inhalants	Volatile solvents
Nicotine	Tobacco
Opioids	Opioids
Phencyclidine	
Sedatives, hypnotics or anxiolytics	Sedatives or hypnotics
Polysubstance	Multiple drug use
Other	

* The order of entries in the classification has been amended to show parallels with DSM-IV.

Table 18.3 Criteria for substance abuse (DSM-IV) and harmful use (ICD–10)	
DSM-IV	**ICD–10**
A A maladaptive pattern of substance use leading to clinically significant impairment or distress, as manifested by one (or more) of the following occurring within a 12-month period	A A pattern of psychoactive substance use that is causing damage to health; the damage may be to physical or mental health
(1) Recurrent substance use resulting in a failure to fulfil major role obligations at work, school, or home	
(2) Recurrent substance abuse in situations that are physically hazardous	
(3) Recurrent substance abuse-related legal problems	
(4) Continued substance abuse despite having persistent or recurrent social or interpersonal problems caused by or exacerbated by the effects of the substance	
B Has never met the criteria for substance dependence for this class of substance	

Source: Peachey and Loh (1994).

Table 18.4 Criteria for dependence in DSM-IV and ICD–10

DSM-IV	ICD–10
A Diagnosis of dependence should be made if three (or more) of the following have been experienced or exhibited at any time in the same 12-month period	A Diagnosis of dependence should be made if three or more of the following have been experienced or exhibited at some time during the last year
(1) Tolerance defined by either need for markedly increased amounts of substance to achieve intoxication or desired effect, or markedly diminished effect with continued use of the same amount of the substance	(1) A strong desire or sense of compulsion to take the substance
(2) Withdrawal, as evidenced by either of the following: the characteristic withdrawal syndrome for the substance, or the same (or closely related) substance is taken to relieve or avoid withdrawal symptoms	(2) Difficulties in controlling substance-taking behaviour in terms of its onset, termination, or levels of use
	(3) Physiological withdrawal state when substance use has ceased or been reduced, as evidenced by either of the following: the characteristic withdrawal syndrome for the substance, or use of the same (or closely related) substance with the intention of relieving or avoiding withdrawal symptoms
(3) The substance is often taken in larger amounts over a longer period of time than was intended	
(4) Persistent desire or repeated unsuccessful efforts to cut down or control substance use	(4) Evidence of tolerance, such that increased doses of the psychoactive substance are required in order to achieve effects originally produced by lower doses
(5) A great deal of time is spent in activities necessary to obtain the substance, use the substance, or recover from its effects	(5) Progressive neglect of alternative pleasures or interests because of psychoactive substance use and increased amount of time necessary to obtain or take the substance or to recover from its effects
(6) Important social, occupational, or recreational activities given up or reduced because of substance use	(6) Persisting with substance use despite clear evidence of overtly harmful consequences (physical or mental)
(7) Continued substance use despite knowledge of having had a persistent or recurrent physical or psychological problem that was likely to have been caused or exacerbated by the substance	

are dependent on alcohol. The term alcoholism, if it is used at all, should be regarded as a shorthand way of referring to some combination of these four conditions. However, since these specific terms have been introduced fairly recently, the term alcoholism has to be used in this chapter when referring to the older literature. At this point it is appropriate to examine the *moral* and *medical* models of alcohol misuse.

The moral and medical models

According to the moral model, if someone drinks too much, he does so of his own *free will*, and if his drinking causes harm to himself or his family, his actions are *morally bad*. The corollary of this attitude is that public drunkenness should be *punished*. In many countries this is the official practice; public drunks are fined and if they cannot pay the fine, they go to prison. Many people now believe that this approach is too harsh and unsympathetic. Whatever the humanitarian arguments, there is little practical justification for punishment, since there is little evidence that it influences the behaviour of excessive drinkers.

According to the medical model, a person who misuses alcohol is *ill* rather than wicked. Although it had been proposed earlier, this idea was not strongly advocated until 1960 when Jellinek published an influential book, *The disease concept of alcoholism*. The disease concept embodies three basic ideas:

- Some people have a *specific vulnerability* to alcohol misuse.

- Excessive drinking progresses through well-defined stages, at one of which the person can *no longer control* his drinking.

- Excessive drinking may lead to *physical and mental disease* of several kinds.

One of the main consequences of the disease model is that attitudes towards excessive drinking become more humane. Instead of blame and punishment, medical treatment is provided. The disease model also has certain disadvantages. By implying that only certain people are at risk, it diverts attention

from two important facts. First, anyone who drinks a great deal for a long time may become dependent on alcohol. Second, the best way to curtail the misuse of alcohol may be to limit consumption *in the whole population*, and not just among a predisposed minority.

Excessive alcohol consumption

In many societies the use of alcohol is sanctioned and even encouraged by sophisticated marketing techniques. Therefore the level of drinking at which an individual is considered to demonstrate excessive alcohol consumption is a somewhat *arbitrary concept*, usually defined in terms of the level of use associated with significant risk of alcohol-related health and social problems. It is usually expressed in units of alcohol consumed per week (Austoker 1994) (Table 18.5).

Whilst there is reason to suppose that anyone may become dependent on alcohol if he or she drinks a sufficiently large amount for long enough, because of substantial individual variation no exact threshold can be specified. However, *women are more sensitive than men* to the harm-inducing effects of alcohol.

Table 18.5 Alcohol consumption in men and women and risk of social and health problems

Alcohol intake (units/week)	Risk of problems
Men 0–21 Women 0–14	Low
Men 22–50 Women 15–35	Increasing, particularly in smokers
Men >50 Women >35	High, particularly in smokers

Source: Austoker (1994).

Table 18.6 Alcohol content of some beverages

Beverage	Approximate alcohol content (%)	Grams alcohol per conventional measure	Units of alcohol per conventional measure (approximate)
Beer and cider			
Ordinary beer	3	16 per pint 12 per can	2 per pint 1.5 per can
Strong beer	5.5	32 per pint 24 per can	4 per pint 3 per can
Extra-strong beer	7	40 per pint 32 per can	5 per pint 4 per can
Cider	4	24 per pint	3 per pint
Strong cider	6	32 per pint	4 per pint
Wine			
Table wine	8–10	8 per glass 56 per bottle	1 per glass 7 per bottle
Fortified wines (sherry, port, vermouth)	13–16	8 per measure 120 per bottle	1 per measure 15 per bottle
Spirits (whisky, gin, brandy, vodka)	32	8–12 per single measure 240 per bottle	1–1.5 per measure* 30 per bottle

* Somewhat larger measures are used in Scotland and Northern Ireland (12 grams).

Adapted from the Royal College of Physicians (1987, p. 6).

If the concept of excessive alcohol consumption is to be understood and accepted, it is necessary to explain the units in which it is assessed. In everyday life, this is done by referring to conventional measures such as pints of beer or glasses of wine. These measures have the advantage of being widely understood, but they are imprecise because both beers and wines vary in strength (Table 18.6). Alternatively, consumption can be measured as the amount of alcohol (expressed in grams). This measure is precise and useful for scientific work, but is difficult for many people to relate to everyday measures.

For this reason, the concept of a *unit of alcohol* has been introduced for use in health education. A unit can be related to everyday measures for it corresponds to half a pint of beer, one glass of table wine, one conventional glass of sherry or port, and one single bar measure of spirits. It can also be related to average amounts of alcohol (see Table 18.6); thus on this measure a can of beer (450 ml) contains nearly 1.5 units, a bottle of table wine contains about 7 units, a bottle of spirits about 30 units, and 1 unit is about 8 g of alcohol.

Epidemiological aspects of excessive drinking and alcohol misuse

Epidemiological methods can be applied to the following questions concerning excessive drinking and alcohol misuse.

- What is the annual per capita consumption of alcohol for a nation as a whole, and how does this vary over the years and between nations?

- What is the pattern of alcohol use of different groups of people within a defined population?

- How many people in a defined population misuse alcohol?

- How does alcohol misuse vary with such characteristics as sex, age, occupation, social class, and marital status?

Unfortunately, we lack reliable answers to these questions, partly because different investigators have used different methods of defining and identifying alcohol misuse and 'alcoholism', and partly because excessive drinkers tend to be evasive about the amounts that they drink and the symptoms that they experience.

Consumption of alcohol in different countries

In the UK, the annual consumption of alcohol per adult (calculated as absolute ethanol consumption) doubled between 1950 and 1980 but has now flattened off. The average annual consumption per adult is around 7.5 litres. Consumption in Europe is a generally higher than this, particularly in France (about 13 litres annually). More recently, economic and political changes in the former Soviet Union and other parts of eastern Europe have been accompanied by striking increases in alcohol consumption and associated mortality (Cockerham 1997).

Current changes in the UK can be usefully considered in a historical perspective. For example, in Great Britain between 1860 and 1900 the consumption of alcohol was about 10 litres of absolute alcohol per head of population over 15 years old. Consumption then fell until the early 1930s, reaching about 4 litres per person over 15 years per annum. Consumption then increased slowly until the 1950s when it began to rise more rapidly.

These changes have been accompanied by alterations in the kinds of alcoholic beverages consumed. In Britain in 1900 beer and spirits accounted for most of the alcohol drunk; in 1980 the consumption of wine had risen about four times and accounted for almost as much of the consumption of alcohol as did spirits, though most alcohol was still consumed as beer.

Drinking habits in different groups

Surveys of drinking behaviour generally depend on self-reports, a method that is open to obvious errors. Enquiries of this kind have been conducted in several countries including the UK and the USA.

Such studies show that the highest consumption of alcohol is generally amongst *young men* who are *unmarried, separated, or divorced*. However, over the last 15 years drinking by women has increased. In 1992, men in the UK drank on average 15.9 units of alcohol a week (about 8 pints of beer), while women drank about a third of this amount. The alcohol consumption of 27% of men and 11% of women exceeded recommended limits; therefore these subjects could be considered at risk of developing an alcohol-related disorder, including alcohol dependence. Six per cent of men and 2% of women drank more than 50 units a week (Austoker 1994).

The prevalence of alcohol misuse

This can be estimated in three ways: from hospital admission rates, from deaths from alcoholic cirrhosis, and by surveys in the general population.

Hospital admission rates These give an inadequate measure of prevalence because a large proportion of excessive drinkers do not enter hospital. In the UK, admissions for problems related to alcohol misuse account for 10% of all psychiatric admissions. In France, Germany, and Eire the figure is almost 30%. More recent trends to treat patients with alcohol problems outside hospital are likely to result in a decline in these figures. Alcohol misuse also figures prominently in admissions to general hospitals, where screening questionnaires identify alcohol misuse in about 20–30% of male admissions and 5–10% of female admissions (Chick 1994).

Deaths from alcoholic cirrhosis About 10–20% of people who drink alcohol excessively develop cirrhosis of the liver, and there are correlations in a population between rates of liver cirrhosis and mean alcohol consumption. Therefore deaths from cirrhosis can be used as a means of estimating rates of alcohol misuse. Rates of mortality from liver cirrhosis are showing a decline in a number of developed countries. For example, over the last 10 years in southern Europe there has been a sustained decrease in deaths from cirrhosis, probably as a result of sustained fiscal, law enforcement, and health promotion policies (Gual and Colom 1997).

General population surveys One method of ascertaining the rate of problem drinking in a population is by seeking information from general practitioners, social workers, probation officers, health visitors, and other agents who are likely to come in contact with heavy drinkers. Another approach is the community survey in which samples of people are asked about the amount they drink and whether they experience symptoms.

Two recent epidemiological investigations in the USA (the Epidemiological Catchment Area Programme and the National Comorbidity Survey) suggested a combined 1-year prevalence rate for alcohol misuse and dependence of 7–10%. The corresponding lifetime risks were about 14–20% (Kessler *et al.* 1994; Regier *et al.* 1994b).

A general population survey of UK households found a 1-year prevalence of alcohol dependence of 4.7% (Meltzer *et al.* 1994). However, surveys based on households are likely to miss certain groups at high risk of alcohol misuse and dependence. The UK Psychiatric Morbidity Surveys also sampled separately from homeless populations and from those in institutions such as prisons. Among people living in night shelters or sleeping rough, 40% were found to drink more than 50 units of alcohol a week and 36% of those sleeping rough were estimated to have severe alcohol dependence (Gill *et al.* 1996). High rates of alcohol misuse were also found in prisoners, especially among white men (Singleton *et al.* 1997).

In a cross-national study of ten different cultural regions, lifetime prevalence rates for alcohol misuse and dependence varied from about 0.5% in Shanghai to 22% in Korea (Helzer and Canino 1992). Whilst there are undoubtedly wide variations between countries in the real prevalence of alcohol-related disorders, some of the apparent differences may stem from contrasting cultural perspectives on what constitutes alcohol misuse and the extent to which people chose to reveal their drinking habits to investigators.

Alcohol misuse and population characteristics

Gender Rates of alcohol misuse and dependence are consistently higher in men than in women but the ratio of affected men to women varies markedly across cultures. In Western countries, about three times as many men as women suffer from alcohol misuse and dependence, but in Asian and Hispanic cultures over ten times as many men are affected (Helzer and Canino 1992). In the National Comorbidity Survey in the USA, the 1-year prevalence of alcohol misuse and dependence in men (14.1%) was almost three times that in women (5.3%) (Kessler *et al.* 1994). Similarly, in the UK Psychiatric Morbidity Survey, prevalence of alcohol dependence was three times higher among men than among women (Meltzer *et al.* 1994).

Age We have seen that the heaviest drinkers are *men in their late teens or early twenties*. In most cultures the prevalence of alcohol misuse and dependence is lower in those aged over 45 years (Helzer and Canino 1992; Meltzer *et al.* 1994). Recent studies suggest that the homeless young are at considerably greater risk of misusing alcohol and other substances (Gill *et al.* 1996).

Ethnicity and culture The followers of certain *religions* which proscribe alcohol, for example, Islam, Hinduism, and the Baptist Church, are less likely than the general population to misuse alcohol. It is also worth noting that Afro-Caribbeans in the UK and blacks in the USA are less likely to drink excessively than the white population and therefore have a lower rate of alcohol-related disorders (Kessler *et al.* 1994).

In some instances, the low consumption of alcohol in a particular ethnic group may be due to a *biologically determined* lack of tolerance to alcohol. For example, Asians and Orientals with a particular variant of the isoenzyme of aldehyde dehydrogenase experience flushing, nausea, and tachycardia due to accumulation of acetaldehyde when they drink alcohol. Such subjects are likely to be at reduced risk of excess drinking and the consequent development of alcohol-related disorders. Thus, although the aldehyde dehydrogenase variant that causes the flushing reaction was present in 35% of the general Japanese population, it was found in only 7% of Japanese patients with alcoholic liver disease (Shibuya and Yoshida 1988).

Occupation The risk of alcohol misuse is much increased among several *occupational groups* chefs, kitchen porters, barmen, and brewery workers, who have easy access to alcohol, executives and salesmen who entertain on expense accounts, actors and entertainers, seamen, and journalists and printers. *Doctors* are another important group with an increased risk of problem drinking, and they are often particularly difficult to help (Chick 1992).

The syndromes of alcohol dependence and alcohol withdrawal

Patients are described as alcohol dependent when they meet the criteria for *substance dependence* described in Table 18.4. The presence of withdrawal phenomena are not necessary for the diagnosis of dependence and substantial minority of subjects who meet dependence criteria do not experience any withdrawal phenomena when their intake of alcohol diminishes or stops. However, about 5% of dependent subjects experience severe *withdrawal symptomatology* including *delirium tremens* and *grand mal seizures*.

Course of alcohol dependence

Schuckit *et al.* (1993) reviewed the course of over 600 men with alcohol dependence who received in-patient treatment at a single facility in the USA between 1985 and 1991. These subjects showed a general pattern of *escalation of heavy drinking* in their late twenties followed by evidence of serious *difficulties in work and social life* by their early thirties. In their middle to late thirties, following the perception that they could not *control their drinking*, subjects experienced increasing social and work problems together with a significant *deterioration in physical health*.

The alcohol withdrawal syndrome

Withdrawal symptoms occur across a spectrum of severity, from mild anxiety and sleep disturbance to the life-threatening state known as *delirium tremens*. The symptoms generally occur in people who have been drinking heavily for years and who maintain a high intake of alcohol for weeks at a time. The symptoms follow a drop in blood concentration. They characteristically appear on waking, after the fall in concentration during sleep. *Dependent drinkers* often take *a drink on waking* to stave off withdrawal symptoms. In most cultures, *early-morning drinking* is diagnostic of dependency. With increasing need to stave off withdrawal symptoms during the day, the drinker typically becomes *secretive* about the amount consumed, hides bottles, or carries them in a pocket. Rough cider and cheap wines may be drunk regularly to obtain the most alcohol for the least money.

The earliest and commonest feature of alcohol withdrawal is acute *tremulousness* affecting the hands, legs, and trunk ('the shakes'). The sufferer may be unable to sit still, hold a cup steady, or do up buttons. He is also *agitated* and easily startled, and often dreads facing people or crossing the road. *Nausea, retching, and sweating* are frequent. *Insomnia* is also common. If alcohol is taken, these symptoms may be relieved quickly; if not, they may last for several days.

As withdrawal progresses, *misperceptions* and *hallucinations* may occur, usually only briefly.

Objects appear distorted in shape, or shadows seem to move; disorganized voices, shouting, or snatches of music may be heard. Later there may be *epileptic seizures*, and finally after about 48 hours *delirium tremens* may develop (Victor and Adams 1953) (see below).

Other alcohol-related disorders

The different types of damage – *physical*, *psychological*, and *social* – that can result from alcohol misuse are described in this section. A person who suffers from these disabilities may or may not be suffering from alcohol dependence.

Physical damage

Excessive consumption of alcohol may lead to physical damage in several ways. First it can have a *direct toxic effect* on certain tissues, notably the *brain* and *liver*. Second, it is often accompanied by *poor diet* which may lead to deficiency of *protein* and *B vitamins*. Third, it increases the risk of *accidents*, particularly head injury. Fourth, it is accompanied by general neglect which can lead to increased *susceptibility to infection*.

Physical complications of alcohol misuse occur in several systems of the body. *Alimentary disorders* are common, notably liver damage, gastritis, peptic ulcer, oesophageal varices, and acute and chronic pancreatitis. *Damage to the liver*, including fatty infiltration, hepatitis, cirrhosis, and hepatoma, is particularly important.

Cirrhosis

For a person who is dependent on alcohol, the risk of dying from liver cirrhosis is almost *ten times greater* than the average. However, only about 10–20% of alcohol-dependent people develop cirrhosis. The vulnerability to alcohol-induced liver disease may be influenced by *genetic differences* in the enzymes that metabolize alcohol. For example, the incidence of liver disease was higher in those excess alcohol users with a particular polymorphism for *alcohol dehydrogenase* (Sherman *et al.* 1993).

Nervous system

Alcohol also damages the nervous system. Neuropsychiatric complications are described later; other neurological conditions include *peripheral neuropathy, epilepsy*, and *cerebellar degeneration*. The last of these is characterized by unsteadiness of stance and gait, with less effect on arm movements or speech. Rare complications are optic atrophy, central pontine myelinolysis, and *Marchiafava-Bignami syndrome*. The last of these results from widespread demyelination of the corpus callosum, optic tracts, and cerebellar peduncles. Its main features are dysarthria, ataxia, epilepsy, and marked impairment of consciousness; in the more prolonged forms, dementia and limb paralysis occur. *Head injury* is also common in alcohol-dependent people.

Cardiovascular system

Alcohol misuse is associated with *hypertension* and increased risk of *stroke*. Paradoxically, men who drink moderate amounts of alcohol (up to about 20 units a week) appear less likely than non-drinkers to die from coronary artery disease (see Goldberg *et al.* 1999). Alcohol misuse has also been linked to the development of certain cancers, notably of the mouth, pharynx, oesophagus, and liver.

Other physical complications of consumption of alcohol are too numerous to detail here. Examples include anaemia, myopathy, episodic hypoglycaemia, haemochromatosis, cardiomyopathy, vitamin deficiencies, and tuberculosis. They are described in textbooks of medicine, for example the *Oxford textbook of medicine* (Weatherall *et al.* 1995).

Mortality

Not surprisingly, the *mortality rate* is increased in those who misuse alcohol. Follow-up investigations have studied mainly middle-aged men in whom overall mortality is at least *twice the expected rate*. Mortality in *alcohol-dependent women* appears substantially *higher than this* (Harris and Barraclough 1998). In a study of 99 married men who had attended a specialist alcohol problems clinic in London, Marshall *et al.* (1994) found that 44 subjects had died during 20-year follow-up. The mortality rate in the moderately alcohol-dependent subjects was almost three times the expected value, whilst in those classified as severely dependent it was increased almost 4.5 times. The major causes of death were diseases of the circulatory system, and cancer. However, six deaths were caused by injury or poisoning, of which at least three were due to suicide.

Even allowing for the fact that heavy drinkers also tend to be heavy smokers, alcohol itself is almost certainly responsible for a substantial part of this increased mortality. In the UK it is estimated that excess alcohol consumption leads to about 33 000 premature deaths a year, mainly from cardiovascular disorders, cirrhosis, accidents, and cancer (Austoker 1994; Ashworth and Gerada 1997).

Damage to the fetus

There is evidence that a *fetal alcohol syndrome* occurs in some children born to mothers who drink excessively. In France, Lemoine *et al.* (1968) described a syndrome of *facial abnormality, small stature, low birth-weight, low intelligence, and overactivity*. In a 10-year follow-up of children with fetal alcohol syndrome, Spohr *et al.* (1993) found that, whilst the characteristic craniofacial malformations decreased with time, many subjects had evidence of persisting mental retardation.

In a large prospective study in France (Kaminski *et al.* 1976), women who drank about 400 ml of wine (or equivalent of other drinks) daily were not found to have babies with higher rates of congenital malformation or neonatal mortality. However, the women had more than the expected number *of stillbirths*, and their babies' *birth-weights were lower*. Compared with other mothers, those who drank excessively were older, more often unmarried, of lower social status, and of greater parity, and they smoked more. They also had more bleeding in early pregnancy. When allowance was made for these factors, the authors still found that alcohol independently affected birth-weight, placental weight, and stillbirths.

It seems reasonable to conclude that, among the offspring of some mothers who drink excessively, there is a syndrome of the kind mentioned above, but that it occurs infrequently and only when the mother has been drinking heavily during pregnancy. When mothers drink excessively, though less heavily than this, their infants appear to have lower birth-weights and smaller stature than others. Long-term effects on development have also been observed. At the moment it is not known if there is, in fact, a 'safe level' of alcohol consumption during pregnancy (Allebeck and Olsen 1998).

Psychiatric disorders

Alcohol-related psychiatric disorders fall into four groups:

- intoxication phenomena
- withdrawal phenomena
- toxic or nutritional disorders
- associated psychiatric disorders.

Intoxication phenomena

The severity of the symptoms of alcohol intoxication correlate approximately with the blood concentration. As noted above, there is much individual variation in the psychological effects of alcohol, but certain reactions such as lability of mood and belligerence are more likely to cause social difficulties. At high doses, alcohol intoxication can result in serious adverse effects such as falls, respiratory depression, inhalation of vomit, and hypothermia.

The *molecular mechanisms* that underlie the acute effects of alcohol are not clear. An influential view has been that alcohol interacts with neuronal membranes to *increase their fluidity*, an action also ascribed to certain anaesthetic agents. This action gives rise to more specific changes in the release of a range of neurotransmitters leading to the characteristic pharmacological actions of alcohol. For example, the pleasurable effects of alcohol use could be mediated by release of *dopamine and opioids* in mesolimbic forebrain, whilst the anxiolytic effects could reflect facilitation of brain *gamma-aminobutyric acid* (GABA) activity (Nutt 1999).

The term *idiosyncratic alcohol intoxication* has been applied to marked maladaptive changes in behaviour, such as aggression, occurring within minutes of taking an amount of alcohol insufficient to induce intoxication in most people (with the behaviour being uncharacteristic of the person). In the past, these sudden changes in behaviour were called pathological drunkenness, or *manie à potu*, and the descriptions emphasized the explosive nature of the outbursts of aggression. There is doubt, however, whether behaviour of this kind really is induced by small amounts of alcohol. The term idiosyncratic alcohol intoxication does not appear in DSM-IV or ICD-10.

Memory blackouts or *short-term amnesia* are frequently reported after heavy drinking. At first the events of the night before are forgotten, even though consciousness was maintained at the time. Such memory losses can occur after a single episode of heavy drinking in people who are not dependent on alcohol; if they recur regularly, they indicate habitual excessive consumption. With sustained excessive drinking, memory losses may become more severe, affecting parts of the daytime or even whole days.

Withdrawal phenomena

The general withdrawal syndrome has been described earlier under the heading of alcohol dependence. Here we are concerned with the more serious psychiatric syndrome of *delirium tremens*.

Delirium tremens This occurs in people whose history of alcohol misuse extends over several years. Following alcohol withdrawal there is a dramatic and rapidly changing picture of disordered mental activity, with *clouding of consciousness, disorientation* in time and place, and *impairment of recent memory*. Perceptual disturbances include *misinterpretations of sensory stimuli* and *vivid hallucinations*, which are usually visual but sometimes occur in other modalities. There is severe *agitation*, with restlessness, shouting, and evident fear. *Insomnia* is prolonged. The hands are *grossly tremulous* and sometimes pick up imaginary objects, and truncal ataxia occurs. *Autonomic disturbances* include sweating, fever, tachycardia, raised blood pressure, and dilatation of pupils. *Dehydration and electrolyte disturbance* are characteristic. Blood testing shows *leucocytosis* and *impaired liver function*.

The condition lasts 3 or 4 days, with the symptoms characteristically being worse at night. It often ends with deep prolonged sleep from which the patient awakens with no symptoms and little or no memory of the period of delirium. Delirium tremens carries a *significant risk of mortality* and should be regarded as a medical emergency.

Toxic or nutritional conditions

These include *Korsakov's psychosis* and *Wernicke's encephalopathy* (see also Chapter 14) and *alcoholic dementia*, which is described next.

Alcoholic dementia In the past there has been disagreement as to whether alcohol misuse can cause dementia. This doubt may have arisen because patients with general intellectual defects have been wrongly diagnosed as having Korsakov's psychosis. However, it is now generally agreed that chronic alcohol misuse can cause cognitive impairment, particularly in tests of *frontal lobe function* (see O'Malley and Krishnan-Sarin 1998).

Attention has also been directed to the related question of whether chronic alcohol misuse can cause structural brain atrophy. Both CT scanning and magnetic resonance imaging (MRI) have shown that excess alcohol consumption is associated with *enlarged lateral ventricles*. Furthermore, MRI scans have shown focal deficits with *loss of grey matter* in both cortical and subcortical areas. Subcortical changes are more likely to be found in patients with Korsakov's syndrome. Thinning of the *corpus callosum* has also been reported in patients with alcohol dependence. Functional brain imaging reveals decreased blood flow and glucose metabolism in cortical regions; however, these changes may be secondary to loss of cerebral tissue.

Many of the changes noted above occur in patients without obvious neurological disturbance, though, as note above, psychological testing usually reveals deficits in *cognitive function*. The changes in brain structure and cognitive impairment seen in excessive drinkers remit to some extent with cessation of alcohol use; however, many abnormalities can still be detected after long periods of abstinence. (For a review of the effect of alcohol on structural and functional brain imaging see Besson 1993 and Chick 1997.)

Studies of this kind suggest that alcoholic dementia is more common than was previously supposed, and it should be searched for carefully in every problem drinker. Older patients appear to be more at risk than younger ones with a similar length of heavy drinking, and those who have been drinking without respite seem to be more at risk than people who have periods in which they reduce their drinking. Women appear to be more vulnerable than men to alcohol-induced cognitive impairment (Mann *et al.* 1992).

Associated psychiatric disorder

Personality deterioration As the patient becomes more and more concerned with the need to obtain alcohol, interpersonal skills and attendance to usual interests and responsibilities may deteriorate. These changes in social and interpersonal functioning should not be confused with personality disorder, which should be diagnosed only when the appropriate features have been clearly present prior to the development of alcohol dependence.

Mood disorder The relationship between alcohol consumption and mood is complex. On the one hand, some depressed patients drink excessively in an attempt to improve their mood; on the other hand, excess drinking may induce persistent depression or anxiety. In hospital populations major depression frequently coexists with alcohol misuse and dependence, but in community samples the relationship is weaker, particularly for men. Davidson and Ritson (1993) concluded that the most common reason for depressive symptomatology in alcohol-dependent subjects was *adjustment disorder or alcohol-induced mood disorder*.

Suicidal behaviour Suicide rates amongst alcoholics are higher than among non-alcoholics of the same age.

Kessel and Grossman (1965) found that 8% of alcoholics admitted for treatment killed themselves within a few years of discharge. The rate of suicide in alcohol-dependent people is increased about sixfold (Harris and Barraclough 1997). In a study of 50 alcohol misusers who had committed suicide, Murphy *et al.* (1992) identified a number of risk factors for suicidal behaviour, including continued drinking, co-morbid major depression, serious medical illness, unemployment, and poor social support. Suicide among alcohol misusers is discussed further on p. 551. Here it is worth noting that suicide in young men is associated with a high rate of substance misuse, including alcohol.

Impaired psychosexual function Erectile dysfunction and delayed ejaculation are common. These difficulties may be worsened when drinking leads to marital estrangement, or if the wife develops a revulsion for intercourse with an inebriated partner.

Pathological jealousy Excessive drinkers may develop an overvalued idea or delusion that the *partner is being unfaithful*. This syndrome of pathological jealousy is described on p. 389.

Alcoholic hallucinosis This is characterized by *auditory hallucinations*, usually voices uttering insults or threats, occurring in clear consciousness. The patient is usually distressed by these experiences, and appears anxious and restless. The hallucinations are not due to acute alcohol withdrawal and can indeed persist after several months of abstinence. There has been considerable controversy about the aetiology of the condition. Some follow Kraepelin and Bonhoffer in regarding it as a rare organic complication of alcoholism; others follow Bleuler in supposing that it is related to schizophrenia.

Benedetti (1952) made a retrospective survey of 113 cases of alcoholic hallucinosis and divided them into 90 cases of less than 6 months' duration (acute cases) and the remaining chronic group. Among the former he found no evidence of a link with schizophrenia as judged by family history.

However, he did find evidence of an organic cause, in that about half had experienced memory disorders. Despite this, the condition cleared up without residual defect. Among the cases that had lasted 6 months, nearly all went on for much longer, despite abstinence. Half developed the typical picture of schizophrenia and half developed amnesic syndromes or dementia. More recent reviewers have concluded that alcoholic hallucinosis is an alcohol-induced organic psychosis, which is distinct from schizophrenia and has a good prognosis if abstinence can be maintained (see Stober 1999).

In both DSM-IV and ICD-10, *alcoholic hallucinosis* is subsumed under the heading of *substance-induced psychotic disorder*.

Social damage

Family problems

Excessive drinking is liable to cause profound social disruption particularly in the family. Marital and family tension is virtually inevitable. The *divorce rate* amongst heavy drinkers is high, and the wives of such men are likely to become anxious, depressed, and socially isolated; the husbands of '*battered*' *wives* frequently drink excessively, and some women admitted to hospital because of self-poisoning blame their husband's drinking. The home atmosphere is often detrimental to the children because of quarrelling and violence, and a drunken parent provides a poor role model. Children of heavy drinkers are at risk of developing emotional or behaviour disorders, and of performing badly at school.

Work difficulties and road accidents

At work, the heavy drinker often progresses through declining efficiency, lower-grade jobs, and repeated dismissals to lasting unemployment. There is also a strong association between *road accidents* and *alcohol misuse*. In the USA in 1990, 44 529 people were killed in traffic accidents, with alcohol being involved in 41% of these fatalities (Zobeck *et al.* 1994).

Crime

Excessive drinking is also associated with *crime*, mainly petty offences such as larceny, but also with fraud, sexual offences, and crimes of violence including murder. Studies of recidivist prisoners in England and Wales have shown that many of them had serious drinking problems before imprisonment. It is not easy to know how far alcohol causes the criminal behaviour and how far it is just part of the lifestyle of the criminal. In addition, there is a link between certain forms of alcohol misuse and *antisocial personality disorder* (see below and p. 168).

The causes of excessive drinking and alcohol misuse

Despite much research, surprisingly little is known about the cause of excessive drinking and alcohol dependence. At one time it was believed that certain people were particularly predisposed, either through personality or an innate biochemical anomaly. Nowadays this simple notion of specific predisposition is no longer held. Instead, alcohol misuse is thought to result from a variety of interacting factors which can be divided into individual factors and those in society.

Individual factors

Genetic factors

Alcohol use Twin studies provide an opportunity to investigate the role of genetic and familial factors in patterns of alcohol use. A study employing this approach has suggested that liability to lifetime alcohol use is *environmentally determined*. However, the risk *of illicit, under-age drinking* has strong genetic determinants (Maes *et al.* 1999).

Alcohol misuse and dependence Most genetic studies of alcoholism have investigated subjects with evidence of physiological alcohol dependence. If less severe diagnostic criteria are involved, for example, fairly broadly defined alcohol misuse, the relative genetic contribution is somewhat less (Kendler *et al.* 1994).

It is well established that alcohol dependence *aggregates in families*. If this is partly the result of genetic factors (rather than social influences in the family), rates of dependence should be higher in monozygotic (MZ) than dizygotic (DZ) twins. Generally, results of MZ-DZ comparisons have shown a *higher MZ concordance* for alcohol dependence in male and female twins (Kendler *et al.* 1994; Heath *et al.* 1997). These studies have suggested that about 50–60% of the liability to develop alcohol dependence may result from genetic factors.

Support for a genetic explanation also comes from investigations of *adoptees*. A number of studies have indicated an increased risk of alcohol misuse and dependence in the adopted-away sons of alcohol-dependent biological parents than in the adopted-away sons of non-alcohol-dependent biological parents. Such studies suggest a genetic mechanism but do not indicate its nature.

Adoption studies in Sweden have led to the suggestion that there are two separate kinds of alcohol dependence, which have been called *type 1 and type 2* (Cloninger *et al.* 1987). Type 2 alcoholism is strongly genetic, has an early age of onset and is associated with criminality and sociopathic disorder in both adoptee and biological father. By contrast, type 1 alcoholism has a later age of onset and is only mildly genetic (Gurling and Cook 1999).

If a genetic component to aetiology were confirmed, it would still be necessary to discover the mechanism. The latter might be biochemical, involving the metabolism of alcohol or its central effects, or psychological, involving personality. In addition, it is important to note that a predisposition to misuse alcohol and develop dependence will be expressed only if a person consumes excessive amounts of alcohol. Here non-genetic familial factors are likely to play a major role (Ball and Murray 1994).

Allelic association studies have also been applied to alcohol misuse, particularly the alleles of the dopamine D_2 receptor. Results of studies have been contradictory, perhaps because of the variance of D_2 receptor polymorphisms between different ethnic groups. This can make it difficult to match control and patient samples appropriately. However, it seems possible that there is a significant association between possession of the A1 allele of the dopamine D_2 receptor and alcohol dependence, at least in certain populations. More recently, collaborative studies screening the entire human genome have indicated potential loci predisposing to alcohol dependence on several chromosomes, particularly chromosome 4 (see Gurling and Cook 1999).

Other biological factors

Several possible biochemical factors have been suggested to predispose to alcohol misuse and dependence, including abnormalities in alcohol dehydrogenase or in neurotransmitter mechanisms. As mentioned above, a significant proportion of Oriental subjects, who possess a particular allele of the isoenzyme aldehyde dehydrogenase, develop unpleasant reactions to alcohol and therefore are much less likely to misuse it.

The *sons of men with alcohol dependence* are at increased risk of developing alcohol dependence themselves, and a number of studies have attempted to find biological abnormalities that may antedate and predict the development of alcohol dependence in these subjects. A variety of impairments have been described, including abnormal performance on cognitive tasks and on the P300 visual evoked response, which is a measure of visual information processing (Berman and Noble 1993). There is also reasonably consistent evidence that sons of alcohol-dependent men are less sensitive to the acute intoxicating effects of alcohol (Heath *et al.* 1999). Presumably, if subjects experience less subjective response to alcohol, they may tend to drink more, thus putting themselves at risk of developing alcohol dependence. While plausible, this hypothesis is not supported by direct evidence.

Learning factors

Alcohol use Children tend to follow their parents' drinking patterns and from an early age boys tend to be encouraged to drink more than girls. Non-genetic familial factors appear to be important in determining levels of alcohol use. Nevertheless, it is not uncommon to meet people who are abstainers although their parents drank heavily. It has been proposed that an *expectation of positive effects of alcohol* in childhood correlates with the degree of subsequent alcohol use (Berman and Noble 1993).

Alcohol dependence It has also been suggested that learning processes may contribute in a more specific way to the development of alcohol dependence. For example, recent formulations that combine biochemical and cognitive approaches emphasize the role of *dopamine release in mesolimbic pathways* in mediating *incentive learning*. In this way drugs such as alcohol which increase dopamine levels in this brain region stimulate *motivational behaviours* focused on the need to secure further drug supplies. These behaviours may be outside conscious control and are difficult to extinguish (see Robbins and Everitt 1999).

Personality factors

Little progress has been made in identifying personality factors that contribute to alcohol misuse and dependence. In clinical practice it is common to find that excessive alcohol consumption is associated with *chronic anxiety*, a pervading sense of inferiority, or self-indulgent tendencies. However, many people with personality problems of this kind do not resort to excessive drinking or become alcohol dependent. More recent surveys have emphasized the role of personality traits that lead to *risk taking* and *novelty seeking* (Berman and Noble 1993). It seems likely that these characteristics apply to those with antisocial personality disorder who are known to be at increased risk of misusing alcohol and developing alcohol dependence. However, the majority of alcohol-dependent subjects do not have an antisocial personality disorder.

Psychiatric disorder

Alcohol misuse is commonly found in conjunction with other psychiatric disorders and sometimes appears to be secondary to them. For example, some patients with *depressive disorders* take to alcohol in the mistaken hope that it will alleviate low mood. Those with anxiety disorders, particularly *panic disorder* and *social phobia*, are also at risk. Alcohol misuse is also seen in patients with bipolar disorder and schizophrenia.

Alcohol consumption in society

There is now general agreement that rates of alcohol dependence and alcohol-related disorders are correlated with the *general level of alcohol consumption* in a society. Previously it had been supposed that levels of intake amongst excessive drinkers were independent of the amounts taken by moderate drinkers. The French demographer Ledermann (1956) challenged this idea, proposing instead that the distribution of consumption within a homogeneous population follows a logarithmic normal curve. If this is the case, an increase in the average consumption must inevitably be accompanied by an increase in the number of people who drink an amount that is harmful.

Although the mathematical details of Ledermann's work have been criticized, there are striking correlations between average annual consumption in a society and several indices of alcohol-related damage among its members. For this reason, it is now widely accepted that the proportion of a population drinking excessively is largely determined by the average consumption of that population.

What then determines the average level of drinking within a nation? *Economic*, *formal*, and *informal* controls must be considered. The *economic control* is the price of alcohol. There is now ample evidence from the UK and other countries that the real price of alcohol (i.e. the price relative to average income) profoundly influences a nation's drinking. Also, heavy drinkers as well as moderate drinkers reduce their consumption when the tax on alcohol is increased.

The main *formal controls* are the *licensing laws* but these do not seem to influence drinking behaviours in a consistent way when comparisons are made between different countries. *Informal controls* are the *customs and moral beliefs* in a society that determine who should drink, in what circumstances, at what time of day, and to what extent. Some communities seem to protect their members from alcohol misuse despite general availability of alcohol; for example, alcohol-related problems are uncommon among Jews even in countries with high rates in the rest of the community. For a detailed discussion of economic and social aspects of alcohol consumption see Edwards (1994).

Recognition of alcohol misuse

Detection

Only a small proportion of alcohol misusers in the community are known to specialized agencies. When special efforts are made to screen patients in medical and surgical wards, between *10 and 30%* are found to misuse alcohol, with the rates being highest in accident and emergency wards (Chick 1994).

Alcohol misuse often goes undetected because subjects conceal the extent of their drinking. However, doctors and other professionals often do not ask the right questions. It should be a standard practice to ask all patients – medical, surgical, and psychiatric – about their alcohol consumption. It is useful to ask four questions:

◆ Have you ever felt you ought to *cut down* on your drinking?

◆ Have people *annoyed you* by criticizing your drinking?

◆ Have you ever felt *guilty* about your drinking?

◆ Have you ever had a drink first thing in the morning (an 'eye-opener') to steady your nerves or get rid of a hangover?

These questions are known as *CAGE*, from the initial letters of the words cut, annoyed, guilty, and eye-opener. Two or more positive replies are said to identify alcohol misuse (see p. 152). Some patients will give false answers, but others find that these questions provide an opportunity to reveal their problems.

In a comparative study of alcohol-dependent subjects and non-dependent controls, the CAGE questionnaire was more effective at detecting the presence of alcohol dependence than routine laboratory blood tests such as the GGT level and the mean corpuscular volume (MCV) (Girela *et al.* 1994).

The next requirement is for the doctor to be suspicious about 'at-risk' factors. In general practice, alcohol misuse may come to light as a result of problems in the *marriage and family*, at *work*, with *finances*, or with *the law*. The wife may complain of the husband's boastfulness, lack of consideration, sexual dysfunction, or aggressiveness towards herself and the children. The alcohol misuser is likely to have many more *days off work* than the moderate drinker, and repeated absences on Monday are highly suggestive. The at-risk occupations (see p. 543) should also be remembered.

In hospital practice, the alcohol-dependent subject may be noticed if he develops *withdrawal symptoms* after admission. Florid delirium tremens is obvious, but milder forms may be mistaken for an acute organic syndrome, for example, in pneumonia or postoperatively.

In both general and hospital practice, at-risk factors include physical disorders that may be alcohol related. Common examples are *gastritis*, *peptic ulcer*, and *liver disease*, but others such as *neuropathy* and *seizures* should be borne in mind. *Repeated accidents* should also arouse suspicion. Psychiatric at-risk factors include anxiety, depression, erratic moods, impaired concentration, memory lapses, and sexual dysfunction. Alcohol misuse should be considered in all cases of *deliberate self-harm*.

Drinking history

If any of the above factors raise suspicion about alcohol misuse, the next stage is to take a *comprehensive drinking history* (Box 18.1). This should be carried out sensitively, with understanding that the patient may have difficulty giving a clear history. The clinician should aim to build up a picture of what and how much the patient drinks throughout a *typical day* for example, when and where does he have the *first drink of the day*? The patient should be

---

Box 18.1 Alcohol use history

- Describe typical day's drinking. What time is first drink of the day?
- When did daily drinking start?
- Presence of withdrawal symptoms in morning or after abstinence
- Previous attempts at treatment
- Medical complications
- Patient's attitude towards drinking

---

asked how he feels if he goes without a drink for a day or two, and how he feels on *waking*. This can lead on to enquiries about the typical features of dependence and the range of physical, psychological and social problems associated with it.

To get an idea of the duration of alcohol problems, key points in the history may include establishing when the patient first began *drinking every day*, when he began drinking *in the mornings* and when, if ever, he first experienced *withdrawal symptoms*. It is useful to ask about periods of abstinence from alcohol, what factors helped maintain this state of affairs and what led to a resumption of drinking. This can lead on to enquiries about past attempts at *treatment*.

It is necessary to gain a clear understanding of the patient's own view of his drinking behaviour, because there are a number of possible treatment goals. In this situation the patient's *attitude* to his problems plays a key role in deciding which approaches are likely to be most beneficial (see section on motivational interviewing).

Laboratory tests

Several laboratory tests can be used to detect alcohol misuse, though none gives an unequivocal answer. This is because the more sensitive tests can give 'false positives' when there is disease of the liver, heart, kidneys, or blood, or if enzyme-inducing drugs, such as anticonvulsants, steroids, or barbiturates, have been taken. However, abnormal values point to the possibility of alcohol misuse. Only the three most useful tests are considered here.

Gamma-glutamyl-transpeptidase (GGT) Estimations of GGT in blood provide a useful screening test. The level is raised in *about 70% of alcohol misusers*, both men and women, whether or not there is demonstrable liver damage. The heavier the drinking, the greater is the rise in GGT.

Mean corpuscular volume (MCV) MCV is raised above the normal value in about *60% of alcohol misusers*, and more commonly in women than in men. If other causes are excluded, a raised MCV is a strong pointer to excessive drinking. Moreover, it takes several weeks to return to normal after abstinence.

Blood alcohol concentration A high concentration does not distinguish between an isolated episode of heavy drinking and chronic misuse. However, if a person is not intoxicated when the blood alcohol concentration is well above the legal limit of driving, he is likely to be unusually tolerant of alcohol. This tolerance suggests persistent heavy drinking. Alcohol is eliminated rather slowly from the blood and can be detected in appreciable amounts for 24 hours after an episode of heavy drinking.

The treatment of alcohol misuse (Box 18.2)

Early detection and treatment

Early detection of excessive consumption of alcohol and alcohol misuse is important because treatment of established cases is difficult, particularly when dependence is present. Many cases can be detected early *by general practitioners, physicians, and surgeons* when patients seek treatment for another problem. If counselling is given to such patients during their stay in a medical ward, their alcohol consumption is found to be reduced a year later (Chick 1994).

Brief intervention in primary care

General practitioners are well placed to provide early treatment of alcohol problems, and they are likely to know the patient and his family well. It is often effective if the general practitioner gives

Box 18.2 **Approach to treatment of alcohol misuse**

- Raise awareness of problem
- Increase motivation to change
- Withdraw alcohol (or controlled drinking)
- Support and advice
- Cognitive–behaviour therapy (social skills, relapse prevention)
- Marital therapy
- Alcoholics Anonymous
- Medication (disulfiram, acamprosate)

Box 18.3 Motivational interviewing

- Express empathy
- Avoid arguing
- Detect and 'roll with' resistance
- Point out discrepancies in history
- Raise awareness about contrast between drug user's aims and behaviour

Source: Bruce (2000)

simple advice in a frank matter-of-fact way, but with tact and understanding.

Brief intervention studies in general practice have shown that 5–10 minutes of *simple advice* by a general practitioner plus an educational leaflet can lead to a mean reduction of about 25% in alcohol intake over the next year and a corresponding reduction of about 45% in the proportion of excessive drinkers (Austoker 1994). Whilst such results may not be achieved in more severely affected patients, nevertheless they are important because excessive alcohol consumption without obvious dependence is more common and contributes more to social and economic cost.

Motivational interviewing

Patients with problems of alcohol misuse, particularly those detected by screening methods, may be unsure whether or not to engage in treatment programmes. An appropriate interviewing style, particularly during the first assessment, can help to persuade the patient to engage in a useful review of their current pattern of drinking.

Confrontation is avoided in motivational interviewing, and a *less directive* approach is taken during which patients are helped to assess the balance of the positive and negative effects of alcohol on their lives. The clinician can help in this exercise by providing feedback to the patient on the personal risks that alcohol poses both to them and to their

family, together with a number of options for change. The aim of motivational interviewing is to persuade the patients to argue their own case for changing their pattern of substance use (Box 18.3) (For a review of motivational interviewing and its role in the treatment of substance misuse in general see Miller and Rollnick 1991.)

Treatment plans for more established alcohol misuse and dependence

Where patients have significant alcohol-related disorders, particularly in the presence of alcohol dependence, treatment may need to be more intensive. Any intervention should be preceded by a full assessment and should include a *drinking history* and an appraisal of current *medical, psychological,* and *social problems.* An intensive and searching enquiry often helps the patient gain a new recognition and understanding of his problem, and this is the basis of treatment. As noted above, however, it is important to *avoid confrontation* as this will only alienate someone who is likely to have very mixed feelings about the prospect of life without alcohol. It is usually desirable to involve the husband or wife in the assessment, both to obtain additional information and to give the spouse a chance to unburden feelings.

An explicit treatment plan should be worked out with the patient (and spouse, if appropriate). There should be specific goals and the patient should be required to take responsibility for realizing them. These goals should deal not only with the *drinking problem*, but also with any accompanying problems in *health, marriage, job*, and *social adjustment*. In the early stages they should *be short term* and *achievable*, for example, complete abstinence for 2 weeks. In this way the patient can be rewarded by early achievement.

Longer-term goals can be set as treatment progresses. These will be concerned with trying to change factors that precipitate or maintain excessive drinking, such as tensions in the family. In drawing up this treatment plan, an important decision is whether to aim at *total abstinence* or at limited consumption of alcohol (*controlled drinking*).

Total abstinence versus controlled drinking

The disease model of alcoholism proposes that an alcohol-dependent person must become totally abstinent and remain so, since a single drink would lead to relapse. Alcoholics Anonymous have made this a tenet of their approach to treatment.

The issue of abstinence versus controlled drinking remains unresolved. A prevalent view is that controlled drinking may be a feasible goal for people whose alcohol misuse has been detected early and who are not dependent or physically damaged. Abstinence is a better goal for others and those who have attempted controlled drinking unsuccessfully. While there are few controlled studies of this issue, recent investigations have supported the idea that controlled drinking can be a realistic goal in patients without alcohol dependence and lesser levels of alcohol-related disorders (World Health Organization Brief Intervention Group 1996) If controlled drinking is to be attempted, then the doctor should advise the patient clearly about safe levels (see p. 539).

Withdrawal from alcohol

For patients with the dependence syndrome, withdrawal from alcohol is an important stage in treatment which should be carried out carefully. In the less severe cases, withdrawal may be at home provided there is adequate support and clinical monitoring. This should involve *daily assessment* by the general practitioner, practice nurse, or specialist alcohol worker to check the patient's physical state and supervise medication. However, any patient likely to have severe withdrawal symptoms, especially if there is a history of *delirium tremens* or *seizures*, should be admitted to hospital.

The extensive research on pharmacological treatment for alcohol withdrawal has been systematically reviewed by Mayo-Smith and colleagues (1997). The most important concern is the prevention of major complications of withdrawal such as seizures or delirium tremens; treatment with benzodiazepines is usually the most suitable choice.

Benzodiazepines differ in their duration of action (see p. 656). Whilst the longer-acting compounds may carry the risk of oversedation in the elderly or in those with significant liver disease, they also have the advantage of smoother withdrawal and generally better relief of withdrawal symptoms. *Chlordiazepoxide* is often used. A typical out-patient regimen would be 20–30 mg four times daily, reducing over 5 days. In more severe cases, particularly in-patients, diazepam in a starting dose of 30–50 mg daily may be preferred because it can be administered parenterally. If convulsions occur, larger doses of benzodiazepines should be used.

Chlormethiazole was frequently used in the management of alcohol withdrawal but is now not recommended because of its toxicity when combined with alcohol. However, it may be needed for the most severe withdrawal states where intensive in-patient medical monitoring is available. *Antipsychotic drugs* lower the seizure threshold and their use is generally unnecessary; in established delirium tremens, however, the presence of hallucinations and delusions may require the use of low-dose, high-potency agents such as haloperidol. *Vitamin supplements*, particularly thiamine, should also be given to prevent the Wernicke-Korsokov syndrome (p. 412).

Psychological treatment

As noted above, *provision of information and advice* about the effects of excessive drinking is an important first stage in treatment. The information given should relate to the specific problems of the individual patient, both those that have occurred already and those likely to develop if drinking continues. The technique of *motivational interviewing* can be useful (see p. 553).

Group therapy This has probably been the most widely used treatment for problem drinkers. Regular meetings are attended by about 10 patients and one or more members of staff. The aim is to enable patients to observe their own problems mirrored in other problem drinkers and to work out better ways of coping with their problems. They gain confidence, whilst members of the group jointly strive to reorganize their lives without alcohol.

Until recently, the most common plan of treatment in specialist alcohol units was an in-patient programme of group therapy lasting about 8 weeks; this treatment could be preceded by detoxification if required. However, because of the lack of evidence that this kind of intensive treatment approach is particularly beneficial (see below), most clinics now offer a broader range of care including out-patient and day-patient programmes that utilize a variety of psychotherapeutic approaches including marital and family therapy and cognitive–behavioural methods of treatment (see below). Group therapy is discussed further on p. 747.

Cognitive–behavioural therapy Cognitive–behavioural methods of treatment tackle the drinking behaviour itself rather than the presumed underlying psychological problems. Such approaches stress the role of *education* and the improvement of *social and interpersonal skills* as these relate to alcohol misuse (see Grabowski and Schmitz 1998).

For example, it may be helpful to identify situational or interpersonal triggers that cause an individual to drink excessively, and then to plan and rehearse new methods of coping with these situations. This is called *relapse prevention*. The use of *cue exposure* to alcoholic drinks, without subsequent consumption, may also lessen the risk of subsequent relapse when subjects have to contend with the ready availability of alcohol in social settings. It is important for the patient to appreciate that a *lapse* in drinking behaviour does not have to progress to a full-blown *relapse*. Many patients who misuse alcohol have general deficiencies in problem-solving skills, and appropriate training may help reduce relapse rates. Where patients are in a relatively stable relationship with a partner, *behavioural marital therapy* (see p. 754) can produce improvements in drinking behaviour as well as marital adjustment (for a review of psychological treatments see Chick 2000).

Pharmacological treatments to help maintenance of abstinence

Disulfiram Disulfiram (*Antabuse*) acts by blocking the oxidation of alcohol so that acetaldehyde accumulates. Some patients find it useful because the anticipation of an unpleasant reaction acts as a deterrent to impulsive drinking. The reaction includes facial flushing, throbbing headache, hypotension, palpitations, tachycardia, and nausea and vomiting. In vulnerable patients, cardiac arrhythmias and collapse may occur.

The main contraindications to the use of disulfiram are a history of heart failure, coronary artery disease, hypertension, psychosis, and pregnancy. Patients should be given clear verbal and written instructions along with a list of substances to be avoided that contain alcohol. Common side-effects are drowsiness, bad breath, nausea, and constipation. Disulfiram is given in a single dose of 800 mg on the first day of treatment, reducing over 5 days to 100–200 mg daily.

The efficacy of disulfiram depends on *compliance*. The treatment is likely to be more successful if a partner or health worker is able to supervise compliance. In general, disulfiram appears to lower drinking frequency but without necessarily improving abstinence (Garbutt *et al.* 1999).

Acamprosate (calcium acetyl homotaurinate) Acamprosate is described an 'anti-craving' agent and produces modest but useful reductions in drinking behaviour in alcohol-dependent subjects. It is believed to act by stimulating GABA inhibitory neurotransmission and decreasing the excitatory effects of glutamate. At least nine good quality randomized controlled trials have shown that following detoxification, acamprosate increases non-drinking days from about 30% to 50% over 1 year of treatment. Abstinence rates are approximately doubled although the majority of treated patients do return to some form of drinking (Garbutt *et al.* 1999).

The usual dose of acamprosate is two tablets (each 333 mg) three times daily with meals. In lighter subjects (>60 kg), four tablets daily are recommended. Acamprosate is not metabolized in the liver and is excreted by the kidney. It therefore is unlikely to cause drug interactions. Adverse effects include diarrhoea, and, less frequently, nausea, vomiting, and abdominal pain. Skin rashes may occur as can fluctuations in libido.

Naltrexone The opioid antagonist, naltrexone, is believed to block some of the reinforcing effects of alcohol and in this way decrease the likelihood of relapse after detoxification. Studies have not consistently documented an effect of naltrexone to decrease drinking behaviour. Unsurprisingly, its efficacy is greater where compliance is better. Its effects may also be enhanced by concomitant cognitive–behaviour therapy (Garbutt *et al.* 1999). Side-effects of naltrexone treatment include headache, dizziness, and weight loss.

Antidepressant drugs Antidepressant medication is useful in patients who experience persistent symptoms of major depression after detoxification. Some studies have suggested that selective serotonin reuptake inhibitors (SSRIs) such as citalopram and fluvoxamine can reduce drinking in non-depressed alcohol-dependent patients but not all studies are in accord (see Chick 2000).

Other agencies concerned with drinking problems

Alcoholics Anonymous (AA) This is a self-help organization founded in the USA by two alcoholic men, a surgeon and a stockbroker. It has since spread to most countries of the world. Members attend group meetings, usually twice weekly on a long-term basis. In crisis they can obtain immediate help from other members by telephone.

The organization works on the firm belief that abstinence must be complete. At present there are about 1200 groups in the UK.

Alcoholics Anonymous does not appeal to all problem drinkers because the meetings involve an emotional confession of problems. However, the organization is of great value to some problem drinkers, and anyone with a drink problem should be encouraged to try it.

A treatment approach similar to that provided by Alcoholics Anonymous coupled with encouragement to attend Alcoholic Anonymous meetings was one of the psychological therapies employed in project MATCH (see below). All treatments were effective and patients with fewer psychiatric problems at entry tended have a better outcome with the Alcoholic Anonymous type of treatment.

Al-Anon This is a parallel organization providing support for the spouses of excessive drinkers. Al-Ateen does the same for their teenage children.

Councils on alcoholism These are voluntary bodies that coordinate available services in an area and train counsellors. They advise problem drinkers and their families where to obtain help, and provide social activities for those who have recovered.

Hostels These are intended mainly for homeless problem drinkers. They provide rehabilitation and counselling. Usually abstinence is a condition of residence.

Results of treatment

A number of investigations have combined results from different treatment centres. The Rand Report (Armor *et al.* 1976) describes a prospective study of 45 treatment centres in the USA, of which eight were followed for 18 months. Only a quarter of the patients remained abstinent for 6 months, and fewer than 10% for 18 months. However, at 18 months 70% of patients had reduced their consumption of alcohol. Patients with a better outcome had received more intensive treatment, but the form of treatment made no difference.

In a controlled trial with 100 male alcoholics, Edwards *et al.* (1977) compared simple advice with intensive treatment that included introductions to Alcoholics Anonymous, medication, repeated interviews, counselling for their wives, and, where appropriate, in-patient treatment as well. The advice group received a 3-hour assessment together with a single session of counselling with the spouse present. The two groups were well matched. After 12 months there was no significant difference between them in drinking behaviour, subjective ratings, or social adjustment (Orford and Edwards 1977).

Similar findings with regard to drinking behaviour were reported by Chick *et al.* (1988) who found that at a 2-year follow-up there was no difference in stable abstinence rates between patients who received a minimal treatment intervention, consisting mainly of advice, and those offered a broad range of therapies, including in-patient care and group therapy. However, the group offered the broad range of therapies suffered *less alcohol-related harm*, particularly in relation to family life.

Some have argued that abstinence rates by themselves do not provide a useful measure of treatment outcome. For example, whilst subjects may still be drinking, the amount consumed may decrease. This can be associated with reductions in aspects of alcohol-related harm as shown by the study by Chick *et al.* (1988). From this viewpoint, harm reduction, even where people continue to drink, is a worthwhile achievement. The principles of the harm-reduction approach have been applied to the misuse of other substances (see below).

Interest in the effectiveness of structured psychological treatments has been reinforced by Project MATCH, a large randomized controlled trial of three psychological treatments for alcohol problems (Project MATCH Research Group 1997). The three treatments studied were a cognitive–

behavioural intervention, a motivational therapy and a treatment that aimed to help people make use of the '12 step' philosophy of Alcoholics Anonymous. The main aim of the study was to attempt to find patient characteristics that predicted response to particular treatments. There were no important differences between the treatments and few strong correlations were found between effectiveness and patient characteristics. However, in general, the outcome was favourable and the authors concluded that structured psychological treatments of various kinds were helpful in the management of alcohol misuse.

There are likely to be factors within the patient that will predict a good response to a number of different kinds of treatment. There is some disagreement as to what these factors are, but the following generally predict a better prognosis whatever treatment is used: good insight into the nature of the problems; social stability in the form of a fixed abode, family support, and ability to keep a job; ability to control impulsiveness, to defer gratification, and to form satisfactory emotional relationships.

Prevention of alcohol misuse and dependence

In seeking to prevent excessive drinking and alcohol-related disorders, two approaches are possible. The first is to improve the help and guidance available to the individual, as already described. The second is to introduce social changes likely to affect drinking patterns in the population as a whole. It is with this second group that we are concerned here. Consumption in a population might be reduced by four methods:

♦ *the pricing of alcoholic beverages.* Putting up the price of alcohol would probably reduce the consumption (see above).

♦ *advertising.* Controlling or abolishing the advertising of alcoholic drinks might be another preventive measure. It is unclear how far advertising encourages use of particular brands of alcohol rather than overall consumption.

◆ *controls on sale.* Another preventive measure might be to control sales of alcohol by limiting hours or banning sales in supermarkets. While relaxation of restrictions has been shown to lead to increased sales of alcohol in some countries, it does not follow that increased restrictions would reduce established rates of drinking. However, there is evidence that a higher minimum age of legal drinking is associated with decreased alcohol consumption, car accidents, and suicide in recent school leavers (see Links 2000).

◆ *health education.* It is not known whether education about alcohol misuse is effective. Little is known as to how attitudes are formed or changed. Although education about alcohol seems desirable, it cannot be assumed that classroom lectures or mass media propaganda would alter attitudes. In general, programmes tailored to the target audience that use a multifaceted approach to focus on healthy lifestyles are more acceptable. Combining this approach with treatment and advice may be particularly effective (Rawaf 1998).

Other substance use disorders

Under this heading we shall consider the use and misuse of substances other than alcohol. Although these substances include agents such as volatile substances (inhalants), the general term *drug* will be employed because it is in common use. In this discussion the term *misuse* will be applied to what is classified as *harmful use* in ICD-10 and *abuse* in DSM-IV (Table 18.3).

Epidemiology

Illicit drug use

The *National Household Survey on Drug Abuse* (NHSDA) in the USA in 1991 found that 37% of the whole adult population had used at least one illicit drug in their lifetime, whilst 13% had used illicit substances in the past year and 6% in the previous month (National Institute on Drug Abuse 1991; Kaplan *et al.* 1994). Use was highest in unemployed people in the age range 18–25. The most commonly used illicit drug was *cannabis*.

In a survey of 7722 school pupils aged 15 and 16 in the UK, Miller and Plant (1996) found that 42% said that they had at some time tried illicit drugs, mainly cannabis. This cross-sectional study does not provide information on regular use, though it indicates that *experimentation* with illicit drugs is common among young people in this age group. There was a strong association between *cigarette smoking* and the use of cannabis. Boys were more likely to have used an illicit drug than girls but the differences were not large (43% of the boys and 38% of the girls reported having used cannabis). In relation to previous surveys of young people in the UK, the rate of experimentation with illicit drugs has risen in recent years. A significant number of young people in the UK are part of the 'club scene' where polydrug misuse is common. About a quarter of 18-year-olds have used two or more illegal drugs (see Robson 2000).

There are differing national temporal trends in illicit drug use. Problems associated with substance misuse in general appear to be growing in developing countries. A recent survey of teenagers in the UK found that self-reported use of illicit drugs had declined by about 5% since 1995 (Plant and Miller 2000).

Drug misuse and dependence

Little is known for certain about the *prevalence* of different types of drug misuse and drug dependence. In the UK, information comes from several sources: *criminal statistics*, mainly based on offences involving the use and misuse of illicit drugs, *special surveys*, and *hospital admissions*. The UK Home Office for many years kept a national register of persons notified by doctors as dependent on certain drugs, but the register was discontinued in 1997. None of these sources is satisfactory since much drug misuse goes undetected.

Reported national prevalence rates of drug misuse and drug dependence vary widely, partly because different methods of ascertainment have been used. The National Comorbidity Survey in the USA (Kessler *et al.* 1994) found that the 1-year prevalence for drug misuse and drug dependence (excluding alcohol misuse) was 3.6%, whilst the lifetime prevalence was 11.9%. The 1-year prevalence of drug misuse and dependence in men (5.1%) was more than twice that in women (2.2%).

In the UK Psychiatric Morbidity Survey, 2.2% of adults living in private households met criteria for drug dependence (Meltzer *et al.* 1994). Men were twice as likely to be drug dependent as women and drug dependence was most common amongst young adults, especially men aged 16–24. Among the homeless population sampled (Gill *et al.* 1996), 24% of people sleeping rough met criteria for drug dependence. The sample for *prisoners* in the UK showed the highest rates of drug use with the majority of subjects reporting a history of illicit drug use (Singleton *et al.* 1997). Among remand prisoners, 51% of men and 54% of women reported dependence on drugs before coming into prison, whereas among sentenced prisoners, 43% of men and 41% of women reported drug dependence.

Rates of drug misuse and dependence are high in disadvantaged areas of large cities. Adolescents are at risk, particularly around school-leaving age. A high proportion of attenders at drug-dependence clinics in large cities are unemployed with few stable relationships and leading disorganized lives. However, many young drug users remain in employment and apparently regard their drug taking as part of recreational activity for their particular peer group.

Causes of drug misuse

There is no single cause of drug misuse. It is generally argued that three factors are important:

- availability of drugs
- a vulnerable personality
- adverse social environment.

The widespread *availability* of illicit drugs means that occasional use in a young person can no longer be regarded as abnormal behaviour. Relative to the numbers of people experimenting with drugs on an occasional basis, the numbers who develop significant problems is low (Robson 2000). However, about 10% of those who experiment with drugs will go on to develop problems with them.

Once regular drug-taking has started, *pharmacological factors* play a role in determining misuse and dependence. Studies of the aetiology of misuse of substances other than alcohol are still at an early stage. For example, it is unclear whether similar risk factors predict misuse of a range of substances, including alcohol, or whether there is some specificity in the mechanisms, which leads certain individuals to misuse particular substances (Berman and Noble 1993).

Availability of drugs

People can misuse and become dependent on drugs by three routes:

- by taking drugs that can be *bought legally* without prescription. Nicotine is an obvious contemporary example, and in the nineteenth century much dependence on opioids arose from taking freely available remedies containing morphia. (Alcohol dependence is also acquired in this way, but we are not concerned here with that problem.)

- by taking drugs *prescribed by doctors*. In the first part of the twentieth century much of the known dependence on opioids and barbiturates in Western countries was of this kind; more recently, benzodiazepine dependence was often acquired in this way.

- by taking drugs that can be obtained only from *illicit sources* ('street drugs').

Personal factors

Of those who experiment with drugs, the users who go on to develop problems appear to have some degree of personality vulnerability before taking drugs. They may live in disrupted families and have started taking drugs at a relatively young age. Associated behaviours include a *poor school record*, *truancy*, or *delinquency*. Traits such as *sensation seeking* and *impulsivity* are also common. Many of those who misuse drugs report depression and anxiety, but it is seldom clear whether these are the causes or the consequences of drug misuse and dependence. Some give a history of mental illness or personality disorder in the family.

Social environment

The risk of drug misuse is greater in societies that *condone drug use* of one sort or another. Within the immediate group, there may be *social pressures* for a young person to take drugs to achieve status. Thus drug use by individuals is influenced by the substance use of their peers. There are also links between drug misuse and indices of social deprivation such as *unemployment and homelessness* (Gill *et al.* 1996).

Neurobiology of drug use, misuse, and dependence

Many subjects use drugs without misusing them, and not all drug misusers become drug dependent. Therefore it is useful to study the biological mechanisms underlying drug use, misuse, and dependence separately. Drugs are used and misused because they have the ability to serve as *positive reinforcers*, i.e. they increase the frequency of behaviours that lead to their use (Robbins and Everitt 1999). Drugs act as positive reinforcers because they cause positive subjective experiences such as euphoria or reduction in anxiety.

An important neurological substrate that mediates such effects is the *midbrain dopamine system*, whose cell bodies originate in the ventral tegmental area and innervate the forebrain, particularly the *nucleus accumbens*. It has been proposed that these dopamine pathways form part of a physiological reward system, which has the property of increasing the frequency of behaviours that activate it. Therefore it is of interest that administration of different kinds of drugs of misuse, including alcohol, nicotine, and opioids, to animals increases dopamine release in the nucleus accumbens. This suggests that activation of midbrain dopamine

pathways may be a common property of drugs that have a propensity to be used and misused. While this hypothesis may explain in part the social use of particular drugs, it does not account for the misuse of drugs in some circumstances. Presumably this is a consequence of interactions between the pharmacological properties of the drug, the biological disposition and personality of the user, and the social environment.

Dependence on drugs has traditionally been described as either psychological or physiological. In DSM-IV, dependence is separated into whether or not it is *physiological* in nature. *Physiological dependence* is diagnosed when a substance user demonstrates either *tolerance* to the pharmacological effects of the drug or a characteristic *withdrawal syndrome* when use of the drug is diminished. A cardinal feature of both physiological and non-physiological dependence is desire for the drug and drug-seeking behaviour. These features probably result from the continued need to obtain the reinforcing properties of the drug, as described above. Learning and conditioning factors are likely to be important here (Robbins and Everitt 1999).

It is important to note that, even in non-physiological dependence, phenomena such as craving and dysphoria are associated with altered brain function. For example, in experimental studies the discontinuation of cocaine after a period of administration results in a sharp decline in dopamine release in the nucleus accumbens. It is possible that such an effect could correspond clinically to symptoms such as anhedonia and a desire to obtain more supplies of the drug.

The phenomena of *tolerance* and *withdrawal* are believed to be a result of neuroadaptive changes in the brain. These are part of a homeostatic process that counteracts the acute pharmacological effects that occur when a drug is administered. For example, many drugs that are misused for their anxiolytic and hypnotic properties, such as barbiturates, benzodiazepines, and alcohol, have, among their acute pharmacological effects, the ability to *enhance brain GABA function*. During continued treatment with these agents, adaptive changes occur in GABA and benzodiazepine receptor sensitivity that tend to offset the effect of the drugs to facilitate GABA neurotransmission. Such an effect could account for the phenomenon of tolerance, with the result that an individual needs to take more of the drug to produce the same pharmacological effect.

If the drug is abruptly discontinued, persistence of the adaptive changes in receptor function could lead to a sudden decline in GABA activity. In fact, many of the clinical features of withdrawal from anxiolytic drugs, such as anxiety, insomnia, and seizures, can be explained on the basis of *diminished brain GABA* function. Such an effect can also explain the well-known phenomenon of cross-tolerance between anxiolytics and hypnotics and alcohol, which makes it possible, for example, to treat alcohol withdrawal with a benzodiazepine.

Similar kinds of adaptive changes have been proposed to account for the tolerance and withdrawal phenomena seen with other drugs of misuse. For example, whilst acute administration of opioids decreases the firing of noradrenaline cell bodies in the brainstem, tolerance to this effect occurs during repeated treatment, probably because of adaptive changes in the sensitivity of opioid receptors. If opioids are now suddenly withdrawn, there is a sudden increase in the firing of noradrenaline neurons and in the release of noradrenaline in terminal regions. Increased noradrenergic activity may account for several of the clinical features of acute opioid withdrawal, including sweating, tachycardia, hypertension, and anxiety. These studies have led to the use of the noradrenaline autoreceptor agonists clonidine and lofexidine in the management of opioid withdrawal (see p. 568).

While the positive reinforcing actions of drugs are seen as the major factor in promoting continued drug use, withdrawal effects are also likely to play a part because they are invariably unpleasant and individuals are likely to try to prevent them by taking more drug. It is worth noting that for many months following the cessation of a clear-cut withdrawal syndrome, dependent subjects may experience a sudden intense desire to consume the drug. Often, particular *psychological and social stimuli* previously associated with drug use may trigger intense craving associated with symptoms resembling a withdrawal state. It has been proposed that a single exposure to the drug during this period may rapidly lead to a full relapse, the so-called *reinstatement effect*. An analogous effect has been shown in previously drug-dependent animals where a single priming dose of the drug concerned can lead to a full recovery of drug-seeking behaviours that had previously been extinguished. For reviews of brain mechanisms involved in drug misuse and their implications for treatment see Nutt (1996) and Robbins and Everitt (1999).

Adverse effects of drug misuse

Drug misuse has many undesirable effects both for the individual and society.

Physical health

Drug misuse can lead people to neglect their health in addition to the direct physical consequences of the substance itself. These are discussed in more detail under the heading of individual drugs.

Intravenous drug use poses particular health risks. This practice is very common with opioid use, but barbiturates, benzodiazepines, amphetamines, and

Table 18.7 Some consequences of intravenous drug misuse

Local
Vein thrombosis
Infection of injection site
Damage to arteries
Systemic
Bacterial endocarditis
Hepatitis B and C
HIV infection

other drugs may be taken in this way. Intravenous drug use has important consequences, some local and others general (Table 18.7).

The most serious complications of intravenous drug use include *HIV infection* and *hepatitis*. Rates of HIV infection among UK drug users are lower than those found in some other European countries and some attribute this to the vigorous harm reduction policies in the UK (methadone prescribing, needle exchanges, and education for drug users). However, hepatitis C is a recent concern as preliminary studies suggest that this infection has a prevalence of between 50 and 80% amongst UK users who inject drugs. Rates of hepatitis B are lower but still significant (30–50%).

Drug misuse in pregnancy and the puerperium

Often drug misusers do not take up health-care services until late into the pregnancy, which increases the health risk to both mother and baby. When a pregnant woman misuses drugs, the *fetus* may be affected. When drugs are taken in early pregnancy, there is a risk of increased rates of *fetal abnormality*. *Opioids* may directly decrease *fetal growth*. When drugs are taken in late pregnancy, the fetus may become *dependent* on them. The risk of fetal dependence is great with heroin and related drugs, and after delivery the neonate may develop serious withdrawal effects requiring skilled care. If the mother continues to take drugs after delivery, the infant may be *neglected*. Intravenous drug use may lead to infection of the mother with HIV or other conditions that can affect the fetus.

Psychiatric co-morbidity

There is a strong association between between substance misuse, particularly with dependence, and psychiatric co-morbidity (often described as *dual diagnosis*). For example, patients with substance misuse often have additional diagnoses of personality disorder, depression, and anxiety. Sometimes symptoms of mood disturbance may be a direct result of drug use. For example, patients who use stimulants can experience depression subsequently (Curran and Travill 1997).

In other cases the relationship is more complex with premorbid psychiatric disorder interacting with substance misuse. Thus patients with primary psychiatric disorders such as schizophrenia, bipolar disorder, and sociopathic personality disorder frequently misuse alcohol and illicit drugs. This practice increases the morbidity of the underlying disorder and heightens the risk of violence and self-harm (see Lowe 1999). It has been argued that patients with significant co-morbid substance misuse and psychiatric disorder may require access to specialist 'dual-treatment' services (see Johnson 1997) because of their particular problems in terms of continued engagement with services and risk of violence.

Social consequences of drug misuse

There are three reasons why drug misuse has undesirable social effects:

- Chronic intoxication may affect behaviour adversely, leading to unemployment, motoring offences, accidents, and family problems including neglect of children.

- Illicit drugs are generally expensive, the user may cheat or steal to obtain money.

- Drug misusers often keep company with one another, and those with previously stable social behaviour may be under pressure to conform to a group ethos of antisocial or criminal activity.

Diagnosis of drug misuse

It is important to diagnose drug misuse early, at a stage when *dependence* may be less established and behaviour patterns less fixed, and the complications of intravenous use may not have developed. Before describing the clinical presentations of the different types of drugs, some general principles will be given. The clinician who is not used to treating people who misuse drugs should remember that he is in the unusual position of trying to help a patient who may be attempting to deceive him. Patients misusing heroin may overstate the daily dose to obtain extra supplies for their own use or for sale to others. Also, many patients *take more than one drug* but may not say so. It is important to try to corroborate the patient's account of the amount he takes by asking detailed questions about the duration of drug-taking, and the cost and source of drugs; by checking the story for internal consistency, and by external verification whenever possible.

Physical signs

Certain physical signs lead to the suspicion that drugs are being injected. These include *needle tracks and thrombosis of veins*, especially in the antecubital fossa, wearing garments with long sleeves in hot weather, and scars. Intravenous use should be considered in any patient who presents *with subcutaneous abscesses or hepatitis.*

Behavioural signs

Behavioural changes may also suggest drug misuse. These include absence from school or work and occupational decline. Dependent people may also neglect their appearance, isolate themselves from former friends, and adopt new friends in a drug culture. Minor criminal offences, such as petty theft and prostitution, may also be indicators.

Medical presentation

Dependent people may come to medical attention in several ways. Some declare that they are dependent on drugs. Others conceal their dependency, and ask for controlled drugs for the relief of pain such as renal colic or dysmenorrhoea. It is important to be particularly wary of such requests from temporary patients. Others present with drug-related complications, such as cellulitis, pneumonia, serum hepatitis, or accidents, or for the treatment of acute drug effects, overdose, withdrawal symptoms, or adverse reactions to hallucinogenic drugs. A few are detected during an admission to hospital for an unrelated illness.

Taking a drug history

When taking a *drug history* (Box 18.4) from a patient who is misusing drugs, the doctor should ask the patient to describe his drug use the

---

> **Box 18.4 Drug-use history**
>
> - Age of starting drug misuse (including alcohol and nicotine)
> - Types and quantities of drugs taken (including alcohol and nicotine)
> - Frequency of misuse and routes of administration
> - Overdose
> - Abstinence and relapse triggers
> - Symptoms experienced when drugs unavailable
> - Medical complications
> - Psychiatric and forensic history
>
> Source: Department of Health 1999b

---

previous day and also to describe a *typical drug-using day* (which drug, how often, and which route of use). A typical week can be described if drugs are not used every day. The doctor should ask about craving, withdrawal symptoms, and other features of the dependence syndrome such as increased tolerance to the drug and the priority of drug seeking over other duties and pleasures. The patient should be asked specifically about *risky behaviour* such as dangerous injecting (into groin or neck or infected injection sites), and sharing injection equipment.

A *chronological history* of the development of use of each drug can then be taken. Useful milestones can include the first use of the drug, when the patient began to use the drug daily, when withdrawal symptoms were first experienced, and when the patient first injected drugs. A history of sharing injection equipment will be important in estimating the risk of *HIV or hepatitis.*

If the patient has had periods of *abstinence*, it is useful to ask which influences helped them achieve this and what factors led to *relapse*. A history of complications should include adverse effects of the drug itself as well as complications of the route of administration. Any history of accidental overdose should also be elicited. The patient should be asked about family, occupational, and legal problems. Any past history of treatment should be elicted. There are several possible goals in the treatment of drug misusers. Abstinence is one but safer drug use (*harm reduction*) may be a more realistic aim for many. It is therefore important to obtain the patient's views on their drug use and the changes they would like to make.

Laboratory diagnosis

Whenever possible, the diagnosis of drug misuse should be confirmed by *laboratory tests*. Urine testing is most commonly used, as it is easier and less invasive than repeated blood testing. However, blood and hair analysis can be useful in certain circumstances. The laboratory should be provided with as complete a list as possible of drugs that are likely to have been taken, including those prescribed (for a review of laboratory investigations see Wolff *et al.* 1999).

Prevention, treatment, and rehabilitation – general principles

Prevention

Because treatment is difficult, considerable effort should be given to *prevention*. For many drugs, important preventive measures such as restricting availability and lessening social deprivation depend on government, not medical, policy. The reduction of overprescribing by doctors is important, especially with benzodiazepines and other anxiolytic drugs.

Whilst education programmes by themselves do not seem effective in prevention, it is important that *information* about the dangers of drug misuse should be available to young people in the school curriculum and through the media. Another aspect of prevention is the identification and treatment of family problems that may contribute to drug-taking. In all these preventive measures, the general practitioner has an important role.

Treatment

Motivation and change

When drug misuse has begun, treatment is more effective before *dependence* is established. At this stage, as at later stages, the essential step is to *motivate* the person to control his drug-taking. This requires a combination of advice about the likely effects of continuing misuse and help with any concurrent psychological or social problems. The techniques of motivational interviewing (Miller and Rollnick 1991) (see p. 553 and Box 18.3) may be useful here. The *stages of change model* described by Prochaska and Diclemente (1986) can help the clinician to encourage motivation effectively (Box 18.5).

Aims of treatment

The main aim of the treatment of the drug-dependent person is the *withdrawal* of the drug of dependence. However, drug withdrawal (or detoxification) by itself has no effect on long-term

---

Box 18.5 Stages of change model

Pre-contemplation
  Misuser does not believe there is a problem, though others recognize it.

Contemplation
  Individual weighs up pros and cons and considers that change might be necessary.

Decision
  Point reached where decision is made to act (or not to act) on issue of substance misuse.

Action
  User chooses a strategy for change and pursues it.

Maintenance
  Gains are maintained and consolidated. Failure may lead to relapse.

Relapse
  Return to previous pattern of behaviour. However, relapse may be a positive learning experience, with lessons for the future.

outcome (Vaillant 1988), and so this process should be part of a *wider treatment programme*. If withdrawal cannot be achieved, continued prescribing of certain drugs, for example, opioids, may be considered as part of a *harm reduction* programme (see below). In addition, psychological treatment and social support are required. At this point in the chapter, the general principles of treatment are outlined. In later sections, treatment specific to individual drugs will be considered.

Treatment setting

In the UK, drug misusers are treated in a variety of settings. Most clinics are associated with psychiatric treatment facilities based in psychiatric hospitals or community bases. In-patient care is provided in psychiatric hospitals, in psychiatric units in general hospitals, or in a small number of specialist in-patient units. Individual counselling, group therapy, and therapeutic communities are provided by a variety of charitable organizations. General practitioners may manage drug-dependent patients with the support of specialist services and models of shared care between primary and secondary services are currently being developed (Department of Health 1999b). *All doctors in the UK treating drug misusers for their drug problems should provide information on the standard form to their local Regional Drug Misuse Database.* Contact numbers are in the *British National Formulary*.

Physical complications

The complications of self-injection may need treatment in a general hospital. They include accidental overdose, skin infections, abscesses, septicaemia, hepatitis, and HIV infection. Drug misusers will also need help with general health issues such as nutrition and dental care. Immunization against hepatitis B may be advisable.

Principles of withdrawal

The withdrawal of misused drugs is sometimes called *detoxification*. For many drugs, particularly opioids, withdrawal may be most effectively carried out in hospital (see below). Withdrawal

from stimulant drugs and benzodiazepines can often be an out-patient procedure provided that the doses are not very large and that barbiturates are not taken as well. Nevertheless, the risk of depression and suicide should be remembered.

Drug maintenance

Some clinicians undertake to prescribe certain drugs to dependent people who are not willing to give them up. The usual procedure is to prescribe a drug which has a slower action (and therefore is less addictive) than the 'street' drug. Thus methadone is prescribed in place of heroin and diazepam in place of temazepam. When this procedure is combined with help with social problems and a continuing effort to bring the person to accept withdrawal, it is called *maintenance therapy*.

The rationale of this approach is twofold:

- Prolonged prescribing will remove the need for the patient to obtain 'street' drugs, and will thereby reduce the need to steal money and associate with other drug-dependent people.

- Social and psychological help will make the person's life more normal so that he will be better able to give up drugs eventually.

Maintenance drug treatment is used particularly for people with *opioid dependence*. If maintenance drug therapy is used, it should be remembered that some drug-dependent people convert tablets or capsules into material for injection, which is a particularly dangerous practice. Also, some attend a succession of general practitioners in search of supplementary supplies of drugs. They may withhold information about attendance at clinics or pose as temporary residents.

Some patients who receive maintenance drugs achieve a degree of social stability, but others continue heavy drug misuse and deteriorate both medically and socially. Subjects on maintenance methadone are more likely to be retained in treatment than those in drug-free programmes. This may be important because the length of time spent in treatment, regardless of type, is the best predictor of favourable outcome. (The use of methadone maintenance treatment in the management of opioid dependence is considered in more detail below.)

Harm reduction

The increase in HIV and hepatitis C infection has emphasized the importance of *harm-reduction programmes* (Strang 1993), of which prescribing maintenance may be one component. Such programmes have the aim of increasing the number of substance misusers who enter and comply with treatment. The aim is to identify intermediate treatment goals, which though short of total abstinence, nevertheless reduce the risk of drug misuse to the individual and society. For example, even if subjects continue to misuse drugs, the risk of hepatitis and HIV infection can be lessened by appropriate education and practical help. Such interventions may lead to drug misuse using safer routes of drug administration or sterile injection equipment. Counselling and screening for hepatitis and HIV may also be worthwhile and hepatitis B vaccination should be offered to non-immune patients.

Psychological treatments

Some drug-dependent patients are helped by simple measures such as counselling. In many units, group psychotherapy is provided to help patients develop insight into personal and interpersonal problems. Some patients benefit from treatment in a therapeutic community in which there can be a frank discussion of the effects of drug-taking on the person's character and relationships within the supportive relationship of the group (see p. 753 for an outline of community therapy).

Cognitive–behavioural methods of treatment as described for the management of alcohol misuse (see p. 555) are also helpful (Grabowski and Schmitz 1998). The aim of such treatment is to increase recreational and personal skills so that the individual becomes less reliant on drugs and the drug culture as a source of satisfaction. Involvement of family and partners is often helpful.

As with alcohol dependence, the technique of *relapse prevention* (p. 555) can be used to identify, in advance, situations that contain triggers for drug use; in this way alternative methods of coping can be planned. It has already been mentioned that when a drug misuser is confronted with a situation that contains personal cues for drug use, he can experience acute discomfort associated with a *strong desire* to use the drug. The technique of cue exposure aims, through repeated exposure, to desensitize drug misusers to these effects and thus improve their ability to remain abstinent.

Rehabilitation

Many drug takers have great difficulty in establishing themselves in normal society. The aim of rehabilitation is to enable the drug-dependent person to leave the drug subculture and to develop new social contacts. Unless he can do this, any treatment is likely to fail.

Rehabilitation may be undertaken after treatment in a therapeutic community (see p. 753). Patients first engage in work and social activities in sheltered surroundings, and then take greater responsibility for themselves in conditions increasingly like those of everyday life. Hostel accommodation is a useful stage in this gradual process. Continuing social support is usually required when the person makes the transition to normal work and living.

Misuse of specific types of drug

Opioids

This group of drugs includes morphine, heroin, codeine, and synthetic analgesics such as pethidine, methadone, and dipipanone. The pharmacological effects of opioids are mediated primarily through interaction with specific opioid receptors, with morphine and heroin being quite selective for the μ-opioid receptor type. The medical use of opioids is mainly for their powerful analgesic actions; they are misused for their euphoriant and anxiolytic effects.

In the past morphine was misused widely in Western countries, but has been largely replaced as a drug of misuse by *heroin*, which has a particularly powerful euphoriant effect, especially when taken intravenously.

Epidemiology

The NHSDA survey in the USA estimated that at least 1.3% of Americans had used heroin at least once in their lives, with the highest rate (1.8%) in the 18–25-years age group. There may be about half a million people with opioid dependence in the USA (Kaplan *et al.* 1994). When the UK Home Office Addicts Index was still in operation, the numbers of subjects registered in 1997 was about 40 000. Of course many more users were not registered.

Use and misuse

The data from the USA indicate that many people use heroin without becoming dependent on it. However, there is no doubt that repeated heroin use can lead to the rapid development of *dependence* and marked *physiological tolerance*. As well as the intravenous route, opioid users may employ other methods of administration, for example, *subcutaneous administration* ('skin-popping') or *sniffing* ('snorting'). Heroin may also be heated on a metal foil and inhaled ('chasing the dragon'). Heroin users may change their customary method of drug administration from time to time. From the perspective of harm reduction, methods that avoid intravenous administration are preferable.

Clinical effects

As well as *euphoria and analgesia*, opioids produce respiratory depression, constipation, reduced appetite, and low libido. Tolerance develops rapidly, leading to increasing dosage. Tolerance does not develop equally to all the effects, and constipation often continues when the other effects have diminished. When the drug is stopped, tolerance diminishes rapidly so that a dose taken after an interval of abstinence has greater effects than it would have had before the interval. This loss of tolerance can result in dangerous – sometimes fatal – respiratory depression when a previously tolerated dose is resumed after a drug-free interval, for example, after a stay in hospital or prison.

Withdrawal from opioids

Withdrawal symptoms include intense craving for the drug, restlessness and insomnia, pain in muscles and joints, running nose and eyes, sweating, abdominal cramps, vomiting, diarrhoea, piloerection, dilated pupils, raised pulse rate, and disturbance of temperature control. These features usually begin about 6 hours after the last dose, reach a peak after 36–48 hours, and then wane. Withdrawal symptoms rarely threaten the life of someone in reasonable health, though they cause great distress and so drive the person to seek further supplies.

Methadone

Methadone is approximately as potent, weight for weight, as morphine. It causes cough suppression, constipation, and depression of the central nervous system and of respiration. Pupillary constriction is less marked. The withdrawal syndrome is similar to that of heroin and morphine, and is at least as severe. Because methadone has a long half-life (1–2 days), symptoms of withdrawal may begin only after 36 hours and reach a peak after 3–5 days. For this reason, methadone is often used to replace heroin in patients dependent on the latter drug.

The natural course of opioid dependence

Longer-term follow-up studies of opioid misusers have revealed that in most the disorder appears to run a chronic relapsing and remitting course with a significant mortality (10–15%) over 10 years. Nevertheless, up to 50% of opioid users have been found to be abstinent at 10-year follow-up, which suggests a trend towards natural remission in survivors (Robson 1992).

Deaths are not infrequently due to accidental overdosage, often related to loss of tolerance after a period of enforced abstinence. Suicide is also a common cause of death. Deaths from HIV infection and hepatitis have also become more frequent in recent years. Pointers to a good outcome include substantial periods of employment and marriage (Vaillant 1988).

Abstinence is often related to changed circumstances of life. This point is reflected in the report of 95% abstinence among soldiers who returned to the USA after becoming dependent on opioids during service in the Vietnam War (Robins 1993). This finding is consistent with the observation that a change in residence following discharge from in-patient or residential care is associated with increased rates of abstinence (Robson 1992).

Prevention

Because dependence develops rapidly and treatment of dependent opioid misusers is unsatisfactory, preventive measures (see p. 564) are particularly important with this group of drugs.

Treatment of crisis

Opioid misusers present in crisis to a doctor in three circumstances. First, when their *supplies have run out*, they may seek drugs either by requesting them directly or by feigning a painful disorder. Although withdrawal symptoms are very unpleasant, so that the misuser will go to great lengths to obtain more drugs, they are not usually dangerous to an otherwise healthy person. Therefore it is best to offer drugs only as the first step of a planned maintenance or withdrawal programme. This programme is described in the following sections. The second form of crisis is *drug overdose*. This requires medical treatment, directed particularly to any respiratory depression produced by the drug. The third form of crisis is an *acute complication of intravenous drug usage* such as local infection, necrosis at the injection site, or infection of a distant organ, often the heart or liver.

Planned withdrawal (detoxification)

The severity of withdrawal symptoms depends on psychological as well as pharmacological factors. Therefore the *psychological management* of the patient during withdrawal is as important as the drug regimen. The speed of withdrawal should be discussed with the patient to establish a timetable which is neither so rapid that the patient will not collaborate, nor so protracted that the state of dependence is perpetuated. During withdrawal, much personal contact is needed to reassure the

patient; the relationship formed in this way can be important in later treatment.

When the dose is low, opioids can be withdrawn rapidly while giving symptomatic treatment for the withdrawal effects. Drugs such as *loperamide* or *metoclopramide* can be useful for gastrointestinal symptoms. *Non-steroidal analgesics* may be useful for aches and pains. Another drug that may be useful is the α_2-adrenoceptor antagonist, *lofexidine*. Lofexidine has a similar action to clonidine but causes less hypotension. Some studies suggest that it is as effective in ameliorating the withdrawal syndrome as methadone (Bearn *et al.* 1996).

When the daily dose of heroin is high, it may be necessary to prescribe an opioid, reducing the dose gradually. This can be done most effectively if heroin is replaced by *methadone*, which has a more gradual action. The difficulty is to judge the correct dose of methadone because patients often lie about their dosage of heroin, either overstating it in the hope of ensuring that the withdrawal regimen will be gradual or understating it in an attempt to avoid censure. In addition, as noted below, the strength of street drugs varies.

Methadone should be given in a liquid form to be taken by mouth. The initial methadone dose is normally between 10 and 40 mg daily depending on the patient's usual consumption. Users with evidence of opioid tolerance may require dosing at the higher end of this range. If 4 hours after an initial dose there is evidence of withdrawal symptoms, a supplementary dose may be given but caution should be employed because methadone is long acting and accumulation and toxicity could result.

Although 10 mg of pharmaceutical heroin is about equivalent to 10 mg of methadone, street heroin varies in potency in different places and at different times. Therefore, if possible, advice about the equivalent dose of methadone should be obtained from a doctor experienced in treating drug dependence. The rate of methadone reduction depends on the clinical circumstances and the patient's clinical responses. The most rapid regimen may take about 10 days to 3 weeks but slower reductions over several months may sometimes be appropriate. As the dose falls, reduction should be more gradual.

Pregnancy and opioid dependence

The babies of women who misuse opioids are more likely than other babies to be *premature* and of *low birth-weight*. They may also show withdrawal symptoms after birth, including irritability, restlessness, tremor, and a high-pitched cry. These signs appear within a few days of birth if the mother was taking heroin, but are delayed if she was taking methadone, which has a longer half-life in the body. Low birth-weight and prematurity are not necessarily related directly to the drug, since poor nutrition and heavy smoking are common among heroin misusers. Women in *methadone maintenance programmes* have pregnancies with a better outcome than those who are not (Ward *et al.* 1999).

Later effects have been reported, with the children of opioid-dependent mothers being more likely, as toddlers, to be overactive and to show poor persistence. However, these late effects may result from the unsuitable family environment rather than from a lasting effect of the intrauterine exposure to the drug.

Maintenance treatment for opioid dependence

As described above, withdrawal from opioids is the preferred treatment option, but if this is not possible, *maintenance treatment*, usually with methadone, may lessen the physical and social harm associated with the intravenous use of illicit drug supplies. The principle of this treatment is explained on p. 565. Instead of heroin, methadone is prescribed as a liquid preparation formulated to discourage attempts to inject it.

Methadone maintenance treatment has been extensively evaluated (for a review see Ward *et al.* 1999). There is good evidence from randomized studies that methadone maintenance decreases the use of illicit opioids and reduces criminal activity. In addition, subjects in methadone maintenance programmes show less risky injecting behaviours and lower rates of HIV infection.

Methadone doses of 20–40 mg daily have been widely advocated as appropriate for maintenance treatment, but there is some evidence that higher doses (50–120 mg daily) are associated with lower rates of illicit opioid use and improved retention in the therapeutic programme (Strain *et al.* 1999). The latter is associated with an improved therapeutic outcome. The best approach is probably to have a flexible dosing policy, bearing in mind the potential toxicity of methadone in subjects whose tolerance is unknown or hard to assess. Generally it is better to start treatment with lower doses initially (not more than 40 mg daily) and increase over a number of weeks, titrating against the presence of withdrawal symptoms. It should be remembered that methadone levels will go on increasing for about 5 days following the last dosage adjustment. (For practical advice on methadone treatment see Department of Health 1999b).

Evaluation of methadone clinics has shown that the more effective programmes have methadone maintenance treatment rather than abstinence as a primary goal of therapy. The more effective clinics were also characterized by high-quality counselling and a wide range of medical services (see Ward *et al.* 1999).

Other drugs may also be helpful in the maintenance treatment of opioid dependence. The agonist, *lambda-alpha-acetylmethadol (LAAM)* and the mixed agonist/antagonist, *buprenorphine* are equivalent in their effects to methadone in reducing illicit opioid use. Both allow dosing every other day. The long duration of action of LAAM can result in inadvertent accumulation and toxicity. The mixed agonist/antagonist properties of buprenorphine makes this less of a problem (see Valmana *et al.* 1999).

Naltrexone is a long-acting opioid antagonist which is used to help prevent relapse in detoxified opioid dependent subjects. While naltrexone treatment may have a role in certain dependent subjects with high motivation, its benefit in the wider community of opioid users is more doubtful (Ward *et al.* 1999). Naltrexone is also used in a procedure known as *rapid opioid detoxification* in conjunction with heavy sedation and sometimes general anaesthesia. The safety and efficacy of this procedure are not established (Spanagel 1999).

Therapeutic community methods

These forms of treatment aim to produce abstinence by effecting a substantial change in the patient's *attitudes and behaviour*. Drug-taking is represented as a way of avoiding pre-existing personal problems and as a source of new ones. Group therapy and communal living are combined in an attempt to produce greater personal awareness, more concern for others, and better social skills. In most therapeutic communities, some of the staff have previously been dependent on drugs and are often better able than other staff to gain the confidence of the patients in the early stages of treatment.

Anxiolytic and hypnotic drugs

The most frequently misused drugs of this group are now the *benzodiazepines*. *Barbiturates* are little prescribed and misuse has fallen. Other drugs of this group that are currently misused include chlormethiazole and chloral. The clinical effects of these drugs are thought to result from their ability to facilitate brain *GABA function*. Benzodiazepines produce these effects by binding to a specific benzodiazepine receptor.

Benzodiazepines

These drugs were in therapeutic use for many years before it became apparent that their prolonged use could lead to tolerance and dependence with a characteristic *withdrawal syndrome*. The withdrawal syndrome includes:

◆ *anxiety symptoms* – anxiety, irritability, sweating, tremor, sleep disturbance;

◆ *altered perception* – depersonalization, derealization, hypersensitivity to stimuli, abnormal body sensations, abnormal sensation of movement;

◆ *other features (rare)* – depression, psychosis, seizures, delirium tremens.

Epidemiology Benzodiazepine use is extremely widespread; for example, it has been estimated that about 10% of the population of Europe and the USA use benzodiazepines as anxiolytics or hypnotics. Over the last few years the prescription of benzodiazepines for anxiety has shown a decline. Most long-term users are older women; however, there is a significant misuse problem in younger people, often associated with intravenous administration and *polysubstance misuse*. A significant proportion of people who are *dependent on alcohol* are also dependent on benzodiazepines.

Dependence Dependence on benzodiazepines often results from prolonged medical use but may also result from the availability of benzodiazepines as street drugs because of their euphoriant effects and calming effects. The withdrawal syndrome closely resembles the anxiety symptoms for which the drugs are usually prescribed; hence if symptoms appear after the dose of benzodiazepine has been reduced, the doctor may revert to a higher dosage in the mistaken belief that these symptoms indicate a persistent anxiety disorder. It has been estimated that about one-third of subjects who take a benzodiazepine at therapeutic doses for more than 6 months may become dependent (Lader 1994).

Treatment Treatment of dependence usually consists of gradual withdrawal over at least 8 weeks combined with supportive counselling (Lader 1994). Withdrawal appears to be more severe from benzodiazepines that have *short half-lives and high potency* at the benzodiazepine receptor. For this reason it is often suggested that patients on such compounds should be switched to longer-acting drugs such as diazepam before withdrawal is attempted. For patients who have difficulty withdrawing with these measures, anxiety management may be useful (see p. 225).

Current advice is that the dose of benzodiazepine be lowered by about one-eighth (range, one tenth to one quarter) every fortnight. However, if a patient experiences troublesome withdrawal symptoms, the dose can be maintained or even temporarily increased until symptoms settle. When patients have been misusing benzodiazepines and taking very high doses, it may be difficult to identify an appropriate starting dose. In general, patients should not be given more than 40–60 mg diazepam daily. This dose should gradually be reduced by about half over 6 weeks (Department of Health 1999b).

Many patients experience their most troublesome withdrawal symptoms once the benzodiazepine dose has been fully tapered off. Symptoms usually subside over the next few weeks, although the time course can be irregular and some symptoms such as muscle spasm may not appear until other features of withdrawal have largely disappeared. A few patients continue to experience withdrawal-like symptoms for months or even years after cessation of benzodiazepines ('prolonged withdrawal syndrome').

Prevention The prevention of benzodiazepine dependence lies in the restriction of prescribing. *Psychological treatments* are effective for most anxiety disorders (see p. 225) and non-pharmacological approaches to insomnia are also beneficial (p. 661). If benzodiazepines are prescribed, it should be for the short-term relief of symptoms that are severely disabling or distressing. In some patients who are already long-term users, the balance of benefit and risk will favour continued prescribing, but patients should be regularly reviewed and the daily dose of diazepam should not exceed 30 mg (Department of Health 1999b). Advice from a general practitioner can be sufficient to persuade between 20 and 40% of long-term benzodiazepine users to reduce their daily dose or discontinue treatment. See Lader (1994) for further information about benzodiazepine dependence.

Barbiturates

Barbiturate prescribing has greatly diminished over the last decade as newer anxiolytic and antidepressant agents are preferred. Thus illicit use is becoming rare. Previously many people dependent on barbiturates began taking the drug because it had been prescribed as a hypnotic. Some barbiturates reached young drug misusers who administered them intravenously by dissolving capsules. Polysubstance misuse with barbiturates was common.

Withdrawal Abrupt withdrawal of barbiturates from a dependent person is dangerous. It may result in a delirium, like that after alcohol withdrawal, and may lead to seizures and sometimes to death through cardiovascular collapse. Hence if it is necessary to withdraw a person who has been taking doses substantially in excess of the therapeutic range, in-patient detoxification is advisable. If, however, a patient has been taking a therapeutic dose, slow out-patient withdrawal may be considered.

Maintenance treatment This may be considered for some elderly patients who have taken barbiturates for a long time. The barbiturate is replaced by a benzodiazepine and continued efforts are made to reduce the dose gradually. In most cases, withdrawal can be achieved eventually.

Cannabis

Cannabis is derived from the plant *Cannabis sativa*. It is consumed either as the dried vegetative parts in the form known as marijuana or grass, or as the resin secreted by the flowering tops of the female plant. Cannabis contains several pharmacologically active substances of which the most powerful psychoactive member is δ-9-*tetrahydrocannabinol*. It seems likely that the pharmacological effects of cannabinols are mediated through interaction with a specific cannabinoid receptor in the central nervous system. The endogenous ligand for these receptors is probably anandamide (see Adams and Martin 1996).

Epidemiology In some parts of North Africa and Asia, cannabis products are consumed in a similar way to alcohol in Western society. In North America and Britain the intermittent use of cannabis is widespread. For example, it has been estimated that about one-third of the population of the USA have used cannabis at least once in their lifetimes and

13% are current users. About 60% of the adult population aged 26–34 reported some lifetime use of cannabis (National Institute on Drug Abuse 1991). It appears that most users do not take any other illegal drug, but some are given to high consumption of alcohol.

Clinical effects The effects of cannabis vary with the dose, the person's expectations and mood, and the social setting. Users sometimes describe themselves as 'high' but, like alcohol, cannabis seems to exaggerate the pre-existing mood, whether exhilaration or depression. Users report an increased enjoyment of aesthetic experiences and distortion of the perception of time and space. There may be reddening of the eyes, dry mouth, tachycardia, irritation of the respiratory tract, and coughing. Cannabis intoxication presents hazards for car drivers.

Adverse effects No serious adverse effects have been proved among those who use cannabis intermittently at small doses. Although there is no positive evidence of teratogenicity, cannabis has not been proved safe in the first 3 months of pregnancy. Inhaled cannabis smoke irritates the respiratory tract and is potentially carcinogenic.

The most common adverse psychological effect of acute cannabis consumption is *anxiety*. Mild paranoid ideation is also not uncommon. At higher doses, toxic confusional states and occasionally psychosis in clear consciousness may rarely occur. It is not certain how far psychotic reactions are a consequence of a predisposition in the individual, rather than a specific reaction to the pharmacological action of the drug.

Cannabis and schizophrenia The question as to whether chronic cannabis use can predispose to schizophrenia is controversial. Andreasson *et al.* (1987) followed up 45 570 Swedish conscripts for 15 years. They found that the relative risk of developing schizophrenia was 2.5 times greater in subjects who used cannabis, and the relative risk for heavy users was six times greater. Whilst these data suggest that cannabis could be a risk factor for the development of schizophrenia, it is also possible that those predisposed to develop schizophrenia are also predisposed to misuse cannabis. It is better established that cannabis can modify the course of an established schizophrenic illness, with evidence from a number of studies that users are more likely to experience psychotic episodes and relapse (Hall and Solowij 1998).

It is also said that chronic use of cannabis can lead to a state of apathy and indolence (an amotivational state). However, this proposal has not been confirmed by epidemiological studies. It is possible that the symptoms and signs of the amotivational state could reflect chronic intoxication (see Hall and Solowij 1998).

Tolerance and dependence There is evidence that tolerance to cannabis can occur in subjects exposed to high doses for a prolonged period of time, but it is much less evident in those who use small or intermittent dosing. Withdrawal from high doses gives rise to a syndrome of irritability, nausea, insomnia, and anorexia. These symptoms are generally mild in nature. The epidemiological data show that the vast majority of cannabis users do not misuse the drug or become dependent on it. For a review of the adverse effects of cannabis use see Hall and Solowij (1998).

Stimulant drugs

These drugs include *amphetamines*, related substances such as phenmetrazine, and methylphenidate. *Cocaine* is also a stimulant drug, but is considered separately in the next section. Amphetamines have been largely abandoned in medical practice, apart from their use for the hyperkinetic syndrome of childhood (p. 831) and for narcolepsy (p. 440). The psychomotor stimulant effects of amphetamines are believed to result from their ability to release and block the re-uptake of dopamine and noradrenaline.

Epidemiology Amphetamines are probably the most commonly used stimulant in the UK, although cocaine is more commonly used in the USA. A survey in the USA estimated that 7% of the population had used an amphetamine at least once in their lives. The highest level of use was among those aged 18–25, of whom 9% reported using amphetamines at least once, whilst 1% described themselves as current users. It should be noted that in the USA, 3,4-methylenedioxymethamphetamine (MDMA), a mixed amphetamine and hallucinogen (see below), is classified as an amphetamine derivative, and a considerable proportion of reported amphetamine use is probably accounted for by this drug (Kaplan *et al.* 1994).

In the UK, about 10–15% of young people have tried amphetamines by the age of 19. About 10% of those presenting to specialist drug misuse services use amphetamine as their main drug whilst a further 10% use it as a secondary drug usually in conjunction with opiates. Almost half of these users were injecting amphetamine and thereby exposed to the health risks of intravenous administration (see Seivewright and McMahon 1996).

In the past, most addiction to stimulant drugs arose from injudicious prescribing. However, most amphetamines are now illicitly synthesized and used as a 'street drug', known as 'speed' or 'whizz'. As well as being taken orally or intravenously, amphetamines can also be 'snorted' (taken like snuff). A pure form of amphetamine ('ice'), can be smoked or injected. It is said to produce particularly powerful effects.

Clinical effects Apart from their immediate effect on mood, the drugs produce over-talkativeness, over-activity, insomnia, dryness of lips, mouth, and nose, and anorexia. The pupils dilate, the pulse rate increases, and blood pressure rises.

With large doses there may be *cardiac arrhythmia*, severe hypertension, cerebrovascular accident, and occasionally circulatory collapse. At increasingly high doses, neurological symptoms such as seizures and coma may occur. Acute adverse psychological effects of amphetamines include dysphoria, irritability, insomnia, and confusion. Anxiety and

---

> **Box 18.6 Some complications of amphetamine and cocaine misuse**
>
> *Medical*
>
> Cardiovascular – hypertension, stroke, arrhythmias, myocardial infarction
>
> Infective – abscesses, septicaemia, hepatitis, HIV
>
> Obstetric – reduced fetal growth, miscarriage, premature labour, placental abruption
>
> Other – weight loss, dental problems, epilepsy, general neglect
>
> *Psychiatric*
>
> Anxiety, depression, antisocial behaviour, paranoid psychosis

---

panic can also be present. *Obstetric complications* include miscarriage, premature labour, and placental abruption (Box 18.6).

Amphetamine-induced psychosis Prolonged use of high doses of amphetamines may result in repetitive stereotyped behaviour, for example, repeated tidying. A *paranoid psychosis* that has been likened to paranoid schizophrenia may also be induced by prolonged high doses. The features include persecutory delusions, auditory and visual hallucinations, and sometimes hostile and dangerously *aggressive behaviour* (Connell 1958). Usually the condition subsides in about a week, but occasionally it persists for months. It is not certain whether these prolonged cases are true drug-induced psychoses, schizophrenia provoked by the amphetamine, or merely coincidental. Whatever the nature of the association, it is not uncommon for patients with amphetamine misuse to present to general psychiatric services.

Tolerance and dependence From the epidemiology of amphetamine use, it seems that many recreational users do not progress to misuse and dependence. In more persistent users tolerance to amphetamines leads to users taking higher doses of the drug. A withdrawal syndrome ('crash') of varying severity follows cessation of amphetamine use. In mild cases it consists mainly of low mood and decreased energy. In some cases, particularly in heavy users, depression can be severe, and accompanied by anxiety, tremulousness, lethargy, fatigue, and nightmares. Craving for the drug may be intense and *suicidal ideation* prominent. Dependence on amphetamines can develop quickly. Dependence on stimulant drugs may be recognized from the history of overactivity and high spirits alternating with inactivity and depression. Whenever amphetamine use is at all likely, a urine sample should be taken for analysis as soon as possible because these drugs are quickly eliminated.

Prevention and treatment Prevention of amphetamine misuse depends on restriction of the drugs and careful prescribing. Doctors should be wary of newly arrived patients who purport to suffer from narcolepsy.

Treatment of acute overdoses requires sedation and management of hyperpyrexia and cardiac arrhythmias. Most toxic symptoms, including paranoid psychoses, resolve quickly when the drug is stopped. An antipsychotic drug may be needed to control florid symptoms, but if this medication can be avoided the differential diagnosis from schizophrenia will be easier.

The treatment of amphetamine dependence is difficult because craving for the drug can be intense. *Abstinence* is the usual goal and to achieve this a full range of social and psychological interventions may be needed (see above). Benzodiazepines may be helpful for managing acute distress occasioned by a severe withdrawal syndrome, and antidepressants may be needed for a persistent depressive disorder. Abstinence-based programmes are not suitable for all misusers and in view of the considerable harm that is associated with severe intravenous misuse, some specialist centres undertake maintenance treatment with oral amphetamine. The use of the practice is not fully tested but may achieve the goal of harm reduction in carefully selected situations (see Bruce 2000).

Cocaine

Cocaine is a central nervous stimulant with effects similar to those of amphetamines (described above). It a particularly powerful positive reinforcer in animals and causes strong dependence in humans. These latter effects probably stem from the ability of cocaine to block the re-uptake of dopamine into presynaptic dopamine terminals. This leads to substantial increases in extracellular levels of dopamine in the nucleus accumbens and consequent activation of the physiological 'reward system' (Robbins and Everitt 1999).

Cocaine is administered by injection, by smoking, and by sniffing into the nostrils. The latter practice sometimes causes perforation of the nasal septum. In 'freebasing', chemically pure cocaine is extracted from the 'street' drug to produce 'crack', which has a very rapid onset of action, particularly when inhaled.

Epidemiology In 1991, 12% of Americans reported lifetime use of cocaine, with 3% having used the drug in the previous year but fewer than 1% in the previous month. The highest rate of use in the previous month (2%) was in those aged 18–25 (see National Institute on Drug Abuse 1991; Kaplan *et al.* 1994). Cocaine use in the USA has been associated with high levels of violent crime. The incidence of cocaine use in the UK has increased over the last decade, but to a lesser extent than that seen in the USA. For example, only 4% of drug misusers presenting to specialist services use cocaine as their primary drug of misuse but over 10% use it in conjunction with opioids (Seivewright and McMahon 1996).

Clinical effects The psychological effects of cocaine include excitement, increased energy, and euphoria. This can be associated with grandiose thinking, impaired judgement, and sexual disinhibition. Higher doses can result in visual and auditory hallucinations. *Paranoid ideation* may lead to *aggressive behaviour*. More prolonged use of high doses of cocaine can result in a paranoid psychosis with violent behaviour. This state is usually short-lived but may be more enduring in those with a pre-existing vulnerability to psychotic disorder (Strang 1993). Formication ('cocaine bugs'), a feeling as if insects are crawling under the skin, is sometimes experienced by cocaine misuse.

The physical effects of cocaine include increases in pulse rate and blood pressure. Dilatation of the pupils is often prominent. Severe adverse effects of cocaine use include *cardiac arrhythmias*, *myocardial infarction*, *myocarditis*, and *cardiomyopathy*. Cocaine use has also been associated with cerebrovascular disease, including cerebral infarction, subarachnoid haemorrhage, and transient ischaemic attacks. Seizures and respiratory arrest have been reported. *Obstetric complications* include miscarriage, placental abruption, and premature labour.

Tolerance and dependence In persistent users, tolerance to the effects of cocaine develops and a withdrawal syndrome similar to that seen following withdrawal of amphetamines can occur. After acute cocaine use, the 'crash' consists of dysphoria, anhedonia, anxiety, irritability, fatigue, and hypersomnolence. If the preceding cocaine use has been relatively mild, such symptoms resolve within about 24 hours. After more prolonged use, the symptoms are more severe and extended, and are associated with intense craving, depression, and occasionally severe *suicidal ideation*. Craving for cocaine can re-emerge after months of abstinence, particularly if the subject is exposed to psychological or social cues previously associated with its use.

Treatment Acute intoxication may require sedation with benzodiazepines or, in severe cases, an antipsychotic agent such as haloperidol. Concurrent medical crises such as seizures or hypertension should be managed in the usual way.

As with amphetamines, the treatment of cocaine dependence is difficult because of the intense craving associated with abstinence from the drug. For moderate cocaine users it may be sufficient to provide psychological and social support on an outpatient basis. Heavy and chaotic users with strong dependence will need more intensive management,

perhaps as in-patients (Strang *et al.* 1993). There is some evidence where dependence and craving are severe that treatment with the tricyclic antidepressant desipramine may be helpful in promoting abstinence (Withers *et al.* 1995).

Various psychotherapeutic programmes may also be effective in subjects with cocaine dependence. The evidence suggests that cognitive–behavioural approaches, including relapse prevention, produce rather better results than simple counselling (Higgins *et al.* 1993). Cue exposure (see above) may also have a role (Strang 1993). As far as individual treatment programmes are concerned, it is worth noting that subjects who misuse cocaine often misuse other drugs such as opioids and alcohol.

MDMA (ecstasy)

The recreational use of *3,4 methylenedioxymethamphetamine (MDMA)* or 'ecstasy' has increased rapidly over the last decade. Ecstasy is a synthetic drug classified in the DSM-IV substance list as a hallucinogen. However, it has stimulant as well as mild hallucinogenic properties. It is usually taken in tablet or capsule form in a dose of about 50–150 mg. Given in this way, its effects last for about 4–6 hours. Like amphetamines, ecstasy increases the release of dopamine but it also releases 5-hydroxytryptamine (5-HT), which may account for its hallucinogenic properties.

Clinical effects Ecstasy produces a positive mood state with feelings of euphoria, sociability, and intimacy. It also produces sensations of newly discovered insights and heightened perceptions. The physical effects of ecstasy include loss of appetite, tachycardia, bruxism, and sweating. Tolerance to successive doses of ecstasy develops quickly. Weekend users describe a midweek 'crash' in mood which may represent withdrawal effects (Curran and Travill 1997).

Adverse reactions Rarely, ecstasy can cause severe adverse reactions, and deaths due to hyperthermia and its complications have been reported in healthy young adults. Hyperthermia probably results from the effect of ecstasy in increasing brain 5-HT release, together with the social setting in which the drug is customarily taken (crowded parties with prolonged and strenuous dancing). Deaths have also been reported through cardiac arrhythmias, though pre-existing cardiac disease may have played a role. Intracerebral haemorrhage has occurred in ecstasy users, probably as a consequence of hypertensive crises. Cases of toxic hepatitis could reflect impurities in manufacture (Solowij 1993).

The use of ecstasy has been associated with acute and chronic paranoid psychoses but, as with other drug-induced psychotic states, it is not clear how far such disorders represent idiosyncratic reactions of vulnerable individuals. There are also reports of 'flashbacks', which are the recurrence of abnormal experiences weeks or months following drug ingestion. Such effects have been reported with other hallucinogens (see below).

In experimental animals, including primates, repeated treatment with ecstasy produces *degeneration of 5-HT nerve terminals* in cortex and forebrain. Therefore it is possible that such effects could occur in humans, and brain-imaging studies show changes in serotonin transporter binding consistent with 5-HT neuronal damage (McCann *et al.* 1998). Whether such a change could be associated with long-term neuropsychological or psychiatric sequelae is not known.

Prevention and harm reduction Although the risk of serious harm following acute ecstasy use appears to be low, it is important to inform potential users about the acute risks and the *potential long-term hazard of neurotoxicity*. Consumption of large doses and pre-existing psychiatric disorder are likely to be associated with increased risk of adverse reactions. Education may also help users to avoid heatstroke by encouraging breaks from dancing and the consumption of sufficient replacement fluid during vigorous exercise.

Hallucinogens

Hallucinogens are sometimes known as psychedelics, but we do not recommend this term because it does not have a single clear meaning. The term psychotomimetic is also used because the drugs produce changes that bear some resemblance to those of the functional psychoses. However, the resemblance is not close, and so we do not recommend this term.

The synthetic hallucinogens include *lysergic acid diethylamide (LSD)*, dimethyl tryptamine, and methyldimethoxyamphetamine. Of these drugs, LSD is encountered most often in the UK. Hallucinogens also occur naturally in some species of mushroom, and varieties containing *psilocybin* are consumed for their hallucinogenic effects. The mode of action of hallucinogenic drugs is unclear, but most act as partial agonists at *brain 5-HT$_{2A}$ receptors*.

Epidemiology Trends in both the USA and Europe suggest that misuse of hallucinogens is increasing. For example, between 1988 and 1997 the proportion of US high school students reporting lifetime hallucinogen use rose from 7.7 to 13.6%. Similar figures apply in the UK (see Abraham 2000).

Clinical effects The effects of LSD have been most studied and will be described here. The physical actions of LSD are variable. There are initial sympathomimetic effects: heart rate and blood pressure may increase and pupils dilate. However, overdosage does not seem to result in severe physiological reactions.

In predisposed subjects, the hypertensive effects of hallucinogens can cause adverse myocardial and cerebrovascular effects. The psychological effects develop during a period of 2 hours after LSD consumption and generally last from 8 to 14 hours. The most remarkable experiences are distortions or intensifications of sensory perception. There may be confusion between sensory modalities (synaesthesia), with sounds being perceived as visual or movements experienced as if heard. Objects may be seen to merge with one another or move rhythmically. The passage of time appears to be slowed and experiences seem to have a profound meaning.

A distressing experience may be distortion of the body image, with the person sometimes feeling that he is outside his own body. These experiences may lead to *panic with fears of insanity*. The mood may be exhilaration, distress, or acute anxiety. According to early reports, behaviour could be unpredictable and extremely dangerous, with the user sometimes injuring or killing himself through behaving as if he were invulnerable. Since then there may have been some reduction in such adverse reactions, possibly because users are more aware of the dangers and take precautions to ensure support from other people during a 'trip'.

Whenever possible, adverse reactions should be managed by 'talking down' the user, explaining that the alarming experiences are due to the drug. If there is not time for this, an anxiolytic such as *diazepam* should be given and is usually effective. Tolerance to the psychological effects of LSD can occur, but a withdrawal syndrome has not been described. Dependence may occur in long-term and heavy users, but is rare (Kaplan *et al.* 1994).

It has been argued that use of LSD can cause long-term abnormalities in thinking and behaviour or even schizophrenia. The evidence for such an association is dubious (Kaplan *et al.* 1994). However, flashback, i.e. the recurrence of psychedelic experience weeks or months after the drug was last taken, is a recognized event. This experience may be distressing and occasionally requires treatment with an anxiolytic drug.

Phencyclidine

Phencyclidine is sufficiently different from the hallucinogens in its actions to require a separate description. It can be synthesized easily, and is taken by mouth, smoked, or injected. Phencyclidine was developed as a disassociative anaesthetic, but its use was abandoned because of adverse effects such as delirium and hallucinations. It is related to the currently used anaesthetic agent ketamine.

Both phencyclidine and ketamine antagonize neurotransmission at *N-methyl-D-aspartate (NMDA) receptors*, which may account for their hallucinogenic effects. The psychological effects of ketamine in healthy volunteers have been used to model some of the clinical symptoms and cognitive changes seen in patients with schizophrenia (Krystal *et al.* 1999).

Phencyclidine is widely available in the USA but is little used in the UK. Most users of phencyclidine also use other drugs, particularly alcohol and cannabis. Ingestion of phencylcidine may be inadvertent because it is often added to other 'street' drugs to boost their effects.

Clinical effects Small doses of this drug produce drunkenness, with analgesia of fingers and toes, and even anaesthesia. Intoxication with the drug is prolonged, with the common features being agitation, depressed consciousness, aggressiveness and psychotic-like symptoms, nystagmus, and raised blood pressure. With high doses there may be ataxia, muscle rigidity, convulsions, and absence of response to the environment even though the eyes are wide open. Phencyclidine can be detected in the urine for 72 hours after it was last taken.

With serious overdoses, an adrenergic crisis may occur with hypertensive heart failure, cerebrovascular accident, or malignant hyperthermia. Status epilepticus may appear. Fatalities have been reported, due mainly to hypertensive crisis but also to respiratory failure or suicide. Other people may be attacked and injured. Chronic use of phencyclidine may lead to *aggressive behaviour* accompanied by memory loss. Tolerance to the effects of phencyclidine occurs, though withdrawal symptoms are rare in humans. Dependence occurs in chronic users (Kaplan *et al.* 1994).

Treatment of phencyclidine intoxication Treatment of acute intoxication is symptomatic, according to the features listed above. *Haloperidol*, or *diazepam*, or both, may be given. Caution should be employed if using benzodiazepines alone because of the risk of further behavioural disinhibition. *Chlorpromazine* should be avoided because it may increase the anticholinergic effects of phencyclidine and worsen mental state. Hypertensive crisis should be treated with antihypertensive agents such as phentolamine. Respiratory function needs to be carefully monitored because excessive secretions may compromise the airway in an unconscious patient.

Volatile substances (solvents, inhalants)

The misuse of *volatile substances (also known as solvents)* is not new but public concern about widespread misuse was first apparent in the USA in the 1950s. Similar concerns emerged in the UK in the early 1970s. Although public interest has waned since then, there is a continuing high level of volatile substance misuse, particularly amongst *adolescents*.

The pharmacological actions of volatile substances in the central nervous system are not clear but, like alcohol, they may increase the fluidity of neuronal cell membranes and could also increase brain GABA function (Kaplan *et al.* 1994).

Epidemiology Volatile substance misuse is a worldwide problem. In the NHSDA survey, about 5% of the American population had used volatile substances at least once in their lives, but fewer than 1% had used them in the past month (National Institute on Drug Abuse 1991). In the UK, up to a fifth of young people have tried sniffing volatile substances (Miller and Plant 1996). Volatile substance misuse is very prevalent among the very young homeless populations in South American countries.

Volatile substance use occurs mainly in *young men*. Use is more common in those from lower socioeconomic backgrounds. Most of the young people known to use volatile substances do so as a group activity, and only about 5% are solitary users. There is some evidence that a subgroup of volatile substance users have antisocial personalities and are likely to use and misuse multiple substances. However, the epidemiological data suggest that most who use volatile substances do so only a few times and then abandon the practice (Dinwiddie 1994).

Substances used and methods of use The volatile substances used are mainly solvents and adhesives (hence the name 'glue sniffing'), but also include many other substances such as petrol, cleaning fluid, aerosols of all kinds, agents used in fire extinguishers, and butane. Toluene and acetone are frequently used. In this chapter the term 'volatile substance' will be used to describe all these various substances. The methods of ingestion depend on the substance; they include inhalation from tops of bottles, beer cans, cloths held over the mouth, plastic bags, and sprays. Volatile substance use may be associated with taking other illicit drugs or with tobacco or alcohol consumption, which can be heavy.

Clinical effects The clinical effects of volatile substances are similar to those of alcohol consumption. The central nervous system is first stimulated and then depressed. The stages of intoxication are similar to those of alcohol: euphoria, blurring of vision, slurring of speech, incoordination, staggering gait, nausea, vomiting, and coma. Compared with alcohol intoxication, volatile substance intoxication develops and wanes rapidly (within a few minutes, or up to 2 hours). There is early disorientation and two-fifths of cases may develop hallucinations, which are mainly visual and often frightening. This combination of symptoms may lead to serious accidents.

Adverse effects Volatile substance misuse has many severe adverse effects, of which the most serious is *sudden death*. These fatalities occur during acute intoxication, and over the last 10 years about 100 such deaths have occurred annually in the UK (Ives 2000). About half the deaths are due to the direct toxic effects of the volatile substance, particularly cardiac arrhythmias and respiratory depression. The rest are due to trauma, asphyxia (plastic bag over head), or inhalation of stomach contents.

Chronic users may show evidence of *neurotoxic effects* and severe and disabling peripheral neuropathy has been described in teenager misusers. Other neurological adverse effects, particularly associated with toluene, include impaired cerebellar function, encephalitis, and dementia. Volatile substance misuse can also damage other organs including liver, kidney, heart, and lungs.

Gastrointestinal symptoms include nausea, vomiting, and haematemesis.

Tolerance and dependence Dependence can develop if use is regular, but physical withdrawal symptoms are unusual. When such symptoms occur they usually consist of sleep disturbance, irritability, nausea, tachycardia, and, rarely, hallucinations and delusions. With sustained use over 6–12 months, tolerance can develop.

Diagnosis The diagnosis of acute volatile substance intoxication is suggested by several features: glue on the hands, face, or clothes; chemical smell on the breath; rapid onset and waning of intoxication; disorientation in time and space. Chronic misuse is diagnosed mainly on an admitted history of habitual consumption, increasing tolerance, and dependence. A suggestive feature is a facial rash ('glue-sniffers rash') caused by repeated inhalation from a bag.

Treatment As noted above, for many users experimentation with volatile substances is a temporary phase which does not appear to lead to persistent misuse or dependence. Advice and support may well be sufficient for such subjects. However, a significant subgroup of those who misuse volatile substances also misuse other substances such as alcohol and opioids. Such subjects are more likely to have an antisocial personality disorder and to have experienced a chaotic and abusive family life. Treatment of this group is difficult, and a full range of psychological and social treatments is likely to be needed (see above). There is no specific pharma-cotherapy for volatile substance misuse, but associated psychiatric disorders such as depression may require treatment in their own right.

Prevention Prevention of volatile substance misuse may best be directed at the large numbers of young people who experiment with volatile substances through curiosity or peer pressure. Policies include the restriction of sales of volatile substances to children and adolescents. Education, particularly concerning the risk of severe injury and death (which can, of course, occur in occasional or first-time users), seems worthwhile. Wider social measures such as the provision of improved recreational facilities have also been advocated. For a review of volatile substance misuse see Ives (2000).

Further reading

Department of Health (1999). *Drug misuse and dependence – Guidelines of clinical management*. HMSO, London. (Current practice guidelines for assessment and treatment of drug misuse.)

Miller, W. R. and Rollnick, S. (1991). *Motivational interviewing: preparing people to change addictive behaviour*. Guilford Press, London. (Account of how best to motivate drug misusers to change their drug habit.)

Robson, P. (1999). *Forbidden drugs*. Oxford University Press, Oxford. (Readable account of illicit drugs, reasons for use and treatment of misuse.)

Vaillant, G. (1995). The natural history of follow-up alcoholism revisited. Harvard University Press, Harvard. (Careful longitudinal study of young men with alcohol dependence.)

Problems related to sexuality and gender identity

Problems related to sexuality and gender identity

This chapter is concerned with four topics related to sexuality and gender: sexual orientation, sexual dysfunction, abnormalities of sexual preference, and disorders of gender identity.

◆ *Sexual orientation* refers to the various aspects of sexual attraction towards members of the opposite or the same sex.

◆ *Sexual dysfunction* denotes impaired or dissatisfying sexual enjoyment or performance. Such conditions are common.

◆ *Abnormalities of sexual preference* are uncommon, but they take many forms and therefore require relatively more space than the more common sexual dysfunctions.

◆ *Gender identity* is a person's sense of being male or female. When this sense of identity is at variance with the anatomical sex, the person is said to have a gender identity disorder.

To decide what sexual activities are abnormal requires an understanding of the wide variations that exist in normal sexual functioning. The chapter begins with an account of these variations. No account is given of sexual physiology; readers seeking information on this subject are referred to Bancroft (1989) or Levin (2000).

Variations in sexual behaviour

Human sexual behaviour is very varied. It is not known what determines this variation but it is likely that it has biological and social determinants. Compared with the behaviour of other primates, human sexual behaviour is less tied to biological factors; for example, it is not limited to a periods of oestrus. Also the biologically deter-

mined sexual signals related to the breasts, pubic hair, buttocks, and lips are augmented in many cultures by the use of make-up, perfumes, and clothing. In other cultures, clothing is used to hide these innate sexual signals by covering the arms, legs, and, in some societies, the women's faces. Moreover, man's artistic abilities are used to produce erotic images and writing that increase sexual arousal.

Social rules control the range of sexual behaviours that may be expressed. Sexual relations between family members are widely prohibited by social rules and also in law. Sexual relations with unrelated minors are also widely forbidden, though ages of consent vary in different societies. Some sexual behaviours that were generally condemned in the past are now widely accepted. For example, in the late nineteenth century, masturbation was condemned in many countries as sinful and also harmful to health; now it is widely accepted as normal. In ancient Greece, homosexual relations were widely accepted; at the present time, they are generally accepted though condemned by some religions groups. Clinicians need to be aware of these variations in sexual behaviour and attitudes, and refrain from imposing their own values and attitudes on their patients.

Surveys of sexual behaviour

One way to discover what sexual behaviours are common is to ask people. The first major investigation was carried out by the group led by American biologist Alfred Kinsey (Kinsey *et al.* 1948, 1953). The surveys were large (12 000 males and 8000 females), but the subjects were not representative of the general population. Thus, although the results were valuable in showing the range of sexual behaviour, the estimates of frequency could not be generalized. This is even more the case now since the surveys were carried out in the 1950s and sexual attitudes and behaviour have changed in many ways since then.

Two recent surveys give a more representative picture of current sexual behaviour in the USA and the UK. Whilst similar findings might be expected in countries with comparable cultures, the results should not be generalized too widely.

In the *US survey* (Michael *et al.* 1994), 3194 English-speaking adults were interviewed. About 20% of those approached refused to be interviewed and although this is a generally satisfactory response rate for this kind of study, it is possible that those who refused had sexual attitudes and behaviour different from those of the rest. The main findings were:

- Men thought about sex more often than did women. Half the men reported sexual thoughts several times a day; most women reported sexual thoughts a few times a week or less.

- The percentages of men and women reporting various frequencies of sexual intercourse were: none in the last year, 14%; a few times in the last year, 16%; a few times a month, 40%; 2–3 times a week, 26%; more than this, 8%.

- A third of females aged 18–60 said they were uninterested in sex

- The most appealing sexual activity was vaginal intercourse (80%), followed by watching the partner undress (50% of males; but 30% of females).

- Oral sex was common: 68% of women had given it and 73% had received it at some time.

- Anal sex was said to be unappealing by 73% of men and 87% of women.

- Frequency of intercourse was related inversely to age, and to the length of time that the couple had been together. It was not related to race, education, or religion. However, reported sexual practices did vary with race and social class.

The *UK survey* concerned 18 876 adults (Wellings *et al.* 1994). Although the findings were similar to those of the US survey, they should be interpreted cautiously since, of those approached, nearly 30% refused to be interviewed. The mean frequency of intercourse of those in their twenties was about 5 per month falling to 2 per month in those aged 55–59. Oral sex was the most common sexual activity after vaginal intercourse. Anal intercourse was infrequent: only 14% of males and 13% of females said that they had practised it.

Homosexual intercourse has been less studied than heterosexual intercourse but it is probably no less variable. With the obvious exception of vaginal intercourse, it includes all the sexual activities described by heterosexual people, including oral-genital contact and mutual masturbation. For males, it may include anal intercourse, and for women the use of an artificial phallus. Sexual partners may exchange roles in these acts, or one partner may be always passive and the other always active.

Apart from these survey results, it is widely accepted that many sexual activities that are regarded as abnormal when they are the preferred form of sexual behaviour, are practised widely as a minor component of both heterosexual and homosexual activity, for example, painful stimulation, or wearing certain clothes to increase arousal.

Sexual orientation

Kinsey *et al.* (1948) found that people cannot be divided sharply into those with homosexual and those with heterosexual orientation. Between people who are exclusively heterosexual and those who are exclusively homosexual is a continuum of people who experience in varying degrees both homosexual and heterosexual attraction and fantasies, who engage in varying mixtures of homosexual and heterosexual behaviour and relationships, and who adopt various degrees of homosexual and heterosexual lifestyles. For this and other reasons, Klein *et al.* (1985) suggested that sexual orientation should be assessed against six criteria: sexual attraction, sexual fantasies, sexual behaviour, affectional relationship preference, lifestyle, and self-identification. The expression of homosexual and heterosexual behaviour varies in the same person with age and with circumstances. The potential for bisexual attraction and behaviour seems to be greater in adolescence than in adult life. Also, homosexual behaviour is more likely to be expressed when heterosexual behaviour is unavailable, for example in prisons; and more likely to be suppressed when religious beliefs or the attitudes in the society are strongly disapproving.

In the study referred to above, Kinsey *et al.* (1948) estimated that 10% of men were 'more or less exclusively homosexual' for at least 3 years, and that 4% of men were exclusively homosexual throughout their lives. Kinsey *et al.* (1953) reported that 4% of single women were continuously homosexual from the ages of 20 to 35. Neither study was of a representative sample of the population, and subsequent estimates suggest that the true figure may be nearer 3% of men and 1% of women (Gagnon and Simon 1973; Laumann *et al.* 1994).

Lifestyle is an aspect of sexual orientation that varies according to cultural factors. Nevertheless, in most societies the majority of homosexual and heterosexual people have similar lifestyles. Other homosexual people prefer work and leisure activities that are more often chosen by members of the opposite sex. A small minority of homosexual people adopt the mannerisms and dress resembling, sometimes in an exaggerated way, those of the opposite sex. (Unlike transsexual people, they do this while recognizing that their gender corresponds to their anatomical sex.) Most people of either sexual orientation seek lasting relationships, but in either group a promiscuous minority seek a series of brief sexual experiences.

Self-identification also varies considerably among people of the same sexual orientation. Some exclusively homosexual people experience strong feelings of identity with other homosexuals and seek their company in preference to that of heterosexuals, for example in clubs or bars.

Determinants of sexual orientation

The determinants of sexual orientation are not known. Several theories have been proposed, concerned with: genetic factors, hormonal influences, neuroanatomical differences, and psychological factors.

Genetic determinants

Twin and adoption studies

Several investigators have reported that MZ twins are more often alike in respect of homosexuality than are DZ twins (Kallmann 1952; Eckhert *et al.* 1986; Bailey and Pillard 1991; King and McDonald 1992). These findings are compatible with a genetic aetiology, but could also arise if the early environment of MZ twins is more similar in crucial ways than that of DZ twins. Adoption studies could exclude this possibility. However, there is no conclusive investigation of this kind although Eckhert *et al.* (1986) reported that of the two male twin pairs, reared apart, one pair was concordant for homosexuality, and of the four female twin pairs, none was concordant.

Chromosome studies

No convincing evidence has been reported of chromosome differences in either male or female homosexuals. Although a linkage with chromosome Xq28 has been reported (Hamer *et al.* 1993), the methodology of the study has been criticized (Baron 1993) and the finding was not confirmed in a subsequent study (Rice *et al.* 1999).

Hormonal theories

Research with animals suggests that the intrinsic pattern of the mammalian brain is female, and that the development of male brain characteristics depends on androgen production by the fetus. In animals, male or female brain characteristics are inferred from differences in reproductive behaviour, such as mounting by the male and the lordosis of the sexually receptive female. It is uncertain whether information about the neural control of these mating behaviours can be extrapolated to the wider issues of human sexual orientation. Moreover, although male animals engage at times in sexual behaviour with other males, exclusively homosexual behaviour probably occurs only in humans.

If prenatal hormonal levels determine sexual orientation, there should be an excess of people with homosexual orientation among males with syndromes of prenatal androgen deficiency or insensitivity, and among females with syndromes involving androgen excess. No such increase has been observed among men with androgen deficiency or insensitivity (Byrne and Parsons 1993). However, an increased rate of homosexual orientation has been reported among women with congenital virilizing adrenal hyperplasia (Money *et al.* 1984; Byrne and Parsons 1993). The interpretation of this finding is uncertain because these females are born with masculinized external genitalia, and it is possible that sexual orientation in adult life was affected by this feature rather than by a direct effect of hormones on the brain.

Neuroanatomical differences

There have been reports of differences, between homosexual and heterosexual men, in the structure of the hypothalamus (LeVay 1991) and suprachiasmatic nucleus (Swaab and Hoffman 1990), but these studies have been criticized on technical grounds (Byrne and Parsons 1993).

Psychological causes

Theories about psychological causes of sexual orientation derive mainly from psychoanalytical studies. These studies are of single cases or of highly selected groups of homosexual people, and they rely on the unconfirmed recollections by adults of events in early childhood. The theories generally suppose that homosexual orientation among males is determined by poor relationships with the parents in early childhood: a distant relationship with, or prolonged absence of the father; or an overprotective mother. It is supposed that either can interfere with the development of a

heterosexual orientation. Similarly, homosexual orientation among females is supposed to result from problems in early relationships with a mother who is rejecting or indifferent (Wolff 1971). These ideas have not been supported by evidence obtained by methods of enquiry other than psychoanalytical approaches.

Psychological problems related to sexual orientation

Most people of either sexual orientation are contented and have a stable relationship with a partner. However, people may consult doctors about four kinds of problem related to sexual orientation. Many of these problems are related to public attitudes, religious convictions, and personal beliefs that conflict with the person's sexual orientation.

Uncertainty about sexual orientation

Shy and sexually inexperienced young men may seek advice because they are uncertain of their sexual orientation. They can be helped by sympathetic discussion in which they are allowed time to reflect on their situation.

Problems in adolescence

Young people who have realized that they are partly or predominantly homosexual may be uncertain about the implications for their lives especially if they encounter intolerant attitudes. Some of these young people are bullied at school. A study of American school students showed a higher rate of suicide intent and suicide attempts among male homosexual students than heterosexuals. The corresponding rates among females were not increased (Remafedi *et al.* 1998).

Some young people ask whether their sexual orientation is likely to change as they grow older. There are no reliable data, but it seems that a person who has reached adult life without experiencing heterosexual attraction or fantasies is unlikely to develop these later.

Problems in early adult life

People of either sexual orientation may ask for help with emotional disorders related to sexual or social relationships, or when their sexual urges conflict with religious or other beliefs. Some homosexual people ask for help with problems related to the unfavourable attitudes of other people. Some homosexual women marry and then seek advice, often at the suggestion of the spouse, about dysfunction in heterosexual intercourse.

Problems in middle age

People of either sexual orientation who have not formed a stable sexual relationship may become lonely and depressed if they do not have close friends and family. Men who have depended previously on casual sexual experiences may find these harder to arrange as they grow older and may turn towards prostitutes.

Other problems

Other problems are often related to fears of sexually transmitted diseases, nowadays most often the possibility of having contracted AIDS, or a positive result of testing for HIV. People with these problems require appropriate medical treatment and counselling.

Problems of sex and gender identity

Classification of problems of sex and gender identity

In both DSM-IV and ICD-10 problems of sex and gender identity are classified in three groups:

- sexual dysfunction;
- disorders known as paraphilias in DSM-IV and disorders of sexual preference in ICD-10;
- gender identity disorders.

In DSM-IV these conditions are grouped together under the heading of sexual and gender identity disorders. In ICD-10 they appear in two parts of

the classification: sexual dysfunction are in F5, 'physiological dysfunction associated with mental or behavioural factors'; disorders of sexual preference and of gender identity are in F6, 'abnormalities of adult personality and behaviour'. The two classifications are shown side by side in Table 19.1. In both systems each of the three main categories is classified further. *Sexual dysfunctions* are divided according to the stage of the sexual response that is mainly affected: disorders of sexual desire; disorders of sexual arousal; disorders of orgasm. There are also categories for the painful conditions vaginismus and dyspareunia. The slight differences in terminology between DSM-IV and ICD-10 are shown in Table 19.1.

Paraphilias (abnormalities of sexual preference) are subdivided in the two classifications. The only substantial difference is that DSM-IV has a category for the uncommon disorder known as frotteurism, a condition which in ICD-10 would be classified under 'other abnormalities of sexual preference'.

Gender identity disorders are divided in DSM-IV, but not in ICD-10, into those in children and those in adolescents and adults.

Sexual dysfunctions

In men sexual dysfunction refers to repeated impairment of normal sexual interest and/or performance. In women it refers more often to a repeated unsatisfactory quality to the experience; sexual intercourse can be completed, but without enjoyment. What is regarded as normal sexual intercourse, and therefore what is thought to be impaired or unsatisfactory, depends in part on the expectations of the two people concerned. For example, one couple may regard it as normal that the woman is regularly unable to achieve orgasm, whilst another may seek treatment.

As explained above, problems of sexual dysfunction are classified into those affecting:

- sexual desire and sexual enjoyment,
- the genital response (erectile impotence in men, lack of arousal in women), and

Table 19.1 Classification of sexual and gender identity disorders

DSM-IV	ICD–10
Sexual dysfunction	*Sexual dysfunction not caused by organic disorders**
Sexual desire disorders	Lack or loss of sexual desire
Hypoactive sexual desire disorder	
Sexual aversion disorder	Sexual aversion and lack of sexual enjoyment
Sexual arousal disorder	
Female sexual arousal disorder	Failure of genital response
Male erectile disorder	
Orgasm disorders	Orgasmic dysfunction
Female orgasmic disorder	
Male orgasmic disorder	
Premature ejaculation	Premature ejaculation
Sexual pain disorders	
Dyspareunia	Non-organic dyspareunia
Vaginismus	Non-organic vaginismus
Sexual dysfunction due to a general medical condition	Excessive sexual drive
Paraphilias	*Disorders of sexual preference***
Exhibitionism	Exhibitionism
Fetishism	Fetishism
Frotteurism	–
Paedophilia	Paedophilia
Sexual masochism	Sadomasochism
Sexual sadism	
Voyeurism	Voyeurism
Transvestic fetishism	Fetishistic transvestism
Gender identity disorders	*Gender identity disorders****
In children	
In adolescents and adults	

*   In ICD–10 sexual dysfunction is part of F5, behavioural syndromes associated with physiological disturbances and physical factors.

** In ICD–10 disorders of sexual preference are part of F6, disorders of adult personality and behaviour (to aid comparison with DSM-IV, the order in which the disorders appear has been changed from that in the text of ICD–10).

***In ICD–10 gender identity disorders are part of F6.

◆ orgasm (premature or retarded ejaculation in men, orgasmic dysfunction in women).

A further group includes problems resulting in pain: vaginismus and dyspareunia in women, and painful ejaculation in men. It should be remembered that sexual function is not always disclosed directly but may be revealed during enquiries about another complaint, such as depression or poor sleep, or gynaecological symptoms.

Prevalence of sexual dysfunctions

In the USA, a random probability sample of 3442 people aged 18–59 were asked about sexual problems. It is not clear whether the problems recorded by the investigators would have met diagnostic criteria for the corresponding sexual dysfunction. The reported rates are shown in Table 19.2.

In the UK, Dunn *et al.* (1998) carried out a postal survey of four general practices, and a stratified random sample of the adult general population. The mean age of the respondents was 50 years. A third of the men and two-fifths of the women reported a current sexual problem. Erectile dysfunction and premature ejaculation were the most common problems among the men. Vaginal dryness and infrequent orgasm were the most common problems among the women. Half of those with a problem reported that they would have liked help, but only one in ten had received it.

In an early survey by Kinsey *et al.* (1948), total and persisting erectile dysfunction was reported by 1.3% of American men aged under 35, 6.7% aged under 50, and 18.4% aged under 60. More recently, Felderman *et al.* (1994) reported the interview responses of 1290 randomly selected males. Some degree of impotence was reported by 52% of males aged 40–70 years. Factors associated with reported impotence included: increasing age; diabetes, heart disease, and hypertension; cigarette smoking and excessive alcohol intake; and depression.

Among women attending a sex clinic, impaired sexual interest was described by about half and orgasmic dysfunction by about 20% (Hawton 1985). In about a third of couples seen for treat-

Table 19.2 Reported frequency of sexual dysfunctions among 3442 American men and women aged 18–59 years*	
Males	
Lack of sexual interest	16%
Erectile difficulties	29%
Premature ejaculation	17%
Anxiety about performance	17%
Females	
Lack of sexual interest	33%
Sex not pleasurable	21%
Unable to reach orgasm	24%
Pain on coitus	14%

*Data from Lauman *et al.* (1994).

ment, both partners have a problem, usually low libido in the woman and premature ejaculation in the man. Sexual dysfunction is found in about 10% of psychiatric out-patients (Swan and Wilson 1979).

General causes of sexual dysfunction

Sexual dysfunction arises from varying combinations of a poor general relationship with the partner, low sexual drive, ignorance about sexual technique, and anxiety about sexual performance. Other important factors are physical illness, depressive and anxiety disorders, medication, and alcohol or drug abuse. Some of these factors will now be considered. When assessing aetiology in an individual patient, it is important to recognize that both psychological and physical factors are often present.

Low sexual drive

Sexual drive varies between people but the reason for this is not known. Endocrine factors have been suggested because in the male the increasing sexual drive at puberty is related to an increased output of androgens. Castration, treatment with oestrogens, or the administration of anti-androgenic drugs also reduce sexual drive in the male. However, no convincing association has been shown between androgens and low sexual drive in men seeking help for this problem. Also, treatment with androgens does not usually increase sexual drive in men with normal endocrine function. Small doses of androgens increase sexual drive in women (Hawton 1985).

Anxiety

Anxiety is an important cause of sexual dysfunction. Sometimes anxiety is an understandable consequence of an earlier frightening experience such as a man's failure in his first attempt at intercourse, or a woman's experience of sexual abuse or assault. Sometimes the anxiety relates to frightening accounts of sexual relationships received from parents or other people. Psychoanalysts suggest that anxiety about sexual relationships originates from even earlier experiences, namely failure to resolve the oedipal complex in boys or the corresponding attachment to the father in girls (see p. 116). Such ideas are difficult to test.

Physical illness and surgical treatments

Sexual dysfunction sometimes dates from a period of abstinence associated with pregnancy or childbirth, or from the debilitating effects of physical illness (Table 19.3). Of the diseases that have a direct effect on sexual performance, *diabetes mellitus* is particularly important. Between a third and a half of diabetic men experience erectile dysfunction as a result of either neuropathology affecting the autonomic nerves mediating erection or vascular disorders. Impaired ejaculation also occurs. Some diabetic women may be affected in a corresponding way, although this is less certain (see Webster 1994 for a review). Sexual dysfunction after *myocardial infarction* may result from anxiety and medication side-effects rather than from physical causes (H. A. Taylor 1999). Most of the associations between physical disease or its treatment and sexual dysfunction are obvious. Nevertheless, doctors often fail to think of the sexual conse-

Table 19.3 Medical and surgical conditions commonly associated with sexual dysfunction
Medical
Endocrine
Diabetes, hyperthyroidism, myxoedema, Addison's disease, hyperprolactinaemia
Gynaecological
Vaginitis, endometriosis, pelvic infections
Cardiovascular
Angina pectoris, previous myocardial infarction
Respiratory
Asthma, obstructive airways disease
Arthritic
Arthritis from any cause
Renal
Renal failure with or without dialysis
Neurological
Pelvic autonomic neuropathy, spinal cord lesions, stroke
Surgical
Mastectomy
Colostomy, ileostomy
Oophorectomy
Episiotomy, operations for prolapse
Amputation
Modified from Hawton and Oppenheimer (1983).

quences of disease and the (often unexpressed) problems that result.

Effects of medication

Several drugs have side-effects that involve sexual function (Table 19.4). The most important drugs are antihypertensives (especially adrenoceptor antagonists), antipsychotics (especially thioridazine), monoamine oxidase inhibitors, and specific serotonin re-uptake inhibitors. Anxiolytics, seda-

Table 19.4 Some drugs that may impair sexual function
Therapeutic agents
Antihypertensives
Diuretics, spironolactone, sympatholytics, α-blockers, β-blockers
Antidepressants
Tricyclics, monoamine oxidase inhibitors, specific serotonin re-uptake inhibitors
Mood regulators
Lithium
Anxiolytics and hypnotics
Benzodiazepines
Antipsychotics
Especially thioridazine
Hormonal agents
Anabolic steroids, corticosteroids, oestrogens
Misused substances
Tobacco, alcohol, cocaine, marijuana

Table 19.5 Assessment of sexual dysfunction
Define the problem (ask both partners)
Origin and course
With other partners?
Sexual drive
Knowledge and fears
Social relationships generally
Social relations between the partners
Psychiatric disorder
Substance misuse
Medical illness; medical or surgical treatment
Why seek help now?
Physical examination
Laboratory tests -see text
(Special tests for erectile function)

tives, and hormones have more effect on the sexual activity of men than of women. Apart from these prescribed drugs, the excessive use of alcohol and street drugs impairs sexual performance.

General approach to the assessment of patients with sexual dysfunction

History taking

Whenever possible, the sexual partner should be interviewed as well as the patient. The two should be seen separately, and then together. The following enquiries are important (see Table 19.5).

- *Define the problem* as it appears to each partner. Details should not be omitted because the interviewer feels embarrassed.
- *Origin and course* Has the problem always been present or did it start after a period of normal functioning?

- *Has the problem occurred with more than one partner?* Each partner should be asked this question separately.
- *Strength of sexual drive* is assessed by asking each partner separately about frequency of intercourse and masturbation, about sexual thoughts, and about feelings of sexual arousal.
- *Knowledge of sexual technique and anxiety about sex* Possible sources of misinformation and anxiety are considered by asking about the family's attitude to sex, and the extent of sex education and sexual experience. Each partner should be asked about the sexual technique of the other.
- *Social relationships with the opposite sex* Is either partner shy or socially inhibited?
- *The couple's social relationship* Some couples ask for help with sexual problems which are the result and not (as they suggest) the cause of marital conflict.
- *Psychiatric disorder* Is there a psychiatric disorder in either partner, especially depressive

disorder, which might account for the sexual problem, directly or through the drugs used to treat it (see Table 19.4)?

♦ *Misuse of alcohol or drugs* See above.

♦ *Physical illness and medical or surgical treatment* With particular attention to the factors listed in Tables 19.3 and 19.4.

♦ *Why have they sought help now?* The sexual problem may have increased, or one partner may have refused to continue with the relationship.

Physical examination and special investigations

Physical examination If the general practitioner or another specialist has not already done so, a physical examination should be carried out (see Table 19.6).

Laboratory tests should be arranged in appropriate cases; for example, fasting blood sugar, testosterone, sex-hormone-binding globulin, luteinizing hormone, and prolactin in men with erectile dysfunction.

General approaches to the treatment of sexual dysfunction

Before directing treatment to the sexual problem, it is important to consider whether *couple therapy* is more appropriate because the sexual problem is secondary to a problem in the relationship. If it is appropriate to focus treatment on the sexual problem, *advice and education* may be all that is needed.

If *sex therapy* is appropriate, it should be directed to both partners whenever possible. The usual approach, which owes much to the original work of Masters and Johnson (1970), has four characteristic features:

♦ the partners are treated together;

♦ they are helped to communicate better, about their sexual relationship;

♦ they receive education about the anatomy and physiology of sexual intercourse;

♦ they take part in a series of 'graded tasks'.

Table 19.6 Important points in the physical examination of men presenting with sexual dysfunctions

General examination (directed especially to evidence of diabetes mellitus, thyroid disorder, and adrenal disorder)

Hair distribution

Gynaecomastia

Blood pressure

Peripheral pulses

Ocular fundi

Reflexes

Peripheral sensation

General examination

Penis: congenital abnormalities, foreskin, pulses, tenderness, plaques, infection, urethral discharge

Testicles: size, symmetry, texture, sensation

Prostate – in men aged over about 50 years

Adapted from Hawton (1985).

Masters and Johnson held that two other factors were important. The first was that treatment should be intensive, for example, seeing both partners every day for up to 3 weeks. The second was that treatment should be carried out by a man and a woman working as co-therapists. It has been shown that neither of these additional factors is essential; good results can be obtained when treatment is given once a week and when only one therapist sees the couple.

Treatment as a couple Although better results are obtained when the couple are treated together, some help can be given to a patient who has no regular partner. Such patients can at least discuss their difficulties and possible ways of overcoming them. Discussion of this kind can sometimes help to overcome social inhibitions.

Communication Communication is not only the ability to talk freely about specific sexual problems; it is also concerned with increasing understanding of the other person's wishes and feelings. Each partner may believe that the other should know instinctively how to give pleasure during intercourse, so that failure to please is attributed to lack of concern or affection rather than to ignorance. Such failure can be overcome by helping the partners to express their own desires more frankly.

Education Education stresses the physiology of the sexual response. For example, if the problem is anorgasmia in the woman, the doctor may explain the longer time needed for a woman to reach sexual arousal, and may emphasize the importance of foreplay, including clitoral stimulation, in bringing about vaginal lubrication. Suitably chosen sex education books can reinforce the therapist's advice. Such counselling is often the most important part of the treatment of sexual dysfunctions.

Graded tasks These begin with tender physical contact. The couples are encouraged to caress any part of the other person's body except the genitalia in order to give enjoyment (Masters and Johnson call this the 'sensate focus'). Next, the couple may engage in mutual masturbation, but not in penetration at this stage. At both stages, the partners are encouraged to discover the experience most enjoyed by the other person and then to provide this experience. They are strongly discouraged from checking their own state of sexual arousal because this checking generally has an inhibiting effect. Such checking is a common habit in people with sexual disorder, and has been called the 'spectator role'. Graded tasks are not only directly beneficial; they also help to uncover hidden fears or areas of ignorance that need to be discussed.

For further information about sexual therapy for couples, see Crowe (1998).

Results of sex therapy

There have been few adequately controlled studies of sex therapy. The general methods described above are followed by a successful outcome, using broad criteria, in about a third of cases, and by worthwhile improvement in a further third (Heinman and LoPiccolo 1983; Hawton *et al.* 1986). Improvement at the end of treatment are maintained for months (Heinman and LoPiccolo 1983), but may not be sustained 3 years after therapy (De Amicis *et al.* 1985). Outcome is better among patients who engage wholeheartedly in treatment. The results seem to be as good in problems of long duration as in others (Hawton *et al.* 1986).

Types of sexual dysfunction

Lack or loss of sexual desire (hypoactive sexual desire disorder)

Description and causes Complaints of diminished sexual desire are much more common among women than among men. The term lack of sexual desire indicates that the condition has been present since the start of sexual activity. The term loss of sexual desire indicates that the condition developed after a period when sexual desire was normal. Loss may be global or situational.

Global lack of desire suggests a biologically determined low level of sexual drive, or homosexual orientation when the complaint relates to heterosexual intercourse.

Global loss of desire suggests a medical or psychiatric cause. Medical causes include low testosterone, high prolactin, systemic disease, and the side-effects of medication. Psychiatric causes include depressive disorder, the consequences of sexual trauma, and severe intrapsychic conflict leading to inhibition. Loss of desire after a depressive disorder usually returns to the previous level as the disorder resolves, but occasionally it persists.

Situational loss of desire often reflects general problems in the relationship between the sexual partners.

Special aspects of assessment Sexual desire is assessed by asking about:

◆ *imagery* the frequency and nature of sexual imagery and dreams;

◆ *desire* for and *frequency* of sexual behaviour, with a partner or alone.

Potential causes are assessed by asking about:

◆ relationship problems: loss of affection, anger, etc.;

◆ sexual orientation, sexual preferences;

◆ tiredness, anxiety, depression;

◆ past sexual experiences causing fear or disgust.

The *medical causes* listed above should be considered, including testosterone and prolactin measurement in selected cases.

For a review of the assessment of sexual desire disorders see Rosen and Leiblum (1987).

Treatment Because there is little research evidence, treatment is based on clinical experience. Any psychiatric or medical causes should be treated. Couple therapy, cognitive therapy or counselling may be chosen, depending on the psychiatric cause. Testosterone may increase desire in patients who have low levels of bioavailable testosterone but there is no evidence from controlled trials of sustained increase of sexual desire in patients with low sexual desire and normal testosterone levels.

Sexual aversion disorder

Sexual enjoyment is sometimes replaced by a positive aversion to genital contact. When this aversion is persistent or severe and accompanied by avoidance of almost all genital sexual contact with a sexual partner, the condition is classified as sexual aversion disorder. The causes of the condition are not well understood; they seem to be similar to the psychological causes of hypoactive sexual desire disorder. Assessment and treatment is similar to that for hypoactive sexual desire disorder.

Specific sexual fears

A few women are made extremely anxious by specific aspects of the sexual act, such as being touched on the genitalia, the sight or smell of seminal fluid, or even kissing. Despite these specific fears, they may still enjoy other parts of sexual intercourse. Assessment and treatment

follows the general approach described on pp. 591 and 592.

Female sexual arousal disorder

Lack of sexual arousal in the female appears as reduced vaginal lubrication. This reduction may be due to:

◆ inadequate sexual foreplay by the partner;

◆ lack of sexual interest; or

◆ anxiety about intercourse.

After the menopause, hormonal changes may lead to reduced vaginal secretions. Assessment and treatment follow the general approach described on pp. 591 and 592.

Male erectile disorder

This condition is the inability to reach an erection or to sustain it long enough for satisfactory coitus. It may be present from the first attempt at intercourse (primary) or develop after a period of normal function (secondary). It is more common among older than younger men (in contrast with premature ejaculation, see below).

Causes *Primary cases* may occur through a combination of low sexual drive and anxiety about sexual performance. *Secondary cases* may arise from diminishing sexual drive in the middle-aged or elderly, loss of interest in the sexual partner, anxiety, depressive disorder, and organic disease and its treatment. A few cases are due to abnormalities of the vascular supply to the penile erectile tissue, including reduced arterial perfusion, increased venous leakage, and Peyronie's disease (Kirby *et al.* 1991).

Assessment The following aspects of the general assessment are particularly important:

◆ Has there been a previous period of normal function? Erectile failure may be a transient disorder arising at times of stress, or may reflect loss of interest in the sexual partner.

◆ Has the failure occurred with more that one partner?

◆ Does erection occur during foreplay?

◆ Does erection occur on waking or in response to masturbation? Erection in these circumstances suggests psychological causes.

◆ Is there evidence of alcohol or drug abuse (ask the partner as well as the patient)?

◆ Are there possible effects of any medication?

Special tests for erectile dysfunction When aetiology is uncertain after history taking, physical examination, and blood tests, several special investigations may be considered. The *Rigiscan* helps to assess penile tumescence and rigidity. Measurements can be made during exposure to visual sexual stimuli, in response to a vibrator, or during sleep. These tests help to differentiate between psychogenic and neurological impairment. If vascular impairment is suspected, *Doppler ultrasound* and/or *duplex ultra-sonography* may help to identify arterial or venous dysfunction. *Intracavernosal prostaglandin* produces a penile response if there is vascular capability. More specialized investigations may be indicated when vascular surgery appears to be indicated. For a review see Althof and Seftel (1995).

Treatment Any reversible causes should be treated. Psychological causes may respond to appropriate *cognitive or psychodynamic therapy*, although temporary relapses may occur (Hawton 1986).

◆ *Oral medication* Sildenafil inhibits the breakdown of cyclic GMP by a specific cyclic GMP phosphodiesterase. Since the drug potentiates the action of cyclic GMP greater than stimulates its production, it facilitates rather than initiates sexual arousal. Care should be taken to observe the manufacturer's advice about contraindications, side-effects, and interactions with other drugs. (For further information about sildenafil see Goldstein *et al.* 1998.) Before the introduction of sildenafil, the main oral medication for male erectile disorder was yohimbine, an α2-adrenergic blocker.

◆ *Treatment for vascular or neurogenic causes* Several treatments are available for patients with impotence due to vascular or neurogenic abnormalities, including those secondary to diabetes. These methods include drugs, vacuum devices, the surgical correction of vascular abnormalities, and penile prostheses.

◆ *Intracavernosal injections* of the smooth muscle relaxant papaverine, or the α-receptor blocker phenoxybenzamine, produce erection and have been used to treat impotence (Virag 1982; Padma-Nathan *et al.* 1987), as have injections of prostaglandins (Lee *et al.* 1988). Alprostadil is a newer drug available for intracavernosal injection (Linet and Ogrinc 1996). Small doses of the chosen drug are given at first, and increased gradually. When an appropriate dose has been determined, patients are taught to inject themselves. (Doses are not given here because the treatment should be learned from a doctor experienced in its use.) Overdose can lead to prolonged erection, which may require the aspiration of blood and the injection of an α1-agonist such as phenylephrine (Kirby 1994).

◆ *Intraurethral treatment* Alprostadil can be administered by the intraurethral route (see Padma-Nathan *et al.* 1997) as well as by the intracavernosal route described above.

◆ *Vacuum devices* can be tried for patients who do not respond to intracavernosal drug injections (Witherington 1989). The penis is placed in a surrounding cylinder in which the pressure is reduced; an erection follows, and is maintained by applying a restricting band to the base of the penis before the cylinder is removed. Although this procedure is generally effective in producing an erection, it is disliked by many patients.

◆ *Surgical methods* have been used to treat erectile disorder resulting from proven vascular abnormalities. Microsurgery can be used to revascularize the corpora cavernosa when there are stenoses or occlusions in the arteries. Short-term improvement rates of about 50% have been reported in selected cases (Goldstein

1986). An alternative approach is to insert a penile prosthesis, which may be semirigid or capable of being inflated before intercourse

For a review of treatments for erectile dysfunction see Wylie (1998), or Ralph and McNicolas (2000).

Female orgasmic dysfunction

Whether failure to reach orgasm regularly is regarded as a disorder depends on the attitudes of society and of the individual. Many women do not regularly reach orgasm during vaginal intercourse but do so in response to clitoral stimulation. A much quoted early survey found that about 25% of women have no orgasm during intercourse for the first year of marriage (Gebhard *et al.* 1970) but it is not known whether this finding applies to current marriages.

Causes This disorder arises from normal variations in sexual drive, poor sexual technique by the partner, lack of affection for the partner, tiredness, depressive disorder, physical illness, and the effects of medication.

Assessment In addition to the general assessment, the following questions are important:

♦ Has the woman ever achieved orgasm?

♦ If so, during intercourse with another partner, or masturbation, or in response to a particular fantasy?

Medication such as SSRIs, other antidepressants, and antihypertensives are possible causes.

Treatment Graduated practice in masturbation is reported to lead to orgasm in women who have never achieved orgasm (Riley and Riley 1978). Alternatively, the partner is encouraged to use the sensate focus technique of sex therapy. Whichever approach is chosen, help should be given with any relationship, or personal psychological problems.

Male orgasmic disorder

This term refers to serious delay in, or absence of, ejaculation. Usually the problem occurs only during coitus, but it may also occur during mastur-

bation. It is usually associated with a general psychological inhibition about sexual relations, but it may be caused by drugs including antipsychotics, monoamine oxidase inhibitors, and specific serotonin uptake inhibitors.

Premature ejaculation

This term refers to habitual ejaculation before penetration or so soon afterwards that the women has not gained pleasure. It is more common among younger than older men, especially during their first sexual relationships.

Causes This disorder is so common in sexually inexperienced young men that it can be regarded as a normal variation. When it persists, it is often because of fear of failure.

Treatment Psychological causes should be treated with the general approach described on p. 592. If the partner is willing, this disorder can be treated with the 'squeeze technique'. When the man indicates that he will soon have an orgasm, the woman grips the penis for a few seconds and then releases it suddenly. Intercourse is then continued. An alternative 'start-stop' method has been described in which the woman attempts to regulate the amount of sexual stimulation during intercourse. Similar techniques can be used during masturbation. In the 'quiet vagina' technique, the penis is contained within the vagina for increasing periods without any movement, before the man ejaculates. It is important to understand the woman's point of view thoroughly before asking her to assist in such treatment.

SSRIs and other antidepressants delay ejaculation, whether this is normal or premature. However, the effect is generally lost when the medication stops. If used at all, medication should not be the first line of treatment, and should be combined with psychological measures.

Sexual pain disorders

Dyspareunia This term refers to pain on intercourse. Such pain has many causes. Pain experienced after partial penetration may result from impaired lubrication of the vagina, from scars or other painful lesions, or from the muscle spasm of vaginismus. Pain on deep penetration strongly suggests pelvic pathology such as endometriosis, ovarian cysts and tumours, or pelvic infection, though it can be caused by impaired lubrication associated with low sexual arousal.

Vaginismus Vaginismus is spasm of the vaginal muscles which causes pain when intercourse is attempted, in the absence of a physical lesion causing pain. The spasm is usually part of a phobic response to penetration, and may be made worse by an inexperienced partner. Spasms often begin as soon as the man attempts to enter the vagina; in severe cases it occurs even when the woman attempts to introduce her own finger. Severe vaginismus may prevent consummation of marriage. So-called 'virgin wives' may have a generalized fear and guilt about sexual relationships rather than a specific fear of penetration. Some women with vaginismus are married to passive men who have low libido and are able to accept their wives' refusal to permit full sexual relations (Dawkins 1961; Friedman 1962). Low libido in the man then becomes evident when the treatment has reduced the woman's problem.

Points of special relevance in the sexual history include:

- the circumstances that provoke spasm (intercourse, tampon, partner's finger, patient's own finger);
- the partner's sexual technique;
- any history of traumatic sexual experience.

Treatment is by the general sex therapy techniques described above with emphasis on a ban on vaginal intercourse. Fears are treated with cognitive or psychodynamic approaches, and the woman is helped to desensitize herself gradually by inserting first her finger and then dilators of increasing size.

Pain on ejaculation This problem is uncommon. The usual causes are urethritis or prostatitis. Sometimes no cause is found.

Sexual dysfunction among the physically handicapped

Physically handicapped people have sexual problems arising from several sources:

- *specific effects* of the physical handicap on sexual function, for example, disease of the nervous system affecting the autonomic nerve supply;
- *general effects* such as tiredness, and pain;
- *fears* about the effects of intercourse on the handicapping condition;
- *lack of information* about the sexual activities of other people with the same disability.

Much can be done to help disabled people by overcoming fears and discussing the forms of sexual activity that are possible despite their disability, and, if appropriate, adapting the methods already described for treating sexual dysfunction.

Abnormalities of sexual preference (paraphilias)

The study of these disorders in the past

For centuries, abnormalities of sexual preference were regarded as offences against the laws of religion rather than conditions that doctors should study and treat. The systematic investigation of these disorders began in the 1870s. Krafft-Ebing (1840–1902), a professor of psychiatry in Vienna, wrote a systematic account of paraphilias in his book *Psychopathia sexualis*, first published in 1886. Soon afterwards, Schrenck-Notzing (1895) reported successful treatment with therapeutic suggestion. In England, Havelock Ellis (1859–1939) wrote extensively about sexual disorders.

The concept of abnormal sexual preference

This concept has three aspects:

- *social* the behaviour does not conform to some generally accepted view of what is normal. The accepted view is not the same in every society or at every period of history; for example, regular masturbation was regarded as abnormal by many medical writers in Victorian England.

- *harm* that might be done to another person involved in the sexual behaviour. Intercourse with young children or extreme forms of sexual sadism are examples.

- *suffering* experienced by the person himself. This suffering is related to the attitudes of the society in which the patient lives (for example, attitudes to cross-dressing), to conflict between the person's sexual urges and his moral standards, and to the person's awareness of harm or distress caused to others.

General considerations

Mode of presentation

Abnormalities of sexual preference may come to medical attention in various ways, and the doctor should be aware of the different modes of presentation.

Direct requests for help

A doctor may be consulted directly by the person with the abnormalities. He may be asked to help by the spouse or other sexual partner, sometimes because the behaviour has just been discovered, and sometimes because known behaviour has become more frequent and can be tolerated no longer.

Indirect presentations

Sometimes the problem is presented as sexual dysfunction, and the abnormality of sexual preference is discovered only in the course of history taking.

As a forensic problem

A doctor may be asked for an opinion about a patient charged with an offence arising from an abnormality of sexual preference. Offences of this kind include the stealing of clothes by fetishists, indecent exposure, the behaviour of a 'peeping Tom', appearing in public in clothes of the opposite sex, sexual assaults upon children, and rape. With one exception, these offences are discussed below in relation to the corresponding abnormality of sexual preference. The exception is rape, with is considered with other sexual offences in Chapter 26.

The role of psychiatrists

There are different opinions about the extent to which doctors should attempt to alter abnormal sexual preferences. There seems to be no reason why doctors should not try to help people who wish to alter unusual patterns of sexual behaviour, but they should not try to impose treatment on people who do not want it. How to decide who really wants psychiatric help is a difficult point that is taken up later in this chapter.

Pornography

The reading of pornography is not a sexual disorder but it is considered here because doctors may be asked about the effects of such publications. Since some of the publications are designed for people with disorders of sexual preference, this is a convenient point at which to consider the topic. It is not known whether these publications merely provide a harmless outlet for sexual impulses, including those that might otherwise be inflicted on another person, or whether they increase such impulses and so encourage paraphilias and increase sexual offences. The question has been approached in several ways.

Epidemiological studies have attempted to relate the numbers of sexual offences to changes in the law on pornography. Winnick and Evans (1996) studied arrest data for a variety of offences during a period when American state pornography laws were operative, and a period when they were not.

During the period without enforcement, the explicitness and quantity of sexual materials increased. Similar outcomes have been described in Denmark, but the results are not conclusive and they do not reveal the effects on individuals.

Clinical experience with the paraphilias suggests that the reading of pornographic literature can increase related fantasies experienced during sexual arousal. However, it is not known whether the strengthening of sexual fantasies in this way increases the likelihood of enacting them. It is possible that pictorial material could promote solitary sexual release and so reduce the involvement of others in the person's paraphilia.

Public policy on these important matters, like many others, has to be decided on limited scientific information. Without more definite evidence, it seems appropriate that pornographic material relating sexual activity to violence or to children should not be available to young people whose sexual development is incomplete. The arguments put forward for more general restrictions are that pornographic publications debase women, that some put children at risk of exploitation during the making of the material and in other ways, and that it has not been proved that the material is harmless.

Advice to individuals

Doctors may be asked what effect pornographic material, discovered by a wife or parent, may have on a husband or adolescent son. Doctors should explain the different points of view and the uncertainty of the scientific evidence. They should indicate that the effects are likely to differ in different people, and offer to interview the person. If the person's sexual life is reviewed thoroughly, some useful advice can generally be given. Such advice should extend to broader aspects of personal relationships and not merely to the effects of the pornographic material.

Types of abnormality of sexual preference

Abnormalities of sexual preference can be divided into two groups: abnormalities of the 'object' of the person's sexual interest, and abnormalities in the preference of the sexual act. Abnormalities of the sexual 'object' include fetishism, paedophilia, transvestic fetishism, zoophilia, and necrophilia. Abnormalities of preference of the sexual act include exhibitionism, voyeurism, sadism, masochism, and autoerotic asphyxia.

General aspects of the assessment of abnormalities of sexual preference

Assessment is often in the context of possible or actual legal proceedings. It is important therefore to explain the relation of the interview to any proceedings, explain confidentiality and its limits, and obtain necessary consent to the interview. Leading questions may be needed to help the patient reveal some problems, but any information obtained in this way should be checked by asking for examples of the behaviour in question. People seen for the assessment of abnormality of sexual preference often have more that one kind of abnormal preference (Abel and Osborn 2000), though they may not volunteer this information when first interviewed. It may need more than one interview before the patient feels able to confide the full extent of the sexual problems. Whenever possible, an interview should be arranged, with the patient's consent, with any regular sexual partner, and with other informants who may assist with, for example, the assessment of personality.

Assessment includes a psychiatric history and should include the following steps:

◆ *exclude mental illness*, especially when the abnormal sexual preference comes to notice for the first time in middle age or later. Abnormal sexual preference is sometimes secondary to dementia, alcoholism, depressive disorder, or mania. These illnesses probably release the behaviour in a person who has previously experienced the corresponding sexual fantasies but controlled them.

- *detail the sexual behaviour.* Obtain details of the normal and of the abnormal sexual behaviour, currently and in the past. Remember that, as noted above, it is not uncommon for patients to have more than one form of abnormal sexual preference.

- *describe the wider significance of the behaviour.* Find out what part the abnormal sexual preference is playing in the patient's life other than as a source of sexual arousal. It may be a comforting activity that helps to ward off feelings of loneliness, anxiety, or depression. If so, unless other means are found to deal with such feelings, treatment that reduces the abnormal sexual preference may worsen the patient's emotional state.

- *assess motivation.* Motives are often mixed for seeking treatment. Patients who have little wish to change their sexual behaviour may consult a doctor because of pressure from a sexual partner, a relative, or the police. Such people may hope to be told that no treatment will help, so as to justify the continuation of their paraphilia. Others seek help when they are depressed and feel guilty about their behaviour. Strong wishes for change, expressed during a period of depression, may fade quickly as normal mood returns. Strong motivation is important whatever the proposed mode of treatment, so its assessment is important.

- *psychophysiological assessment.* Some specialists use penile plethysmography or polygraphy to assess sexual interests (see Abel and Osborn 2000). In the former, changes in penile circumference are measured while the patient views visual material or listens to audiotapes. Positive responses can be discussed with the patient who may confirm the interest. However, the method is of limited value because patients can produce false-negative responses by directing attention away from the stimuli, and may falsely deny positive responses. Polygraphy, measuring several physiological variables, can also reflect sexual arousal to stimuli. It has limitations similar to those of penile plethysmography. These methods are not part of routine assessment.

General aspects of the management of abnormalities of sexual preference

Some aspects of management apply to all kinds of abnormality of sexual preference. These aspects are described here. Management specific to a particular disorder is described below with the other aspects of the disorder.

Agreeing the aims

The aim of treatment should be discussed with the patient: whether it is to control, or if possible give up, the behaviour, or to adapt better to the behaviour so that less guilt and distress are felt. In considering these aims, the doctor will have to take into account whether any psychological or physical harm is being caused to other people. At this early stage it is important to make clear that, whatever the aim, treatment will require considerable effort on the part of the patient.

Aiding adjustment

If the agreed aim is better adjustment, treatment will be by counselling designed to explore the patient's feelings and to help him to identify the problems caused by his sexual practices and to find ways of reducing them. If the agreed aim is change, the first step is to find ways of improving ordinary heterosexual relationships. Treatment is directed to any anxieties that are impeding social relationships with the opposite sex. Attention is then directed to any sexual inadequacy using the methods outlined earlier in this chapter. Usually, these two steps are the most important part of treatment.

Anticipating problems from abstinence

Some patients occupy much of their time in preparing for the sexual act (for example, fetishists may spend many hours searching for a particular kind of women's underclothes). As already noted, the behaviour often becomes a way or warding off feelings of loneliness or despair. To safeguard against distress, the patient must be helped to develop leisure activities, to seek new friends, and to find other ways of coping with unpleasant emotions.

Reducing the paraphilia

Only when these steps have been taken should attention be directed to ways of suppressing the unwanted sexual behaviour. Sometimes the preceding steps are enough to strengthen the patient's capacity to control himself, but additional help is often needed.

Masturbation fantasies about the paraphilia maintain the abnormal sexual behaviour. Therefore the patient should be encouraged to keep any abnormal fantasies out of mind while masturbating, and to try to imagine normal heterosexual intercourse instead. If he cannot dismiss the abnormal fantasies, he should try to modify them progressively so that the sexual themes become less abnormal and increasingly concerned with ordinary heterosexual intercourse.

Hormonal treatment

Most patients with paraphilias are men, and for some, treatment to reduce androgen levels is a helpful adjunct to psychological treatment. Generally, cyproterone acetate, a testosterone antagonist, is used Europe for this purpose, and medroxyprogesterone acetate is used in the USA. Both have been reported to benefit some exhibitionists and paedophiles (see Murray 1998).

Behavioural treatment

Behavioural treatment has been used to reduce the paraphilia directly, and also to help indirectly by treating any sexual inadequacy. Several direct methods have been tried. Advice about changing masturbation fantasies (described above) are sometimes regarded as a behavioural technique. *Covert sensitization* makes an immediate link in imagination between paraphiliac thoughts and urges, and

humiliating adverse consequences that are normally delayed such as discovery by family or arrest. In smell or taste aversion, an unpleasant odour or taste is associated with the paraphilic fantasies. The long-term efficacy of these techniques has not been demonstrated convincingly.

Relapse prevention focuses on the situations in which paraphiliac urges are likely to be experienced. Patients are encouraged to identify these situations and to avoid them. Particular attention is paid to the earliest stages of the chain of behaviour leading up to the paraphilias, for example an action by the patient which regularly makes his wife angry, and thus provides an excuse to go to a place where the paraphilia may be stimulated. For a review of psychological treatments for paraphilias, see Wylie (1994).

Legal considerations

Many people with abnormal sexual preferences appear before the courts. Sanctions such as a suspended sentence or probation order can sometimes help the patient to gain control of his own behaviour. However, doctors should not agree to treat patients who are referred against their wishes. Sexual offences are considered further on p. 911–15.

Types of abnormality of preference for the sexual object

These abnormalities involve preferences for an 'object' other than another adult in the achievement of sexual excitement. The alternative 'object' may be inanimate, as in fetishism and transvestic fetishism, or may be a child (paedophilia) or an animal (zoophilia).

Fetishism

In sexual fetishism, the preferred or only means of achieving sexual excitement are inanimate objects or parts of the human body that do not have direct sexual associations. The disorder shades into normal sexual behaviour; it is not uncommon for men to be aroused by particular items of clothing, such as stockings, or by parts of the female body that do not have direct sexual associations, such as the hair. The condition is abnormal when the behaviour takes precedence over the usual patterns of sexual intercourse.

Prevalence Sexual fetishism as the sole or preferred means of sexual arousal is uncommon, but no exact figures are available for the rate in the community.

Description Fetishism usually begins in adolescence. It occurs almost exclusively among men, although a few cases have been described among women. Most fetishists are heterosexual but some are homosexual – 20% according to Chalkley and Powell (1983). The objects that can evoke sexual arousal are many and varied, but for each person there is usually a small number of objects or classes of objects. Among the more frequent are rubber garments, women's underclothes and high-heeled shoes, and, for homosexual fetishists, men's shoes (Weinberg *et al.* 1994). Sometimes the object is an attribute of a person (partialism), for example, lameness or deformity, or a part of the human body, such as the hair or foot, or the absence of a part through amputation (apotemnophilia). The texture and smell of objects is often as important as their appearance, for example furs, velvet, rubber garments, and polished leather. Contact with the object causes sexual excitement, which may be followed by solitary masturbation or by sexual intercourse incorporating the fetish if a willing partner or paid prostitute is available.

Fetishists may spend much time seeking desired objects. Some buy them, others steal – for example, underclothes from a washing line. When the 'object' is an attribute of a person, many hours may be spent in searching for and following a suitable woman, for example, a woman with a limp. Fetishists often hoard fetish objects such as women's shoes or underclothes, or pictures of such objects.

Aetiology The cause is unknown but several theories have been proposed:

◆ *Conditioning* Fetishism was the first sexual disorder for which a theory of association learning was put forward. Binet (1877) suggested that the condition arose by a chance coming together of sexual excitation and the object that becomes the fetish object.

◆ *Psychoanalytical theories* These suggest that sexual fetishism arises when castration anxiety is not resolved in childhood, and the man attempts to ward off this anxiety by maintaining in his unconscious mind the idea that women have a penis (Freud 1927). In this view, each fetish is a symbolic representation of a phallus. Although some fetishes can be interpreted in this way, others require tortuous interpretations if the general hypothesis is to be sustained (Stekel 1953). In any case, the general idea does not convincingly explain most cases, and there is no objective evidence to support the theory.

◆ *Brain dysfunction* Over the years, occasional cases have been reported in which fetishism is associated with EEG evidence of temporal lobe dysfunction (e.g. Epstein 1961) or with frank epilepsy (e.g. Mitchell *et al.* 1954). However, there is no evidence of such associations in most cases, and the reported cases may be chance associations.

◆ *Maintaining factors* However fetishism arises, clinical experience suggests that it is maintained, in part, by inhibited expression of normal sexual behaviour, for example, by shyness or fears, and by the reinforcing effects of sexual release during actual or imagined contact with the fetish object.

Prognosis There are no reliable follow-up data. Clinical experience suggests that fetishism in adolescents and young adults often diminishes or ceases when satisfying heterosexual relationships have been established. The prognosis appears to be worse for solitary single men who are shy with women and without a sexual partner than for those who are younger and socially better adjusted. The prognosis is generally worse when the behaviour is frequent and has persistently broken social conventions and legal barriers. Legal proceedings instituted for the first time may increase motivation to control the behaviour.

Treatment There are case reports of successful treatment by *psychoanalysis* and by *behaviour therapy* but no controlled trials. Clinical experience indicates that the *general measures* earlier in the chapter are generally as effective as either of these special techniques. Treatment with the *anti-androgen*, cyproterone acetate, has been advocated for paraphilic patients with intense and frequent sexual desire (Gijs and Gooren 1996) but there is insufficient evidence to judge its efficacy.

Transvestic fetishism

In ICD-10 this condition is known as fetishistic transvestism. The term transvestic fetishism is used here because it indicates a similarity to the cases of sexual fetishism in which the object is an article of clothing. Transvestic fetishism varies from the occasional wearing of a few articles of clothing of the opposite sex to complete cross-dressing. Transvestic fetishism is rare among women (almost all women who cross-dress are transsexual or lesbian). For this reason, the description below applies to men.

Prevalence Estimates of the percentage of the population who have ever cross-dressed vary from 1.5% to 10%.

Description The person usually begins to put on articles of women's clothing at about the time of puberty. He usually starts by putting on only a few garments, but as time goes by he adds more until eventually he may dress entirely in clothes of the other sex. Transvestic fetishists generally experience sexual arousal when cross-dressing and the behaviour often terminates with masturbation. Sexual arousal is more frequent in younger people. It may diminish as they grow older, so that the person dresses mainly to feel feminine. Sometimes the clothes are worn in public, either underneath male outer garments or in some cases without such precautions against discovery.

Unlike the transsexuals described later, transvestic fetishists have no doubt that their gender conforms with their external sexual characteristics. Most are heterosexual. Many transvestic fetishists have heterosexual partners. Most of those seen by psychiatrists hide the behaviour from their partner. If the partner has discovered the behaviour, most express distress and disgust but a few assist in obtaining the clothing. Brown (1994) surveyed wives who were aware of their partner's fetishistic transvestitism. They had been married for a mean of 13 years and had known of the cross-dressing for a mean of 9 years. They were no more likely than the general population to have had lesbian experiences, but a quarter reported at least occasional sexual arousal to the partner's cross-dressing. The latter were more accepting of the partner's cross-dressing.

Aetiology The cause is unknown. There are several theories, all unsupported by evidence:

- *Genetic factors* There is no convincing evidence that the chromosomal sex or hormonal make-up of transvestic fetishists is abnormal. Despite a report of three cases in one family (Liakos 1967), transvestic fetishism is not familial and there is no evidence that it is inherited.

- *Brain dysfunction* Although occasional associations with temporal lobe dysfunction have been reported (Davies and Morgenstern 1960; Epstein 1960), there is no evidence for such an association in the majority.

- *Conditioning* It is suggested that the causes of transvestic fetishism resemble those proposed above for fetishism (see above).

- *Psychoanalytical theories* These are similar to those concerning fetishism, namely that the transvestic fetishist is creating a 'phallic woman' (himself in woman's clothes) to allay castration anxiety.

Prognosis There are no reliable follow-up studies. Clinical experience suggests that most cases persist for years, becoming less severe as sexual drives decline in middle age or later. However, there are wide variations in outcome, and the comments made earlier about the prognosis of fetishism apply here as well. A minority of transvestic fetishists gradually develop the idea that they are women: they continue to cross-dress but without sexual arousal, so that they resemble transsexual people (see p. 608).

Treatment There is no specific treatment for transvestic fetishism. Management is with the general procedures described on p. 600.

Paedophilia

Paedophilia is repeated sexual activity (or fantasy of such activity) with prepubertal children as a preferred or exclusive method of obtaining sexual excitement. It is almost exclusively a disorder of men. Paedophilia has to be distinguished from intercourse with young people who have passed puberty but not yet reached the legal age of consent (which differs between legislations). Paedophilia is not concerned with the borderline of legal consent but with intercourse between an adult and a prepubertal child.

Prevalence There is no reliable information about the prevalence of paedophilia. From the existence of child prostitution in some countries and the ready sale of pornographic material depicting sex with children, it appears that interest in sexual relationships with children is not rare. However, paedophilia as an exclusive form of sexual behaviour is probably uncommon.

Description Paedophiles usually choose a child aged between 6 years and puberty, but some prefer a very young child. The child may be of the opposite sex (heterosexual paedophilia) or the same sex (homosexual paedophilia). Some paedophiles approach children within their extended family, or those who are in their professional care; others befriend unrelated children. Although most paedophiles seen by doctors are men of middle age, the condition is established early in life. There is no evidence that an established interest in adult sexual partners changes to an interest in child partners. With younger children, fondling or masturbation is more likely than full coitus, but sometimes children are injured by forcible attempts at penetration. There are rare and tragic cases of paedophilia associated with sexual sadism. (Sexual abuse of children is described on p. 858.)

Differential diagnosis Paedophilia has to be distinguished from exhibitionism towards young girls (in which no attempt is made to engage in direct sexual contact). Sexual contact with children may be sought by people with subnormal intelligence, dementia, and alcoholism.

The child Most of the females involved in paedophilia are aged between 6 and 12 years, most of the male children involved in homosexual paedophilia are somewhat older. Of the children involved in cases of paedophilia coming to the attention of the law, many have cooperated in sexual activity more than once with the same or another adult. Most of these children have been involved through fear rather than interest; a small minority are promiscuous and delinquent.

The *effects on the child* of sexual abuse are considered on p. 859.

Aetiology This is unknown. Paedophiles often have a marked incapacity for relationships with adults and fears of relationships with women.

Prognosis In the absence of reliable information from follow-up studies, prognosis has to be judged in individual patients by the length of the history, the frequency of the behaviour, the absence of other social and sexual relationships, and the strengths and weaknesses of the personality. Behaviour that has been frequently repeated is likely to persist despite efforts at treatment.

Treatment There is no evidence that any treatment is effective. Paedophiles who are genuinely motivated to control their impulses may be helped by support and problem-solving counselling. Attempts to treat those convicted of sex offences are considered on p. 912.

For a review of paedophilia, see McConaghy (1998).

Other abnormalities in the preference of sexual object

Zoophilia Zoophilia, otherwise called bestiality or bestiosexuality, is the use of an animal as a repeated and preferred or exclusive method of achieving sexual excitement. It is uncommon and rarely encountered by doctors.

Necrophilia In this extremely rare condition sexual arousal is obtained through intercourse with a dead body. Occasionally there are legal trials of men who murder and then attempt intercourse with the victim. No reliable information is available about the causes or prognosis of this extreme form of abnormal sexual preference.

Types of abnormality in the preference for the sexual act

The second group of abnormalities of sexual preference involves variations in the behaviour that is carried out to obtain sexual arousal. Generally, the acts are directed towards other adults, but sometimes children are involved (for example, by some exhibitionists).

Exhibitionism

Exhibitionism is the repeated exposing of the genitals to unprepared strangers for the purpose of achieving sexual excitement but without any attempts at further sexual activity with the other person. The name exhibitionism was suggested by Lasègue (1877). (This technical use of the term is clearly different from its everyday sense of self-display.)

Prevalence This is not known. Exhibitionists make up about a quarter of sexual offenders dealt with in the courts (Rosen 1979). Almost all are men, except for a very few women exhibitionists who repeatedly expose the breasts and an even smaller number who expose the genitalia.

Description Amongst exhibitionists seen by doctors, most are aged 20–40 years and two-thirds are married (Gayford 1981). In some, the urge to exhibitionism is persistent; in others it is episodic. The act of exposure is usually preceded by a feeling of mounting tension. Most exhibitionists choose places from which escape is easy. The exhibitionist often steps out from a hiding place, and exposes his penis; sometimes, instead of hiding, he conceals his exposed penis, for example, behind a newspaper which he suddenly removes. Occasionally the exhibitionist appears nude. Some masturbate during exposure; others do this afterwards. The exhibitionist seeks to evoke a strong emotional reaction from the other person. Whatever this reaction may be, it is interpreted by the exhibitionist as sexual interest, though it is in fact shock, fear, or even laughter. This distorted interpretation is accompanied by a state of intense excitement.

As a broad generalization, two groups of exhibitionists can be described. The first group includes men of inhibited temperament who struggle against their urges and feel much guilt after the act; they sometimes expose a flaccid penis. The second group includes men who have aggressive traits, sometimes accompanied by features of antisocial personality disorder. They usually expose an erect penis, often while masturbating. They gain pleasure from any distress they cause and often feel little guilt.

In the UK, if a man is brought to court because of exhibitionism, he is charged with the offence of indecent exposure (see Chapter 26, p. 912). About four-fifths of men charged with indecent exposure are exhibitionists (as defined at the beginning of this section).

Exhibitionism and the making of obscene phone calls There is uncertainty about the relationship between exhibitionism and the making of obscene phone calls by men who talk to women about sexual activities while masturbating. It has been suggested (Tollison and Adams 1979) that these obscene callers are also exhibitionists, but it is not easy to identify them in order to study their psychopathology.

Aetiology The cause of exhibitionism is unknown. Psychoanalytical theories suggest failure to resolve Oedipal conflict or a general inhibition of relationships with women. In an influential paper, Rickles (1950) suggested some exhibitionists describe unduly close relationships with their mothers and a poor relationship with ineffectual fathers. However, these accounts are retrospective, and may not reflect the actual circumstances of the patient's upbringing. Also, many people describe similar experiences in childhood, but do not become exhibitionists.

Exhibitionism that starts in middle or old age is occasionally associated with organic disease of the brain or alcoholism. It is possible that these conditions reduce previously effective control of urges to exhibitionism.

Prognosis There is no reliable follow-up information. Men who exhibit only once do not fall within the definition of the disorder. Clinical experience suggests a variable outcome for the rest. Among men who exhibit repeatedly but only at times of stress, the prognosis depends on the likelihood of the stressors returning. Exhibitionists who repeat often, and not solely at times of stress, are likely to persist with the behaviour for years despite treatment by psychiatrists or punishment by the courts. In keeping with these clinical impressions, the evidence from the courts is that the reconviction rate for indecent exposure is low after a first conviction but high after a second conviction. Although a history of exhibitionism is given by some men who commit rape, it seems that most exhibitionists do not go on to commit violent sexual acts nor do they interfere with children (Rooth 1973).

Treatment Any associated psychiatric disorder such as depressive disorder, alcoholism, or dementia should be sought and treated appropriately if found. Many treatments have been tried specifically for exhibitionism, including psychoanalysis, individual and group psychotherapy, and covert sensitization. There is no satisfactory evidence that any of these treatments is generally effective. A practical approach combines counselling and behavioural techniques. Counselling deals with the effects of exhibitionistic behaviour and with problems in personal relationships. Behavioural techniques are concerned with self-monitoring to identify circumstances that trigger the behaviour and to help the person avoid them. Cyproterone acetate and related drugs have been used to reduce the sex drive, but are not recommended because of uncertain results and problems of gynaecomestia and depression with long-term use. The general measures described on p. 600 can be tried, though without high expectation of success. For further information about exhibitionism, see Abel and Osborn (2000).

Sexual sadism

Sadism is named after the Marquis de Sade (1774–1814) who inflicted extreme cruelty on women for sexual purposes. Sexual sadism is achieving sexual arousal, habitually and in preference to heterosexual intercourse, by inflicting pain on another person, by bondage, or by humiliation.

Prevalence Inflicting pain in fantasy or practice is a not uncommon accompaniment of other forms of sexual behaviour. Sex shops sell chains, whips, and shackles, whilst some pornographic magazines provide pictures and descriptions of sadistic sexual practices. Sexual sadism as a predominant sexual practice is probably uncommon, but its frequency is not known.

Description Beating, whipping, and tying are common forms of sadistic activity. Repeated acts may be with a partner who is a masochist or a prostitute who is paid to take part. Sadism may be a component of homosexual as well as heterosexual acts. The acts may be symbolic, with little actual damage, and some involve humiliation rather than injury. However, at times, serious and permanent injuries are caused. Extreme examples are the rare 'lust murders', in which the killer inflicts serious repeated injuries – usually stabbings and mutilations – on the genitalia of his victim. In these rare cases, ejaculation may occur during the sadistic act or later by intercourse with the dead body (necrophilia). An historically significant description is given by Hirschfeld (1944).

Aetiology This is not known. Psychoanalytical explanations draw attention to the association between love and aggressive feelings that is supposed to exist in the young child's early relationship with his parents. Behavioural formulations rely on association learning. Neither explanation is satisfactory.

Prognosis There is no reliable follow-up information. Clinical experience suggests that, once established, the behaviour is likely to persist for many years.

Treatment No treatment has been shown to be effective in clinical trials. Men who have committed serious injury are dealt with by legal means. The risks must not be underestimated when potentially dangerous behaviour has been planned or has taken place.

Sexual masochism

Sexual masochism is achieving sexual excitement, as a preferred or exclusive practice, through the experience of suffering or humiliation. As a predominant activity it differs from the common use of minor painful practices as an accompaniment to sexual intercourse. The condition is named after Leopold von Sacher-Masoch (1836–1905), an Austrian novelist, who described sexual gratification from the experience of pain.

Prevalence Fantasies of being beaten or humiliated are sufficiently common among males to create a demand for pornographic literature on this theme, and for prostitutes who enable the man to act out his fantasies. Established sexual masochism is probably uncommon, though no exact information is available.

Description The suffering may take the form of being beaten, trodden upon, bound, or chained, or the enactment of various symbolic forms of humiliation, for example, dressing as a child and being punished. Masochism, unlike most other sexual deviations, occurs in women as well as in men. It may occur in homosexual as well as heterosexual relationships. Some masochists desire dangerous behaviours such as strangulation, a practice that can increase sexual excitation through the resulting partial anoxia (see also auto-erotic asphyxia, p. 608).

Aetiology This is not known. Conditioning theory suggests that it arises as a result of association between sexual arousal and beatings received as punishment around puberty. Psychoanalytical theory suggests that masochism is sadism turned inwards, and therefore is explicable in the same way as sadism (see above). Neither theory is supported by evidence.

Prognosis There is no reliable follow-up information. Clinical experience suggests that, once established as a preferred form of sexual behaviour, masochism is likely to persist for many years.

Treatment Psychoanalysis and behavioural treatments have been proposed but neither has been shown to be effective. General measures (see p. 600) can be tried, without high expectation of success.

Voyeurism

Many men are sexually excited by observing others engaged in intercourse. Voyeurism is observing the sexual activity of others repeatedly as a preferred means of sexual arousal. The voyeur also spies on women who are undressing or without clothes, but does not attempt sexual activity with them. Voyeurism is usually accompanied or followed by masturbation. Recently, voyeurs have used video cameras to observe women undressed or engaging in sexual activities (Simon 1997).

Voyeurism is a disorder of heterosexual men whose heterosexual activities are usually inadequate. Although the voyeur usually takes great care to hide from the women he is watching, he often takes considerable risks of discovery by other people. Hence most voyeurs are reported by passers-by, and not by the victim.

Aetiology Among adolescents voyeuristic activities are not uncommon as an expression of sexual curiosity, but they are usually replaced by direct sexual experience. The voyeur continues to watch because he is shy, socially awkward with girls, or prevented from normal sexual expression by some other obstacle. Psychoanalytical explanations follow the general lines described above for other sexual disorders. Behavioural theories seek an explanation in terms of chance associations between a first experience of peeping and sexual arousal. Neither theory is supported by evidence.

Prognosis No reliable information is available.

Treatment No treatment has been shown to be effective in clinical trials. It is reasonable to try the general measures described earlier in this chapter.

Other abnormalities of preference of the sexual act

Auto-erotic asphyxia Autoerotic asphyxia is the practice of inducing cerebral anoxia to heighten sexual arousal while masturbating. Asphyxia is usually induced by partial strangulation with cords or by plastic bags placed over the head. The practice occurs almost exclusively in men. It is hazardous and may lead to death. The act may be accompanied by the use of objects to produce anal stimulation, by the use of fetish objects, or by cross-dressing. The person may look at himself in a mirror or photograph himself, or he may apply bondage, for example by tying the ankles. Few people who practise auto-erotic asphyxia seek help from doctors. Most information about the condition comes from forensic studies of persons who have died during the act although occasional cases have been studied in life (e.g. Quinn and Twomey 1998). For further information see Blanchard and Hucker (1991) or Hucker (1990).

Frotteurism In frotteurism, the preferred form of sexual excitement is by rubbing the male genitalia against another person, or by fondling the breasts of an unwilling participant, who is usually a stranger, generally in a crowded place such as an underground train.

Coprophilia, coprophagia, sexual urethism, and urophilia In coprophilia, sexual arousal is induced by thinking about or watching the act of defecation and this is the preferred sexual activity; in coprophagia arousal follows the eating of faeces. In sexual urethism, which occurs mainly in women, erotic arousal is obtained by stimulation of the urethra. Urophilia refers to sexual arousal obtained by watching the act of urination, being urinated upon, or drinking urine.

The prevalence of these disorders is not known, but some are sufficiently common to demand provision from prostitutes. Further information can be found in Allen (1969) and Tollison and Adams (1979).

Abnormalities of gender identity

Transsexualism

Transsexual people are convinced that they are of the gender opposite to that indicated by their chromosomes. They have an overpowering wish to live as a member of the gender group opposite to their anatomical sex, and seek to alter their bodily appearance and genitalia.

In the past, the condition was called eonism because it was exemplified by the Chevalier d'Eon de Beaumont. In psychiatric literature, the condition was mentioned by Esquirol in 1838 and described in more detail by Krafft-Ebing in 1886 (see Krafft-Ebing 1924). In the 1960s, the attention of doctors and the public was directed to the condition by a number of striking reports and by a publication by Benjamin (1966).

Terminology

The terms transsexual male and transsexual female are used in different ways. Transsexual people generally prefer the usage in which transsexual female refers to people identified at birth as male, but experiencing themselves as female; transsexual males are people who were identified at birth as female but experience themselves as male. In the medical literature transsexual male is often used to denote people identified at birth as males but experiencing themselves as female. In the following account, we generally use the terms male to female transsexual, and female to male transsexual as they describe the sequence of events in the person's life. Thus male to female transsexuals are people who were identified at birth as male, but who later experience themselves as female. Some transsexual people object to the use of the word transsexual, as a noun. When the word transsexual is used in this way in the following account, it denotes a transsexual person, just as heterosexual is widely used as a noun to denote a heterosexual person.

Some transsexual people consider that their condition should not be listed as a psychiatric disorder. However, it is listed in both ICD and DSM, and this listing may assist some transsexual people who request treatment since in many countries treatment under a state health scheme or private insurance is restricted to disorders listed in one of the classifications of diseases.

Prevalence

Epidemiological data are difficult to obtain. A survey in the Netherlands gave the prevalence of gender identity disorder in adults as 1 per 10 000 born male and 1 per 30 000 born female (Kesteren *et al.* 1996). Among those seeking help at clinical centres, male to female transsexual people exceed female to males by 3 to 1 and 4 to 1 (Green 2000a).

Description

Transsexual people have a strong conviction of belonging to the sex opposite to that to which they were assigned, usually starting before puberty. Parents sometimes report that, as children, these people preferred the company and pursuits of children of the opposite anatomical sex, although such a history is not invariable. However, follow-up studies of effeminate boys have found that they more often grow up as homosexual than as transsexual adults (see Green 1974).

By the time that medical help is requested, most transsexual people have started to cross-dress. In contrast with transvestic fetishists, male to female transsexuals cross-dress to feel more like a woman, not to produce sexual arousal. Benjamin (1966, p. 21) wrote:

the transvestist looks on his sex organ as an organ of pleasure, and the transsexual turns from it in disgust.

(Contrast also homosexual men who dress as women to attract other male homosexuals.) Make-up is worn and the hair is arranged in a feminine style; facial and body hair are usually removed by electrolysis. These people develop feminine gestures, alter the pitch of voice, and seek changes in social role.

Many transsexual people are greatly distressed by their predicament. Depression is common, and some make suicide attempts. About a third marry but about half of these become divorced (Roth and Ball 1964).

Male to female transsexuals often ask for help in altering the appearance of the breasts and external genitalia. Usually the first requests are for oestrogens to enlarge the breasts. Later requests may be for surgery to the breasts, castration and removal of the penis, and operations to create an artificial vagina. These people are greatly distressed and some threaten self-castration or suicide if they cannot have surgery. These threats are sometimes acted upon.

Female to male transsexuals adopt masculine dress, voice, gestures, and social behaviour. They wish to have intercourse in the role of male with a heterosexual woman (and not with a female homosexual). Some ask for mastectomy or hysterectomy, and a few hope for plastic surgery to create an artificial penis.

Aetiology

The causes of this condition are unknown. The following factors have been investigated:

Genetic causes Transsexuals have normal sex chromosomes, and there is no convincing evidence of a genetic cause.

Early upbringing There is no convincing evidence that transsexuals have been brought up in the gender role opposite to their anatomical sex. As noted above, most boys with gender identity disorder grow up as homosexual rather than transsexual adults.

Endocrine causes No definite endocrine abnormality has been found in adult transsexuals. It has been suggested that transsexualism might result from hormonal abnormalities during intrauterine development. When pregnant rhesus monkeys are given large doses of androgens, their female infants behave more like males during play (Young *et al.* 1964). Also, female children with adrenogenital syndrome, who are exposed to large amounts of androgen before and after birth, have been reported to show boyish behaviour in childhood (Ehrhardt *et al.* 1968). However, they do not grow up as transsexual. A high rate of polycystic ovarian disease has been reported in female to male transsexuals (Bosinski *et al.* 1997). However, very few of the patients with this ovarian condition have gender identity disorder (Green 2000a).

Differences in brain structure The volume of the central subdivision of the bed nucleus of the stria terminalis is larger in men than in women. One study of six post-mortem brains from male to female transsexuals found the size of the nucleus similar to that in described in women (Zhou *et al.* 1995). The brains were collected over a 10-year period before the anatomical study and it has been suggested that in this period there may have been artefactual shrinkage of the nucleus (Green 2000a).

Transition from transvestism In a minority of male to female transsexual people, the condition begins after many years of transvestic fetishism. These people start by cross-dressing to obtain sexual excitement, but the resultant arousal gradually diminishes. At the same time, they gradually become convinced that they are women.

Course

There is no reliable information about the course of untreated transsexuals. Clinical experience suggests that they change little over many years. It is uncertain whether the rate of suicide among transsexuals is increased. A follow-up of 318 male to female and 117 female to male transsexuals did not find an increased rate (Cole *et al.* 1997) but more studies are needed.

Treatment

First stages Treatment generally follows the guidelines of the Harry Benjamin International Gender Dysphoria Association (International Gender Dysphoria Association 1985). The following account summarizes the steps; for further information see the original publication or Green (2000a).

◆ *Agreeing a plan* Transsexual people have often decided what treatment they require and may be impatient to obtain it. They may regard psychiatric assessment as an unnecessary obstacle in the path to hormonal treatment and surgery. Sometimes patients threaten suicide or self-mutilation if their own timetable is not met. Such threats should always be taken seriously as an indication of great distress, and a need for immediate help. Nevertheless, it should be explained that certain stages have to be gone through.
The first is to demonstrate the psychological stability that is essential if the person is to succeed in the transition that is sought.
To help establish this stability, the person needs to pass through the 'real life test' (see below). If possible, this test should be supervised by a doctor with special experience in the problem.

◆ *Psychological treatment* Transsexual people are unlikely to seek treatment to reduce their conviction about their gender, nor is there any evidence that psychological treatment can bring about this change. Psychological treatment should be offered to those who are willing to accept it, with the aim of listening to the person's distress and helping with alternative ways of coping.

The 'real life test' A male to female transsexual person has to become accustomed to appearing, speaking, and behaving as a woman. Facial hair is often removed by electrolysis or laser treatment and voice training may be required. The test requires the person to live in the new gender role continuously for at least 1 year, and preferably for two. During this time the person has to be employed full time in work or as a student. (The criterion of full-time employment may be difficult to meet at times of high unemployment.) Appropriate hormone treatment (see below) is prescribed during this year. At the end of the year, patients who can demonstrate to an assessment panel that they are better adjusted in the new gender role than in the old, may be considered for surgery.

Hormonal treatment *Oestrogens* may be prescribed to produce breast enlargement. The effects of oestrogen on breast development are as variable in genetic males as they are in genetic females, but in most cases fat increases around the hips and buttocks, giving a more female appearance. Prolonged oestrogen treatment carries the risk of deep vein thrombosis (van Kesteren *et al.* 1997). Malignant breast tumours have been reported (e.g. Symmers 1968), but there were no cases in a recent series of 816 male to female transsexuals (van Kesteren *et al.* 1997).

Androgens may be prescribed to female to male transsexual patients. The voice deepens, hair increases on the face and body, menstruation ceases, the clitoris enlarges, and the sex drive increases. These changes are generally more pronounced than the changes in male to female transsexual patients taking oestrogen. Prolonged use of androgens carries the risk of liver damage.

Surgery Patients who have successfully passed the previous stages of treatment may be considered for surgery. Because there is uncertainty about the long-term outcome of surgical treatment (see

below), opinions differ about this treatment. Decisions should be taken jointly by psychiatrist and a surgeon, each with special experience of the treatment of this condition.

For a male to female patient, possible surgical procedures include mammoplasty, penectomy, orchidectomy, and the creation of vagina-like structure. The latter is constructed from penile skin, with the addition of other skin or large intestine.

For a female to male patient, surgical procedures include mastectomy, ovariectomy, and phalloplasty. In the latter, a 'microphallus' is formed from the clitoris (already enlarged by androgens), or from skin taken from another part of the body (see Green 2000a).

Help for the family Transsexual patients are often married and may have children. Spouses, and especially children, require help in coming to terms with the effects of the changes in the patient on their own lives. Concerns may be expressed about the possibility of gender role problems in the children. Green (1998) studied 34 children with a transsexual parent and found no instances of gender identity disorder.

Outcome More than a dozen follow-up studies have been reported, but none has been able to compare patients allocated randomly to surgery or no surgery. A review of the English language literature over a 10-year period found that 90% of male to female transsexual were reported to have had a successful outcome of sex reassignment surgery (Green and Fleming 1991). However, this figure must be viewed cautiously because of possible bias in selection and loss from follow-up (see Green 2000a). In one study (Mate-Kole *et al.* 1990), 40 patients were selected for surgery, and then allocated alternately to treatment within 3 months, or treatment after 2 years. Two years after their operation the first group had lower scores for neurotic symptoms and somewhat better work adjustment than the group that was still waiting for the operation. However, Meyer and Reter (1979) compared operated patients with unoperated ones and found a similar rate of improvement in the two groups. However, this finding cannot be generalized since the groups were not randomly assigned, only half the patients were assessed at follow-up, and the follow-up period was longer for operated patients.

Dual-role transvestism

This term is used in ICD-10 to describe people who wear clothes of the opposite sex but are neither transvestic fetishists (seeking sexual excitement) nor transsexuals (wishing a change of gender and sexual role). Instead they enjoy cross-dressing in order to gain temporary membership of the opposite sex.

Gender identity disorder of adolescence and adulthood – non-transsexual type

This term is used in DSM-IV to denote people who have passed puberty and feel a persistent or recurrent discomfort or sense of inappropriateness about their assigned gender identity. They cross-dress persistently or repeatedly, or imagine themselves doing this, but are not sexually excited by these actions or fantasies nor preoccupied with change in their primary or secondary sex characteristics.

Gender identity disorders in children

Parents more often seek advice about effeminate behaviour in boys than about masculine behaviour in small girls (it is not clear whether such behaviour in girls is less frequent or more socially acceptable). Effeminate boys prefer girlish games and enjoy wearing female clothing. The outcome amongst these boys is variable; some develop normal male interests and activities. Most boys with gender disorder in childhood become homosexual men. Further information is given by Green (2000b).

Other aspects of sexual behaviour

Rape and incest are discussed in Chapter 26 on forensic psychiatry.

Ethical problems in the diagnosis and treatment of disorders of sexuality and gender

Any of the ethical problems associated with the practice of psychiatry can arise when sexual disorders are treated but the following are especially likely to cause difficulty.

The professional relationship

When sexual problems are the main topic of the interviews, there is an increased risk that the relationship between patient and therapist will become sexualized. Medical codes of practice contain an absolute prohibition against a sexual relationship with a patient because this exploits the patient and undermines the general trust in doctors.

Confidentiality

Problems may arise when one sexual partner reveals information to the therapist and refuses to allow it to be passed to the other partner, even though it is relevant. The problem can usually be avoided if a full history is taken from both partners before deciding whether sex therapy is an appropriate treatment, and if the therapist does not see the partners separately after therapy has started.

Diagnosis, stigmatization, and responsibility

It has been objected that to give a psychiatric diagnosis to a pattern of sexual behaviour has two undesirable consequences. First, it can stigmatize the person; second, it can excuse behaviour that is morally wrong. Both problems are a reminder that the concept of diagnosis was developed mainly to assist with questions about treatment. It cannot be applied uncritically to other problems including those of responsibility.

Many people with the behaviour diagnosed as gender identity disorder argue that the diagnosis stigmatizes them because it implies that the behaviour is pathological rather than a normal variation. A similar objection was made in the past about homosexual behaviour at a time when it was viewed as a disorder (which is no longer the case). The question about transsexualism is still the subject of debate. In such debate a clear distinction has to be made between medical evidence and religious prohibitions – even though the two may, at times, coincide. For example, in the late nineteenth century, masturbation was regarded as morally wrong, and also medically harmful. The practice was condemned by the church and treated by doctors.

Some people argue that to diagnose certain kinds of sexual behaviour as a disorder excuses the person from responsibility for the effects of his behaviour. However, whilst the diagnosis of a disorder allows the person to adopt the sick role (see p. 203), this role does not absolve the patient from all responsibilities. Indeed, it adds the responsibility to seek treatment, and does not remove the responsibility of not doing harm to other people.

Further reading

Bancroft, J. (1989). *Human sexuality and its problems*, 2nd edn. Churchill Livingstone, Edinburgh. (Although somewhat out of date in its details until a 3rd edition appears, the account of normal sexual function and sexual disorders is valuable.)

Gelder, M. G., López-Ibor, J. J. Jr, and Andreasen, N. C. (eds) (2000). *The new Oxford textbook of psychiatry*, Section 4.11: Sexuality, gender identity, and their disorders. Oxford University Press, Oxford. (The four chapters in this section include an account of normal sexual function.)

Golombek, S. and Fivush, R. (1998). Gender development. Chapter 2. In *Psychosexual disorders* (eds H. Freeman, I. Pullen, G. Stein, and G. Wilkinson). Gaskell, London.

Hawton, K. (1985). *Sex therapy: a practical guide*. Oxford University Press, Oxford. (Although written in 1985, this remains a valuable guide to the sex therapy techniques used in psychiatric practice.)

CHAPTER 20

Psychiatry of the elderly

Psychiatry of the elderly

Introduction

Older people with mental health problems present particular challenges which the practice and organization of old age psychiatry services have to take into account. They are often physically, as well as mentally, frail and this affects presentation and course. On the other hand, they have the advantage of a rich history to tell and a lifetime's experience of responding to fortune and adversity.

When considering psychiatric disorder in the elderly, the clinician must be able to collect and integrate information from a variety of sources, and to produce a management plan which takes account of physical and social needs, as well as the psychological. This plan is likely to involve the cooperation of several professionals. It is in this clinical complexity that much of the challenge and fascination of old age psychiatry lies.

Demography

In 1993, 6% of the world's population was over 65 years of age. However, in the more developed countries the proportion was about 14%, whilst in less developed countries it was 4% (United Nations 1993). Less developed countries have higher birth rates, but the expectation of life at birth is substantially lower than in developed countries: 60 years compared to 73. In the UK, life expectancy at birth has increased from 41 in 1840 to 46 in 1900, 69 in 1950, and 76 in 1990 (OPCS 1993).

Table 20.1 and Figure 20.1 show that the difference in age structure of the population is changing; the proportion of older people in less developed countries is increasing much faster than it is in developed countries. As many illnesses, such as

most of the dementias, occur more frequently with increasing age, all countries will be faced with the problem of managing large numbers of mentally ill older people.

The effects of ageing

Physical changes in the brain

The *weight* of the human brain decreases by approximately 5% between the ages of 30 and 70 years, by a further 5% by the age of 80, and by another 20% by the age of 90. As well as these changes, the *ventricles enlarge* and the *meninges thicken*. There is some *loss of nerve cells*, though this is relatively minor and selective. There may also be a reduction

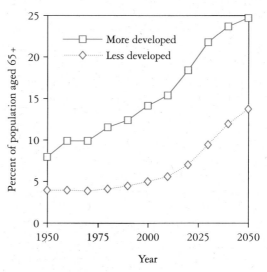

Figure 20.1 Percentage of the population aged 65+ for more developed and less developed countries. Data from 1996 United Nations population estimates and projections. From Jorm A. F. 2000.

Table 20.1 Percentage change in population of the world, 1975–2000			
Age	Total	% Change 1975–2000	
		Developed	Less developed
<15	57.6	20.2	72.6
15–24	41.8	8.6	50.0
25–34	56.5	4.2	75.0
35–44	72.2	16.9	95.0
45–54	74.5	33.2	104.2
55–64	64.5	30.5	86.7
65–74	68.9	33.2	104.2
75–79	84.3	53.4	121.2
>80	91.7	64.7	138.0

Source: UN (1988).

in dendritic processes. Magnetic resonance studies have shown a *decrease in cortical grey matter* with white matter relatively unchanged. *Cerebral blood flow* in the thalamus and in the frontal and temporal lobes also appears to decrease with age (Buchsbaum and Siegel 1994).

In old age, the cytoplasm of nerve cells accumulates a pigment called *lipofuscin*, which is probably made up of degraded cellular components. There are also changes in the components of the neuronal cytoskeleton. A protein called tau, which plays a role in linking neurofilaments and microtubules, can accumulate to produce paired helical filaments that form *neurofibrillary tangles* in, and destroy, some nerve cells. In normal ageing neurofibrillary tangles are usually confined to a small number of cells in the hippocampus and entorhinal cortex.

In addition to neurofibrillary tangles, the normal ageing brain can also contain *senile plaques* which are collections of neuritic processes aggregated together in an irregular spherical form, sometimes with a central core of extracelluar amyloid at the centre. There are also 'diffuse' plaques. Senile plaques also contain paired helical filaments composed of tau protein. All plaques contain

amyloid. The distribution of senile plaques in the normal ageing brain is rather wider than that of neurofibrillary tangles, and can occur in both the neocortex and amygdala as well as in the hippocampus and entorhinal cortex. A small proportion of brains from non-demented old people contain *Lewy bodies*. These are intracellular inclusion bodies with a laminated appearance, usually confined to the substantia nigra and locus ceruleus. For a review of the neuropathology of normal ageing see Esiri and Nagy (2002).

The psychology of ageing

Assessment of cognitive function in the elderly is complicated by the frequent presence of physical ill health, particularly by sensory deficits.

Longitudinal studies suggest that *intellectual function*, as measured by standard intelligence tests, shows a significant decline only in later old age. A characteristic pattern of change occurs with psychomotor slowing and impairment in the

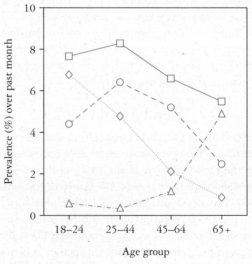

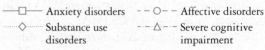

Figure 20.2 Prevalence of mental disorders across age groups: data are 1-month prevalence rates from the Epidemiologic Catchment Area Study using DSM-III criteria. From Jorm A. F. 2000.

manipulation of new information. By contrast, tests of well-rehearsed skills such as verbal comprehension show little or no age-related decline.

Short-term memory, as measured by the digit span test, for example, does not change in the normal elderly. Tests of *working memory* show a gradual decrease in capacity, so that the elderly perform significantly less well than the young if attention has to be divided between two tasks or if the material has to be processed additionally in some way. The elderly can usually recall remote events of personal significance with great clarity. Despite this, their long-term memory for other remote events shows a decline; for a review see Morris (1997). Overall, there appears to be a balance between losses in flexible problem solving with age and the benefits of accumulated wisdom derived from experience.

As well as these cognitive and motor changes, there are important alterations in *personality and attitudes*, such as increasing cautiousness and rigidity.

Physical health

In addition to a general decline in functional capacity and adaptability with ageing, chronic degenerative conditions are common. As a result, the elderly consult their family doctors frequently and occupy half of all general hospital beds. These demands are particularly large in those aged over 75. Medical management is often made more difficult by the presence of more than one disorder, the consequent increased risk of side-effects of treatment, and by psychiatric and social problems (Kane 1985).

Sensory and motor disabilities are frequent among elderly people. In a study in Jerusalem (Davies and Fleischchman 1981), difficulties in seeing were reported by 54% of 70–74-year-olds, and by 69% of those aged over 80. The corresponding figures for other disabilities were as follows:

- difficulty in hearing, 34% and 50%;
- difficulty in walking, 29% and 62%;
- difficulty in talking, 9% and 22%.

Studies by the World Health Organization show that although the reported prevalence of these disorders differs somewhat in other countries, the figures from Jerusalem are fairly representative (Davies 1986).

Social circumstances

For most people, ageing brings with it profound changes in social circumstances.

Retirement affects not only income but also social status, time available for leisure, and social contacts. In developed countries, governments have tended to encourage retirement at progressively earlier ages. In the UK, nearly half of all men over 65 were economically active in 1931, compared with a quarter in 1961 and only 8% in 1991 (Henretta 1994). Countries with the highest per capita incomes have the lowest economic participation rates in those aged 55 and over.

Loss of income is a serious problem facing the elderly. Of those aged over 65 in the European Commision Age and Attitudes survey, 44% thought that financial worry was the main problem facing older people. In 1991, a third of pensioners in the UK had incomes less than half the national average.

Social isoloation

Older people in developed countries are much more likely to live alone than those elsewhere. In the UK, 37% of those over 65 lived alone in 1993, compared with a similar proportion in Scandinavia and the USA, 7% in Chile and 3% in China. The figure in the UK has increased rapidly in the second half of this century: in 1851 it was 7%, and in 1921, 11%. However, evidence suggests that for many older people, living alone is not seen as a problem and is aided by slowly increasing pensioner incomes and greater availability of suitable housing. Many see family, friends, and neighbours regularly and provide as much support as they receive. In the 1993 European Commission survey, 44% of older Europeans relatives saw a relative every day. This figure was highest in southern Europe and lowest in northern Europe,

			Marital status		
Age	Sex	Single	Married	Wid/Div	All
65–74	M	9.2	0.4	2.9	1.4
	F	6.3	0.4	1.8	1.4
75–84	M	15.6	1.7	8.0	4.3
	F	13.7	2.2	8.0	7.0
>85	M	31.6	6.9	21.1	15.6
	F	36.1	12.5	27.8	27.6

Table 20.2 **Elderly people resident in institutions (%) by marital status, Britain, 1991**

Source: Grundy (1996), from 1991 census data.

but, interestingly, reported loneliness showed the same pattern, being highest in countries with the highest levels of family contact. Although almost all older people live at home, the proportion living in institutions rises with age and being single (Table 20.2).

Other factors

Not only does the number of elderly people change with time, but there are marked changes in experiences and expectations with successive cohorts. In Europe, the generation born in the early decades of the twentieth century mostly received only basic education, had large families, worked long hours in unprosperous conditions and experienced two world wars. Those who survived had considerable resilience and powers of endurance. By comparison, those born 50 years later grew up mostly in more affluent circumstances, with more education, and with higher expectations. In the UK and most parts of Europe there have been rapid recent changes in ethnic composition and in household structure. All these factors will affect demands on both health and social services in the future (Royal Commission on Long Term Care 1999).

Psychiatric disorders of the elderly

Epidemiology

Kay *et al.* (1964) carried out the first systematic prevalence study of psychiatric disorder amongst elderly people in the general population, including those living at home as well as those living in institutions, in an area of Newcastle-upon-Tyne. The findings have been broadly replicated in subsequent surveys. In this and subsequent studies there have been problems of case definition and case finding. It is particularly difficult to distinguish mild dementia from the effects of normal ageing or from life-long poor cognitive performance due to low intelligence or lack of education.

Other surveys have shown a high prevalence of psychiatric disorder among elderly people in sheltered accommodation and in hospital. A third of the residents in old people's homes have significant cognitive impairment. In general hospital wards, a third to a half of the patients aged 65 or over suffer from some form of psychiatric illness.

It has frequently been reported that general practitioners are unaware of many of the psychiatric problems amongst elderly people living in the community. Moreover, the presentation of such disorders to general practitioners and psychiatrists is determined as much by social factors as by a change in the patient's mental state. For example, there may be a sudden alteration in the patient's environment, such as illness of a relative, or a bereavement. Sometimes an increasingly exhausted or frustrated family decide that they can no longer continue to care for an old person. At other times there is an element of manipulation by relatives who are trying to rid themselves of an unwanted responsibility.

Epidemiology is discussed further when individual syndromes are considered later in this chapter. Reviews of epidemiological methods and findings have been provided by Jorm (2000) and Prince (2002).

Dementia in the elderly

In this book, the main account of dementia is given in Chapter 14. This section is concerned only with those forms that are especially frequent in the elderly.

Although there are references in classical literature, dementia in the elderly has been recognized by modern medicine since the French psychiatrist Esquirol described *démence senile* in his textbook *Des maladies mentales* (Esquirol 1838). Esquirol's description of the disorder was in general terms, but it can be recognized as similar to the present-day concept (Alexander 1972). Kraepelin distinguished dementia from psychoses due to other organic causes such as neurosyphilis, and he divided it into presenile, senile, and arteriosclerotic forms. In an important study, Roth (1955) showed that dementia in the elderly differed from affective disorders and paranoid disorders in its poorer prognosis. ICD-10 introduced a new category of mild cognitive disorder (MCD) but its validity is not proven (Christensen *et al.* 1995).

Epidemiology

There has been extensive research on the prevalence of dementia with several meta-analyses of pooled data (Figure 20.3). Prevalence rises steeply with age, up to the age of 90. Alzheimer's disease and vascular disease are the two major causes but their

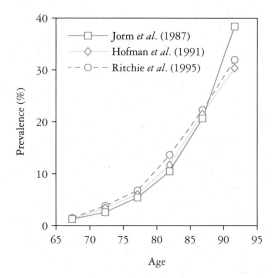

Figure 20.3 Prevalence rates for dementia across age groups: data from three meta-analyses. From Jorm A. F. 2000.

relative importance differs from country to country. In Europe, North America, and Australasia, Alzheimer's disease is the more common. However, vascular dementia is apparently more prevalent in a number of countries in the Far East. There is much less information about other parts of the world. A recent community-based neuropathology study (Neuropathology Group of the Medical Reserch Council Cognitive Function and Aging Study 2001) suggests difficulties in correlating conventional diagnostic criteria and neuropathology. Alzheimer's type and vascular pathology were the major pathological correlates of cognitive decline, but most patients had mixed disease. There were no clear thresholds that predicted dementia status.

Alzheimer's disease

The general clinical features of the dementia syndrome have been described on p. 405; the clinical features of Alzheimer's disease in the elderly are considered here. The condition is common and important in the elderly, and its features are characteristic (though not discriminating enough to allow accurate diagnosis from other forms of dementia).

Epidemiology

Alzheimer's disease is the most common form of dementia in the elderly. Point prevalence rates for populations over 65 years old range from 2 to 7% for moderately or severely affected people. It is difficult to agree diagnostic criteria for mild levels of disease, so that estimates of the prevalence in this group are unreliable. Prevalence rates are generally higher in institutional populations. Age-specific prevalence rates approximately double with every additional 5 years of age from about 1% at 65, rising to about 8–10% at age 80 and 30–40% at age 90. Alzheimer's disease is rare before age 60. See Jorm (2000, 2002) for reviews of epidemiology.

Clinical features

The first evidence of the condition is often minor forgetfulness which may be difficult to distinguish from normal ageing. The condition progresses gradually for the first 2–4 years, with increasing memory disturbance and lack of spontaneity.

Language is affected, with difficulty in finding words or naming objects, and impairments in the ability to construct fluent and informative sentences. Visuospatial skills may be affected with difficulties in tasks such as copying pictures or learning the way round unfamiliar environments, for example, on holiday or in an unfamiliar house. Disorientation in time gives rise to poorly kept appointments and changes in the diurnal pattern of activity.

Mood changes are common, more than half of sufferers experiencing depressive symptoms. Hallucinations occasionally occur in the late stages of Alzheimer's disease, but florid visual hallucinations earlier in the course of a dementia suggest Lewy body dementia. Delusions include the very common belief that items have been stolen (however, as this idea often arises from the patient's forgetfulness it is questionable whether it is helpful to regard this as a true delusion), as well as more developed persecutory or other beliefs.

Behaviour

Changes in behaviour are common and are of particular concern to carers. Patients may be restless and may wake at night, disorientated and perplexed. Motor activity may increase in the evening ('sundowning'), and eventually the sleep–wake cycle may become totally disorganized. Aggression is common, both verbal and physical, and often takes the form of resistance to help with personal care. Serious physical violence to others is rare. Both increases and reductions in level of activity are common, involving varying degrees of purposefulness. 'Wandering' can refer to a variety of different behaviours (Hope 1994), but patients may place themselves at risk by going into unsafe environments. Patients with dementia may under- or overeat, with associated change in weight and nutritional state. Changes in sexual behaviour occur, usually with reduction in drive, although sexual disinhibition occasionally occurs, requiring careful management.

Self-care and social behaviour decline, although some patients maintain a good social facade despite severe cognitive impairment, particularly if carers are able to assist with these functions.

Course

In the early stages of Alzheimer's disease, the clinical features are modified by the premorbid personality, and any personality defects tend to be exaggerated. In the middle and later stages of the illness, cognitive and non-cognitive impairments become more obvious. Neurological abnormalities including focal signs of parietal lobe dysfunction (such as dysphasia or dyspraxia) and frontal impairment, as indicated by decreased verbal fluency, personality change, and loss of emotional control, are common. Incidental physical illness may cause a superimposed delirium resulting in a sudden deterioration in cognitive function, which usually improves when the physical illness has been treated but may sometimes be permanent.

Differential diagnosis

The differential diagnosis of dementia is discussed on p. 417. Alzheimer's disease is distinguished clinically from multi-infarct dementia on the basis of additional features of the latter syndrome, such as stepwise progression, fluctuating course, and focal motor signs. However, post-mortem studies indicate that these clinical criteria are not always reliable. Patients with Lewy body dementia may show hallucinations, a greater degree of fluctuation in cognitive impairment, unexplained falls, and are more likely to have a concomitant extrapyramidal disorder (see p. 625).

Brain imaging can be helpful in supporting the diagnosis of Alzheimer's disease. CT scanning may show enlarged lateral ventricles and atrophy of medial temporal structures, and serial examination may reveal evidence of disease progression. Structural magnetic resonance imaging may demonstrate atrophy in specific structures such as the hippocampus. Studies of cerebral metabolism and blood flow with positron emission tomography (PET) and single-photon emission tomography (SPET) characteristically reveal bilateral deficits in posterior parietal and temporal cortex (Buchsbaum et al. 1991; Jobst et al. 1992).

Neuropathology

The pathological changes in late onset Alzheimer's disease are the same as those in the presenile form of the disease. On gross examination the brain is shrunken with widened sulci and enlarged ventricles. There is neuronal loss together with proliferation of astrocytes and increased gliosis. Silver staining shows senile plaques throughout the cortical and subcortical grey matter, and also neurofibrillary tangles and granulovacuolar degeneration. In comparison with the normal elderly brain, the senile plaques and neurofibrillary tangles are more numerous, particularly in limbic regions, and have a more widespread distribution. For example, both plaques and tangles may be found in subcortical structures such as Meynert's nucleus and the locus ceruleus which have diffuse projections to the cortex (Esiri and Nagy 2002). Plaques

consist of an amyloid core surrounded by dystrophic neurites. The amyloid appears to be derived from peptides which arise from the amyloid precursor protein (APP). Neurofibrillary tangles are composed of paired helical filaments made of a protein – tau.

The degree of cognitive impairment in Alzheimer's disease correlates with the synaptic loss and the number of neurofibrillary tangles (Arriagada et al. 1992). Amongst recent research, Förstl et al. (1993) found correlations between behavioural disturbance, lower brain weight, density of cortical neurofibrillary tangles, and neuronal loss in the hippocampus and Meynert's nucleus.

Aetiology and molecular neurobiology

In certain rare pedigrees, usually those with an early onset of illness, an autosomal dominant mode of inheritance can be discerned. Mutations identified in several locations include: (1) APP gene on chromosome 21; (2) Presenilin 1 on chromosome 14; (3) Presenelin 2 on chromosome 14.

First-degree relatives of patients with late onset Alzheimer's disease have a risk of developing the disorder which is three times that of the general population. Most cases appear to be clinically sporadic without a family history. However, it is inappropriate to attempt to differentiate 'familial' and sporadic groups; all seem to be due to an interaction of genetic vulnerability and environmental factors (head injury, educational achievement, pre-morbid intelligence, and several drugs including non-steroidal anti-inflammatory agents and statins).

In addtion to the three deterministic genes there is a fourth genetic factor, apolipoprotein E (APOE), a susceptibility locus that accounts for approximately half of late onset Alzheimer's disease. There is a strong association between late-onset Alzheimer's disease and the $\varepsilon 4$ allele of apoliprotein E which is found in both the senile plaques and neurofibrillary tangles. The gene for apolipoprotein E4 is located on chromosome 19 and has a frequency of 0.3–0.5 in Alzheimer patients compared with 0.1–0.15 in age-matched controls.

Exactly how APOE ε4 and the AOPE4 influence the pathophysiology of Alzheimer's disease is unknown but it appears to determine ealier onset. In vitro and animal model studies stronly suggest that brain apolipoprotein E is a multifunctional molecule with roles in amyloid deposition and many other cellular mechanisms (Saunders 2000). In addition, the ε4 allele is a risk factor for hyper-cholesterolaemia and coronary artery disease as well as for Alzheimer's disease (Owen *et al.* 1994). For a review of genetic risk and the significance for advising relatives see Liddell *et al* (2001).

The suggestion that *aluminium* may be a con-tributory environmental cause of Alzheimer's disease has been controversial it now has little support.

The amyloid cascade hypothesis

In 1984 the protein deposited in blood vessels in Alzheimer's disease was shown to be a peptide known as β-amyloid, idential to the amyloid plaques. It is derived from a protein APP, the gene for which is coded on chromosome 21. This discovery, together with the seminal finding in 1991 of a rare mutation in the parent APP gene, resulted in the amyloid cascade hypothesis, which remains the dominant molecular model for the disorder. Most workers now agree that a major, perhaps the central, pathogenic event is an increased formation of β-amyloid, specifically the 42 amino acid variant which is preferentially deposited in the plaques. This metabolic abnor-mality can arise for a number of different reasons, including many rare mutations. It is still contro-versial how the amyloid pathology relates to the tau protein and neurofibrillay tangles, but the consensus is in favour of the tangles being secondary to the protein (Nøslund *et al.* 2000).

Much research has concentrated on under-standing the metabolism of APP and the formation of β-amyloid peptide. At least three secretase enzymes cleave APP; they may be identical with the presenilins. The importance of APP and β-amyloid is emphasised by the important experi-mental finding that transgenic mice carrying APP mutations developed Alzheimer's pathology, as well as by the findings of research seeking to apply knowledge to therapeutic development either by attempts to inhibit beta or gamma secretase or by immunisation with β-amyloid.

Neurotransmitter changes: the cholinergic hypothesis

Neurochemical studies in Alzheimer's disease have shown a widespread loss of several neurotransmit-ters, particularly in association areas of cerebral cortex and hippocampus. The cells of origin of several of these neurotransmitters, for example, noradrenaline and 5-hydroxytryptamine (5-HT), are located in subcortical nuclei which can them-selves be subject to the pathological changes of Alzheimer's disease. Observations of this type, together with studies of the more conspicuous role of acetyl choline in animal and human behaviour, led to the *cholinergic hypothesis* that cognitive impairment of Alzheimer's disease is due to disorder primarily affecting cholinergic neurones. "Studies have resulted in the discovery of an asso-ciation between a decline in learning and memory, and a deficit in excitatory amino acid (EAA) neuro-transmission, together with important roles for the cholinergic system in attentional processing and as a modulator of EAA neurotransmission" (Francis *et al.* 1999). Even though the cholinergic hypothesis was a over-simplification of abnormalities in several neurotransmitter substances, it has led to pharmacological interventions to correct the loss of cholinergic pre-synaptic function.

Treatment

Initial efforts to develop treatment were based on the cholinergic hypothesis. The widespread nature of neurotransmitter deficits in Alzheimer's disease suggests that it will be difficult to devise a replace-ment treatment. Nevertheless, there is some evidence (Francis *et al.* 1999) that increasing acetylcholine function may benefit cognitive func-tion in some patients (see p. 628).

The most promising treatment strategy involves approaches to retarding, halting, or preventing the formation or accumulation of β-amyloid plaques. Despite some encouraging results no current therapy has been shown to halt or reverse the underlying disease process (Emilien *et al.* 2000). Another recent and innovative approach involves immunization with the pathological β-amyloid peptide itself to generate an immune response targeted agains the amyloid plaques in the brain (Schenk *et al.* 2000).

See Lovestone (2000) for a review of Alzheimer's disease.

Dementia with Lewy bodies

In the past decade, a type of dementia with a relatively distinct pathology and clinical course has been described under the terms dementia with Lewy bodies (DLB), Lewy body dementia, cortical Lewy body disease, diffuse Lewy body disease, Lewy body variant of Alzheimer's disease, and dementia associated with Lewy bodies. *Dementia with Lewy bodies* (DLB) has now, by consensus, been agreed to be the correct term (McKeith *et al.* 1996).

Lewy bodies have been recognized for many years in the substantia nigra of patients with Parkinson's disease, but more recently a characteristic form of dementia has been noted in association with Lewy bodies in the cerebral cortex. Neuropathological autopsy studies have found DLB in 15–25% of all cases, suggesting that it may be the second most frequent cause of dementia after Alzheimer's disease. It is not yet clear whether Lewy body dementia is a distinct syndrome from dementia occurring in patients with pre-existing Parkinson's disease. See Perry *et al.* (1997) and McKeith (2000) for reviews.

Clinical features

Lewy body dementia is a progressive dementing illness which can be distinguished clinically from Alzheimer's disease by its fluctuating course, the occurrence of marked visual hallucinations, and motor features of parkinsonism. Lewy body dementia is associated with repeated falls, syncope, transient loss of consciousness, delusions, auditory hallucinations, and extreme sensitivity to the extrapyramidal effects of antipsychotic drugs. The diagnosis is less likely in the presence of stroke or other physical illness which may account for these clinical features (McKeith *et al.* 1996).

Histopathology

The characteristic histopathological feature of Lewy body dementia is the presence of Lewy bodies in cerebral cortex and substantia nigra. Senile plaques may be present but neurofibrillary tangles are absent. Like Alzheimer's disease, Lewy body dementia is associated with widespread reductions in choline acetyltransferase in the neocortex and there is also some loss of dopamine from the caudate nucleus.

Vascular dementia

In the past, the dementia caused by cerebrovascular disease was referred to as 'atherosclerotic' psychosis. Following the separation of distinct syndromes of psychiatric disorder in late life (Roth 1955), it became apparent that dementia was often associated with multiple infarcts of varying size, mostly caused by thromboembolism from extracranial arteries, and Hachinski *et al.* (1974) suggested the now superseded term multi-infarct dementia (MID).

Recent research has shown that patients with multi-infarct dementia are a subgroup of a larger group of patients with dementia due to vascular disease, and the term vascular dementia is now preferred. The pathogenic mechanisms are very varied, and include large or small vessel arteriosclerosis, embolus, vasculitis, amyloid angiopathy, and intracranial haemorrhage.

For a review of the pathology of vascular dementia see Esiri and Nagy (2002), and for diagnostic criteria see Roman *et al.* (1993).

Epidemiology

Vascular dementia is slightly more common in men than in women. The prevalence increases with age, approximately doubling every 5 years. There appear to be geographical differences, with especially high rates of vascular dementia reported in China, Japan, and the Russian Federation (Henderson 1994).

Clinical picture

Onset, which is usually in the late sixties or the seventies, may follow a cerebrovascular accident and is often more acute than that of Alzheimer's disease. Emotional and personality changes may appear first, followed by impairments of memory and intellect that characteristically progress in steps. Depression is frequent, and episodes of emotional lability and confusion are common, especially at night. Fits or minor episodes of cerebral ischaemia are usual at some stage. Insight is often maintained to a late stage. Behavioural retardation and anxiety are more common than in Alzheimer's disease.

The course of vascular dementia is usually a stepwise progression, with periods of deterioration that are sometimes followed by partial recovery for a few months. About half the patients die from ischaemic heart disease, and others from cerebral infarction or renal complications. From the time of diagnosis the life span varies widely but averages about 4–5 years. Most studies show somewhat shorter survival in vascular dementia than in Alzheimer's disease.

Diagnosis

The diagnosis is difficult to make with confidence unless there is a clear history of strokes or definite localizing signs. Suggestive features are patchy psychological deficits, erratic progression, and relative preservation of the personality. On physical examination there are usually signs of hypertension and of arteriosclerosis in peripheral and retinal vessels, and there may be neurological signs such as pseudobulbar palsy, rigidity akinesia, and brisk reflexes. See Erkinjuntti (2000) for a review.

The assessment of dementia in the elderly

The assessment of dementia in the elderly follows the principles that apply to assessment of dementia at other ages. These principles are described on p. 415.

Dementia has to be differentiated from:

◆ delirium

◆ depressive disorders

◆ paranoid disorders.

Delirium is suggested by impaired and fluctuating consciousness, and by perceptual misinterpretations and hallucinations (see p. 403). The differentiation of dementia from *affective disorders* and *paranoid states* is discussed later in this chapter (pp. 632). It is important to be aware that subjective complaints of cognitive decline are more likely to be associated with anxiety and depression than with dementia (Jorm *et al.* 1994). It should be remembered that hypothyroidism may be mistaken for dementia.

In the assessment of dementia it is important to look for the treatable causes, although they are rare. The term treatable in relation to dementia usually means arrestable rather than reversible; the effect of treatment may stop the progression of the dementia but it seldom results in a return to premorbid function. Treatable causes include:

◆ normal pressure hydrocephalus

◆ operable tumours

◆ hypothyroidism

◆ neurosyphilis

◆ deficiency of vitamin B12 and folate.

Whilst B12 and folate can cause dementia, this is rare, and in most elderly demented patients low B12 and folate levels are caused by poor nutrition.

Physical investigations may include a full blood count, a biochemical screen including thyroid and liver functioning, B12 and folate, syphilis serology, urine analysis and culture, chest radiography, and ECG. If physical illness is suspected, additional investigations may be required.

The role of *imaging* is developing rapidly in the investigation of the dementias. *CT scanning* is relatively widely available, and may be useful to exclude potentially reversible causes of dementia such as brain tumours, subdural haemorrhage or normal pressure hydrocephalus, and to provide positive evidence of the type of dementia. *MR imaging* offers a high level of structural resolution, but the procedure is less well tolerated than CT by some patients. *Radioisotope scanning* (SPET and PET) may also be useful in distinguishing different types of dementia, but is less widely available. As with any patient, the extent of physical investigation required should be assessed in each case.

It is important to make some assessment of the extent of cognitive impairment in all patients. Standardized instruments are valuable in quantifying this, but do not replace a clinical assessment of mental state. Psychometric testing may be useful in comparing current functioning with premorbid state, as assessed by educational, employment, and social achievements. Schedules such as the Mini-Mental State Examination (MMSE, see p. 68) are widely used. These are useful measures of current state that help in the planning of treatment and monitoring of change. Serial measurements can provide better evidence of decline, but the assessor must be aware of the test-retest reliability of his methods.

In skilled hands, more sophisticated psychometric testing has an important though limited role (Hodges 1994). Common obstacles to testing include confusion, lack of motivation, sensory handicaps, and the length of time required for patients to become accustomed to the test procedure. The main uses of psychometric assessment are to assist in:

◆ clarification of diagnosis;

◆ prediction of outcome;

◆ identifying the need of support and intervention;

◆ monitoring change.

Psychometric testing is now used less frequently than in the past. It is seldom used to differentiate cognitive impairment from functional illness; for this purpose clinical assessment is generally preferred.

For a detailed review of the diagnosis and management of dementia, see Wilcock *et al.* (1999).

The treatment of dementia in the elderly

Principles of management and the organization of services are discussed later. Here treatments specific to the dementias will be considered. Successful dementia care is based on the idea that people with dementia should to be regarded first and foremost as persons with similar needs to any other people, albeit presenting the individuals and organizations caring for them with considerable problems in understanding and responding appropriately to their needs (Kitwood 1997).

The first concern is to *treat any treatable physical disorder*. If the latter is the primary cause, the dementia may be arrested. Even if the physical disorder is not a direct cause of dementia, the treatment of the former may lead to improvement in the patient's condition.

Behavioural changes ranging from mild disturbance of sleep or appetite to aggression and motor restlessness occur frequently in patients with dementias. Medication should be considered but older people, particularly those with cognitive impairments are especially sensitive to the adverse effects of drugs, and it is important to consider the causes (for example, pain or fear) and non-pharmacological strategies of management before using drugs. Reducing restlessness can be an important first step when the patient is cared for at home by the family, since they are likely to be worn down by this behaviour. CBT-based family intervention can be helpful in reducing the burdens on carers (Marriott *et al.* 2000). For a review of psychosocial interventions see Kasl-Godley and Gatz (2000).

A wide range of drugs has been used for the management of agitation, although there are few well-designed trials in this area. Antidepressants, anxiolytics, and antipsychotic drugs may all have a place. However, in the USA, legislation prohibits the use of neuroleptics for the treatment of agitation and restlessness in patients in nursing homes. Antipsychotic drugs may also be required for paranoid delusions, and antidepressants for severe depressive symptoms. Patients with Lewy body dementia have been reported to be particularly sensitive to the adverse effects of antipsychotic drugs. Newer neuroleptics, such as risperidone, appear to be effective with fewer side-effects (Katz *et al.* 1999). See Alexopoulos *et al.* (1998) for guidelines for the treatment of agitation associated with dementia.

Specific treatment

A wide variety of drugs have been proposed as possible agents in the treatment of Alzheimer's disease. Trials with cholinergic precursors (e.g. lecithin), stimulators of synthesis of acetylcholine, directly acting cholinomimetics and cerebral vasodilators (e.g. naftidrofuryl) have been generally disappointing. There is considerable research continuing into the possibility of interfering with the biochemical pathways by which amyloid protein and paired helical filaments are formed and into other neurochemical mechanisms such as nerve growth factors, in the hope that this may lead to drugs which prevent or retard the progression of the disease. However, several cholinesterase inhibitors have now been licensed in the USA and Europe (e.g. donepezil and rivastigmine), and clinical trials show that these have a limited but definite effect on cognitive and other impairments in Alzheimer's

Table 20.3 Some clinical features distinguishing between delirium and dementia*

Feature	Delirium	Dementia†
Clinical course		
Mode of onset	Acute or subacute (hours or days)	Chronic (usually several years)
Fluctuations	Frequent and rapid (in hours)	Slow changes (months)
Conscious level		
Attention	Markedly reduced	Reduced in severe cases
Arousal	Increased or decreased	Usually normal
Alertness	Reduced in severer cases	Normal
Cognitive changes		
Delusions	Fleeting, poorly systematized	If present, often consistent
Hallucination	Common (usually visual)	Infrequent (both visual and verbal)
Orientation	Usually impaired	Impaired in proportion to severity
Motor features		
Abnormal movements	Tremor and myoclonus	Usually absent
Psychomotor activity	Usually abnormal: increased or decreased	Usually normal
Dysgraphia	Usually present	Absent in mild cases
Autonomic features	Abnormalities often present	Normal (except that postural hypotension is common

* Note that the terminal phase of dementia may be indistinguishable from a chronic delirium.

† The features in this column refer to mild to moderate cases of dementia

Adapted from Fairweather and Stewart (2001)

disease (Cummings 2000). There is no specific treatment for vascular dementia apart from the control of risk factors (e.g. hypertension and diabetes mellitus), low-dose aspirin, and, if indicated, surgical treatment of carotid artery stenosis (see Iversen 2000). See Fleminger (2000) and Rabins *et al.* (1999) for reviews of the management of dementia.

Delirium

Delirium is common in the elderly. Surveys of elderly patients admitted to medical and geriatric wards show that up to a fifth suffer delirium.

The clinical features and management of delirium are discussed on p. 405 (see also Lindesay 2000a; Fairweather and Stewart 2002). In this section, Table 20.3 summarizes the main clinical features distinguishing between delirium and dementia. It should be remembered that delirium is often superimposed on dementia and may account for sudden unexplained deterioration in dementia. The course is frequently a subclinical infection, such as of the urinary tract, treatment of which results in a marked improvement.

Mood disorders

Depressive disorder

Depressive disorders are common in later life, and depressive symptoms are even more frequent. However, the first onset of depressive disorder becomes less common after the age of 60, and rare after the age of 80. A systematic review of community-based studies found an average prevalence of clinically relevant depression of 13.5% for those aged 55 or over, of which 9.8% was classed as minor and 1.8% as major. Prevalences were higher in women and among older people living in adverse circumstances (Beekman *et al.* 1999). Rates of major depression depend on the setting. Koenig and Blazer (1992) reported the following rates: 0.4–1.4% in the community, 5–10% among medical out-patients, 10–15% among medical in-patients, and 15–20% among nursing home patients. It seems that many depressive disorders in elderly patients are frequently not detected by their general practitioners. The incidence of suicide increases steadily with age, and suicide in the elderly is usually associated with depressive disorder.

See Jorm (2000) for a review of epidemiology.

Clinical features

There is no clear distinction between the clinical features of depressive disorders in the elderly and those in younger people, but some symptoms are often more striking in the elderly. Post (1972) reported that a third of depressed elderly patients had severe retardation and agitation. Abas *et al.* (1990) found evidence of cognitive impairment in 70% of elderly patients with a depressive disorder. The pattern suggested impairment on tasks demanding effort, for example, learning and memory, indicating the importance of poor concentration (Austin *et al.* 1992).

Depressive delusions concerning poverty and physical illness are common, and occasionally there are nihilistic delusions such as beliefs that the body is empty, non-existent, or not functioning (see Cotard's syndrome, p. 275). Hallucinations of an accusing or obscene kind may occur. Depression itself is sometimes not conspicuous and may be masked by other symptoms, particularly hypochondriacal complaints. Depressive disorder in the elderly should always be considered when the patient presents with anxiety, hypochondriasis, or confusion.

A small proportion of retarded depressed patients present with 'pseudodementia', i.e. they have conspicuous difficulty in concentration and remembering, but careful clinical testing shows that there is no major defect of memory.

Course and prognosis

Before the introduction of ECT, many depressive disorders in the elderly lasted for years. Nowadays considerable improvement within a few months can be expected in about 85% of admitted patients; the remaining 15% do not recover completely. However, *long-term follow-up* shows a less encouraging picture. Post (1972) reported that patients who recovered in the first few months fell into three groups: one-third remained completely well for 3 years, another third suffered further depressive disorders with complete remissions; and the remaining third developed a state of chronic invalidism punctuated by depressive disorders. More recent studies have generally found a similar outcome.

Factors predicting a good prognosis for depression in old age are:

◆ onset before the age of 70;

◆ short duration of illness;

◆ good previous adjustment;

◆ absence of disabling physical illness;

◆ good recovery from previous episodes.

Poor outcome is associated with the severity of the initial illness, presence of organic cerebral pathology, poor compliance with antidepressant medication, and severe life events in the follow-up period. Physical illness is an important factor determining the outcome of treatment.

Murphy *et al*. (1988) found that depressed patients had a significantly higher mortality than matched controls and that the difference was not entirely due to differences in physical health between the groups when first seen. As explained in Chapter 17 on suicide and deliberate self-harm, suicide is frequent in elderly depressives (Jacoby 2000a).

Despite the poor outlook for depressive disorder in the elderly, only a small number of the patients develop dementia (Roth 1955; Post 1972).

Aetiology

In general, the aetiology of depressive disorders of first onset in late life almost certainly resembles the aetiology of similar disorders at younger ages. However, *genetic factors* may be of less significance. For first-degree relatives, the risk is 4–5% with elderly probands, as against 10–12% with young and middle-aged probands (Mendlewicz 1976). However, the recent evidence is complex in that age of onset and whether the depressive illness is of the recurrent or non-recurrent type appear to be independent variables. This means that up to a third of those with late-onset depression may give a family history of depression.

It might be expected that the *loneliness and hardship* of old age would be important predisposing factors for depressive disorder. Surprisingly, there is no convincing evidence for such an association (Murphy 1982). Indeed, Parkes *et al*. (1969) even found that the association between bereavement and mental illness no longer held in the aged.

Although *neurological and other physical illnesses* are slightly more frequent among depressed compared with non-depressed elderly patients, there is no evidence that they have a specific aetiological role. Instead, such illnesses appear to act as non-specific precipitants.

Differential diagnosis

It is sometimes difficult to distinguish between *depressive pseudodementia* and *dementia*. It is essential to obtain a detailed history from other informants and to make careful observations of mental state and behaviour. In depressive pseudodementia, a history of mood disturbance usually precedes the other symptoms. The depressed patient's unwillingness to answer questions during mental state examination can usually be distinguished from the demented patient's failure of memory. In dementia impairment is global; depressed patients are likely to have partial deficits. Psychological testing is often said to be useful, but it requires experienced interpretation and it usually adds little to skilful clinical assessment. At times, dementia and depressive illness coexist. If there is real doubt, a trial of antidepressant treatment may be appropriate.

Less frequently, depressive disorder has to be differentiated from a *paranoid disorder*. When persecutory ideas occur in a depressive disorder, the patient usually believes that the supposed persecution is justified by his wickedness (see p. 275). Particular diagnostic difficulty may occur with the small group of patients who suffer from schizoaffective illness in old age (see p. 631).

Treatment

The principles of the treatment of depressive disorders are the same as for younger adults. They are described in Chapter 11 (p. 316). With elderly patients it is especially important to be aware of the risk of suicide. Any intercurrent physical disorder should be thoroughly treated.

Antidepressants are effective, but should be used cautiously, perhaps starting with half the normal dosage and adjusting this in relation to side-effects and response. The aim is to start with a lower dose, to achieve a therapeutic dose more slowly than for a young adult, and to be aware that the therapeutic dose might be lower (especially with tricyclics). Some psychiatrists prefer to start treatment with a tricyclic antidepressant; others prefer specific serotonin re-uptake inhibitor (SSRI) antidepressants or newer combined serotonin and noradrenaline re-uptake inhibitors because they have fewer side-effects and are less cardiotoxic. Although it is appropriate to start drug treatment cautiously, it is equally important to ensure that an adequate final dose is achieved.

For patients who do not respond to the full dose of an antidepressant, it may be necessary to use a combination of drugs as in younger patients (see p. 318). However, before changing treatment it should be remembered that the compliance with drugs is often poor in elderly patients.

ECT is usually appropriate for depressive disorder with severe and distressing agitation, suicidal ideas and behaviour, life-threatening stupor, or failure to respond to drugs. If the patient is unduly confused after ECT, treatments should be given at longer intervals (see p. 641). If a patient has previously responded to antidepressants or ECT, but does not respond in the present episode, undetected physical illness is a likely cause.

After recovery, full-dosage antidepressant medication should be continued for at least several months, as in younger patients (see p. 321). The evidence suggests that in older people treatment should continue for considerably longer and possibly permanently (Old Age Depression

Interest Group 1993). See Baldwin (2000, 2002) for reviews of mood disorder in the elderly.

Mania

Mania accounts for between 5 and 10% of affective illnesses in old age. Unlike depressive disorder, mania does not increase in incidence with age. Broadhead and Jacoby (1990), in the first prospective study of mania in old age, found that the clinical picture was the same as in younger patients but that a depressive episode, immediately after the manic episode occurs more frequently in older patients.

Management is similar to that described for younger patients (p. 322). Lithium prophylaxis is valuable, but the blood levels should be monitored with special care and should be kept at the lower end of the therapeutic range used for younger patients. See Shulman (2002) for a review of mania in old age.

Schizoaffective disorder

In a study of patients aged over 60 admitted to hospital, Post (1971) found that 4% had schizoaffective disorders (i.e. disorders with a more or less equal mixture of the symptoms of schizophrenia and mood disorder) or a schizophrenic illness followed by a mood disorder or vice versa. Intermediate and long-term outcomes were less favourable for these conditions than for depressive disorder. The treatment of this disorder in the elderly is the same as that for younger patients (see p. 343).

Anxiety disorders and personality disorder

In later life, emotional disorders are seldom causes for referral to a psychiatrist, although this may be largely because of non-presentation by patients and lack of recognition or referral by general practitioners.

In general practice, Shepherd *et al.* (1966) found that, after the age of 55, the incidence of new cases of neurosis (i.e. anxiety disorder) declined; however, the frequency of consultations with the general practitioner for neurosis did not fall – presumably as a result of chronic or recurrent cases. Surveys in the general population indicate that after the age of 65 some new cases of emotional disorder appear, with a prevalence of cases of at least moderate severity of about 12% (Kay and Bergmann 1980). Anxiety disorders among the elderly are often non-specific, with symptoms of both anxiety and depression. Hypochondriacal symptoms may be prominent. Dissociative and conversion disorder, obsessional disorder, and phobic disorders are less common. It is now evident that all anxiety disorders are clinically much more important than had been previously recognized. For a review see Lindesay (2000b, 2001). For a review of anxiety see Stanley and Beck (2000).

Personality disorder is an important predisposing factor in most anxious elderly patients. Physical illness is a frequent precipitant, and retirement, bereavement, and change of accommodation are other causes.

In differential diagnosis it is important to differentiate between chronic anxiety (present continuously or intermittently) and new symptoms. It is wise to consider that the latter may be due to a depressive disorder until proved otherwise.

Personality disorder causes many problems for elderly patients and their families (Holroyd 2000). Paranoid traits may become accentuated with the social isolation of old age, sometimes to the extent of being mistaken for a paranoid disorder (see below).

Abnormal personality is one of the causes of the *senile squalor syndrome*, in which elderly people become isolated and neglect themselves in filthy conditions. Such gross self-neglect is often associated with social isolation and physical illness, and is associated with a high mortality after hospital admission. It is often difficult to decide when to intervene and when to use compulsory powers.

Criminal behaviour is unusual in the elderly (Fazel and Jacoby 2002). In England and Wales in 1989 about 1% of males found guilty of indictable offences were aged 60 and older, whereas 36% were aged under 21.

The treatment of anxiety disorders and personality disorders in old age is generally similar to that in younger adult life. It is essential to treat any physical disorder.

Schizophrenia-like and paranoid states in the elderly

Kraepelin introduced the term paraphrenia in 1909 to describe patients with chronic delusions and hallucinations without the characteristic personality deterioration of dementia praecox. Mayer (later known as Mayer-Gross) followed up these patients and, over 10 years later, found that just under half showed a typical schizophrenic decline. In 1955, Roth introduced the term late paraphrenia for paranoid conditions starting after the age of 60 'in a setting of well preserved personality and affective response'. Although other terms such as 'persistent persecutory states' and 'late-onset schizophrenia' have been suggested, late paraphrenia is still widely used. However, this term is slowly being abandoned in favour of others which will appear in future versions of ICD and DSM. 'Late schizophrenia' will refer to psychoses of onset between 40 and 50 years of age, whereas 'very-late-onset-schizophrenia-like-psychosis' will cover psychoses arising after 60 years of age (Howard *et al.* 2000). The use of this term does not prejudge the question of whether very-late-onset-schizophrenia-like psychosis is essentially paranoid schizophrenia of delayed onset or a distinct entity.

Neither ICD-10 nor DSM-IV has a clear and unequivocal place for late paraphrenia. In both systems cases have to be fitted into one of several categories according to the pattern and duration of symptoms, paranoid schizophrenia, delusional disorder, and schizoaffective disorder.

Patients with 'very-late-onset-schizophrenia-like-psychosis' form approximately 10% of admissions to psychiatric wards for the elderly. There are no good data on the prevalence in the community because it is difficult to identify all cases of a condition in which many sufferers keep their experience to themselves for as long as they can and are unlikely to cooperate with 'doorstep' interviews.

Aetiology

A number of aetiological factors have emerged from research into late paraphrenia compared with aged-matched controls. *Premorbid personality* of people with late paraphrenia is characterized by poor adjustment, as suggested by lower marriage and child-bearing rates. Many patients have good work and social records. However, they tend to form fewer close personal relationships than others of their generation and to be prickly, querulous, and unapproachable.

Cooper *et al.* (1974) found that *conductive deafness* of onset in earlier middle life, a factor which increases social isolation, was significantly more common in late paraphrenia.

A consistent finding in late paraphrenia is an *excess of females* over males in a ratio of about 7:1. This compares with younger schizophrenic patients who tend to show a more or less equal sex distribution over the period of risk.

Genetically, patients with late paraphrenia occupy an intermediate position between the unaffected population and those with schizophrenia of earlier onset. In one study (Kay 1972), the risk of schizophrenia in first-degree relatives was found to be 3.4% in late paraphrenics compared with 5.8% in young schizophrenics and less than 1% in the general population.

Clinical features

The predominant clinical feature of late paraphrenia is delusional thought. Delusions are mostly of persecution, usually more commonplace and narrowly centred than those found in paranoid schizophrenia of earlier life. Thus, where a younger paranoid schizophrenic patient may assert a plot by extraterrestial beings, an older late paraphrenic is more likely to complain that the neighbours are plotting to kill her or impugning her sexual virtue.

Hallucinations are characteristic in late paraphrenia. The most common are auditory; tactile and olfactory hallucinations are not infrequent, but visual hallucinations are rare. Naguib and Levy (1987) observed mild cognitive impairment in late paraphrenic patients compared with controls, but this finding may have been due to factors such as medication, poor concentration, or coincidental organic cerebral disease. Holden (1987) followed up patients with late paraphrenia and found the outcome to be heterogeneous with some developing dementia. Although there are these differences between some cases of late paraphrenia and paranoid schizophrenia, other cases are closely similar.

Treatment

Some 50–75% of patients with late paraphrenia may show a full or partial response to antipsychotic drugs. Although it is uncommon for symptoms to remit completely, the delusional beliefs usually become encapsulated so that patients can often return to the premorbid level of functioning. Follow-up usually requires the help of a community psychiatric nurse who should strike a balance between seeing the patient regularly and persuading him to accept medication, and appearing too intrusive so that the patient refuses treatment. The premorbid personality factors described above make it necessary to try hard to win patients' trust so that they are more likely to comply with treatment. They may be more willing to accept medication as helping with a stressful situation rather than as a specific treatment of a psychiatric illness. Many patients have to be admitted to hospital to start treatment. See Howard (2000) and Howard and Levy (2002) for reviews.

Abuse and neglect of the elderly

Abuse and neglect of the elderly by other family members is often overlooked. The types of abuse are physical, psychological, and financial, through violation of rights, and by active and passive neglect. Women are more often affected than men, and those who have physical illness or psychiatric disorder are most at risk. Abuse is usually by a relative and is often repeated. It may take the form of neglect or forced confinement, which may be shown in failure to thrive. Also, property may be misused. Dementia and the demands it makes of carers may predispose to abuse (Hirsch and Vollhardt 2002).

Organization of services

National policies for the provision of services for the elderly differ widely. In the USA, emphasis has been placed on care in hospitals and nursing homes. In Europe, Canada, and Australasia, there has been varying emphasis on social policies to provide sheltered accommodation and care in the community. In this section, services in the UK will be described as an example. Health, social, and voluntary services will be described separately, although good care depends on close collaboration at all levels, from strategic planning to the coordinated provision of care to each individual patient.

Health services

Primary health care

In the UK, general practitioners, together with district nurses, manage most of the problems of mentally ill older people without referring them to specialists. However, as already mentioned, general practitioners do not detect all the psychiatric problems of the elderly at an early stage, nor do they always provide all the necessary long-term medical supervision. These problems are partly due to lack of awareness of the significance of psychiatric illness among the elderly, and partly to the provision of a service in which doctors respond to requests from patients rather than seeking out their problems. Some old age psychiatry services will only accept referrals from a general practitioner,

but increasingly referrals may be accepted directly from any source, though liaison with the general practitioner will always be important. In a few areas, general practices themselves employ community psychiatric nurses (CPNs), though it is more usual for CPNs to be part of secondary care (hospital-based) teams.

Old age psychiatry services

The organization of psychiatric services varies in different localities, since it reflects the local styles of service providers, local needs, and the extent of provision for this age group by general psychiatric services, as well as national policies. Nevertheless, there are some general principles of planning. The aims should be to maintain the elderly person at home for as long as possible, to respond quickly to medical and social problems as they rise, to ensure coordination of the work of those providing continuing care, and to support relatives and others who care for the elderly person at home. There should be close liaison with primary care, other hospital specialists who may be involved, with social services, and with voluntary agencies. A multidisciplinary approach should be adopted with a clinical team that may include psychiatrists, psychologists, community psychiatric nurses, and social workers. Some members of the team should spend more of their working day in patients' homes and in general practices than in the hospital. The contributions of the various parts of a service will now be considered.

In the UK, specialist (secondary) care for older people with mental health problems includes both assessment and treatment of acute conditions, and long-term care. Old age psychiatry services may offer assessment and treatment either in the patient's home (domiciliary care), or in day hospitals, or in in-patient units.

Domiciliary psychiatric care

Increasingly, assessments and treatments are offered in the patient's own home, which is both more convenient for the patient and offers a more relevant assessment of the difficulties facing the patient and carers. Community psychiatric nurses act as a bridge between primary care and specialist services. The nurses may assess referrals from general practitioners, monitor treatment in collaboration with general practitioners and the psychiatric services, and take part in the organization of home support for the demented elderly.

Out-patient clinics

Out-patient clinics have a smaller part to play in providing care for the elderly than for younger patients because assessment at home is particularly important for old people. However, such clinics are convenient for the assessment and follow-up of mobile patients. There are advantages when these clinics are staffed jointly by medical geriatricians and old age psychiatrists. In some areas, memory clinics have been developed for the specialist assessment of patients with early memory problems (Wilcock *et al.* 1999).

Day hospitals

Although some treatments can be provided at home, others may require the patient to attend a day hospital, where a high level of stimulation and social interaction can also be provided. In the 1950s, day care began in geriatric hospitals. A few years later the first psychiatric day hospitals for the elderly were opened. Psychiatric day hospitals should provide a full range of diagnostic services and offer both short-term and continuing care for patients with functional or organic disorders, together with support for relatives. A much smaller number of patients will need to be admitted to in-patient units for assessment and treatment.

In-patient units

In-patient teams should be able to provide multi-disciplinary assessment and treatment of patients with severe mental health problems. In addition to psychiatrists and psychiatric nurses, teams may include occupational therapists, psychologists, speech and language therapists, physiotherapists, social workers, health care assistants, and others. There is substantial variation in different areas as to the composition of the team and as to whether patients with functional illnesses are cared for separate from or together with those with organic disorders.

Geriatric medicine

There is inevitably some overlap in the characteristics of patients treated by units for geriatric medicine and those treated in psychiatry units. Both types of unit are likely to treat patients with a dementia, although old age psychiatry units are more likely than geriatric units to treat patients with functional psychiatric disorders.

In the past there was considerable concern that many patients were 'misplaced' and therefore received poor treatment, stayed too long in hospital, and had an unsatisfactory outcome. Research has generally not confirmed these concerns. For example, Copeland *et al.* (1975) found that although 64% of patients admitted to geriatric hospitals were psychiatrically ill, only 12% appeared to be wrongly placed. Moreover, the outcome of these misplaced patients did not appear to be affected adversely: it seems that many patients can be cared for equally well in either type of hospital. The optimal placement of the rest depends on the relative predominance of behavioural or physical disorder. Medical and psychiatric teams need to cooperate closely if all patients are to receive appropriate treatment.

Long term hospital care

In many countries, most elderly psychiatric patients are still treated in the wards of psychiatric hospitals. However, the nature of the care provided is more important than the type of institution in which it is given. The basic requirements are opportunities for privacy and the use of personal possessions, together with occupational and social therapy. Provided that these criteria are met, long-term hospital care can be the best provision for very disabled patients. Increasingly in the UK, hospital provision of long-term care has been reduced (with some increase in the level of community care), and long-term care is largely provided outside hospital in residential and nursing homes. There is an active debate on how long-term care should be funded, since care provided by the NHS is free whilst care provided through the social services is means tested (Royal Commission on Long Term Care 1999).

Community care

Care provided in a person's home may come from a number of different agencies, the general practitioner and district nurse, the community mental health team (a multidisciplinary team, often linked closely with a psychiatric hospital, but whose members work largely in the community), the social services, and the voluntary sector. It is important that the care provided by these different agencies is coordinated, and in the UK, the Care Programme Approach is intended to improve coordination by making a single person, the key worker, responsible for ensuring that appropriate assessment, care planning, and review takes place.

Social services

Domiciliary services

In addition to medical services, domiciliary services include home helps, meals at home, laundry, telephone, and emergency call systems. In the UK, local authorities both provide and commission these services; they also support voluntary organizations and encourage local initiatives such as good neighbour schemes and self-help groups. In a random sample of nearly 500 people aged 65 and over living at home, Foster *et al*. (1976) found that 12% were receiving domiciliary services but a further 20% still needed them. Although these provisions are increasing, so are the numbers of those requiring them. Bergmann *et al*. (1978) have argued that if resources are limited, more should be directed to patients living with their families than to those living alone. This is because the former can often remain at home if they receive such help, whereas many of the latter require admission before long, even when extra help is given.

Day care

In the UK, whilst the health services provide psychiatric day hospitals for assessment and treatment, day-care provisions by social services include day centres and social clubs. They also often involve voluntary sector organizations such as Age Concern and the Alzheimer's Disease Society. They can assist severely demented patients who do not require regular medical or nursing care. All arrangements depend crucially on adequate transport facilities.

Residential and nursing care

Older people may need a variety of social service accommodation, ranging from entirely independent housing through sheltered housing schemes, where there may be some communal provision, often including access to a warden, to residential or nursing homes where there are staff available at all times. There is a need for special housing for the elderly, conveniently sited and easy to run. Ideally, the elderly should be able to transfer to more sheltered accommodation if they become more disabled, without losing all independence or moving away from familiar places. In many communities in the UK, there is still not enough variety of accommodation offering a range of independence. Provision of this kind is better in many parts of Europe, the USA, and Australasia (Grundy 1987).

'Continuing care' refers to the provision of homes where staff are available on site at all times. In residential homes, the needs of residents for assistance with personal care can be met by care assistants with relatively little training, whereas in nursing homes residents will have need for regular nursing care, and therefore the staff will include a substantial number of trained nurses. Some, but not all, nursing homes specialize in the care of older people with mental health problems.

In the UK, local social services are responsible for providing residential homes and other sheltered accommodation, although many independent organizations and charities also provide residential homes for older people. The growth of continuing care provision in the private sector has had some advantages in encouraging a greater variety of facilities, but in some places undue emphasis on the cost rather than the standard of care, together with a lack of coordinated planning, has made it difficult to develop integrated local services to meet the needs of the elderly. Over the past two decades there has been a steady rise in the level of disability of residents in residential homes.

Other countries have different systems of care and elderly people with similar problems receive different forms of care. For example, there are considerably more hospital beds per unit of population for the elderly in Scandinavia than in the UK; there are also more residential places which are more varied and of better quality, and generally offer greater privacy and freedom of choice.

In the USA in the past, the main emphasis in long-term care was on nursing homes, but this is changing to a wider range of provisions. However, many of these provisions are privately funded and the less well off elderly are unable to afford them. Further difficulties have arisen from the closure of state psychiatric hospitals, limitation of the number of nursing home beds, and restrictions of Medicare and Medicaid funding. Despite an increasing interest in the psychiatric care of the elderly, it is unlikely that resources will increase to keep pace with the rate of increase of the number of the elderly.

In the USA, the care of those aged 65 accounts for approximately one-third of all health-care expenditure, with two-thirds being financed by the federal government, principally by Medicare. Unfortunately, the low rates of reimbursement compared with the fees usually expected mean that it is difficult for the elderly to obtain appropriate out-patient psychiatric care and there are few home visits.

Voluntary services

As indicated above, voluntary agencies play a large role in the provision of facilities and support to patients, their families, and carers. It is essential that their contributions are integrated with health and social service provisions.

Informal carers

Informal carers are those unpaid relatives, neighbours, or friends who look after disabled (usually demented) elderly persons at home. The term differentiates these people from formal carers such as paid home helps and district or community psychiatric nurses. Informal carers provide substantially more care to older people than do the statutory services, and their role in the overall provision of care should not be underestimated. Most informal carers of older people are (in descending order of frequency) spouses, adult daughters, or sons. About twice as many women as men are informal carers. About half of all informal carers are themselves elderly.

Several studies have shown that patients suffering from dementia place the greatest stress on carers (Baumgarten *et al.* 1994). In general, the more severe the dementia, the greater the strain. Incontinence, behavioural disturbance at night, and aggression are the most distressing problems for carers. As assessed by the General Health Questionnaire, many carers have symptoms as severe as those of a psychiatric case. Symptoms diminish when the patient has moved to permanent residential care (Morris *et al.* 1988; Henderson 1990).

Accurate assessment of carers' needs is important (see Table 20.4), and in the UK, social services now have a statutory responsibility to provide this, where requested. Time should be spent with family carers in giving advice about the care of patients and discussing their problems. Such support can help families avoid some of the frustration and anxiety of caring for elderly relatives. Published guides are useful. Other practical help may include day-care or holiday admissions, and laundry and meal services to the home. With such assistance many patients can remain in their own homes without imposing an unreasonable burden on their families. The assessment of need and carer support may often need to be multidisciplinary; both community psychiatric nurses and care managers (social workers) play essential roles in coordinating these services, supporting relatives, and providing direct nursing care.

Management of mental health problems in the elderly

Table 20.4 Support for carers
Levin (1997) made the following 10 key recommendations for comprehensive support for carers:
1. early identification of dementia (the role of primary care practitioners is vital);
2. comprehensive medical and social assessment of identified cases;
3. timely referrals between agencies, for example, from general practitioner to old age psychiatrist;
4. continuing reviews of each patient's needs, and backup for carers;
5. active medical treatment for any intercurrent illness;
6. the provision of information, advice, counselling for carers;
7. regular help with household and personal care tasks;
8. regular breaks for carers, for example, by providing day care and respite care for the patient;
9. appropriate financial support;
10. permanent residential care when this becomes necessary.

Principles of assessment

The purpose of assessment is broadly to develop a plan of care which will assist the patient and those involved in caring for him to ensure that the care provided is as good as circumstances will allow. This will usually extend beyond a strictly medical understanding of the patient's conditions and its medical treatment to include assessment of the wider psychosocial situation, taking account not only of the patient's needs but also those of carers and other involved people. On some occasions it may be that diagnostic information is all that is required, although more usually there will be wider management questions.

The referral

It is important to establish at the outset what prompted the referral, and what is hoped to be gained from it. This may well require information to be collected even before the patient is seen, not least in order to establish the most useful way to approach the assessment. In any one case, each person involved in care may have different, and possibly conflicting, needs.

Informants

Many old people seen by psychiatrists are unable to give complete or reliable information about themselves. Frequently there is a partner or other close relative living with the patient, but in other cases it may be necessary to talk to neighbours or friends. It may be useful to spend considerable time telephoning relatives or others who may be able to give information about family history or previous personality. Many patients seen for the first time will already be well known to their primary care physician and to other professionals and it is essential to consult them.

Where to assess the patient

In the UK, most old age psychiatrists prefer to assess patients *in their own homes*. This enables much essential information about the patient's ability to function at home to be gained, and avoids the patient appearing excessively disorientated simply because of the disturbing effect of having to travel to a hospital for assessment in an unfamiliar environment. It is also likely to make it easier to interview other members of the family, and to assess the level of support from neighbours or outside carers, who may be prepared to be available at the patient's home at the time of the assessment.

Old age psychiatrists may also be asked to assess patients on *general hospital wards*. Although this will normally provide much less information about the patients circumstances, it has the advantage of making close liaison with the hospital team possible. Conditions on hospital wards are often unfavourable for a quiet, private interview, but it is important to spend time reading the notes carefully, talking to nursing and other staff, and then requesting the use of an office or side room in which to see the patient. Even if the family or other carers cannot be present, it may be possible to telephone them. Increasingly, some patients with early cognitive impairments are being offered assessments in a *memory clinic*, usually in a hospital out-patient setting. For some patients this offers advantages of a systematic and detailed assessment, and enables relevant further investigations and follow-up to be arranged as efficiently as possible. Similar principles apply to assessment in *residential and nursing homes.*

Whatever the setting in which the assessment takes place, a wide range of information needs to be collected. The elements of the history and examination are not different from those in other areas of psychiatry, but great emphasis will need to be placed on the effect that the symptoms are having on the patient's life and level of function, the impact of this on others, the source and extent of support from both informal and professional carers, and on concurrent physical problems.

The history

The information required about the medical and psychiatric history is the same as in younger patients. However, it may be necessary to piece it together from accounts given by the patient and by other informants. It is of particular importance to obtain a clear medical history and to determine past and present medication.

Mental state

A great deal can be learned from the appearance of the patient, the home environment, and from behaviour during the assessment.

Cognitive examination is important and many psychiatrists use standardized questionnaires, such as the Mini-Mental State Examination (MMSE) (see p. 68). No standard questionnaire is adequate by itself; the questionnaire needs to be supplemented by questions covering the main areas of cognitive function.

Physical assessment

Since physical problems are extremely common, the psychiatrist needs to be able to conduct a physical examination. Laboratory investigations are important for admitted patients and others with significant psychiatric disorder (for investigation of dementia see p. 626).

Assessment of carers' needs

Most elderly people with mental disorders live in their own homes and are cared for by family or, occasionally, by good neighbours or friends. The considerable burden on such carers should be assessed (Table 20.4). For a review of the assessment of patients and carers see Jacoby (2000b).

Principles of treatment

Essentially, the psychiatric treatment of the elderly resembles that of other adults, but there are differences in emphasis. If practicable, treatment at home is generally preferable to that in hospital, not only because most elderly people want to be at home, but also because they are likely to function best there. Home treatment requires a willingness on the part of the doctor to be flexible and responsive to changing needs, to arrange a plan with the family, to organize appropriate day care or help, and to admit the patient to hospital should it become necessary. Ethical and legal issues may need to be considered (Box 20.1).

An important part of the old age psychiatrist's role is to work with others to develop *comprehensive collaborative care* which addresses as many of the patient's problems as possible, and this is likely to involve close liaison with the GP, social services, and often voluntary agencies.

Older people often suffer from *multiple disabilities*, and much may be achieved by minimizing the

Confidentiality in relation to information from carers

Confidentiality of information about financial circumstances

Consent to treatment

- Capacity to consent to physical and psychological treatment
- Advance directives
- Decisions 'not to treat'

Damaging behaviour

Management of financial affairs

- Nominating another to take responsibility (Power of Attorney)
- Procedures to enable others to take responsibility

Entitlement to drive a car

Research (see Chapter 6)

Priority setting resource allocation for the elderly

impact of any of these which can be improved. The treatment of physical disorders, however minor, can also benefit the mental state; for example, a urinary tract infection may cause mild delirium which adds to the features of dementia and improves with treatment. Mobility should be encouraged and physiotherapy is often helpful. A good diet should be arranged. For a review of treatment of the elderly see Oppenheimer (2000).

Physical treatment

Use of drugs

Substantially more psychotropic and non-psychotropic drugs are prescribed for the elderly than for younger people. *Drug-induced morbidity* is a major medical problem, partly because the pharmacokinetics of drugs are different in old people. Most problems arise with drugs used to treat cardiovascular disorders (hypotensives, diuretics, and digoxin) and those acting on the central nervous system (antidepressants, hypnotics, anxiolytics, antipsychotics, and antiparkinsonian drugs).

It is essential to restrict the number of drugs to avoid harmful drug interactions and prudent to start with small doses, and to increase doses slowly. Medication should be reviewed regularly and kept to a minimum.

Compliance with treatment is a problem in elderly patients, especially in those who live alone, have poor vision or are confused. The drug regimen should be as simple as possible, medicine bottles should be labelled clearly, and memory aids, such as packs containing the drugs to be taken on a single day with daily dose requirements, should be provided. If possible, drug taking should be supervised and the patient's response watched carefully. In these aspects of treatment, as in many others, domiciliary care plays a vital part.

Despite the need for caution in prescribing, elderly patients should not be denied effective drug treatment, especially for depressive disorders. Antidepressant medication should be started cautiously and increased gradually.

Poor sleep

Many elderly people sleep poorly, and about 20% of those aged over 70 take hypnotics regularly. Simple measures, such as avoidance of stimulants before going to bed, taking exercise earlier in the day, having a warm drink, not going to bed until completely ready for sleep (see p. 439) are helpful. It is important to treat any specific physical or other causes of sleeplessness and also to review existing medication to identify drugs that may be increasing sleeplessness.

Hypnotic drugs often cause adverse side-effects in the elderly, notably daytime drowsiness leading to confusion, falls, incontinence, and hypothermia. Some psychiatrists consider that benzodiazepines are specially liable to cause delirium; chlormethiazole, chloral, dichloralphenazone, and trazodone in low doses are useful as alternatives. If a hypnotic is essential, the minimum effective dose should be used and the effects monitored carefully. For a review of the treatment of sleep disturbance see Martin *et al* (2000).

Electroconvulsive therapy

ECT is one of the most effective treatments for serious depressive disorder in the elderly. In patients with cognitive impairment, ECT may be followed by temporary memory impairment and confusion so that longer intervals between treatments are advisable. Particular attention should be paid to the physical health of elderly patients undergoing this treatment, and physically frail patients should be assessed by an experienced anaesthetist before receiving ECT. Advanced age is not a contraindication for ECT.

Psychological treatment

Supportive therapy with clearly defined aims is often helpful, and joint interviews with the spouse are sometimes required. *Family therapy* is increasingly widely used. Interpretative psychotherapy is seldom appropriate for the elderly.

Cognitive and behavioural treatments are increasingly used in the treatment of elderly psychiatric patients (Thompson *et al.* 1987; Fisher and Carstensen 1990). Behavioural methods have been used with demented patients to reduce problems in continence, eating behaviours, or social skills. Memory aids such as notebooks and alarm clocks have been used to assist patients with memory disorder.

Reality orientation therapy, *reminiscence therapy*, and *validation therapy* were all developed for elderly patients in particular, but are perhaps more successful in encouraging positive attitudes amongst carers than in producing identifiable behavioural outcomes (Holden and Woods 1995). See Woods and Charlesworth (2002) for a review of psychological assessment and treatment.

Psychosocial treatment

Some patients can achieve independence through measures to encourage self-care, and domestic skills, and to increase social contacts. More severely impaired patients can benefit from an environment in which individual needs and dignity are respected and each person retains some personal possessions. Disorientation can be reduced by the general design of the ward and the use of aids such as colour codes on doors. For those living at home, a domiciliary occupational therapist may be helpful in advising on environmental or other modifications which will help the patient to live in a more independent way.

Legal and financial issues

Financial affairs

Older people, particularly those with mental health problems, may have difficulty in managing their financial affairs. In the UK, if the issues are relatively simple, for example, involving only a state pension and benefits, the person can request that someone else, known as an appointee, collects these benefits on his behalf. Alternatively, while the person still has mental capacity to understand what is involved, he can make an Enduring Power of Attorney in favour of one or more others. The attorney then has authority to carry out any financial transaction on behalf of that person. If the donor of the power subsequently becomes mentally unable to manage his own affairs, the attorney may continue to do so on his behalf (in the UK, provided the arrangement is registered with the Court of Protection). Sometimes a person becomes mentally incapable of managing his affairs without having made any formal arrangement for someone else to act on his behalf; under these circumstances, an application supported by medical evidence of incapacity may be made to the Court of Protection for a receiver to be appointed to manage his affairs. It is important to note that all these provisions apply only to financial affairs, and do not carry any authority to make treatment decisions on behalf of the patient.

Driving

A common practical problem is the inability of older patients with early cognitive impairment to drive safely. Doctors generally have an obligation, which overrides confidentiality, to inform authorities responsible for the provision of driving licences.

Testamentary capacity

In England and Wales, in order to execute a valid will, the testator must be of 'sound disposing mind' at the time at which the will is made. The criteria for this are:

- that he must understand that he is giving his property to one or more objects of his regard;
- that he understands and recollects the extent of his property; and
- that he understands the nature and extent of the claims on him both of those he is

including and those he is excluding from his will.

See Posenor and Jacoby (2001) for a review. See also p. 82.

Further reading

Gelder, M. G., López-Ibor Jr, J. J., and Andreason, N. C. (eds) (2000). *The new Oxford textbook of psychiatry*, Section 8: The psychiatry of old age. Oxford University Press, Oxford.

Jacoby, R. and Oppenheimer, C. (eds) (2002). *Psychiatry in the elderly*, 3rd edn. Oxford University Press, Oxford. (An essential reference work with authoritative chapters by leading research workers. An excellent source of further references.)

CHAPTER 21

Drugs and other physical treatments

Drugs and other physical treatments

This chapter is concerned with the use of drugs and other physical treatments such as electroconvulsive therapy and psychosurgical procedures. Psychological treatments are the subject of Chapter 22. This separation, although convenient when treatments are described, does not imply that the two kinds of therapy are to be thought of as exclusive alternatives when an individual patient is considered; on the contrary, many patients require both. In this book, the ways of combining treatments are considered in other chapters where the treatment of individual syndromes is discussed. It is important to keep this point in mind when reading this chapter and the next.

Our concern is with clinical therapeutics rather than basic psychopharmacology, which the reader is assumed to have studied already. An adequate knowledge of the mechanisms of drug action is essential if drugs are to be used in a rational way, but a word of caution is appropriate. The clinician should not assume that the therapeutic effects of psychotropic drugs are necessarily explained by the pharmacological actions that have been discovered so far. For example, substantial delay in the effects of antidepressant and antipsychotic drugs suggests that their actions on transmitters, which occur rapidly, are only the first steps in a chain of biochemical changes.

This caution does not imply that a knowledge of pharmacological mechanisms has no bearing on psychiatric therapeutics. On the contrary, there have been substantial advances in pharmacological knowledge since the first psychotropic drugs were introduced in the 1950s, and it is increasingly important for the clinician to relate this knowledge to his use of drugs.

History of physical treatments

Physical treatments have been applied to patients with psychiatric disorders since antiquity, though, in retrospect, the most that could be claimed for the best of these interventions is that they were relatively harmless. Of course, the same holds for the management of patients with general medical disorders, for which similar treatments, such as bleeding and purging, were often used regardless of diagnosis. It is wise not to be too censorious about the treatment of disorders of which the aetiology is still largely unknown, but to bear in mind that 'it may well be that in a hundred years current therapies, psychotherapies as well as physical therapies, will be looked upon as similarly uncouth and improbable' (Kiloh *et al.* 1988).

Historically, physical treatments can be divided into two main classes:

◆ those that were aimed at producing a direct change in a *pathophysiological process*, usually by some alteration in brain function;

◆ those that were aimed at producing symptomatic improvement through a *dramatic psychological impact*.

The latter interventions were often based on philosophical theories about the moral basis of madness. For example, many physicians appear to have followed the proposal of Heinroth (1773–1843) that insanity was the product of evil and personal wrongdoing. Accordingly, restraint with chains and corporal punishment were seen as appropriate remedies. Other physical treatments, such as the spinning chair introduced by Erasmus Darwin (1731–1802), seemed designed to produce a general 'shock to the system', and perhaps thereby interrupt the morbid preoccupations of the patient. A less arduous regimen was the use of continuous warm baths, often given in combination with cold packs. This treatment was recommended by clinicians as distinguished as Connolly (1794–1866) and Kraepelin (1856–1926), and was still in use at the Bethlem Hospital in the 1950s.

Drugs that produce changes in the function of the central nervous system, such as opiates and anticholinergic agents, have been used in the treatment of mental disorders for hundreds of years. Whilst some of these drugs may sometimes have had calming effects, they were of no specific value in the treatment of psychiatric disorders. Often a physical treatment was used, not because of proven efficacy, but because it was recommended by an eminent and vigorous physician. Also, the assessment of efficacy depended almost entirely on uncontrolled clinical observation.

In 1933, about 10 years after the isolation of insulin by Banting and Best, Sakel introduced *insulin coma treatment* for psychosis (Sakel 1938). A suitable dose of insulin was used to produce a coma, which was terminated by either tube feeding or intravenous glucose. A course of treatment could include up to 60 comas. Not surprisingly, serious side-effects were common, and a mortality of at least 1% could be expected depending on the standard of the clinic and on the physical state of the patient. Insulin coma treatment was rapidly taken up throughout Europe and many specialized treatment units were built. There was a great improvement in the morale of patients and staff because of the belief that this dramatic treatment could cure symptoms of some of the most serious psychiatric disorders.

There were always some doctors who doubted the efficacy of insulin coma treatment. Their doubts were reinforced by a controlled trial by Ackner and Oldham (1962), who found that, in patients with schizophrenia, insulin coma was no more effective than a similar period of unconsciousness induced by barbiturates. This study was published about the time when chlorpromazine was introduced, and

both factors led to a rapid decline in the use of insulin coma treatment. It should be noted that some controlled studies did not exclude the efficacy of insulin treatment in some circumstances, and a number of workers continued to maintain that it was effective. Therefore it is interesting that recent experimental studies have shown that insulin administration causes striking changes in the release of monoamine neurotransmitters in the brain. Perhaps the main lesson to be learned from insulin coma treatment is that the introduction of a new medical treatment should be preceded by adequate controlled trials to determine whether it is therapeutically more effective or safer than current therapies (see Chapter 6). This lesson is particularly important in psychiatry because the aetiology of some disorders may be obscure and outcome may vary widely, even amongst patients with the same clinical syndrome.

Electroconvulsive therapy (ECT) was introduced about the same time as insulin coma treatment. Unlike the latter, ECT has retained a place in current clinical practice. The rationale for convulsive therapy was a postulated antagonism between schizophrenia and convulsions such that the one would exclude the other. This view is erroneous in so far as schizophrenia-like illnesses are more common in patients with temporal lobe epilepsy than would be expected by chance (see p. 436). Astute clinical observation, in combination with controlled trials, has shown that ECT is effective in the acute treatment of severe mood disorders. Thus, even though the rationale for the introduction of ECT was incorrect and its mode of action remains unclear, controlled trials have confirmed that, in carefully defined clinical situations, ECT is a safe and effective treatment (see p. 706).

The action of *lithium* in reducing mania was a chance finding by Cade (1949) who had been investigating the effects of urates in animals and had decided to use the lithium salt because of its solubility. Lithium is a toxic agent, and so Cade's important observations did not make a significant impact on clinical practice until the following decade, when controlled trials showed that lithium was effective in both the acute treatment of mania and the prophylaxis of recurrent mood disorders.

Other agents that revolutionized psychopharmacology were introduced about this time (Box 21.1). Their efficacy and their indications were first recognized through clinical observation, and were subsequently confirmed by controlled clinical trials. None of these agents was introduced on the basis of an aetiological hypothesis. Indeed, such aetiological hypotheses as there are in biological psychiatry have been largely derived from knowledge of the mode of action of effective drugs. Thus the dopamine receptor antagonist properties of antipsychotic drugs have given rise to the dopamine hypothesis of schizophrenia, whilst the action of tricyclic antidepressants and monoamine oxidase inhibitors (MAOIs) in facilitating the effects of noradrenaline and 5-hydroxytryptamine (5-HT) has led to the various monoamine hypotheses of mood disorders.

The last 30 years have brought a period of consolidation in psychopharmacology. Clinical trials have

been widely used to refine the indications of particular drug treatments and to maximize their risk/benefit ratios. New compounds have continuously become available; most have been derived from previously described agents, and so their range of activity is not strikingly different from that of their predecessors. In general, however, the newer agents are better tolerated and sometimes safer – developments which are important for clinical practice.

There may now be grounds for more optimism about the prospects for advances in psychopharmacology. For example, there is rapidly increasing knowledge about chemical signalling in the brain. Numerous neurotransmitters and neuromodulators interact with specific families of receptors, many of which exist in a number of different subtypes. Several of these receptors have been cloned, and selective ligands for them are becoming available. There is increasing knowledge as to how these chemical messengers may modify behaviour through their interactions with specific brain regions and distributed neuronal circuits.

New compounds are likely to differ from current drugs in their range of behavioural effects. These new preparations are likely to lead to important new developments in psychopharmacology. Given the complex causes of psychiatric disorders, it seems likely that detailed knowledge of aetiology and pathophysiology may lag behind advances in therapeutics. Of course, this disparity is not uncommon in general medicine. It serves to reinforce the importance of *randomized clinical trials* in the assessment of new psychopharmacological treatments.

General considerations

The pharmacokinetics of psychotropic drugs

Before psychotropic drugs can produce their therapeutic effects, they must reach the brain in adequate amounts. How far they do so depends on their absorption, metabolism, excretion, and passage across the blood-brain barrier. A short review of these processes is given here. The reader who has not studied them before is referred to the chapter on pharmacokinetics in Grahame-Smith and Aronson (2000). The following processes are important:

- absorption
- distribution
- metabolism
- excretion.

Absorption

In general, psychotropic drugs are easily absorbed from the gut because most are *lipophilic* and are not highly ionized at physiological pH values. Like other drugs, they are absorbed faster from an empty stomach, and in reduced amounts by patients suffering from intestinal hurry or malabsorption syndrome.

Distribution

Psychotropic drugs are distributed in the plasma where most are largely bound to proteins; thus diazepam, chlorpromazine, and amitriptyline are about 95% bound. They pass easily from the plasma to the brain because they are highly lipophilic. For the same reason, they enter fat stores, from which they are released slowly long after the patient has ceased to take the drug.

Metabolism

Most psychotropic drugs are *metabolized in the liver*. This process begins as the drugs pass through the liver in the portal circulation on their way from the gut. This 'first-pass' metabolism reduces the amount of available drug, and is one of the reasons why larger doses are needed when a drug such as chlorpromazine is given by mouth than when it is given intramuscularly. The extent of this liver metabolism differs from one person to another. It is altered by certain other drugs which, if taken at the same time, induce liver enzymes (for example, carbamazepine) or inhibit them (for example, selective serotonin re-uptake inhibitors [SSRI]).

Some drugs, such as carbamazepine, induce their own metabolism, especially after being taken for a long time. Not all drug metabolites are inactive; for example, chlorpromazine is metabolized to a 7-hydroxy derivative, which has therapeutic properties, as well as to a sulphoxide, which is inactive. Because chlorpromazine, diazepam, and many other psychotropic drugs give rise to many metabolites, measurements of plasma concentrations of the parent drug alone are a poor guide to therapeutic activity.

Excretion

Psychotropic drugs and their metabolites are excreted mainly through the *kidney*. When kidney function is impaired, excretion is reduced and a lower dose of drug should be given. Lithium is filtered passively and then partly reabsorbed by the same mechanism that absorbs sodium. The two ions compete for this mechanism; hence reabsorption of lithium increases when that of sodium is reduced. Certain fractions of lipophilic drugs such as chlorpromazine are partly excreted in the bile, enter the intestine for the second time, and are then partly reabsorbed, i.e. a proportion of the drug is recycled between intestine and liver.

Measurement of circulating drug concentrations

As a result of individual variations in the mechanisms described above, plasma concentrations after standard doses of psychotropic drugs vary substantially from one patient to another. Tenfold differences have been observed with the antidepressant drug nortriptyline. Therefore it might be expected that measurements of the plasma concentration of circulating drugs would help the clinician. With the exception of lithium, however, this practice is rarely helpful. There are a number of reasons for this:

- Many psychotropic drugs are bound extensively to plasma proteins; however, only their plasma-free fractions are pharmacologically active. Most assays measure the total concentration of drug in plasma (i.e. free and bound), and therefore do not necessarily provide a reliable estimation of the amount of drug available to produce a therapeutic effect.

♦ Many drugs have active metabolites, some of which have therapeutic effects while others do not. Some assays are too specific, measuring only the parent drug but not its active derivatives; others are too general, measuring active and inactive metabolites alike.

♦ It seems likely that the therapeutic effects of many psychotropic drugs may be associated with *adaptive responses* of neurons to the presence of the drug. These cellular adaptive responses depend on many factors, particularly perhaps on the properties of the neurons concerned. Therefore it would not be surprising if drug-induced adaptive changes in the neuron did not correlate in a straightforward way with levels of the drug in plasma.

Pharmacodynamic measures

As an alternative to these assays, it may be possible to measure the pharmacological property, which is thought to be responsible for the therapeutic effect of a particular drug. For example, positron emission tomography can be used to measure directly the degree of brain dopamine receptor blockade produced by antipsychotic drugs during treatment. Such information has proved valuable in improving dosage regimens of drugs such as haloperidol. However, these pharmacodynamic measures have not yet been able to identify why some patients do not respond to medication. For example, the degree of dopamine receptor blockade is the same in patients who respond to antipsychotic drugs as in those who do not (Geaney *et al.* 1992).

Plasma half-life

Plasma concentrations of drugs vary throughout the day, rising immediately after the dose and falling at a rate that differs between individual drugs and individual people. The rate at which a drug level declines after a single dose varies from hours with lithium carbonate to weeks with slow-release preparations of injectable neuroleptics. Knowledge of these differences allows more rational decisions to be made about appropriate intervals between doses.

The concept of *plasma half-life* is useful here. The half-life of a drug in plasma is the time taken for its concentration to fall by a half, once dosing has ceased. With most psychotropic drugs, the amount eliminated over time is proportional to plasma concentration and in this case it will take approximately five times the half-life for the drug to be eliminated from plasma. Equally, when dosing with a drug begins, it will take five times the half-life for the concentration in plasma to reach steady state. This can be important when planning treatment. For example, MAOIs should not be given with SSRIs. Therefore if a patient is taking sertraline, which has an elimination half-life of about 26 hours, it will be important to leave at least five times the half-life (a week is recommended) before starting MAOI treatment. When sertraline treatment begins, the plasma concentrations will continue to rise for about a week before reaching a steady state.

Drug interactions

When two psychotropic drugs are given together, one may interfere with or enhance the actions of the other. Interference may arise through alterations in absorption, binding, metabolism, or excretion (*pharmacokinetic interactions*), or by interaction between the pharmacological mechanisms of action (*pharmacodynamic interactions*).

Pharmacokinetic interactions

Interactions affecting *drug absorption* are seldom important for psychotropic drugs, although it is worth noting that absorption of chlorpromazine is reduced by antacids. Interactions due to *protein binding* are also uncommon, although the chloral metabolite trichloroacetic acid may displace warfarin from albumin. Interactions affecting *drug metabolism* are of considerable importance. Examples include the inhibition of the metabolism of sympathomimetic amines by MAOIs and the increase in the metabolism of chlorpromazine and tricyclic antidepressants by carbamazepine, which induces the relevant *cytochrome P450 enzymes* (see below). Interactions affecting *renal excretion* are mainly important for lithium, the elimination of which is decreased by thiazide diuretics.

Cytochrome P450 enzymes There have been significant developments in the understanding of the *microsomal cytochrome P450 enzyme system*. These enzymes are located mainly in the liver but also in other tissues including gut wall and brain. Their role is to detoxify exogenous substances such as drugs and their activity can be increased or decreased by concomitant drug administration. This can give rise to clinically important drug interactions (see Richelson 1998).

The various P450 enzymes are encoded by separate genes which gives rise to a somewhat complex nomenclature (see Figure 21.1). Importantly, several new antidepressants, particularly selective SSRIs, potently inhibit P450 enzymes (see Table 21.11).

Pharmacodynamic interactions

Pharmacodynamic interactions are exemplified by the *serotonin syndrome* in which drugs that potentiate brain 5-HT function by different mechanisms (for example, SSRIs and MAOIs) can combine to produce dangerous 5-HT toxicity (see p. 688).

As a rule, a single drug can be used to produce all the effects required of a combination; for example, many antidepressant drugs have useful anti-anxiety effects. It is desirable to avoid combinations of psychotropic drugs whenever possible; if a combination is to be used, it is essential to know about possible interactions. The *British National Formulary* provides a useful guide.

Drug withdrawal

Many psychotropic drugs do not achieve useful therapeutic effects for several days or even weeks. After drugs have been stopped, there is often a comparable delay before their effects are lost. Psychotropic and, indeed, many other classes of drugs produce neuroadaptive changes during repeated administration. Tissues therefore have to readjust when drug treatment is stopped; this readjustment may appear clinically as a *withdrawal*

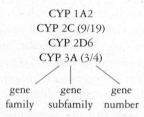

Figure 21.1 Key cytochrome (CYP) P450 isoenzymes in psychotropic drug metabolism.

or abstinence syndrome. Characteristic abstinence syndromes have been described for antidepressants and anxiolytics while sudden discontinuation of lithium can provoke a 'rebound' mania. It is important to be able to distinguish withdrawal syndromes from relapse of the disorder being treated. In addition, the risk of abstinence symptoms makes it prudent to withdraw psychotropic drugs slowly wherever possible.

General advice about prescribing

Use well-tried drugs

It is good practice to use well-tried drugs with therapeutic actions and side-effects that are thoroughly understood. The clinician should become familiar with a small number of drugs from each of the main classes. In this way he can become used to adjusting the dosage and recognizing side-effects. Well-tried drugs are usually less expensive than new preparations.

Give an adequate dose

Having chosen a suitable drug, the doctor should prescribe it in *adequate doses*. He should not change the drug or add others without a good reason. In general, if there is no therapeutic response to one established drug, there is no likelihood of a better response to another that has very similar pharmacological properties (provided that the first drug has been taken in adequate amounts). However, since the main obstacle to adequate dosage is usually side-effects, it may be appropriate to change to a drug with a different pattern of side-effects – for example, from a tricyclic antidepressant to an SSRI or vice versa.

Use drug combinations cautiously

Some drug companies market tablets that contain a mixture of drugs, for example, tricyclic antidepressants with a small dose of a phenothiazine. These mixtures have little value. In the few cases when two drugs are really required, it is better to give them separately so that the dose of each can be adjusted independently.

Occasionally, drug combinations are given deliberately in the hope of producing interactions that will be more potent than the effects of either drug taken alone in full dosage (for example, a tricyclic antidepressant with a MAOI). This practice, if it is to be used, is best carried out by specialists because the adverse effects of combinations are much less easy to predict than those of single drugs.

Dosing and treatment duration

When a drug is prescribed, it is necessary to determine the dose, the interval between doses, and the likely duration of treatment. The dose ranges for commonly used drugs are indicated later in this chapter. Ranges for others will be found in the manufacturers' literature, the *British National Formulary*, or a comparable work of reference. Within the therapeutic range, the correct dose for an individual patient should be decided after considering the severity of symptoms, the patient's age, and weight, and any factors that may affect drug metabolism (for example, other drugs being taken or renal disease).

Next, the interval between doses must be decided. Psychotropic drugs have often been given three times a day, even though their duration of action is such that most can be taken once or twice a day without any undesirable fall in plasma concentrations between doses. Less frequent administration has the advantage that out-patients are more likely to be reliable in taking drugs. In hospital, less frequent drug rounds mean that nurses have more time for psychological aspects of treatment. Some drugs, such as anxiolytics, are required for immediate effect rather than continuous action; they should not be given at regular intervals but shortly before occasions on which

symptoms are expected to be at their worse. The duration of treatment depends on the disorder under treatment; it is considered in the chapter dealing with the clinical syndrome.

Explain treatment to patient

Before giving a patient a first prescription for a drug, the doctor should explain several points. He should make clear what effects are likely to be experienced on first taking the drug, for example, drowsiness or dry mouth. He should also explain how long it will be before therapeutic effects appear and what the first signs are likely to be, for example, improved sleep after starting a tricyclic antidepressant. He should name any serious effects that must be reported by the patient, such as coarse tremor after taking lithium. Finally, he should indicate how long the patient will need to take the drug. For some drugs such as anxiolytics, the latter information is given to discourage the patient from taking them for too long; for others, such as antidepressants, it is given to deter the patient from stopping too soon.

Compliance, concordance, and collaboration

Many patients do not take the drugs prescribed for them. This problem is greater when treating out-patients, but also occurs in hospital where some patients find ways of avoiding drugs administered by nurses.

If a patient is to comply with medication of any kind, he must be convinced of the need to take it, free from unfounded fears about its dangers, and be aware of how to take it. Each of these requirements presents particular problems when the patient has a psychiatric disorder. Thus patients with schizophrenia or seriously depressed patients may not be convinced that they are ill or they may not wish to recover. Deluded patients may distrust their doctors, and hypochondriacal patients may fear dangerous side-effects. Anxious patients often forget the prescribed dosage and frequency of their drugs. Therefore it is not surprising that many psychiatric patients do not take their drugs in the prescribed way. It is important for the clinician to pay attention to this problem. Time spent in discussing the patient's concerns is time well spent, for it often increases compliance. Written instructions can be a valuable adjunct.

It is increasingly recognized that the successful and safe use of medication requires an essentially *collaborative* relationship between patient and doctor. Some have proposed that the term *concordance* should therefore be preferred to *compliance*, which carries the implicit assumption that the patient's job is to obey instructions (Mullen 1997).

Whatever the term used, it is clearly important to recognize that the use of drug treatment, particularly in psychiatry, requires a thorough understanding of the *patient's attitude* to the illness as well its treatment. The used of a cognitive strategy that helps patients weigh advantages and disadvantages of drug treatment ('compliance therapy') has been shown to improve the outcome in patients with schizophrenia (Kemp *et al.* 1996).

Ethical aspects of drug prescription

The ethical issues in this complex area have been reviewed by Brown and Pantelis (1999).

- The basis of ethical prescribing is the *practitioner's comprehensive knowledge of risk and benefits of drug therapies*. This will be derived from evidence-based approaches where possible.

- The doctor-patient relationship is the appropriate framework through which this knowledge is communicated to the patient

- The therapeutic partnership between patient and doctor must lead to *true informed consent*, which includes the right of competent patients to refuse treatment.

Difficulties arise where the evidence base of treatment is lacking and where there is uncertainty what approach to pursue. Here the clinician has the responsibility to use clinical guidelines, where available, and also to advise treatments that would be supported by peer opinion. The clinician should also support the right of patients to genuinely effective treatment where this is being hindered by cost constraint and other economic factors.

Prescribing for special groups

Children and the elderly

Children seldom require medication for psychiatric problems. When they do require it, doses should be adjusted appropriately by consulting an up-to-date work of reference (such as the *British National Formulary*). For elderly patients, who are often sensitive to side-effects and may have impaired renal or hepatic function, it is important to start with low doses.

Pregnant women

There are special problems about prescribing psychotropic drugs in pregnancy because of the risk of *teratogenesis*. Information about the teratogenic risk of individual drugs can be obtained from the relevant manufacturer and the *British National Formulary*, although available evidence is often scanty or difficult to interpret. The practitioner and patient have the difficult task of weighing this information against the risk of managing the illness without medication (Cohen and Rosenbaum 1998). For this reason, it is prudent where possible to advise women of child-bearing age who require psychotropics to avoid pregnancy until the need for the drug treatment is over.

Anxiolytics and antidepressants

Anxiolytic drugs are seldom essential in early pregnancy, and psychological treatments can usually be used. If medication is needed, in general, *benzodiazepines* have not been shown to be teratogenic although one meta-analysis has shown an increased risk of oral clefts after first trimester exposure. If an *antidepressant drug* is required, it is probably better to use a long-established preparation such as *imipramine* and *amitriptyline* for which there is no evidence of a teratogenic effect after many years of use. There is also reasonable experience with *fluoxetine*, which does not appear to be associated with an increased risk of major malformations. The rate of minor malformations may be increased, however (Wisner *et al.* 1999).

Antipsychotic drugs and mood stabilizers

It is seldom necessary to start *antipsychotic drugs* in early pregnancy. There is little evidence that high-potency agents such as *haloperidol* carry an increased teratogenic risk. However, there may be a higher rate of congenital malformations in babies exposed to lower potency agents such as *chlorpromazine*. There is little information on the teratogenic risk of newer antipsychotic agents.

Lithium treatment early in pregnancy has been associated with cardiac abnormalities in the fetus, particularly *Ebstein's anomaly*; therefore, women considering pregnancy have been recommended to discontinue lithium before conceiving. Similarly, women who become pregnant whilst taking lithium have usually been advised to stop the treatment. However, recent epidemiological studies have suggested that whilst the relative risk of Ebstein's anomaly is increased at least tenfold in infants exposed to lithium in the first trimester, the absolute risk is still fairly low, *between 0.05 and 0.1%*. Withdrawal of lithium carries a high risk of relapse in women with bipolar illness and the balance of risk to mother and baby may therefore suggest continuation of lithium treatment during pregnancy in some cases. *Anticonvulsant drugs* such as *carbamazepine* and *valproate* are increasingly used as mood stabilizers. However, both these agents are associated with an increased risk of neural tube defects as well as excessive neonatal bleeding.

Neonatal toxicity

Exposure to psychotropic drugs in the later stages of pregnancy can give rise to *neonatal toxicity* either through the presence of the drug or a withdrawal syndrome. For example, it has been reported that among babies born to mothers who have been receiving *tricyclic antidepressants* there may be withdrawal reactions including tremulousness, vomiting, poor feeding, and seizures. Direct anticholinergic effects such as gastrointestinal stasis and bladder distension have also been reported. These reactions, whilst clearly problem-

atic, appear to settle quickly without causing lasting sequelae.

There is also a possibility that late exposure to *fluoxetine* and *sertraline* may be associated with an increased risk of neonatal complications including jitteriness, hypoglycaemia, poor muscle tone, and respiratory difficulties (Wisner *et al.* 1999). The perinatal toxicity associated with *lithium* use includes 'floppy baby syndrome' with cyanosis and hypotonicity whereas *benzodiazepine* treatment can result in impaired temperature regulation together with breathing and feeding difficulties.

Animal studies suggest that fetal exposure to psychotropic medication can cause *longer-term abnormalities in brain development and behaviour*. Thus far, however, a limited number of human studies have not detected such effects in children followed up for the first few years of life (Cohen and Rosenbaum 1998).

Breast-feeding

Psychotropic drugs should be prescribed cautiously to women who are *breast-feeding* (Llewellyn and Stowe 1998). *Diazepam* and other *benzodiazepines* pass readily into breast milk and may cause sedation and hypotonicity in the infant. Antipsychotic drugs and antidepressants also enter breast milk, although rather less readily than diazepam. *Sulpiride*, however, is excreted in significant amounts and should be avoided. Similarly, *doxepin* may accumulate in the infant and cause oversedation. *Fluoxetine* and its metabolites could also accumulate, but *fluvoxamine* and *sertraline* are present in only very small amounts in breast milk.

Lithium salts enter the milk freely, and serum concentrations in the infant can approach those of the mother so that breast-feeding requires great caution. However, the amounts of *carbamazepine* and *valproate* in breast milk are considered too low to be harmful. A general issue is that, even when the concentration of a particular drug in breast milk is low and no detectable clinical effect upon the infant can be discerned, it is nevertheless possible that subtle longer-term effects on brain development and behaviour could occur. For this reason, some authorities recommend that women receiving psychotropic medication should not breast-feed at all. A more pragmatic view is provided by the *British National Formulary*.

What to do if there is no therapeutic response

The first step is to find out whether the patient has been taking the drug in the correct dose. He may not have understood the original instructions, or may be worried that a full dose will produce unpleasant side-effects. Some patients fear that they will become dependent if they take the drug regularly. Other patients may have little wish to take drugs for the reasons discussed above. If the doctor is satisfied that the drug has been taken correctly, he should find out whether the patient is taking any other drug (such as carbamazepine) which could affect the metabolism of the psychotropic agent. Finally, he should review the diagnosis to make sure

that the treatment is appropriate before deciding whether to increase the dose. Failure to respond adequately to psychotropic medication is a common reason for psychiatric referral. Specific pharmacological approaches for individual disorders are discussed in the relevant chapters.

The classification of drugs used in psychiatry

Drugs that have effects mainly on mental symptoms are called *psychotropic*. Psychiatrists also use *antiparkinsonian agents*, which are employed to control the side-effects of some psychotropic drugs.

Psychotropic drugs are conventionally divided into different classes, as shown in Table 21.1, but the therapeutic actions of particular compounds are not confined to one diagnostic category. For example, SSRIs are classified as antidepressants and

Table 21.1 Classification of clinical psychotropic drugs

Class of drug	Examples of classes	Indications
Antipsychotic	Phenothiazines	Acute treatment of schizophrenia and mania, prophylaxis of schizophrenia
	Butyrophenones	
	Substituted benzamides	
Antidepressant	Tricyclic antidepressants MAOIs SSRIs	Major depression (acute treatment and prophylaxis), anxiety disorders, obsessive-compulsive disorder (SSRIs)
Mood stabilizer	Lithium	Acute treatment of mania
	Carbamazepine	Prophylaxis of recurrent mood disorder
Anxiolytic	Benzodiazepines	Generalized anxiety disorder
	Azapirones (buspirone)	
Hypnotic	Benzodiazepines	Insomnia
	Cyclopyrrolones (zopiclone)	
Psychostimulant	Amphetamine	Hyperkinetic syndrome of childhood
		Narcolepsy

are effective in the treatment of major depression, but they also produce useful therapeutic effects in anxiety states, obsessive–compulsive disorders, and eating disorders. Of course, this breadth of effect does not mean that the latter syndromes are forms of depression. It merely emphasizes that the neuropsychological consequences of facilitating brain 5-HT function may provide beneficial effects in a variety of psychiatric disorders.

Whilst there is considerable understanding of the pharmacological actions of psychotropic drugs, little is known about the neuropsychological consequences of these pharmacological actions and about the ways in which neuropsychological changes are translated into clinical benefit in different diagnostic syndromes. At present, therefore, the best plan is to classify drugs according to their major therapeutic use but to bear in mind that the therapeutic effects of different classes of drugs *may overlap considerably.*

The main groups of drugs will now be reviewed in turn. For each group, an account will be given of therapeutic effects, pharmacology, principal compounds available, pharmacokinetics, unwanted effects (both those appearing with ordinary doses and the toxic effects of unduly high doses), and contraindications. General advice will also be given about the use of each group in everyday clinical practice, but specific applications to the treatment of individual disorders will be found in the chapters dealing with those conditions. Drugs that have a limited use in the treatment of a single disorder, for example, *disulfiram* for alcohol problems, are discussed in the chapters dealing with the relevant clinical syndromes.

Anxiolytic drugs

Anxiolytic drugs, particularly *barbiturates* and *benzodiazepines*, have been prescribed widely and often inappropriately. Before prescribing anxiolytic drugs it is always important to seek the causes of anxiety and to try to modify them. It is also essential to recognize that a degree of anxiety can motivate patients to take steps to reduce the problems that are causing it. Hence removing all anxiety in the short term is not always beneficial to the patient in the long run. Anxiolytics such as benzodiazepines are most useful when given for a short time, either to tide the patient over a crisis or to help him tackle a specific problem.

Tolerance is a particular problem with barbiturates and benzodiazepine-like anxiolytic drugs, and physical dependence can develop. Because the benzodiazepines are still widely used anxiolytics, they will be considered first. *Antidepressants* are increasingly used to treat specific anxiety syndromes but their therapeutic actions differ in important ways from benzodiazepine-like drugs. Their indications in the treatment of anxiety disorders will be considered here but their detailed pharmacology is discussed in the section on antidepressant drugs (p. 675). When reading this section, it is important to keep in mind that psychological treatments are effective in the management of anxiety disorders and have certain advantages over drug treatment, including more sustained efficacy after treatment cessation.

Benzodiazepines

Pharmacology

Benzodiazepines have several actions:

♦ anxiolytic

♦ sedative and hypnotic

♦ muscle relaxant

♦ anticonvulsant.

Their pharmacological actions are mediated through specific receptor sites located in a supramolecular complex with *gamma-aminobutyric acid (GABA) receptors.* Benzodiazepines enhance GABA neurotransmission, thereby altering indirectly the activity of other neurotransmitter systems such as those involving noradrenaline and 5-HT.

Compounds available

Many different benzodiazepines are available. They differ both in the potency with which they interact with benzodiazepine receptors and in their plasma half-life (Box 21.2). In general, *high-potency benzodiazepines* and those with *short half-lives* are

Box 21.2 **Half-lives of some drugs acting at GABA/benzodiazepine receptor complex**

Diazepam	20–100 h*
Chlordiazepoxide	5–30 h*
Lorazepam	8–24 h
Temazepam	5–11 h
Zaleplon	1–1.5 h
Zopiclone	4–6 h
Zolpidem	1.5–2 h
Chlormethiazole	4–6 h (4–12 h in elderly)
Chloral	6–8 h

*Active metabolite

more likely to be associated with dependence and withdrawal. Benzodiazepines with short half-lives (less than 12 hours) include lorazepam, temazepam, and lormetazepam.

Because of problems with dependence, long-acting compounds are preferable for the management of anxiety, even if such treatment is to be given intermittently on an 'as required basis'. The long-acting benzodiazepines include drugs such as diazepam, chlordiazepoxide, alprazolam, and clonazepam. *Diazepam* is rapidly absorbed and can be used both for the continuous treatment of anxiety and for treatment 'as required'. *Alprazolam*, a high-potency benzodiazepine, is effective in the treatment of panic disorder. This therapeutic efficacy is not confined to alprazolam because equivalent doses of other high-potency agents such as *clonazepam* are also effective.

Flumazenil is a benzodiazepine receptor antagonist that produces little pharmacological effect by itself but blocks the actions of other benzodiazepines. Therefore it may be useful in reversing acute toxicity produced by benzodiazepines but carries a risk of provoking acute benzodiazepine withdrawal. Flumazenil is available only for intravenous use.

Pharmacokinetics

Benzodiazepines are rapidly absorbed. They are strongly bound to plasma proteins but, because they are lipophilic, pass readily into the brain. They are metabolized to a large number of compounds, many of which have therapeutic effects of their own; temazepam and oxazepam are among the metabolic products of diazepam. Excretion is mainly as conjugates in the urine.

Benzodiazepines with short half-lives, such as temazepam and lorazepam, have a 3-hydroxyl grouping, which allows a one-step metabolism to inactive glucuronides. Other benzodiazepines, such as diazepam and clorazepate, are metabolized to long-acting derivatives, such as desmethyl-diazepam, which are themselves therapeutically active.

It is now common practice to give benzodiazepines (often in combination with low-dose antipsychotic drugs) to produce a rapid calming effect in psychosis. In this situation, benzodiazepines may be given parenterally and it is worth noting that the absorption of diazepam following intramuscular injection is poor, and lorazepam should be preferred if this route of administration is used.

Unwanted effects

Benzodiazepines are well tolerated. When they are given as anxiolytics, their main side-effects are due to the sedative properties of large doses, which can lead *to ataxia and drowsiness* (especially in the elderly) and occasionally to *confused thinking and amnesia*. Minor degrees of drowsiness and of impaired coordination and judgement *can affect driving skills* and the operation of potentially dangerous machinery; moreover, people affected in this way are not always aware of it. For this reason, when benzodiazepines are prescribed, especially those with a longer action, patients should be advised about these dangers and about the potentiating effects of alcohol. The prescriber should remember that these effects are more common among elderly patients and those with impaired renal or liver function.

Although in some circumstances benzodiazepines reduce tension and aggression, they can also lead to a *release of aggression* by reducing inhibitions in people with a tendency to aggressive behaviour. In this they resemble alcohol. This possible effect should be remembered when prescribing to those judged to be at risk of child abuse or to any person with a previous history of impulsive aggressive behaviour.

Toxic effects

Benzodiazepines have few toxic effects. Patients usually recover from large overdoses because these drugs do not depress respiration and blood pressure as barbiturates do. Even so, fatal overdoses of benzodiazepines have occasionally been reported.

Drug interactions

Benzodiazepines, like other sedative anxiolytics, potentiate the effects of alcohol and of drugs that depress the central nervous system. Significant respiratory depression has been reported in some patients receiving combined treatment with benzodiazepines and clozapine.

Dependence and withdrawal

It is now generally agreed that *physical dependence* develops after prolonged use of benzodiazepines. The frequency depends on the drug and the dosage, and has been estimated as between 5 and 50% among patients taking the drugs for more than 6 months (Petursson and Lader 1984; Schweizer and Rickels 1998).

Dependence is associated with a *withdrawal syndrome* characterized by apprehension, insomnia, nausea, and tremor, together with heightened sensitivity to perceptual stimuli. In severe cases, epileptic seizures have been reported. Since many of these symptoms resemble those of anxiety disorder, it can sometimes be difficult to decide whether the patient is experiencing a benzodiazepine withdrawal syndrome or a recrudescence of the anxiety disorder for which the drug was prescribed originally.

Withdrawal symptoms generally begin within 2–3 days of stopping a short-acting benzodiazepine and within 7 days of stopping a long-acting one. The symptoms generally last for 3–10 days. Withdrawal symptoms seem to be more frequent after drugs with a short half-life than after those with a long half-life. If benzodiazepines have been taken for a long time, it is best to withdraw them gradually over several weeks (Committee on the Review of Medicines 1980; Schweizer and Rickels 1998). If this is done, withdrawal symptoms can be minimized or avoided (see p.570).

Azapirones (buspirone)

Indications and pharmacology

The only drug in the azapirone class currently marketed for the treatment of anxiety is *buspirone* (see Cowen 1997). Buspirone is effective in the treatment of generalized anxiety disorder but is not helpful in the treatment of panic disorder. Unlike the benzodiazepines, the anxiolytic effects of buspirone take several days to develop. It is also important to note that buspirone cannot be used to treat benzodiazepine withdrawal.

Pharmacologically, buspirone has no affinity for benzodiazepine receptors but stimulates a subtype of 5-HT receptor called the *5-HT$_{1A}$ receptor*. This receptor is found in high concentration in the raphe nuclei in the brainstem where it regulates the firing of 5-HT cell bodies. Administration of buspirone lowers the firing rate of 5-HT neurons and thereby decreases 5-HT neurotransmission in certain brain regions. This action may be the basis of its anxiolytic effect.

Pharmacokinetics and unwanted effects

Buspirone has poor systemic availability because it has an extensive first-pass metabolism. The side-effect profile differs from that of benzodiazepines. For example, buspirone treatment does not cause sedation but instead is often associated with *lightheadedness*, *nervousness*, and *headache* early in treatment. There is little evidence that tolerance and dependence occur during buspirone use, although such a judgement must always be made with circumspection.

Drug interactions

Buspirone is relatively free from significant drug interactions, but in combination with MAOIs has been reported to cause raised blood pressure.

Antidepressant drugs

Antidepressant drugs usually ameliorate the anxiety that accompanies depressive disorders. Tricyclic antidepressants have also been shown to be as effective as benzodiazepines in the management of both *generalized anxiety* and *panic disorder* whether or not significant depressive symptoms are present. Similarly, both SSRIs and MAOIs are effective in the treatment of panic disorder, but the selective noradrenaline uptake inhibitor maprotiline is not. Recent studies have also shown that SSRIs are effective in the treatment of *social phobia* and *obsessive–compulsive disorder* (see Cowen 1997; Fineberg 1999).

The therapeutic profile of antidepressant drugs in the treatment of anxiety differs significantly from that of benzodiazepines. The time of onset of effect is much slower with antidepressants and, particularly in panic disorder, there may be an *exacerbation of symptoms* early in treatment. However, the ultimate therapeutic effect of antidepressants is as least as great and they are less likely to produce cognitive impairment (Nutt and Bell 1997). In addition, the use of antidepressants is not associated with tolerance and dependence though, as noted above, sudden cessation of treatment can cause abstinence symptoms.

Antipsychotic drugs

These drugs are sometimes prescribed for their anxiolytic effects. In low doses that do not lead to side-effects (for example, flupenthixol, 1.0 mg), they are generally no more effective than benzodiazepines. Nevertheless, antipsychotic drugs have a small place as anxiolytics in the treatment of two groups of patients – those with persistent anxiety who have become dependent on other drugs, and those with aggressive personalities who respond badly to the disinhibiting effects of other anxiolytics. However, even low-dose antipsychotic treatment, if maintained, is not free from the risk of *tardive dyskinesia*.

Beta-adrenoceptor antagonists

These drugs relieve some of the autonomic symptoms of anxiety, such as tachycardia, almost certainly by a peripheral effect. They are best reserved for anxious patients whose main symptom is palpitation or tremor, particularly in social situations. An appropriate drug is *propranolol* in a dose of 20–40 mg three times a day. Contraindications are heart block, systolic blood pressure below 90 mmHg or a pulse rate of less than 60/minute, and a history of bronchospasm. Beta-adrenoceptor antagonists precipitate heart failure in a few patients and should not be given to those with atrioventricular node block as they decrease conduction in the atrioventricular node and bundle of His. They can exacerbate Raynaud's phenomenon and hypoglycaemia in diabetics.

Barbiturates and other sedative anxiolytics

In the past, barbiturates were widely used as anxiolytics. Although effective, they readily cause *dependency* and they should not be used as anxiolytics. Propanediols such as meprobamate also have no advantage over benzodiazepines and are more sedative in doses needed to relieve anxiety.

Unwanted effects resemble those of the benzodiazepines and generally appear at doses nearer to the anxiolytic dose. Barbiturates may produce *irritability*, *drowsiness*, and *ataxia*. In large doses, the toxic effects of sedative anxiolytics are to depress respiration and reduce blood pressure. This is a particular problem with the barbiturates. The interactions of these drugs with others resemble those of the benzodiazepines. In addition, barbiturates interact with *coumarin* drugs and reduce their anticoagulant action. They also increase the metabolism of *tricyclic antidepressants* and some *antibiotics*. The effects of withdrawal resemble the effects of withdrawing benzodiazepines, described above, but are *more severe*. After stopping barbiturates, the effects are particularly marked in the form of psychological tension, sweating, tremor, irritability, and, after large doses, seizures. Hence barbiturates should not be stopped suddenly if the dose has been substantial.

Advice on management

Before an anxiolytic drug is prescribed, the cause of the anxiety should always be sought. In addition, it is helpful to classify the nature of the anxiety disorder because this can have implications for drug treatment. It is worth remembering that whilst medication is undoubtedly helpful in the treatment of anxiety syndromes, *psychological treatments* are also effective and are often preferred by patients. In practice, medication tends to be used when psychological treatments are not readily available or have not been successful.

For most patients with *generalized anxiety symptoms*, attention to life problems, an opportunity to talk about their feelings, and reassurance from the doctor are enough to reduce anxiety to tolerable levels. If an anxiolytic is needed, a benzodiazepine should be given for a short time – seldom more than 3 weeks – and withdrawn gradually. It is important to remember that dependency is particularly likely to develop among people with alcohol problems. If the drug has been taken for several weeks, the patient should be warned that he may feel tense for a few days when it is stopped.

A compound such as *diazepam* is suitable for both the intermittent treatment of anxiety and continuous treatment throughout the day. The use of diazepam on an 'as needed' basis usually means that lower total doses are consumed and the risk of tolerance and dependence is diminished. For longer-term treatment of severe generalized anxiety, *antidepressant medication* may be more appropriate.

Antidepressants are often helpful in the treatment of *panic disorder*, although the risk of early symptomatic worsening must be remembered and explained to the patient. The use of small doses early in treatment (for example, 10 mg imipramine, 5 mg paroxetine) can be helpful (Nutt and Bell 1997). High-potency benzodiazepines

such as *alprazolam* and *clonazepam* are effective in panic disorder but can cause cognitive impairment and withdrawal problems. They may be helpful, however, in patients who do not respond to other treatments. *MAOI treatment* has a similar indication (Nutt and Bell 1997).

Other anxiolytic drugs should be kept for the specific purposes outlined above: beta-adrenoceptor antagonists for control of palpitations and tremor caused by anxiety, low-dose antipsychotic drugs for patients who respond badly to the disinhibiting effects of sedative anxiolytics (for example, abnormally aggressive patients) or patients who have become dependent upon them.

Hypnotics

Hypnotics are drugs used to improve sleep. Many anxiolytic drugs also act as hypnotics, and they have been reviewed in the previous section. Hypnotic drugs are prescribed widely and often continued for too long. This reflects the frequency of insomnia as a complaint. For example, about 10% of the UK population suffer from insomnia unrelated to specific events or other disorders (Chevalier *et al.* 1999). Insomnia is reported more often by women and the elderly. Effective psychological treatments are available for the management of insomnia and they appear to have a more sustained duration of action than hypnotics (Morin *et al.* 1999).

Pharmacology

The ideal hypnotic would increase the length and quality of sleep without residual effects the next morning. It would do so without altering the pattern of sleep and without any withdrawal effects when the patient ceased to take it. Unfortunately, no drug meets these exacting criteria. It is not easy to produce drugs that affect the whole night's sleep and yet are sufficiently eliminated by morning to leave behind no sedative effects (Shneerson 1999).

Most prescribed hypnotics *enhance the action of GABA* either through interaction with the benzodiazepine receptor or other adjacent sites located on the GABA macromolecular complex.

Antihistamines and low doses of sedating anti-depressants such as amitriptyline are also used to facilitate sleep.

Compounds available

Nowadays the most commonly used hypnotics are *benzodiazepines* or non-benzodiazepine ligands which act at or close to the benzodiazepine receptor site. These include *zopiclone*, *zolpidem* and *zaleplon*. The actions of these drugs can be reversed by the benzodiazepine receptor antagonist, flumazenil. Among other available hypnotic agents are *chloral hydrate* (or its derivatives), *chlormethiazole*, and *sedating antihistamines* (the latter are often present in 'over the counter' preparations).

Of the benzodiazepines, the shorter-acting compounds such as temazepam and lormetazepam are appropriate as hypnotics because of their relative lack of hangover effects the next day (Box 21.2). Other benzodiazepines that have been marketed as hypnotics, such as flurazepam and nitrazepam, have a long duration of action and produce significant impairments in tests of cognitive function on the day following treatment.

Zopiclone is a cyclopyrrolone. Zopiclone produces fewer changes in sleep architecture than benzodiazepine hypnotics. It is relatively free of daytime hangover and performance impairment and also is reported to be less liable to produce tolerance and dependence that benzodiazepines. However, cases have been reported. The most common side-effect is a *bitter after-taste* following ingestion, but behavioural disturbances including *confusion*, *amnesia*, and *depressed mood* have been reported.

Zolpidem is an imidazopyridine. It has a very short duration of action and, like zopiclone, has little effect on sleep architecture or daytime performance. Its possible adverse effects include *nausea*, *dizziness*, *headaches*, and *diarrhoea*.

Zaleplon is a pyrazolopyrimidine. It has the shortest duration of action of all currently marketed hypnotics (about 1 hour) and is recommended for 'as needed' use in patients who wake in the middle of the night and cannot fall asleep again. Further evaluation of zaleplon's longer-term

adverse effect profile (including the risk of dependence) is needed

Other hypnotic drugs that facilitate GABA include *chloral hydrate*, which is sometimes prescribed for children and old people. It is a gastric irritant and should be diluted adequately. *Chloral* is also available in tablet form. *Chlormethiazole edisylate* is a hypnotic drug with anticonvulsant properties. It has often used to prevent withdrawal symptoms in patients dependent on alcohol. For this reason, it is sometimes thought, mistakenly, to be a suitable hypnotic for alcoholic patients. This belief is wrong because the drug is as likely as any other hypnotic drug to cause dependency and can cause *respiratory depression* when combined with alcohol. It retains a place in the treatment of insomnia in the elderly because of its short duration of action. Unwanted effects *include sneezing*, *conjunctival irritation*, and *nausea*.

Unwanted effects

As well as specific side-effects of individual compounds noted above, all hypnotics have a number of general problems associated with their use. One of the most important is the presence of *residual effects*, which are experienced by the patient on the next day as feelings of being *slow* and *drowsy*. This is accompanied by deficits in daytime performance. Such effects are less apparent with the shorter-acting compounds noted above. Other problems include the *development of tolerance* in which the original dose of the drug has progressively less efficacy and '*rebound*' insomnia on withdrawal, which makes preparations difficult to stop. *Tolerance* is less of a problem with sedating antidepressants, but such drugs have long half-lives accompanied by residual psychomotor effects the next day.

Interactions

The most important interaction of hypnotic drugs is with *alcohol* where a potentiated effect can be seen. The interaction between *chlormethiazole and alcohol* is particularly dangerous and can result in death from respiratory failure. For this reason there must be adequate supervision if the drug is used during withdrawal of alcohol. It should not be prescribed for alcoholics who continue to drink. Hypnotics will also potentiate the effect of other drugs with sedating actions such as some antidepressant and antipsychotic agents.

Advice on management

Before prescribing hypnotic drugs, it is important to find out whether the patient is really sleeping badly and, if so, why. Many people have unrealistic ideas about the number of hours they should sleep. For example, they may not know that length of sleep often becomes shorter in middle and late life. Others take 'cat naps' in the daytime, perhaps through boredom, and still expect to sleep as long at night. Some people ask for sleeping tablets in anticipation of poor sleep for one or two nights, for example when travelling. Such temporary loss of sleep is soon compensated by increased sleep on subsequent nights, and any supposed advantage in alertness after a full night's sleep is likely to be offset by the residual effects of the drugs. If a drug is justifiable in these circumstances, it should be a *short-acting benzodiazepine* or *zopiclone* or *zolpidem*.

Among the common causes of disturbed sleep are excessive caffeine or alcohol, pain, cough, pruritus, and dyspnoea, and anxiety and depression. When any primary cause is present, this should be treated, not the insomnia. Often simple 'sleep hygiene' measures may be helpful (Box 21.3). If, after careful enquiry, a hypnotic appears to be essential, it should be prescribed for a few days only. The clinician should explain this to the patient, and should warn him that a few nights of restless sleep may occur when the drugs are stopped, but this restlessness will not be a reason for prolonging the prescription.

The prescription of hypnotics for children is not justified, except for the occasional treatment of night terrors and somnambulism. Hypnotics should also be prescribed with particular care for the elderly, who may become confused and get out of bed in the night, perhaps injuring themselves. Many patients are started on long periods of dependency on hypnotics by the prescribing of 'routine

---

Box 21.3 Some sleep hygiene measures

- Get to bed and get up about the same time each day.
- Avoid caffeine-containing drink and food in the evening.
- Avoid alcohol late in the evening.
- Avoid daytime 'napping'.
- If you cannot sleep, get up and occupy yourself until you feel sleepy.

---

night sedation' in hospital. Prescription of these drugs should not be routine; it should be a response only to a real need, and should be stopped before the patient goes home.

Antipsychotic drugs

This term is applied to drugs that reduce psychomotor excitement and control symptoms of psychosis. Alternative terms for these agents are *neuroleptic* and *major tranquillizer*. None of these names is wholly satisfactory. Neuroleptic refers to the side-effects rather than to the therapeutic effects of the drugs and major tranquillizers does not refer to the most important clinical action. The term antipsychotic is used here because it appears in the *British National Formulary*.

The main therapeutic uses of antipsychotic drugs are to reduce *hallucinations*, *delusions*, *agitation*, and *psychomotor excitement* in schizophrenia, mania, or psychosis secondary to a medical condition. The drugs are also used prophylactically *to prevent relapses* of schizophrenia. The introduction of chlorpromazine in 1952 led to substantial improvements in the treatment of schizophrenia and paved the way to the discovery of the many psychotropic drugs now available.

Pharmacology

Antipsychotic drugs (Table 21.2) share the property of *blocking dopamine receptors*. This may account for their therapeutic action, a suggestion supported by the close relationship between their potency in

Table 21.2 **A list of antipsychotic drugs**
Phenothiazines with aliphatic side-chain
Chlorpromazine
Promazine
Phenothiazines with piperidine side-chain
Thioridazine
Pipothiazine
Phenothiazines with piperazine side-chain
Trifluoperazine
Fluphenazine
Thioxanthines
Flupenthixol
Clopenthixol
Butyrophenones
Haloperidol
Droperidol
Diphenylbutylpiperidines
Pimozide
Dibenzodiazepines
Clozapine
Olanzapine
Substituted benzamides
Sulpiride
Amisulpride
Benzisoxazole
Risperidone

blocking dopaminergic receptors *in vitro*, and their therapeutic strength.

Dopamine receptors are of several biochemical and morphological subtypes (Baldesserini and Tarazi 1996; Jaber *et al.* 1996). Most antipsychotic drugs bind strongly to dopamine D_2 receptors, and this action appears to account for both their antipsychotic activity and their propensity to cause movement disorders. Positron emission tomography (PET) studies suggest that an antipsychotic effect is obtained when D_2 receptor occupancy lies between 60 and 70%. Higher levels are associated with extrapyramidal movement disorders (see Kapur 1999).

Distinction between typical and atypical antipsychotic drugs

The term *atypical* antipsychotic agent has been introduced to distinguish newer antipsychotic drugs from conventional agents such as chlorpromazine and haloperidol. Whilst the definition of the term 'atypical' varies in the literature, a fundamental property of an atypical antipsychotic is the ability to produce an antipsychotic effect *without causing extrapyramidal side-effects* (Stahl 1999). This definition is not free of difficulty; for example, haloperidol prescribed in sufficiently low doses may also have this effect. However, it is true to say that atypical antipsychotic agents have a lower likelihood of producing extrapyramidal side-effects through their usual therapeutic range.

Another property sometimes attributed to atypical antipsychotic drugs is improved efficacy against *positive* and *negative* symptoms of psychosis relative to typical agents. Whilst this is true of the prototypic atypical antipsychotic, clozapine, it is not clear how far more recently developed compounds meet this exacting criterion (Stahl 1999). Whether atypical antipsychotic drugs may *improve cognitive performance* in patients with schizophrenia is a topic of active investigation (Sharma 1999).

Pharmacology of typical (conventional) antipsychotics (Figure 21.2)

All these drugs are effective dopamine receptor antagonists but many possess additional pharmacological properties which influence their *adverse effect profile*.

Phenothiazines Phenothiazines fall into three groups:

♦ Aminoalkyl compounds such as *chlorpromazine* antagonize α_1-adrenoceptors, histamine H_1-receptors and muscarinic cholinergic receptors. Blockade of α_1-adrenoceptors and histamine H_1-receptors gives chlorpromazine a sedating

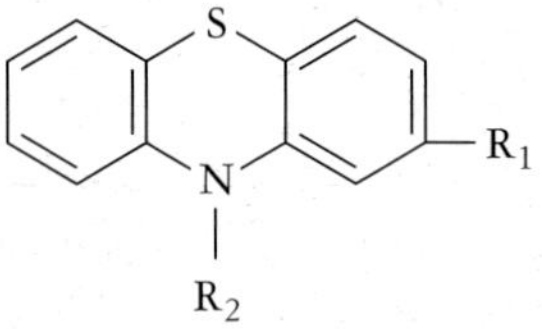

The basic phenothiazine structure

Type of compound	Example	R$_1$	R$_2$
Aminoalkyl	Chlorpromazine	— Cl	— (CH$_2$)$_3$ — N $\begin{array}{c} \diagup CH_3 \\ \diagdown CH_3 \end{array}$
Piperidine	Thioridazine	— SCH$_3$	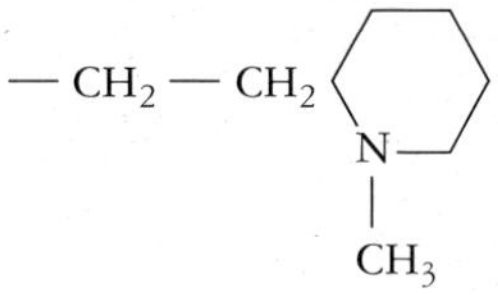 — CH$_2$ — CH$_2$ (piperidine ring, N—CH$_3$)
Piperazine	Trifluoperazine	— CF$_3$	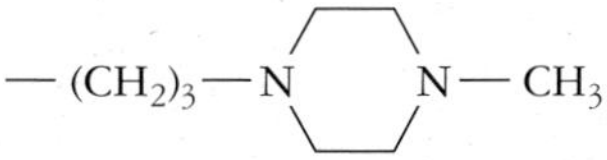 — (CH$_2$)$_3$—N (piperazine) N— CH$_3$
	Fluphenazine	— CF$_3$	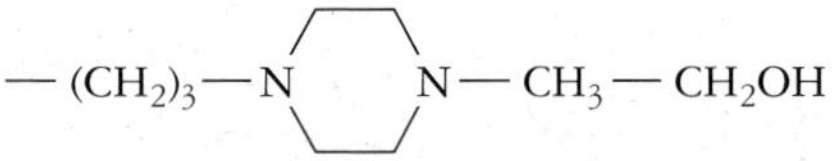 — (CH$_2$)$_3$—N (piperazine) N— CH$_3$ — CH$_2$OH

Flupenthixol,
a thioxanthine

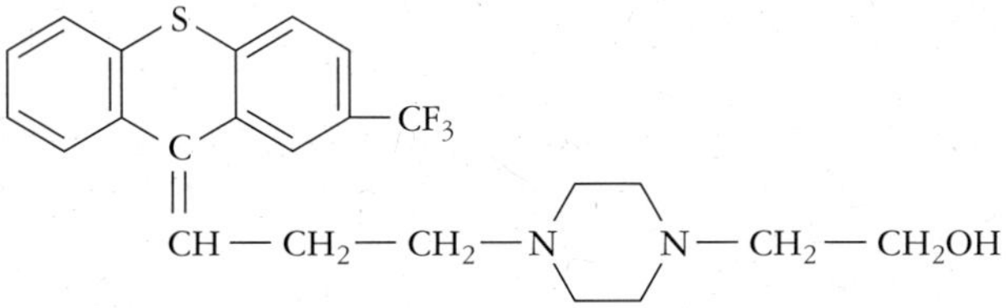

Haloperidol,
a butyrophenone

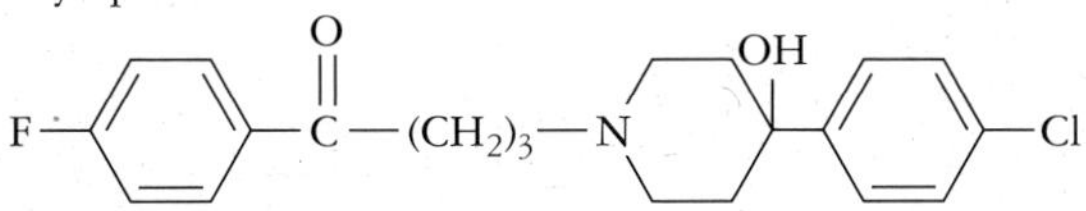

Figure 21.2 Some typical antipsychotic drugs.

profile, while α_1-adrenoceptor blockade also causes hypotension. The anticholinergic activity may cause dry mouth, urinary difficulties, and constipation, while on the other hand offsetting the liability to produce extrapyramidal effects.

- Piperidine compounds such as *thioridazine* are similar to chlorpromazine but are very potent muscarinic antagonist with a correspondingly low incidence of movement disorders.

- Piperazine compounds such as *trifluoperazine* or *fluphenazine* are the most selective dopamine receptor antagonists, the least sedating and the most likely to produce extrapyramidal effects.

Thioxanthenes and butyrophenones Thioxanthines such as *flupenthixol* and *clopenthixol* are similar in structure to the phenothiazines. The therapeutic effects are similar to those of the piperazine group. Butyrophenones such as *haloperidol* have a different structure but are clinically similar to the thioxanthenes. They are potent dopamine receptor antagonists with few effects at other neurotransmitter receptors. They are not sedating but have a high propensity to cause extrapyramidal side-effects.

Pharmacology of atypical antipsychotic drugs (Figure 21.3, Table 21.3)

Atypical antipsychotic drugs have a diverse pharmacology but currently two main groupings can be

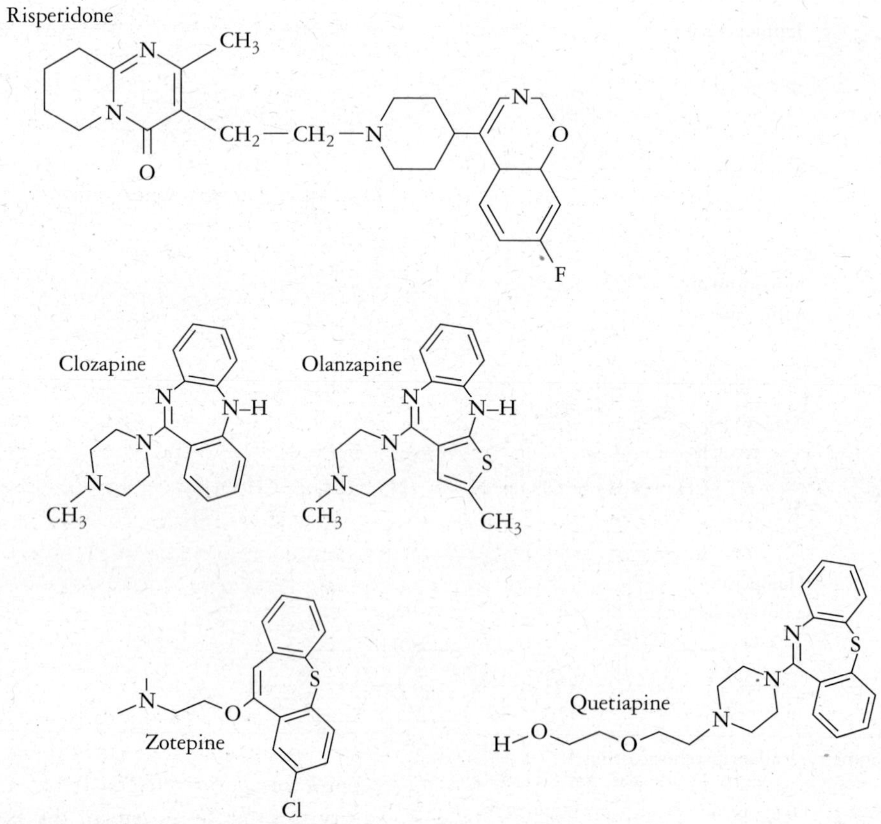

Figure 21.3 Some atypical antipsychotic drugs.

Table 21.3 Atypical antipsychotics

Drug	EPS*	Prolactin	Weight gain	Adverse effects
Amisulpride	+	↑	+	Insomnia, agitation, nausea, constipation, Q-T prolongation (rare)
Sulpiride	+	↑	+	Insomnia, agitation, abnormal liver function tests
Clozapine	0	0	+++	Agranulocytosis – white cell monitoring mandatory, myocarditis and myopathy (rare), fatigue, drowsiness, dry mouth, sweating, tachycardia, postural hypotension, nausea, constipation, ileus, urinary retention, seizures, diabetes
Olanzapine	+/0	0	+++	Somnolence, dizziness, oedema, hypotension, dry mouth, constipation, diabetes
Quetiapine	0	0	++	Somnolence, dizziness, postural hypotension, dry mouth, abnormal liver function tests, Q-T prolongation (transient)
Risperidone	+	↑	++	Insomnia, agitation, anxiety, headache, impaired concentration, nausea, abdominal pain
Zotepine	+	↑	+++	Constipation, dry mouth, insomnia, sleepiness, tiredness

*EPS, extrapyramidal symptoms: 0, not present; +, sometimes; ++, often; +++, can be excessive.

discerned. On the one hand are *substituted benzamides* such as *sulpiride* and *amisulpride*. These drugs are highly selective D_2 receptor antagonists which, for reasons that are not well understood, seem less likely to produce extrapyramidal movement disorders. They also lack sedative and anticholinergic properties.

5-HT$_2$-D$_2$ receptor antagonists The other major group of atypical antipsychotic drugs possess *5-HT$_2$ receptor antagonist properties*. In other aspects, for example, potency of dopamine D_2 receptor blockade, these drugs differ significantly from one another (Richelson 1999). *Risperidone* is a potent antagonist at both 5-HT$_2$ receptors and dopamine D_2 receptors.

It also possess α_1-adrenoceptor blocking properties, which can cause mild sedation and hypotension. *Zotepine* has a similar pharmacological profile to risperidone but has a somewhat low selectivity for 5-HT$_2$ over D_2 receptors. It is also a stronger antihistamine, making it more likely to cause weight gain (Prakash and Lamb 1998).

Olanzapine is a slightly weaker D_2 receptor antagonist than risperidone but has anticholinergic and histamine H_1 receptor blocking activity. This gives it strong sedating effects. *Quetiapine* has modest 5-HT$_2$ receptor antagonist effects with even weaker D_2 receptor antagonist effects. It has a very low propensity to produce movement disorders (Stahl 1999).

Sertindole is a potent 5-HT$_2$ receptor antagonist with weak D$_2$ receptor antagonist effects. Sertindole produces clinically significant effects of the QT interval in the electrocardiogram and its use is currently suspended. *Ziprasidone* is another 5-HT$_2$ and D$_2$ receptor antagonist currently in clinical development. It differs from the other 5-HT$_2$/D$_2$ receptor antagonists described here because its also binds to 5-HT$_{1A}$ receptors and is a noradrenaline re-uptake inhibitor (Davis and Markham 1997). The clinical profile of ziprasidone is still being investigated but somnolence and dizziness are the most common side-effects and it causes relatively little weight gain.

To some extent these latter drugs were designed to reproduce the pharmacological profile of *clozapine*, which was the first antipsychotic agent to show definite benefit in the treatment of patients whose psychotic symptoms had failed to respond to conventional agents. In addition, clozapine has a low liability to produce movement disorders and is therefore usually regarded as the prototypic atypical antipsychotic drug (Kane *et al.* 1988). Clozapine is a *weak dopamine D$_2$ receptor antagonist but has a high affinity for 5-HT$_2$ receptors*; it also binds to a variety of other neurotransmitter receptors including histamine H$_1$, 5-HT$_2$, α$_1$-adrenergic and muscarinic cholinergic receptors (Richelson 1999).

The pharmacological basis for the increased efficacy of clozapine is not well understood. It is clear, however, that the use of clozapine is associated with a high risk of *leucopenia*, which restricts its use to patients who do not respond to or who are intolerant of other antipsychotic drugs. The haematological monitoring of clozapine treatment is discussed below.

Depot antipsychotic drugs

Slow-release preparations are used for patients who need to take antipsychotic medication to prevent relapse but cannot be relied on to take it regularly. These 'depot' preparations include the esters *fluphenazine decanoate, flupenthixol decanoate, zuclo-* *penthixol decanoate, haloperidol decanoate,* and *pipothiazine palmitate.* All are given intramuscularly in an oily medium. Zuclopenthixol acetate reaches peak plasma levels within 1–2 days and has a shorter duration of action than other depots. It is used for the immediate control of acute psychosis but its superiority to ordinary intramuscular injections is not established (see D. Taylor 1999). A slow release injection of risperidone is now available

Pharmacokinetics

Antipsychotic drugs are well absorbed, mainly from the jejunum. When they are taken by mouth, part of their hepatic metabolism is completed as they pass through the portal system on their way to the systemic circulation (first-pass metabolism). Antipsychotic drugs are *highly protein bound*.

With the exception of *amisulpride*, which is excreted unchanged by the kidney, antipsychotic drugs are extensively metabolized by the liver to produce a range of active and inactive metabolites. Following administration of chlorpromazine, for example, about 75 metabolites have been detected in the blood or urine. This complex metabolism has made it difficult to interpret the clinical significance of plasma concentrations of most antipsychotics; hence the latter are seldom used in everyday clinical work. The half-life of most antipsychotic drugs (around 20 hours) is sufficient to allow once-daily dosing. *Quetiapine*, however, has a half-life of about 7 hours, and twice-daily dosing is recommended.

The pharmacokinetic profile of *depot preparations* differs substantially from standard preparations. For all compounds except zuclopenthixol acetate, several weeks is needed for steady-state drug levels to be reached in plasma (Table 21.4). This means that relapse after treatment discontinuation is likely to be similarly delayed.

Drug interactions

Antipsychotic drugs potentiate the effects of other *central sedatives*. They may delay the hepatic metabolism of tricyclic antidepressants and antiepileptic

Table 21.4 Some pharmacokinetic properties of depot antipsychotic drugs

Depot	Time to peak plasma level (days)	Time to steady state (weeks)	Usual frequency of administration (weeks)	Equivalent dose (mg)
Flupenthixol decanoate	7–10	8	2	40
Fluphenazine decanoate	1–2	8	2	25
Haloperidol decanoate	3–9	12	4	100
Pipothiazine palmitate	9–10	8–12	4	50
Zuclopenthixol decanoate	4–7	8	2	200
Risperidone slow release injection	28	6	2	25

drugs, leading to increased plasma levels of these latter agents. The *hypotensive* properties of chlorpromazine and thioridazine may enhance the effects of *antihypertensive drugs* including ACE inhibitors.

Antipsychotic drugs, particularly *pimozide* and *thioridazine, can increase the QT interval* and should not be given with other drugs likely to potentiate this effect, such as anti-arrhythmics, astemizole and terfenadine, cisapride and tricyclic antidepressants. There are also reports of increased risk of cardiac arrhythmias when pimozide has been combined with clarithromycin and erthyromycin. *Clozapine* should not be given with any agent likely *to potentiate its depressant effect on white cell count* such as carbamazepine, co-trimoxazole, and penicillamine. *SSRIs* slow the hepatic metabolism and increase blood levels of several antipsychotic drugs including haloperidol, risperidone, and clozapine.

Unwanted effects

The many different antipsychotic drugs share a broad pattern of unwanted effects that are mainly related to their *antidopaminergic, antiadrenergic,* and *anticholinergic* properties (see Table 21.5). Details of the effects of individual drugs will be found in the *British National Formulary* or a similar work of reference. Here we give an account of the general pattern, with examples of the side-effects associated with a few commonly used drugs.

Extrapyramidal effects

These are related to the antidopaminergic action of the drugs on the *basal ganglia*. As already noted, the therapeutic effects may also derive from the antidopaminergic action, though presumably at mesolimbic and mesocortical sites. Atypical agents produce a more effective dopamine receptor blockade at the latter sites than at the basal ganglia.

The effects on the extrapyramidal system fall into four groups (see Barnes and Spence 2000):

- *Acute dystonia* occurs soon after treatment begins, especially in young men. It is observed most often with butyrophenones and with the piperazine group of phenothiazines. The main features are torticollis, tongue protrusion, grimacing, and opisthotonos, an odd clinical picture which can easily be mistaken for histrionic behaviour. It can be controlled by an *anticholinergic agent* given carefully by intramuscular injection.

- *Akathisia* is an unpleasant feeling of physical restlessness and a need to move, leading to an inability to keep still. It usually occurs in the first 2 weeks of treatment with antipsychotic drugs, but may begin only after several months. *Akathisia is not reliably controlled by antiparkinsonian drugs*, but β-adrenoceptor antagonists and short-term treatment with benzodiazepines may be helpful. The best

Table 21.5 Some unwanted effects of antipsychotic drugs

Antidopaminergic effects
  Acute dystonia
  Akathisia
  Parkinsonism
  Tardive dyskinesia

Antiadrenergic effects
  Sedation
  Postural hypotension
  Inhibition of ejaculation

Anticholinergic effects
  Dry mouth
  Reduced sweating
  Urinary hesitancy and retention
  Constipation
  Blurred vision
  Precipitation of glaucoma

Other effects
  Cardiac arrhythmias
  Weight gain
  Amenorrhoea
  Galactorrhoea
  Hypothermia

strategy is to reduce the dose of antipsychotic drug, if possible.

♦ *Parkinsonian syndrome* is characterized by akinesia, an expressionless face, and lack of associated movements when walking, together with rigidity, coarse tremor, stooped posture, and, in severe cases, a festinant gait. This syndrome often does not appear until a few months after the drug has been taken, and then sometimes diminishes even though the dose has not been reduced. The symptoms can be controlled with *antiparkinsonian drugs*.

However, it is not good practice to prescribe antiparkinsonian drugs prophylactically as a routine, because not all patients will need them. Moreover, these drugs themselves have undesirable effects in some patients; for example, they occasionally cause an acute organic syndrome, and may worsen or unmask concomitant *tardive dyskinesia*.

♦ *Tardive dyskinesia* is particularly serious because, unlike the other extrapyramidal effects, it does not always recover when the drugs are stopped. It is characterized by *chewing and sucking movements, grimacing, choreoathetoid movements*, and possibly *akathisia*. The movements usually affect the face, but the limbs and the muscles of respiration may also be involved. Whilst the syndrome is seen occasionally among patients who have not taken antipsychotic drugs, it is more common among those who have taken antipsychotic drugs for a number of years. It is also sometimes seen in patients taking dopamine receptor blockers for other indications, for example, metoclopramide for chronic gastrointestinal problems.

Epidemiology of tardive dyskinesia Tardive dyskinesia is more common among *women, the elderly*, and patients who have *diffuse brain pathology*. A diagnosis of *mood disorder* is also a risk factor (Kane 1999). In about half the cases, tardive dyskinesia disappears when the drugs are stopped. Estimates of the frequency of the syndrome vary in different series, but it seems to develop in about 20% of schizophrenic patients with schizophrenia treated with long-term antipsychotic drugs.

Pathophysiology of tardive dyskinesia The cause of tardive dyskinesia is uncertain, but it could be *supersensitivity to dopamine* resulting from prolonged dopaminergic blockade. This explanation is consistent with the observations that tardive dyskinesia may be aggravated in three ways:

♦ frequently by stopping the antipsychotic drugs;

◆ by the action of anticholinergic *antiparkinsonian drugs* (presumably by upsetting further the balance between cholinergic and dopaminergic systems in the basal ganglia); and

◆ by L-dopa and apomorphine in some patients.

However, there are other observations that do not readily fit this explanation. For example, ligand binding studies do not show clear relationships between dopamine receptor binding and the presence of tardive dyskinesia (see Barnes and Spence 2000).

Treatment of tardive dyskinesia Many treatments for tardive dyskinesia have been tried but none is universally effective. Therefore it is important to reduce its incidence as far as possible by limiting long-term antipsychotic drug treatment to patients who really need it. At the same time, a careful watch should be kept for abnormal movements in all patients who have taken antipsychotic drugs for a long time. If dyskinesia is observed, the antipsychotic drug should be stopped if the state of the mental illness allows this.

Although the dyskinesia may first worsen after stopping the drug, in many cases it will improve over several months. If the dyskinesia persists after this time or if the continuation of antipsychotic medication is essential, a trial can be made of an atypical agent with weaker dopamine receptor antagonist properties. This can sometimes lead to remission of the disorder. Other agents that have been tried include vitamin E, although the evidence for its efficacy is conflicting (Lohr and Lavori 1998). Preliminary data suggest that the incidence of tardive dyskinesia is less with *atypical antipsychotic agents* such as clozapine, olanzapine, and risperidone than with haloperidol (Beasley *et al.* 1999; Jeste *et al.* 1999). However, cases still occur, albeit at a lower level.

Anti-adrenergic effects

These include sedation, postural hypotension with reflex tachycardia, nasal congestion, and inhibition of ejaculation. The effects on blood pressure are particularly likely to appear after intramuscular administration, and may appear in the elderly whatever the route of administration.

Anticholinergic effects

These include dry mouth, urinary hesitancy and retention, constipation, reduced sweating, blurred vision, and, rarely, the precipitation of glaucoma.

Other effects

Cardiac conduction defects Cardiac arrhythmias are sometimes reported. ECG changes are more common in the form of *prolongation of the QT* and T-wave blurring. The use of *pimozide* has been associated with serious cardiac arrhythmias. Cautious dose adjustment with ECG monitoring is recommended. A recent survey also suggested that thioridazine and droperidol might be relatively more likely to produce QT prolongation (Reilly *et al.* 2000). Subsequently droperidol was withdrawn by the manufacturers and the indications for thioridazine greatly restricted.

Depression Depression of mood had been said to occur, but this is difficult to evaluate because untreated patients with schizophrenia may have periods of depression. It is certainly possible that excessive dopamine receptor blockade in the mesolimbic forebrain could be associated with anhedonia and loss of drive, which could then resemble depressive or negative symptoms of schizophrenia.

Endocrine and metabolic changes Some patients *gain weight* when taking antipsychotic drugs, especially chlorpromazine and atypical agents such as olanzapine, zotepine, and clozapine (Table 21.3). Clozapine and olanzapine are associated with an increased risk of type II diabetes (Koro *et al.* 2002) *Galactorrhoea* and *amenorrhoea* are induced in some women by high prolactin levels and it is possible that low libido and sexual dysfunction may also result. Some atypical agents do not increase prolactin levels significantly (Table 21.3).

Hypothermia and eye problems In the elderly, *hypothermia* is an important unwanted effect. Some antipsychotic drugs, particularly lower potency agents, such as chlorpromazine and clozapine, *lower seizure threshold* and can increase the frequency of seizures in epileptic patients. Prolonged *chlorpromazine* treatment can lead to *photosensitivity* and to accumulation of pigment in the skin, cornea, and lens. *Thioridazine* in exceptionally high dose (more than 800 mg/day) may cause *retinal degeneration*.

Sensitivity reactions Phenothiazines, particularly *chlorpromazine*, have been associated with cholestatic jaundice, but the incidence is low (about 0.1%). Blood cell dyscrasias also occur rarely with antipsychotic drugs, but are most common with clozapine. Skin rashes can also occur.

Adverse effects of clozapine

The use of clozapine is associated with a significant risk of *leucopenia* (about 2–3%), which can progress to agranulocytosis. Weekly blood counts for the first 18 weeks of treatment and at 2-weekly intervals thereafter are mandatory. After a year, the frequency of blood sampling may be lowered to monthly. With this intensive monitoring, the early detection of leucopenia can be followed by immediate withdrawal of clozapine and by reversal of the low white cell count. This procedure greatly reduces, but does not eliminate, the risk of progression to agranulocytosis. It is usually recommended that clozapine be used as the sole antipsychotic agent in a treatment regimen. Clearly, it is wise to avoid concomitant use of drugs such as *carbamazepine*, which may also lower the white cell count.

Because of its relatively weak blockade of dopamine D_2 receptors, clozapine is unlikely to cause extrapyramidal movement disorders, including tardive dyskinesia. It does not increase plasma prolactin; hence galactorrhoea does not occur. However, its use is associated with *hypersalivation, drowsiness, postural hypotension, weight gain, and hyperthermia. Seizures* may occur at higher doses. Clozapine is a sedating compound, and cases of respiratory and circulatory embarrassment have been reported during combined treatment with clozapine and benzodiazepines. Rarely, fatal *myocarditis* and *myopathy* have been reported (Kilian *et al.* 1999). The weight gain may be responsible for an increased risk of diabetes mellitus (Henderson *et al.* 2000).

The neuroleptic malignant syndrome

This rare but serious disorder occurs in a small minority of patients taking antipsychotic drugs, especially high-potency compounds. Most reported cases have followed the use of antipsychotic agents for schizophrenia, but in some cases the drugs were used for mania, depressive disorder, and psychosis secondary to a medical condition. *Combined lithium and antipsychotic* drug treatment may be a predisposing factor. The overall incidence is probably about 0.2% of patients treated with antipsychotic drugs (see Kohen and Bristow 1996).

The onset is often, but not invariably, in the first 10 days of treatment. The clinical picture includes the rapid onset (usually over 24–72 hours) of severe *motor, mental, and autonomic disorders*. The prominent motor symptom is generalized muscular hypertonicity. Stiffness of the muscles in the throat and chest may cause dysphagia and dyspnoea. The mental symptoms include akinetic mutism, stupor, or impaired consciousness. Hyperpyrexia develops with evidence of autonomic disturbances in the form of unstable blood pressure, tachycardia, excessive sweating, salivation, and urinary incontinence.

In the blood, *creatinine phosphokinase (CPK)* levels may be raised to very high levels, and the white cells increased. Secondary features may include pneumonia, thromboembolism, cardiovascular collapse, and renal failure. The mortality rate appears to be declining over recent years but can be of the order of 10%. The syndrome lasts for 1–2 weeks after stopping an oral neuroleptic but may last two to three times longer after stopping long-acting preparations. Patients who survive are usually without residual disability.

The differential diagnosis includes encephalitis, and in some countries heat stroke. Before the introduction of antipsychotic drugs, a similar disorder was reported as a form of catatonia sometimes called acute lethal catatonia.

The condition can probably occur with any antipsychotic agent, but in many reported cases the drugs used have been haloperidol or fluphenazine. Cases have also been reported with atypical antipsychotic drugs, including clozapine. The cause could be related to excessive dopaminergic blockade, though why this should affect only a minority of patients cannot be explained.

Treatment is symptomatic; the main needs are to stop the drug, cool the patient, maintain fluid balance, and treat intercurrent infection. No drug treatment is certainly effective. *Diazepam* can be used for muscle stiffness. *Dantrolene*, a drug used to treat malignant hyperthermia, has also been tried. *Bromocriptine*, *amantadine*, and L-*dopa* have been used, but with insufficient cases for a definite statement about their value. Some patients require intensive care unit support to maintain respiration and deal with renal failure.

Some patients who developed the syndrome on one occasion have been given the same drug again safely after the acute episode has resolved. Nevertheless, if an antipsychotic has to be used again, it is prudent to restart treatment cautiously with a low-potency drug or an atypical agent, used at first in low doses. At least 2 weeks should elapse before antipsychotic drug treatment is reinstated.

Contraindications

There are few contraindications to antipsychotic medication and they vary with individual drugs. Before any of these drugs is used, it is important to consult the *British National Formulary* or a comparable work of reference. Contraindications include myasthenia gravis, Addison's disease, glaucoma (where compounds have significant anticholinergic activity), and, in the case of clozapine, any evidence of bone marrow depression. For patients with liver disease, chlorpromazine should be avoided and other drugs used with caution. Caution is also required when there is renal disease, cardiovascular disorder, epilepsy, or serious infection. Patients with parkinsonism sometimes require antipsychotic medication to deal with psychotic states induced by dopaminergic agents; an atypical agent is preferable in these circumstances. Antipsychotic drugs can produced severe movement disorders and changes in consciousness in some patients with dementia, particularly *Lewy body dementia*.

Dosage

Doses of antipsychotic drugs need to be adjusted for the individual patient and changes should be made gradually. Doses should be lower for children, the elderly, patients with brain damage or epilepsy, and the physically ill. The dosage of individual drugs can be found in the *British National Formulary* or a comparable work of reference or in the manufacturer's literature.

PET imaging studies

There is a growing trend for lower doses of antipsychotic drugs to be recommended. This is based in part on studies with PET which have demonstrated that adequate dopamine D_2 receptor blockade (in the basal ganglia at least) can be obtained with *low doses* of conventional antipsychotic drugs (about 5 mg haloperidol, for example) (Table 21.6) (Farde *et al.* 1989; Kapur *et al.* 1999).

Such doses produce an adequate antipsychotic effect in the majority of patients. Higher doses may cause further calming but are also likely to be associated with significant adverse effects, some of which may be serious (for example, cardiac arrhythmias). A view of growing influence is that the combination of modest doses of antipsychotic drugs with a benzodiazepine is a safer and more effective means of producing rapid sedation than high doses of antipsychotic drugs (see Marder *et al.* 2000).

Antipsychotic drugs and risk of sudden death

The association of *sudden unexplained death* with antipsychotic drug treatment is a matter of continuing debate. Patients with schizophrenia treated with antipsychotic drugs appear to have higher rates of cardiac arrest and ventricular arrythmias than controls. This could be due to the illness or to treatment (Hennessy *et al.* 2002). However, antipsychotic drugs are known to alter *cardiac conduction*, and drugs such as chlorpromazine also produce hypotensive effects. An association between high doses of *pimozide* (often in the setting of a recent dose increase) and sudden unexplained death led to a reduction in the recommended maximum daily dose to 20 mg (Committee on the Safety of Medicines 1995). Whilst the relationship between high doses of antipsychotic drug treatment and sudden death is not well established, it is clearly prudent to use as low a dose of an antipsychotic

Table 21.6 Dosage and D_2 receptor blockade of some antipsychotic drugs

Drug	Relative dose (oral)	Maximum BNF dose (mg)	D_2 receptor occupancy *in vivo* (%) [daily dose (mg)]*
Chlorpromazine	100	1000	80 [200]
Thioridazine	100	600	75 [300]
Trifluoperazine	5	NA	80 [10]
Haloperidol	2	30	80 [4]
Flupenthixol	1	18	74 [10]
Sulpiride	200	2400	74 [800]
Clozapine	60	900	65 [600]
Risperidone	2	16	75 [4]
Olanzapine	8	20	75 [15]

NA, Not available.

* Farde *et al.* (1989); Nyberg and Farde (2000).

drug as the clinical circumstances permit. For a review of this area and the question of high-dose antipsychotic drug treatment see Royal College of Psychiatrists (1993).

An indication of the relative dosage of some commonly used drugs taken by mouth is given in Table 21.6. Some practical guidance on the most frequently used drugs is given in the next section.

Advice on management

Use in emergencies

Medication Antipsychotic drugs are used to control psychomotor excitement, hostility, and other abnormal behaviour resulting from schizophrenia, mania, or organic psychosis. If the patient is very excited and is displaying abnormally aggressive behaviour, the aim should be to bring the behaviour under control as quickly and safely as possible. *Chlorpromazine* (orally or intramuscularly) has previously been recommended for this purpose, but it has the disadvantage of producing autonomic side-effects such as hypotension. Current practice favours the use of low doses of drugs such as *haloperidol* (2–5 mg) or *lorazepam* (1–4 mg) singly

or if necessary in combination. (Chambers and Druss 1999; Taylor *et al.* 1999).

These drugs can be given orally or parenterally (diazepam is poorly absorbed intramuscularly). The intravenous route should be used only in exceptional circumstances. If haloperidol is used, an anticholinergic agent will reduce the risk of acute movement disorder. (National Institute of Clinical Excellence 2002). It is important to check for possible respiratory depression, particularly in the elderly or those with concomitant physical illness. It is also wise to have the benzodiazepine antagonist *flumazenil* available.

Another possibility is to use a medium-acting depot preparation such as *zuclopenthixol acetate* (Accuphase), which produces sedation shortly after its adminstration and has a duration of action of 1–2 days. Whilst this regimen may be useful in some circumstances, it does not permit the careful titration of dose against clinical response as described above. For this reason it should not usually be given to patients whose tolerance of antipsychotic drugs is not established (Royal College of Psychiatrists 1993).

Diagnosis and clinical management There are several other practical points in the management of the acutely disturbed patient that can be dealt with conveniently here. Although it may not be easy in the early stages to differentiate between mania and schizophrenia as causes of the disturbed behaviour, it is necessary to try to distinguish them from psychosis secondary to medical conditions and from outbursts of aggression in abnormal personalities. Among medical conditions it is important to consider post-epileptic states, the effects of head injury, transient global amnesia, and hypoglycaemia.

People with personality disorder may act in an extremely abnormal way when subjected to stressful events, especially if they have taken alcohol or other drugs. When overactive behaviour is secondary to an organic cause, it may be necessary to treat it symptomatically, but any drugs must be given cautiously and the primary disorder should be treated whenever possible. If the patient has been drinking alcohol, the danger of potentiating the sedative effects of antipsychotic drugs and benzodiazepines should be remembered. Similarly, antipsychotic drugs that may provoke seizures should be used with caution in post-epileptic states.

In order to make a diagnosis, a careful history should be taken from an informant as well as from the patient. It is unwise to be alone with a patient who has already been violent, at least until a diagnosis has been made. The interviewer should do his best to calm the patient. Provided that it seems safe and help remains at hand, he should disengage anyone who is restraining the patient physically. If medication is essential and the patient refuses to accept it, compulsory powers must be acquired by involving the relevant part of the Mental Health Act before applying treatment. If a calming injection is required, having obtained the necessary legal authority, the doctor should assemble enough helpers to restrain the patient effectively. They should act in a swift and determined way to secure the patient; half measures are likely to make him more aggressive. After the patient has become calmer, blood pressure and respiration should be monitored.

Drug treatment of the acute episode

When any necessary emergency measures have been taken, or from the beginning in less urgent cases, treatment with *moderate doses* of an oral antipsychotic drug should be started. An appropriate prescription would be haloperidol 4–12 mg daily in divided doses, chlopromazine 150–300 mg daily, riperidone 2–4 mg daily or olanzapine 10 mg daily.

In the early stages of treatment, the amount and timing of doses should be adjusted if necessary from one day to the next, until the most acute symptoms have been brought under control. Thereafter, regular once- or twice-daily dosage is usually appropriate. A careful watch should be kept for *acute dystonic reactions* in the early days of treatment. Watch should also be kept for *parkinsonian* side-effects as treatment progresses; if they appear, an antiparkinsonian drug should be given (see next section). For the elderly or physically ill, appropriate observations of temperature and blood pressure should be made to detect hypothermia or postural hypotension.

Whilst patients often become more settled a few days after starting antipsychotic drugs, improvement in psychotic symptoms is usually slow, with resolution often taking a number of weeks. Again, current trends are to maintain the dose of antipsychotic drugs at a modest steady level and not to escalate the dose in the hope of speeding up the rate of improvement. For patients in whom agitation and distress continue to cause concern, it may be appropriate to add short-term intermittent treatment with a *benzodiazepine* rather than increase the dose of antipsychotic agent.

Atypical antipsychotic drugs As noted above, *atypical antipsychotic agents* are less likely to produce extrapyramidal movement disorders than conventional agents. However, meta-analyses suggest that this advantage is less if the typical drug (usually haloperidol) is given in low dose (4–12 mg daily) (National Schizophrenia Guideline Group 1999).

Current advice is that *atypical antipsychotic drugs* should be preferred in patients with a *first episode* of illness and in other patients demonstrating *inadequate therapeutic response* or adverse effects such as *movement disorders* or *hyperprolactinaemia. Clozapine* is indicated for patients who are intolerant to or who do not respond to other atypical agents (National Institute for Clinical Excellence 2002).

Some authorities believe that the use of atypical agents will result in improved compliance with medication in the longer-term and less deterioration in cognitive function. Follow up studies will be needed to test these important possibilities.

It should be noted that some authorities believe that atypical antipsychotic drugs should be given as first-line treatment because their improved tolerability will lead to better long-term compliance and improved cognitive function. Longer-term studies are needed to test these proposals.

Drug treatment after the acute episode

Episodes of mania and acute psychosis secondary to medical conditions usually subside within weeks. However, patients with schizophrenia often require treatment for many months or years. Such maintenance treatment can be a continuation, often in a smaller dose, of the oral medication used to bring the condition under control.

Use of depot preparations Where patients do not take their drugs reliably, one of the intramuscular depot preparations may be useful. At the start of treatment a small test dose is given to find out whether serious side-effects are likely with the full dose (D. Taylor 1999). The appropriate maintenance dose is then established by observation and careful follow-up. As noted earlier, depot preparations have long half-lives, and therefore it may take *several weeks* for maximum plasma concentrations to be reached. This has implications for the rate at which dose increases and decreases should be made, and also for the tapering of doses of oral antipsychotic medication once depot treatment has started.

It is important to find the *smallest dose* of medication that will control the symptoms; since this may diminish with time, regular reassessment of the remaining symptoms of illness and the extent of side-effects is needed. It is not necessary to give *antiparkinsonian drugs* routinely; if they are needed, it may be only for some days after the injection of the depot preparation (when the drug plasma concentrations are highest).

Antiparkinsonian drugs

Although these drugs have no direct therapeutic use in psychiatry, they are often required to control the *extrapyramidal side-effects* of typical antipsychotic drugs.

Pharmacology

Of the drugs used to treat idiopathic parkinsonism, currently only the *anticholinergic compounds* are used for drug-induced extrapyramidal syndromes. These drugs are antagonists of *muscarinic cholinergic receptors* both centrally and in the periphery. Some also possess *antihistaminic* properties.

Preparations available

Many anticholinergic drugs are available and there is little to choose between the compounds. However, some authorities suggest that the use of agents more selective for the M_1 *subtype* of the muscarinic receptor, for example, *biperiden*, may be associated with fewer peripheral anticholinergic effects (Cunningham Owens 1998). Other preparations employed include *procyclidine* and *benzhexol. Orphenadrine* and *benztropine* have combined antihistaminic and anticholinergic properties.

Pharmacokinetics

Limited data are available. Anticholinergic drugs appear to be well absorbed and are extensively metabolized in the liver. They are highly protein bound. Their half-lives are generally between 15 and 20 hours.

Unwanted effects

In large doses these drugs may cause an *acute organic syndrome*, especially in the elderly. Their anticholinergic activity can summate with those of antipsychotic drugs so that glaucoma or retention of urine in men with enlarged prostates may be precipitated. Drowsiness, dry mouth, and constipation also occur. These effects tend to diminish as the drug is continued. Some studies have found that concomitant treatment with anticholinergic drugs can attenuate the therapeutic effect of antipsychotic drug treatment (Johnstone *et al.* 1983).

Orphenadrine may be more toxic than other anticholinergic drugs in overdose whereas *benztropine* has been associated with heat stroke (Cunningham Owens 1998). All anticholinergic drugs can exacerbate tardive dyskinesia but are probably not a predisposing factor in its development (see Barnes and Spence 2000).

Drug interactions

Antiparkinsonian drugs can induce *drug-metabolizing enzymes* in the liver, so that plasma concentrations of antipsychotic drugs are sometimes reduced. As noted above, anticholinergic agents can potentiate the effects of other drugs with anticholinergic activity such as chlorpromazine and amitriptyline.

Advice on management

As noted already, anticholinergic drugs should not be given routinely because they may increase the manifestation of tardive dyskinesia. It has also been pointed out that patients receiving injectable long-acting antipsychotic preparations usually require anticholinergic drugs for only a few days after injection, if at all. There have been reports of *abuse* and *dependence* on anticholinergic drugs, possibly resulting from a mood-elevating effect.

If anticholinergic drugs are required, *biperiden* (2–12 mg daily) or *procyclidine* (5–30 mg daily) are appropriate for routine use. These drugs are usually given in a thrice-daily dosing regimen, although their half-lives would suggest that less frequent dosing should be possible. It is best not to give anticholinergic drugs in the evening because of the possibility of excitement and *sleep disruption*.

Antidepressant drugs

Currently used antidepressant drugs can be divided into three main classes, depending on their acute pharmacological properties:

◆ *monoamine re-uptake inhibitors* Compounds that inhibit the re-uptake of noradrenaline and/or 5-HT (tricyclic antidepressants, SSRIs, selective noradrenaline and serotonin re-uptake inhibitors (SNRIs), and selective noradrenaline re-uptake inhibitors (NARIs).

◆ *monoamine oxidase inhibitors (MAOIs)* Compounds that deactivate monoamine oxidase irreversibly (phenelzine and tranylcypromine) or reversibly (moclobemide).

◆ *5-HT$_2$ receptor antagonists* These drugs (mirtazepine, nefazodone, and trazodone) have complex effects on monoamine mechanisms but share the ability to block 5-HT$_2$ receptors.

In the broad range of major depression, these drugs are of equivalent efficacy. The main distinctions between them are in their *adverse effects, toxicity, and cost* (Table 21.7). These three classes of drugs will be considered in turn after some comments on the possible mechanism of action of antidepressants.

Mechanism of action

The acute effect of re-uptake inhibitors and of MAOIs is to enhance the functional activity of noradrenaline and/or 5-HT. These actions can be detected within hours of the start of treatment and yet the antidepressant effects of drug treatment can be delayed for several weeks. For example, it has been suggested that at least 6 weeks should elapse before an assessment of the effects of an antidepressant drug can be made in an individual patient.

To some extent, this delay in the onset of therapeutic activity may be due to pharmacokinetic factors. For example, the half-life of most tricyclic antidepressants is around 24 hours, which means that steady state in plasma drug levels will be reached only after 5–7 days. However, it seems unlikely that this can account completely for the lag in antidepressant activity.

Table 21.7 Groups of antidepressant drugs

Drug	Advantages	Disadvantages
Tricyclic anti-depressants	Well studied No serious long-term toxicity Useful sedative effect in selected patients Inexpensive	Cardiotoxic*, dangerous in overdose Anticholinergic side-effects Cognitive impairment Weight gain during longer-term treatment
SSRIs SNRI	Lack cardiotoxicity: relatively safe in overdose Not anticholinergic No cognitive impairment Relatively easy to give effective dose	Long-term toxicity not fully evaluated Gastrointestinal disturbance, sexual dysfunction May worsen sleep and anxiety symptoms initially Greater risk of drug interaction Expensive‡
Trazodone Mianserin Mirtazepine	Lack cardiotoxicity†, relatively safe in overdose Not anticholinergic Useful sedative effect in selected patients	Daytime drowsiness Cognitive impairment Less well established efficacy in severe depression Expensive

* Lofepramine has important differences from conventional tricyclic antidepressants.

† Cardiac arrhythmias have rarely been reported with trazodone.

‡ Generic fluoxetine now available.

An important feature of both noradrenaline and 5-HT pathways is that the cell bodies in the midbrain possess *inhibitory autoreceptors*, stimulation of which decreases cell firing. Drugs that acutely increase synaptic neurotransmitter levels of noradrenaline and 5-HT (such as tricyclics and MAOIs) indirectly activate these autoreceptors through dendritic release of noradrenaline and 5-HT. This action diminishes cell body firing and attenuates the increase in neurotransmission caused by the antidepressant drug.

Biochemical and behavioural studies have indicated that, as antidepressant treatment is continued for several days, the autoreceptors on noradrenaline and 5-HT cell bodies become *subsensitive*. The effect of this is to free noradrenergic and 5-HT neurons from inhibitory feedback control, and to restore the firing rate of the cell bodies to normal levels despite the presence of increased synaptic concentrations of noradrenaline and 5-HT. This would be expected to increase further the ability of antidepressant drugs to augment noradrenaline and 5-HT function.

These findings suggest that the clinical effects of antidepressant treatment result from an increasing potentiation of noradrenaline and 5-HT neurotransmission over time. Recent experimental studies have suggested that increased monoamine function can lead to activation of *intracellular second messengers* such as cyclic AMP and this in turn results in increased elaboration of *neurotropic factors* required for neuronal function and survival. This model proposes that the effects of antidepressants are expressed ultimately at the level of synaptic plasticity and remodelling (see Duman *et al.* 1997).

Tricyclic antidepressants

Pharmacology

Tricyclic antidepressants have a three-ringed structure with an attached side chain. A useful distinction is between compounds that have a terminal methyl group on the side chain (*tertiary amines*) and those that do not (*secondary amines*). In general, compared with the secondary amines, tertiary amines (for example, amitriptyline, clomipramine, and imipramine) have a higher affinity for the 5-HT uptake site and are more potent antagonists of α_1-adrenoceptors and muscarinic cholinergic receptors. Therefore, in clinical use, tertiary amines are more sedating and cause more anticholinergic effects than secondary amines (for example, desipramine, nortriptyline, and protriptyline).

Tricyclic antidepressants inhibit the re-uptake of both 5-HT and noradrenaline. They also have *antagonist activities at a variety of neurotransmitter receptors*. In general, these receptor-blocking actions have been thought to cause adverse effects (Table 21.8), though some investigators have argued that the ability of some tricyclics to antagonize brain 5-HT$_2$ receptors may also mediate some of their therapeutic effects. Tricyclics have quinidine-like *membrane-stabilizing effects*, and this may explain why they impair cardiac conduction and cause high toxicity in overdose.

Pharmacokinetics

Tricyclic antidepressants are well absorbed from the gastrointestinal tract, and peak plasma levels occur 2–4 hours after ingestion. Tricyclics are subject to significant first-pass metabolism in the liver and are highly protein bound. The free fraction is widely distributed in body tissues. In general, the elimination half-life of tricyclics is such that it is unnecessary to give them more than once daily.

Tricyclics are metabolized in the liver by hydroxylation and demethylation; it is noteworthy that demethylation of tricyclics with a tertiary amine structure gives rise to significant plasma concentrations of the corresponding secondary amine. There can be substantial (10–40-fold) differences in plasma tricyclic antidepressant levels between individual subjects when fixed-dose regimens are employed.

Plasma monitoring of tricyclic antidepressants Despite a considerable research effort, the role of plasma level monitoring in the use of tricyclics is not well established. In general, it has been difficult to show a consistent relationship between plasma level and therapeutic response. The possible reasons for this have been discussed above. However, there is some agreement (though the studies are not all in accord) that plasma levels of *nortriptyline* demonstrate a

Table 21.8 Some adverse effects of tricyclic antidepressants

Pharmacological action	Adverse effect
Muscarinic receptor blockade (anticholinergic)	Dry mouth, tachycardia, blurred vision, glaucoma, constipation, urinary retention, sexual dysfunction, cognitive impairment
α_1-Adrenoceptor blockade	Drowsiness, postural hypotension, sexual dysfunction, cognitive impairment
Histamine H$_1$ receptor blockade	Drowsiness, weight gain
Membrane-stabilizing properties	Cardiac conduction defects, cardiac arrhythmias, epileptic seizures
Other	Rash, oedema, leucopenia, elevated liver enzymes

curvilinear relationship with clinical outcome. The highest response rates occur with plasma concentrations in the range of 50–150 ng/ml, and above this level the response rate may actually decline.

However, the relationship between clinical response during amitriptyline treatment and total plasma levels of amitriptyline and nortriptyline is not clear, with different studies reporting variously a linear relationship, a curvilinear relationship, and no relationship at all.

There is some evidence that high levels of tricyclic antidepressants are more likely to be associated with toxic side-effects such as *delirium*, *seizures*, and *cardiac arrhythmias*. The risk of such side-effects is minimized if total plasma levels of tricyclic antidepressants are *lower than 300 ng/ml* (Burke and Preskorn 1999). In this context it is worth noting that a small proportion of patients who metabolize drugs slowly may develop significantly increased plasma levels of tricyclics while taking routine clinical doses.

Overall, plasma-level monitoring has a useful but rather limited role in the management of tricyclic antidepressant treatment (Table 21.9). Plasma monitoring may be useful to assess *compliance* and is often helpful in patients who *have not responded* to what are usually adequate tricyclic doses, particularly if increases in dose above 225 mg daily are contemplated. Finally, plasma level monitoring is useful in patients with *coexisting medical disorders*, especially if there is a possibility of *drug interaction*. For example, in patients with seizure disorders, it is prudent to maintain plasma tricyclic levels within the usual range for the particular compound being used because tricyclics *lower the seizure threshold*. An additional level of complexity is added by the effects of coadministered antiepileptic drugs which can increase or lower plasma tricyclic levels through pharmacokinetic interactions.

Compounds available

These include amitriptyline, amoxapine, clomipramine, desipramine, dothiepin, doxepin, imipramine, lofepramine, nortriptyline, protriptyline,

Table 21.9 Indications for plasma monitoring of tricyclic antidepressants

To check compliance

Toxic side-effects at low dose

Lack of therapeutic response

Coexisting medical disorder (e.g. epilepsy)

Possibility of drug interaction

and trimipramine. Some of these are sufficiently distinct from amitriptyline and imipramine to be worth separate mention.

Amoxapine is a fairly selective inhibitor of noradrenaline uptake but, unusually for a tricyclic antidepressant, produces significant *blockade of dopamine D_2 receptors*. The combined effect of amoxapine to increase noradrenaline neurotransmission and antagonize D_2 receptors has led to suggestions that this compound may be particularly useful in the treatment of depressive psychosis when combined treatment with antidepressant and antipsychotic drugs is often required. However, the use of a single preparation to produce a combined pharmacological effect limits prescribing flexibility. Furthermore, as might be expected, the D_2 receptor blocking properties of amoxapine may result in extrapyramidal disorders (Rudorfer and Potter 1989).

Clomipramine is the most potent of the tricyclic antidepressants in inhibiting the re-uptake of 5-HT; however, its secondary amine metabolite, desmethylclomipramine, is an effective noradrenaline re-uptake inhibitor. In studies of depressed inpatients, the antidepressant effect of clomipramine was found to be superior to that of the SSRIs citalopram and paroxetine (Danish University Antidepressant Group 1990). Unlike other tricyclic antidepressants, clomipramine is also useful in ameliorating the symptoms of *obsessive–compulsive disorder* (whether or not there is a coexisting major depressive disorder) (p. 247).

Lofepramine is a tertiary amine which is metabolized to desipramine; however, during lofepramine treatment, desipramine levels are probably too low to contribute significantly to the therapeutic effect. Lofepramine is a fairly selective inhibitor of noradrenaline re-uptake, and has fewer anticholinergic and antihistaminic properties than amitriptyline. Lofepramine has been widely compared with other tricyclic antidepressants and in general its antidepressant efficacy appears equivalent (Anderson 1999).

Lofepramine is not sedating; early in treatment it can be experienced as activating, an effect which some depressed patients find unpleasant. Similarly, impaired sleep does not usually improve until the underlying depression remits. The most important feature of lofepramine is that, unlike conventional tricyclics, it is not *cardiotoxic in overdose.* This means that lofepramine is likely to be safer than other tricyclics for patients with cardiovascular disease, though caution is still recommended. There have been reports of *hepatitis* in association with lofepramine, but it is not clear whether the incidence is greater than with other tricyclic antidepressants.

Maprotiline is often referred to as a quadricyclic antidepressant because the tricyclic nucleus is supplemented by an ethylene bridge across the middle ring. It is the most selective noradrenaline uptake inhibitor of the tricyclic antidepressants currently available, and has moderate antihistaminic properties but rather less anticholinergic effects than imipramine. It is not well established whether maprotiline is more effective than placebo for depression, but in comparative studies with reference tricyclics its therapeutic activity appears equivalent.

The use of maprotiline at doses above 200 mg has been associated with a *higher incidence of seizures* than is usual during tricyclic treatment (Curran and de Pauw 1998). Therefore a dose range of 75–150 mg daily has been recommended, and the co-prescription of other drugs that may lower the seizure threshold, such as phenothiazines, should be approached with caution. Maprotiline has effects on the heart that are similar to those of conventional tricyclics, and in overdose it is at least as toxic.

Unwanted effects of tricyclic antidepressants

These are numerous and important (see Table 21.8).

- ◆ *Autonomic* Dry mouth, disturbance of accommodation, difficulty in micturition leading to retention, constipation leading rarely to ileus, postural hypotension, tachycardia, and increased sweating. Retention of urine, especially in elderly men with enlarged prostates, and worsening of glaucoma are the most serious of these effects; dry mouth and accommodation difficulties are the most common. Nortriptyline and lofepramine have relatively fewer anticholinergic side-effects.

- ◆ *Psychiatric* Tiredness and drowsiness with amitriptyline and other sedative compounds; insomnia with desipramine and lofepramine; acute organic syndromes; mania may be provoked in manic-depressive patients.

- ◆ *Cardiovascular effects* Tachycardia and hypotension occur commonly. The electrocardiogram frequently shows prolongation of PR and QT intervals, depressed ST segments, and flattened T-waves. Ventricular arrhythmias and heart block develop occasionally, more often in patients with pre-existing heart disease.

- ◆ *Neurological* Fine tremor (commonly), incoordination, headache, muscle twitching, epileptic seizures in predisposed patients, and, rarely, peripheral neuropathy.

- ◆ *Other* Allergic skin rashes, mild cholestatic jaundice, and, rarely, agranulocytosis; weight gain and sexual dysfunction are also common.

- ◆ *Withdrawal effects* Tricyclic antidepressants should be withdrawn slowly if at all possible. Sudden cessation may be followed by nausea, anxiety, sweating, gastrointestinal symptoms, and insomnia.

Toxic effects

In overdosage, tricyclic antidepressants produce a large number of effects, some of which are extremely serious. Therefore urgent expert treatment in a general hospital is required, but the psychiatrist should know the main signs of overdosage. These can be listed as follows. The cardiovascular effects include *ventricular fibrillation, conduction disturbances, and low blood pressure*. Heart rate may be increased or decreased depending partly on the degree of conduction disturbance. The respiratory effects lead to *respiratory depression*. The resulting hypoxia increases the likelihood of cardiac complications. Aspiration pneumonia may develop.

The central nervous system complications include agitation, twitching, convulsions, hallucinations, delirium, and coma. Parasympathetic effects include dry mouth, dilated pupils, blurred vision, retention of urine, and pyrexia. Most patients need only supportive care, but cardiac monitoring is important and arrhythmias require urgent treatment by a physician in an intensive care unit. Tricyclic antidepressants delay gastric emptying, and so gastric lavage is valuable for several hours after the overdose. Lavage must be carried out with particular care to prevent aspiration of gastric contents; if necessary, a cuffed endotracheal tube should be inserted before lavage is attempted.

Antidepressants and heart disease

The cardiovascular side-effects of tricyclic drugs, noted above, coupled with their toxic effects on the heart when these drugs are taken in overdose, have led to the suggestion that tricyclic antidepressant drugs may be dangerous in patients with heart disease. Indeed, patients with abnormal cardiac function do seem to be more at risk of orthostatic hypotension and heart block during treatment.

Some of the newer antidepressants, particularly the SSRIs, appear safer in patients with cardiac disease. With the availability of safer drugs it is probably wise not to use tricyclic antidepressants for patients with clinical or electrocardiographic evidence of cardiac disease (see D. L. Evans *et al.* 1999). A recent epidemiological study found a higher risk of myocardial infarction in patients maintained on tricyclics than those on SSRIs with an increase in relative risk of 2.2 (95% CI 1.2–3.8) (Cohen *et al.* 2000).

Antidepressants and epilepsy

Most classes of antidepressants lower the seizure thresholds to some extent. This can lead to an increased risk of seizures in patients who have epilepsy or are predisposed to it. In general, SSRIs, nefazodone, and trazodone are believed less likely to lower the seizure threshold than tricyclics. MAOIs are also said not to lower seizure threshold.

Another complication is that antidepressant drugs can cause pharmacokinetic interactions with anticonvulsants in various ways. For example, SSRIs and nefazodone can increase carbamazepine levels whereas valproate can elevate tricyclic concentrations. Before prescribing an antidepressant with an anticonvulsant, it is prudent to check possible interactions in the *British National Formulary* (see also Table 21.11).

Interactions with other drugs

- Tricyclic antidepressants antagonize the hypotensive effects of α_2-adrenoceptor agonists such as *clonidine* but can be safely combined with thiazides and angiotensin-converting enzyme (ACE) inhibitors.

- The ability of tricyclics to block noradrenaline re-uptake can lead to hypertension with systemically administered noradrenaline and adrenaline.

- Tricyclics should not be used in conjunction with *anti-arrhythmic drugs*, particularly *amiodarone*.

Plasma levels of tricyclics can be *increased* by numerous other drugs including cimetidine, sodium valproate, calcium channel blockers and SSRIs. Tricyclics may increase the action of warfarin. Interactions of *tricyclic drugs with MAOIs* are considered later.

Contraindications

Contraindications include agranulocytosis, severe liver damage, glaucoma, prostatic hypertrophy and significant cardiovascular disease. The drugs must be used cautiously in epileptic patients, in the elderly.

Clinical use of tricyclic antidepressants

In the use of tricyclics the old adage is recommended that it is best to get to know one or two drugs well and stick to them. It is probably sufficient to be familiar with one sedating compound (for example, amitriptyline) and one less sedating drug (for example, nortriptyline). Other tricyclics can then be reserved for special purposes; for example, lofepramine can be used for patients who present the risk of overdose, whilst clomipramine can be reserved for patients in whom a depressive disorder is related to an obsessional illness.

The prescribing of amitriptyline can be taken as an example. At the outset it is important to explain to patients that, whilst side-effects may be noticed early in treatment, any improvement in mood may be delayed for a week or more, and therefore it is important to persist. Early signs of improvement may include better sleep and a lessening of tension. Common side-effects should be mentioned because a forewarned patient is more likely to continue with medication.

The usual practice of starting with a *low dose* of amitriptyline and building up is probably wise, because side-effects are generally milder and patients are more likely to develop tolerance to them. The starting dose will depend to some extent on the patient's age, weight, physical condition, and history of previous exposure to tricyclics; daily doses of 25–50 mg for an out-patient and 50–75 mg for an in-patient would be reasonable. The whole dose can be given at night about 1–2 hours before bedtime because the sedative effects of the drug will help sleep.

Patients should be *reviewed frequently* in the first few weeks of treatment when support and advice are helpful both to maintain morale and to ensure compliance with medication. Often the clinician can detect improvements in rapport and initiative early in treatment. It can then be useful to discuss these changes with the patient. The dose of amitriptyline to be aimed is about 125 mg daily or above. With careful monitoring and encouragement, this dose can usually be reached over 2 weeks.

In some patients, *side-effects* limit the rate of dosage increase, but if there is clinical improvement it is reasonable to settle for lower doses. In general, side-effects should not be greater than the patient can comfortably tolerate.

For patients who show little or no improvement, it is usually advisable to continue amitriptyline for 4 weeks at the maximum tolerated dose before deciding that the drug is ineffective.

Some patients respond only to *higher doses* (up to 300 mg daily), and cautious increases towards this level are warranted provided that side-effects are tolerable. In doses above 225 mg daily, it is wise to *monitor plasma tricyclic levels* and the *electrocardiogram* before each further dosage increase.

Plasma tricyclic concentrations have to be interpreted in the context of a patient's clinical condition, but generally *levels above 450 ng/ml* are more likely to be associated with severe toxic reactions. In patients with concomitant medical disorders, a limit of *300 ng/ml* may be more appropriate (Burke and Preskorn 1999).

In the ECG it is important to note any evidence of impaired cardiac conduction, for example, *lengthening of the QT interval* and the appearance of bundle branch block or arrhythmias. Because of the half-life of amitriptyline, each dose increase will take about a week to reach steady state. If the patient has not improved, and if he cannot tolerate an increase in dose or fails to respond to higher doses, then other treatments should be considered. Some possible strategies are outlined in Chapter 11 on mood disorders (see p. 318).

Maintenance and prophylaxis

If patients respond to amitriptyline, they should be maintained on treatment for at least 6 *months* because continuation therapy greatly reduces the risk of early relapse. The same dose of amitriptyline should be maintained if possible, but if side-effects become a problem the dose can be lowered until tolerance is again satisfactory.

It is often not clear when antidepressant drug treatment should be withdrawn, because in some patients depression is a recurrent disorder. Long-term prophylactic treatment may then be justified.

Obviously the risk of recurrence increases with the number of episodes that the patient suffers, but other clinical and biochemical predictors of relapse are not well established. It has been reported that, if patients have been entirely free of depressive symptoms for at least 16 weeks, they are most likely to do well when drug treatment is withdrawn (Prien and Kupfer 1986).

Selective serotonin reuptake inhibitors (SSRIs)

Pharmacological properties

Five SSRIs – citalopram, fluoxetine, fluvoxamine, paroxetine, and sertraline – are available at present for clinical use in the UK. SSRIs are a structurally diverse group, but they all *inhibit the re-uptake of 5-HT* with high potency and selectivity. None of them has an appreciable affinity for the noradrenaline uptake site, and present data suggest that they have a low affinity for other monoamine neurotransmitter receptors.

Pharmacokinetics

In general, SSRIs are absorbed slowly and reach peak plasma levels after about 4–8 hours, although citalopram is absorbed more quickly. The half-lives of citalopram, fluvoxamine, paroxetine, and sertraline are between 20 and 30 hours, whereas the half-life of fluoxetine is 48–72 hours. The SSRIs are primarily eliminated by hepatic metabolism. Fluoxetine is metabolized to norfluoxetine, which is also a potent 5-HT uptake blocker and has a half-life of 7–9 days. Sertraline is converted to desmethylsertraline, which has a half-life of 2–3 days and is 5–10 times less potent than the parent compound in inhibiting the reuptake of 5-HT. The contribution of desmethylsertraline to the antidepressant effect of sertraline during treatment is unclear.

Efficacy of SSRIs in depression

The SSRIs have been extensively compared with placebo and with reference tricyclic antidepressants. The SSRIs are all clearly *superior to placebo* and are *generally as effective as tricyclics* in the treatment of major depression (see Anderson 1999). Most comparative studies have been of moderately depressed out-patients and there has been concern that SSRIs may be less effective than conventional tricyclic antidepressants for more severely depressed patients, particularly in-patients (Anderson 1999). For example, the Danish University Antidepressant Group (1990) found that clomipramine was significantly more effective than either paroxetine or citalopram for depressed inpatients.

Unwanted effects of SSRIs

The *adverse effects* of SSRIs differ significantly from those of tricyclic antidepressants. A major difference is that SSRIs are *less cardiotoxic than tricyclic antidepressants* and are generally much *safer in overdose*, though concerns have been raised about the safety of citalopram in this respect. SSRIs also *lack anticholinergic effects* and are not sedating. Side-effects can be grouped as follows (Table 21.10):

◆ *Gastrointestinal* Nausea (in about 20% of patients, though it may resolve with continued administration), dyspepsia, bloating, flatulence, and diarrhoea. Unlike tricyclic antidepressants, SSRIs are not usually associated with weight gain.

◆ *Neuropsychiatric* Insomnia, daytime somnolence, agitation, tremor, restlessness, irritability and headache. SSRIs have also been associated with seizures and mania, although they are probably less likely than tricyclics to produce the latter effects. By contrast, *extrapyramidal side-effects* such as parkinsonism and akathisia are more common during treatment with SSRIs than with tricyclics. In particular, paroxetine has been associated with *acute dystonias* in the first few days of treatment.

◆ *Other Sexual dysfunction* including ejaculatory delay and anorgasmia are common during SSRI treatment. Sweating, headache, and dry mouth are also reported. Cardiovascular side-effects are rare with SSRIs, but some reduction in pulse rate may occur and postural hypotension has been reported. Fluoxetine has been associated with skin rashes and, rarely, a more generalized allergic reaction with arthritis. SSRIs have been associated with a *low sodium state* secondary to inappropriate ADH secretion, especially in the elderly. As with tricyclic antidepressants, elevation of liver enzymes can occur but is generally reversible on treatment withdrawal. Recent evidence suggests that SSRIs may increase the risk of *upper gastrointestinal bleeding*.

- *Suicidal behaviour* There have been anecdotal reports that fluoxetine treatment may be associated with *hostile and suicidal behaviour*. While meta-analyses of controlled trials of fluoxetine have found no increase in suicidal ideation or suicidal acts, as compared with placebo or tricyclic antidepressants, it is likely that some of the reported cases of restlessness and suicidal behaviour associated with fluoxetine are attributable to *akathisia* (Power and Cowen 1992).

Interactions with other drugs

Pharmacodynamic interactions The most serious interaction yet reported is where simultaneous administration of SSRIs and MAOIs has provoked a *5-HT toxicity syndrome* ('the serotonin syndrome') with agitation, hyperpyrexia, rigidity, myoclonus, coma, and death (for further details see the section on MAOIs). Other drugs that increase brain 5-HT function must be used with caution in combination with SSRIs; they include lithium and tryptophan, which have been reported to be associated with mental state changes, myoclonus, and seizures. Serotonin toxicity can also occur if SSRIs are combined with 5-HT receptor agonists such as sumatriptan.

SSRIs may potentiate the induction of extrapyramidal movement disorders by antipsychotic drugs, although this effect could be partly due to a pharmacokinetic interaction whereby SSRIs increase plasma levels of certain antipsychotic drugs (see below).

Pharmacokinetic interactions SSRIs can produce substantial inhibition of some hepatic cytochrome P450 enzymes and can decrease the metabolism of several

---

Table 21.10 Side-effects of SSRIs

Gastrointestinal	*Common* nausea, appetite loss, dry mouth, diarrhoea, constipation, dyspepsia
	Uncommon vomiting, weight loss
Central nervous system	*Common* headache, insomnia, dizziness, anxiety, fatigue, tremor, somnolence
	Uncommon extrapyramidal reaction, seizures, mania
Other	*Common* sweating, delayed orgasm, anorgasmia
	Uncommon rash, pharyngitis, dyspnoea, serum sickness, hyponatraemia, alopecia

---

other drugs, thereby elevating their plasma levels (Table 21.11). Examples where clinically important reactions have been reported include tricyclic antidepressants, antipsychotic agents, including clozapine and risperidone, anticonvulsants, and warfarin. *Citalopram* and *sertraline* cause fewer reactions of this nature.

The clinical use of SSRIs in depression

Some authorities recommend that SSRIs should be used as the initial treatment in major depression; whilst others believe that (unless specifically contraindicated) tricyclic antidepressants should be used for this purpose because more is known about their efficacy and adverse effects and they are significantly cheaper. In clinical trials, the rate of drop-out due to adverse effects is modestly but significantly lower with SSRIs than tricyclics; this difference may be greater in routine clinical practice (see Anderson 1999). Economic analyses of the cost-benefit of SSRIs compared to tricyclics have given conflicting results (see Crott and Gilis 1998).

In general, it seems reasonable to use tricyclic antidepressants as initial treatment for severely depressed patients, particularly in-patients and those with depressive psychosis. SSRIs are suitable

Table 21.11 Inhibition of P450 enzyme by antidepressant drugs

	CYP 1A2	CYP 2D6	CYP 2C9	CYP 2C19	CYP 3A/4
Inhibitors	Fluvoxamine (+++)	Fluoxetine (+++)	Fluoxetine (+++)	Fluvoxamine (+++)	Nefazodone (++)
		Paroxetine (+++)	Fluvoxamine (+++)	Fluoxetine (++)	Fluvoxamine (+)
		Sertraline (+)		Venlafaxine (+)	Fluoxetine (+)
Some substrates (plasma level (increased)	Olanzapine Clozapine Haloperidol Tricyclic anti-depressants Theophylline	Tricyclic anti-depressants Nefazodone Venlafaxine Haloperidol Thioridazine Risperidone Clozapine Olanzapine	Warfarin Tolbutamide Phenytoin	Tricyclic anti-depressants Diazepam Propranolol Omeprazole	Terfenadine Astemizole Cisapride Benzodiazepines Carbamazepine Quetiapine Clozapine

Inhibition: +++, strong; ++, modest; +, mild.

alternatives to tricyclics for patients who may be vulnerable to anticholinergic effects or cardiotoxicity.

Particularly when the *risk of suicide* is significant and when supervision of medication is not assured, the lower acute toxicity of SSRIs makes them preferable to conventional tricyclic antidepressants. The *lack of sedation* makes SSRIs useful for outpatients who are striving to maintain their usual social and work activities. SSRIs may also be preferable for patients who gain *excessive weight* with tricyclic antidepressants. As mentioned above, depression in association with *an obsessional disorder* is an indication for treatment with an SSRI or clomipramine (Box 21.4).

Although the overall efficacy of individual SSRIs does not differ significantly, there are a few clinical distinctions which are worth considering (Edwards and Anderson 1999) (Table 21.12). *Fluvoxamine* appears to have *higher drop-out rates* from trials and may be somewhat less well tolerated. *Fluoxetine* has the most *activating effect* and also has a distinctive

Box 21.4 Indications for SSRI treatment in depression

◆ Concomitant cardiac disease*
◆ Intolerance of anticholinergic effects
◆ Significant risk of deliberate overdose
◆ Likelihood of excessive weight gain
◆ Sedation undesirable
◆ Depression and obsessive–compulsive disorder

* SSRIs are safer than tricyclic antidepressants but should be used with caution.

pharmacokinetic profile in relation to its *long-acting metabolite* which has a half-life of about a week. On the one hand, this results in a potential for troublesome *drug interactions* several weeks after fluoxetine has been stopped. For example, at least 5 weeks should elapse between stopping fluoxetine and starting an MAOI. On the other hand, this slow tapering of plasma concentration results in

Table 21.12 Contrasts between SSRIs

Drug	Risk of pharmacokinetic interaction*	Discontinuation syndrome	Other
Citalopram	Low	Not commonly reported	May be less safe in overdose
Fluoxetine	High	Rare	Increased risk of agitation, slower onset of action
Fluvoxamine	High	Common	Less well tolerated
Paroxetine	High	Common	Acute dystonia early in treatment
Sertraline	Moderate	Common	May have dopaminergic effects

*Based on inhibition of cytochrome P450 enzymes.

fluoxetine being the least likely of the SSRIs to cause a *withdrawal syndrome*.

In treating depressive disorder, dosing is easier with SSRIs than with tricyclic antidepressants because most SSRIs can be started at a standard dose that can often be maintained throughout treatment. For example, although fluoxetine has been given in doses of up to 80 mg daily, there is little evidence of increasing therapeutic efficacy above the 20 mg dose.

As with tricyclic antidepressant treatment, patients starting SSRIs should be warned about likely *side-effects*, including nausea and some restlessness during sleep. A number of patients become more anxious and agitated during SSRI treatment; therefore it is important to explain that such effects are sometimes experienced during treatment but do not mean that the underlying depression is worsening. If patients persist with treatment, anxiety and agitation usually diminish, *but short-term treatment with a benzodiazepine* may be helpful, particularly if sleep disturbance is a problem. Small doses of *trazodone* (50–150 mg) may also help sleep, although there are occasional reports of serotonin toxicity with this combination (Mir and Taylor 1999).

As with tricyclic antidepressants, when patients respond to SSRIs there is good evidence that *contin-uing treatment* for several months lowers the rate of relapse. In addition, placebo-controlled studies have shown that SSRIs are effective in the prophylaxis of recurrent depressive episodes. SSRIs should not be stopped suddenly as there have been reports of *withdrawal reactions* (insomnia, nausea, agitation, dizziness) after the cessation of treatment, particularly with paroxetine (Rosenbaum 1998; Edwards and Anderson 1999).

Monoamine oxidase inhibitors (MAOIs)

MAOIs were introduced just before the tricyclic antidepressants but their use has been less widespread because of both troublesome *interactions with foods and drugs* and uncertainty about their *therapeutic efficacy*. More recent controlled studies have shown that in adequate doses MAOIs are useful antidepressants, often producing clinical benefit in depressed patients who have *not responded* to other medication or ECT. In addition, MAOIs can be useful in *refractory anxiety states* (see Nutt and Bell 1997; Cowen 1999).

These beneficial effects have to be weighed against the need to adhere to *strict dietary and drug restrictions* in order to avoid reactions with tyramine and other sympathomimetic agents. In practice this means that MAOIs are very rarely used as first-line treatment.

Pharmacological properties

MAOIs inactivate enzymes that oxidize noradrenaline, 5-HT, dopamine, and tyramine, and other amines that are widely distributed in the body as transmitters, or are taken in food and drink or as drugs. Monoamine oxidase (MAO) exists in a number of forms that differ in their substrate and inhibitor specificities.

From the point of view of psychotropic drug treatment, it is important to recognize that there are two forms of MAO (type A and type B), which are encoded by separate genes. In general, *MAO-A* metabolizes intraneuronal *noradrenaline and 5-HT*, whereas both *MAO-A* and *MAO-B* metabolize *dopamine and tyramine*.

Compounds available

Phenelzine is the most widely used and widely studied compound. *Isocarboxazid* is reported to have fewer side-effects than phenelzine, and can be useful for patients who respond to the latter drug but suffer from its side-effects of hypotension or sleep disorder. *Tranylcypromine* differs from the other compounds in combining the ability to inhibit MAO with an *amphetamine-like stimulating effect* which may be helpful in patients with anergia and retardation. Some patients, however, have become dependent on the stimulant effect of tranylcypromine. Moreover, compared with phenelzine, tranylcypromine is more likely to give rise to hypertensive crises, though less likely to damage the liver. For these reasons, tranylcypromine should be prescribed with particular caution.

Moclobemide is the most recently developed MAOI to be marketed. It differs from the other compounds in *selectively binding* to MAO-A, which it inhibits in a *reversible* way. This results in a lack of significant interactions with foodstuffs and a quick offset of action (Da Prada *et al.* 1994) (see below).

Pharmacokinetics

Phenelzine, isocarboxazid, and tranylcypromine are rapidly absorbed and widely distributed. They have short half-lives (about 2–4 hours), as they are quickly metabolized in the liver by acetylation, oxidation, and deamination. People differ in their capacity to acetylate drugs; for example, in the UK, approximately 60% of the population are 'fast acetylators' who would be expected to metabolize hydrazine MAOIs more quickly than 'slow acetylators'. Some studies have shown a better clinical response to phenelzine in 'slow acetylators', but this finding has not been consistently replicated. However, it may underlie the observation that the best response rate with MAOIs occurs in studies that have used *higher dose ranges*, presumably because even patients who metabolize MAOIs quickly will receive an adequate dose.

Phenelzine, isocarboxazid, and tranylcypromine bind irreversibly to MAO-A and MAO-B by means of a covalent linkage. Hence, the enzyme is permanently deactivated and MAO activity can be restored only when new enzyme is synthesized. Thus, despite their short half-lives, irreversible MAOIs cause a *long-lasting inhibition of MAO*.

In contrast with these compounds, moclobemide binds reversibly to MAO-A. This compound has a short half-life (about 2 hours), and therefore its inhibition of MAO-A is brief, declining to some extent even during the latter periods of the thrice-daily dosing regimen. Full MAO activity is restored *within 24 hours of stopping moclobemide*; with the irreversible MAOIs, 2 weeks or more may be needed for synthesis of new MAO.

Efficacy of MAOIs in depression

For many years MAOIs were in relative disuse because several studies, in particular a large controlled trial by the Medical Research Council (Clinical Psychiatry Committee 1965), found phenelzine no better than placebo in the treatment of depressive disorders. It seems likely that the doses of MAOIs were too low in these early investigations; in the Medical Research Council study the maximum dose of phenelzine was 45 mg daily as against the current practice of doses up to 90 mg daily if side-effects permit. Subsequent studies have shown that in this wider dose range MAOIs are *superior to placebo* and are *generally equivalent to tricyclic antidepressants* in their therapeutic activity (Paykel 1990).

Investigations in the USA have confirmed early clinical impressions that MAOIs may be of particular value in the treatment of *atypical depression* (Quitkin *et al.* 1989) (see p. 275). It also seems that MAOIs are more effective than tricyclic antidepressants for patients with *bipolar depression* if the clinical features include hypersomnia and anergia (Himmelhoch *et al.* 1991).

Partly because of the concept that MAOIs are effective in atypical depression, it is often said that they are less effective than tricyclics in the treatment of more typical depressive disorders with characteristic vegetative changes. However, if adequate doses are given, MAOIs seem to be effective in the treatment of endogenous depression (Paykel 1990). There is also good evidence that they may be beneficial for depressed patients who *do not respond to tricyclics and other re-uptake inhibitors*, whether or not the depression has endogenous features (Cowen 1999).

Unwanted effects

These include dry mouth, difficulty in micturition, postural hypotension, confusion, mania, headache, dizziness, tremor, paraesthesia of the hands and feet, constipation, and oedema of the ankle. Hydrazine compounds can give rise to hepatocellular jaundice (Box 21.5).

Interactions with foodstuffs

Some foods contain *tyramine*, a substance that is normally inactivated by MAO in the liver and gut wall. When MAO is inhibited, tyramine is not broken down and is free to exert its *hypertensive effects*. These effects are due to release of noradrenaline from sympathetic nerve terminals with a consequent elevation in blood pressure. This may reach dangerous levels and may occasionally result in *subarachnoid haemorrhage*. Important early symptoms of such a crisis include a severe and usually throbbing headache.

The incidence of hypertensive reactions is about 8% in patients taking MAOIs, even in those who

> ### Box 21.5 Adverse effects of MAOIs
>
> **Central nervous system**
> - Insomnia, drowsiness, agitation, headache, fatigue, weakness, tremor, mania, confusion, convulsions (rare)
>
> **Autonomic**
> - Blurred vision, difficulty in micturition, sweating, dry mouth, postural hypotension, constipation
>
> **Other**
> - Sexual dysfunction, weight gain, peripheral neuropathy (pyridoxine deficiency), oedema, rashes, hepatocellular toxicity (rare), leucopenia (rare)

have received dietary counselling (Davidson 1992). Therefore regular reminders about dietary restrictions may be helpful, particularly in patients on longer-term treatment (Box 21.6). There have been reports of many foods being implicated in hypertensive reactions with MAOIs, but many of these have cited single cases and hence are of uncertain validity. Another complication is that the tyramine content of a particular food item may vary, as may the susceptibility of an individual patient to a hypertensive reaction. If a forbidden food has been consumed on one occasion without adverse effects, this does not preclude a future reaction.

It is notable that about four-fifths of all reported reactions between foodstuffs and MAOIs, and nearly all the deaths, have followed the *consumption of cheese*. Hypertensive reactions should be treated with parenteral administration of an α_1-adrenoceptor antagonist, such as *phentolamine*. If this drug is not available, *chlorpromazine* can be used. Recently, the use of oral *nifedipine* has been advocated. Whatever treatment is given, blood pressure must be monitored carefully.

Moclobemide and tyramine reactions

Tyramine is metabolized by both MAO-A and MAO-B. Experimental studies have shown that the hypertensive effect of oral tyramine is potentiated

Box 21.6 **Foods to be avoided during MAOI use**

- All cheeses except cream, cottage, and ricotta cheeses
- Red wine, sherry, beer, and liquors
- Pickled or smoked fish
- Brewer's yeast products (for example Marmite, Bovril, and some packet soups)
- Broad bean pods (such as Italian green beans)
- Beef or chicken liver
- Fermented sausage (for example, bologna, pepperoni, salami)
- Unfresh, overripe, or aged food (for example pheasant, venison, unfresh dairy products)

Box 21.7 **Clinical features of the serotonin syndrome**

Neurological
  Myoclonus, nystagmus, headache, tremor, rigidity, seizures
Mental state
  Irritability, confusion, agitation, hypomania, coma
Other
  Hyperpyrexia, cardiac arrhythmias, death

much less by moclobemide than by non-selective MAOIs (Da Prada *et al.* 1994). In patients taking moclobemide, the dose of tyramine required to produce a significant pressor response is above 100 mg. Even a five-course meal with wine would be unlikely to result in a tyramine intake of more than 40 mg.

Tyramine has relatively little effect in patients receiving moclobemide because MAO-B (present in the gut wall and liver) is still available to metabolize much of the tyramine ingested. Another factor may be that the interaction between moclobemide and MAO-A is reversible, thus allowing displacement of moclobemide from MAO when tyramine is present in excess.

Interactions with drugs

Patients taking MAOIs must not be given drugs whose metabolism depends on enzymes that are affected by the MAOI. These drugs include *sympathomimetic amines* such as *adrenaline, noradrenaline,* and *amphetamine,* as well as *phenylpropanolamine* and *ephedrine* (which may be present in proprietary cold cures). *L-Dopa* and *dopamine* may also cause hypertensive reactions. Local anaesthetics often contain a sympathomimetic amine, which should also be avoided. *Opiates, cocaine,* and *insulin* can also be involved in dangerous interactions. Sensitivity

to *oral antidiabetic* drugs is increased, with consequent risk of hypoglycaemia. The ability of MAOIs to cause postural hypotension can increase the *hypotensive effects* of other agents. Finally, the metabolism of carbamazepine, phenytoin, and other drugs broken down in the liver *may be slowed.*

The serotonin syndrome A number of drugs that potentiate brain 5-HT function can produce a severe *neurotoxicity syndrome* when combined with MAOIs. The main features of this syndrome are shown in Box 21.7). It is worth noting that some of these symptoms resemble the neuroleptic malignant syndrome (see p. 670) with which 5-HT neurotoxicity is occasionally confused (Sternbach 1991). In view of the interactions between dopamine and 5-HT pathways, it is possible that similar mechanisms may be involved.

Current clinical data suggest that combination of *MAOIs* with *SSRIs, venlafaxine, and clomipramine* is contraindicated. The combination of MAOIs with L-tryptophan has also been reported to cause 5-HT toxicity. Adverse reactions have been reported between the 5-HT$_{1A}$ receptor agonist, *buspirone,* and MAOIs. The use of 5-HT$_1$ receptor agonists, such as *sumatriptan,* should be avoided. Use with caution the combination of *lithium* with MAOIs seems safe and is often effective in patients with resistant depression.

If a 5-HT syndrome develops, all medication should be stopped and supportive measures instituted. In theory, drugs with 5-HT receptor antagonist properties such as cypropeptadine or propranolol may be helpful, but formal studies have not been carried out (see Mir and Taylor 1999).

Combination of MAOIs with tricyclic antidepressants The combined use of MAOIs and tricyclic antidepressants fell into disuse because of the severe reactions associated with the 5-HT syndrome. Current views are that combination therapy is safe provided that the following rules are followed:

♦ Clomipramine and imipramine are not used. The most favoured tricyclics in combination with MAOIs are amitriptyline and trim-ipramine.

♦ The MAOI and tricyclic are started together at low dosage, or the MAOI is added to the tricyclic (adding tricyclics to MAOIs is more likely to provoke dizziness and postural hypotension).

The advantages and disadvantages of combined tricyclic and MAOI therapy have not been fully established. On the one hand, patients taking tricyclics with MAOIs are less likely to suffer from *MAOI-induced insomnia*; on the other hand, they are more likely to experience *postural hypotension* and troublesome *weight gain*. The combination is said to be useful in patients with *resistant depression*. Although formal studies have not been carried out in this patient group, there are case reports of patients for whom combined MAOI-tricyclic treatment was successful when either treatment alone had not been helpful. Low doses of *trazodone* (50–150 mg) are also used to ameliorate MAOI-induced insomnia; present experience suggests that this combination is well tolerated, although there are occasional reports of adverse effects that could represent serotonin toxicity.

Contraindications

These include liver disease, phaeochromocytoma, congestive cardiac failure, and conditions that require the patient to take any of the drugs that react with MAOI.

Clinical use of MAOIs in depression

Because of the potential danger of drug interactions and the need for a tyramine-free diet, irreversible MAOIs are rarely used as first-line antidepressant agents. The exception may be when patients have previously shown a favourable response to these drugs as against other classes of antidepressants. Even in atypical depression, for which MAOIs may well be superior to tricyclic antidepressants, it is probably better to try an SSRI first because many patients will respond to this approach.

The clinical use of phenelzine can be taken as an example. Treatment should start with 15 mg daily increasing to 30 mg daily in divided doses (with the final dose not later than 3.00 p.m.) in the first week. Patients should be given *clear written instructions about foods to be avoided* (see below) and should be warned to take no other medication unless it has been specifically checked with a pharmacist or doctor who knows that the patient is taking MAOIs. As always, patients should be warned about the delay in therapeutic response (up to 6 weeks) and about common side-effects (sleep disturbance, dizziness).

In the second week, the dose of phenelzine can be increased to 45 mg daily. At this stage a greater increase to 60 mg may produce a quicker response, but it is also associated with more adverse effects. Accordingly, if feasible, it is better to find out whether an individual patient will respond to lower doses (about 45 mg) before increments are made (up to 90 mg daily). If patients do not respond to 45 mg, the dose can be increased by 15 mg weekly if side-effects permit.

The response to MAOIs can often be sudden; over the course of a day or two the patient suddenly feels better. If there are signs of *overactivity* or *excessive buoyancy* in mood, the dose can be reduced and the patient monitored for signs of developing hypomania. Side-effects likely to be particularly troublesome are insomnia and postural hypotension. Insomnia is best managed by lowering the dose of MAOI if feasible. Otherwise, the addition of a benzodiazepine or trazodone (50–150 mg at night) can be helpful, although the latter drug can sometimes increase problems of dizziness and postural hypotension.

Postural hypotension can be a disabling problem with MAOIs. Again, dose reduction is worth considering. Various measures have been suggested, for example, the use of support stockings, an increase in salt intake, or even the use of a mineralocorticoid. Of course, the latter two measures have their own adverse effects.

Withdrawal from MAOIs

Patients who respond to MAOIs have often suffered from disabling depression for many months or even years. For such patients the usual practice is to continue therapy for at least 6 months to a year. With MAOIs (but not tricyclic antidepressants), it is wise to lower the dose if the patient can tolerate the reduction without relapsing. Sudden cessation of MAOIs can lead to *anxiety* and *dysphoria*. Even gradual withdrawal can be associated with increasing anxiety and depression.

Clinical experience indicates that it is more difficult to stop MAOI than tricyclic antidepressant treatment. An explanation for this difference may be that MAOIs may produce *physical dependence* in some patients; another possible explanation is that MAOIs are given to patients with chronic disabling disorders who frequently relapse. It is emphasized that, because of the time taken to synthesize new MAO, *2 weeks should elapse* between the cessation of irreversible MAOI treatment and the easing of dietary and drug restrictions.

Treatment with reversible type A MAOI inhibitors

In their freedom from tyramine reactions and their quick offset of activity, the reversible type A MAOIs, such as *moclobemide*, have clear advantages over conventional MAOIs. As with all newer antidepressants, however, the therapeutic efficacy of moclobemide, particularly in more severely depressed patients, is not as well established and may be questionable (Anderson 1999). Also, it is not yet known whether moclobemide will prove effective for patients with the various forms of atypical depression and tricyclic-resistant

depression for which conventional MAOIs can be useful.

The starting dose of moclobemide is 150–300 mg daily, which can be increased to 600 mg over a number of weeks. Moclobemide is better tolerated than tricyclic antidepressants or irreversible MAOIs, but side-effects such as nausea and insomnia occur in about 20–30% of patients.

Drug interactions of moclobemide

Moclobemide should not be combined with *SSRIs*, *venlafaxine* or *clomipramine* because a serotonin syndrome may result. Caution is needed with *sumatriptan*. Like the irreversible MAOIs, moclobemide may react adversely with *opiates*. Similarly, moclobemide may potentiate the pressor effects of *sympathomimetic amines*; therefore combined use should be avoided. Moclobemide should not be combined with *L-dopa* because of the risk of hypertensive crisis. *Cimetidine* delays the metabolism of moclobemide.

Other antidepressant drugs

Other antidepressant drugs are available for use in the UK. Their mechanism of action is such that they cannot easily be grouped with tricyclic antidepressants, SSRIs, or with MAOIs. These drugs also have differing adverse-event profiles. Therefore they are discussed individually below.

Mianserin

Mianserin is a quadricyclic compound with complex pharmacological actions. It has weak noradrenaline re-uptake inhibiting effects, and is a fairly potent antagonist at several 5-HT receptor subtypes, particularly 5-HT$_2$ receptors. Mianserin is also a competitive antagonist at histamine H$_1$ receptors and α_1- and α_2-adrenoceptors. The latter action leads to an increase in noradrenaline cell firing and release. It is not a muscarinic cholinergic antagonist and is not cardiotoxic. Because of these various actions, mianserin has a *sedating profile*, but it is not anticholinergic and is relatively *safe in overdose*.

Pharmacokinetics Mianserin is rapidly absorbed, and the peak plasma concentration occurs after 2–3 hours. Its half-life is 10–20 hours, and the entire daily dose can be given in a single administration at night.

Efficacy Controlled trials have shown that mianserin is *superior to placebo* in the management of depression, and comparative studies against imipramine and clomipramine have shown no difference in effect. These studies are difficult to assess because of the wide range of doses that have been used. Many early studies of mianserin used doses of 30–60 mg daily, whereas much higher doses of up to 200 mg daily have sometimes been advocated for in-patients.

Unwanted effects The main adverse effects of mianserin are *drowsiness* and *dizziness*, though these effects can be lessened by starting at a modest dosage and then increasing gradually. Significant cognitive impairment is more likely with mianserin than with SSRIs. *Weight gain* is a common problem. Dyspepsia and nausea have also been reported. Like tricyclics, mianserin appears to lower seizure threshold to some extent. Postural hypotension occurs occasionally.

The most serious adverse effect of mianserin is lowering of the white cell count, and *fatal agranulocytosis* has been reported. These adverse reactions occur more commonly in elderly patients. It is recommended that a blood count be obtained before starting mianserin treatment, and that the white cell count be monitored monthly for 3 months after treatment has started. Rare side-effects of mianserin include arthritis and hepatitis.

Drug interactions Mianserin can potentiate the effect of other central sedatives. There is a theortical risk that mianserin could reverse the effects of α_2-adrenoceptor agonists such as clonidine.

Mirtazapine

Mirtazapine is an analogue of mianserin with a generally similar pharmacological profile but a weaker affinity for α_1-adrenoceptors. It is said that this permits mirtazapine to activate 5-HT as well as noradrenaline neurons. Like mianserin, mirtazepine has a *sedating profile* (Fawcett and Barkin 1998). *Mirtazepine is known as a noradrenaline- and serotonin-specific antidepressant (NASSA).*

Pharmacokinetics Mirtazapine is well absorbed with peak plasma levels being reached between 1 and 2 hours. The half-life is about 16 hours and the daily dose can be given at night. Mirtazapine is extensively metabolized by the liver and has only minor inhibitory effects on cytochrome P450 isoenzymes.

Efficacy Mirtazapine has demonstrated clinical efficacy in both *placebo-controlled and comparator trials* with SSRIs and tricyclic antidepressants in moderate to severely depressed patients. The effective dose is usually between 30 mg and 45 mg daily. Some have advocated that mirtazapine treatment should be instituted directly at a dose of 30 mg at night rather than a lower intermediate dose because at the higher dose excessive sedation may be actually less common. The theoretical reason given for this is that at the higher dose the powerful antihistaminic action of mirtazapine should be mitigated by activation of noradrenaline pathways (Fawcell and Barkin 1998).

Unwanted effects The common adverse effects of mirtazapine are attributable to its potent antihistaminic actions and include *drowsiness* and *dry mouth*. *Increased appetite* and *body weight* are also common. Thus far leucopenia does not appear more common with mirtazapine than with other antidepressants. The data sheet, however, recommends that physicians be vigilant for possible signs that might reflect low white cell count.

Drug interactions Mirtazapine may potentiate other centrally acting sedatives. As with mianserin, there is a theoretical risk that mirtazapine could reverse the effect of α_2-adrenoceptor agonists.

Trazodone

Trazodone is a triazolopyridine derivative with complex actions on 5-HT pathways. Studies *in vitro* suggest that trazodone has some weak 5-HT re-uptake inhibiting properties which are probably not manifest during clinical use; for example, repeated administration of trazodone does not lower platelet 5-HT content.

Trazodone has antagonist actions at 5-HT_2 receptors but its active metabolite, *m*-chlorophenylpiperazine (*m*-CPP), is a 5-HT receptor agonist. Therefore the precise balance of effects on 5-HT receptors during trazodone treatment is difficult to determine and may depend on relative blood levels of the parent compound and metabolite. Trazodone also blocks post-synaptic α_1-adrenoceptors. Overall it has a distinct *sedating profile*.

Pharmacokinetics Trazodone has a short half-life (about 4–14 hours). It is metabolized by hydroxylation and oxidation, with the formation of a number of metabolites including *m*-CPP. During treatment, plasma levels of *m*-CPP may exceed those of trazodone itself.

Efficacy Several controlled studies have shown that trazodone in doses of 150–600 mg is *superior to placebo* in the treatment of depressed patients. Trazodone also appears to have equivalent antidepressant activity to reference compounds such as imipramine. Many of these studies were carried out in moderately depressed out-patients, and the efficacy of trazodone relative to other antidepressants is not well established (see Anderson 1999).

Some workers have maintained that the efficacy of trazodone is improved if treatment is started at low doses (50 mg) and increased slowly to 300 mg over 2–3 weeks. Despite the short half-life of trazodone, once-daily adminstration of the drug is often sufficient. The drug is usually given in the evening to take advantage of its sedative properties. Doses above 300 mg daily are usually better given in divided amounts. Lower doses (50–150 mg) are sometimes used in combination with SSRIs and MAOIs to ameliorate the sleep-disrupting effects of the latter agents.

Unwanted effects The major unwanted effect of trazodone is *excessive sedation*, which can result in significant cognitive impairment. *Nausea* and *dizziness* are also reported, particularly if the drug is taken on an empty stomach. The α_1-adrenoceptor antagonist properties of trazodone may *lower blood pressure* to some extent, and postural hypotension has been reported. Trazodone is less cardiotoxic than conventional tricyclics, but there are reports that *cardiac arrhythmias* may be worsened in patients with cardiac disease. Nevertheless, trazodone is less toxic in overdose than tricyclic antidepressants.

The most serious side-effect of trazodone is *priapism*. This reaction is seen rarely (about 1 in 6000 male patients). It can cause considerable problems, requiring the local injection of noradrenaline agonists such as adrenaline or even surgical decompression. Long-term sexual dysfunction has sometimes resulted. It is recommended that male patients be warned of this potential side-effect and advised to seek medical help urgently if persistent erection occurs.

Drug interactions As with all sedative antidepressants, trazodone may potentiate the sedating effects of alcohol and other central tranquillizing drugs. Studies in animals have raised the possibility that trazodone could attenuate the hypotensive effect of clonidine, but it is not known whether such an interaction occurs in humans.

Nefazodone

Nefazodone is related to trazodone but lacks α_1-adrenoceptor antagonist properties and is therefore *not sedating*. Like trazodone, it is a 5-HT_2 receptor antagonist and has rather modest 5-HT re-uptake blocking properties and is metabolized to the 5-HT receptor agonist, *m*-CPP (see Horst and Preskorn 1998).

Pharmacokinetics Nefazodone is rapidly absorbed and undergoes extensive first-pass metabolism. It is highly protein bound. The principal metabolites are *m*-CPP and hydroxynefazodone, which has similar pharmacological properties to nefazodone. Both nefazodone and hydroxynefazodone have relatively short half-lives (2–4 hours) which makes twice-daily dosing necessary.

Efficacy Controlled trials in patients with major depression have shown that in doses of 400 mg and greater, nefazodone is *more effective than placebo* and generally *equal in therapeutic activity* to comparator drugs such as SSRIs and tricyclic antidepressants (Rickels *et al.* 1994). A recent placebo-controlled investigation in depressed in-patients showed good efficacy of nefazodone in this setting (Feighner *et al.* 1998). Nefazodone is usually given in two divided doses starting at 100–200 mg daily with titration to 400 mg daily after 1–2 weeks. The maximum dose is 600 mg daily.

Unwanted effects Nefazodone is generally well tolerated with the most common side-effects being *headache, loss of energy, dizziness, dry mouth, nausea,* and *somnolence.* It appears less cardiotoxic than tricyclic antidepressants and is probably *safer in overdose.* Nefazodone is less likely than the SSRIs to cause anxiety, insomnia, and sexual dysfunction. There are reports of severe hepatic reactions linked to nefazodone treatment and the drug has been withdrawn in the UK and some other countries.

Drug interactions Nefazodone inhibits cytochrome P450 3A4. It should therefore not be given with other drugs that are substrates for this enzyme and which also have a low acute toxicity, for example, terfenadine, astemizole, and cisapride (see Table 21.11). Nefazadone also elevates plasma levels of carbamazepine, haloperidol, benzodiazepines, and digoxin. The risk of cardiomyopathy with simvastatin may be increased by nefazodone.

Reboxetine

Reboxetine is a morpholine and is structurally related to fluoxetine. It is a *selective noradrena-line re-uptake inhibitor (NARI)* with no clinically significant effects on other neurotransmitter receptors.

Pharmacokinetics After oral administration reboxetine reaches peak plasma levels after about 2 hours. Its half-life is around 13 hours and twice-daily administration is recommended. Reboxetine is metabolized by the liver where it is a substrate for cytochrome P450 CYP3A.

Efficacy Reboxetine has shown efficacy in *placebo-controlled trials* and against active comparators including tricyclic antidepressants and SSRIs (Burrows *et al.* 1998). It is claimed that reboxetine produces better improvement in social function in depressed patients than fluoxetine (Dubini *et al.* 1997) but this possibility requires further study. The usual dose of reboxetine is 4 mg twice daily with a maximum dose of 12 mg daily.

Unwanted effects Despite its low affinity for muscarinic receptors, reboxetine produces adverse effects characteristic of cholinergic receptor blockade, presumably through interactions of noradrenergic and cholinergic pathways. The most common side-effects are *dry mouth, constipation, sweating,* and *insomnia. Urinary hesitancy, impotence, tachycardia,* and *vertigo* are also occasionally described.

Drug interactions Limited information is available. It is recommended that reboxetine should not be given with other agents that might *potentiate noradrenaline function,* such as MAOIs, or increase blood pressure, such as ergot derivatives. Plasma reboxetine levels might be increased by drugs that inhibit cytochrome P450 3A4, such as some antifungal agents, fluvoxamine, and macrolide antibiotics.

Venlafaxine

Venlafaxine is a phenylethylamine derivative which produces a *potent blockade of 5-HT re-uptake* with somewhat lesser effects on noradrenaline. In this respect the pharmacological properties of venlafaxine resemble those of clomipramine to some extent;

however, unlike clomipramine and other tricyclic antidepressants, venlafaxine has a negligible affinity for other neurotransmitter receptor sites and so lacks sedative and anticholinergic effects (Horst and Preskorn 1998). Venlafaxine has therefore been classified as a *selective serotonin and noradrenaline re-uptake inhibitor (SNRI)*.

Pharmacokinetics Venlafaxine is well absorbed, achieving peak plasma levels about 1.5–2 hours after oral administration. The half-life of venlafaxine is 3–7 hours but it is metabolized to desmethylvenlafaxine which has essentially the same pharmacodynamic properties as the parent compound and a half-life of 8–13 hours. Venlafaxine needs to be administered twice daily. A new formulation of venlafaxine (venlafaxine XL) has an extended release profile with a time maximum plasma level of about 6 hours. This gives a long apparent half-life (about 15 hours) but the drug is still quickly eliminated. Once-daily dosing is possible with this preparation.

Efficacy Venlafaxine has been studied in both in-patients and out-patients with major depression and compared with placebo and active comparators. Current studies suggest that it *is more effective than placebo* and at least of equal efficacy to other available antidepressant drugs including tricyclic antidepressants (see Anderson 1999). Some individual studies and meta-analyses suggest that venlafaxine is more effective than SSRIs particularly for those severely depressed patients (Clerk *et al.* 1994; Smith *et al.* 2002).

Venlafaxine has a wider dosage range than SSRIs, from 75 to 375 mg daily in two divided doses or up to 225 mg of the extended release preparation given as a single dose. The antidepressant efficacy of venlafaxine appears more robust at higher doses, which may also confer a faster onset of action. However, higher doses are associated with a greater incidence of adverse effects. The usual starting dose of venlafaxine is 75 mg daily, which may be sufficient for many patients. Upward titration can be considered where there is insufficient response, or if a faster onset of therapeutic activity is needed.

Unwanted effects The adverse effect profile of venlafaxine resembles that of SSRIs, with the most common adverse effects being *nausea, headache, somnolence, dry mouth, dizziness*, and *insomnia. Anxiety* and *sexual dysfunction* may also occur. Venlafaxine occasionally causes *postural hypotension*, but in addition, dose-related *increases in blood pressure* can occur. Blood pressure monitoring is advisable in patients receiving more than 150 mg venlafaxine daily. Like SSRIs, venlafaxine can lower plasma sodium levels.

Similarly to SSRIs, sudden discontinuation of venlafaxine has been associated with symptoms of *fatigue, nausea, abdominal pain*, and *dizziness*. It is recommended that patients who received venlafaxine for 6 weeks or more should have the dose reduced gradually over at least a 1-week period and longer if possible. Preliminary evidence suggest that venlafaxine is less toxic in overdose than tricyclic antidepressants.

Drug interactions Unlike the SSRIs, venlafaxine appears to produce little effect on hepatic drug-metabolizing enzymes and therefore should be less likely to inhibit the metabolism of co-administered drugs. Like other drugs that potently inhibit the uptake of 5-HT, venlafaxine should not be given concomitantly with *MAOIs* because of the danger of a toxic serotonin syndrome. It is also recommended that 14 days should elapse after the end of MAOI treatment before venlafaxine is started and that 7 days should elapse after venlafaxine cessation before MAOIs are given.

L-Tryptophan

L-Tryptophan is a naturally occurring amino acid, present in the normal diet; about 500 mg of tryptophan is consumed daily in the typical Western diet. Most ingested tryptophan is used for protein synthesis and the formation of nicotinamide nucleotides; only a small proportion (about 1%) is synthesized to 5-HT via 5-hydroxtryptophan (5-HTP). Tryptophan hydroxylase, the enzyme that catalyses the formation of 5-HTP from L-tryptophan, is normally unsaturated with tryptophan.

Accordingly, increasing tryptophan availability to the brain increases 5-HT synthesis.

Pharmacokinetics L-Tryptophan is rapidly absorbed, with plasma levels peaking about 1–2 hours after ingestion. It is extensively bound to plasma albumin. The amount of L-tryptophan available for brain 5-HT synthesis depends on several factors, including the proportion of L-tryptophan free in plasma, the activity of tryptophan pyrrolase, and the concentration of other plasma amino acids that compete with L-tryptophan for brain entry (for a review of these mechanisms see Bender 1982).

Efficacy There is only weak evidence that L-tryptophan has antidepressant activity when given alone, though it may be superior to placebo in moderately depressed out-patients. There is rather better evidence that L-tryptophan combined with MAOI treatment can enhance the antidepressant effects of MAOIs. Similar synergistic effects have been reported in some studies of L-tryptophan combined with tricyclics, though overall the therapeutic benefit of this combination is inconsistent.

Unwanted effects L-Tryptophan is generally well tolerated, although *nausea* and *drowsiness* soon after dosing are not unusual. In recent years, however, the prescription of L-tryptophan has been associated with the development of a severe scleroderma-like illness, the *eosinophilia-myalgia syndrome (EMS)*, in which there is a very high circulating eosinophil count (about 20% of peripheral leucocytes) with severe muscle pain, oedema, skin sclerosis, and peripheral neuropathy. Fatalities have been reported.

It is now reasonably well established that EMS is not caused by L-tryptophan itself but rather by a *contaminant* formed in the manufacturing process used by a particular manufacturer (Kilbourne *et al.* 1996). L-Tryptophan remains available for the treatment of *severe refractory depression*, when it can be used as an *adjunct* to other antidepressant medication (see. for example, Barker *et al.* 1987). Patients receiving L-tryptophan require close supervision, including monitoring for possible symptoms of EMS and regular blood eosinophil counts. L-Tryptophan should be withdrawn if there is any evidence that EMS may be developing.

Drug interactions The only significant drug interactions of L-tryptophan are with drugs that also increase brain 5-HT function. Thus, while administration of *L-tryptophan with MAOIs* may produce clinical benefit, there are also reports that this combination may lead to 5-HT neurotoxicity as described above. Similarly, the combination of *L-tryptophan with SSRIs* has been reported to cause myoclonus, shivering, and mental state changes (Sternbach 1991).

St Johns Wort

St Johns Wort is an extract from the plant, *Hypericum perforatum*. It has been used in medicine for centuries for numerous indications including burns, arthritis, snakebite, and depression. The active principles are probably derived from six major product groups including *hypericins* and *hyperforins*. The pharmacology of St John's Wort is complex but animal experimental and some human studies indicate that it potentiates aspects of monoamine neurotransmission (see Nathan 1999).

Efficacy There have been numerous trials of St Johns Wort, although these are difficult to interpret because the preparations and dosages have been difficult to standardize. In addition, the trials have been carried out in mild to moderately depressed subjects. However, recent meta-analyses have indicated that daily doses of total hypericum of 0.4–2.7 mg are *more effective than placebo* in this patient group (Linde *et al.* 1996). Trials against comparator antidepressants, usually tricyclics, have generally shown no difference, although doses of tricyclics in these studies have been low (Philipp *et al.* 1999). There are few data on long-term efficacy.

Adverse effects and drug interactions St John's Wort is well tolerated with the most common side-effects being *gastrointestinal disturbance*, *dizziness*, and *tiredness*. Cases of mania during treatment have been described. Photosensitivity is also rarely reported. Hypericum extracts may *induce hepatic enzymes* and there are reports that St John's Wort treatment was associated with lowered levels of theophylline, cyclosporin, digoxin, and ethinyloestradiol. Finally, St Johns Wort may cause *serotonin neurotoxicity* when combined with SSRIs and other 5-HT potentiating drugs (see Ernst 1999).

Mood-stabilizing drugs

Several agents are grouped under this heading such as *lithium* and a number of anticonvulsant drugs including *carbamazepine* and *sodium valproate*. These three drugs are effective in the *prevention* of recurrent affective illness and also in the *acute treatment of mania*. Lithium also has useful antidepressant effects in some circumstances, but the antidepressant activity of carbamazepine and sodium valproate is less well established (Shelton 1999). More recently introduced anticonvulsants such as *lamotrigine* and *gabapentin* are also being explored for their mood-stabilizing properties.

Lithium

Placebo-controlled trials have shown that lithium is effective in a number of conditions (see Soares and Gershon 1998):

- for the acute treatment of mania;
- for the prophylaxis of unipolar and bipolar mood disorder;
- as an augmentation therapy in resistant depression;
- in the prevention of aggressive behaviour in patients with learning disabilities.

Mechanism of action

Animal studies have shown that lithium has important effects on the intracellular signalling molecules or 'second messengers' that are activated when a neurotransmitter or agonist binds to a specific receptor. At clinically relevant doses, lithium inhibits the formation of *cyclic adenosine monophosphate* (cAMP) and also attenuates the formation of various *inositol lipid-derived mediators*. Through these actions lithium could exert profound effects on a wide range of neurotransmitter pathways, many of which use the above messenger systems (for a review see Lenox and Hahn 2000).

Pharmacokinetics

Lithium is rapidly absorbed from the gut and diffuses quickly throughout the body fluids and cells. Lithium moves out of cells more slowly than sodium. It is removed from plasma by *renal excretion* and by entering cells and other body compartments. Therefore there is a rapid excretion of lithium from the plasma, and a slower phase reflecting its removal from the whole-body pool.

Like sodium, lithium is filtered and partly reabsorbed in the kidney. When the proximal tubule absorbs more water, lithium absorption increases. Therefore *dehydration* causes plasma lithium concentrations to rise. Because lithium is transported in competition with sodium, more is reabsorbed by the kidney when sodium concentrations fall. This is the mechanism whereby *thiazide diuretics* can lead to toxic concentrations of lithium in the blood.

Dosage and plasma concentrations

Because the therapeutic and toxic doses are close together, it is essential to measure plasma concentrations of lithium during treatment. Measurements should first be made after 4–7 days, then weekly for 3 weeks, and then, provided that a satisfactory steady state has been achieved, once every 6 weeks. Subsequently, lithium levels are often very stable, and plasma monitoring can be carried out at intervals of 2–3 months unless there are clinical indications for more frequent monitoring.

After an oral dose, plasma lithium levels rise by a factor of two or three within about 4 hours. For this reason, concentrations are normally measured approximately *12 hours* after the last dose, usually just before the morning dose, which can be delayed for an hour or two if necessary. It is important to follow this routine because published information about lithium concentrations refers to the level

12 hours after the last dose, and not to the 'peak' reached in the 4 hours after that dose. If an unexpectedly high concentration is found, it is important to establish whether the patient has inadvertently taken the morning dose before the blood sample was taken.

Previously, the accepted range for prophylaxis was 0.7–1.2 mmol/l measured 12 hours after the last dose. However, current trends are to maintain lithium at *lower plasma levels* (0.5–0.8 mmol/l), because this decreases the burden of side-effects. Some studies suggest that patients with lower lithium levels (0.4–0.7 mmol/l) experience more affective illness during maintenance treatment than patients with higher levels (0.8–1.0 mmol/l). However, this is not a consistent finding (see Ferrier *et al.* 1999b).

In practice, it seems that many patients can be managed satisfactorily if their lithium levels are kept in the 0.4–0.7 mmol/l range. However, if a patient's course is unstable, it may be worthwhile maintaining slightly higher lithium levels if side-effects permit.

In the treatment of acute mania, plasma concentrations below 0.8 mmol/l appear to be ineffective and a range of 0.8–1.2 mmol/l is probably required. Serious toxic effects appear with concentrations above 2.0 mmol/l, though early symptoms may appear above 1.2 mmol/l.

A number of delayed-release preparations of lithium are now available, but their pharmacokinetics *in vivo* do not differ significantly from those of standard lithium carbonate preparations. *Liquid formulations* of lithium citrate are available for patients who have difficulty in taking tablets.

Lithium may be administered once or twice daily. Frequency of administration does not appear to affect urine volume. In general, it is more convenient to take lithium as a single dose at night, but patients who experience gastric irritation on this regimen may be helped by divided daily dosage.

Unwanted effects (Table 21.13)

A mild *diuresis* due to sodium excretion occurs soon after the drug is started. Other common effects include *tremor* of the hands, *dry mouth*, a *metallic taste*, feelings *of muscular weakness*, and *fatigue*.

Some degree of mild *polyuria* is common in patients taking lithium, probably because lithium blocks the effect of antidiuretic hormone (ADH) on the renal tubule. This is rarely of clinical significance, but a few patients show progression to a *diabetes insipidus-like syndrome* with pronounced polyuria and polydipsia. This may necessitate withdrawal of lithium treatment although the use of lower plasma lithium levels may cause the syndrome to remit.

Some patients, especially women, gain some *weight* when taking the drug. Persistent fine tremor, mainly affecting the hands, is common, but coarse tremor suggests that the plasma concentration of lithium has reached toxic levels. Most patients adapt to the fine tremor; for those who do not, propanolol up to 40 mg three times daily may reduce the symptom. Both *hair loss* and coarsening of hair texture can occur.

Thyroid gland enlargement occurs in about 5% of patients taking lithium. The thyroid shrinks again if thyroxine is given while lithium is continued and it generally returns to normal a month or two after lithium has been stopped. Lithium interferes with thyroid production, and *hypothyroidism* occurs in up to 20% of women patients with a compensatory rise in thyroid-stimulating hormone.

Tests of thyroid function should be performed every 6 months to help to detect these changes, but these intermittent tests are no substitute for a continuous watch for suggestive clinical signs, particularly *lethargy* and substantial *weight gain*. If hypothyroidism develops and the reasons for lithium treatment are still strong, thyroxine treatment should be added. Lithium has also been associated with elevated serum calcium levels in the context of *hyperparathyroidism*. This is occasionally associated with severe depression, making distinction from the underlying mood disorder difficult.

Reversible ECG changes also occur. These may be due to displacement of potassium in the myocardium by lithium for they resemble those of hypokalaemia, with T-wave flattening and inversion or

Table 21.13 Some adverse effects of lithium, carbamazepine and valproate

	Lithium	Carbamazepine	Valproate
Neurological	Tremor, weakness, dysarthria, ataxia, impaired memory, seizures (rare)	Dizziness, weakness, drowsiness, ataxia, headache, visual disturbance	Tremor, sedation
Renal/fluid balance	Increased urine output with decreased urine concentrating ability. Thirst, diabetes insipidus (rare), oedema	Acts to increase urine concentrating ability. Low sodium states, oedema	Increased plasma ammonia
Gastrointestinal/hepatic	Altered taste, anorexia, nausea, vomiting, diarrhoea, weight gain	Anorexia, nausea, constipation, hepatitis	Anorexia, nausea, vomiting, diarrhoea, weight gain, hepatitis (rare), pancreatitis (rare)
Endocrine	Decreased thyroxine with increased TSH. Goitre, hyperparathyroidism (rare)	Decreased thyroxine with normal TSH	Menstrual disturbances
Haematological	Leucocytosis	Leucopenia, agranulocytosis (rare)	Low platelet count. Abnormal platelet aggregation
Dermatological	Acne, exacerbation of psoriasis	Erythematous rash	Hair loss
Cardiovascular	ECG changes (usually clinically benign)	Cardiac conduction disturbances	

widening of the QRS. They are rarely of clinical significance. Other changes include a reversible *leucocytosis* and occasional papular or maculopapular *rashes*. There is some uncertain evidence that prolonged treatment may lead to *osteoporosis* in women.

Effects on *memory* are sometimes reported by patients, who complain particularly of everyday lapses of memory such as forgetting well-known names. It is possible that this impairment of memory is caused by the mood disorder rather than by the drug itself, but there is also evidence that lithium can be associated with impaired performance on certain cognitive tests.

Long-term effects on the kidney As noted above, lithium treatment decreases *tubular concentrating ability* and can occasionally cause diabetes inspidus. In addi-

tion, there have been reports that over many years of treatment lithium can sometimes cause an increasing and in some cases *irreversible decline* in tubular function. This may be more likely in patients with higher plasma concentrations of lithium and where concomitant psychotropic medication has been employed (Bendz *et al.* 1994).

Several follow-up studies have examined the effect of longer-term lithium maintenance treatment on *glomerular function*. In general, any decline in glomerular function is usually mild and related to lithium intoxication (Johnson 1998). However, there are occasional case reports of substantial glomerular decline and even frank *renal failure* in lithium-treated patients when other causes of nephrotoxicity appear to be absent (see Gitlin 1993).

With the current trends towards long-term prophylaxis of mood disorders, it is clearly wise to monitor plasma *creatinine* levels regularly. It seems likely that the risk of nephrotoxicity will be minimized by maintaining plasma lithium levels at the *lower end* of the therapeutic range provided that they are therapeutically effective for the individual patient.

Toxic effects

These are related to dose. They include *ataxia, poor coordination of limb movements, muscle twitching, slurred speech, and confusion.* They constitute a serious medical emergency for they can progress through *coma* and *fits* to *death*.

If these symptoms appear, lithium must be stopped at once and a high intake of fluid provided, with extra sodium chloride to stimulate an osmotic diuresis. In severe cases, renal dialysis may be needed. Lithium is rapidly cleared if renal function is normal so that most cases either recover completely or die. However, cases of permanent neurological damage despite haemodialysis have been reported.

As noted earlier (p. 653), lithium can increase *fetal abnormalities*, particularly of the heart, although the magnitude of the individual risk is low. The decision whether or not to continue with lithium treatment during pregnancy must therefore be carefully weighed. Important factors include the likelihood of affective relapse if lithium is withheld and the difficulty that could be experienced in managing an episode of affective illness in the individual woman.

If pregnant patients continue with lithium, plasma levels should be monitored closely. Ultrasound examination and fetal echocardiography are valuable screening tests as the pregnancy progresses. Patients with a history of *bipolar disorder* have a substantially *increased risk* of psychotic relapse in the post-partum period. In such patients it may be worth considering the introduction of lithium shortly after delivery to provide a prophylactic effect. However, significant concentrations of lithium can be measured in the plasma of breast-fed infants which may make bottle-feeding is advisable (see p. 653).

Drug interactions (Box 21.8)

Because of the narrow therapeutic index of lithium, *pharmacokinetic* drug interactions are of major clinical importance. *Pharmacodynamic* interactions may involve potentiation of *5-HT promoting agents*, leading to a serotonin syndrome. In addition, therapeutic plasma levels of lithium can be associated with *neurotoxicity* in the presence of certain other centrally acting agents.

ECT and surgery It is possible that the continuation of lithium during *ECT* may lead to neurotoxicity. If feasible, lithium treatment should be suspended or plasma levels reduced during ECT because the customary overnight fast beforehand may leave patients relatively dehydrated the following

---

Box 21.8 Some drug interactions of lithium

Pharmacokinetic

Increased lithium levels

- Diuretics (frusemide safest)
- Non-steroidal anti-inflammatory drugs (aspirin/sulindac safest)
- Antibiotics (spectinomycin/metronidazole)

Decreased lithium levels

- Theophylline
- Sodium bicarbonate

Pharmacodynamic

5-HT neurotoxicity

- SSRIs (can be used safely with care)
- 5-HT$_1$ agonists

Extrapyramidal side-effects enhanced

- Antipsychotic agents, metoclopramide, domperidone

Enhanced neurotoxicity

- Carbamazepine, calcium channel blockers, methyldopa

morning. If possible, lithium treatment should be discontinued before *major surgery* because the effects of *muscle relaxants* may be potentiated. However, the risk of acute withdrawal and 'rebound' mania must be considered (see below).

Lithium withdrawal

In some studies, abrupt *lithium withdrawal* has been associated with the rapid onset of mania (Mander and Loudon 1988). Undoubtedly there is an increased risk of recurrent mood disorder after lithium discontinuation, probably because lithium is an effective prophylactic agent and because it is used for disorders with a high risk of recurrence. However, there is probably also a lithium withdrawal syndrome with 'rebound' mania, although this may be restricted to patients with bipolar disorder.

The risk of rapid relapse is lessened if lithium is *discontinued slowly* over a period of several weeks (Faedda *et al.* 1993). Even patients who have remained entirely well for many years may experience a further episode of affective disorder after lithium discontinuation. Most of these subjects will respond to the reintroduction of lithium (Tondo *et al.* 1997).

Contraindications

These include renal failure or recent renal disease, current cardiac failure or recent myocardial infarction, and chronic diarrhoea sufficient to alter electrolytes. Lithium should not be prescribed if the patient is judged unlikely to observe the precautions required for its safe use. This includes a propensity to discontinue it suddenly against advice.

The management of patients on lithium

Preparation A careful routine of management is essential because of the effects of therapeutic doses of lithium on the thyroid and kidney, and the toxic effects of excessive dosage. The following routine is one of several that have been proposed and can be adopted safely. Successful treatment requires attention to detail, and so the steps are set out below at some length.

Before starting lithium, a *physical examination* should be carried out, including the measurement of blood pressure. It is also useful to *weigh* the patient.

Blood should be taken for estimation of *electrolytes*, serum *creatinine*, and a *full blood count*. When a particularly thorough evaluation is indicated, *creatinine clearance* is carried out, with an 18-hour collection usually being adequate. *Thyroid function tests* are also necessary. If indicated, an ECG and pregnancy tests should be performed as well.

If these tests show no contraindication to lithium treatment, the doctor should check that the patient is not taking any drugs that might interact with lithium. A careful explanation should then be given to the patient. He should understand the possible early toxic effects of an unduly high blood level, and also the circumstances in which this can arise, for example, during intercurrent gastroenteritis, renal infection, or the dehydration secondary to fever. He should be advised that if any of these arise, he should stop the drug and seek medical advice.

It is usually appropriate to include another member of the family in these discussions. Providing *printed guidelines* on these points is often helpful (either written by the doctor, or in one of the forms provided by pharmaceutical firms). In these discussions a sensible balance must be struck between alarming the patient by overemphasizing the risks and failing to give him the information that he needs to take a responsible part in the treatment.

Starting treatment Lithium should normally be prescribed as the carbonate, and treatment should begin and continue with a *single daily dose* unless there is gastric intolerance, in which case divided doses can be given. If the drug is being used for prophylaxis, it is appropriate to begin with 200–400 mg mg daily in a single dose. The lower is appropriate where patients are taking concomitant medication such as SSRIs that might interact with lithium.

Blood should be taken for lithium estimations every week and adjusting the dose until an appropriate concentration is achieved. A lithium level of 0.4–0.7 mmol/l (in a sample taken 12 hours after the last dose) may be adequate for prophylaxis, as explained above; if this is not effective, the previously accepted higher range of 0.8–1.0 mmol/l should be used. In judging response, it should be remembered that several months may elapse before lithium achieves its full effect.

Continuation treatment As treatment continues, lithium estimations should be carried out every *6–12 weeks*. It is important to have some means of reminding patients and doctors about the times at which repeat investigations are required. Computerized databases may be helpful in this respect. *Every 6 months*, blood samples should be taken for electrolytes, urea, and creatinine, a full blood count, and the thyroid function tests listed above. If two consecutive thyroid function tests a month apart show evidence of *hypothyroidism*, lithium should be stopped or L-thyroxine prescribed. Troublesome *polyuria* is a reason for attempting a reduction in dose, whilst severe persistent polyuria is an indication for specialist renal investigation including tests of concentrating ability. A persistent *leucocytosis* is not uncommon and is apparently harmless. It reverses soon after the drug is stopped.

When lithium is given, the doctor must keep in mind the *interactions* that have been reported with psychotropic and other drugs (see above). It is also prudent to watch for toxic effects with extra care if *ECT* is being given. If the patient requires an anaesthetic for any reason, the anaesthetist should be told that the patient is taking lithium; this is because, as noted above, there is some evidence that the effects of muscle relaxant may be potentiated.

Lithium is usually continued for at least a year, and often for much longer. The need for the drug should be reviewed once a year, taking into account any persistence of mild mood fluctuations, which suggest the possibility of relapse if treatment is stopped. Continuing medication is more likely to be needed if the patient has previously had several episodes of mood disorder within a short

time, or if previous episodes were so severe that even a small risk of recurrence should be avoided.

Some patients have taken lithium continuously for 15 years or more, but there should always be compelling reasons for continuing treatment for more than 5 years. As noted above, lithium should be withdrawn slowly, over a number of months if possible. Patients should be advised not to *discontinue lithium suddenly* on their own initiative.

Carbamazepine

Carbamazepine was originally introduced as an *anticonvulsant* and was found to have useful effects on mood in certain patients. Subsequently it was found to be beneficial in many bipolar patients, including those who had proved *refractory to lithium*. There is reasonable evidence that carbamazepine is effective in the management of *acute mania* and also in the *prophylaxis* of *bipolar disorder*. However, by current standards many of the studies have significant methodological deficiences (see Dardennes *et al.* 1995; Post *et al.* 1997).

Carbamazepine may also have some benefit in the treatment of *drug-resistant bipolar depression*, but it does not have an established role in the prophylaxis of recurrent unipolar depression (Shelton 1999).

Like certain other anticonvulsants, carbamazepine blocks *neuronal sodium channels*. It is unclear whether this action plays a role in the mood-stabilizing effects.

Pharmacokinetics

Carbamazepine is slowly but completely absorbed and widely distributed. It is extensively metabolized, with at least one metabolite, carbamazepine epoxide, being therapeutically active. The half-life during long-term treatment is about 20 hours. Carbamazepine is a strong *inducer of hepatic microsomal enzymes* and can lower the plasma concentrations of other drugs.

Dosage and plasma concentrations

The dosage of carbamazepine in the treatment of mood disorders is similar to that used in the treatment of epilepsy, within the range of 400–1600 mg daily. Treatment is usually given in divided doses twice daily, because this practice may improve tolerance. No clear relationship has been established between plasma carbamazepine concentrations and therapeutic response, but it seems prudent to monitor levels (about 12 hours after the last dose) and to maintain them in the usual anticonvulsant range as a guard against toxicity.

Unwanted effects (Table 21.13)

Side-effects are common at the beginning of treatment. They include *drowsiness, dizziness, ataxia, diplopia, and nausea*. Tolerance to these effects usually develops quickly. A potentially serious side-effect of carbamazepine is *agranulocytosis*, though this complication is very rare (variously estimated from 1 in 10 000 to 1 in 125 000 patients).

A *relative leucopenia* is more common, with the white cell count often falling in the first few weeks of treatment, though usually remaining within normal levels. Rashes occur in about 5% of patients. Elevations in *liver enzymes* may also occur and, rarely, *hepatitis* has been reported. Carbamazepine can cause disturbances of *cardiac conduction* and therefore is contraindicated in patients with pre-existing abnormalities of cardiac conduction.

Carbamazepine lowers plasma *thyroxine concentrations*, but thyroid-stimulating hormone levels are not elevated and clinical hypothyroidism is unusual. Carbamazepine has also been associated with *low sodium states*. The unwanted effects of carbamazepine are compared with those of lithium and valproate in Table 21.13.

Drug interactions

Carbamazepine *increases the metabolism* of many other drugs including tricyclic antidepressants, benzodiazepines, haloperidol, oral contraceptive agents, thyroxine, warfarin, other anticonvulsants, and some antibiotics. A similar mechanism may underlie the *decline in plasma carbamazepine* levels that occur after the first few weeks of treatment.

Carbamazepine levels may be *increased* by SSRIs, nefazodone, and erythromycin. The pharmacodynamic effects and plasma levels of carbamazepine may be increased by some calcium-channel blockers such as diltiazem and verapamil. Conversely, carbamazepine may decrease the effect of certain other calcium-channel antagonists such as felodipine and nicardipine. *Neurotoxicity* has been reported when *carbamazepine and lithium* have been combined even in the presence of normal lithium levels. The manufacturers of carbamazepine recommend that combination of carbamazepine with *MAOIs* be avoided. However, there are case reports of these drugs being used safely together. It is possible that some MAOIs may increase plasma carbamazepine levels.

Clinical use of carbamazepine

The usual indication for carbamazepine is:

◆ the prophylactic management of bipolar illness in patients for whom lithium treatment is ineffective or poorly tolerated;

◆ in the treatment of patients with *frequent mood swings* and *mixed affective states* for which carbamazepine may be more effective than lithium;

◆ added to lithium treatment in patients who have shown a partial response to the latter drug; in these circumstances it is important to remember that this combination can cause neurotoxicity;

◆ in the acute treatment of mania, again usually as an alternative or addition to lithium (see Post *et al.* 1998).

If clinical circumstances permit, it is preferable to start treatment with carbamazepine slowly at a dose of 100–200 mg daily, increasing in steps of 100–200 mg twice weekly. Patients show wide variability in the blood levels at which they experience adverse effects; accordingly, it is best to titrate the dose against the side-effects and the clinical response.

Because of the risk of a *lowered white cell count*, it is prudent to monitor the count in the first 3 months of treatment. Patients should be instructed to seek help urgently if they develop a fever or other sign of infection. When patients have responded to the addition of carbamazepine to lithium, it is possible subsequently to attempt a cautious lithium withdrawal. However, the current clinical impression is that, for many patients, the maintenance of mood stability requires continuing treatment with both drugs.

Sodium valproate

Like carbamazepine, sodium valproate was first introduced as an anticonvulsant. In recent years there has been increasing interest in using the drug in the management of mood disorders.

There have been several controlled studies indicating that valproate is effective in the *acute management of mania*. As yet there is less clear evidence that valproate is effective in *longer-term prophylaxis* of bipolar disorder. However, a recent randomized trial by Bowden *et al.* (2000) showed a marginal benefit for valproate over lithium and placebo in bipolar patients over a 1-year follow-up. There have been numerous case studies and open studies that have reported useful prophylactic effects of valproate in patients *unresponsive to lithium and carbamazepine*, including those with rapid cycling mood disorders (Bowden 1998; Keck *et al.* 1998).

Valproate is a simple branch-chain fatty acid with a mode of action that is unclear. However, there is some evidence that it can slow the breakdown of the *inhibitory neurotransmitter GABA*. This action could account for the anticonvulsant properties of valproate, but whether it also underlies the psychotropic effects is unclear.

Pharmacokinetics

Valproate is rapidly absorbed, with the peak plasma concentrations occurring about 2 hours after ingestion. It is widely and rapidly distributed and has a half-life of 8–18 hours. Valproate is metabolized in the liver to produce a wide variety of metabolites, some of which have anticonvulsant activity. Unlike carbamazepine, valproate does not induce hepatic microsomal enzymes and, if anything, tends to delay the metabolism of other drugs.

Dosing and plasma concentrations

Valproate can be started at a dose of 400–600 mg daily, which may be increased once or twice weekly to a range of 1–2 g daily. Plasma levels of valproate do not correlate well with either the anticonvulsant or the mood-stabilizing effects, but it has been suggested that efficacy in the treatment of acute mania is usually apparent when plasma levels are *greater than 50 µg/ml*.

Unwanted effects (Table 21.13)

Common side-effects with valproate include *gastrointestinal disturbances, tremor, sedation, and tiredness*. Other troublesome side-effects include *weight gain* and *transient hair loss* with changes in texture on regrowth.

Patients taking valproate may have some elevation *in hepatic transaminase enzymes*; provided that this increase is not associated with hepatic dysfunction, the drug can be continued while enzyme levels and liver function are carefully monitored. However, there have been several reports of fatal *hepatic toxicity* associated with the use of valproate; most of these cases have occurred in children taking multiple anticonvulsant drugs. Valproate must be withdrawn immediately if vomiting, anorexia, jaundice, or sudden drowsiness occur.

Valproate may also cause *thrombocytopenia* and may inhibit platelet aggregation. *Acute pancreatitis* is another rare but serious side-effect, and increases in plasma *ammonia* have also been reported. Other possible side-effects include *oedema, amenorrhoea*, and *rashes*.

Drug interactions

Valproate potentiates the effects of central sedatives. It has been reported to increase the side-effects of other anticonvulsants (without necessarily improving anticonvulsant control). It may *increase plasma levels* of phenytoin and tricyclic antidepressants.

Clinical use

At present valproate can be considered as maintenance treatment for patients with *refractory bipolar disorder* who do not respond to either lithium or carbamazepine or who are intolerant of these drugs. Valproate has recently received a licence for the acute treatment of mania in the UK.

The efficacy of valproate in the acute treatment of mania has been established by several controlled trials. It produces a quicker onset of action than lithium and carbamazepine because it can be dosed at high levels initially. For example, a therapeutic effect can be apparent with a day or two employing a loading dose of valproate of 20 mg/kg. Valproate may be more effective than lithium in the management of patients with *mixed affective states* (Keck *et al.* 1998).

In terms of prophylaxis, valproate seems more effective in the prevention of manic than depressive episodes. It has not been established whether valproate is valuable in the management of resistant depression. It has often been used in combination with lithium for patients who have shown a partial response to lithium, and this combination appears to be safe. Valproate has also been used in combination with carbamazepine. For patients who continue to show episodes of mood disturbance, valproate can be combined with antidepressant or antipsychotic drugs.

Lamotrigine

Lamotrigine is a triazine derivative which blocks voltage-dependent *sodium channels* and reduces excitatory neurotransmitter release, particularly that of *glutamate*. Lamotrigine is licensed in the UK as a monotherapy and adjunctive treatment for epilepsy.

Lamotrigine is not licensed for the treatment of mood disorders but there are open studies showing therapeutic benefit when it has been added to the medication of patients with *bipolar illness refractory to standard treatments*. In these studies lamotrigine has improved symptomatology in all phases of the disorder (see Bowden 1998). In addition, a placebo-controlled trial showed that lamotrigine was effective as a monotherapy in the treatment of *bipolar depression* (Calabrese *et al.* 1999).

Pharmacokinetics

Following oral administration, lamotrigine is rapidly absorbed with peak plasma levels occurring after about 1.5 hours. The drug is extensively metabolized by the liver but does not induce cytochrome P450 enzymes. Its half-life is about 30 hours. A plasma therapeutic range has not been identified.

Adverse effects

Skin eruptions, usually maculopapular in nature, occur in about 3% of patients and may be associated with fever. They are most common in the first few weeks of treatment and their incidence can be reduced by careful initial dosing (see below). Other side-effects include *nausea, headache, diplopia, blurred vision, dizziness, ataxia, and tremor*. Very serious adverse effects such as *angioedema, Stevens–Johnson syndrome* and *toxic epidermal necrolysis* have been reported rarely.

Drug interactions

Plasma levels of lamotrigine can be lowered by drugs that induce hepatic-metabolizing enzymes such as *carbamazepine*. Combination of carbamazepine and lamotrigine can also cause neurotoxicity. Lamotrigine levels are increased by concomitant administration of *valproate*.

Clinical use

Until more data are available, lamotrigine should be used in bipolar disorder only when more familiar agents have proved unsuccessful (Porter *et al.* 1999). Lamotrigine may then be helpful as an *adjunctive therapy*, paying due attention to the drug interactions noted above. Lamotrigine may also be useful in the treatment of *bipolar depression*, again when standard agents are poorly tolerated or unsuccessful. It is presumed that lamotrigine will be less likely to produce mania or rapid cycling in bipolar patients than conventional antidepressants, but this has yet to be clearly established.

When initiating lamotrigine treatment, to minimize the risk of rash, it is important to follow the *dosage recommendations in the British National Formulary* (25 mg daily for the first 2 weeks, followed by 50 mg daily for the next 2 weeks). The usual therapeutic dose in bipolar disorder is between 50–300 mg daily.

Gabapentin

Gabapentin was developed as a structural analogue of GABA. Despite its structural relationship to GABA, its anticonvulsant mechanism of action is uncertain, although it does increase *GABA turnover* in the brain.

Gabapentin is licensed as an adjunctive treatment for seizure disorders and is not licensed for the treatment of mood disorders. There are published case series showing benefit when gabapentin has been used as an adjunctive therapy in patients with *bipolar disorder resistant to standard medication regimens* (Keck *et al.* 1998; Young *et al.* 1999). Gabapentin has a *sedating* profile and may also have *anxiolytic* properties.

Pharmacokinetics

After oral absorption peak, plasma levels of gabapentin are reached after 2–3 hours. Gabapentin is not metabolized by the liver and is excreted entirely by the kidney. Its half-life is about 5–7 hours and thrice-daily dosing is recommended.

Unwanted effects

The most common side-effects of gabapentin are *somnolence, dizziness, fatigue, and nystagmus.* No serious adverse effects have been reported.

Drug interactions

Probably because of its lack of hepatic metabolism, thus far no significant pharmacokinetic interactions of gabapentin with other medications have been described. It may potentiate the effects of other central sedatives.

Clinical use

As with lamotrigine, gabapentin can be considered in patients with bipolar disorder who have *not responded* to standard therapies (Porter *et al.* 1999). Gabapentin has a wide dosage range but the usual dose in bipolar illness is between 600 mg and 2400 mg daily. Sedative and anxiolytic effects are often apparent at lower doses.

Psychostimulants

This class of drugs includes mild stimulants, of which the best known is *caffeine*, and more powerful stimulants such as *amphetamine* and *methylphenidate*. Pemoline has intermediate effects. *Cocaine* is a powerful psychostimulant with a particularly high potential for inducing dependence (see p. 574). It is useful as a local anaesthetic but has no other clinical indications. Psychostimulants *increase the release* and *block the re-uptake* of dopamine and noradrenaline.

Indications

Amphetamines were used for numerous conditions in the past, but they are now prescribed much less frequently because of the high risk of dependence. They are not appropriate for the treatment of obesity. In adults the agreed indication for amphetamines is *narcolepsy*. Methylphenidate is used to treat *the hyperkinetic syndrome of childhood*.

In the past, amphetamines were widely prescribed for the treatment of depression, but they have been superseded by the antidepressant drugs. Some specialists, mainly in the USA, believe that psychostimulants may have a role either as sole agent or in combination with other antidepressant drugs for patients with *refractory depressive disorder* (see Cowen 1998a). Also, there is some interest in using psychostimulants for *elderly depressed patients with concomitant medical illness* (Olin and Masand 1996). A blanket proscription of psychostimulant treatment in depression therefore seems unjustified. However, psychostimulants should be used only by practitioners with special experience in the psychopharmacological management of resistant depression.

The main preparations are dexamphetamine sulphate, given for narcolepsy in divided doses of 10 mg daily increasing to a maximum of 50 mg daily in steps of 10 mg each week, and methylphenidate, which has similar effects.

Unwanted effects

These include restlessness, insomnia, poor appetite, dizziness, tremor, palpitations, and cardiac arrhythmias. Toxic effects from large doses include disorientation and aggressive behaviour, hallucinations, convulsions, and coma. Persistent abuse can lead to a paranoid state similar to paranoid schizophrenia. Amphetamines can cause severe hypertension in combination with MAOIs and to a lesser extent with tricyclic antidepressants. They are contraindicated in cardiovascular disease and thyrotoxicosis.

Other physical treatments

Electroconvulsive therapy (ECT)

History

Convulsive therapy was introduced in the late 1930s on the basis of the mistaken idea that epilepsy and schizophrenia do not occur together. It seemed to follow that induced fits should lead to improvement in schizophrenia. However, when the treatment was tried it became apparent that the most striking changes occurred not in schizophrenia but *in severe depressive disorders*, in which it brought about a substantial reduction in chronicity and mortality (Slater 1951).

At first, fits were produced either by using cardiazol (Meduna 1938) or by passing an electric current through the brain (Cerletti and Bini 1938). As time went by, electrical stimulation became the rule. The subsequent addition of brief anaesthesia and muscle relaxants made the treatment safe and acceptable.

Indications

This section summarizes the indications for ECT (Box 21.9). Further information about the efficiency of the procedure will be found in the chapters dealing with the individual psychiatric syndromes.

ECT is a rapid and effective treatment for *severe depressive disorders*. In the Medical Research Council trial (Clinical Psychiatry Committee 1965) it acted faster than imipramine or phenelzine, and was more effective than imipramine in women and more effective than phenelzine in both sexes.

Box 21.9 Indications for ECT

Major depression
- Not responding to antidepressant drugs
- With psychotic symptoms
- With failure to eat and drink
- With depressive stupor
- With high suicide risk

Schizoaffective depression

Catatonic schizophrenia

Mania not responding to drug treatment

Post-partum affective psychosis

These findings accord with the impression of many clinicians, and with the recommendations of this book, that ECT should be used mainly when it is essential to bring about improvement quickly. Therefore, the strongest indications are an immediate *high risk of suicide, depressive stupor, or danger to physical health* because the patient is not drinking enough to maintain adequate renal function.

Placebo-controlled trials of ECT, in which workers in the UK played a pre-eminent role, confirmed that ECT is particularly effective for patients with depressive psychosis or definite psychomotor disturbance (Buchan *et al.* 1992). In addition, other clinical studies indicate that treatment with ECT can be beneficial in depressed patients for whom antidepressant medication has been *unsuccessful* (Prudic *et al.* 1990).

ECT is also effective in the treatment of the *affective psychoses that follow childbirth*. These puerperal psychoses often present with mixed affective features that can be difficult to resolve quickly with psychotropic drug treatment. ECT may often prove rapidly effective for such patients, a matter of some importance in the early development of the relationship between mother and baby.

ECT is also effective in the treatment of *mania* (Mukherjee *et al.* 1994; Small *et al.* 1996), but is generally reserved for patients who do not respond to drug treatment or for those whose manic illness is severe, requiring high doses of antipsychotic drugs.

On the basis of clinical case studies, it has long been held that ECT is useful in the treatment of *acute catatonic states* and *schizoaffective disorders*. Controlled studies have also shown that ECT is effective in patients with acute schizophrenia with predominantly positive symptoms. In these studies ECT is effective not only for affective symptoms but also for positive symptoms such as *delusions* and *thought disorder* (Brandon *et al.* 1985). In general, however, ECT adds little to the effects of adequate doses of antipsychotic drugs, though it probably produces a greater rate of symptomatic improvement in the short term.

The role of ECT is unclear for patients with schizophrenia whose positive symptoms do not respond to antipsychotic medication. Several older studies suggest that ECT does not improve the negative symptoms of schizophrenia. The current evidence for the efficacy of ECT for different psychiatric disorders is well discussed in the ECT handbook of the Royal College of Psychiatrists (1995).

Mode of action

Role of the seizure Presumably, the specific therapeutic effects of ECT must be brought about through physiological and biochemical changes in the brain. The first step in identifying the mode of action must be to find out whether the therapeutic effect depends on the seizure, or whether other features of the treatment are sufficient, such as the passage of the current through the brain and the use of anaesthesia and muscle relaxants.

Clinicians have generally been convinced that the patient does not improve unless a convulsion is produced during ECT procedure. This impression has been confirmed by several double-blind trials which, taken together, show that ECT is strikingly more effective than a full placebo procedure that includes anaesthetic and muscle relaxant (see Buchan *et al.* 1992).

This evidence does not necessarily support the notion that a full seizure is the sufficient and neces-sary therapeutic component of ECT, and recent studies have shown that this notion is incorrect. Modern ECT machines deliver brief pulses of electrical current that enable a seizure to be induced by administration of relatively low doses of electrical energy. With this mode of administration, both *electrode placement* and *electrical dosage* can have profound effects on the therapeutic efficacy of ECT (see Sackheim *et al.* 1993). In particular, it appears that the *amount by which the applied electrical dose exceeds the seizure threshold of the individual patient* is an important determinant of both efficacy and cognitive side-effects of ECT. Furthermore, the seizure threshold varies greatly (about 15-fold) between individuals.

This situation has important implications for the practical management of ECT when the clinician's aim is to find the best balance between *therapeutic efficacy* and *cognitive side-effects* (see below). From a theoretical viewpoint, however, it can be concluded that an important determinant of ECT efficacy is how far the applied electrical energy *exceeds the seizure threshold* of the individual patient.

Neurochemical effects of ECT Electrical seizures in animals produce many biochemical and electrophysiolog-ical changes, and therefore it is difficult to identify the processes that are important in the antidepres-sant effect of ECT. It is of interest that some of the changes in brain monoamine pathways found in rodents after ECT (for example, *downregulation of noradrenaline β-adrenoceptors*) resemble those found are after antidepressant drug treatment. In addi-tion, both ECT and antidepressants increase the expression of *dopamine D_2 receptors* in the nucleus accumbens, which could be associated with im-provements in motivational behaviour. In the case of ECT, this may involve interaction with *gluta-matergic pathways* (see S. E. Smith *et al.* 1997).

During a course of ECT, the seizure threshold of patients tends to *increase*. This change occurs more with bilateral than with unilateral electrode place-ment, suggesting that the processes underlying the seizure threshold change could be important in the therapeutic action of ECT in depression. From this viewpoint ECT can be regarded as an anticonvulsant treatment, and it is therefore intriguing that various antiepileptic compounds, such as carbamazepine and sodium valproate, are now known to be useful in the treatment of severe mood disorders.

Physiological changes during ECT

If ECT is given without atropine premedication, the pulse first slows and then rises quickly to 130–190 beats/min, falling to the original resting rate or beyond towards the end of the seizure before a final less marked tachycardia lasting several minutes. Marked increases in blood pressure are also common and the systolic pressure can rise to 200 mmHg. Cerebral blood flow also increases by up to 200%.

Unilateral or bilateral ECT

As discussed above, with the newer brief pulse machines there are clinically important differences in antidepressant effects between *low-dose right unilateral ECT* and *low-dose bilateral ECT*. The current advice of the Royal College of Psychiatrists (1995) is that *low-dose treatment* (about 50% above seizure threshold) with *bilateral electrode placement* provides the best combination of therapeutic efficacy and minimal post-treatment cognitive impairment.

The problem with this advice is that it is not easy to know what is 'low dose' for an individual patient, that is, how far above seizure threshold a particular dose of current may be. It is possible to determine this in the first treatment session by starting with a very low dose and gradually increasing this until a fit occurs; this, is called 'dose titration'.

More recent studies of this issue have concluded that:

- high-dose right unilateral ECT (titrated to a dose five times greater than seizure threshold) is as effective as low-dose bilateral ECT and causes less cognitive impairment;
- high fixed-dose right unilateral ECT (about 400 millicoulombs) is more effective than moderately (2.5 times) suprathreshold right unilateral ECT;

- cognitive impairment with right unilateral ECT also increases as dose exceeds seizure threshold but is less than any form of bilateral ECT.

These data suggest that that the most appropriate electrode placement for ECT is right unilateral with dose titrated to about five times above initial seizure threshold. This is likely to give the best overall combination of efficacy and lower cognitive impairment (see McCall *et al.* 2000; Sackheim *et al.* 2000).

Unwanted effects after ECT

Subconvulsive shock may be followed by anxiety and headache. ECT can cause a brief *retrograde amnesia* as well as loss of memory for up to 30 minutes after the fit. *Brief disorientation* can occur, particularly with bilateral electrode placement. *Headache* can also occur. Some patients complain of confusion, nausea, and vertigo for a few hours after the treatment, but with modern methods these unwanted effects are mild and brief.

A few patients complain of *muscle pain*, especially in the jaws, which is probably attributable to the relaxant. There have been a few reports of sporadic major seizures in the months after ECT, but these may have had other causes. Occasional damage to the teeth, tongue, or lips can occur if there have been problems in positioning the gag or airway. Poor application of the electrodes can lead to *small electrical burns*. *Fractures*, including crush fractures of the vertebrae, have occurred occasionally when ECT was given without muscle relaxants.

All these physical consequences are rare provided that a good technique of anaesthesia is used and the fit is modified adequately. Other complications of ECT are rare and mainly occur in people suffering from physical illness. They include *cardiac arrhythmia, pulmonary embolism, aspiration pneumonia, and cerebrovascular accident*. Prolonged apnoea is a rare complication of the use of muscle relaxants. Rarely, *status epilepticus* may occur in predisposed subjects or in those taking medication that prolongs seizure duration.

Since the introduction of ECT, there has always been concern as to whether it may cause *brain damage*. When ECT is given to animals in the usual clinical regimen, there is no evidence that brain damage occurs. Also, structural imaging studies in patients have been reassuring on this point (Devanand *et al.* 1994).

Memory disorder after ECT

Short-term effects As already mentioned, the immediate effects of ECT include loss of memory for events shortly before the treatment (*retrograde amnesia*), and impaired retention of information acquired soon after the treatment (*anterograde amnesia*). These effects depend on both electrode placement (unilateral versus bilateral) and electrical dose; electrode placement appears to be the more important factor.

Controlled studies indicate that the *anterograde amnesia* produced by ECT is *temporary*. Sackheim *et al.* (1993) found either no differences in memory tests or some improvements in the weeks after ECT. Depressive disorders substantially impair cognitive function, and many patients report their memory as subjectively* much improved after ECT (Sackheim *et al.* 1993). Also, several studies have found no significant differences in memory tests between ECT-treated patients and controls who had not received ECT (see Weeks *et al.* 1980).

Long-term effects Possible long-term effects of ECT on memory take two forms. First, some patients describe loss of *memories for personal and impersonal remote events* (retrograde amnesia for remote events). For example, Squire *et al.* (1981) found that after bilateral ECT, in particular, there was a patchy loss of memory for some personal events, television programmes or major news items. More recently, Lisanby *et al.* (2000) found that 2 months after ECT there was some persistent loss of remote memories for impersonal events, which were more marked than those for personal events. Bilateral ECT caused more deficts in this respect than unilateral ECT.

The other possible complication is decreased ability to *learn new information* (long-term anterograde amnesia). For example, in a study of former patients who were complaining that they had suffered permanent harm to memory from ECT given in the past, Freeman *et al.* (1980) found that these patients did worse than controls on some tests in a battery designed to test memory. However, they also had residual depressive symptoms, and so it is possible that continuing depressive disorder accounted for the memory problems. It seems reasonable to conclude that, when used in the usual way, *ECT is not usually followed by persisting anterograde memory disorder* and where this does occur it is mild and may be accounted for by concurrent depressive symptomatology.

The mortality of ECT

The death rate attributable to ECT was estimated to be *3–4 per 100 000 treatments* by Barker and Barker (1959). This is similar to that seen with general anaesthesia in general medical conditions. The risks are related to the anaesthetic procedure and are greatest in patients with cardiovascular disease. When death occurs it is usually due to *ventricular fibrillation* or *myocardial infarction*.

Contraindications

The contraindications to ECT are any medical illnesses that increase the risk of anaesthetic procedure by an unacceptable amount, for example, respiratory infections, serious heart disease, and serious pyrexial illness. Other contraindications are diseases likely to be made worse by the *changes in blood pressure and cardiac rhythm* that occur even in a well-modified fit; these include serious heart diseases, recent myocardial infarction, cerebral or aortic aneurysm, and raised intracranial pressure.

Mediterranean and Afro-Caribbean patients who might have *sickle cell trait* need additional care that oxygen tension does not fall. Extra care is also required with diabetic patients who take insulin. Although risks rise somewhat in old age, so do the risks of untreated depression and drug treatment.

Adverse effects, including increased cognitive impairment, have been reported when ECT has been given with *lithium*. *SSRIs* have been associated with prolonged seizures during ECT. Some anaesthetists prefer not to anaesthetize patients taking *MAOIs*, but ECT can, in fact, be given safely to patients receiving MAOI therapy.

Technique of administration

In this section we outline the technical procedures used at the time of treatment. Although the information in this account should be known, it is important to remember that ECT is a *practical procedure* that must be learned by apprenticeship as well as by reading. Much useful information is given in the ECT handbook of the Royal College of Psychiatrists (1995).

ECT clinic ECT should be given in pleasant safe surroundings. Patients should not have to wait where they can see or hear treatment given to others. There should be waiting and recovery areas separate from the room in which treatment is given, and adequate emergency equipment should be available including a sucker, endotracheal tubes, adequate supplies of oxygen, and facilities to carry out full resuscitation. The nursing and medical staff who give ECT should receive *special training*.

Arrival of patient The first step in giving ECT is to put the patient at ease and to check his identity. The case notes should then be seen to make sure that there is a valid consent form. The drug sheet should be checked to ensure that the patient is not receiving any drugs, such as MAOIs, that might complicate anaesthetic procedures. It is also important to check for evidence of drug allergy or adverse effects of previous general anaesthetics. The drug sheet should be available for the anaesthetist to see. A full physical evaluation should have been carried out by the patient's treating doctor. Specialist advice should be sought when there may be medical contraindications to ECT.

Electrode placement A decision about electrode placement should have been made by the treating doctor prior to treatment. In using unilateral treatment, it

is important to apply the electrodes to the *non-dominant hemisphere*. In right-handed people, the left hemisphere is nearly always dominant; in left-handed people, either hemisphere may be dominant. Hence, if there is evidence that the patient is not right-handed, it is usually better to use bilateral electrode placements.

In all cases the patient should be watched carefully after the first application of ECT. *Marked confusion*, especially with dysphasia, for more than 5 minutes after the return of consciousness suggests that the dominant side has been chosen inadvertently. In such an event, either the opposite side should be stimulated subsequently, or bilateral placement should be used instead.

Anaesthetic procedures The next steps are to make sure that the patient has taken nothing by mouth for at least 5 hours, and then, with the anaesthetist, to remove dentures and check for loose or broken teeth. Finally, the record of any previous ECTs should be examined for evidence of delayed recovery from the relaxant (due to deficiency in pseudocholinesterase) or other complications.

An anaesthetist should be present when ECT is given (though this cannot always be achieved in developing countries). Suction apparatus, a positive-pressure oxygen supply, and emergency drugs should always be available. A tilting trolley is also valuable. As well as the psychiatrist and anaesthetist, at least one nurse should be present.

There is some debate as to whether atropine pretreatment helps to prevent vagal arrhythmias and dry excess bronchial secretion. There is little evidence that atropine in usual dosage is useful for these purposes, and the current advice of the Royal College of Psychiatrists (1995) is that atropine should not be given routinely. If an anticholinergic agent is required to dry secretions, glycopyrrolate should be used because it does not cross the blood-brain barrier.

Anaesthesia for ECT is best induced with *methohexitone*, a short-acting barbiturate. However, this agent is becoming increasingly difficult to obtain. Alternatives are *propofol, etomidate* or *thiopentone* but

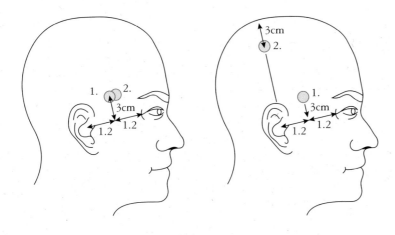

| Bitemporal (BT) | Right unilateral (RU) | Figure 21.4 ECT electrode placements. |

all have some drawbacks (Freeman 1999). *Propofol* is probably the most widely used in day-case anaesthesia but it can *decrease seizure length* during ECT and has also been associated with *delayed convulsions*, *delayed recovery*, and *anaphylaxis*.

The induction agent is followed immediately by a *muscle relaxant* (often suxamethonium chloride) from a separate syringe, although the same needle can be used. The anaesthetist is responsible for the choice of drugs and should also ensure that the lungs are well oxygenated before a mouth gag is inserted.

Application of ECT While the anaesthetic is being given, the psychiatrist checks both the *dose of electricity* and the *electrode placement* that has been prescribed for the patient. The skin is cleaned in the appropriate areas and moistened electrodes are applied. (If good electrical contact is to be obtained, it is also important that grease and hair lacquer are removed by ward staff before the patient is sent for ECT.) While dry electrodes can cause skin burns, it is also important to remember that excessive moisture causes shorting and may prevent a seizure response.

Although enough muscle relaxant should have been given to ensure that convulsive movements are minimal, a nurse or other assistant should be ready to restrain the patient gently if necessary. The

electrodes are now secured firmly. For unilateral ECT, the first electrode is placed on the non-dominant side, 3 cm above the midpoint between the external angle of the orbit and the external auditory meatus. The second is *at least 10 cm* away from the first, vertically above the meatus of the same side (see Figure 21.4). A wide separation of the electrodes increases the efficacy of unilateral ECT (see Lock 1999). The stimulus is then given.

A constant current apparatus should be used. These machines are preset to deliver a fixed amount of charge. For *fixed-dose right unilateral ECT* the initial dose should be set at 400 millicoulombs and subsequently adjusted according to clinical efficacy and cognitive side-effects. However dose-titration offers advantages in terms of individualizing the dose for each patient (see above).

For *bilateral ECT*, electrodes are on opposite sides of the head, each 3 cm above the midpoint of the line joining the eternal angle of the orbit to the external auditory meatus – usually just above the hairline (Figure 21.4). As discussed above, when using bilateral electrode placement, the present practice is to administer a dose of electricity that is only modestly (about 50%) above the seizure threshold for the individual.

The seizure threshold for ECT is best determined by *dose titration* (see above and Lock 1999).

Otherwise an appropriate dose can be estimated from the fact that two-thirds of the population have seizure thresholds between 100 and 200 millicoulombs. In addition, seizure thresholds are higher in men than in women, and increase with age. For example, a reasonable starting dose for a male patient under 40 who is to receive bilateral ECT, would be 150 millicoulombs.

Subsequently this dose could be adjusted depending on the length of seizure, the cognitive side-effects, and clinical response. The dose might be increased if the seizure were short or absent, or if there were no improvement after several treatments. Conversely, troublesome post-ECT cognitive disturbance would indicate that the dose of electricity should be reduced.

It is important to note that seizure duration may *decrease* during a course of ECT because repeated treatment tends to increase seizure threshold. Thus, if a dose of electricity initially produced a seizure of satisfactory duration, it may subsequently need to be increased.

The seizure It is essential to observe carefully for evidence of seizure. If satisfactory muscle relaxation has been achieved, the seizure takes the following form. First the muscles of the face begin to twitch and the mouth drops open; then the upper eyelids, thumbs, and big toes jerk rhythmically for about half a minute. It is important not to confuse these convulsive movements with muscle twitches due to the depolarization produced by suxamethonium.

EEG monitoring has been used to check whether a seizure has been induced, but the records can be difficult to interpret because of the muscle artefact produced by direct stimulation of the frontalis muscle. An alternative is to *isolate one forearm from the effects of the muscle relaxant.* This can be done by blowing up a blood pressure cuff to above systolic pressure before the relaxant is injected; this pressure is maintained during the period in which the seizure should occur and then released.

Seizure activity can then be observed in the muscles of the isolated part of the arm. When judging the appropriate cuff pressure, it is important to remember that systolic pressure rises during the seizure; if the cuff is not at sufficient pressure the relaxant will pass into the forearm at this stage.

There is no direct correlation between treatment outcome and duration of seizure activity, but it is recommended that the dose of electricity be adjusted to achieve a seizure duration of *between 20 and 50 seconds.* This duration is recommended because short seizures are likely to be therapeutically ineffective whereas long seizures are more likely to be associated with cognitive disturbance.

Psychotropic drugs may alter seizure threshold and seizure duration. For example, most antidepressant and antipsychotic drugs lower seizure threshold, whilst benzodiazepines and carbamazepine have the reverse effect.

Recovery phase After the seizure, the lungs are oxygenated thoroughly with an airway in place. The patient remains in the care of the anaesthetist and under close nursing observation until breathing resumes and consciousness is restored. During recovery, the patient should be turned on his side and cared for in the usual way for anyone recovering from an anaesthetic after a minor surgical procedure. A qualified nurse should be in attendance to supervise the patient and reassure him. Meanwhile the psychiatrist makes a note of the date, type of electrode placement, drugs used, and amount of current, together with a brief description of the fit and any problems that have arisen. When the patient is awake and orientated, he should rest for an hour or so on his bed or in a chair.

If ECT is given to a day patient, it is especially important to make certain that no food or drink has been taken before he arrives at the hospital. He should rest for several hours and should not leave until it is certain that his recovery is complete; he should leave in the company of a responsible adult, preferably by ambulance, and certainly not riding a bicycle or driving a car.

Failed stimulations The most important problem, apart from those relating to the anaesthetic procedure, is failure to produce a clonic convulsion (a tonic jerk produced by the current must not be mistaken for a seizure). If it is certain that no seizure has appeared, checks should be made of the machine, electrodes, and contact with the skin. The possibility of shorting due to excess moisture on the scalp should also be considered. If all these are excluded, the patient may have either an unusually high resistance to the passage of current through the extracranial tissues and skull, or a high convulsive threshold. The charge can then be increased by 50% and a further stimulus given.

Frequency and number of treatments

In the UK, ECT is usually given twice a week, although in urgent cases three applications may be used in the first week. In general, thrice-weekly ECT has *little therapeutic advantage* over a twice-weekly regimen, and may produce more cognitive impairment.

Decisions about the length of a course of ECT have to depend on clinical experience since relevant information is not available from clinical trials. *A course of ECT is usually from six to a maximum of 12 treatments.* Progress should be reviewed at least once a week; there is usually little response until two or three treatments have been given, after which increasing improvement takes place. If the response is more rapid than this, fewer treatments may be given. If there has been no response after six to eight treatments, the course should usually be abandoned since it is unlikely that more ECT will produce useful change.

It is important that, whereas ECT may produce striking benefit in depressed patients, there is *a high relapse rate* unless continuation therapy with antidepressant medication is undertaken. Sometimes the choice of antidepressant drug can be difficult because if a patient does not respond to an adequate dose of an antidepressant drug prior to ECT, continuing the same drug after the course of ECT is completed *may not provide a useful prophylactic effect* (Sackheim *et al.* 1990). Thus, if a patient

has required ECT because of non-response to antidepressant medication, it is good practice to consider a different class of antidepressant drug or else lithium carbonate in the continuation and prophylactic phases of drug treatment.

A few patients respond well to ECT but continually relapse even when maintained on multiple drug therapy. In these circumstances some practitioners give *maintenance ECT* at a reduced frequency, such as fortnightly or monthly. Patients receiving continuing ECT require careful monitoring of both mood and cognitive state (Scott *et al.* 1991).

Medicolegal issues including consent to ECT

Before a patient is asked to agree to ECT, it is essential to *explain the procedure* and indicate its *expected benefits* and *possible risks* (especially the possible effects on memory). Written informations sheets can be particularly helpful (Royal College of Psychiatrists 1995).

Many patients expect severe and permanent memory impairment after treatment and some even expect to receive unmodified fits. Once the doctor is sure that the patient understands what he has been told, the latter is asked to sign a standard form of consent. The patient should understand that consent is being sought for the whole course of ECT and not just for one treatment (although he can, of course, withdraw consent at any time). All this is the doctor's job – he should not delegate it to other staff.

If a patient refuses consent or is unable to give it because he is in a stupor or for other reasons, and if the procedure is essential, further steps must be considered in the UK. The first is to decide whether there are grounds for involving the appropriate section of the Mental Health Act (see Appendix). The section does **not allow** anyone to give consent on behalf of the patient, but it does establish formally that he is mentally ill and in need of treatment. In England and Wales, the opinion of a second independent consultant is required by the Mental Health Act 1983. Readers working elsewhere should find out the relevant legal requirements.

If the decision is made in this careful way, it is rare for patients to question the need for treatment once they have recovered. Instead, most acknowledge that treatment has helped, and they understand why it was necessary to give it without their expressed consent.

Ethical aspects of ECT

As for drug treatment, the key issue for a competent patient is the concept of *full informed consent*. Generally ECT is widely regarded as a safe and effective treatment, a view supported by randomized controlled trials. However, it is important that patients be warned about the possibility of loss of remote memories outlined above. In addition, with medication-resistant patients, the issue of relapse should be discussed.

ECT in the case of non-competent patients raises difficult issues. Usually, in these circumstances ECT is needed to treat a patient whose life is placed at risk through their illness. The legal safeguards for patients are outlined above but the clinician has the duty to explain to the patient and their family the reasons for the action taken. Merskey (1999) emphasizes the value of 'a scrupulous fiduciary approach'.

Bright light treatment

The use of *phototherapy*, or *artificial bright light*, as a psychiatric treatment was first studied systematically by Rosenthal *et al.* (1984). These workers used bright light to treat patients with the newly identified syndrome of *seasonal affective disorder*. Since then, phototherapy has become the mainstay of treatment of *winter depression*, particularly in patients with *atypical depressive features* such as hyperphagia and hypersomnia (Rodin and Thompson 1997).

Mechanism of action

The light-dark cycle is believed to be one of the most important 'Zeitgebers' regulating circadian and seasonal rhythmicity in mammals. Initially, phototherapy was believed to ameliorate the symptoms of winter depression by extending the photoperiod. This was based on the view that patients with winter depression were particularly sensitive to the effects of short winter days and that bright light treatment produced a day length equivalent to that of summer.

More recent formulations have suggested that the antidepressant effect of bright light may be attributable to a *phase advance in circadian rhythm*. This is supported by the fact that controlled trials show that in most patients morning phototherapy is more effective than evening phototherapy. However, other studies have shown that bright light given at midday is also therapeutically effective. It is difficult to devise a truly plausible placebo condition for bright light treatment and some have argued that the antidepressant effects of bright light may be mediated in large measure by placebo effects, particularly patient expectation (Avery 1998).

Equipment

A conventional light box contains fluorescent tubes mounted behind a translucent plastic diffusing screen. The tubes provide an output that can vary between 2500 and 10 000 lux. Light sources producing 10 000 lux are more expensive but may allow a *reduced duration of exposure* (30 minutes compared with 120 minutes) to secure a therapeutic effect.

Phototherapy has also been administered using *head-mounted units* or *light visors*. These instruments are attached to the head and project light into the eyes, allowing subjects to remain mobile while receiving treatment. Whilst light visors are more convenient to use than light boxes, results from placebo-controlled trials of light visors have proved disappointing and their use is not currently recommended.

Therapeutic efficacy and indications

The major indication for light therapy is seasonal affective disorder where patients experience winter depressions. Numerous controlled trials have shown that bright light treatment is more effective than placebo in patients with winter depression, particularly if they experience:

- increased sleep
- carbohydrate craving
- afternoon slump in energy.

Patients with more *typical melancholic symptoms*, for example, weight loss and insomnia, do less well with phototherapy as a sole treatment even where the disorder is seasonal in nature.

Phototherapy may also be of benefit in other disorders characterized by depressed mood and appetite changes, for example, *premenstrual syndrome* and *bulimia nervosa*. The literature contains a number of controlled trials in such disorders where light treatment has improved ratings of depression. However, the difficulty of distinguishing specific and placebo effects of bright light makes the current data difficult to interpret.

Adverse effects

Generally, phototherapy is well tolerated although mild side-effects occur in up to 45% of patients early in treatment. These include *headache, eye strain, blurred vision, eye irritation, and increased tension*. Insomnia can also occur, particularly with late evening treatment. Rare adverse events that have been reported include *manic mood swings* and *suicide* attempts, the latter putatively through light-induced alerting and energizing effects prior to mood improvement. Whether these rare events are actually adverse reactions to light is uncertain. There is no evidence that phototherapy employed in recommended treatment schedules causes ocular or retinal damage.

Clinical use of phototherapy

Since the best established indication for phototherapy is seasonal affective disorder, the following account will describe the use of bright light treatment in winter depression. One of the major practical difficulties in phototherapy is the time needed to administer the treatment. For this reason, a 10 000 lux light box may be preferred because the daily duration of therapy can be reduced to 30–45 minutes. It seems likely that cool-white light and full-spectrum light have equivalent clinical efficacy but because cool-white light is free of ultraviolet light it is theoretically safer.

The evidence suggests that bright light treatment of winter depression is most effective when administered in the early morning. However, treatments given at other times of day including the evening may prove beneficial and can be more convenient for individual patients. In an initial trial, therefore, it is best to recommend early morning treatment but to advise the patient that the exact timing of therapy can eventually represent a balance of therapeutic efficacy and practical convenience. Treatment should not be given late in the evening because of the possibility of *sleep disruption*.

Early morning phototherapy should start within a few minutes of awakening. Subjects should allow an initial duration of treatment of 30 minutes with a 10 000 lux light box or two hours with 2500 lux equipment. They should seat themselves about 30–40 cm away from the light-box screen. They should not gaze at the screen directly but face it at an angle of about 45 degrees and glance across it once or twice each minute.

The antidepressant effect of light treatment can appear within *a few days* but in controlled trials longer periods – up to 3 weeks – can be needed before the therapeutic effects of bright light exceed those of placebo treatment. As noted above, mild side-effects are common in the early stages of treatment but usually settle without specific intervention. If they are persistent and troublesome, the patient can sit a little further away from the light source or reduce the duration of exposure. Exposure should also be reduced if elevated mood occurs.

Once a therapeutic response has occurred, it is necessary to *continue phototherapy* up to the point of natural remission, otherwise relapse will occur. It may be possible, however, to lower the daily duration of treatment. Phototherapy may also be started in advance of the anticipated episode of depression as this appears to have a *prophylactic effect*.

Neurosurgery for psychiatric disorders (psychosurgery)

History of procedure

Psychosurgery refers to the use of *neurosurgical procedures* to modify the symptoms of psychiatric illness by operating on either the nuclei of the brain or the white matter. Psychosurgery began in 1936 with the work of Moniz whose operation consisted of an extensive cut in the white matter of the frontal lobes (*frontal leucotomy*). This extensive operation was modified by Freeman and Watts (1942) who made smaller coronal incisions in the frontal lobes through lateral burr holes.

Although their so-called standard leucotomy was far from standardized anatomically, and although it produced unacceptable *side-effects* (see below), the procedure was widely used in the UK and other countries. There was enthusiasm for the initial improvements observed in patients, but this was followed by growing evidence of *adverse effects including intellectual impairment, emotional lability, disinhibition, apathy, incontinence, obesity, and epilepsy.*

These problems led to a search for more restricted lesions capable of producing the same therapeutic benefits without these adverse consequences. Some progress was made, particularly with the incorporation of *stereotactic techniques* (see Fenton 1999) but at the same time advances in pharmacology made it possible to use drugs to treat the disorders for which surgery was intended.

The term for psychosurgery is now often replaced with the phrase 'neurosurgery for psychiatric disorders'. This change in terminology is intended to emphasize:

- the techniques involved now involve placement of localized lesions in specific cerebral sites;
- the treatment is for specific psychiatric conditions (treatment-resistant major depression and obsessive–compulsive disorder) and not for primary behavioural disturbance.

Indications

Thus far there have been no controlled trials to test the value of these operations. If such surgery is used

---

> ### Box 21.10 Stereotactic procedure used in psychosurgery
>
> *Subcaudate tractotomy*
> Lesion made beneath the head of each caudate nucleus, in the rostral part of the orbital cortex
> *Cingulotomy*
> Bilateral lesions within the cingulate bundles
> *Limbic leucotomy*
> Subcaudate tractotomy combined with cingulotomy – suggested for obsessive compulsive disorder
> *Capsulotomy*
> Bilateral lesions in anterior limb of internal capsule – suggested for obsessive compulsive disorder

at all, it should be only after the most thorough and persistent attempts to produce improvement with other forms of treatment. If this is done, the requirement for psychosurgery will be extremely small.

The current indications for psychosurgery are considered to be *intractable mood disorder* and *obsessive–compulsive disorder*.

Types of operation

Nowadays the older 'blind' operations have been replaced by stereotactic procedures that allow the lesions to be placed more accurately (Box 21.10). Serious adverse effects appear to be rare (Table 21.14).

Effectiveness

In the absence of controlled trials, assessment has been in the form of long-term *follow-up studies*. For example, Poynton *et al.* (1995) described a cohort of 23 severely ill treatment resistant patients, 16 of whom had major depression and 5 bipolar disorder. They underwent stereotactic subcaudate tractotomy and were followed up prospectively. At 1 year of follow-up, 13 of the patients had shown either a very good or good response with the remainder experiencing intermediate benefit or no change.

No serious physical sequelae of the operation were reported. However, detailed neuropsychological testing showed changes in the pattern of

Table 21.14 Adverse effects of stereotactic psychosurgery

Acute

- Operative mortality (less than 0.1%)
- Haemorrhage, hemiplegia (less than 0.3%)
- Transient confusion, lethargy

Long-term

- Epilepsy (1–2%)
- Frontal lobe syndrome (very rare)
- Personality changes (usually mild)

cognitive function. For example, there were improvements in some tests requiring speed and attention but deterioration on others such as the Stroop task which depend on intact frontal lobe function.

Follow-up studies of patients with obsessive–compulsive disorder show somewhat lower rates of improvement of about 40%. However, some patients show significant benefit, which is not usually apparent in subjects matched for severity of illness and followed up naturalistically (Hay *et al.* 1993).

Clinical use

The operation should never be carried out until the effects of several years of vigorous treatment have been observed. If this rule is followed, the operation will hardly be used. In fact, only about 20 psychosurgical operations a year are currently carried out in the UK (about one-third the annual rate in the 1980s). If the operation is to be considered at all, it should only be for chronic intractable obsessional disorder and severe chronic depressive disorders in older patients. There is no clear justification for psychosurgery for anxiety disorders or schizophrenia. For a less conservative view the reader should consult Sachdev and Sachdev (1997) and Marino and Cosgrove (1997).

Ethical issues

The ethical issues concerning the use of psychosurgery have been discussed by Merskey (1999). The brain is the organ of judgement and decision making but it is regarded ethically permissible to operate, for example, on a brain tumour, if a patient gives consent. The situation with regard to psychosurgery is different because the tissue which is lesioned is not overtly diseased. This distinction, however, is not clear cut. Surgeons not infrequently operate on non-diseased tissue (for example, cosmetic surgery). The practical problems for psychosurgery (which distinguish it from ECT) are as follows:

- the lack of randomized studies to show that it is effective;
- the irreversibility of the procedure;
- the potentially serious nature of some of the adverse effects.

For these reasons it seems ethically appropriate that psychosurgery should be offered only to competent patients who are able to give full informed consent. Determining competence may, of course, be difficult in a patient with chronic severe mood disorder. In the UK, this has led to the development of safeguards under Section 57 of the 1983 Mental Health Act.

Transcranial magnetic stimulation

The use of transcranial magnetic stimulation (TMS) rests on the principle that if a conducting medium such as the brain is adjacent to a magnetic field, a current will be induced in the conducting medium. In TMS, an electromagnetic coil is placed on the scalp. Passage of high-intensity pulses of current in the coil produces a powerful magnetic field [typically about 2 tesla (T)], which results in current flow in neural tissue and neuronal depolarization. Neuropsychological effects of TMS are particularly likely when pulse of current are delivered rapidly, so-called *repetitive TMS or rTMS*. If the stimulation occurs more quickly than once per second (1 Hz), it is called *fast rTMS*.

Uses of TMS

TMS has been used for many years in clinical neurophysiology to explore, for example, the integrity of motor cortex after stroke. In research settings, TMS is used to localize the cortical substrates of specific neuropsychological functions. For example, short-term verbal recall can be disrupted by rTMS administered over left temporal cortex.

Clinically rTMS has been used to relieve *depressive states*. Initially, studies used fast rTMS applied to left prefrontal cortex. In some, but not all studies, rTMS applied daily for 1–2 weeks was more effective than sham control treatment. However, other investigations have employed different kinds of electromagnetic coil, stimulation parameters, and site of coil application. For example, Klein *et al.* (1999) found antidepressant effects of slow rTMS given daily to the right prefrontal cortex. Thus there is still uncertainty about the extent of therapeutic effect of rTMS in depression, the best way to achieve it, and the length of time for which it is likely to persist.

TMS has also been employed in treatment studies of other disorders such as mania and obsessive–compulsive disorder. Findings in these conditions are still preliminary (see George *et al.* 1999).

Adverse effects of TMS

The use of single-pulse TMS in neurophysiological studies has not raised significant safety concerns. The major hazard with rTMS is the risk of inducing *seizures*. This is greater with fast rTMS than slow rTMS. Current safety protocols, which adjust the amount of magnetic stimulation in relation to the motor threshold of the individual, appear to have greatly reduced the likelihood of fits although subjects with risk factors (for example, family history of epilpepsy) are generally excluded from TMS studies of healthy volunteers.

Minor side-effects are more common and include *muscle tension headaches*, and sufficient noise to cause short-term changes in *hearing threshold*. This can be prevented by the use of earplugs (by both subjects and investigators). rTMS appropriately localized also has the potential to disrupt cognitive function but thus far changes have been short-lived. There is insufficient knowledge to know whether there might be any long-term sequelae to the brain or other organs from the high-intensity magnetic field generated during TMS. No specific hazard has been revealed by current follow-up studies.

For a discussion of the current status of TMS in psychiatry readers should consult George *et al.* (1999).

Further reading

Leonard, B. E;.(1997). *Fundamentals of pychopharmacology*. John Wiley, Chichester. (Overview of mechanisms of psychotropic drug action clearly linked to CNS neuropharmaoclogy.)

Stahl, S. M. (2000). *Essential psychopharmacology*. Cambridge University Press, Cambridge. (Well illustrated account of basic and clinical use of psychotropic drugs.)

CHAPTER 22

Psychological treatment

Psychological treatment

This chapter is concerned with various kinds of counselling, psychotherapy, behavioural and cognitive therapies, and certain related techniques. The subject is large, and the chapter will be easier to follow if the reader's attention is drawn to various points about the organization of the chapter:

- The account in this chapter should be read in conjunction with the general advice on physical treatment (Chapter 21) and on the provision of services (Chapter 23).

- This chapter includes advice on the general value of the various treatments, but advice about the value of the treatments in specific disorders is given in the chapters concerned with the relevant disorders.

- Psychological treatments are often combined with medication. Appropriate ways of doing this are also considered in the chapters concerned with the relevant disorders.

- Because many different techniques of treatment are described here, none can be described in detail and suggestions for further reading are given in several places in the chapter.

- Although outline descriptions of technique are given in several places, supervised experience is required before any of these treatments can be used with patients.

- Psychological treatments for sexual disorders are described in Chapter 19.

The word psychotherapy is used in two ways. In the first usage, psychotherapy denotes all forms of psychological treatment, including counselling and cognitive–behaviour therapy treatments. In the second usage, psychotherapy excludes coun-selling and cognitive–behaviour therapy. We have generally used the words psychological treatment for the broad sense of the term, and in using the word psychotherapy, have qualified it to indicate a precise meaning, for example, for brief dynamic psychotherapy. The treatments considered in this chapter are listed in Table 22.1, which also shows the general structure of the chapter.

How psychological treatments developed

The use of psychological healing is as old as the practice of medicine. Parallels have been drawn between aspects of modern techniques and the ceremonial healing carried out in some of the temples of ancient Greece. However, in the history of psychiatric treatment, psychological treatment starts in the nineteenth century with developments in hypnosis. These developments begin with the activities of Anton Mesmer (1734–1815), a Viennese physician who believed that magnetic forces could be used to alter the functions of the body. These forces could, he believed, arise from actual magnets or from the 'animal magnetism' present in the body of the therapist. Mesmer believed, therefore, that the curative effect of animal magnetism could be enhanced by the use of physical magnets (Block 1980). Mesmer's theories were not generally accepted by the medical profession, but a Manchester doctor, James Braid, gave a more physiologically plausible explanation of the phenomena. Braid drew parallels between the states produced by mesmerism and sleep, and for this reason suggested the name hypnosis. He also showed that therapeutic effects could be obtained without the use of magnets (Braid 1843).

Treatment with hypnosis became popular in France, where a disagreement arose about its mechanism of action. In Nancy, A. A. Liebeault (1823–1904) and Hippolyte Bernheim (1837–1919) considered that hypnosis was a normal state, allied to sleep that could be induced in most people, and that its effects were brought about through suggestion. Bernheim's book *Suggestive therapeutics* (Bernheim 1890) described the use of suggestion to treat hysteria and other neurotic conditions, as well as painful afflictions and gastro-

intestinal problems. The alternative view was championed by Jean Martin Charcot (1825–1893) who practised neurology at the Salpetriere hospital in Paris. Charcot maintained that hypnosis was a pathological state which occurred only in patients with hysteria.

The main alternative to hypnosis was 'persuasion', a method in which symptoms and other problems were explained and discussed without any attempt to increase suggestibility. An important proponent of this approach was Paul Dubois, a Swiss professor of neuropathology, whose book *The psychic treatment of nervous disorders*, published in

1904 (and translated into English as Dubois 1909) was widely influential. Dubois taught that although hypnosis had some limited value for hysteria, persuasive treatment was more appropriate for other neuroses.

In the late nineteenth century, most neuroses were treated by neurologists and when Freud began practice as a neurologist he saw many neurotic patients. To improve his therapeutic skills, he visited France to study hypnosis (see Freud 1892). He visited Bernheim in Nancy and in Paris he watched Charcot's demonstrations of hypnosis in hysterical patients. When he returned to Vienna, Freud tried hypnosis with some of his neurotic patients and at first was pleased by its results. However, he could not maintain these early successes and he began to use hypnosis in a new way. Thus in 1889, he described the case of Emmy von N, in which he used hypnosis not to change symptoms directly, but to release the emotion associated with the repressed ideas that he believed to be the cause of the symptoms (Greenson 1967).

Freud then remembered that Bernheim had shown that patients could recall forgotten events without hypnosis and he asked his patients to do so while they shut their eyes and he placed his hands on their forehead (Breuer and Freud 1893–5, pp. 109, 279). Next Freud discovered that recall was as effective when the patient simply lay on a couch while the therapist kept out of sight. In this way the method of free association developed. Freud found how to encourage free associations, and comment on their significance, and learned how to achieve the appropriate intensity of relationship with his patients. His discoveries became the basic technique of psychoanalysis and subsequently of a larger group of dynamic psychotherapies. (They are described briefly on p. 744–6. The interested reader is recommended to read one of the accounts written by Freud himself (Freud 1895a, 1895b, 1923). Freud's theories of mental functioning are summarized in this book on p. 114–17.)

Gradually, psychoanalytical and related techniques became more widely used than hypnosis and persuasion. Freud published striking accounts of his new treatment and elaborated his theories in increasingly complex ways. He attracted a group of followers, but some came to disagree with the further developments of his ideas, and formed their own 'schools' of dynamic psychotherapy. These developments are now described briefly; more information will be found in the chapter by Holmes (2000) or the book by Munroe (1955).

Alfred Adler left Freud in 1910. He rejected the libido theory (see p. 116) and pointed instead to the influence of social factors in development. In his therapeutic technique, called individual analysis, he tried to understand how the patient's lifestyle had developed, and he focused on current problems. Adler's theories lacked the ingenuity and interest of Freud's ideas, and his treatment was not used widely. However, his ideas can be seen as the basis for the influential dynamic-cultural school of American analysts (see below). For more information about Adler's contributions see Ansbacher and Ansbacher (1964).

While Adler emphasized the real problems in the patient's life, *Carl Jung* was more concerned with the inner world of fantasy. In his form of psychotherapy he emphasized the interpretation of unconscious material as represented in dreams and artistic productions, although he did not neglect the contemporary. Jung believed that part of the unconscious was common to all people (the 'collective' unconscious) and was expressed in universal images called archetypes (Fordham 1990). Despite this emphasis on the unconscious, the relationship between therapist and patient in Jungian analysis is less one-sided than in psychoanalysis in that the therapist is more active and reveals more about himself. For more information about Jung's ideas see Storr (2000).

The *neo-Freudian* school of analysis developed in the USA in the 1930s. Its members accepted that the origins of character and of neurosis are in childhood but did not accept that libido development was of crucial importance. Instead, family and wider social factors were judged more important. Three important figures in this school were Karen Horney and Erich Fromm (both refugees from Nazi

Box 22.1 The neo-Freudians

Karen Horney took issue with Freud's view of the psychological development of women, especially the concept of 'penis envy'. For Horney, anxiety in childhood arose from the experience of being insignificant, helpless, and threatened. This anxiety was normally overcome by the experience of being brought up by loving parents, and in some children who lacked this experience, anxiety persists and defences develop against it. These defences include striving for affection, striving for power, and excessive submissiveness. Horney summarized the difference between her treatment and Freud's methods as follows: 'I differ from Freud in that after the recognition of the neurotic trends, while he primarily investigates their genesis I primarily investigate their actual functions and their consequences.' (Horney 1939, p. 282)

Erich Fromm also rejected Freud's theory of instinctual development as a cause of neurosis. He accepted the importance of family influences in shaping character, and drew attention to wider cultural influences. Fromm was generally concerned more with social than with clinical issues, and his ideas did not greatly influence therapy.

Harry Stack Sullivan, unlike Fromm, was more interested in therapy than in theory. His treatment centred on the relationship between analyst and patient, and the discussion of everyday social encounters. Patient and therapist were more equal than in Freudian analysis, and Sullivan preferred pointed questions and provocative statements to interpretations based on theory (Sullivan 1953).

concept of the 'object', a term that can refer both to an emotionally important person (for example, a parent) and to the internal psychological representation of that person. Klein used this concept to explain how, in the early stages of development, an infant experiences these 'objects' and the instinctual feelings of love and hatred that accompany them. The theory cannot be tested directly, and its details are difficult to accept, but the general approach and the concept of 'objects' has been widely influential. For an outline of Klein's theories see Segal (1963), and for an account of Klein's technique of analysis of children see Klein (1963).

Attachment theory originated in the work of *John Bowlby*, a British analyst. The theory is based on the idea that infants need a secure relationship with their parent, and that insecure attachments can lead to emotional problems in later life. These ideas had a considerable effect on the care of children, for example, by drawing attention to the need to maintain contact with the parents when a child is admitted to hospital.

Brief psychodynamic psychotherapy This development can be traced to the work of Ferenczi, who foresaw the need to develop treatments shorter than psychoanalysis. He did this by setting time limits, making the role of the therapist less passive, and planning the main themes of treatment. These innovations have found their way into the brief dynamic psychotherapy used today. (see p. 744).

The development of cognitive–behaviour therapy

Interest in a treatment based on scientific psychology can be traced to Janet's (1925) methods of re-education, to Watson and Rayner's (1920) use of learning principles in the treatment of children's fears, and to the use in the 1930s of aversion therapy for alcoholism. However, the origins of current cognitive–behaviour therapy were in the 1950s. At that time, psychologists working at the Maudsley Hospital in London were disillusioned with the extravagant claims made for psychoanalysis and by its unscientific approach. They

Germany who settled in the USA in 1930s) and Harry Stack Sullivan. Their contributions are summarized in Box 22.1.

The object relations school developed in Britain in the 1930s and 1940s. It originated from the work of Melanie Klein who enlarged Freud's theories about early infant development. She also suggested ways in which psychoanalytical techniques could be adapted for use with children by interpreting their play as if it were the equivalent of the utterances of adult patients. Klein developed the

began to use learning principles in the treatment of patients with phobic disorders in the hope that the lessons learned with these conditions might indicate how learning principles could be applied more widely. At about the same time, Joseph Wolpe, a psychiatrist working in South Africa, wrote an influential book, *Psychotherapy by reciprocal inhibition* (Wolpe 1958), in which he described a widely applicable treatment for neurotic disorders, also based on learning theory. In the USA, Skinner (1953) suggested that the principles of operant conditioning could be used in the treatment of psychiatric disorders.

Wolpe's ideas were adopted in the UK where they fitted well with the initiatives at the Maudsley Hospital, but in the USA there was at first more interest in methods based on operant conditioning. Later the approaches converged, and similar methods are now used in these two countries and elsewhere. From the beginning there was a strong emphasis on the evaluation of the new treatment methods. The first clinical trial, to compare desensitization with individual and group dynamic psychotherapy, was reported in 1978 (Gelder *et al.* 1978). By current standards, the trial had many shortcomings but it was followed by many more, carried out with increasing sophistication, so that there is now a strong evidence base for most of the behavioural methods now in use, whilst those whose claimed effects were not confirmed by evidence have fallen out of use.

Cognitive therapy began, in the USA, with the work of A. T. Beck, a psychiatrist who had become dissatisfied with the results of psychoanalytical psychotherapy and sought an alternative way of treating depressed patients. He was struck by the recurring themes in the thinking of these patients, for example, about personal failure, and he suggested that these themes were part of the primary disorder and had to be changed. Beck devised an ingenious way of challenging and altering these beliefs and other cognitions of depressed patients (see p. 741).

A second source of ideas leading to cognitive therapy was a group of US psychologists who had

become dissatisfied with operant conditioning methods in which the mind was regarded as a 'black box' and thoughts and feelings were ignored. For example, Meichenbaum (1977) proposed that the recurrent thoughts of people with emotional disorders played a part in maintaining their distress, and suggested how they might be controlled. These approaches and those of Beck were taken up by other psychologists and psychiatrists, and integrated with previous work on behaviour therapy as the current methods of cognitive–behaviour therapy (described below). The strong evidence base, the clearly described procedures, and the relatively brief treatment time of cognitive–behaviour therapies have caused them to be the preferred psychological treatment for many disorders.

Classification of psychological treatments

There are so many kinds of psychological treatment that it is useful to group them in a simple classification. Various classifications have been proposed, of which two will be considered here, followed by a simple scheme used here to help readers relate the treatments to their use in most health-care systems.

The first, and simplest way of classifying psychological treatments is in terms of the *number of patients taking part*. Treatments are grouped into those carried out with one patient (individual treatments), with couples and families, and with small and large groups. The choice between individual, marital, family, or group therapy, is considered later in the chapter. At this stage, it can be said that individual treatment is usually chosen when the treatment needs to be tailored to the particular problems of the patient, or when group discussion would cause distress, either because of the nature of the problem (for example, a sexual deviation) or because of social anxiety. Couple therapy may be chosen when relationship problems are an important contributory cause of psychiatric disorder. Family therapy may be chosen when the difficulties of a child or adolescent are part of a wider problem in the family. Group treatment may be chosen when several patients require similar treatment (for example, exposure treatment for agoraphobia), or when the contributions of other group members will be helpful (for example, to help alcohol abusers view their problems more objectively).

The second way of classifying psychological treatments is in terms of *complexity* into three groups:

♦ *Counselling* These are the least complex treatments, and they are provided by all health professionals. They are used for the less severe emotional problems, and to help people adjust to stressful situations or make difficult decisions (for example, whether to terminate a pregnancy).

♦ *Moderately complex psychological treatments* are provided by all psychiatrists, and by appropriately trained members of other professions. This group includes less specialized cognitive–behaviour therapies and some of the brief dynamic psychotherapies. These treatments are used to treat anxiety disorders and eating disorders, some of the less severe mood disorders, often as part of a plan that includes medication and social measures.

♦ *Complex psychological treatments* are provided by specialists who usually work mainly with the technique. This group includes the more complex forms of psychodynamic and cognitive–behaviour therapy. The treatments are used to treat the more severe or complex disorders, alone or as part of a wider plan of management.

Within a health service, psychological treatments are used for several reasons. They are the principal treatment for some psychiatric disorders, alone or with medication. Counselling, crisis intervention and cognitive–behaviour therapies are used in this way when they have been shown to be effective in clinical trials. Dynamic psychotherapy is now used mainly to modify factors that are thought to increase the risk of relapse or recurrence of a disorder, for example, to help overcome low self-esteem. In the past, dynamic psychotherapy was used to treat many conditions that would now be called 'subthreshold', that is, emotional problems that are distressing but are not severe or lasting enough to meet diagnostic criteria for a psychiatric disorder. Within a health service these problems are now treated usually with counselling, and the use of psychodynamic methods for this purpose is now mainly in private practice.

Common factors in psychological treatment

Research on psychological treatment has shown that, for many conditions, different methods achieve results which are similar and greater than those of no treatment. This finding suggests that in these cases the features that the psychotherapies share are more important than their differences. This conclusion was reached many years ago by Jerome Frank (1967) who suggested that the important common features are: the therapeutic relationship, listening sympathetically, allowing the release of emotion, providing information, providing a rationale for the patient's condition, restoring morale, using prestige suggestion, and forming a relationship. These features are shown in Box 22.2.

Transference and counter-transference

When the therapeutic relationship becomes intense it develops in ways that are called transference and counter-transference.

Transference is an unrealistic element of the therapeutic relationship which becomes increasingly strong as treatment progresses. Transference is especially strong when the patient reveals personal problems that in other circumstances would be revealed only to someone in an intimate relationship with the patient, such as a close relation or

Box 22.2 Common factors in psychotherapy

The therapeutic relationship This is generally thought to be the most important of the common factors in psychotherapy. However, it may become too intense with resulting problems (see text).

Listening By listening intently, the therapist shows concern for the patient's problems and begins to develop the helping relationship in which the patient feels understood.

Release of emotion Emotional release can be helpful at the beginning of treatment, but repeated release is seldom useful. Intense and rapid emotional release is called *abreaction*.

Restoration of morale Many patients have suffered repeated failures, and no longer believe that they can help themselves. By improving morale, the therapist helps the patient begin to help himself.

Providing information Distressed patients may remember little of what they have been told about their condition because their concentration is poor. Information should be as simple as possible and expressed clearly. It may be necessary to explain important points more than once, or write them down.

Providing a rationale All forms of psychological treatment provide reasons for the patient's condition, and this adds to the patient's confidence. The reasons may be stated directly by the therapist (as in short-term psychotherapy), or suggested indirectly through questions and interpretations (as in much long-term psychotherapy).

Advice and guidance These are part of all psychotherapy. In brief therapies, the advice and guidance is given directly; in long-term treatments the patient is made to seek the answers, but may still be guided – less obviously – in deciding which are right.

Suggestion Although, with the exception of hypnosis, suggestion is not deliberately increased in psychological treatments, all psychological treatment contains an element of suggestion. This suggestive element contributes to improvement in the early stages of treatment but it does not usually last long.

friend. This feature of the situation leads the patient to experience intimacy in the relationship with the therapist. Since the psychotherapist does not reveal personal details, the patient constructs a picture of the therapist by drawing on experience of another person with whom he has experienced a similarly close relationship, and this person is usually one of the parents. When this happens, patients can be said to have transferred, to the therapist, feelings and attitudes from their relationship with the parents. This process is called transference. When the transferred feelings are good, transference is said to be positive; when the transferred feelings are bad, the transference is said to be negative. Just as feelings toward a parent are mixed, so transference has both positive and negative components, which may involve a complex mixture of love, hate, envy, and jealousy.

In psychotherapy, therapists have to be genuinely concerned about their patients' most intimate problems and yet remain impartial and professional. Even with special training, therapists cannot always achieve this ideal combination of concern and detachment. They may then respond in ways that are not simply a reflection of their patients' personal qualities but also a displacement onto their patients of ideas and feelings related to other figures in the therapists' own lives. This process is called *counter-transference*. (The reader should note that some writers include in counter-transference realistic as well as unrealistic feelings and attitudes towards the patient.)

Transference can assist treatment but it may also impede it. Transference may lead to excessive dependency expressed in attempts to prolong interviews, requests for extra appointments, and behaviour demanding additional care, such as threats of suicide. Dependency may also make it difficult to bring treatment to an end due to a recrudescence of symptoms, and demands for further treatment. If dependency is noticed early and discussed with the patient, further difficulties can often be prevented. At the same time, patients can learn more about themselves by understanding the true origins of their feelings and behaviour.

Counter-transference problems arise when therapists become inappropriately involved in their patients' problems or inappropriately angry with them. These problems will be recognized earlier, when therapists scrutinize their feelings and recognize their origins in their personal experience. It is partly for this reason that training for intensive psychotherapy often includes an examination of links between the therapist's past experiences and his current emotional reactions.

Transference and counter-transference develop most strongly in long-term psychological treatments, and in psychoanalysis, transference is used as tool of therapy (see p. 746). However, transference and counter-transference are relevant in every kind of psychological treatment. Therapists overlook this fact at their peril.

Counselling and crisis intervention

Counselling

In everyday usage, the word counselling denotes the giving of advice. As a technical term, it denotes a wider procedure concerned with emotions as well as with knowledge. There are many techniques of counselling, each used for a variety of problems, and in a variety of settings (for example, general medical practice, as part of psychiatric care, and in a student health service).

Counselling incorporates the non-specific factors shared by all kinds of psychotherapy (see Box 22.2). In all techniques, the relationship between the counsellor and the person counselled is important. The relative importance of giving information, allowing the release of emotion, and thinking afresh about the situation vary according to the purpose of counselling. In the past much counselling used the *client-centred approach* in which the counsellor takes a passive role. He gives little information and largely restricts his interventions to comments on the emotional content of the client's utterances; for example, instead of asking for clarification of facts, he might say 'that seems to make you angry' (reflection of feelings). The technique has been largely

replaced, in health-care systems, by the more structured and focused procedures (reviewed below), since these are generally agreed to be more effective. They are, however, still used by some of the many counsellors working independently.

Approaches to counselling

Problem-solving counselling is a highly structured form of counselling, suitable for patients whose problems are clearly related to stressful circumstances. It is mentioned first in this section because it is widely applicable to conditions in which life problems are exacerbating or maintaining a disorder. The basic counselling techniques are combined with a systematic approach to the resolution of problems. The patient is helped to:

- identify and list problems that are causing distress;
- consider what practicable courses of action might solve or reduce each problem;
- select one problem, and try out the course of action that appears most feasible and likely to succeed;
- review the results of the attempt to solve the problem and then either choose another problem for solution if the first action has succeeded, or choose another course of action if the first has not succeeded.

This approach has been shown to be effective for the less severe forms of mood disorder (Catalan *et al.* 1991; Mynors-Wallace *et al.* 1995).

Interpersonal counselling was developed by Klerman *et al.* (1987) from interpersonal therapy (which is described on p. 732), but has many similarities to the problem-solving approach. Attention is focused on current problems in personal relationships within the family, at work, and elsewhere. These problems are considered under four headings: *loss, interpersonal disputes, role transitions, and interpersonal deficits.* Using a problem-solving approach similar to that described above, the therapist encourages patients to consider alternative ways of coping with their difficulties, and to try these out between sessions of treatment. The method has been shown to be effective for patients in primary care presenting with minor mood disorders (Klerman *et al.* 1987).

Psychodynamic counselling places more emphasis on the influence of past experience on the development of current behaviour, mediated in part through unconscious processes. It is influenced by object relations theory, that is, by the idea that previous relationships leave lasting traces which affect self-esteem, and may result in maladaptive patterns of behaviour. The patient's emotional reactions to the counsellor are considered to be a source of information about problems in other relationships. These approaches can be combined with the problem-solving methods described above. This form of counselling is used, for example, in student health centres where the developmental approach fits well with problems that although manifest at university, often originated in experiences before the student entered university. Psychodynamic counselling has been described by Jacobs (1988). It has not been evaluated as thoroughly as the other two approaches.

Counselling for specific purposes

Counselling to relieve acute distress

Here initial emphasis is given to emotional release, and to ways of coping with the immediate problems. When this approach is used for survivors of disasters, who are encouraged to recall the distressing events, it is called *debriefing*. Evidence from clinical trials indicates that debriefing does not improve the outcome of survivors, and that methods using cognitive techniques may be more helpful (see p. 194).

Counselling for relationship problems

Counselling for relationship problems helps couples to talk constructively about problems in their relationship. The focus is on the need for each partner to understand the point of view, needs, and feelings of the other, and to identify positive aspects of the relationship as well as those causing conflict.

Grief counselling

Grief counselling focuses on working through the stages of grief (see p. 208). It combines an opportunity for emotional release (including in appropriate cases, the expression of anger), information about the normal course of grieving, encouragement to engage in final acts such as viewing the body and disposing of clothing, and advice about the practical problems of living without the deceased person. (Grief counselling is considered further on p. 210.)

Counselling for the late effects of trauma

Clinical experience strongly suggests that nondirective and unstructured approaches should not be used since they may result in the recollection of distressing experience without enabling the person to deal adequately with the resulting emotions or to do the necessary cognitive processing. Cognitive or psychodynamic methods appear to be more suitable, but they, too, require careful planning and skilful management.

Counselling about risks

Counselling about risks is exemplified by counselling about genetic risks and about the risks of sexually transmitted disease. The essential steps are to give information about the risks, provide an opportunity for reflection on the impact of the various outcomes, and to help the person decide how best to respond.

Counselling in primary care

In primary care, many patients with minor psychiatric disorders are treated by practice counsellors who have training in counselling but are not members of the medical, nursing, or social work professions. These counsellors used various methods but many employ non-directive techniques. The average number of sessions is about seven, and the average length of each session is about 50 minutes (Sibbald *et al.* 1996a). There have been few controlled evaluations of this treatment, and those that have been reported have methodological problems. Three of four recent studies found no difference between the outcomes of counselling and routine care by the general practitioner (Boot *et al.* 1994; Hemmings 1997; Harvey *et al.* 1998); the fourth found greater change in symptoms in the counselled group but there were problems in the randomization of cases, and there was no follow-up (Friedli *et al.* 1997). Patients who received counselling generally took less medication than patients treated by the general practitioner, so that counselling can be an alternative treatment for those who do not wish to be treated with drugs. Most of the counselling in these studies was non-directive, and it is possible that better results would be obtained with problem-solving techniques (see p. 728).

Crisis intervention

This treatment helps patients cope with a crisis in their lives, and to learn effective ways of dealing with future difficulties. The approach is used, for example, after the break-up of a relationship. It can be used also in the aftermath of natural disasters such as floods and earthquakes, but cognitive methods (see below) are now often preferred in these circumstances. Crisis intervention, which originated in the work of Lindemann (1944) and Caplan (1961), is based on Caplan's description of four stages of coping (Caplan 1961):

- emotional arousal with efforts to solve the problem;
- if these fail, greater arousal leading to a disorganization of behaviour;
- trials of alternative ways of coping;
- if there is still no resolution, exhaustion and decompensation.

Crisis intervention seeks to limit the reaction to the first stage, or if this has been passed before the person seeks help, to avoid the fourth stage.

Problems leading to crisis

These can be divided usefully into:

- *loss problems* such as the loss of a person through death or separation, or the loss of a body part or the function of an organ;

- *role changes* such as entering marriage, parenthood, or a new job with added responsibilities;
- problems in *relationships* such as those between sexual partners, or between parent and child;
- *conflict* problems, which are usually difficulties in choosing between two undesirable alternatives.

Crisis intervention methods

The methods generally resemble interpersonal counselling (p. 728) and problem-solving counselling (p. 728), though with a greater emphasis on reducing arousal. Treatment starts as soon as possible after the crisis and is brief, usually a few sessions over days or a few weeks. The approach is collaborative, involving the patient fully, and often including family or close friends. The focus is on current problems, although relevant past events are also considered. Patients in crisis have a high level of emotional arousal, which interferes with problem solving, and the first aim of treatment is to reduce this level. Usually this can be achieved with reassurance and an opportunity to express emotions, but occasionally anxiolytic medication is required for a few days. Although the general approach is that patients should help themselves, in this first stage some arrangements may have to be made for them, for example, arrangements for the care of children.

The second stage of crisis intervention resembles the problem-solving counselling described above. The patient's problems and assets are assessed carefully. The patient is encouraged to suggest alternative solutions and to choose the most promising. The therapist's role is to encourage, prompt, and question. He does not formulate problems or suggest solutions directly but helps the patient to do so himself. The patient should discover general methods of coping that will be useful for solving future problems.

Indications

Clinical experience suggests that crisis intervention is most valuable for well-motivated people with stable personalities who are facing major but transitory difficulties; in other words, those who are most likely eventually to cope on their own. Crisis intervention is used, especially, after deliberate self-harm arising in response to a social crisis.

Supportive psychotherapy

Supportive psychotherapy is used to relieve distress or to help a person to cope with difficulties, when problem-solving approaches are unlikely to succeed. It is used, for example, for some patients with chronic mental or physical illness and as part of the care of the dying (see p. 206). As a general rule, supportive treatment should not be used unless more active forms of intervention have failed or are highly unlikely to succeed.

Supportive therapy is based on the common factors of psychological treatment (see Box 22.2). Its basic elements are a therapeutic relationship, listening, allowing the release of emotions, explaining, encouraging hope, and persuasion. The various components will be considered briefly.

- *The therapeutic relationship* is used to sustain patients. It is important to avoid dependence since the treatment often has to be long lasting; but if patients are severely handicapped or have dependent personalities, it may be difficult to achieve this aim. If dependence cannot be avoided, it should be directed as far as possible to the group of staff caring for the patient and not to any individual. The risk of dependence will be less if, from the beginning, it is agreed with patients how much time can be allocated for the support.
- *Listening* As in all forms of psychological treatment, patients should feel that they have their doctor's full attention and sympathy while he is with them, and that their concerns are being taken seriously.
- *Emotional release* can be helpful in the early stages of supportive treatment. However, repeated release of emotions is unlikely to be beneficial, except when a new problem has

arisen, for example, in a progressive physical illness.

- *Information and advice* are important but their timing should be considered carefully. Information should always be accurate, but it is not necessary to explain everything at the first session. Indeed, patients with serious and incurable illness may need to receive information gradually, coping with parts before they face the whole extent of their problems. Most patients indicate, directly or indirectly, how much they wish to be told on each occasion.
- *Encouraging hope* is important but premature or unrealistic reassurance can destroy a patient's confidence in the carers. Reassurance should be offered only when the patient's concerns have been fully understood. Reassurance must, of course, be truthful and patients who find that they have been deceived lose the basic trust on which supportive therapy depends. When a patient asks about prognosis, the therapist can give a range of outcomes, including the most optimistic that can be foreseen. Even with the most difficult problems, a positive approach can often be maintained by encouraging patients to build on their remaining assets and opportunities.
- *Persuasion* In supportive treatment, patients should generally decide to take actions themselves as a result of their understanding the situation. Nevertheless, it is sometimes appropriate for doctors to use their powers of persuasion to help patients to take some necessary step, for example, to continue to cope despite a temporary exacerbation of their condition.

Supportive treatment need not always be provided by a health professional. Self-help groups give valuable support to some patients and to relatives. Indeed, this form of support is sometimes more effective than support from a doctor since it is given by people who have struggled with the same problems as the patient. An account of supportive treatment is given by Bloch (1986).

Interpersonal psychotherapy

Interpersonal psychotherapy was developed as a structured psychological treatment for the interpersonal problems of depressed patients (Klerman *et al.* 1984). The method has a wider application to other disorders in which similar problems are maintaining behaviour, for example, eating disorders. It is characterized by its approach rather than its techniques, which overlap with those of other kinds of psychotherapy.

The treatment is highly structured. The number and content of treatment sessions are planned carefully. The initial assessment period lasts one to three sessions. Interpersonal problems are considered under four headings:

- bereavement and other loss
- role disputes
- role transitions
- 'interpersonal deficits' such as loneliness.

Problems are considered by reference to specific situations and alternative ways of coping are evaluated. Clear goals are set and progress towards them is monitored. New coping strategies are tried out in homework assignments.

In the middle phase of treatment, specific methods are used for each of the four kinds of problem listed above. For grief and other problems of loss, the methods resemble those described under grief counselling (p. 729). For interpersonal disputes, patients are helped to identify clearly the issues in the dispute, as well as any differences between their own values and those of the other person. They are helped to negotiate with the other person and to recognize their own contributions to problems that they ascribe to that person. Problems of role transition are dealt with in a similar way. Interpersonal deficits are discussed by analysing present relationship problems and the patient's previous attempts to overcome them, and by discussing alternatives. In the final two or three sessions, patients are helped to anticipate future problems and consider how they might overcome them.

Several clinical trials have shown that interpersonal therapy is effective for depressive disorders (see p. 309) and bulimia nervosa (see p. 453). In one study, the extent to which there was a focus on interpersonal themes was significantly related to the reduction of relapse of recurrent major depression (Frank *et al.* 1991).

For an account of interpersonal therapy, see Weissman *et al.* (1999).

Cognitive–behaviour therapy

All psychiatric disorders have cognitive and behavioural components and these features have to change if the patient is to recover. With most treatments, the change comes about indirectly but cognitive–behaviour therapy is designed to change cognitions and behaviour directly. Cognitive–behaviour therapy differs from dynamic psychotherapy, in that it is not concerned with the way in which the disorder developed. Instead the focus is on the factors which are maintaining the disorder at the time of treatment.

Most behavioural techniques are concerned with factors that provoke or maintain psychiatric disorders. Provoking factors are most obvious in the phobic disorders, but are important, though less obvious, in other disorders. For example, in bulimia nervosa, episodes of excessive eating may be provoked by situations which cause the patient to feel inadequate. Avoidance is a common maintaining factor, which is important in phobic and other anxiety disorders, which prevents the extinction of anxiety response to provoking situations. Many behaviours are *maintained by their consequences*. For example, escape from an anxiety-provoking situation is followed by a fall in anxiety, and this fall reinforces the phobic avoidance. Increased attention is another powerful reinforcer of behaviour. For example, a child's noisy and unruly behaviour will be reinforced if the parents pay more attention when the child behaves in this way than when he is quiet and well behaved.

Most cognitive therapy focuses on two kinds of disturbed thinking: intrusive thoughts ('automatic

Box 22.3 Three types of illogical thinking

Over-generalization Patients draw general conclusions from single instances (for example, he does not love me so no one will ever love me).

Selective abstraction Patients focus on a single unfavourable aspect of a situation but ignore favourable aspects.

Personalization Patients blame themselves for the consequences of the actions of other people.

thoughts') and dysfunctional beliefs and attitudes ('dysfunctional assumptions'). Automatic thoughts provoke an immediate emotional reaction, usually of anxiety or depression. Dysfunctional beliefs and attitudes determine the way in which situations are perceived and interpreted.

Three factors maintain dysfunctional beliefs and attitudes. First, patients *attend selectively* to evidence that confirms these beliefs and attitudes, and ignore or discount evidence that contradicts them. For example, patients with social phobias attend more to the critical behaviour of others, than to signs of approval. Second, people *think illogically*. They do this in several ways, of which three are especially relevant to cognitive therapy, are shown in Box 22.3.

The third factor that maintains dysfunctional beliefs and attitudes is *safety behaviour*. People develop this kind of behaviour as a way of reducing their immediate concerns but the long-term effect is to perpetuate the concerns. For example, a patient who believes that she will faint during a panic attack, may tense her muscles every time she feels anxious. She continues to believe that she will faint, even though she has not done so in hundreds of attacks, because she is convinced she would have fainted had she not tensed her muscles on each occasion.

General features of cognitive–behaviour therapy

Certain features characterize cognitive behavioural treatments:

- *The patient as an active partner* The patient takes an active part in treatment, with the therapist acting as an expert advisor who asks questions, and offers information and guidance.

- *Attention to provoking and maintaining factors* Patients keep daily records to identify factors which precede or follow the disorder and may be provoking or maintaining it. This kind of assessment is sometimes called the *ABC approach*, the initials referring to antecedents, behaviour, and consequences.

- *Treatment as experiment* Therapeutic procedures are usually presented as experiments which, even if they fail to produce improvement, will help the patient find out more about his condition.

- *Homework assignments* Patients practise new behaviours between sessions with the therapist, or carry out experiments to test explanations suggested by the sessions. Box 22.4 contains an example of a behavioural experiment.

- *Highly structured sessions* At each session, progress since the last session is reviewed, including any homework. New topics are considered, the following week's homework is planned, and the main points of the session are summarized.

- *Monitoring of progress* Assessment of progress does not rely solely on the patient's verbal account but typically includes the checking of daily record kept by the patient, and sometimes formal rating scales. (See Clark 2000 for a list of rating scales suitable for use in cognitive–behaviour therapy of anxiety disorders.)

Box 22.4 **Patient's record of a behavioural experiment by an agoraphobic patient**

Situation Shopping in a crowded supermarket

My predictions

I shall panic and feel dizzy.

Unless I tense my stomach muscles and breath deeply, I shall faint.

Experiment When anxious, do not tense stomach muscles or breathe deeply.

Outcome

I did panic quite badly. I felt dizzy but less so than usual.

I did not faint.

What I learnt I did not faint even though I had a severe panic and I did nothing to prevent fainting. I seem to be wrong in thinking I shall faint whenever I panic. Also tensing and deep breathing may not be having the effect I supposed. My therapist could be right in thinking that deep breathing makes me more dizzy.

What I should do next Repeat the experiment next time I go shopping.

Table 22.2 **Topics to be considered in assessment for cognitive-behaviour therapy**

1. Description of each problem including behaviour, thoughts and emotions

   Where it occurs most often

   Common prior events

   The patient's response to these events

   What follows the problem

2. Factors that make the problem better or worse

3. Maintaining factors

   Avoidance

   Safety behaviours (see text)

   Selective attention

   Maladaptive beliefs

   The responses of others

♦ *Treatment manuals* are often available describing the procedures and the way in which they are to be applied. Manuals ensure that different therapists use procedures that are closely similar to those shown to be effective in clinical trials.

Assessment for cognitive–behaviour therapy

Topics to be covered

As well as a full psychiatric history, certain additional topics are addressed.(see Table 22.2) For each of the presenting problems, the interviewer obtains an account of the antecedents, the behaviour, and the consequences (the ABC approach described above). Note that the term behaviour is used here in a wide sense to include thinking and emotion, as well as actions. By considering the sequence ABC on several occasions, regular patterns of thinking and responding are identified. The assessor is particularly concerned with patients' reasons for holding their beliefs, since this knowledge is essential in planning how arrange experiences that will negate and change the beliefs.

Sources of information for the assessment

Self-monitoring Patients record their thoughts and behaviours over a period of days or weeks. The record is made as soon as possible after the events, so that important details are not forgotten. The record includes symptoms, thoughts, emotions, and actions; the date and time of day at which they occurred. The situation and events immediately preceding the problem are noted as well as those occurring at the time, and afterwards.

Observations during treatment sessions Patients may be asked to imagine situations in which problems arise, and report the accompanying thoughts and emotions. Also, symptoms like those of the disorder may be produced in another way, for example, symptoms resembling those of panic may be produced by hyperventilation, and accompanying thoughts and emotions are noted. This technique is often used in treating panic disorder (see p. 741).

Special interviewing Although some patients are aware of their maladaptive beliefs and can describe them, other patients need help to do so. *Laddering* is one way of doing this: a series of questions is asked, each about the answer to the previous question. For example, a patient with an eating disorder might be asked what would happen if she were to gain weight; she might answer that she would lose her friends. The next question would ask why she would lose friends and she might reply that she is unlikeable, and that thin people are more popular and attractive than others.

The formulation

The information obtained in these ways and from the usual psychiatric history are combined in a formulation of:

♦ the type of events that provoke symptoms (for example, opening a conversation);

♦ any special features of the events (for example, speaking to a female of the same age);

♦ background factors (for example, a previous broken relationship; and

♦ maintaining factors.

The formulation is discussed with the patient. Some therapists present it diagrammatically on a whiteboard so that it can be built up step by step, and if necessary modified in the course of the discussion.

Behavioural techniques

There are many behavioural techniques therapy, some for a single disorder (for example, the enuresis alarm, p. 738), others used for a variety of disorders (for example, exposure, see below). The following account concerns the more commonly used methods. The reader is reminded that evidence for the efficacy of a treatment in a particular psychiatric disorder is considered in the chapter dealing with that disorder.

Relaxation training

This treatment is the simplest behavioural technique. It is useful for subthreshold states of anxiety and for stress-related disorders, such as initial insomnia and mild hypertension (Brauer *et al.* 1979). In the original method, known as progressive relaxation, patients are trained to relax individual muscle groups one by one, and to regulate breathing (Jacobson 1938). The technique is lengthy and simpler procedures are available for routine clinical use (see, for example, Bernstein and Borkovec 1973). A rapid but intensive method – applied relaxation – was developed by Öst (1987b) for use in anxiety disorders where it has been shown to have worthwhile effects. Whatever the method, patients can learn partly from tape-recorded instructions or in a group to reduce the time needed from the therapist. Relaxation has to be practised regularly between the training sessions and many patients lack the motivation to sustain this for long enough.

For a review of relaxation training see Glaister (1982).

Exposure

Exposure is used to reduce avoidance behaviour, especially in the treatment of phobic disorders. For simple phobias, exposure alone is often sufficient but for the other phobic disorders it is usually combined with cognitive procedures (see p. 740). Exposure can be carried out in two main ways: *in practice*, that is in the actual situations that provoke anxiety; or *in imagination*, that is while imagining the phobic situations vividly enough to induce anxiety. In either procedure, exposure can be gradual, starting with situations that provoke little anxiety and progressing slowly through increasingly more difficult ones (*desensitization*); or it can be intensive from the start (*flooding*). The usual form of exposure is usually carried out with a speed and intensity between these extremes, and when possible, in practice rather than in imagination (see below).

Desensitization

The steps in desensitization are as follows. First, a list is compiled of situations that provoke increasing amounts of anxiety (*a hierarchy*). The list usually has about 10 items, chosen so that there is an equal increment of anxiety between the items. This aim is sometimes difficult to achieve, in which case the severity of anxiety of certain items may be adjusted by introducing modifying factors. For example, the anxiety response to a situation may be less if the person has a trusted companion. Sometimes the anxiety-provoking situations seem so diverse that they cannot form a single hierarchy; for example, an agoraphobic patient may fear visiting the hairdresser, going to the cinema, and attending a teacher-parent evening. In such cases, a unifying fear should be sought, for example, the fear of being unable to leave a situation without embarrassment. When no common theme exists, two hierarchies are constructed.

Patients then imagine and/or enter the situations on the hierarchy while relaxing. Relaxation is used both to reduce the anxiety response, and to make imagery more vivid. Patients imagine or enter each item on the hierarchy, while relaxing, until they can do this without anxiety. The procedure is repeated with each item on the hierarchy. Desensitization in imagination is used when exposure to the actual situation is impractical, for example phobia of flying, and in post-traumatic stress disorder. Otherwise exposure in practice is generally more effective.

Flooding

Patients enter situations near the top of the hierarchy from the start of treatment, and remain in there until the anxiety has diminished. The process is repeated with other near-maximal stimuli. When successful, this procedure leads to a rapid reduction of anxiety, but many patients find the experience distressing. As the technique has not been shown to be more effective than desensitization, it is used infrequently.

Exposure in everyday practice

Most exposure treatment is carried out in a way intermediate in speed and intensity between those used in desensitization and flooding. Sessions last about 45 minutes. The patient enters a feared situation every day, either alone or with a relative or friend. If anxiety does not diminish, it may be necessary to start again with items lower on the hierarch. Some patients fail to progress because they have formed a habit of disengagement from anxiety-provoking situations by thinking of other things. Such patients should be helped to change this behaviour so that progress can be made.

Exposure with response prevention

This technique is used to treat obsessional rituals. Patients refrain from carrying out rituals despite their strong urges to do so (response prevention). If the restraint continues for long enough (usually at least an hour), the urge diminishes. As treatment progresses, these urges are deliberately increased by encouraging the patient to enter situations that provoke rituals and have previously been avoided (exposure). At first, patients are accompanied by the therapist and reassured while they strive to prevent the rituals, but with practice they are able to do this on their own. Sometimes the therapist reassures the patient on the first few occasions by carrying out the exposure procedure himself, a procedure called 'modelling'.

The therapist begins by explaining the rationale of treatment and agreeing targets for exposure with the patient. A target might be to touch a 'contaminated' object such as a door handle, and not to wash the hands during the next hour. A more advanced target might be to do all the household dusting without washing the hands until the task is completed. Patients need to feel confident that every task will be agreed in advance and that they will never be faced with the unexpected. Response prevention generates substantial anxiety at first, but patients usually tolerate this if they know that it will decline.

Obsessional thoughts accompanying rituals generally improve as the rituals are brought under control. Obsessional thoughts without rituals are more difficult to treat. *Habituation training* is a form of mental exposure treatment: patients dwell on the obsessional thoughts for long periods or listen repeatedly to a tape-recording of the thoughts spoken aloud for an hour or more. (A second technique for obsessional thoughts, *thought stopping*, is described below under distraction techniques (p. 739).

Social skills training

Some aspects of social behaviour can be regarded as skills that can be learned, for example, making eye contact, or starting a conversation. These skills can improved through modelling, guided practice, role play and video-feedback. The training is useful mainly for socially inadequate people, and as part of a wider programme of rehabilitation for people with chronic mental disorder.

Assertiveness training

Assertiveness training is a particular kind of social skills training designed for people who have difficulty in being appropriately assertive. Patients enact social encounters in which moderate self-assertion would be appropriate, for example, being ignored by a gossiping shop assistant. By a combination of coaching, modelling, and role reversal, patients are encouraged to practise appropriate verbal and non-verbal behaviour, and to judge the level of self-assertion appropriate to various situations. The account of these methods given by Rimm and Masters (1979) is still useful.

Anger management

This treatment follows the general lines of social skills training, while focusing on situations which provoke anger. Patients are helped to discover and practise alternative ways of dealing with such situations, such as delaying a response until anger can be brought under control. They are also helped to discover the situations that lead to anger, and any attitudes which lead them to feel anger that is out of any proportion to an objective assessment of the situation. Factors that reduce restraints on anger are also considered, especially the use of alcohol.

Self-control techniques

All behavioural treatments aim to increase patients' control over their own behaviour. Self-control techniques attempt to do this directly without the intermediate step of changing thoughts or emotions as would be done in cognitive therapy. Self-control techniques are based on operant conditioning principles, and on Bandura's (1969) studies of the role of self-reward in the control of social behaviour. The techniques are useful when the behaviour is potentially controllable but the patient has found it difficult to achieve this. Overeating and excessive smoking are examples of such behaviours.

Self-control treatment begins with *self-monitoring*, that is, the keeping of daily records of the problem behaviour and the circumstances in which it appears. For example, patients who overeat can be asked to record what they eat, when they eat, and any associations between eating, stressful events, and mood states. Keeping such a record is in itself a powerful stimulus to self-control for patients who have previously avoided facing the true extent of their problem, or are unaware of the factors that control it. Later, the daily records of the behaviour are used to assess progress.

Achievements to be awarded are agreed with each patient (*self-evaluation*). It is often useful to devise a system of reward points that can be accumulated to earn a material reward. Thus a woman might award herself a point for each day that she keeps to her diet, and buy herself new shoes when she reaches a pre-agreed number of points.

Self-control methods are usually part of a wider programme of treatment, for example, of a cognitive–behaviour programme for eating disorders (see p. 742).

Contingency management

Contingency management, like self-control techniques, is concerned with providing rewards for desired behaviour and removing reinforcement from undesired behaviour. However, instead of relying on self-monitoring and self-reinforcement, in contingency management another person monitors the behaviour, and provides the reinforcers. The latter are usually social reinforcers such as indications of approval or disapproval, or enjoyable activities earned by accumulating points. Contingency management has four stages:

- *Define and record the behaviour* The behaviour to be changed is defined and another person (usually a nurse, spouse, or parent) is trained to record it; for example, a mother might count the number of times a child with learning difficulties shouts loudly.
- *Identify the stimuli and reinforcements* Stimuli for the behaviour are identified among the events that regularly precede it. Thus the abnormal behaviour of one person may be provoked repeatedly by the actions of another. Aggressive behaviour in children and in adults is often provoked in this way. Reinforcers are identified by recording the events that immediately follow the behaviour. Often these reinforcing consequences are not obvious to the people involved; for example, parents may be unaware that by paying more attention to their child when he shouts than at other times, they are reinforcing the shouting.
- *Change the reinforcement* Reinforcement is directed away from the problem behaviours and to desired behaviours; for example, parents are helped to attend less when their child shouts than when he is quiet.
- *Monitor progress* As treatment progresses, records are kept of the frequency of the problem behaviours and of the desired behaviours.

Contingency management is used most often as part of a more general programme. The term *token economy* is used when contingency management is applied to a group of patients living together in a ward or hostel. Although used in the past, token economies are seldom used now because the changes are limited and do not generalize to other situations. (Practical details of contingency management have been described by Rimm and Masters 1979.)

Enuresis alarms

This treatment was developed specifically for nocturnal enuresis (see p. 847). In the original method, two metal plates separated by a pad were placed under the sheets of the bed (the pad and bell method). If the child passed urine in his sleep, the pad became moist and its resistance fell, allowing electric contact between the metal plates, which are wired to a battery and a bell or buzzer. Nowadays a small sensor attached to the pyjamas can replace the plates and pad. The noise of the alarm wakes the child, who must then rise to empty his bladder. After this procedure has been repeated on several nights, the child wakes before his bladder empties involuntarily. Eventually he sleeps through the night without being enuretic. The waking from sleep before passing urine can be understood as the result of classical conditioning. It is less easy to understand how the treatment leads to an uninterrupted dry night. The procedure is considered further on p. 847.

Eye movement desensitization and reprocessing

This treatment was developed for post-traumatic stress disorder. There are three components:

- exposure using imagined images of the traumatic events;
- a cognitive component in which patients attempt to replace negative thoughts associated with the images, with positive ones; and
- saccadic eye movements induced by asking the patient to follow rapid side-to-side movements of the therapist's finger.

It is claimed that the last, unusual, component, assists in the 'processing' of the cognitions associated with the traumatic events (Shapiro 1995). When compared with exposure therapy and 'stress inoculation training', eye movement desensitization and reprocessing was less effective (Devilly and Spence 1999). When the full procedure was compared with the exposure and cognitive components without the eye-movement component, there was no difference in outcome, suggesting that any therapeutic effect is not due to eye movement (Pitman *et al*. 1996). For a review see Shepherd *et al.*, 2000.

Dialectic behaviour therapy

Linehan *et al.* (1994) developed this method as a treatment for patients who repeatedly harmed themselves, and who had borderline personality disorder. The treatment is highly structured and it has been described in a manual. Despite its name, the techniques are as much related to problem solving (see p. 728) as to other behavioural techniques reviewed in this section. Patients learn problem-solving techniques for dealing with stressful events, including ways of improving social skills and of controlling anger and other emotions. Treatment is intensive with individual and group sessions and access by telephone to the therapist between sessions, and lasts for up to a year. For further information see Linehan (1993).

Behavioural techniques no longer in general use

Biofeedback

This technique assists patients to be aware of changes in a bodily function, such as blood pressure, over which they otherwise have little or no control. Information about the function is presented in an easily understood form such as a tone of varying pitch or a visual display. The person then tries to alter the function, usually in an indirect way such as relaxing. Biofeedback is not in general use because it has not been proved that it adds to the effects of relaxation alone. The technique may be of some value when normal sensory information has been lost, for example, after spinal injury (Brudny *et al.* 1974). For further information see Basmajian (1983) or Stroebel (1985).

Aversion therapy

Aversion therapy was one of the earliest behavioural techniques, having been developed in the 1930s as a treatment for alcohol dependence. Negative reinforcement was used to suppress unwanted behaviour, but the method fell out of use because of two problems. First, negative reinforcement has only temporary effects on behaviour. Second, the use of negative reinforcement causes ethical problems. Although patients consent to the use of the negative stimuli, the therapist is nevertheless using something which, in other circumstances, might be used for punishment. The problem of separating treatment from punishment is particularly difficult with disorders which are, or could be, the subject of legal proceedings.

Negative practice

Negative practice is another early technique, introduced by Dunlap (1932) as a treatment for tics and habit disorders. The technique is based on experiments showing that repeated massed practice causes reactive inhibition of the behaviour (Hull 1943). Patients repeat the problem behaviour frequently, and over long periods. Any beneficial effects are short lived.

Cognitive techniques

Techniques used to change cognitions

Four methods are commonly used to bring about change in cognitions:

- *Distraction*, that is, focusing attention away from distressing thoughts. This is done by attending to something in the immediate environment (for example, the objects in a shop window); or by engaging in a demanding mental activity (such as mental arithmetic); or by producing a sudden sensory stimulus (for example, snapping a rubber band on the wrist). The last technique is called 'thought stopping'.

- *Neutralizing* The emotional impact of anxiety-provoking thoughts can be reduced by rehearsing a reassuring response, for example, 'my heart is beating fast because I feel anxious, not because I have heart disease'. To make it easier to focus on reassuring thoughts, patients may carry a 'prompt card' on which the reassuring thoughts are written.

◆ *Challenging* is used to change maladaptive thoughts and beliefs. It is not enough to present evidence to the contrary because (as noted above) such thoughts and beliefs often persist because people think in illogical ways. They over-generalize from single instances, and they pay more attention to evidence that supports their beliefs than evidence that contradicts them (Beck 1976). The therapist provides information but he also tries to reveal and undermine the illogical ways of thinking by asking questions. Some useful questions are shown in Box 22.5.

◆ *Reassessing* Some beliefs persist because patients overestimate the extent of their responsibility for events that have multiple determinants. Patients can reassess their role by constructing *pie charts* that shows all the determinants. For example, a mother who feels responsible for ensuring that every member of her family is content would make a 'pie chart' showing the contribution of all the factors that determine their state of mind (events at school or at work, relationships with friends, the weather, etc). By allocating appropriate sectors to each of these factors before entering her own contribution, she discovers that the room for the latter is less than she supposed.

Cognitive–behaviour therapy for anxiety disorders

In this treatment, cognitive techniques are combined with exposure (see p. 735). The importance of exposure varies with the amount of avoidance behaviour, being greater in the phobic disorders and less important in generalized anxiety disorders.

Three kinds of cognition are considered in treatment: general concerns about the effects of being anxious (*fear of fear*); concerns about specific symptoms, for example, fears that palpitations are a sign

---

> ### Box 22.5 Useful questions for challenging beliefs
>
> What is the evidence for this thought?
>
> Is there an alternative way of looking at the situation?
>
> How might other people think in the situation?
>
> Are you focusing on what you felt rather than on what happened?
>
> Are you forgetting relevant facts?
>
> Are you focusing on irrelevant matters?
>
> Are you overestimating how likely this is?
>
> Are you applying to yourself, higher standards than you would apply to others?
>
> Are you thinking in black and white terms when you should consider shades of grey?
>
> Are you overestimating your responsibility for the outcome?
>
> What is the worst that could happen, and how bad would that be?
>
> What if the worst should happen? How bad would it be? Could you cope?
>
> Are you underestimating what you can do to deal with the situation?
>
> Adapted from Clark (2000)

---

of heart disease (*fear of symptoms*), and concerns that other people will react unfavourably to the patient (*fear of negative evaluation*). The balance of these cognitions varies in the different anxiety disorders. In social phobia, fears of negative evaluation are particularly important, as are concerns about blushing and trembling. In agoraphobia, fear of fear is particularly important (usually as thoughts that the person will faint, die, or lose control), together with fears about the symptoms of a panic attack. Such cognitions are modified in the ways listed above, that is, by giving information about the physiology of anxiety, and by questioning their logical basis. Information about the physiology of anxiety helps patients to attribute symptoms such as dizziness and palpitations to the correct cause, instead of to physical illness such as heart disease (a common concern of these patients). The logical basis of the fears is questioned by reviewing the patient's own evidence for the beliefs and suggesting ways in which he can test these and alternative explanations.

For *panic disorder*, treatment is focused on the characteristic fears that physical symptoms of anxiety are evidence of serious physical disease (see p. 240). These fears, which often relate to heart disease, create a vicious circle in which anxiety symptoms such as tachycardia generate more anxiety, which further increases the physical symptoms. Vigorous heart action and other symptoms feared by the patient may be induced by voluntary hyperventilation or by strenuous exercise. Symptoms produced in these ways usually trigger the anxious thoughts and, thereby lead to anxiety. This demonstration that physical symptoms lead to anxious thoughts, which in turn lead to anxiety, helps patients to understand how a vicious circle of anxiety can lead to a panic attack. Patients then monitor the thoughts that precede naturally occurring panic attacks, to find out whether these attacks arise through the same mechanism. Attention is also given to safety behaviours as described on p. 733, and to any dysfunctional beliefs which make ordinary situations stressful (see p. 733).

In *post-traumatic stress disorder*, attention is given to the intrusive visual images that characterize the condition. Patients imagine the situations repeatedly as in systematic desensitization (see above). Also they try to change the content of the images progressively and in small steps to ones that are less distressing. They are helped in integrating and processing the fragmentary and distressing recollections of the traumatic events. Treatment for post-traumatic stress disorder is considered further on p. 198.

For further information about cognitive treatment of generalized anxiety disorder see Clark (2000).

Cognitive–behaviour therapy for depressive disorders

Cognitive therapy for depressive disorders was the first effective form of cognitive therapy, and was developed by A. T. Beck (1976). It is a complex procedure which combines behavioural and cognitive techniques, with an emphasis on changing ways of thinking. Cognitive therapy for depression, is intended to alter three aspects of the thinking of depressed patients: negative intrusive thoughts, assumptions that render ordinary situations stressful, and errors of logic that allow these assumptions to persist despite evidence to the contrary. Behavioural and cognitive procedures are used to bring about these changes.

Patients identify intrusive thoughts (for example, 'I am a failure') by writing down their thoughts at times of low mood. Dysfunctional assumptions are discovered by the therapist by questioning the patient using questions from Box 22.5. A typical assumption of a depressed patient is 'unless I always try to please other people, they will not like me'. Activities are also recorded and each marked with a P if it was pleasurable and a M if the patient felt a sense of mastery and achievement.

If the patient is severely depressed and inactive, treatment begins with an activity schedule to increase activities identified as leading to pleasure and mastery. The schedule also helps to bring a sense of order and purpose into the patient's life and reduces the need to make decisions, which are difficult for someone who is severely depressed.

If the patient is less severely depressed, treatment begins with an explanation of the cognitive model and an attempt to control intrusive thoughts. This is done through distraction (see p. 739) and by neutralizing the intrusive thoughts with a reassuring alternative (for example, 'because I think something it will not necessarily happen'). It is often helpful to use a prompt card (p. 740) to help the patient concentrate on the positive statement. As treatment proceeds, depressive cognitions are challenged using the techniques described in Box 22.5.

Certain points are particularly important when depressed patients are treated:

- *Reviewing evidence* Depressed patients are particularly prone to focus on evidence that supports their negative ideas and overlook evidence that contradicts them. The therapist helps patients give appropriate weight to the positive evidence.

- *Considering alternatives* Depressed patients are likely to reject alternatives suggested by the therapist. Instead the therapist helps the patient consider alternatives by asking questions such as: What do you think that another person would think about this situation? What would you think if another person had done what you have done? (See Box 22.5 for other appropriate questions.)

- *Considering consequences* Patients are helped to see the consequences of thinking negative thoughts; for example, the thought that everything is hopeless may prevent them from attempting small changes that could be beneficial.

- *Considering errors of logic* This is done in the usual way (see p. 740), by encouraging the patient to ask himself questions such as: 'Am I thinking in black and white terms?' 'Am I drawing too wide conclusions from this single event?' 'Am I blaming myself for something for which I am not responsible?' 'Am I exaggerating the importance of events?' These questions are asked about specific ideas and situations.

- *Behavioural experiments* are used to make predictions and provide evidence relevant to the patient's assumptions.

As treatment comes to an end, more attention is given to underlying assumptions since these can lead to relapse. The technique of laddering (p. 735) helps to uncover them. Useful further questions include:

- 'In what ways is this idea helpful?'
- 'In what ways is it unhelpful?'

- 'What alternatives are there?'

For a more detailed account of cognitive therapy for the depressed patient, see Fennell (2000).

Cognitive–behaviour therapy for bulimia nervosa

The treatment of bulimia nervosa by cognitive–behaviour therapy is based on the idea that the central problems are excessive concern about shape and weight, and low self-esteem. This concern leads to extreme dieting, which makes the control of eating more difficult and leads to binge-eating. Self-induced vomiting, sometimes combined with abuse of laxatives and diuretics, prevents weight gain and also reduces restraint on overeating, leading to more binges and a greater tendency to diet. In this way a vicious circle is set up which can be interrupted by (i) restoring a regular pattern of eating three meals a day, (ii) increasing restraint on binge-eating, and (iii) discussing ideas about shape, weight, and self-esteem.

The therapist attends first to the disordered pattern of eating before attempting to modify cognitions. He explains the cognitive model and relates it to the patient's experience. He emphasizes the importance of regular meals, the causal role of long periods of fasting, and the ill-effects of repeated vomiting, and of repeatedly taking laxatives and diuretics. Patients keep records of what they eat, when they eat, and when they induce vomiting or take laxatives and diuretics. The situations that provoke binge-eating are recorded. With this information, patients are more able to control the urge to overeat and, subsequently, the bouts of vomiting. Patients are more likely to control their eating successfully if:

- meals are eaten in a place separate from that in which food is prepared or stored;

- a limited amount of food is available at each meal, for example two slices of bread are put on the table but not a whole loaf;

- a small amount of food is left on the plate and then thrown away, in order to mark the end of the meal; and

◆ a shopping list is made in advance and purchases of food are limited strictly to the list.

The therapist strongly discourages frequent checking of weight and of appearance, since both habits maintain the disorder.

Because patients often binge when they are unhappy, lonely, or bored, they are helped to find other ways of dealing with these feelings. For example, they might seek out friends or listen to music. Vomiting usually stops when binges are under control. The dangers of abuse of laxatives and diuretics are explained, and patients are encouraged strongly to throw away all such drugs.

When eating is under better control, attention turns to cognitions. Patients record these together with the eating behaviour. Relevant cognitions are concerned not only with body shape and weight but also with self-esteem. Examples of these cognitions are:

◆ to be fat is to be a failure;

◆ dieting is a sign of strong will and self-control;

◆ it is necessary to be thin to be happy and successful.

Such beliefs persist because of the illogical ways of thinking described above (p. 733), namely selective use of evidence, over-generalization from limited instances, all or none reasoning, and overestimation of the person's contribution to events with multiple causes. The questioning used to identify cognitions and illogical thinking resembles that described in Box 22.5. Some patients with bulimia nervosa may have a distorted body image, and this cannot usually be changed directly by cognitive procedures. However, the distortion often diminishes as the other symptoms are brought under control.

For further information about cognitive–behaviour therapy for bulimia nervosa see Fairburn *et al.* (1993).

Cognitive–behaviour therapy has not been shown to be effective in *anorexia nervosa*. However some of the underlying principles can be applied in management (see p. 450).

Cognitive–behaviour therapy for hypochondriasis

The approach is twofold: to identify behaviours that maintain the disorder, and to change hypochondriacal ideas directly. The relevant behaviours are repeatedly seeking reassurance, which relieves anxiety briefly but reinforces the concerns in the longer term, and checking bodily functions (for example, counting the pulse rate) or structure (for example, palpating for lumps). Hypochondriacal ideas are approached along the lines described above in relation to cognitive–behaviour therapy for anxiety and depressive disorders, using questioning and behavioural experiments. For further information see Salkovskis and Bass (1997).

Cognitive–behaviour therapy for schizophrenia

There are two approaches. The aim of the first is to reduce stressors that may be exacerbating the disorder, or provoking individual symptoms, especially hallucinations. The methods are similar to those developed to treat anxiety disorders, namely distraction and other alternative ways of dealing with stressful situations. Patients are helped to cope with hallucinations, for example, by distancing themselves and repeating statements that neutralize their effects.

The aim of the second approach is to challenge delusions. This approach is directed to secondary delusions, especially those that seem to have developed to explain hallucinations. The therapist encourages the patient to regard the delusions as beliefs rather than facts, and to discuss alternatives. In questioning the basis of the delusions, the therapist has to be careful not to appear to be challenging them directly. Instead he tries to persuade the patient to consider the consequences of holding the delusion and what would be the consequences of thinking in another way. The therapist then tries to reformulate the delusion as a way of making sense of certain experiences, which can be understood in terms of the knowledge the patient had at the time but should now be reconsidered. Patients selected for their willingness to reconsider their delusions are likely to differ in other ways from the majority of schizophrenic patients and it is not known how much the changes reported with this treatment are brought about by this rather than resulting from the method of selection.

For further information see Birchwood and Spencer (2000).

Cognitive therapy for personality disorder

A. T. Beck suggested that the techniques he had developed for the treatment of depressive disorders could be adapted for personality. He described beliefs and ways of thinking that characterize each type of personality disorder. Each disorder can be considered in terms of the person's self-view, views of others, general beliefs, perceived threats, main strategies for coping, and primary affective responses. Beck also suggested a 'schema' characteristic of each type of personality disorder and made up of statements that can be challenged in treatment. For example, the schema for histrionic personality disorder includes the following statements:

- 'unless I captivate people, I am nothing';
- 'to be happy, I need other people to admire me';
- 'I must show people that they have hurt me'.

Schemas are challenged using the general techniques of cognitive therapy (see p. 740 and Box 22.5). As yet the treatment has not been evaluated as fully as the other cognitive treatments described in this section. For more information about the general use of cognitive therapy for personality disorders, see Beck and Freeman (1990). For information about its use with borderline personality disorder see Layden et al. (1993).

Individual dynamic psychotherapies
Brief insight-oriented psychotherapy

This kind of psychotherapy reconstructs the origins of a psychiatric disorder in early life experience of the patients, and seeks for unconscious factors that account for the abnormal thinking, emotions, and behaviour. It aims to produce limited but worthwhile changes within 6–9 months, with sessions once a week. This period is called brief in contrast to the much longer psychoanalytical treatment (see p. 746). The treatment is focused upon specific problems; hence the alternative term *focal psychotherapy*. The procedures can be summarized as follows.

Starting treatment

The initial assessment is important and should not be hurried. As well as identifying indications and contraindications (discussed below), the aim is to identify the problems that are to be the focus of treatment. This focus and the length of treatment are agreed with the patient. Usually, some problems remain at the end of treatment, and this possibility is explained at the start. The therapist also explains the general aim of linking past and present behaviour patterns. He indicates that the therapist's role is to help patients find their own solutions to their problems, not to do it for them. From the start, an atmosphere is created in which the patient feels involved, listened to, and safe to speak about ideas and fantasies that he has not previously revealed to anyone.

Subsequent sessions

In these patients are encouraged to:

- give specific examples of the selected problems, and consider how they thought, felt, and acted at the time;
- talk freely about emotionally painful subjects, within the limits of topics agreed with the therapist;

- be prepared to express ideas and feelings even if they seem illogical or shameful;

- review their own part in any difficulties that they ascribe to other people;

- look for common themes in their problems and their responses to situations;

- consider how present patterns of behaviour began, what function they served in the past, and why they may be continuing;

- consider alternative ways of thinking and behaving in the situations that cause difficulties;

- try out new and more adaptive ways of behaving and responding to emotions.

The therapist responds to the emotional as well as to the intellectual content of the patient's utterances (for example, 'it sounds as though you felt angry when this happened'). He helps the patient to examine feelings that previously have been denied, and to think about past situations in which similar feelings were experienced. The therapist pays as much attention to patients' non-verbal behaviour as to their words, because discrepancies between the two often point to problems that have not been expressed directly. The therapist maintains the focus, that is, he avoids problem areas which are too complex to deal with in the agreed time.

The therapist may make *interpretations*, for example, hypotheses linking present or past events and behaviours. Other interpretations concern defence mechanisms which could include, for example, blocks in recall during the sessions, or ways in which the patient unconsciously protects himself from unpleasant feelings in his daily life.

The therapist is alert to the development of *transference and counter-transference* (see p. 726). Transference may reveal how the patient responds to other people at the present time, or how he responded to his parents in childhood. In brief therapy, counter-transference is usually taken to include both appropriate and inappropriate responses by the therapist to the patient's emotional state.

A therapist who has insight into his own reactions will understand the patient's situation better, whereas a therapist who lacks this insight will be less objective. Because such insights are difficult to achieve, therapists often work with a supervisor who can help to identify the counter-transference. Some therapists undergo a period of personal psychotherapy to understand better how events in their past determine their responses to their parents.

Ending treatment

To ensure that treatment ends on time, realistic goals should be chosen and the focus should remain on these goals. Also, potential problems related to termination should be discussed from an early stage. As the end of treatment approaches, patients should feel that they have a better understanding of the chosen problems and should be more confident about dealing with them. It is often useful to ease the termination of treatment by arranging a few follow-up appointments spaced over 2 or 3 months.

Indications

Because there is no satisfactory, adequate evidence from randomized clinical trials, the indications for short-term dynamic psychotherapy have to be based on clinical experience. Treatment appears to be more useful for emotional and interpersonal problems than for specific psychiatric disorders. Indications include low self-esteem, and recurrent problems in forming intimate relationships. Patients are more likely to benefit if they are willing to bring about change though their own efforts, are able to look honestly at their own motives, and have a problem that can be conceptualized in psychodynamic terms. Patients should have adequate social support and be capable of putting a stop to self-exploration when the sessions end.

Contraindications

These include obsessional or hypochondriacal disorders, severe mood disorder, schizophrenia, and a personality disorder, especially one leading to acting out of problems.

See Ursano and Ursano (2000) for a concise account of the theories and methods of brief individual dynamic psychotherapy, or the books by Sifneos (1979) and Davanloo (1980).

Cognitive-analytical therapy

This treatment uses cognitive therapy techniques (see p. 739) with a framework of psychodynamic understanding. The aim is to combine what has been found useful in the two methods of treatment. In the absence of evidence from randomized clinical trials, the use of cognitive-analytical therapy is based on clinical assessments of its effectiveness; it does not have the evidence base of cognitive therapy methods. Compared with cognitive therapy, attention is focused more on interpersonal behaviours than on symptoms. Compared with brief insight-orientated psychotherapy, the patient has a more active role. Also, there is less emphasis on transference interpretations, and more use of behavioural homework. The methods have not been described in as much detail as is available for many cognitive therapies.

The patient is actively involved from the start by keeping diaries of moods, behaviour, and intrusive thoughts. Through discussion of repeated patterns of behaviour revealed by the diaries, he is helped to identify maladaptive cognitions, for example, the assumption that a person who cares for another, must always give in to the demands of the other. As well as this cognitive approach, patterns of behaviour and thinking are considered from a psychodynamic viewpoint. For example, present maladaptive behaviour is viewed as arising from behaviour that was adaptive when the person was younger.

At the start of treatment, goals are agreed with the patient. The relation of these goals to the patient's attitudes and values is examined so that possible resistances to change are identified. Goals are recorded on a 'target problems list', procedures are agreed that could bring about desired changes, and a time limit is set for therapy. The procedures are written down in an appropriate formulation that links them with the target problems; for example, if the problem is that the person is trying to please everyone, the general procedure would be 'to assert needs appropriately'. Specific examples of general procedures are identified from the patient's diaries, and homework is arranged whereby these specific procedures can be tried out. At the end of treatment, the therapist may write a letter to the patient summarizing what has been learned and encouraging him to continue to practise the new behaviours.

For an account of cognitive-analytical therapy see Ryle (1990).

Long-term individual dynamic psychotherapy

Long-term individual dynamic psychotherapy is a general term referring to many kinds of individual psychotherapy lasting for longer that the 9 months that is often taken as the upper limit of brief dynamic psychotherapy. The longest, most intensive, and best known form is psychoanalysis, and most methods are derived from it. Long-term dynamic psychotherapy is costly, and because its results have not been shown to be better than those of shorter forms of treatment, it is not generally available as part of the health services of most countries. When it is used, it is usually for patients judged unsuitable for short-term psychotherapy, even though it is in these cases that its effects are least certain.

The primary aim of long-term dynamic psychotherapy is to increase insight, defined as 'the conscious recognition of the role of unconscious factors on current experience and behaviour' (Fonagy 2000). Insight requires more than an awareness of these factors; it involves the integration of this knowledge into ways of thinking, feeling and behaving, a process that is called 'working through'. Insight is achieved by bringing to conscious awareness mental contents that were previously outside consciousness, by interpreting their significance, and by linking past experiences with present modes of functioning.

Unconscious material is brought to conscious

awareness through free association, and by examining the content of fantasies and dreams. Analysis of the patient's unrealistic responses to the therapist (the transference) provides further information about unconscious processes. Therapists vary in the extent to which they work with the transference. Analysis of the counter-transference provides further relevant information since it reflects not only the therapist's psychological make-up but also aspects of the patient to which the therapist is responding. The need to understand the counter-transference is one reason why therapists generally undergo personal psychotherapy as part of their training to undertake long-term dynamic psychotherapy.

Attempts to access unconscious material and to increase insight activate *resistance* of three kinds. Resistance by repression blocks access to unconscious material. Transference resistance restricts the intensity of the relationship with the therapist. A negative therapeutic reaction is expressed in new symptoms, which retard progress. Although resistance impedes progress, analysis of resistance can increase insight.

Interpretations are generally regarded as one of the main techniques of this kind of treatment. However, the use of interpretations varies considerably between the various types of long-term dynamic psychotherapy. Interpretations may be concerned with defences, unconscious processes, transference, or the links between past experience and present patterns. Transference interpretations are often used, in keeping with the greater importance of transference in long-term, compared with short-term therapy.

Other ways in which long-term psychodynamic psychotherapy differs from brief dynamic psychotherapy include:

♦ It is less structured; patients are encouraged to talk and associate ideas freely without a specific focus.

♦ The therapist is less active and guides the patient less. He tries to make the material clearer by asking questions, pointing out contradictions, commenting on evasions and resistance, and making interpretations.

♦ Patients are seen more frequently (up to five times a week). This is one of the factors leading to the more intense transference noted above. In psychoanalysis, transference may be increased further by arranging that the therapist sits out of direct vision of the patient who lies on a couch.

For a fuller account of psychoanalysis and other long-term dynamic psychotherapies, see Fonagy (2000).

Results of and indications for long-term dynamic psychotherapy

In general, the research literature does not contradict the impression of experienced clinicians that most patients can be helped as effectively with short-term dynamic therapy as with longer methods. Clinical experience suggests that if long-term therapy is ever appropriate, it is for patients who have long-lasting and complicated emotional difficulties, or significant maturational problems in their personal development. Specific psychiatric disorders respond less well than do problems of personality and relationships. Long-term psychotherapy should not be used with patients with schizophrenia, manic-depressive disorder, or marked paranoid personality traits. Histrionic and schizoid personality disorders, whilst not contra-indications, are particularly difficult to treat.

Group psychotherapy

Small-group psychotherapy

This section is concerned with psychotherapy carried out with a group of about eight patients. Treatment in larger groups is considered later. Small-group psychotherapy is used most often to modify personality problems, and difficulties in interpersonal relationships; as a form of supportive treatment; or to encourage adjustment to the effects physical or mental illness.

How group psychotherapy developed

Group therapy is often said to have originated from the work of Joseph Pratt, an American physician who used 'class methods' to treat patients with pulmonary tuberculosis (Pratt 1908). However, Pratt's classes were limited to support and education. A more obvious precursor of modern group psychotherapy is the work of J. L. Moreno, a Romanian who worked in Vienna before emigrating to the USA, and of Trigant Burrow, an American (Burrow 1927). However, the main roots of group therapy were in the experience of treating war neuroses in the 1940s in the UK.

In the Northfield Military Hospital in England, S. H. Foulkes developed the methods of group analysis (Foulkes and Lewis 1944). His approach was based on psychoanalysis; the therapist or group leader was passive, and used analytical interpretations (Foulkes 1948, p. 136). W. R. Bion, a Kleinian analyst who also worked at Northfield Hospital, developed a different approach (Bion 1961). He focused specifically on the unconscious defences of the group as a whole rather than on the problems of individual members.

Further developments took place in the USA in the 1960s and early 1970s, where so-called action groups were used to provide a more intense form of group experience. Many variations of group technique have developed but it is now generally accepted that the features that the different methods have in common are more important than the differences.

Types of small-group therapy

Pines and Schlapobersky (2000) have suggested a useful classification based on the goals of the group (specific versus non-specific) and the activity of the leader (high versus low). The resulting four categories are therefore:

- *Specific goals – high leader activity*: includes structured programmes for alcohol and drug dependence, as well as cognitive–behaviour therapy carried out in a group;

- *Specific goals – low leader activity*: includes problem solving groups;

- *Non-specific goals – high leader activity*: includes the many kinds of short-term group therapy, as well as psychodrama;

- *Non-specific goals – low leader activity*: includes the various kinds of psychodynamic group such as the Tavistock, eclectic, and interpersonal approaches, and group analytical therapy.

Several of these methods will be discussed below.

Terminology

Groups are often described in terms of their structure, process, and content:

- *Structure* describes the enduring reciprocal relationships between each member of the group and the therapist, and between the members.

- *Process* describes the short-term changes in emotions, behaviours, relationships, and other experiences of the group.

- *Content* refers to the observable events in the group meetings: the themes, responses, and discussions, and the silences.

Therapeutic factors in group therapy

Group treatments share the therapeutic factors common to all kinds of psychological treatment, namely restoring hope, releasing emotion, giving information, providing a rationale, and prestige suggestion (see Box 22.2). In group treatment, there are additional factors not present in individual therapies but common to all kinds of group psychotherapy. These factors are shared experience, support to and from group members, socialization, imitation, and interpersonal learning (see Yalom 1985). These factors are summarized in Box 22.6.

General indications for group therapy

Group or individual therapy?

There is no evidence that the results of group therapy differ in general from those of individual psychotherapy of the same duration and used for

Box 22.6 Curative factors in group therapy

Universality (shared experience) helps patients to realize that they are not isolated and that others have similar experiences and problems. Hearing about experiences is often more convincing and helpful than reassurance from a therapist.

Altruism Supporting others increases the self-esteem of the person giving the support, as well as helping the receiver. Mutual support is one of the factors leading to a sense of belonging to the group.

Group cohesion The feeling of belonging to the group is especially valuable for patients who previously have felt isolated. Group cohesion can sustain the group when problems threaten to destroy it

Socialization is the acquisition of social skills within a group as a result of the comments and reactions members provide about one another's behaviour. Members can try out new social behaviours within the safety of the group.

Imitation is learning from observing and adopting the behaviours of other group members. If the group is run well, patients imitate adaptive behaviours; if it is not run well, they may imitate maladaptive behaviours such as extravagant displays of emotion, or talking in a way that deflects attention from their own emotional problems.

Interpersonal learning is learning from the inter-actions within the group and from practising new ways of interacting. Interpersonal learning is an important component of group therapy.

Recapitulation of the family group As the group proceeds, interactions are increasingly unrealistic and based on past relations between patients and their parents and siblings. This group transference develops eventually in all groups; it is encouraged and used in treatment mainly in treatments using a psychoanalytical approach.

the same problem, or that the results of any one form of group therapy differ from those of the rest. In particular, there is no evidence that encounter groups or action techniques are superior to other methods, and there is some evidence that they can increase symptoms in some patients (Yalom *et al.* 1973).

What problems are suitable?

Group therapy appears to be useful to patients whose problems are mainly in relationships with other people. As in individual psychotherapy, results are generally thought to be better in patients who are young, well-motivated, able to express themselves fluently, and free from severe personality disorder. Groups are often suitable for patients with moderate degrees of social anxiety, presumably because such patients benefit from the opportunity to rehearse social behaviour. (Severe social anxiety is a contraindication.)

General contraindications for group therapy

These are similar to the contraindications for individual psychotherapy (see above), with the addition of severe social anxiety. Also, a group should never include a member whose problems are so unlike those of the others that he may become an outsider or a scapegoat.

Supportive groups

Many of the therapeutic factors present in a group (see Box 22.6) are at work in supportive treatment. In a supportive group, the therapist should encourage self-help and ensure that the experiences of the group members are used positively. He should ensure that relationships do not become too intense, protect vulnerable patients when necessary, and ensure that each member is supported and gives support to other members. The problems that can arise in therapeutic groups (see below) may develop also in supportive groups. The leader of a supportive group should be alert to these potential problems and be capable of dealing with them along the lines described below (p. 751).

Self-help groups

Self-help groups are organized and led by patients or ex-patients who have learned ways of overcoming or adjusting to their difficulties. The other group members benefit from this experience, from the opportunity to talk about their own problems and express their feelings, and from mutual support. Group processes develop as much in these groups as in any other, so it is important that those who lead them have appropriate training and support. Some groups, such as Alcoholics Anonymous, have strict rules of procedure; others have a professional advisor.

There are self-help groups for people who suffer from many kinds of problems, for example, Alcoholics Anonymous (see p. 556), groups to help people lose weight (Weight Watchers), groups for patients with chronic physical conditions such as colostomy, groups for people facing special problems such as parents with a handicapped child, and groups for the bereaved (CRUSE Clubs). Only a few self-help groups have been evaluated. One study found that a self-help group for recently bereaved women was as effective as brief dynamic psychotherapy (Marmar *et al.* 1988).

For a review of self-help groups see Lieberman (1990).

Therapeutic groups

Interpersonal group therapy

Interpersonal group therapy developed particularly from the work of Yalom (see Yalom 1985). Treatment is focused on problems in current relationships and examines the ways in which these problems are reflected in the group. The past is discussed only in so far as it helps to make sense of the present problems.

Stages of treatment

The first stage The group members try to depend on the therapist, seeking expert advice about their problems and about the way they should behave in the group. Before long, some members become disillusioned by the therapist's refusal to solve their problems and miss meetings or come late. Other members leave because they are anxious about talking in the group.

The second stage The remaining members begin to know each other better, they become used to discussing each other's problems, and they begin to seek answers. This is the stage in which most change can be expected. The therapist encourages the examination of current problems and relationships, and comments on the dynamics of the group.

The last stage The group can become dominated by the residual problems of the members who have made least progress and who still show the most dependency. This development should be anticipated by starting to discuss these and other problems of termination several months before the group is due to end.

Preparation for the group

It is useful to prepare patients for their experience in a group by emphasizing the following points:

- The proceedings of the group are *confidential.*

- Members must *attend regularly* and on time, and not leave early.

- They are required to *disclose* their problems and to *show concern* for the problems of others.

- They may experience *initial disappointment* at the lack of rapid change, or frustration at the need to share the time available for speaking.

- The *duration* of the group is explained, together with need to remain until the end.

- The group members *may not meet outside the group*; if this rule is ever broken, it must be reported to the next meeting of the group.

Setting up the group

General considerations A therapeutic group has about eight members when it begins. The members should have some problems in common, and should be able to empathize with each other's difficulties and be willing to assist each other. No member should have problems that set him aside from the rest of the group. Meetings should be held in a room of adequate size, with the chairs arranged in a circle so that all members can see one another. Meetings usually last for 60–90 minutes to allow adequate time for every member to take part; they are usually held once a week and generally continue for 12–18 months. Most groups are *closed*, that is, no new members join after the first few weeks. (Groups that accepts new members are called *open*; such groups are usually supportive or educational.)

One or two therapists? Some groups are run by one therapist, some by co-therapists. The advantage of employing two therapists is that one can help the other to recognize and deal with counter-transference problems (which are as important in group as in individual psychotherapy). The potential disadvantages are that the two therapists may develop different views about the running of the group, or may behave defensively with one another. However, when the therapists trust each other's judgements and if any differences are discussed as they arise, they can provide further insight into the group process. At the start, differences between co-therapists may be discussed outside the group. However, when the group is well integrated, such differences can be discussed within the group, as a way of increasing the members' understanding of interpersonal processes.

Managing the group

The therapist should be aware of five basic issues that are likely to require attention:

- the conflict between each member's wish to be helped and the requirement to help others;
- the conflict between a wish to gain the therapist's approval and the desire to be approved by the other members of the group;
- the process by which members of a group establish a hierarchy of dominance, and the rivalries that this produces;
- the risk that one person may become a scapegoat when the group is dissatisfied;

- the risk that members may be excessively passive and dependent on the therapist instead of working out solutions themselves.

The group therapist's role has been compared to that of the conductor of an orchestra. He helps the members to work in harmony, prevents any one member from dominating the group, and regulates the speed and emotional intensity of the discourse. He also helps the members to understand one another, to accept suggestions, and to see aspects of themselves in other people. If a therapeutic group is working well, members are active, they give and take, and they support each other. They discuss problems constructively and do not blame or scapegoat other members.

Some problems in group therapy

However skilful the therapist, certain problems commonly arise in the course of group therapy:

Formation of sub-groups Some members may form a coalition based on age, social class, shared values, or other characteristics. Because subgroups disrupt the therapeutic process, the therapist should be alert for early signs of such alliances. He should discourage them by asking the group to discuss the reasons for their formation.

Members who talk too much In its early stages the group may welcome a talkative member who relieves the others of the need to speak about themselves. As meetings continue, the group is likely to become dissatisfied with this member for monopolizing time that would be better shared. The therapist should draw attention to this problem at an early stage, before the group rejects the talkative member. Attention can sometimes be drawn to the problem by asking the group why they allow one person to absolve them from the need to speak about themselves.

Members who talk too little The therapist should assist silent members to speak and should therefore understand the reasons for silence. Some patients are generally awkward in company; some are afraid to reveal a specific problem to the group and fear that this problem will be uncovered if they speak; and some are silent because they are angry and dissatisfied with the progress of the group.

Conflict between members The therapist should not take sides in conflicts but should encourage the whole group to discuss the issue in a way that leads them to understand why the conflict has arisen, for example, because a hostile transference has developed.

Avoidance of the focus The usual focus of a group is on the current problems of the members and on the reflection of these problems in the interactions of the group. The past experience of the members is considered in so far as it assists understanding present problems. Sometimes the group members talk excessively about the past as a way of avoiding their present difficulties. When this happens, the therapist can ask questions or use interpretations as an indirect way of bringing the discussion back to the present problems of the members. For example, a woman who dwells inappropriately on past difficulties with her overpowering father, may be asked whether she does this because she feels that one of the men in the group is behaving in a similar way.

Potentially embarrassing revelations A group member may say, for example, that he has been unfairly criticized by a member of the group. The therapist should then help the group to examine the remark constructively to understand whether the feelings relate to past or present experiences outside the group as well as to experiences within it. Such discussions are more useful when they are specific. For example, it is more useful to discuss why a woman feels angry when a particular man in the group offers her advice than to discuss why she has a general problem of anger with men. Consideration of the specific instances will lead to understanding of the wider problem.

To supplement this outline of interpersonal group therapy, the reader is referred to Vinogradov and Yalom (1989), or Block and Aveline (1996).

Group analytical therapy

This technique, which is derived from psychoanalysis, differs from the interpersonal method described above, mainly in the greater use of interpretations about transference and unconscious mechanisms. Instead of agreeing a focus, the therapist encourages 'free floating discussion'. He points out conflicts, preoccupations, and evasions, and makes interpretations. Particular attention is given to transferences to the therapist and between members, which are interpreted as reflecting relations in earlier life with parents and siblings. This knowledge of earlier relationships is then used to understand current problems outside the group. This process leads to questioning of present assumptions, and a greater self-understanding. As the group progresses, the leader becomes less active, and exerts his influence more by example than as an expert, thereby encouraging the allowing the members to take more responsibility for the proceedings

For a fuller account of group analytical therapy, see Pines and Schlapobersky (2000).

Encounter groups and psychodrama (action techniques)

In *encounter groups* the interaction between members is made more intense and rapid in the hope that this will lead to greater change. The encounter can be entirely verbal, using challenging language, or it can include touching or hugging between the participants. Sometimes the experience is intensified further by prolonging the group session for a whole day or even longer (*marathon groups*). Although some participants are helped by encounter groups, many are not, and a few are made worse (Lieberman *et al.* 1973). Adverse effects are more likely in people with substantial emotional disorders, and in groups using the most confrontational methods.

Psychodrama is another form of intensive group experience. The group enacts events from the life of one member, in scenes reflecting either current relationships or those of the family in which the person grew up. The enactment usually provokes strong feelings in the person represented, and often reflects the problems experienced by other members of the group. Members sometimes exchange roles so as to understand better the other person's point of view. The drama is followed by a group discussion. Instead of building a drama round the personal experiences of one member, the action may be concerned with problems that the participants share, for example, how to deal with authority. This method is called *sociodrama*. For an account of psychodrama see Goldman and Morrison (1984) and Holmes and Karp (1991).

Action techniques are now used mainly as an adjunct to other group methods. A session of psychodrama can provide topics for discussion when a group using other methods is failing to make progress. Role reversal can help some patients to view their problems more objectively and perhaps for the first time from the standpoint of other people.

Large-group therapy

Ward groups

This form of group therapy is part of the daily programme of many psychiatric wards. It is also a characteristic component of the programme of a therapeutic community. Large groups usually include all the patients in a treatment unit together with some or all of the staff. At the simplest level, large groups allow patients to express problems of living together. At a more ambitious level, such groups can attempt to change their members, presenting to each member examples of his disordered behaviour or irrational responses. At the same time, support is provided by other members who share similar problems and opportunities for social learning. The group is sometimes used as a kind of governing body that formulates rules and seeks to enforce them. Because large groups can evoke much anxiety, in patients and also in staff, great care should be taken in conducting them. The general principles resemble those of small-group therapy (see above). Special care is needed to prepare new members for the experience, regulate the emotional level of the sessions, protect

vulnerable people, and excuse those too unwell to take part.

Therapeutic communities

In a therapeutic community, every shared activity is viewed as a potential source of change. Members learn about themselves through the reactions of other members and they are able to practise new behaviours and appreciate points of view other than their own. The members live together and take part in frequent group meetings. Maxwell Jones, one of the founders of this form of treatment, referred to it as a living-learning situation (Jones 1968). There are usually 20–30 members of the community and they stay for between 9 and 18 months. The principal features of the regimen are shown in Box 22.7.

The role of the staff is to ensure a basic structure within which members of the community can interact. The amount of staff activity is greater

---

Box 22.7 Principal features of a therapeutic community

Informality There are few rules, and staff dress and behave informally.

Mutual help The members support each other and help others to change.

Permissiveness Members tolerate behaviour that they might not accept elsewhere.

Directness and honesty Members respond directly to distortions of reality and other kinds of self-deception.

Shared decisions Members and staff join in the day-to-day decisions about the running of the unit, and the behaviour of its members, and usually about the admission of new candidates.

Shared activities Members provide some of the 'hotel' services in the community in order that each has a job with responsibilities to other people

Group meetings The whole group meets, usually daily, to discuss any aspect of the life of the community, especially the behaviour of the members and the effect of this on other people.

when there are conflicts and other problems within the unit, and less when the members are able to function effectively. The staff also have to ensure a balance within the unit, protecting the vulnerable and ensuring safety. The staff also arrange that there is a sufficient variety of activities to allow members to find something in which they can work cooperatively, and for which they can take responsibility. Staff also help members to understand their interactions, and ensure that problems are discussed constructively.

Indications and contraindications

It is difficult to assess the value of the therapeutic community method and there is no satisfactory body of evidence from clinical trials. Indications are also uncertain but are thought to include personality disorders of the dyssocial and unstable types, including those associated with previous drug dependence (all communities have a rule of abstinence). Contraindications include severe depression, hypomania, schizophrenia, paranoid personality, and persistent violence. Potential members need to be highly motivated to change, and willing to spend a long time in treatment. These last two requirements make it difficult to compare results of those who remain in treatment with those who remain in treatments that demand less of the patients.

For further information about therapeutic communities see Kennard (1998).

Psychotherapy with couples and families

Couple therapy

Treatment of this kind is usually given either because conflict in a relationship appears to be the cause of emotional disorder in one of the partners, or because the relationship is unsatisfactory or likely to break up, and both partners wish to save it. In the apparently simple step from treating an individual to treating a couple, there is an important conceptual change in that the problem is not thought of as confined to one person but shared between two. The problem is conceived as resulting from the way that the couple interact, and treatment is directed to this interaction. In assessing the interaction, it is useful to examine issues that are important in all relationships, for example, the sharing of values, concern for the welfare and personal development of the partner, tolerance of differences, and an agreed balance of dominance and decision making. It is useful also to bear in mind the three stages of most marriages or other long-term relationships: living together, bringing up children, and readjusting when the children leave home. To avoid imposing values, the therapist adopts a 'target problem' approach, whereby couples are required to identify the difficulties that they would like to put right.

Several techniques of therapy have developed, based on psychodynamic, behavioural, and systems theory approaches, and on a combination of techniques drawn from the last two approaches.

Psychodynamic couple therapy

The central idea is that the behaviour of a married couple is largely determined, from the moment that they choose each other, by unconscious forces. Each person selects a partner who is perceived as completing unfulfilled parts of himself. When the selection is successful, the couple complement one another, but sometimes one partner fails to live up to the (unconscious) expectations of the other. For example, a wife may criticize her husband for failing to show the independence and self-reliance that she lacks herself. Also, each partner may project on the other, unwanted aspects of the self which are split off and denied. For example, a husband may project on to his wife the vulnerability that he feels but cannot accept as part of himself.

The aim of this kind of treatment is to help each partner to understand his own emotional needs and how they relate to those of the other. This may be done in several ways. One therapist may see the couple together, two therapists may see them together (each therapist having a primary concern with one of them), or two therapists may see the patients separately but meet regularly to coordinate their treatments. Therapists take a more active part than they would in the analytical treatment of a single patient. Also, interpretations are concerned more with the relationship between the partners than with transference involving the therapist.

Systems approaches to couple therapy

The focus of treatment is on the hidden rules that govern the behaviour of the couple towards one another, on disagreements about who makes these rules, and on inconsistencies between these two 'levels' of interaction. Important concepts include enmeshment, that is, excessive involvement with the other person, and the idea of a cycle of cause and effect such that neither person is wholly to blame. These ideas are discussed around conflicts arising in the everyday life of the couple, for example, who decides where to go on holiday, and how the couple decide who is to decide this. In this way it is hoped to arrive at a more balanced and more cooperative relationship. Some therapists use *'paradoxical injunctions'*, that is, provocative statements designed to elicit a (beneficial) counter-response that the couple have previously resisted. One or two therapists may take part but the partners are always seen together. The account of the method given by Haley (1963) is still valuable.

Behavioural couple therapy

This form of couple therapy is brief and highly structured. It is based on the principles of operant conditioning. The therapist tries to identify ways in which undesired behaviour between the couple is being reinforced unwittingly by one of its consequences. Each partner is asked to say what alternative behaviours they desire in the other. These behaviours must be described in specific terms, for example 'talk to me for half an hour when you come in from work' rather than 'take more notice of me'. Each partner agrees a way of rewarding the other when the desired behaviour is carried out. The reward could be the expression of approval and affection, or doing something that the partner

desires. This exchange is called 'reciprocity negotiating'. In addition, the couple is helped to communicate more directly, to listen to one another, and to express individual wishes more clearly. Described briefly, the treatment may seem a crude form of bargaining that is remote from a loving relationship. In practice it can enable a couple to cooperate and give up habits of criticism and nagging, with consequent improvement in their feelings for one another. The method has been described by Stuart (1980). Some therapists add cognitive approaches based on the ideas of Beck (1988).

The behavioural-systems couple therapy

The approach described here was developed by Crowe for use with problems of couples encountered in psychiatric practice. It is described in detail by Crowe and Ridley (1990). As the name implies, it has two sets of components. The behavioural components are 'reciprocity negotiating' (see above) and training in communication. The systems components are 'structural moves' (see below), timetables and tasks, and the use of paradox. These components are drawn together progressively, starting with the simplest and adding complexity only when it is clearly necessary. Figure 22.1 shows the order in which the procedures are combined. Behavioural methods are used for simpler cases and the more complex systems procedures are added for couples with more symptoms, less willingness to accept the relationship as the focus of treatment, and more rigid patterns of interaction. The various procedures have been described above.

Treatments last usually for 5–10 sessions over 3–6 months. The therapist has to develop a relationship with both partners without favouring either or taking sides. He maintains a focus on mutual interactions, and helps them to make changes in the way they interact. The therapist's role is more like that of the director of a play than a negotiator. He encourages the couple to speak to each other, not to the therapist, and comments on what they say and do in the sessions. Difficulties

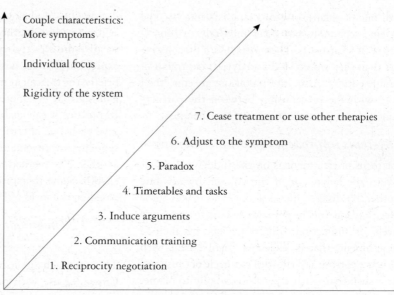

Couple characteristics:
More symptoms

Individual focus

Rigidity of the system

7. Cease treatment or use other therapies

6. Adjust to the symptom

5. Paradox

4. Timetables and tasks

3. Induce arguments

2. Communication training

1. Reciprocity negotiation

Therapist interventions: more need for therapist ingenuity
less reliance on couple's stated goals

Figure 22.1
The alternative levels
of intervention hierarchy.
(Reproduced with
permission from Crowe
2000)

may arise with couples who communicate well about intellectual matters but not about their feelings. In such cases, instead of questioning one person, it is often better to ask the other partner to put the question. For example, 'Could you ask John what he thinks about what you said?' Sessions usually end with a summary message for the couple to consider together when they return home.

Structural moves include requiring disagreement, reversed role play, and sculpting. Couples may be *asked to disagree* about something when one partner dominates the other who habitually gives in to avoid disagreement. The topic does not matter, the aim is to help the passive partner express an opinion forcefully and to help the other to value it. *Role reversal* helps one partner to understand the point of view and experience of the other. In *sculpting,* the partners take up positions, silently, to express some aspect of the relationship without words; for example, one partner may depict the depth of her dissatisfaction with the relationship through a tableau in which the two sit side by side, looking away from one other.

Tasks and injunctions

Systemic tasks concern interactions that occur either too seldom or too often . A timetable is made in which specific times are allocated for the interaction. For example, if the couple do not spend undivided time together, times are agreed at which they will spend time together without any distractions. If one partner returns repeatedly to the same complaint, it is agreed that complaints will be made only at specific times, and that the other will agree to listen at these times.

The use of paradox has been described on p. 755. *Paradoxical injunctions* should be given only after consideration of possible consequences other than the intended one, and in the context of a caring relationship. Often the paradox is to 'prescribe the symptom'. The therapist tells the couple to continue with the problem behaviour, and give a reason that is unacceptable to the couple. Crowe (2000) gives an example in which the therapist tells a chronically depressed and passive wife that she should go in this way because otherwise she and her husband would argue all the time. The intervention was intended to stir the wife into greater activity and assertiveness, which in this case was achieved. The example shows the importance of understanding the personality of each partner before venturing a paradox, which could have an opposite and unfortunate effect in another case. For further information about behavioural-systems couple therapy, see Crowe and Ridley (1990).

Informal approaches

In practice, many couples are helped in more informal ways using the general principles outlined above and restricting interventions to those at the bottom of the hierarchy depicted in Figure 22.1.

Evaluation of couple therapy

The use of couple therapy has to be based mainly on clinical impressions since few clinical trials have been reported. Reviews by Gurman (1979) and Baucom (1998) indicate that marital therapy is better than no treatment, and that the behavioural form of marital therapy was followed by improvement in up to two-thirds of reported cases. Snyder and Wills (1989) found that behavioural and insight-orientated couple therapy had about equal effects. Crowe (1973) compared behavioural treatment for couples with a treatment combining elements of systems theory and interpretation, and with a non-directive approach. Improvement was least with the non-directive approach, and there were no differences in the response to the other two treatments. Clinical impressions suggest that eclectic methods can be a useful part of a wider plan of treatment

Family therapy

Several or sometimes all members of a family members take part in this treatment. Usually both parents are involved, often together with the child whose problems have led the family to seek help. They may be joined by other children, grandparents, or others members of the extended family. The aim of treatment is to improve family functioning, and so to help the identified patient. Since success depends on the collaboration of several people, drop-out rates are high. Whatever their method, family therapists have the following goals for the family:

- improved communication,
- improved autonomy for each member,
- improved agreement about roles,
- reduced conflict, and
- reduced distress in the member who is the patient.

Family therapy dates from the 1950s. It can be traced to two sources: an influential book by Ackerman (1958) called *The psychodynamics of family life*, and the work on communication by Bateson and his colleagues mentioned above. Ackerman's work led to psychodynamic methods of treatment, whilst Bateson's treatments led to the systems approach. The latter approach was developed further in the USA by Salvador Minuchin who advocated a practical approach to resolving problems in his structural family therapy, and in Italy by the Milan school who used hypotheses about the family system to suggest ways of promoting change. These approaches are described briefly below, together with an eclectic approach. The reader will find fuller accounts in the chapter by Bloch and Harari (2000) and the book by Gurman and Kriskern (1991).

Indications and contraindications for family therapy

Family therapy is used mainly in the treatment of problems presented by young people living with their parents. These problems are often related to difficulties in communication between members of the family, or to role problems. In the practice of adult psychiatry, family therapy is often combined with other treatment, for example, antidepressant medication for a depressive disorder, Family therapy is used in treating some young people with anorexia nervosa after weight has been restored by other means (see p. 450). Special kinds of family treatment have been developed to reduce relapses in schizophrenia (see pp. 366 and 370).

Psychodynamic family therapy

This method is based on the idea that current problems in the family originate in the separate past experiences of its individual members, particularly those of the parents. Present problems arise in part from unconscious conflicts within individual members who need to gain insight into these conflicts if they are to change their behaviour. The therapist's task is to help members gain this insight and to understand how their own problems and those of other family members interact. The therapist does this by examining his own relationship with each of the family members. The therapist uses the non-directive method described under individual dynamic psychotherapy (p. 744).

A related approach has been developed by Skynner (1991) using *object relations theory* (see p. 724). Skynner emphasized ways in which the childhood experience of a parent affects the ways that they relate to their own children; for example, a mother who received no adequate mothering may develop a 'projective system', i.e. expectations shaped by her childhood experiences rather than current reality. Projective systems affect the parents' ways of relating to one another as well as to the children. Sometimes a conflict between the projective systems of the parents is resolved by diverting the projections onto the child. By identifying these systems, the therapist helps the family resolve their conflicts.

Structural family therapy

The term family structure refers to a set of unspoken rules that organize the ways in which family members relate to one another. Some rules determine the hierarchy in the family, for example, that parents have more authority and responsibility than children. Some rules determine cooperation in the family, for example, that father and mother share certain tasks and responsibilities, and take on others individually. In some families, both parents set rules for behaviour and admonish children when the rules are broken; in other families, the father is the strict parent. Rules also determine boundaries; sometimes these are broken, for example, when an unhappy wife involves her son in her problems with her husband. In structural family therapy, hypotheses about these rules are often presented to the family in a paradoxical way; for example, 'you seem to be very dependent on your wife; what does she do to make you feel less competent?' Such interventions, which increase family tension in the short term, are intended to bring about change.

Systemic family therapy

Systemic family therapy is concerned with the present functioning of the family, rather than with the past experiences of its members. The therapist's task is to identify the family's unspoken rules, their disagreements about who makes these rules, and their distorted ways of communicating. The therapist helps the family to understand and modify the rules, and to improve communication.

In the *Milan approach* (Palazzoli *et al.* 1978) there are usually 5–10 sessions, spaced at intervals of a month or more ('long brief therapy'). *Circular questioning* is often used to assess the family. In this technique, one person is asked to comment on the relationships of others, for example, the mother may be asked how her husband relates to their son, and others are asked to comment on her response. The purpose is to discover and clarify confused or conflicting views. A hypothesis is then constructed about the family functioning. For example, the boundary between the parent and child subsystems may have been breached, in that one parent has an inappropriately strong alliance with one of the children. Such hypotheses are presented to the family, who are asked to consider them in and between sessions. The family may be asked to try to behave in new ways. Sometimes the therapist provokes change with paradoxical injunctions designed to provoke the family into making changes that they cannot make in other ways. For example, if the patient fears that the parents will separate, the injunction may be designed to make them prove the therapist wrong and so bring them closer.

Criticisms of the systems approach are that they ignore on the one hand the effects of past experience and unconscious motives, and on the other the effects of realistic problems such as unemployment and poverty. A review of ten outcome studies of Milan systemic family therapy (five of which included comparison groups) found it as effective as other kinds of family therapy. There was symptomatic improvement in about two-thirds of patients, and improved functioning in about half the families. Generally, these results were obtained in less than ten sessions (Carr 1991).

Eclectic family therapy

In everyday clinical work, especially with adolescents, it is practicable to use a simple short-term method designed to bring about limited changes in the family. For this purpose, it is appropriate to concentrate on the present situation of the family and to examine how the members communicate with one another. The number of family members taking part is decided on practical grounds; for example, some children may be too young, whilst others may be away from home. The interval between sessions is varied to allow time for the family to work together on the problems raised in treatment.

Assessment

Assessment begins with the family structure which can be summarized as a genogram using conventional symbols (see Figure 22.2). Further questions concern the current and past state of family life, and the roles of the members. Several kinds of questioning may be used: circular questioning (see above); questions about the roles of the members (who takes care of others, who worries most, who decides, etc.); about triadic relationships (for example, what does A do when B criticizes C); and about responses to a previous change (for example, the death of a grandparent).

The therapist tries to answer two questions: how does the family function, and are family factors involved in the patient's problems? Bloch and Harari (2000) have proposed a useful framework in which to consider these questions.

How does the family function?

- *structure* recorded in the genogram: for example, single parent, a step parent, size and age spread of the sibship;
- *changes and events* such as births, deaths, departures, and financial problems;
- *relationships* close, distant, loving, conflictual, etc;
- *patterns of interaction* involving two or more people, for example, a child who sides with one parent against the other.

Are family factors involved in the patient's problems? The family may be:

- *reacting* to the patient's problems – but there may be unrelated problems as well;
- *supporting* the patient;
- *contributing* to the patient's problems, for example, the problems of a daughter who cannot leave her lonely mother.

The answers to these questions lead to a hypothesis about what should and can change.

Intervention

Specific goals for change are agreed with the members of the family, who are asked to consider how any changes will affect themselves and others, and what has prevented the family from making the changes. Paradoxical injunctions may be included but should be made only after the most careful consideration of the range of possible responses. The therapist should remember that interchanges in the sessions are likely to continue when the family return home, and try to ensure that this does not lead to further problems.

Results of family therapy

In a meta-analysis of the results of 19 studies of family therapy, the effect was found to be comparable to that of other forms of psychotherapy. About 75% of patients receiving family therapy

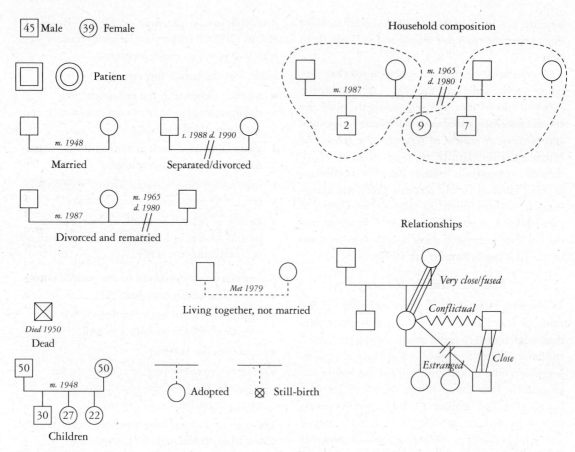

Figure 22.2 Symbols used in the construction of a genogram. (Reproduced with permission from Bloch and Harari 2000)

had a better outcome than similar patients receiving minimal or no treatment. The size of the effect increased during the first year after treatment, remained unchanged for a further 6 months, and then decreased (Markus *et al.* 1990).

For further information about family therapy in psychiatry see Barker (1992), or Bloch and Harari (2000).

Psychotherapy for children

The kinds of psychotherapy discussed so far do not lend themselves to the treatment of young children who lack the necessary verbal skills. In practice there are fewer difficulties than might be expected,

because many emotional problems of younger children are secondary to those of their parents and it is often appropriate to direct psychotherapy mainly to the parents.

Some psychotherapists believe that it is possible to use the child's play as equivalent to the words of the adult in psychotherapy. Klein developed this approach extensively by making frequent analytical interpretations of the symbolic meaning of the child's actions during play, and by attempting to relate these actions to the child's feelings towards his parents. Although ingenious, this approach is highly speculative since there is almost no evidence against which the interpretations can be checked. Anna Freud developed child psychotherapy by a less extreme adaptation of her father's techniques to the needs of the child. She recognized the particular difficulty for child analysis of the child's inability or unwillingness to produce free associations in words. However, she considered that neither play with toys, nor drawing and painting, nor fantasy games could be an adequate substitute. Moreover, she cautioned against the use of uncontrolled play, which may lead to the acting out of aggressive urges in a destructive way. Anna Freud accepted that non-analytical techniques could be helpful for many disorders of development. These techniques include reassurance, suggestion, the giving of advice, and acting as role model (an 'auxiliary ego'). However, for neurotic disorders in childhood, and for the many mixed disorders, she advocated analytical techniques to identify the unconscious content of the disorder and to interpret it in a way that strengthens ego functions. A concise account of Anna Freud's views on child analysis is contained in Freud (1966, Chapters 2 and 6).

In the UK, most psychotherapy for children is eclectic; the therapist tries to establish a good relationship with the child and to learn about his feelings and thoughts, partly through talking and listening, and partly through play. Older children can communicate verbally with adults but younger children can communicate better through actions, including play. The therapist can help children to find words that express thoughts and feelings, and thus can make it easier for them to control and change these thoughts and feelings. However, it is important to ensure that the therapist's interpretations are reflecting the child's own thoughts and not implanting new ideas. Child psychotherapy is discussed further in Chapter 24 on child psychiatry (p. 814).

Other psychological treatments

Treatments of mainly historical interest

Hypnosis

Hypnosis is a state in which the person is relaxed and drowsy, and more suggestible than usual. Enhanced suggestibility leads to diminished sensitivity to painful stimuli, vivid mental imagery, hallucinations, failures of memory, and 'age regression' (behaving as would a much younger person). Although enhanced suggestibility is characteristic of hypnosis, it is not confined to it. Some people respond in a similar way to suggestion when in a state of full alertness (Barber 1962), and there seem to be no phenomena peculiar to the hypnotic state.

Hypnosis can be induced in many ways. The main requirements are that the subject should be willing to be hypnotized and convinced that hypnosis will occur. Most hypnotic procedures contain some combination of a task to focus attention (such as watching a moving object), rhythmic monotonous instructions, and the use of a graduated series of suggestions, for example, that the person's arm will rise. The therapist uses the suggestible state either to implant direct suggestions of improvement or to encourage recall of previously repressed memories.

Indications for hypnosis

Hypnosis is used infrequently in psychiatry. A light trance is used occasionally as a form of relaxation. For this purpose hypnosis has not been shown to be generally superior to relaxation. A deeper trance is used occasionally to enhance suggestion in order to relieve symptoms, especially those of conversion disorder. Although sometimes effective in the short term, this method has not been shown to be superior to suggestion without hypnosis. Also, the sudden removal of symptoms by suggestion under hypnosis can be followed by an increase of anxiety or depression. Hypnosis has been used to aid the recall of memories in psychotherapy, but there is no evidence that this procedure improves outcome. For these reasons the authors do not recommend the use of hypnosis in clinical psychiatry. Readers seeking more information about hypnosis are referred to Wolberg (1977).

Autogenic training

This technique was described by Schultz in 1905 and was in use mainly in continental Europe as a treatment for physical symptoms caused by emotional disorder (Schultz 1932). Patients practise exercises in which they learn to induce feelings of heaviness, warmth, or cooling in various parts of the body, and to slow their respiration. Repeated use of these exercises is supposed to induce changes in autonomic nervous activity and thereby to benefit patients with physical symptoms arising in stress-related and anxiety disorders. It has not been established that autonomic changes after autogenic training differ substantially from those after simple relaxation, nor is there any good evidence that it has a specific therapeutic effect. Interested readers are referred to Schultz and Luthe (1959).

Abreaction

Abreaction (the unrestrained expression of emotion) has long been used to relieve mental distress and some psychiatric symptoms. Although is seldom used today, it is considered here because of its historical interest. Abreaction is part of many forms of religious healing (see below). It was used in psychiatry during the Second World War to bring rapid relief from war neuroses, notably by Sargant and Slater (1940). In civilian practice, abreaction is less effective, perhaps because fewer disorders are the result of overwhelming stress (those that are so caused – the post-traumatic stress disorders – are considered on p. 194). Abreaction can be brought about simply by strong encouragement to relive the traumatic events; but in wartime the procedure was sometimes facilitated by giving a small dose of sedative drug intravenously. For more information about the latter procedure see Sargant and Slater (1963).

Meditation and traditional healing

Meditation

Although not in regular use in psychiatry, meditation is increasingly used by people with minor psychiatric problems as an alternative to psychiatric treatment. There are many methods of meditation, each associated with a different system of belief, but sharing several features. The first is instruction in relaxation and the regulation of breathing. The second is a way of directing attention away from the external world and from the stream of thoughts that would otherwise occupy the mind. Often the person achieves this by repeating a word or phrase (a mantra). The third common feature is the setting aside, from the day's other activities, periods when calm can be restored. Finally, the person joins a group of people who are convinced that the methods work, and encourage each other to practise it. Such group pressure, which is often lacking from hospital-based programmes of relaxation, may explain some of the reported successes of the methods.

There is insufficient evidence to decide the value of meditation. Clinical experience indicates that many of the patients who find them helpful have problems related to a style of life that is too stressful and hurried. For a review of the various forms of meditation and their effects see West (1990).

Traditional healing

There are many kinds of traditional healer but they can be divided into four groups (Jilek 2000):

- *Herbalists* are concerned mainly with plant remedies, some of which are known to contain active ingredients while others appear to be placebos.
- *Medicine men* and women use verbal or ritual methods of healing, sometimes combined with plant remedies. They are believed to have special powers, often of supernatural origin.

◆ *Shamans* use methods like those of medicine men but also enter into altered states of consciousness in which they are believed to communicate with spirits or ancestors, and to recover the abducted souls of people made ill by this supposed loss.

◆ *Diviners* discover and name the cause of illness by interpreting oracles (in clear or in altered consciousness), from the content of dreams, or through some form of communication with ancestors or spirits.

All kinds of traditional healers use methods which are likely to activate the non-specific processes identified as common to many kinds of western psychological treatment (see Box 22.1). In addition, they are aware of the value of naming a condition and answering the questions – 'Why am I afflicted?' and 'Why is this member of our family afflicted?' – thus ending uncertainty and relieving blame and guilt. Some traditional healers use therapeutic suggestion, and many involve the family both in the diagnostic process and in the rituals of treatment. Some employ cleansing or purification rituals to eliminate supposed polluting agents. A few healers use sacrificial rites to appease supernatural beings, sometimes combining these with confession and a promise of changed behaviour. These rituals may be conducted in a group ceremonial involving the wider community as well as the patient and the family. These practices are likely to activate the common factors of group therapy, described in Box 22.6.

Many traditional healers distinguish between 'western' diseases that respond to specific medication, and others in which their procedures help the patient and support the family. There is some scientific evidence that traditional healing is effective for substance abusers (see Jilek 2000) and much anecdotal evidence that it is helpful in minor mental disorders.

For more information about traditional healing and its relevance to psychiatry, see Jilek (2000).

Ethical problems in psychological treatment

Autonomy

The need for informed consent is as great in psychological treatment as in other treatment and to give such consent the patient must understand the nature of the treatment and its likely consequences. This requirement is easily met in cognitive–behaviour therapies which are clearly defined and have been subjected to clinical trial. The course of dynamic psychotherapy and group psychotherapy is less easy to specify at the start, but a broad description should be provided. Such preparation is not only ethically desirable but also likely to improve compliance. A further problem arises when one of the aims of a dynamic psychotherapy is to free the patient from psychological constraints and thereby increase autonomy. In such treatment, it is necessary to review the situation with the patient to ensure that he is fully aware of, and consents to, the new aims and consequences of treatment.

Confidentiality

Group psychotherapy presents special problems of confidentiality. Patients should understand fully the requirement to talk of personal matters in the group but they need to understand equally clearly the requirement to treat as confidential the revelations of other patients. Family therapy presents similar problems, especially if the therapist agrees to see one member outside the family session, and is told of a family secret (relating, for example, to an extramarital affair). When possible, the therapist should refuse to meet individual members in this way but arrange for a colleague to do so when such a meeting seems indicated (for example, if one member is seriously depressed). Similar problems arise in couple therapy.

The problem of when a therapist should reveal confidential material to a third party is the same as in other treatment situations, namely that it is justified when there is a substantial risk to a third party. In the USA, the Tarasoff decision is import- ant (see p. 78).

Exploitation

Patients receiving psychological treatment are vulnerable to exploitation, sometimes because of the experiences that caused them to seek psycho- therapy, but also because of the relationship with the therapist. As in other branches of medicine, exploitation may be financial or sexual. Financial exploitation is a potential problem in private prac- tice in which treatment may be prolonged for longer than is necessary to achieve the patient's goals. Occasionally the exploitation is sexual. In the medical and other caring professions, exploita- tion is prohibited in professional codes of conduct; it is not a matter for utilitarian arguments.

Another form of exploitation is the imposition on the patient of the therapist's values. This may be open and direct, for example, when a therapist imposes his view that termination of pregnancy is morally wrong. Or it may be concealed and indi- rect, for example, when a therapist expresses no opinion but nevertheless gives more attention to the arguments against termination that to those for it. Similar problems may arise, for example, in couple therapy when the therapist's values may affect his approach to the question whether the couple should separate.

In group psychotherapy, one patient may be exploited by another. One patient may bully or scapegoat another within the sessions of treatment, or may seek a sexual relationship between the sessions. The therapist should protect vulnerable patients within the sessions, and make a rule that patients should not meet between the sessions. If they do meet, they should report this to the group at the next session and the matter should be discussed.

Further reading

Bloch, S. (1996). *An introduction to the psychotherapies*, 3rd edn. Oxford University Press, Oxford. (An introduction to the commonly used psychological treatments with a chapter on ethics).

Bateman, A., Brown, D. and Pedder, J. (2000). *Introduction to psychotherapy: an outline of psycho-dynamic principles and practice.* 3rd edn. Tavistock/Routledge, London. (An account of dynamic theory, and practice in individual, couple, family and group formats).

Frank, J. D. and Frank J. B. (1993). *Persuasion and healing*, 3rd edn. Johns Hopkins Press, Baltimore, MD. (A revised version of a landmark account of the non- specific factors in psychotherapy).

Gurman, A. S. and Kriskern, D. P. (1991). *Handbook of family therapy*, 2nd edn. Brunner-Mazel, New York. (A comprehensive work of reference).

Hawton, K., Salkovskis, P. M., Kirk, J. W., and Clark, D. M. (2000). *Cognitive behavioural approaches for adult psychiatric disorders: a practical guide*, 2nd edn. Oxford University Press, Oxford. (An introduction with many valuable practical examples).

Wolberg, L. R. (1995). *The technique of psychotherapy*, 4th edn. Jason Aronson, New York. (A comprehensive work of reference).

Yalom, I. (1995). *The theory and practice of group psychotherapy*, 4th edn. Basic Books, New York. (A comprehensive account with much practical advice).

Psychiatric services

Psychiatric services

The last two chapters dealt with the treatment of individual patients. This chapter is concerned with the provision of psychiatric care for populations. It deals mainly with the needs of and provisions for people aged 18–65.

Services for children are described on pp. 813–17; services for the elderly are described on pp. 634–8; and services for patients with learning difficulties are described on pp. 887–90. The organization of psychiatric services in any country inevitably depends on the organization of general medical services in that country. This chapter will refer specifically to services in the UK, but the principles embodied in these services apply widely.

The chapter begins with an account of the historical development of psychiatric services. This is followed by descriptions of the commonly available psychiatric services and of the problems encountered with these provisions. The chapter ends with a consideration of some innovations designed to overcome these problems.

The history of psychiatric services

Until the middle of the eighteenth century, there were hardly any special provisions for the mentally ill. In England, for example, the only hospital for these patients was the Bethlem Hospital, founded in 1247. In most of continental Europe, there was a similar lack of hospital provision; in the Middle Ages, hospitals in Spain were a notable exception (Chamberlain 1966). Nearly all mentally ill people lived in the community, often with help from Poor Law provisions, or else they were in prison. In England the Vagrancy Act of 1744 made the first legal distinction between paupers and lunatics, and made provision for the treatment of the latter. In response, private provisions for the mentally ill ('madhouses' – later to be called private asylums) were developed mainly for those who could pay for care, but also for some paupers supported by their parishes (Parry-Jones 1972). At about the same time, a few hospitals or wards were established through private benefaction and public subscription. The Bethel Hospital in Norwich was founded in 1713. In London, the lunatic ward at Guy's Hospital was established in 1728, and in 1751, St Luke's Hospital was founded as an alternative to the overcrowded Bethlem Hospital. Then, as now, the value of psychiatric wards in general hospitals was debated (Allderidge 1979).

Moral management

At the end of the eighteenth century, public concern in many countries about the poor standards of private and public institutions led to renewed efforts to improve the care of the mentally ill. In Paris in 1793, Pinel gave an important lead by releasing patients from the chains that were used for restraint. Subsequently he introduced other changes to make the care of patients more humane. In England, similar reforming ideas were proposed by William Tuke, a Quaker philanthropist who founded the Retreat in York in 1792. The Retreat provided pleasant surroundings and adequate facilities for occupation and recreation. Treatment was based on 'moral' (i.e. psychological) management and respect for patients' wishes, in contrast with the physical treatments (usually bleeding and purging) and the authoritarian approach favoured by most doctors at that time.

This enlightened form of care was described several years later by William Tuke's grandson, Samuel, in *A description of the Retreat*, published in 1813. These humane methods were adopted in other hospitals as it became clear that many mentally ill patients could exert self-control and did not require physical restraint and drastic medical treatment.

The asylum movement

Despite such pioneering efforts, in the early years of the nineteenth century many mentally ill people received no care and lived as vagrants or as inmates of workhouses and gaols. Also, there was public concern in England about the welfare of those in care, following reports of scandalously low standards in some private madhouses. This concern led to the County Asylum Act of 1808, which provided for the building of mental hospitals in each of the English counties. Unfortunately, little was done by the county authorities, and in 1845 it was necessary to enact the Lunatics Act, which required the building of an asylum in every county. At first the new asylums provided good treatment in spacious surroundings. Moral management was championed, especially by members of the Non-restraint Movement, which had started with the work of Gardiner Hill at the Lincoln Asylum in 1837 and was developed further by John Conolly at the Middlesex County Asylum, Hanwell. In 1856, Conolly published a significant book, *The treatment of the insane without mechanical restraints*.

Unfortunately, these liberal steps were soon followed by a new restrictive approach. Increasing public intolerance led to the transfer of more and more patients from the community and prisons to the new asylums. Initial optimism about the curability of psychiatric disorder dissipated, as the limitations of moral treatment became apparent. More gloomy views about organic and hereditary causes prevailed. By the 1850s, the problems of overcrowded asylums were evident. Attempts were made to house patients with chronic illness in less restrictive and more domestic surroundings in detached annexes or houses in the grounds of the asylum. Other hospitals returned patients to the community either by boarding them out with a family (a form of care which was practised most successfully at Gheel in Belgium) or by returning them to workhouses. The Lunacy Commissioners, whose role was to oversee the care of the mentally ill, were concerned that these arrangements could lead to abuse, and were opposed to them. Nevertheless, nineteenth-century asylums, even when overcrowded, provided a standard of care for the mentally ill that was lacking elsewhere. Thus the mentally ill were protected from exploitation, and were provided with shelter, food, and general health care. These benefits were counterbalanced by the disadvantages of loss of personal choice and autonomy, and of a monotonous and overprotective regimen that could lead to institutionalism (see p. 769).

Under the increasing pressures of overcrowding and staff shortages, there was less and less time for moral management. Again, a custodial approach was adopted. This change to custodial care was endorsed by the Lunacy Act 1890, which imposed restrictions on discharge from hospital. These custodial arrangements continued into the twentieth century, and their legacy is still seen in the size and structure of the large Victorian hospitals in which most psychiatry was practised until recently. See Jones (1972) and Rothman (1971) for accounts of psychiatric hospitals in the UK and the USA in the nineteenth century.

Arrangements for early treatment

In the UK, the start of a return to more liberal policies was signalled shortly before the First World War, by a substantial gift of money by Henry Maudsley, a wealthy psychiatrist, to provide for a hospital devoted to early treatment. Unfortunately, the war interfered with the project, and the opening of the Maudsley Hospital was delayed until 1923. The hospital provided an out-patient service and voluntary in-patient treatment in surroundings in which teaching and research were carried out.

In the years between the wars, the impetus for change increased. The Mental Treatment Act 1930 repealed many of the restrictions on discharge of patients imposed by the Lunacy Act 1890, and allowed county asylums to accept patients for voluntary treatment. The 1930 Act also encouraged local authorities to set up out-patient clinics and to establish facilities for after-care. Therapeutic optimism increased further as two new treatments were discovered: insulin coma (later abandoned) and electroconvulsive therapy. At the same time, efforts were made to improve conditions in hospitals, to unlock previously locked wards, and to encourage occupational activities. Similar changes took place in other countries.

In most countries, these reforms were halted by the Second World War. Psychiatric hospitals became understaffed as doctors and nurses were recruited to the war effort. They also became overcrowded as some were allocated to the care of the war injured, with the result that their patients had to be relocated among the rest. The effects of the war on an English county asylum have been described by Crammer (1990).

Social psychiatry and the beginning of community care

After the Second World War, several influences led to further changes in psychiatric hospitals. Social attitudes had become more sympathetic towards disadvantaged people. Among psychiatrists, wartime experience of treating 'battle neuroses' had encouraged interest in the early treatment of mental disorder and in the use of group treatment and social rehabilitation. In the UK, the advent of the National Health Service led to a general reorganization of medical services including psychiatry. The introduction of chlorpromazine in 1952 made it easier to manage disturbed behaviour, and therefore easier to open wards that had been locked, to engage patients in social activities, and to discharge some of them into the community.

Despite these changes, services continued to be concentrated on a single site, often remote from centres of population. In the USA, Goffman (1961) argued that state hospitals were 'total institutions', i.e. segregated communities isolated from everyday life. He described such institutions as impersonal, inflexible, and authoritarian. In the UK, Wing and Brown (1970) found that some of the large mental hospitals were characterized by 'clinical poverty' and 'social poverty'. Vigorous methods of social rehabilitation were used to improve conditions in hospital and to reduce the effects of long years of institutional living. Occupational and industrial therapies were used to prepare chronically disabled patients for the move from hospital to sheltered accommodation or to ordinary housing (Bennett 1983). Many long-stay patients were responsive to these vigorous new methods. There was optimism that newly admitted patients could also be helped in these ways.

For patients in the community, day hospitals were set up to provide continuing treatment and rehabilitation, and hostels were opened to provide sheltered accommodation. As a result of all these changes, the numbers of patients in psychiatric hospitals fell substantially in the UK and in other countries. The changes were particularly rapid in the USA. Despite these changes, services were still based in large mental hospitals that were often far from patients' homes. Unfortunately, in many places the provision of community facilities was insufficient for the needs of all newly discharged patients.

Hospital closure

After the initial success of discharging many institutionalized patients, it was optimistically proposed that large asylums could be closed and replaced by small psychiatric units in general hospitals, with support from community facilities. In most countries, the programme of hospital closure took place gradually. A notable exception was Italy, which at first lagged behind most other countries but later made rapid changes. In 1978, the Italian Parliament passed Law 180, which aimed to abolish the mental hospitals and replace them by a comprehensive system of community care. Admission to psychiatric hospitals was prohibited, and there were requirements that psychiatric units be set up in general hospitals and that community services be developed in defined areas. The scheme was based on the work of Franco Basaglia in hospitals in northeast Italy, and on the proposals of the professional and political movement he founded. This movement – Psichiatria Democratica – combined an extreme left-wing political view that patients in psychiatric hospitals were the victims of oppression by the capitalist system with the conviction that severe mental illness was induced by social conditions and not by biological causes. Basaglia's forceful personality and qualities of leadership helped him to succeed in finding new ways of caring for patients in the community. Other workers found it difficult to repeat his successes. The consequences of this sudden change were varied. In those parts of Italy where the reforms were financed adequately and were implemented by enthusiastic staff, the new provisions were successful. In areas where the provision of new facilities was inadequate, there were many problems for patients and their families (Bollini and Mollica 1989).

In the UK and elsewhere, the pace of change was slower, but similar problems arose. Some patients could not manage in the community without intensive support, and even then required repeated readmission to hospital so that the arrangements became known as the 'revolving door policy'. The rehabilitation services had been expected to discharge patients in an improved state, but they found it necessary to provide continuing care for so many that it was difficult to take on new patients. Some discharged patients attended day hospitals for years without further improvement (Gath *et al.* 1973). It became clear that earlier views of the benefits of 'de-institutionalization' had been overoptimistic, and that services outside hospital were inadequate to provide the help needed by discharged patients and their families. Attempts were made to develop more adequate community facilities, a policy known as community care.

The rise of community care

As hospitals closed, psychiatric services had to perform three functions. The first was to treat, in the community, patients with chronic psychiatric disorder who would previously have remained in hospital for many years. The second was to assist primary health services with the detection, prevention, and early treatment of the less severe psychiatric disorders. The third was to treat severe acute psychiatric disorder as far as possible without lengthy admission to hospital and as near as possible to the patient's home. These functions were to be carried out for a defined population. Services were to be comprehensive and deliver continuity of care, and be provided by multidisciplinary teams. These general principles were applied rather differently in the UK and in the USA.

In the UK, emphasis was placed initially on the long-term care of patients with serious psychiatric disorders. In the USA, more emphasis was given to the prevention and early treatment of mental disorder as a way of avoiding admission to hospital. In the USA, the Joint Commission on Mental Illness and Health issued a report in 1961 recommending community treatment, delivered from community mental health centres (CMHCs) staffed from several disciplines. The centres offered psychological and social care and generally placed more emphasis on early intervention with acute problems (crisis intervention) than on the care of patients with chronic psychiatric disorders. This emphasis led to dissatisfaction with the centres as patients discharged from long-term hospital care found their way into private hospitals or prisons, or joined the homeless population of large cities (Goldman and Morrisey 1985).

In the UK and elsewhere, some commonly agreed principles about community services developed from these early experiences:

◆ *Hospital care* Hospital admissions were to be brief, and as far as possible to psychiatric units in general hospitals rather than to psychiatric hospitals. Whenever practicable, patients were to be treated as out-patients or day patients.

- *Rehabilitation* This was to be provided, originally with the hope that most patients would progress to independent living, but subsequently with the more modest aim of preventing further deterioration.
- *Out-reach* Since some of the most vulnerable patients were unwilling to make use of the available care, staff had to take services to patients, and follow them actively.
- *Multidisciplinary teams* Care was to be provided by teams which usually included psychiatrists, community nurses, clinical psychologists, and social workers, all of whom worked in collaboration with members of voluntary groups.
- *Legal reform* In many countries new laws were introduced to limit the uses of compulsory treatment and to encourage alternatives to in-patient care. These reforms also reflected a greater public concern for the rights of the individual.
- *User involvement* Users are increasingly involved in planning their own treatment and the services for populations.

Rates of psychiatric disorder in the community

To determine what psychiatric services are required for a community, it is necessary to know the frequency of mental disorder in the population and the needs for treatment of the people with the disorders identified in this way. Policy decisions have then to be made about the division of care between primary and specialist medical services, between medical and social services, and between people with different kinds of mental disorder. In the National Health Service, priority is given to people with serious mental illness.

It is difficult to determine the exact frequency of mental disorders in a community (for methods of epidemiological research, see p. 118), but approximate estimates are usually sufficient for service planning. Table 23.1 shows two sets of figures, one

Table 23.1 Approximate 1-year prevalence of psychiatric disorder in the community

	US survey* (%)	UK survey† (%)
All disorders	20.0	–
Non-specific neurotic disorder	–	7.7 to 12.4
Anxiety disorders	13.5	4.7
Substance misuse	8.8	6.9
Affective disorders	4.3	2.1
Obsessive–compulsive disorders	1.7	1.2
Schizophrenia	1.0	0.4‡
Somatization	0.1	–

* Data based on Robins and Regier (1991). All rates are for 1-year prevalence.

† Data from Jenkins *et al.* (1997). Rates are for 1-week prevalence except for functional psychosis for which 1-year prevalence is shown.

‡ 'Functional psychosis'.

– Indicates not assessed.

from a large population survey in the USA, the other from a household survey in Great Britain. The higher figure for anxiety disorders in the US survey is balanced by the figure for non-specific neurotic disorder in the UK survey. The other differences may relate to variations in the methods used in the two surveys rather than any major differences in the true population rates.

These and other surveys indicate that psychiatric disorders are common. Amongst persons at risk, about one in five experience one of these disorders in the course of one year. However, many of the conditions are brief anxiety and depressive disorders arising in reaction to stressful circumstances. Anxiety disorders are most frequent, followed by misuse of drugs or alcohol. Mood disorders come next in frequency. Obsessional disorders and schizophrenia are much less frequent.

Rates of psychiatric disorder among primary care attenders

How many affected persons seek help?

Table 23.2 shows that among the adult population of the UK, between 260 and 315 per thousand are found, in community surveys, to have a psychiatric disorder. Not all these people seek medical advice. Some cope on their own, others are supported by family, friends, clergy, or non-medical counsellors. People with substance misuse are particularly likely to consider that they do not need medical help.

Table 23.2 shows that, in the UK where primary care services are well developed, about nine in ten people with a psychiatric disorder attend a general practitioner. The factors which determine whether a person seeks medical help for a psychiatric disorder include:

- the severity and duration of the disorder;

- the person's attitude to psychiatric disorder; some people feel ashamed and embarrassed to ask for help;

- knowledge about possible help; if people do not know what help can be provided, they are less likely to seek help;

- the person's perception of the doctor's attitude to psychiatric disorder; if the doctor is viewed as unsympathetic, the person is less likely to ask for help;

- the attitudes and knowledge of family and friends; if these people are unsympathetic, the affected person may be less likely to seek help.

How many affected persons attend primary care?

Table 23.2 shows that about 230 per thousand of the adult population attend primary care each year with a psychiatric disorder. Put in another way, Shepherd *et al.* (1966) in a seminal paper, estimated that in one year about 10% of adults registered with a general practitioner consult for a condition that is wholly psychiatric, and 5% consult with a disorder with a both psychiatric and physical components.

More recently, Üstün and Sartorius (1995) estimated that about a quarter of attenders in primary care have at least one psychiatric disorder diagnosed by ICD-10 criteria, most being anxiety and depressive disorders.

Strathdee and Jenkins (1996) looked more closely at the frequency of various disorders in primary care and estimated that, for a practitioner with a list of 2000, there would be among the adult attenders:

- 60–100 with depression;

- 70–80 with anxiety;

- 50–60 with situational reactions;

- 2–4 with schizophrenia;

- 6–7 with affective psychosis;

- 4–5 with alcohol or drug dependence.

Similar findings have been reported for children. Among those aged 7–12 years attending primary care, almost a quarter had psychiatric disorder, divided about equally into emotional, conduct, and mixed conduct and emotional disorders (Garralda

Table 23.2 Pathways to care with rates of psychiatric disorder among adults at each level of care*

	Cases per 1000 per annum
In the community (person decides to seek help)	260–315
Attending primary care (GP detects the disorder)	230
Detected in primary care† (GP refers to psychiatric service)	102
Attending psychiatric services (decision to admit)	24
In-patient	6

* Modified from Goldberg and Huxley (1992).

† 'Conspicuous psychiatric morbidity' (see p. 777).

and Bailey 1986). Among adolescents attending general practice, about a third have a psychiatric disorder (Garralda 1994). As with adults, many of the children and adolescents with psychiatric disorder complain of physical symptoms, and in some of these cases the psychiatric disorder is not detected.

How long do the disorders last?

There have been few studies of the duration of the psychiatric disorders among general practice attenders. Mann *et al.* (1981) followed 100 patients with 'neurotic disorder' over a year and found that about 255 recovered quickly, about 50% had an intermittent course, and about 25% had persistent symptoms. On the basis of this and a further follow-up 10 years later (Lloyd *et al.* 1996), Goldberg *et al.* (2000) estimated that about 20% of psychiatric disorders in general practice run a protracted course.

Hidden and conspicuous morbidity

Table 23.2 shows that rather less than half of the disorders present among attenders are likely to be detected. This is because patients do not always reveal the psychiatric symptoms directly (because they are ashamed, or uncertain whether the doctor will be sympathetic) and because some describe only physical symptoms. Factors that affect the rate of detection are discussed below (p. 777).

Assessing need

Need, demand, supply, and utilization

In the simplest terms, need is what people benefit from; demand is what people ask for; supply is what is provided; and utilization is what is used (Thornicroft and Tansella 2000). Some of these simple definitions have to be expanded. Regarding need, who decides what will be beneficial? Psychiatrists, other health professionals, patients, and relatives may have different opinions about the benefits of various measures and the priority to be assigned to each. Patients commonly state their most important aims as financial security, friends, satisfying work, a sexual partner, and freedom from the side-effects of medication. Psychiatrists may give priority to symptom relief and the reduction of risk. Demand is affected by the extent to which people know what services could be provided and by their assessment of the relevance and efficacy of those services. Need is unrelated to cost; utilization is affected by it. Where patients incur no direct cost (as in the National Health Service), utilization is affected by indirect costs such as the requirement to take time from work or pay for childcare while receiving the service. Utilization depends also on the accessibility and acceptability of services provided.

Breakey (2000) has suggested two definitions of need:

- *for individuals* the services which professionals, patients and relatives believe ought to be provided over a relevant time period in order that the patient remains as healthy as is permitted by current knowledge;
- *for populations* the services that a consensus of professionals, consumers, and the informed public believe to be required by a population over a relevant time period for its members to remain or become as healthy as permitted by current knowledge, and measured by objective epidemiological outcomes.

In considering individual patients, psychiatrists use the term unmet need to denote problems for which a patient has not received an adequate trial of a potentially effective intervention (see Marshall 1994).

The assessment of the needs of individuals

Clinical assessment

Every psychiatric evaluation includes an assessment of the needs for treatment, often expressed as a care plan. Primm (1996) has suggested a useful mnemonic for the areas of need (see Table 23.3).

Table 23.3 SHARES: a mnemonic for the areas of need of disabled mentally ill patients

Symptoms

Housing – provision and supervision

Activities of daily living – includes nutrition, self-care and leisure

Recreation, training, and occupation

Employment

Significant others

Adapted from Primm (1996).

Standardized assessment

The following are examples of the several methods available for the assessment of need:

♦ *The Camberwell Assessment of Need*, which is directed especially to the needs of the seriously mentally ill (Phelan *et al.* 1995). Twenty-two domains of need are assessed including accommodation, self-care, psychotic symptoms, physical health, safety, substance use, childcare, and finances.

♦ *The Cardinal Needs Assessment* (Marshall *et al.* 1995), which assesses unmet need (see above).

♦ *The Needs for Care Assessment*, which was developed principally for research (Brewin *et al.* 1987).

♦ *Level of care* An alternative approach is to assign patients to a level of care. Wing (1994) suggested six levels: the lowest for those who need no professional help; the second for those who can be treated in primary care; the remaining levels for those who need specialist care, ranging from out-patient care (level 3) to long-term care, whether in the community or in hospital (level 6).

Assessment of the needs of populations

First, the number of people with each of the various psychiatric disorders is determined by extrapolating from epidemiological studies of similar populations, correcting for any special characteristics of the local population such as a greater number of elderly people or people from ethnic minorities. Estimates of the needs for services of people in each diagnostic group are then applied to these population estimates. These needs will cover the broad range of services appropriate to the various kinds of need. In practice, it is seldom possible to provide for all these needs and priorities have to be set; in the UK, people with serious mental illness have high priority.

Planning a psychiatric service

Locality planning

In most counties, service planning is centred on a geographical area, often called a locality in the UK, a catchment area in the USA, and a sector in Europe. In Europe, sectors vary in size from about 15 000–50 000 in Sweden to 250 000 in Germany (see Thornicroft and Tansella 2000).

Locality planning has advantages since it:

♦ allows for local variations in the population, for example, an unusually large proportion of elderly people;

♦ integrates different parts of the psychiatric services, for example, services for adolescents and adults;

♦ integrates psychiatric and medical services, for example, services for child psychiatry and mental retardation;

♦ integrates medical, social and voluntary services.

Locality planning also has disadvantages:

♦ it may not be cost-effective to provide services for conditions which require specialist care but are of low prevalence, for example, patients needing medium or high security;

- the quality of services may differ between sectors;
- health service and social service sectors may not be co-terminous.

These disadvantages can be reduced by collaboration between sectors in service provision and by the setting of national minimal standards.

The planning process

Thornicroft and Tansella (2000) have listed seven steps in planning services for a locality:

- *Establish principles* This is especially important when planning involves representatives from several professions who may have different values and aims. If these differences are not identified and discussed at the start, the may be the unexpressed reason for failure to reach agreement in later meetings. Thornicroft and Tansella have suggested nine planning principles (see Box 23.1).
- *Set boundaries* to define responsibilities between parts of the psychiatric service (e.g. between general adult services and substance abuse services), between primary and secondary care (e.g. in treating the less severe psychiatric disorders), and between medical and social services (e.g. in the provisions for conduct disordered adolescents).
- *Assess population needs* See above and Table 23.4.
- *Assess current provision* This requires a consideration of the service components listed in Box 23.2. Alternatively, a more formal schedule can be used, for example, the International Schedule of Mental Health Care (World Health Organization 1990).
- *Formulate a strategic plan* with a review of the deficits of the current provisions, a statement of the planned provisions, and short term and long term goals. This plan should be discussed widely and modified appropriately in response to the comments received.

Box 23.1 Nine principles of service planning; the three ACES*

1. *Autonomy* patients should be able to make choices
2. *Continuity* over time and between different parts of the service
3. *Effectiveness* evidence that the intended benefits are achieved
4. *Accessibility* care should be provided where and when it is needed
5. *Comprehensiveness* in relation to the various needs and users
6. *Equity* the distribution of resources, and the way this is decided should be fair and explicit
7. *Accountability* to the users and funders of the service
8. *Coordination* within the mental health service, and between it and other services
9. *Efficiency* the maximum reduction of need from the available resources

Adapted from Thornicroft and Tansella (2000)

- *Implement the plan* as far as resources allow, according to the priorities in the plan.
- *Monitor and review the service* Funds should be identified in the original budget for an evaluation to determine whether changes in services have benefited patients and their families.

Users and relatives should be involved in several of these stages.

The components of a psychiatric service

Because a community psychiatric service supplements the care provided by general practitioners, this account begins with the treatment of psychiatric disorder in primary care.

Box 23.2 Components of a community service*

Out-patient and community services
- Assessment in the community
- Outreach crisis services
- Out-patient services
- Specialist psychological treatments
- General hospital liaison
- Services linked to primary care

Day services
- Training courses
- Rehabilitation
- Sheltered workshops
- Day hospitals
- Self-help groups
- Social clubs
- User groups and advocacy services

In-patient services
- General acute units
- Intensive care units
- Medium secure units

Other residential services
- Hostels: staff awake day and night
- Hostels: with staff sleeping in
- Hostels: with staff on call at night
- Group homes with visiting staff
- Supervised individual accommodation

Services for special groups
- Children and adolescents
- Old age services
- Learning disability services
- Forensic services
- Services for substance misusers

Social and welfare services
- Income support
- Housing support
- Home help/meals

Liaison with other agencies
- Probation/court diversion
- Voluntary agencies

*Modified from Thornicroft and Tansella (2000)

Table 23.4 Estimated need for specialist residential provision per 250 000 total population aged 15–64 years

Type of provision	Number of places	
	Wing (1994)	Strathdee and Thornicroft (1992)
Acute ward	100	50–150
Intensive care/local secure unit	10	5–10
Medium secure unit	4	1–10
'Hotel ward' – staff awake at night	50	40–150
Hostels – staff sleeping in	75	
Hostels – staffed by day only	50	30–120
Group homes – staff visiting	45	48–100
Other supported placements	60	
Total	394	174–540

Services for psychiatric disorder in primary care

Classification of psychiatric disorders in primary care

ICD-10 and DSM-IV were developed for use in psychiatry. They are too detailed for routine use in primary care, and their fine distinctions are seldom helpful in selecting treatment in this setting. The World Health Organization has therefore developed a simpler classification for use in primary care. This classification is described on p. 99. Each diagnosis is linked to a plan of management.

Identification of psychiatric disorders in primary care

The first stage of providing services for psychiatric disorders in primary care is to detect them. This is not a simple matter because, as explained above, some people with a psychiatric disorder do not present with psychiatric symptoms but complain instead of physical symptoms. The latter may be those of a coincidental physical illness or part of the symptoms of the psychiatric disorder, for example, palpitations in an anxiety disorder or tiredness in a depressive disorder. Some patients are aware that they have an emotional problem but describe physical symptoms instead of psychiatric symptoms because they fear that the doctor will not respond sympathetically to psychiatric illness. Other patients are unaware that their physical symptoms have a psychological origin. Goldberg and Huxley (1992) have introduced two useful terms: *conspicuous morbidity* refers to the cases that are detected, *hidden morbidity* refers to the rest. Hidden cases are generally less severe than conspicuous ones.

How accurately the general practitioners identify undeclared psychiatric disorder depends on:

♦ ability to gain the patients' confidence and so enable them to disclose psychiatric problems of which they are aware;

♦ skill in assessing whether physical symptoms are caused by physical or psychiatric illness.

This requires a good knowledge of physical medicine as well as psychiatry.

General practitioners can be trained to increase their ability to identify psychiatric disorder among their patients (Gask 1992).

Disorders treated in primary care

Most psychiatric disorders in primary care attenders can be treated successfully by the general practitioner or another member of the practice team. Examples are most adjustment disorders, the less severe anxiety and depressive disorders, somatization, and some cases of alcohol abuse. The following additional points should be noted; for a fuller account see (Goldberg *et al.* 2000).

Somatizers In primary care, many patients with psychiatric disorder present with physical symptoms. Many of these patients reveal psychiatric symptoms and accept a psychiatric diagnosis when they are interviewed appropriately – *facultative somatizers*. Others continue to deny psychiatric symptoms and reject a psychiatric diagnosis, however skilfully they are examined – *pure somatizers*.

Distressed high users This term is used more in the USA than in the UK where such patients are sometimes referred to as heart-sink patients. The US term is less pejorative, whilst the UK term indicates that the patients are identified more by their effect on their carers rather than by common clinical features. Most of these patients are female and middle aged; about 80% have a present or past psychiatric disorder, usually depression, somatization, or generalized anxiety; and about 60% have a concurrent physical illness (Katon *et al.* 1990). Since most of these patients refuse to be referred to a psychiatric team, the general practitioner has to manage them. One approach is help patients to make links between physical symptoms and stressful life events, leaving out reference to intervening psychological processes, and to consider how life stresses might be reduced.

Disorders referred from primary care to the psychiatric services

Table 23.2 shows that on average about one in four of the patients with psychiatric disorder, identified by general practitioners, is treated by the psychiatric services. This referred group includes patients with severe depressive disorders, schizophrenia, and dementia. General practitioners are more likely to refer patients with other disorders when:

♦ the diagnosis is uncertain;

♦ the condition is severe;

♦ there is a significant suicide risk,

♦ the condition is chronic;

♦ necessary treatment cannot be provided by a member of the primary care team;

♦ previous treatment in primary care has been unsuccessful;

♦ psychiatric services are accessible and responsive;

♦ the patient is willing to attend.

Treatments provided by the primary care team

For acute disorders

Acute problems are generally treated with counselling alone or combined with medication. Some practices also provide simple behavioural treatments. Since general practitioners seldom have time to provide counselling for all those who would benefit from it, the primary care team often includes a counsellor. With additional training, practice nurses can take on this role effectively (Wilkinson *et al.* 1993). The availability of a counsellor has not been shown to reduce the prescribing of psychotropic drugs in the practice (Mynors-Wallis *et al.* 1995; Sibbald *et al.* 1996b); however, medication and counselling often have complementary roles.

For chronic disorders

The respective roles of the general practitioner and the community team should be defined clearly in relation to each patient with chronic mental disorder, and reviewed regularly. For example, in the care of some patients with chronic schizophrenia, the general practitioner might care for physical health, assess general progress, administer and encourage compliance with medication, and support the family. Kendrick *et al.* (1995) found that even with additional training, general practitioners are not very effective in making structured assessments of patients with long-term psychiatric illness. It is generally better that the psychiatric team assess those patients, and agree a plan with the general practitioner. This plan will include elements provided by the psychiatric team, and elements provided by the primary care team, such as the administration of medication, support for the family, and general medical care.

Work in primary care by the psychiatric team

There are four ways in which a psychiatric team can work with the primary care team.

Advise and train general practitioners and their staff

In this style of working, the psychiatrist and other members of the team do not see patients but give advice based on the general practitioner's assessment of patients. The psychiatrist may also hold seminars or case discussions with the primary care staff. This arrangement increases the skills of the members of the primary care team, thus making them more effective in treating similar patients in future. The psychiatric nurse may work similarly with the practice nurses who can play an important part in treating psychiatric disorder.

Assess patients

The psychiatrist assesses patients when the general practitioner is uncertain about diagnosis or treatment. He may do this on his own or jointly with the general practitioner. Patients identified as needing specialist treatment are then referred to a psychiatric out-patient clinic in the usual way.

Assess and treat patients

The psychiatrist works mainly in primary care, seeing most patients at the primary care centre or at home, rather than in the hospital out-patient clinic. Clinical psychologists and psychiatric nurses also work in primary care, providing assessment, counselling, or behavioural treatment. Patients no longer need to visit a psychiatric clinic, but there may be little contact between the psychiatric and primary care teams.

Shared care

This approach fits with the care plan approach used for patients with severe mental illness, but it is not restricted to this group of patients. The general practitioner and the leader of the psychiatric team agree how each team will contribute to an overall plan of management, and a key worker is appointed.

The most appropriate arrangement depends on the needs of the general practitioners, the accessibility of hospital out-patient clinics (generally greater in urban than in rural areas), and the number of primary care centres in which the psychiatrist works (the more centres, the less time for work in each).

Agreeing priorities in primary care

There is debate whether members of the community psychiatry team should accept referrals direct from the general practitioner, or whether referrals should be screened and prioritized by the leader of the psychiatric team leader in order to maintain the team's focus on patients with serious mental disorder. Without screening, community psychiatric nurses may take on large numbers of patients with minor disorders (Warner *et al.* 1993) for whom their work may not be cost-effective (Gournay and Brooking 1994). To avoid conflict, priorities and referral procedures should be agreed at the start of the collaboration between the primary care providers and the community psychiatric team.

Specialist services for acute psychiatric disorder

The patients referred to specialist care

Patients treated by the psychiatric services are a subgroup of people with mental disorder. In some countries patients can go directly to a specialist so that patients treated by the psychiatric services may not be very different from those treated in primary care. In countries such as the UK where the general practitioner acts as the 'gatekeeper' to specialist services, the number and types of patient reaching the psychiatric services depend on:

- the willingness of general practitioners to treat psychiatric disorder;
- the treatment skills and resources of the primary care team;
- patients' willingness to attend for specialist psychiatric advice;
- the general practitioner's criteria for referral to the psychiatric services.

In the UK, most of the patients in contact with the psychiatric services have severe and chronic anxiety disorders and related conditions, severe mood disorder, schizophrenia, or dementia. Among patients particularly likely to be cared for by specialists are those who are suicidal, those who are dangerous to others, and those with dual diagnoses.

Providers of specialist care

In the UK and some other countries, the organization of specialist services is made difficult by a division of responsibilities between different providers with separate funding and different priorities. In the UK, for example, central government provides funds for hospital-based community services, whilst local authorities employ social workers and provide day activities and sheltered accommodation. Voluntary organizations also play a part in providing care. Social services might, for example, assign the highest priority to services for children, whereas psychiatric services might assign the highest priority to patients with serious mental illness, and the voluntary services might have the elderly as their priority. Unless there is close liaison between these various providers, services become uncoordinated and deficient. With planning, the different priorities of the several providers can be taken into account to arrive at a more balanced and comprehensive service.

Provisions for acute specialist care

Specialist care of acute psychiatric disorder requires community teams, supported by out-patient, day-patient, and in-patient provisions.

Assertive Community Treatment

Special arrangements to provide rapid response have been described by Stein and Test (1980) working in the USA. In this approach, called Assertive Community Treatment (ACT), patients with acute psychiatric disorder, who would otherwise be admitted to hospital, are cared for instead by a well-staffed community team. The special features of ACT are:

- staff work with patients as required instead of having individual case lists;
- generous staffing, about one staff member to 10 patients;
- a psychiatrist working specifically with the team;
- services provided in the patients home, or when appropriate, place of work;
- 24-hour availability.

ACT has been described in detail and scales are available to measure the fidelity of a replication to the model (Teague *et al.* 1998).

Stein and Test (1980) compared ACT with standard treatment in which acutely ill patients were admitted to hospital. Over 14 months, symptoms, social functioning, and satisfaction were better in the community group, and bed use was reduced. In Australia, Hoult *et al.* (1983) obtained comparable results with a similar kind of intensive community treatment, and reported that this treatment was less costly than hospital treatment. In the UK, Marks *et al.* (1994) compared routine hospital care

with a form of intensive community treatment, which they called the daily living programme. The study lasted for 3 years, and was concerned with acutely ill patients who had not previously been admitted to hospital. About three-quarters of the community treatment group required an initial brief admission to hospital (average 6 days) before they could be managed in the community. Their stay in hospital was significantly less than that of the control group (average 53 days), and the outcomes for symptoms and social adjustment were slightly better. Deaths from self-harm were not reduced.

A meta-analysis of five randomized trials of ACT or closely similar approaches by Joy *et al.* (1999) showed that, compared with standard care, ACT reduced admission to hospital by about 40% over 1 year without worsening clinical and social outcomes. Burden on families was reduced. One trial reported a homicide by a patient and there was insufficient evidence from the other trials to form a certain assessment of the safety of the approach. Overall costs associated with ACT were less than those of standard care.

Home-based care

Home-based care also aims to assess and treat patients in their homes. However, the psychiatric team is less well staffed than an ACT team, and depends more on collaboration with the primary care teams responsible for the patients. This approach is appropriate for patients with less severe disorders than some of those treated with ACT or admitted to day hospitals (see below). Also, the approach requires well-developed primary care teams, and probably for this reason has been evaluated only in the UK. Two randomized controlled trials (Merson *et al.* 1992; Burns *et al.* 1993) found that admission to hospital was reduced, with no worsening of clinical or social outcome and no evidence of lack of safety. Costs were less than those of the comparison group.

Caution is needed when applying to routine practice the findings of clinical trials in which highly motivated staff work for a limited period

(Audini *et al.* 1994). Also, all the studies confirmed the need for some beds for the treatment of the acute stage of illness; intensive home care can reduce the number of beds needed, but a basic requirement remains.

Out-patient clinics

Although it is often helpful for a psychiatrist to treat patients with acute psychiatric disorders in general practice (see above), work in a central clinic has two important advantages: first, professional staff spend less time travelling and more delivering treatment; second, a senior person is available immediately when less experienced staff need advice. The disadvantages of out-patient clinics are that patients and relatives may have to make long journeys and may be less likely to attend regularly.

Day hospitals

Day hospitals are valuable in two ways in the treatment of acute psychiatric disorder: they can avoid admission to hospital for some patients; and they can shorten in-patient stay by taking over the care of patients when they no longer need the full facilities of an in-patient unit.

For acutely ill psychiatric patients, day care is most appropriate for those who can be with their families in the evening and at weekends. Suitable conditions include depressive disorders of moderate intensity and without substantial risk of suicide, anxiety and obsessional disorders, and some eating disorders. Day care should be planned as carefully as in-patient care, with an active treatment programme specific to each patient's needs. Although the general supportive function of the day hospital has some value, if there is no active programme patients may become dependent and discharge may be delayed.

Diversion to day-hospital care has been compared with admission to hospital for patients with acute psychiatric illness (Creed *et al.* 1990, 1997; Sledge *et al.* 1996). The results indicate that between a third and a half of admissions can be diverted successfully without worsening the clinical or social outcome and with a reduction of the burden on relatives. There are insufficient data to be certain that diversion is as safe as admission, though no evidence that it is not. Direct costs are reduced by between about 20 and 35%. To date the approach has not been widely adopted.

In-patient units

How many places? Although it was originally hoped that a well-resourced provision of community care would greatly reduce the need for in-patient care, it is now recognized that every psychiatric service requires an in-patient unit capable of providing prompt treatment for some acutely ill patients.

The number of beds for patients acute psychiatric required is difficult to determine exactly since it depends on:

- the willingness of families to care for acutely ill relatives;
- the availability psychiatric nurses and other community staff to provide crisis services and 24-hour intensive care in the home;
- facilities for treatment of acute psychiatric disorder outside hospital, such as well-staffed hostels;
- facilities for early discharge of patients from hospital after the acute phase of the disorder; these facilities resemble those under the previous two points above, although it is generally easier to discharge early than to avoid admission.

It has been proposed that a reasonable balance between in-patient and community care can usually be achieved with the number of hospital places shown in Table 23.4, provided that the other facilities mentioned above are in place. The figure of 100 places for acute hospital care per 250 000 total population includes the requirements for both acute disorders and acute exacerbations of chronic disorders in people up to 65 years of age; for patients over this age, the figure excludes dementia. (Provisions for the elderly are discussed on p. 634.) Special provision is required for patients who require intensive nursing during episodes of disturbed behaviour, and for those who may be dangerous to others (some provision for the latter may be provided in a secure unit serving a wider area). See Szmuckler and Holloway (2001) for a review of the needs for beds and other resources in general psychiatry.

When community care was introduced, it was expected that the need for in-patient facilities would be greatly reduced. Experience in England and Wales has not confirmed this expectation: for example, compulsory admissions increased by over 50% between 1990 and 1995 (Department of Health 1996) and ward occupancy rose to almost 100% (Ford *et al.* 1998). These increases arose because of inadequate provision of the alternatives to admission (listed above) for patients who do not need the whole range of services provided in an admission ward, or to speed discharge when the need for full services is at an end (see, for example, Beck *et al.* 1997).

The design of acute in-patient units In their design, in-patient units for acutely ill patients should strike a balance between the patients' needs for privacy and the staff's requirement to observe them. There is a need for secure areas for the most disturbed patients, areas where patients can be alone, and areas where they can interact with others. There should be provisions for occupational therapy, the practice of domestic skills, and recreation. Outdoor space is desirable.

The siting of acute in-patient units In-patient care for acute psychiatric disorders is generally provided as part of a general hospital complex. This siting reduces stigma and provides easy access to general medical services when required. The disadvantages of such siting include the difficulties of providing adequate space for occupational activities and of creating an informal environment suitable for psychiatric care in a hospital designed primarily for the different needs of physically ill patients. Some of these problems can be overcome if the psychiatric unit occupies a separate building within the general hospital complex.

Psychiatric services providing long-term care

Characteristics of patients needing long-term care

Diagnosis

With the exception of the elderly (considered in Chapter 20), most psychiatric patients requiring long-term care have schizophrenia, chronic affective disorders, presenile dementia, or personality disorders associated with aggressive behaviour or substance misuse. Patients who need care in hospital for more than a year are sometimes referred to as the 'new long-stay' (in contrast with the 'old long-stay' who had been resident in hospital for many years before hospital closure programmes were initiated).

Problems

There are several ways of classifying the problems of patients who need long-term psychiatric care. One used approach is to divide the problems into seven groups, three of which are contained in the World Health Organization classification of disablement (see p. 53):

- *symptoms* such as persistent hallucinations, or suicidal ideas;
- *unacceptable behaviours* such shouting obscenities, and threatening or carrying out violent acts;
- *impairments* which are interferences with the functioning of a psychological or physical system, for example, poor memory or lack of drive;
- *disabilities* which are interferences with the activities of the whole person, such as inability to dress;
- *handicaps* which are social disadvantages consequent on disability, for example, inability to work, or to care for children;
- *other social disadvantages* not directly related to disability, such as employment, poverty, and homelessness consequent on the *stigmatizing attitudes* of other people;

◆ *adverse personal reactions* to illness and social disadvantage, such as low self-esteem, hopelessness, denial of illness, or the misuse of drugs.

Wing and Furlong (1986) proposed a useful list of patient characteristics that make it difficult to treat them in the community (see Table 23.5). Patients with severe and persistent problems of this kind need care in a well-staffed hostel, or in hospital which can provide appropriate rehabilitation and security.

Requirements of a community service providing long-term care

If patients with chronic psychiatric disorder are to be treated in the community, it is necessary to provide all the elements of care that they would have received in hospital. In the community seven provisions are required to replace long-term care in hospital:

◆ suitable and well-supported carers;

◆ appropriate accommodation;

◆ suitable occupation;

◆ arrangements to ensure the patient's collaboration with treatment;

◆ regular reassessment, including assessment of physical health;

◆ effective collaboration amongst carers;

◆ continuity of care and rapid response to crises.

Complicated and expensive arrangements are required to make these seven elements available as readily in the community as in hospital. Lack of these arrangements may leave patients homeless, without constructive occupation, inadequately treated, and without a carer. Failure of community care may also leave carers unsupported and family life disrupted. When community care began, it applied mainly to patients who had become institutionalized and compliant after many years in hospital. These patients could be managed in the community without much difficulty. It became evident, however, that some of the patients who had spent less time in hospital were

Table 23.5 Characteristics that make community care difficult
Risk of harm to self and others
Unpredictable behaviour and liability to relapse
Poor motivation and poor capacity for self-management or for performance of social roles
Lack of insight into the need for treatment
Low public acceptability

less compliant, and correspondingly more difficult to manage in the community.

The carers

When patients live at home, *family and friends* are the main carers. They provide much of the help that would be provided by nurses had the patient remained in hospital. For example, they may encourage patients to get up in the morning, maintain personal hygiene, eat regular meals, and occupy themselves constructively. Carers also encourage compliance with treatment. If patients have many problem behaviours, prolonged involvement in care is stressful. Carers may then need support and advice, and sometimes periods of respite.

Volunteer carers play an important part in many systems of community care. Trained volunteers can help to support patients and families, and some charitable organizations employ professional carers such as hostel staff.

Community psychiatric nurses play an essential part in community care by supporting patients and carers, and by evaluating patients, supervising drug therapy, and encouraging social interaction. Evaluation is particularly important for patients whose mental state is unstable and who may act in a threatening or dangerous way when they are more disturbed. One of the problems of community care is that nurses cannot evaluate such patients as frequently as they could have done if the patients had remained in hospital.

Accommodation

Patients discharged from hospital have obvious needs for food and shelter. Many patients live with their families. Some can care for themselves in rented accommodation. Others need more help, which can be provided in three ways.

In lodgings Some people are willing to receive patients with mental disorders as lodgers and to provide them with extra care. This practice works well in some countries but has not been adopted widely in the UK.

In group homes Some patients are able to live in group homes, i.e. houses in which four or five patients live together. The houses may be owned by social or health services or by a charity. The patients are often chronic schizophrenics with social handicaps but few positive symptoms. They are chosen as being able to perform the essential tasks of running the house together, with each using his or her remaining abilities, even though separately unable to complete all the tasks. Patients living in group homes receive regular support and supervision, usually from a community nurse who ensures that arrangements are working well and who encourages patients to take on as much responsibility as possible.

In hostels Much long-term residential care is in hostels. Some patients use hostels as half-way houses from which they move to more independent living. Others need to remain in the hostels for years. In a study of hostel residents, Hewett and Ryan (1975) found that half had remained in the hostel for over 2 years and had reached a plateau in recovery, but most had little behavioural impairment and were working. Although most hostel residents live fairly independent lives, a few of the most disabled require additional care. Levels of supervision can be varied according to the needs of the residents; for example, staff may sleep at night, or they may remain awake as in a hospital ward. The latter arrangement is sometimes called a hospital hotel.

Occupation

Some patients with chronic psychiatric disorders can take on normal employment. Other patients require specially arranged sheltered work, in which they can work productively but more slowly than would be acceptable elsewhere. Such work includes horticulture or the making of craft items. Some patients who cannot meet the requirements of sheltered work may undertake voluntary activities. For those who are more severely handicapped, there is a need for occupational therapy to avoid boredom, understimulation, and lack of social contacts. These occupational activities may be provided in day hospitals or day centres.

Encouraging collaboration with the treatment plan

In hospital, the continuous presence of nurses can ensure compliance with treatment. In community care it is much more difficult to ensure the compliance of poorly motivated patients. It is important that the patient understands the treatment plan. It is often the relatives who undertake this role, and it is important that they understand why the treatment is important as well as the plan of treatment (for example, the dose and timing of medication) and that they know who to inform if the patient departs from the plan. Community nurses have an important role in encouraging compliance with treatment. Patients who object to their plan of treatment should be helped to express their views if necessary by an advocate.

Some patients with chronic psychiatric disorder do not recognize their need for continuing treatment and relapse because they stop taking antipsychotic drugs. In the UK, at the time of writing, there are no compulsory legal powers to require compliance with treatment from patients who are not in-patients. There is a current debate about the best way of dealing with this problem in a way that safeguards patients' rights. The reader should find out the legal and administrative arrangements in the country in which he is working.

Reassessment

Patients living outside hospital require the same regular reassessments that they would have received in a long-stay hospital. Regular reappraisal of the mental state and of compliance with treatment is usually performed by community nurses, with planned but less frequent reassessment by a psychiatrist. Some patients with chronic disorders forget appointments; therefore it is important to have a recall system whereby prompt steps can be taken to re-establish contact as soon as possible. To ensure this arrangement, the psychiatric team needs to work closely with the carers and the general practitioner. It is important to review physical health as well as the psychiatric disorder, because patients with chronic psychiatric disorder may not seek help for physical illness or may not comply with the care that is offered (Brugha *et al.* 1989). Physical assessment is an important part of the general practitioner's contribution to the care of these patients. As noted above, one problem of community assessment is that the frequency of assessment can never be as great as in hospital. Hence it can be difficult to anticipate threatening or dangerous behaviour in patients receiving community care.

Continuity of care

Community care staff need to gain the confidence of their patients to ensure treatment and ask for help if their problems increase. Staff need to know their patients well enough to be able to predict their response to stress and to detect small changes in behaviour that may indicate relapse. These aims cannot be achieved if staff change frequently. Continuity of care is important, and staff should be extra vigilant when care has passed to a new worker.

Response to crisis

Community care staff need to respond quickly to crises. Families and hostel staff accept patients more readily if they know that help will be available quickly in an emergency. Also, readmission to hospital may be avoided by prompt action. Staffing levels need to be adequate for a quick response, preferably by staff who know the patient or else by an emergency team.

Although assertive community treatment was developed for patients with acute illness (see p. 780), it is used more widely to maintain patients with chronic schizophrenia in the community. This use of ACT for this purpose has been assessed in 14 trials (involving 2647 patients) which have been reviewed by Marshall and Lockwood (1998). ACT reduced the number of patients readmitted to hospital, and reduced the amount of hospital care by about 40%. Measures of clinical and social outcome were similar to those of standard care except that the ACT patients were less likely to be homeless. There was insufficient evidence to determine whether ACT was as safe as standard care. A key features of ACT is the high level of staffing and it cannot be assumed that similar results would be obtained with the lower levels and larger case loads obtaining in many routine services.

Working with the family and volunteers

Community care is costly, and in most countries public funds are limited with the result that arrangements often depend on contributions by families and voluntary groups. It is important that these families and voluntary groups are involved in the planning of services, and that there is agreement about their responsibilities and those of professional staff. Without this agreement family members may believe that they are required to take on over-demanding tasks, and professionals may be concerned that volunteers are taking on tasks beyond their capabilities. It is good practice to involve families and voluntary groups in the evaluation of services.

Meeting individual needs: the case management approach

Effective community care requires complicated arrangements involving several professionals as well as relatives and voluntary organizations. The system adopted to ensure that patients receive the necessary services is variously called case management, care management, or the care programme approach. (The last two terms are used more often in the UK.)

The term case (or care) management has been used to describe several rather different procedures. All have five elements in common:

- one person is responsible for the welfare of a patient;
- patients' needs are assessed;
- a plan is made to provide services to meet the needs;
- services are provided;
- the patient and the service delivery are monitored.

The different elements of the various forms of case management can be characterized by dividing them into:

- brokerage in which the managers organize services provided by others but do not provide direct clinical services;
- clinical care management, in which the managers not only arrange the services of other agencies but also provide some treatment for patients, and so have a more direct relationship with them.

The method of case (or care) management adopted in the UK is an amalgam of the types described above; it varies from one place to another. Case management is a plausible way of improving service delivery and has been adopted widely. In England and Wales, it forms part of the requirements of the Community Care Act (1990).

The effectiveness of case (or care) management has been assessed in an analysis of 11 trials involving 1751 patients (Marshall *et al.* 1998). Case management was effective in maintaining contact with patients but it did not reduce admissions – instead admissions increased compared with patients receiving standard care. Despite this, clinical and social outcome of case management was similar to that of patients receiving 'standard' care, which was generally less expensive. Further evaluation is required to discover for which groups case management may be effective (see also Rossler *et al.* 1992).

Supervision registers

Supervision registers are an extension of the case management approach. The intention is to identify, among the patients cared for in the community, those who are especially likely to be aggressive or at high risk for suicide. These and other patients are included in the register when more than usual efforts should be made to respond quickly to crises, to maintain active follow-up, and to seek patients without delay if they fail to keep appointments. Supervision registers alone do little to improve care; they need to be backed by funding sufficient to supply all the needs that have been identified for those on the register. Usually the main need is for intensive individual care and supervision by a member of staff who has a small case load.

Other components of a community care service

Rehabilitation

In psychiatry, the term rehabilitation denotes procedures for helping patients to reach and maintain their best level of functioning. This help may be provided in an in-patient unit, day hospital, or rehabilitation centre. The procedures used in rehabilitation are medical, psychological, occupational, social, and residential.

Medical Most patients in rehabilitation programmes require medication to control symptoms of schizophrenia or of chronic affective disorder.

Psychological Psychological methods include supportive therapy, behavioural programmes, and social skills training (Liberman *et al.* 1986).

Occupational Occupational therapy helps to structure the day and to provide an opportunity for interaction with other people. Good results can be a source of self-esteem, and payment is a further incentive. In the past, occupational therapy was often intended to prepare patients for simple industrial work (see, for example, Wing *et al.* 1964). Now unemployment has increased in many countries and the number of unskilled jobs has decreased, so that opportunities for employment for the handicapped have fallen. For this reason, rehabilitation programmes now include gardening, crafts, cooking, and other activities that can provide a sense of achievement and help unemployed patients use their time constructively.

Social Whenever practicable, handicapped people should be encouraged to join social groups attended by healthy people. Those who cannot achieve this need special clubs and social centres where they can be with other people who have similar difficulties.

In-patient care

For patients with chronic psychiatric disorders, in-patient care may be needed for acute treatment at times of relapse, for intensive rehabilitation, and occasionally for long stay. The basic requirements for an in-patient unit for patients with chronic disorders are broadly similar to those for patients with acute illness (see p. 781). However, since the pace and intensity of treatment is usually slower for patients with chronic disorders than for those with acute disorders, it is generally better to separate the care of the two groups. Secure areas are needed for patients with severely disturbed behaviour, and adequate provision, including outdoor space, should be made for occupational and social activities. Occupational and recreational facilities need not be in the same building, but should be close by. The provisions can be in buildings of a more domestic type than those generally available for patients with acute illness.

Day-hospital care

Day hospitals can play an important part in the care of patients with chronic psychiatric disorder. Patients may attend for assessment and for the supervision of drug treatment, and for occupational and social activities. Since it is difficult to provide simultaneously for the needs of patients with acute disorder and of patients with long-term disorders, it is better to separate activities in different areas of the building or to arrange them at different times.

Out-patient clinics

Out-patient clinics play a smaller part in the care of patients with chronic psychiatric disorders than in the care of those with acute disorders. This is because patients with chronic disorder are more likely to miss booked appointments, and because it is often important to visit their family or other carers. For these reasons, follow-up by a community nurse is more effective for some patients than out-patient care.

The evaluation of community services

Approaches to evaluation

There are two approaches to the evaluation of psychiatric services for a community:

- studies of whole services, and
- studies of particular elements of service, for example day-hospital care.

The two approaches are complementary. Either evaluation requires a clear statement of aims in which inputs, processes, and outcomes are distinguished. Inputs are the resources made available such as the number of beds, or the number of community psychiatric nurses. Processes are the ways that resources are used, for example, the number of in-patient admissions, and length of stay. Outcomes are measures of the effects of the services such as symptom reduction, burden on carers, and suicide rates (see Table 23.6).

Wing and Hailey (1972) suggested six questions that should be asked about the psychiatric services for a population:

- How many patients are in contact with the service?
- What are their needs and those of the relatives?
- Are the services meeting these needs at present?
- How many others, not in contact with the service, also have needs?

Table 23.6 Measures of outcome of psychiatric services
Symptom severity
Ratings of functioning
Measures of disability
Quality of life
Physical morbidity and mortality
Rates of self-harm and suicide
Rates of violent behaviour
Rates of homelessness
Measures of burden on carers
Satisfaction with the services

- What new services, or modifications to existing services, are required to cater for unmet needs?
- Having introduced the new or modified services, are the needs met?

The questions can be asked as a check on an established service, or to examine the effect of a change, such as the closure of a hospital. Questions about the costs can be added to the above list. Such questions are answered through economic analysis.

Sources of data for evaluation

The above questions can be answered with case registers, routine records, and surveys of users and carers. They can be supplemented by specific studies to assess other process or outcome variables.

Case registers

Case registers monitor continuously the number of contacts with the various parts of a service. Such an approach is exemplified in studies of the consequences of closing a psychiatric hospital, resettling its patients, and caring for new cases in the community have been reported in the UK (Leff 1993b) and Italy (Tansella 1991).

Routine records

Routine records can measure inputs, processes, and outcomes. The latter are most difficult to collect routinely. They might include rates at which patients are lost to follow-up, rates of suicide among recently discharged patients, and the number of homeless mentally ill. The value of the last two as indicators of service outcome is limited since both are affected by factors other than the quality of the psychiatric services. In the absence of good outcome indicators, community services are often monitored from routine records of inputs, such as the number of nurses employed or the number of hostel places provided. Process variables are also difficult to monitor. Indices might include the amount of time spent by community nurses with patients who have chronic schizophrenia. However, quality of care depends not only on time spent with each patient but also on what is provided during the sessions.

Clinical audit

Like routine data collection, clinical audit should be continuous, but unlike routine collection, its focus may change from time to time. For example, on one occasion, audit might assess patients' satisfaction with an out-patient clinic, on another the question might be whether clinical guidelines for lithium monitoring are being followed. However, some indicators will be monitored continuously.

Surveys of users and providers

Patients and their relatives, general practitioners, social services, and voluntary agencies have an important perspective on the effectiveness of the services and the need for change.

Specific studies

Special investigations are required to assess certain effects of a service. For example, the results of a formal study of the effects of the closure of a hospital (Leff 1993a) have been used to guide policy on subsequent hospital closures.

Economic evaluation

Economic evaluations of psychiatric care can be divided into macroanalysis dealing with health care systems as a whole, and microanalysis dealing with parts of a system, such as the psychiatric services for a defined population, or a component of such a service (for example, hospital versus day care). Microanalysis examines cost-offset, cost-minimization, cost-effectiveness, cost-benefit and cost-utility.

Cost-offset analysis compares costs incurred in providing a treatment or service with costs saved. Outcome is not measured

Cost-minimization analysis compares two treatments or services known to achieve equal outcomes, in order to find which costs less.

Cost-effectiveness analysis compares two treatments or services of equal cost to find which is more effective. Only one outcome is measured. Problems arise in this and in cost-minimization analysis when different outcome measures do not agree.

Cost-benefit analysis relates costs to benefits, measuring more than one outcome but using a single measure – their monetary value – so that the various benefits can be summed. The approach is attractive but difficult to achieve because it is difficult to agree the monetary value of outcomes such as reduced burden on the family. One approach to valuing a benefit is to ask people to estimate how much (in theory) they would pay to achieve it.

Cost-utility analysis resembles cost-effectiveness analysis but uses a different measure of outcome. Instead of monetary value, improvement in quality of life is assessed, usually as quality-adjusted life years (QUALYs) which combine length and quality of life. Although attractive in principle, such measures are difficult to apply in practice.

An ideal economic analysis would be prospective, compare randomly allocated groups of adequate size, and measure all important costs and outcomes, weighting the latter so that an overall outcome score can be computed. This ideal cannot be achieved when psychiatric services are studied. See Simon *et al.* (1995) as an example of a cost-

economic analysis (of two kinds of medication for depressive disorder). See Weisbrod *et al.* (1980) as an example of cost-benefit analysis (of assertive community treatment for schizophrenia). For a review of economic analysis in psychiatry see Knapp and Chisholm (2000).

Services for patients with special needs

Clinical work and research have identified several groups of patients whose needs cannot be met easily by the usual psychiatric services.

Members of ethnic minorities

Members of ethnic minorities have special needs related to their culture, and many also have needs related to poverty and other social disadvantage. The differences between two ethnic minorities may be greater than those between the first minority group and the general population. There is therefore no single best pattern of service applicable to members of all ethnic minorities. However, the following general points are widely relevant.

Use of the services

Members of ethnic minorities are less likely than other people to use services provided for the majority of the population. They are less likely to consult general practitioners when they have a psychiatric disorder, less likely to accept referral to psychiatric services, and less likely to comply with psychiatric treatment. When members of ethnic minorities ask for help, professional staff are less likely to identify psychiatric disorder, and less able to explain illness and treatment in terms that take account of the beliefs and cultural background of the patients. These and other problems, discussed below, are due not only to limited command of English, but, importantly, to cultural differences.

In the UK, these problems have been studied particularly among people of Asian and Afro-Caribbean origin. People of Asian origin consult their general practitioners more frequently about most conditions than do members of the general population, but consult less about psychiatric symptoms (Murray and Williams 1986; Gillam *et al.* 1989). Some Asian people prefer to seek treatment from a traditional healer when they have a psychiatric disorder (Bhopal 1986). Others consult a general practitioner, but present physical rather than psychiatric symptoms. In some ethnic minorities, referral to a psychiatrist is avoided because it would affect marriage prospects.

Under-recognition of psychiatric disorder

There are two reasons why general practitioners and psychiatric staff may fail to recognize mental disorder in members of ethnic minorities. First, there may be problems of communication, which could partly be overcome by the provision of doctors who are members of the ethnic minority or by providing interpreters to aid other doctors. Second, the presentation of psychiatric disorders may differ between members of ethnic minorities and the general population. As mentioned, people from the Indian subcontinent are more likely than the general population of the UK to complain of physical symptoms when anxious or depressed (Bal 1987).

Problems of diagnosis

People of Afro-Caribbean origin are more likely than members of the general population to be diagnosed as schizophrenic when their behaviour is acutely disturbed (Flaskerud and Hu 1992). It is uncertain how much of this difference reflects a true difference in rates of schizophrenia, and how much is due to misdiagnosis of disturbed behaviour that has other causes, for example, a reaction to stress.

Problems of management.

In England an excess of black people has been observed among patients who are admitted to hospital on a compulsory order (Dunn and Fahy 1990). This finding raises the possibility that different criteria for admission are applied to this group.

Homeless mentally ill people

When hospital closures are planned carefully, few discharged patients become homeless (Leff 1993a; Harrison *et al.* 1994). Nevertheless, surveys have found high rates (30–50%) of chronic psychiatric disorder among the residents of hostels for the homeless in the UK (Priest 1976; Marshall 1989; Marshall and Reed 1992), the USA (Bassuk 1984; Susser *et al.* 1989), and Australia (Herrman *et al.* 1989). Similar high rates (up to 60%) of psychiatric disorder have been found among homeless people and drug misuse is also common in this group.

When people with psychiatric disorder have adopted a vagrant way of life, it is difficult to persuade them to accept treatment or help with accommodation, and many remain on the streets or move to unsatisfactory housing (Marshall and Gath 1992; Caton *et al.* 1993). Carers need patience and persistence, and a willingness to set modest goals. Close liaison between social and medical agencies is essential. For further information, see Craig (2000).

Young people with chronic psychiatric disorder

Most psychiatric patients can be treated by means of a short stay in a psychiatric unit followed by intensive community care. However, there is an important group, composed mainly of young schizophrenic men, who have unremitting illness and need prolonged care. Such patients do not fit well into an acute admission ward and are helped more by treatment in a less stressful environment. Many can be cared for in well-staffed hostels (hostel wards or hospital hostels), provided they can be admitted to an acute psychiatric unit if their disorder relapses (Garety and Morris 1984; Creighton *et al.* 1991). In planning community services, it has to be recognized that many members of this group are likely to require intensive care throughout their lives.

Patients with challenging behaviour

Most of these patients have schizophrenia, often accompanied by personality disorder or the misuse of alcohol or drugs. A few have brain damage. In the past, this small group of patients remained for many years in hospital, where periods of aggressive behaviour could be identified and treated quickly. Most of these patients are now cared for in the community where they require intensive supervision, which is expensive to provide and may not be accepted readily by the patients. Even with intensive supervision, problem behaviours are often difficult to predict when the patient is in the community. The problem is made more difficult because not all violent or otherwise difficult behaviour results from chronic psychiatric disorder. In some patients this behaviour is related to associated personality disorder or substance misuse. It is particularly difficult to prevent or predict episodes of violence in such patients.

Since aggressive behaviour is alarming and may endanger other people, the public tends to judge the effectiveness of a psychiatric service on its ability to care for this small group of patients. They are not managed well in a general psychiatric unit, where their aggressive or unpredictable behaviour may alarm other patients. It is now recognized that special units are needed, designed to meet their special needs. Some of these patients require long-term care in a sheltered and well staffed hostel.

Doctors with psychiatric problems

Although doctors have tried to reduce the stigma associated with psychiatric disorder, many do not seek help if they develop such a disorder themselves. It is helpful to provide special arrangements to enable psychiatrically ill doctors to obtain treatment away from their place of work. If doctors are to seek treatment appropriately, a greater acceptance of psychiatric disorder is required within the medical profession, with appropriate arrangements for after-care and a gradual – and in some cases supervised – return to work. This issue should be discussed openly during medical education and training. When psychiatric disorder is chronic or recurrent, difficult problems are encountered about fitness to practise.

Refugees

Refugees have the general problems of members of ethnic minority groups (described above), together with specific problems consequent upon the experiences that led them to seek refuge in another country. These experiences include persecution, physical injury, torture, or rape; the witnessing of the injury, torture or rape of loved ones; and bereavement. The consequences include general medical as well as psychiatric conditions. The latter are mainly post-traumatic stress disorder and depressive disorder (described on pp. 194 and 291) with culture-specific variations such as a predominance of physical symptoms in depressive disorders.

Refugees need integrated medical and psychiatric care from a team aware of cultural factors. Integrated care is important because general and psychiatric disorders occur together; because refugees often come from cultures in which distress and psychiatric disorder are generally expressed in physical symptoms; and because aid workers are sometimes reluctant to refer refugees to a solely psychiatric service which they think inappropriate for what appears to be a normal response to overwhelming circumstances.

Staff providing services for refugees should be experienced in the treatment of post-traumatic conditions, and should be aided by interpreters. Female members of staff are needed to help female refugees, especially those who have experienced rape. Other staff should have experience in treating children and adolescents. For a review of the psychiatric problems of refugees see Mollica (2000).

Some difficulties with community care

Patients with challenging behaviour

As noted above, the greatest problem in community care is the difficulty of managing patients who have episodes of threatening, aggressive or dangerous behaviour. These patients need well-staffed, long-term, hostel or hospital units providing appropriate security (see above). Until such units are generally available, difficulties will continue in the management of these patients.

The burden on relatives

If members of the family are to take responsibility for patients, by housing them, encouraging adaptive behaviour, supervising medication, and reporting signs of relapse, they need to be well informed, adequately supported, and able to obtain help in an emergency. Such support is time-consuming and expensive, and is not available unless community care is well resourced and the needs of the family are given high priority. Many carers report poor communication from the psychiatric services, for example, about discharge plans. Carers also report difficulty in coping with the negative symptoms and socially embarrassing or aggressive behaviour. Care plans should always consider the possible effects of the patient's illness on any children in the home.

Problems in the distribution of resources

When resources are limited, there is a conflict between the needs of patients with acute and patients with chronic psychiatric disorder. The conflict is most evident in primary care, where the former patients are generally more demanding of care and more responsive to it. The problem has been demonstrated in studies of the allocation of time by community nurses (Wooff and Goldberg 1988; Burns *et al.* 1991), but it is not confined to this professional group.

Problems in the coordination of services

In most countries, long-stay hospital care for patients with chronic psychiatric disorder is provided by a single agency (a hospital authority). Community care requires coordinated action by several agencies, each of which usually has other responsibilities (for example, social services departments have responsibilities for mentally healthy children and elderly people as well as for psychiatric patients). This divided responsibility leads to problems of two kinds – the allocation of resources to the service as a whole, and the availability of specific items of care which are provided by agencies other than the health services (for example, sheltered housing). The problems can be reduced by a coordinating committee with representatives from all the agencies involved in the funding of community care.

Transcultural aspects of service provision

In developing countries, the prevalence and nature of psychiatric disorders is broadly similar to that in developed countries. However, in the developing countries, there is more psychiatric morbidity associated with untreated or inadequately treated physical illness, and there are some differences in the presentation of illnesses, for example, more presentations with physical symptoms.

The pathways to care shown in Table 23.1 are modified in countries whose primary care is less developed than that in the UK. In countries with highly developed private health care, such as the USA, patients can bypass primary care and enter specialist services directly (see Figure 23.1). In such countries, psychologists, social workers, and psychiatrists see many patients who would be treated by the primary care team in the UK.

In many less developed countries, the provision of both primary care and psychiatric services is inadequate. In such countries, many patients who, in other systems of care, would see professional staff, consult traditional healers. These healers are generally valued because their approach accords with cultural beliefs about mental illness (see p. 762). In some countries, medical services work closely with traditional healers. For example, in Zimbabwe a 'defeat depression' campaign

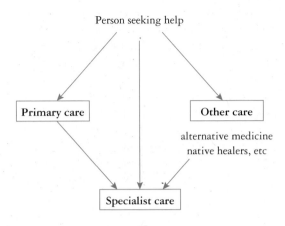

Figure 23.1 Pathways to care.

integrated local beliefs and culturally appropriate counselling with scientific knowledge of psychiatric disorder. The campaign emphasized local causes such as the low status of women and the breakdown of traditional family support systems (Abas *et al.* 1994).

In countries with few specialist psychiatric resources, it is essential to identify priorities. The World Health Organization (1984) identified four such priorities and these still apply:

◆ rapid response to psychiatric emergencies;

◆ provisions for chronic severe psychiatric disorder;

◆ care for psychiatric disorders associated with general medical illness;

◆ care for any high-risk groups found in the country (for example, drug misusers).

The World Health Organization advocates the training of *auxiliary workers* who can supplement the efforts of fully trained staff. Thus in countries with few trained psychiatrists, resources may be used most effectively by improving the skills of nurses who can perform the first-line management of psychiatric disorders, supported by general practitioners. The World Health Organization has recommended that the care of psychiatric problems

should be an important part of the work of all primary care teams (World Health Organization 1978b).

Ethical problems in the provision of psychiatric services

Resource allocation

Problems of resource allocation relate to the ethical principle of distributive justice. There are two kinds of difficulty. The first is to decide the relative needs of people with different disorders and to balance present need (for treatment) with future need (i.e. prevention). The second problem is to decide the relative costs and benefits of different treatments.

In the present state of knowledge, decisions about resource allocation require judgements based of incomplete information, and Daniels and Sabin (1997) have suggested four ways of making the process as acceptable as possible to the majority of the population:

◆ policies for resource allocation should state the procedure to be used, and the criteria for making decisions;

◆ policies should be public documents;

◆ there should be a procedure for challenging both the policies and the decisions;

◆ procedures should be regulated by an external public or voluntary body.

Hope *et al.* (1998) have described how these principles can be put into practice within a UK Health Authority.

Care in the community

Care in the community highlights certain ethical problems that are encountered in all treatment.

Confidentiality

Neighbours may become aware of visits to patients by staff. Outreach programmes may require enquiries about patients who have not kept appointments and who are at high risk of relapse. Care in the community may involve collaboration with housing and other agencies, which are not part of the direct health and social services. These problems need to be anticipated and, when possible, discussed with patients so that advance permission can be obtained. In emergencies, the right to privacy has to be balanced against the risks of harm to the patient or to others if necessary information is not obtained.

Autonomy

Some patients receiving care in the community are poorly motivated and some have a disorder that reduces their competence to make decisions about treatment. Members of the team may need to encourage patients to comply with treatment plans agreed with them when they left hospital. In general, offers of additional help are justified ways of increasing compliance but threats that help will be reduced, are not. Although the limits are often difficult to set, problems can usually be resolved by discussion between members of the community team.

Conflicts of interest

Conflicts arise especially in relation to patients whose care places burdens upon their relatives or other informal carers, and in cases where there is a risk of harm to others. The former conflict of interests may be resolved by discussion between the psychiatrist caring for the patient and the general practitioner or another professional whose primary responsibility is to the carers. The problem of dangerousness is difficult to resolve because it requires first a decision about the level of risk that

is acceptable, and second an assessment of the level of risk (which cannot be made with great accuracy – see p. 924–925). Patients on a supervision register present a particular problem in deciding what is the level of risk that justifies discharge from hospital but at the same time justifies a loss of some civil rights. The ethical problem is the more difficult because even the best available risk assessments inevitably generates false positives, and consequently the restriction of the rights of some people who are not, in fact, dangerous.

Further reading

Breakey, W. R. (Ed.) (1996). *Integrated mental health services*. Oxford University Press, New York. (A comprehensive account written from the U.S. perspective.)

Gelder, M. G., López-Ibor, J. J. Jr, and Andreasen, N. C. (eds) (2000). *The new Oxford textbook of psychiatry*, Part 7: Social psychiatry and service provision. Oxford University Press, Oxford. (The 12 chapters in this part of the textbook review the whole field of community psychiatry, including psychiatry in primary care.)

Goldberg, D. and Huxley, P. (1992). *Common mental disorders: a biosocial model*. Routledge, London. (An account of the development and utility of the important 'filter' model which relates epidemiology to the provision of services.)

Tansella, M. and Thorneycroft, G. (1999). *The mental health matrix*. Cambridge University Press, Cambridge. (Considers the factors that need to be taken into account when planning and providing mental health services for a community.)

Thornicroft, G. and Szmukler, G. (2001). *Textbook of community psychiatry* Oxford University Press, Oxford. (A comprehensive work of reference.)

CHAPTER 24

Child psychiatry

CHAPTER 24
Child psychiatry

The practice of child psychiatry differs from that of adult psychiatry in four important ways:

- *Children seldom initiate the consultation.* Instead, they are brought by a parents, or another adult, who thinks that some aspect the child's behaviour or development is abnormal. Whether a referral is sought depends on the attitudes and tolerance of these adults, and how they perceive the child's behaviour. Healthy children may be brought to the doctor by overanxious and solicitous parents or teachers, whilst in other circumstances severely disturbed children may be left to themselves. A related factor is that psychiatric problems in a child may be a manifestation of disturbance in other members of his family. When a child's problems have previously been contained within the family or school, the child may be referred when another problem, which reduces their capacity to cope with the child, arises in the family or school.

- *The child's stage of development must be considered* when deciding what is abnormal. Some behaviours are normal at an early age but abnormal at a later one. For example, repeated bed-wetting may be normal in a 3-year-old child but is abnormal in a child aged 7. Also, the child's response to life events changes with age. Thus separation from the parents is more likely to affect a younger than an older child.

- *Children are generally less able to express themselves in words.* For this reason, evidence of disturbance often comes from observations of behaviour made by parents, teachers, and others. These informants often give differing accounts, in part because the child's behaviour often varies with his circumstances, and in part because the various informants may have different criteria for abnormality. For this reason, informants should be asked for specific examples of any problem they describe, and asked about the circumstances in which it has been observed.

- Medication is used less in the treatment of children than in the treatment of adults. Instead, there is more emphasis on working with parents and the whole family, reassuring and retraining children, and coordinating the efforts of others who can help children, especially at school. Thus multidisciplinary working is even more important in child than in adult psychiatry. Consequently, treatment is usually provided by a team that includes at least a psychiatrist, psychiatric nurses, a psychologist, and a social worker.

The first part of this chapter is concerned with a number of general issues concerning psychiatric disorder in childhood, including its frequency, causes, assessment, and management. The second part of the chapter contains information about the principal syndromes encountered in the practice of child psychiatry. The chapter does not provide a comprehensive account of child psychiatry. It is an introduction to the main themes for psychiatrists who are undertaking specialist general training. It is expected that they will follow it by reading a specialist text such as one of those listed under further reading on p. 864. Learning disability among children is considered in Chapter 25. Although this is a convenient arrangement, the reader should remember that many aspects of the study and care of learning-disabled children are similar to those described in this chapter.

Normal development

The practice of child psychiatry calls for knowledge of the normal process of development from a helpless infant into an independent adult. In order to judge whether any observed emotional, social, or intellectual functioning is abnormal, it has to be compared with the corresponding normal range for the age group. This section summarizes the main aspects of development that concern the psychiatrist. A textbook of paediatrics should be consulted for details of these developmental phases.

The first year of life

This is a period of rapid development of motor and social functioning. Three weeks after birth, the baby smiles at faces; selective smiling appears by 6 months, fear of strangers by 8 months, and anxiety on separation from the mother shortly thereafter.

Bowlby (1980) emphasized the importance in the early years of life of a general process of attachment of the infant to the parents and of more selective emotional bonding. Although bonding to the mother is most significant, important attachments are also made to the father and other people who are close to the infant. Research has stressed the reciprocal nature of this process and the probable importance of early contacts between the mother (or other carers) and the newborn infant in initiating bonding (Rutter 1995).

By the end of the first year, the child should have formed a close and secure relationship with the mother or other close carer. There should be an ordered pattern of sleeping and feeding, and weaning has usually been accomplished. The child has begun to learn about objects outside himself, simple causal relationships, and spatial relationships. By the end of the first year, the child enjoys making sounds and may say 'mama', 'dada', and perhaps one or two other words.

Year two

This is also a period of rapid development. The child begins to wish to please the parents and appears anxious when they disapprove. He begins to learn to control his behaviour. By now, attachment behaviour should be well established. Temper tantrums occur, particularly if exploratory wishes are frustrated. These tantrums do not last long, and should lessen as the child learns to accept constraints. By the end of the second year he should be able to put two or three words together as a simple sentence.

Pre-school years (2–5 years)

This phase brings a rapid increase in intellectual abilities, especially in the complexity of language. Social development occurs as the child learns to live within the family. He begins to identify with the parents and adopt their standards in matters of conscience. Social life develops rapidly as he learns to interact with siblings, other children, and adults. Temper tantrums continue, but diminish and should disappear before the child starts school. At this age, the child has much curiosity about the environment and may ask a great number of questions.

In children aged 2–5, fantasy life is rich and vivid. It can form a temporary substitute for the real world, enabling desires to be fulfilled regardless of reality. Special objects such as teddy bears or pieces of blanket become important to the child. They appear to comfort and reassure the child, and help sleep. They have been called 'transitional objects'.

The child begins to learn about his own identity. He realizes the differences between males and females in their appearance, clothes, behaviour, and anatomy. Sexual play and exploration are common at this stage.

According to psychodynamic theory, at this stage defence mechanisms develop to enable the child to cope with anxiety arising from unacceptable emotions. These defence mechanisms have been described on p. 188. They include repression, rationalization, compensation, and displacement.

Common problems in early childhood

In children from birth to the beginning of the fifth year, common problems include difficulties in feeding and sleeping, as well as clinging to the parents (separation anxiety), temper tantrums, oppositional behaviour, and minor degrees of aggression.

Middle childhood

By the age of 5, the child should understand his or her identity as boy or girl, and his position in the family. He has to learn to cope with school, and to read, write, and begin to acquire numerical concepts. The teacher becomes an important person in the child's life. At this stage the child gradually learns what he can achieve and what his limitations are. Defence mechanisms, conscience, and standards of social behaviour develop further. According to psychoanalytical theory, this is a period in which psychosexual development is quiescent (the latent period). This notion has been questioned (Paikoff and Brookes-Gunn 1995), and it now seems that in the 5–10-year period sexual interest and activities are present, although they may be concealed from adults.

Common problems in this age group include fears, nightmares, minor difficulties in relationships with peers, disobedience, and fighting.

Adolescence

Adolescence is the growing-up period between childhood and maturity. Among the most obvious features are the physical changes of puberty. The age at which these changes occur is quite variable, usually between 11 and 13 in girls, and 13 and 17 in boys. The production of sex hormones precedes these changes, starting in both sexes between the ages of 8 and 10. Adolescence is a time of increased awareness of personal identity and individual characteristics. At this age, young people become self-aware, are concerned to know who they are, and begin to consider where they want to go in life. They can look ahead, consider alternatives for the future, and feel hope and despair. It is popularly but wrongly believed that emotional turmoil and alienation from the family are characteristic of adolescence (see p. 852).

Peer group relationships are important and close friendships often develop, especially among girls. Membership of a group is common, and this can help the adolescent in moving towards autonomy. Adolescence brings a marked increased in heterosexual interest and activity. At first, tentative approaches are made to the opposite sex. Gradually these become more direct and confident. In late adolescence, there is a capacity for affection towards the opposite sex as well as sexual feelings. How far and in what way sexual feelings are expressed depends greatly on the standards of society and on rules in the family.

Common problems in later childhood and early adolescence

Common problems among children aged from 12 to 16 years include moodiness, anxiety, minor problems of school refusal, difficulties in relationships with peers, disobedience and rebellion including truancy, experimenting with illicit drugs, fighting, and stealing.

Developmental psychopathology

In child psychiatry it is important to adopt a developmental approach for three reasons. First, as explained on p. 797, the child's stage of development determines whether behaviour is normal or pathological; for example, bed-wetting is normal at the age of 3 years but abnormal at the age of 7 years. Second, the effects of life events differ as the child develops; for example, infants aged under 6 months can move to a new caretaker with little disturbance, but children aged 6 months to 3 years of age show great distress when separated from an original caretaker, because an attachment relationship has been formed. After the age of 3 years, attachment bonds are still strong but the child's ability to use language and to understand reduce the effect of a change of caretaker provided that it is arranged sensitively.

The third reason for a developmental approach is that psychopathology may change as the child grows older: anxiety disorders in childhood tend to improve as the child develops; depressive disorders often recur and continue into adult life; conduct disorders frequently continue into adolescence as aggressive and delinquent behaviour, and also commonly as substance abuse – a problem that is less common in younger children.

Continuities and discontinuities from childhood to adulthood depend not only on maturation of the children but also on changes in their environment, especially on changes in the family. An adverse family environment, particularly persistent marital discord, appears to be important, but personality disorder in the parents may be important in causing the marital conflict and the persistent disorder in the child. Conversely, there may be protective factors in the child's environment that reduce some of the continuities between childhood and adult disorder, for example, a close relationship with a caring grandparent. Long-term studies of childhood pathology have been reviewed by Rutter (1996).

Classification of psychiatric disorders in children and adolescents

Both DSM-IV and ICD-10 contain a scheme for classifying the psychiatric disorders of childhood. Disorders of adolescence are classified partly with this scheme, and partly with the categories used in adult psychiatry.

Seven main groups of childhood psychiatric disorders are generally recognized by clinicians and are supported by studies using multivariate analysis (Quay and Werry 1986). The terms used in this book for the seven groups are listed below, with some alternatives in parentheses:

- adjustment reactions;
- pervasive developmental disorders;
- specific developmental disorders;
- conduct (antisocial or externalizing) disorders;

- hyperkinetic (attention-deficit) disorders;
- emotional (neurotic or internalizing) disorders;
- symptomatic disorders.

Many child psychiatric disorders cannot be classified in a satisfactory way by allocating them to a single category. Therefore multiaxial systems have been proposed. ICD-10 has six axes:

1 clinical psychiatric syndromes,
2 specific delays in development,
3 intellectual level,
4 medical conditions,
5 abnormal social situations, and
6 level of adaptive functioning.

In DSM-IV, psychiatric syndrome and specific delays in development are both on axis 1: the other axes are the same as in ICD-10, so that there are five in total. Further information is given by Cantwell and Rutter (1994). This scheme is easy to use, and allows clinicians to record systematically the different kinds of information required in categorizing children's problems.

The DSM-IV and ICD-10 classifications for child psychiatric disorders are shown in Table 24.1. Both schemes are complicated, and so only the main categories are shown in the table. (In this book learning disabilities (mental retardation) in childhood is considered in Chapter 25.) In most ways the two systems are similar; both have categories for specific and pervasive developmental disorders, with the former divided into disorders affecting motor skills, speech and language (communication), and scholastic skills (learning). Both systems have categories for disorders of behaviour, which are divided into conduct (or disruptive behaviour) disorder and attention-deficit (hyperkinetic) disorder. Both systems have a category for anxiety (emotional) disorder (DSM-IV does not provide a separate category for childhood anxiety disorder but uses the adult category instead). Both systems have a category for tic disorders. DSM-IV also has a category for eating and elimination disorders, but ICD-10 classifies these conditions with sleep disorders under 'other

Table 24.1 Classification of childhood psychiatric disorders	
DSM-IV	**ICD–10**
	F8 Disorders of psychological development
Learning disorders	Specific developmental disorders of scholastic skills
Motor skills disorders	Specific developmental disorder of motor function
Communication disorders	Specific developmental disorders of speech and language
Pervasive developmental disorders	Pervasive developmental disorders
	F9 Behavioural and emotional disorders with onset usually occurring in childhood and adolescence
Attention-deficit and disruptive behaviour disorders	Hyperkinetic disorders
	Conduct disorders
	Mixed disorders of conduct and emotions
	Emotional disorders with onset specific to childhood
Tic disorders	Tic disorders
Feeding and eating disorders of infancy – and childhood	–
–	Disorders of social functioning with onset specific to childhood and adolescence
Elimination disorder	–
Other disorders of infancy, childhood, and adolescence	Other behavioural and emotional disorders with onset usually in childhood and adolescence (includes elimination disorders and feeding disorders)

behavioural and emotional disorders'. For further information about classification in child psychiatry see Cantwell and Rutter (1994).

Epidemiology

Behavioural and emotional disorders occur frequently in the general population of children. Estimates vary according to the diagnostic criteria and other methods used, but it appears that rates in the different developed countries are similar. The limited evidence suggests that rates of emotional and behavioural disorders in developing countries are similar to those in developed ones. In the UK, the prevalence of child psychiatric disorder in ethnic minority groups has usually been found to be similar to that in the rest of the population. The exception is a high prevalence of conduct disorder found among West Indian girls (Rutter *et al.* 1974).

The most noteworthy study was carried out more than 30 years ago on the Isle of Wight in the UK. The study was concerned with the health, intelligence, education, and psychological difficulties in all the 10- and 11-year-olds attending state schools in the island – a total of 2193 children (Rutter *et al.* 1970a). Although carried out more than 30 years ago, the findings have generally been confirmed in subsequent research. In the first stage of the enquiry, screening questionnaires were completed by parents and teachers. Children identified in this way were given psychological and educational tests and their parents were interviewed. The 1-year prevalence rate of psychiatric disorder was about 7%, with the rate in boys being twice that in girls. The rate of emotional disorders was 2.5% and the combined rate of conduct disorders together with mixed conduct and emotional disorders was 4%. Conduct disorders were four times more frequent among boys than girls, whereas emotional disorders were more frequent in girls in a ratio of almost 1.5:1. There was no correlation between psychiatric disorder and social class, but prevalence increased as intelligence decreased. It was associated also with physical handicap and especially with evidence of organic brain damage. There was also a strong association between reading retardation and conduct disorder.

A subsequent study using the same methods was carried out in an inner London borough (Rutter *et al.* 1975a, 1975b). Here the rates of all types of disorder were twice those in the Isle of Wight.

The frequency of psychiatric problems varies with age. Richman *et al.* (1982) reported that 7% of 3-year-olds had symptoms amounting to a moderate or severe problem, and a further 15% had mild problems such as disobedience. In the middle years of childhood, rates of psychiatric problems vary in different kinds of area of residence, being twice as high in urban areas (about 25%) than in rural areas (about 12%) (Rutter *et al.* 1975a).

Evidence about adolescence was provided by a 4-year follow-up of the Isle of Wight study (Rutter *et al.* 1976b). At the age of 14, the 1-year prevalence rate of significant psychiatric disorder was about 20%. Prevalence estimates vary between studies (Roberts *et al.* 1998) but most find rates between 15% and 20%.

Studies using DSM criteria find high rates of co-morbidity between childhood disorders. In part this may be because one disorder predisposes to another or because they have common predisposing factors. However, the finding may arise in part because the classification system has gone too far in identifying as distinct disorders, patterns of behaviour that can occur in more than one condition.

The studies considered here were carried out in the UK, but similar findings have been reported elsewhere. For a review see Offord (2000).

Follow-up studies

Mild symptoms and behavioural or developmental problems are usually brief. However, this is not so for the conditions severe enough to be diagnosed as childhood psychiatric disorders, which often persist for several years. Thus in the Isle of Wight Study three-quarters of children with conduct disorder and half of those with emotional disorders at age 10 were still handicapped by these problems 4 years later (Rutter *et al.* 1976b).

The prognosis for adult life has been established in a few long follow-up studies. In an important study, Robins *et al.* (1996) followed up people who had attended a child guidance clinic 30 years previously, and compared them with a control group who had attended the same schools but had not been referred to the clinic. Children with conduct disorder had a poor outcome. As adults they were likely to develop antisocial personality disorder or alcoholism, have problems with employment or marriage, or commit offences. Subsequent studies have shown that children with severe hyperkinetic syndrome are at increased risk of similar outcomes, but only if they have associated problems such as aggression, or severe family problems. Hyperactive children without these other difficulties tend to grow out of their hyperactivity and escape disablement. Some emotional problems starting in childhood have a poor prognosis. Zeitlin (1986) examined the records of people who had attended the same hospital as children and again as adults. He found considerable continuity for many symptoms, especially for depression and obsessional symptoms. Harrington *et al.* (1990) found that depressed adolescents were much more likely than were non-depressed controls to have major depression in adult life. For a review of outcome studies see Rutter (1995).

Aetiology

In discussing the causes of child psychiatric disorders, the principles are similar to those described in the Chapter 5 on the aetiology of adult disorders. Most childhood disorders have multiple causes, with both genetic and environmental components (see Rutter 1999). There is also a developmental aspect; children mature psychologically and socially as they grow up, and their disorders reflect this maturation. In the following paragraphs, four interacting groups of factors will be considered briefly. These are heredity; temperament; physical impairment with special reference to brain damage; and environmental factors in the family, and society. All aspects of aetiology are discussed more fully in the textbook edited by Rutter *et al.* (1994b).

Genetic factors

Children with psychiatric problems often have parents who suffer from a psychiatric disorder. Environmental factors account for a substantial part of this association. However, recent population-based twin studies suggest that there is a significant genetic contribution to many psychiatric disorders, especially hyperactivity and anxiety. These studies suggest that genetic factors are important, not only for emotional and behavioural disorders, but also for the psychological traits that may predispose to these disorders.

The results of individual genetic studies are reviewed later in this chapter; here, some general comments will be made. First, recent studies show the value of using standard criteria for diagnosis, but they also suggest that not all these categories relate closely with the genetic factors in aetiology. For example, the phenotype of autism seems to include some kinds of developmental language disorder, whilst the phenotype of Gilles de la Tourette syndrome seems to include some cases of obsessional disorder. Second, many children have symptoms that qualify for more than one psychiatric diagnosis, for example, depressive disorder and conduct disorder, or eating disorder. As noted above under epidemiology, it is not clear whether this overlap arises because one disorder predisposes to another, or whether they are two manifestations of the same genetic predisposition. Third, it has become clear that single-gene effects may be operating when there is no obvious Mendelian pattern of inheritance. This can arise when many of the affected persons do not have children (for example, in autism), and when the phenotype is very variable so that it is not at first recognized.

The hereditary factors of importance in child psychiatry are polygenic. As in adult life, they interact with psychosocial factors, and genetic investigations may include estimates of environmental factors. There are also indirect genetic influences acting through polygenic control of intelligence and temperament, which in part determine whether situations are experienced as stressful. Methods of genetic investigation are discussed on pp. 126–131, and examples of genetic findings in child psychiatry are given at relevant points in the chapter. In child psychiatry, genetic research has so far been most productive in the study of autism (see p. 826).

For a review of genetic factors in child psychiatry see Rutter *et al.* (1999).

Temperament and individual differences

Many years ago, Thomas *et al.* (1968) carried out an influential longitudinal study in New York. They found that certain temperamental factors detected before the age of 2 might predispose to later psychiatric disorder. In the first 2 years, one group of children ('difficult children') tended to respond to new environmental stimuli by withdrawal, slow adaptation, and an intense behavioural response. Another group ('easy children') responded to new stimuli with positive approach, rapid adaptation, and a mild behavioural response. This group was less likely than the first to develop behavioural disorders later in childhood. The investigators thought that these early temperamental differences were determined both genetically and by environmental factors. Although the validity of the methods in this study, and the significance of the findings, have been questioned (Graham and Stevenson 1987), temperamental factors are still important in discussions of aetiology.

Brain disorder

Although serious physical disease of any kind can predispose to psychological problems in childhood, brain disorders are the most important. In the Isle of Wight Study, about 7% of physically healthy children aged 10–11 years were classified as having psychiatric problems, compared with about 12% of physically ill children of the same age and 34% of children with brain disorders (Rutter *et al.* 1976b). The high prevalence in the latter group was not explained by the adverse social factors known to be associated with the risk of brain disorder. Nor is it likely to have been due to physical disability as such, because rates of psychiatric disorder are less in children equally disabled by muscular disorders. The rate of psychiatric disorder among children with brain damage is related to the severity of the damage, though not closely to the site. It is as common among brain-injured girls as boys, a finding which contrasts with the higher rate of psychiatric disorder among boys in the general population.

Children with brain injury are more likely to develop psychiatric disorder if they encounter adverse psychosocial influences of the kind that provoke psychiatric disorder in children without brain damage (see, for example, the study of children with head injury by Rutter *et al.* 1983).

The theory of minimal brain dysfunction

The observation that defined brain damage was associated with psychiatric disorder led to the suggestion that lesser degrees of damage, insufficient to cause definite neurological signs, could account for otherwise unexplained disorders. The term minimal brain damage was suggested, but was later changed to minimal brain dysfunction after repeated failures to find evidence of any structural changes. It was suggested that this brain dysfunction originated in damage at birth and for a time the phrase 'a continuum of reproductive casualty' (Pasamanick and Knobloch 1966) was used to express this notion. There is an association between histories of abnormal pregnancy, prematurity, and birth asphyxia on the one hand, and psychiatric disorder on the other, but the former factors are also associated with social disadvantage which could be the real cause of the psychiatric disorder. Whilst the concept of minimal brain damage (or dysfunction) has been abandoned, the role of established brain damage is well recognized.

Maturational changes and delayed effects

There are two ways in which the effects of brain lesions are more complex in childhood because the brain is developing:

◆ *Capacity to compensate* The immature brain is more able than the adult brain to compensate for localized damage. For example, even complete destruction of the left hemisphere in early childhood can be followed by normal development of language (Goodman 1987).

◆ *Delayed effects* Early damage may not become manifest as a disorder until a later stage of development when the damaged area takes up a key function. For example, brain injury at birth may not result in seizures until many years later. It has been suggested that there may be similar delays in the behavioural consequences of brain injury.

Lateralized damage and psychopathology

The behavioural effects of lateralized brain damage are less specific in childhood than in adult life. Therefore attempts to explain, for example, educational problems in terms of left- and right-sided damage or dysfunction are unwise, and attempts to use left-brain or right-brain training are unlikely to be helpful.

The consequences of head injury in childhood

Head injury is a common cause of neurological damage in childhood. The form of the disorder is not very specific, partly because the effects of head injury are seldom localized to one area of the brain. Common consequences of severe injury are intellectual impairment and social inhibition. Intellectual impairment is proportional to the severity of the injury, but the relationship of behaviour disorder to the injury is less direct.

Epilepsy as a cause of childhood psychiatric disorder

The relationship between epilepsy and psychiatric disorder in adults is considered on pp. 432–7. In childhood there is a strong association between recurrent seizures and psychiatric disorder. As in adult life, the causal relationship may be of four kinds:

- the brain lesion causing the epilepsy may cause the psychiatric disorder;
- the psychological and social consequences of recurrent seizures may cause the disorder;
- the effects of epilepsy on school performance may cause psychiatric disorder;
- the drugs used to treat epilepsy may cause the disorder through their side-effects.

The *site and the type of epilepsy* seem generally less important, with the exception that temporal lobe epilepsy seems more likely to be associated with psychological disorder. The age of onset of seizures also determines the child's response to epilepsy.

Lead intoxication as a cause of psychological problems

For many years, there has been concern that chronic exposure to lead may impair the developing brain and thereby produce intellectual impairment and behaviour disorder. It is generally accepted that there is an association between IQ and body lead as measured in blood or tooth dentine. However, psychosocial factors could explain the association. Children brought up in poor social conditions may ingest more lead because they play in streets polluted by car exhausts; and IQ is known to be related to social adversity. When social factors are allowed for, it seems that there is still a small but consistent negative association between high lead levels and IQ (Taylor 1991). The possibility of an association between behavioural disorder and lead is even more difficult to investigate because behaviour cannot be measured as precisely as IQ. Cohort studies in several cities in the USA have not given a clear answer to this question (see Taylor 1991 for a review).

Environmental factors

The effect of life events

The concept of life events is useful in child psychiatry as well as in the psychiatry of adult life (see p. 121). Life events may predispose to, or provoke, disorder, or protect against it. Events can be classified by their severity, or their social characteristics, for example, family problems, divorce, or the death of a parent. They can also be classified according to their general significance, for example, as exit events (i.e. separations) or entrance events (i.e. additions to a family by the birth of a sibling).

Some general findings in child psychiatry are that life events have an additive effect, that exit events are associated with anxious and depressive disorders (Goodyer *et al.* 1985), and that events cluster about 4 months before the onset of symptoms (Goodyer *et al.* 1987).

Family influences

As a child progresses from complete dependence on others to independence, he needs a stable and secure family background with a consistent pattern of emotional warmth, acceptance, help, and constructive discipline. Prolonged separation from or loss of parents can have a profound effect on psychological development in infancy and childhood. Poor relationships in the family may have similar adverse effects; overt conflict between the parents seems especially important (Jenkins and Smith 1990).

Shared and non-shared influences.

Investigators have studied the effects of experiences that are shared by all the children in a family, and experiences which are different for the different children. These studies indicate that, with the possible exception of conduct disorders, factors that are not shared are generally more important than are shared factors, as causes of psychiatric disorder in childhood.

Maternal deprivation

The well-known work of Bowlby (1951) led to widespread concern with the effects of 'maternal deprivation'. Bowlby originally suggested that prolonged separation from the mother was a major cause of juvenile delinquency. Subsequently he argued that the early experience or threat of separation from the mother is associated with anxiety or depression in later years (Bowlby 1973, 1980). Also, secure attachments help infants to develop intimacy and trust that will influence their relationships later in life

Since the original formulation of the consequences of maternal deprivation, it has become apparent that the effect of separation depends on many factors. These include the age of the child at the time of separation, his previous relationship with his mother and father, the reasons for the separation, the way in which separation was managed, and the quality of the new care. Also, insecure attachments have been divided into avoidant attachments associated with either rejecting or intrusive care, and resistant or ambivalent attachments associated with inconsistent care. Lack of stimulation in early life and lack of encouragement to learn may result in educational underachievement. It is still thought that poor emotional attachments in early life may result in difficulties in social relationships.

Family risk factors

Family risk factors for psychiatric disorder in childhood are multiple and additive. The risk increases in children of families with severe marital discord, low social status, large size or overcrowding, paternal criminality, and maternal psychiatric disorder. The risk is also increased in children placed in care away from the family. In children with one risk factor, rates of psychiatric disorder are not significantly greater than in children with no risk factors. Children with two risk factors have a fourfold increase in rate of disorder. One in five of children with four risk factors have psychiatric disorder (Garmezy and Mastern 1994).

Protective factors

Protective factors reduce the rate of psychiatric disorder associated with a given level of risk factors. Protective factors include good mothering, strong affectionate ties within the family, sociability and the capacity for problem solving in the child, and support outside the family from individuals, or from the school or church (Werner and Smith 1982; Rutter 1985).

Child-rearing practices

Patterns of child rearing are not clearly related to psychiatric disturbance in the child except when they involve abuse of the child (Rutter and Madge 1976). Physical and sexual abuse (see pp. 855 and 858) are important risk factors.

Effects of alternative child care

Working mothers entrust part of the care of their children to other people. In general, the use of alternative child care does not appear to be a risk factor for psychiatric disorder. Good child care may improve the attachment and language development of children whose mothers are less sensitive to their needs (see NICHD Early Child Care Research Group 1997).

Effects of parental mental disorder

Rates of psychological problems are higher in the children of parents with mental illness than in the children of healthy parents (Rutter 1966). These problems usually involve poor adjustment at home or at school, and often include disruptive behaviour (Orvaschel 1983; Radke-Yarrow *et al.* 1993). The causes are complex, but it is known that depressed mothers involve themselves less with their children, thus providing a less stimulating environment (Gordon *et al.* 1989; Stein *et al.* 1991). Older children of depressed mothers may be depressed, an association that could be determined genetically or through environmental factors. Schizophrenia impairs mothering skills when the mother has psychotic symptoms, negative symptoms, or impairment of affect.

Recently there has been increasing concern about the psychological development of the children of *mothers who misuse alcohol or drugs*. Such children suffer from a series of disadvantages which are related to the effects of drug taking on the mother's care of the child, as well as to features of the mother's personality that led her to take drugs, and to associated social problems. For a review see Hogan (1998).

Effects of divorce

The children of divorced parents have more psychological problems than the children of parents who are not divorced. It is not certain how far these problems precede the divorce and are related to disharmony between the parents, or to the behaviour of one or both parents that contributed to the decision to divorce.

Distress and dysfunction in the children are greatest in the year after the divorce; after 2 years these problems are still present but are generally less severe than those of children remaining in conflictual marriages. There is some evidence that among children brought up by a divorced mother, boys have more problems than girls (Hetherington *et al.* 1985). For a review of the long-term effects of divorce on children, see Wallerstein (1991).

Death of a parent

In children, the response to the death of a parent varies with age. Children aged below 4–5 years do not have a complete concept of death as causing permanent separation. Such children react with despair and anxiety to separation, however caused, and their reaction to bereavement is not different.

Children aged 5–11 years have increasing understanding of death. They usually become depressed and overactive, and may show disorders of conduct. Some have suicidal thoughts and ideas that death would unite them with the lost parent. Suicidal actions are infrequent. In children over the age of 11 years, the response is increasingly like that of adults (see p. 208).

Bereavement may have long-term effects on development, especially if the child was young at the time of the parent's death and if the death was sudden or violent. Outcome probably depends largely on the effects of the bereavement on the surviving parent. Most studies of bereavement in children have been concerned with the death of a parent; few have concerned the death of a sibling. For a review see Black (2000) or Worden (1996).

Social and cultural factors

Although the family is undoubtedly the part of the child's environment with most effect on his development, wider social influences are important as well, particularly in the aetiology of conduct disorder. In the early years of childhood, these social factors act indirectly through their influence on the patterns of family life. As the child grows older and spends more time outside the family, they have a direct effect as well. These factors have been studied by examining the associations between psychiatric disorder and type of neighbourhood and school.

Effects of neighbourhood

Rates of childhood psychiatric disorder are higher in areas of social disadvantage. For example, as already noted (p. 802), the rates of both emotional and conduct disorder were found to be higher in a poor inner London borough than in the Isle of Wight. The important features of inner city life may be lack of play space, inadequate social amenities for older children and teenagers, overcrowded living conditions, and lack of community involvement.

Effects of school

It has long been known that rates of child psychiatric referral and delinquency vary between schools (Power *et al.* 1972; Gath *et al.* 1977). These differences persist when allowance is made for differences in the neighbourhoods in which the children live. It seems that children are less likely to develop psychiatric problems in a school in which teachers praise, encourage and give responsibility to their pupils, set high standards, and organize their teaching well. Factors that seem not to affect rates of psychiatric disorder include the size of the school and the age of its buildings.

Bullying is one of the stressful events that children may encounter ate school. Goodman and Scott (1997, p. 218) define bullying as the repeated and deliberate use of physical or psychological means to hurt another child, without adequate provocation and in the knowledge that the victim is unlikely to retaliate effectively. It seems that between 2 and 8% of children are bullied once or more a week (Goodman and Scott 1997). They may be divided into a passive group, who are insecure and anxious and withdraw when attacked, and a provocative group, who are themselves aggressive directly or by getting others into trouble, and many of whom are aggressive. The bullies are more often boys than girls; boys are more likely to be physically aggressive, girls more likely to exclude their victims or campaign against them. Bullying causes much immediate distress but its long-term effects are not known. Schools can take action to reduce the rates of bullying. For further information see Olweus (1994) or Salmon and West (2000).

Psychiatric assessment of children and their families

The aims of assessment are to obtain a clear account of the presenting problem, to find out how this problem is related to the child's past development and his present life in its psychological and social context, and to plan treatment of the child and family.

The psychiatric assessment of children differs in several ways from that of adults:

◆ *A more flexible approach* With children it is often difficult to follow a set routine: a flexible approach to interviewing is required, though it is still important that information and observations are recorded systematically.

◆ *Interview family members* Both parents should be asked to attend the assessment interview, and it is often helpful to have other siblings present.

◆ *Information from schools* Time can be saved by asking permission to obtain information from teachers before the child attends the clinic. This information should be concerned with the child's behaviour in school and his educational attainments.

Child psychiatrists vary in their methods of assessment. All agree that it is important to see the family together at some stage to observe how they interact. Some psychiatrists do this before seeing the patient alone, others do it afterward. It is generally better to see an adolescent patient on his own before seeing the parents. With younger children the main informants are usually the parents, but children over the age of 6 should usually be seen on their own at some stage. In the special case of suspected child abuse, the interview with the child is particularly important. Whatever the problem, the parents should be made to feel that the interview is supportive and does not undermine their confidence.

Interviewing the parents

Parents should be encouraged to talk spontaneously before systematic questions are asked. The methods of interviewing are similar to those used in adult psychiatry (see Chapter 2). A full list of the items to be included in the history have been listed by Graham (1991), which appears in the Appendix to this chapter. As in adult psychiatry, an experienced interviewer will keep the complete list in mind, while focusing on those relevant to the particular case. It is important to obtain specific examples of general problems, to elicit factual information, and to assess feelings and attitudes. There are several standardized schedules for interviewing parents; they are described in reference books such as Rutter *et al.* (1994b).

Interviewing and observing the child

Because younger children may not be able or willing to express ideas and feelings in words, observations of their behaviour and interaction with the interviewer are especially important; with very young children, drawing and the use of toys may be helpful. With older children, it may be possible to follow a procedure similar to that used with adults, provided care is taken to use words and concepts appropriate to the child's age and background. Several standardized systems of observation have been described for specific purposes. They are described in books of reference such as Rutter *et al.* (1994b).

It is essential to begin by establishing a friendly atmosphere and winning the child's confidence, and asking him what he likes to be called. It is usually appropriate to begin with a discussion of neutral topics such as pets, favourite games, or birthdays, before turning to the presenting problem. When a friendly relationship has been established, the child can be asked about the problem, his likes and dislikes, and his hopes for the future. It is often informative to ask what he would request if given three wishes. Younger children may be given the opportunity to express their concerns and feelings in paintings or play. Children can generally recall events accurately, but they are more suggestible than adults; therefore it is particularly important not to use leading questions in interviewing, and not to suggest actions or interpretations to a child who is being observed at painting or play.

The child's behaviour and mental state should be observed. The items to be noted are listed in the Appendix to this chapter (p. 862). Children who are brought to see a psychiatrist may appear silent and withdrawn at the first meeting; this behaviour

should not be misinterpreted as evidence of depression. At some stage, preferably late in the consultation, a physical examination may be performed, with particular attention to the central nervous system (see Appendix). By the end of the interview an assessment should have been made of the child's stage of development relative to other children of the same age.

Interviewing the family

A family interview can contribute to the assessment of the interactions between family members, but it is not a good way to obtain factual information. The latter is generally obtained better in interviews with the parents or other family members seen on their own. Of the various aspects of family interaction, the psychiatrist will usually be most interested in discord and disorganization, which are the features most closely associated with the development of psychiatric disorder. Patterns of communication between family members are also important.

It is usually best to see the family at the first assessment or soon after this, before the interviewer has formed a close relationship with the patient, or with one of the parents, since this may make it more difficult to interview the others.

The interviewer may begin by asking: 'Who would be the best person to tell me about the problems?' If one member monopolizes the interview, another member should be asked to comment on what has been said. A useful question to stimulate discussion is: 'How do you think that your wife (husband, son) would see the problem?' The interviewer can then ask the wife (husband, son) how they in fact see the problem. As an alternative, family members who are present can be asked what they think an **absent** member would think about the issues.

While observing the family's ways of responding to these and other questions, the interviewer should consider the following:

- Who is the spokesman for the family?
- Who seems most worried about the problem?

◆ What are the alliances within the family?

◆ What is the hierarchy in the family, e.g. who is most dominant?

◆ How well do the family members communicate with one another?

◆ How do they seem to deal with conflict?

Psychological assessment

Measures of intelligence and educational achievement are often valuable. Thus if mental development and achievement are inconsistent with chronological or mental age, or with the expectations of parents or teachers, this may indicate a generalized or specific disorder of development or may indicate a source of stress in disorders of other kinds. Some of the more commonly used procedures are listed in Table 24.2. Projective tests are not recommended because it is difficult to score them reliably and their validity is doubtful.

Other information

The most important additional informants are the child's teachers. They can describe classroom behaviour, educational achievements, and relationships with other children. They may also make useful comments about the family and home circumstances. It is often helpful for a member of the psychiatric team to visit the home. This visit can provide useful information about material circumstances in the home, the relationship of family members, and the pattern of their life together.

Ending the assessment

At the end of the assessment the psychiatrist should explain to the parents – and to the child, depending on age – the result of the assessment and the plan of management. He should explain how he proposes to inform and work with the general practitioner, and seek permission to contact other people involved with the child, such as teachers, or social workers. Throughout, the psychiatrist should encourage questions and discussion.

Formulation

A formulation should be made in every case. This starts with a brief statement of the current problem. The diagnosis and differential diagnosis are discussed next. Aetiological factors are then considered. The developmental stages of the child should be noted, as well as any particular strengths and achievements. An assessment of the problems and the strengths of the family are also recorded. Any further assessments should be specified, a treatment plan drawn up, and the expected outcome recorded.

Court reports

Psychiatrists may be asked to prepare court reports in relation to children. These reports are usually undertaken by specialists in child psychiatry; hence only an outline will be given here. If general psychiatrists are required to make such a report, they should ensure that they are thoroughly aware of the relevant legislation, ask advice from a colleague with relevant special experience, and read a more detailed account of the requirements for Court reports, for example Black *et al.* (1998) or Wolkind (1994), who describe UK practice.

Courts concerned with children obtain evidence from several sources, including social workers, probation officers, community nurses, psychologists, and psychiatrists. In their reports psychiatrists should focus on matters within their expertise, including:

◆ the child's age, stage of development, and temperament and its relevance to the case;

◆ whether the child has a psychiatric disorder;

◆ the child's own wishes about his future, considered in relation to his age and understanding;

◆ the parenting skills of the carers, how far they can meet the child's needs, and other relevant aspects of the family.

Whilst focusing on these matters, the psychiatrist should also be prepared to provide information about the following issues (which are referred to in

Table 24.2 Notes on some psychological measures in use with children and learning-disabled people

Intelligence tests

Stanford-Binet intelligence scale
A revision of the original intelligence test; now seldom used. Provides mental age. Weighted to verbal abilities and this may result in cultural bias. More useful for middle-class patients and for low ability

Weschler intelligence scale for children (WISC III)
Provides a profile of specific verbal and performance ability as well as IQ for children aged 6–14 years; widely used and well standardized; cannot be used for IQ below 40

Weschler pre-school and primary scale of intelligence (WPPSI)
A version of WISC for use with younger children

British ability scales
(4–6.5 years) and with the mentally retarded Twenty-four subscales suitable for 2.5–17 years, and covering six areas: speed of information processing; reasoning; spatial imagery; perceptual matching; short-term memory; retrieval; application of knowledge Analysis can be general or specific

Goodenough-Harris drawing test
A brief test of non-verbal intelligence for children aged 3–10 years

Social development assessments

Vineland social maturity scale
The original development scale recently revised, which has psychometric limitations; covers general self-help, self-help in dressing, self-help in eating, locomotion, communication, self-direction, social isolation, and occupation; provides 'social age'

Adaptive behaviour scales (Nihira)
Rating scales to evaluate abilities and habits in 10 behavioural areas

Gunzburg progress assessment charts
Provides a clear visual display of self-help, communication, social and occupational abilities

Other developmental assessment

Denver development scale
Assessment of gross and fine motor skills, language, and social development; used for children up to 2 years of age

Bayley scales of infant development
Range of items which can be scored on mental and psychomotor development indices; comprehensive and reliable to ages 2 months to 2.5 years

Educational attainment

Neale analysis of reading
Graded test of reading ability, accuracy, comprehension, and rate for age 6 upwards

Schonell graded word reading test
The child reads words of increasing difficulty

Schonell graded word spelling test
The child spells words of increasing difficulty

Tests of mathematical ability
No satisfactory test; use arithmetic subtests of WISC-R, WPPSI, and British ability scales

the Children's Act 1989 of England and Wales – see Harrison 1991):

- the child's physical, emotional, and educational needs;
- the likely effect on the child of any change of circumstances (for example, removal from home, or living with one or other parent after a divorce);
- any harm that the child has suffered or is likely to suffer.

The wishes of the child should be considered in relation to his age and ability to understand the present situation and possible future arrangements, and to relevant factors in the present situation; for example, some abused children maintain strong attachments with the abuser.

Parenting skills are judged partly on the history and reports of other people; they are also judged partly on direct observations of the interactions between the parents and child, including the parent's attachment to the child, sensitivity to cues from the child, and ability to meet the child's needs.

The report is similar in structure to a court report for an adult and presented under the headings shown in Box 24.1.

Children as witnesses

A child's evidence is important in cases of suspected abuse, and occasionally in another kinds of case such as an assault on the mother. When seeking such evidence, the interviewer should be aware of certain points about children's memory and the factors that can influence their accounts.

Memory varies with age, as do the verbal skills required to describe what has been remembered. Children below the age of 3 years seldom have the cognitive and other capacities to produce an account that can be presented in a court of law. Children above the age of 3 years can produce detailed and accurate memories, though they may not be able to describe them clearly without some prompting. Most children above the age of 6 years can use straightforward grammar and syntax

---

Box 24.1 Topics to be addressed in a court report about a child

The *qualifications* of the writer

Who commissioned the report, and what questions were asked

What *written information* was available, and who was interviewed

A summary of the *findings from the interview* (it is not necessary to repeat information contained in social enquiry reports

The writer's *interpretation* of the information from the interviews and written material

In the light of the findings, *comments* on the options before the court, remembering always that it is for the court and not the psychiatrist to determine which option is selected

---

adequately, but their vocabulary is limited and they may be confused by complicated questions. Also, children of this age may expect that an adult who asks a question already knows the right answer since this is how they learn – for example, 'how many flowers did you see in the picture?' Consequently, they may agree with leading questions asked by an adult or, when they cannot remember, make up an answer in the hope that it will be the one wanted by the questioner. A further problem is that young children do not have an accurate sense of the sequencing and timing of events. Finally, the events that children are asked to recall when they are questioned as witnesses are usually frightening and experienced in a state of emotional arousal. Memories of such events are often incomplete, though the recalled fragments may be detailed and vivid.

Thompson and Pearce (2000) suggest the following principles when evidence is obtained from a child:

- allow the child to talk freely asking as few questions as possible;
- obtain the evidence as soon as possible after the event, and if possible before any counselling has taken place;

- try to complete the account on the first occasion since subsequent accounts are likely to be less accurate;
- be aware that the greater the pressure to remember, the less accurate is the account likely to be.

For a review of memory in childhood see Fundudis (1997); for further information about interviewing young children as witnesses see Thompson and Pearce (2000) or Saywitz and Camparo (1998).

Psychiatric treatment for children and families

The role of the primary care team

General practitioners and other members of the primary care team spend much of their time in advising and reassuring parents about children, but they refer only a small proportion of these children to a child psychiatrist or a paediatrician (Bailey *et al.* 1978). General practitioners are more likely to refer certain problems to a paediatrician, for example, developmental difficulties, physical symptoms with a probable psychological cause, and psychological complications of physical illness. Emotional and conduct disorders are more likely to be referred to a child psychiatry clinic. Many of the disorders referred are no more severe than those which the general practitioner manages himself (Gath *et al.* 1977), presumably because the decision to refer depends on other factors such as the wishes of the parents or the family situation.

The psychiatric team

Although the members of the team (doctors, social workers, and psychologists) have special skills, they do not confine themselves to their traditional professional roles when working with children and families. Instead, they take whatever role seems most likely to be helpful in the particular case.

It is usual to adopt a family approach, and to maintain close liaison with other people or agencies working with the child or his family, including paediatricians, child health and social services, teachers, and educational psychologists. Since many childhood problems are evident at school, or lead to educational difficulties, the child's teachers usually need to be involved in treatment. Teachers may require advice about the best way to manage disturbed behaviour, changes may be needed in the child's school timetable, or remedial teaching may be required. Occasionally a change of school is indicated.

In the following sections, brief general descriptions are given of the main kinds of treatment. In the second part of the chapter, further information is given about the management of individual disorders. Further information about treatment in child psychiatry can be obtained from one of the textbooks listed at the end of this chapter.

Medication

Drugs have a limited but increasing place in child psychiatry. The main indications are in the treatment of epilepsy, depressive disorders, obsessional disorders, overactivity syndromes, Gilles de la Tourette syndrome, and, occasionally, nocturnal enuresis (these uses are considered later in this chapter). In all cases, dosages should be checked carefully in the manufacturer's literature or a standard reference book, making sure that the dose is correct for the child's age and body weight.

Psychological treatment

Psychological aspects of management

Whatever the plan of management, children benefit from a warm, secure, and accepting relationship with the therapist. The security of this relationship helps the child to express feelings and to find alternative ways of behaving. For younger children, play with toys can help establish the relationship and provide a medium through which they can express their problems and feelings more effectively than they can with words.

At first, the child often perceives the therapist as an agent of the parents, and expects the therapist to share their attitudes. The child should feel accepted in his own right, and not criticized However, he should not be allowed to feel that anything he does will be approved. It is often advisable to delay discussion of the presenting problems until the child's confidence has been gained by talking about neutral things that interest him.

Children can benefit from support and counselling adapted to their age and understanding Two forms of more elaborate psychological treatment are available, cognitive–behaviour therapy and psychodynamic psychotherapy.

Cognitive–behaviour therapy

Behavioural methods have several applications in child psychiatry. They can be used to encourage new behaviour by positive reinforcement and modelling. This is often done by first rewarding behaviour that approximates to the desired behaviour (shaping), and then giving reinforcement in a more discriminating way. For example, with autistic children, shaping has been used for behavioural problems such as temper tantrums and refusal to go to bed. Punishment is not used in shaping behaviour because its effects are temporary and it is ethically unacceptable. Instead, efforts are made to identify and remove any factors in the child's environment that are reinforcing unwanted behaviour. It is often found that undesired behaviour is being reinforced unwittingly by extra attention given to the child when the behaviour occurs. If the child is ignored at such times and attended to when his behaviour is more normal, beneficial changes often take place. More specific forms of behaviour therapy are available for enuresis (see p. 847) and phobias (see p. 840). Social skills training in a group or in individual sessions may be used for children who have difficulty in relationships with other children and adults. The methods generally resemble those used with adults (see Chapter 22).

Cognitive therapy is useful for older children who can describe and learn to control the ways of thinking that give rise to symptoms and problem behaviours. Older children and adolescents with anxiety disorders and eating disorders can be treated with methods devised for adults. Special techniques have been devised for children with aggressive behaviour (see p. 835).

For a review of the efficacy of cognitive–behaviour therapy in childhood and adolescent depression, see Harrington *et al.* (1998b).

Psychodynamic therapies

Most psychodynamic approaches are based on the methods of Anna Freud and Melanie Klein. Reviews have generally concluded that, whilst many outcome studies have methodological flaws, the better investigations indicate that dynamic psychotherapy is rather more effective than no treatment. However, psychodynamic therapy has not been shown to produce better results than those of counselling or cognitive–behaviour therapy. Consequently, psychodynamic therapies are now used infrequently in the UK (Casey and Berman 1985; Barnett *et al.* 1991).

For a more positive assessment of the value of psychodynamic therapies for children see Fonagy and Target (2000). For an assessment of the general effectiveness of the psychotherapy for children and adolescents, see Weisz *et al.* (1995).

Parent training

Parent training is used to improve the skills of parents with deficient parenting skills, including those who abuse or neglect their children and those with low intelligence. It is also used to assist parents of children with behaviour problems that require special parenting skills, for example, the parents of children with conduct disorder or hyperactivity. Most research has been with parents of children who are oppositional or defiant or have conduct disorders [see, for example, the early studies of Patterson (1982), and the investigations of Webster-Stratton (1991)]. Parent training can be carried out with an educational approach, in which skills of general importance are taught, or with a behavioural approach, in which the specific problems of the particular parent and child are analysed and corrected. In the behavioural approach, use may be made of videotape vignettes showing desirable and undesirable parental responses to children's behaviour. These responses are discussed with the parents of one child, or with a group of parents. Whatever approach is adopted, it is important to take account of the stage of development of the child and of the changing needs of children of different ages.

Studies of the behavioural training of parents have generally found it to be more effective in the short term than less structured approaches, but the long-term benefits have not been established with certainty.

Family therapy

This is a specific form of treatment to be distinguished from the general family approach to treatment, described above. In family therapy, the symptoms of the child or adolescent are considered as an expression of malfunctioning of the family, which is the primary focus of treatment. Several approaches have been used based on behavioural or psychoanalytical systems, or on communication or structural theories. These kinds of therapy are described on pp. 757–60. In practice, most therapists adopt an eclectic approach (see p. 759). The practice of family therapy in child and adolescent psychiatry has been reviewed by Barker (1988).

The *indications* for family therapy are still debated, but most would agreed that such treatment may be appropriate under the following conditions:

♦ the child's symptoms appear to be part of a disturbance of the whole family;

♦ individual therapy is not proving effective; or

♦ family difficulties have arisen during another kind of treatment.

The contraindications for family therapy are that the parents' marriage is breaking up, or the child's problems do not seem to be closely related to family function. It is important that a therapist's interest in family therapy should not prevent a thorough evaluation of the case and the use of other treatments when indicated.

Uncontrolled *evaluations* of family therapy have led to claims that it has substantial effects. Controlled evaluations suggest more modest benefits for children with a wide range of emotional and behavioural disorders. In a study of a mixed group of children with emotional and behavioural disorders, the benefits of Milan Family Therapy for the child were no greater than those of eclectic treatment (Simpson 1990). However, when dynamic family therapy was used for eating disorders in adolescents, the benefits were greater than those of a control treatment (Russell *et al.* 1987). For further information on family therapy, including its evaluation, see Bloch and Harari (2000) and Shadish *et al.* (1995).

Group therapy

Group therapy may be carried out with parents, or with older children and adolescents. Parents may be helped by the opportunity to discuss shared problems of child management or other difficulties. Children may benefit from the support, discussion, and opportunities for modelling adaptive behaviour that form part of group therapy. Group therapy is described on pp. 747–54. The general effectiveness of group therapy for children and adolescents is reviewed by Hoag and Burlingame (1997).

Social work

Social workers play an important role in the care of children with psychiatric disorders and of their families. In the UK, they have statutory duties for the protection of children who are at risk within the family, and who require special care or special supervision. They help parents to improve their skills in caring for their children and to solve problems with finances or accommodation. Social workers carry out family assessments and family therapy, and also provide individual counselling for the child and members of the family.

Occupational therapy

Occupational therapists can play a valuable part in assessment of the child's development, in psychological treatment, and in devising measures to improve parent-child interaction. They work both in day- and in-patient units, and in the community. They work closely with teachers both in assessing and providing therapeutic activities for children.

Special education

Children attending at out-patient clinics, and the smaller number who are day- or in-patients, often benefit from additional educational arrangements. Special teaching may be needed to remedy backwardness in writing, reading, and arithmetic, which is common among children with conduct disorders as well as those with specific developmental disorders.

Substitute care

Residential care

Residential care can be valuable for children with symptoms that result from or are maintained by a severely unstable home environment or extreme parental rejection. Children considered for residential placement often have conduct disorders and severe educational problems. Removal of a child from home should be considered only after every practical effort has been made to improve the circumstances of the family. Residential care may be provided in a foster home, a children's home (in which a group of about 10 children live in circumstances as close as possible to those of a large family), or a residential school.

Residential care is seldom arranged for children under 5 years of age because they have a special need for attachment to parental figures. In general, children who have been in residential care have high rates of psychosocial problems in later childhood and in adult life. As men they most often have problems with the law, whilst as women they most often have unmarried pregnancy and parenting problems. It is not clear how far these problems

relate to the experience of residential care or to previous adverse experiences that led to the residential placement. Reports of the abuse of children placed within care are reminders of the need to ensure good training and supervision of the staff of children's homes and residential schools.

For a review of residential care see Wolkind and Rushton (1994) and Sinclair (2000).

Fostering

Foster care may be of three kinds:

◆ *short-term emergency care*, for example, when a care-giver is ill or when the parents of an autistic child need respite;

◆ *medium-term care*, which may be followed by return home, for example, if the care-giver is receiving treatment for problems that led to neglect or abuse of the child;

◆ *long-term care*, in which the child remains until able to leave independently.

Children in long-term foster care have more problems than children who have been adopted, but it is difficult to determine how far these problems are related to experiences before fostering and how far they are due to the lesser security of fostering as against adoption. Problems seem to be greater when the fostered child is older and when children in the fostering family are of the same age as the fostered child. Children in foster care usually retain some contact with their biological parents. It is not helpful to the child to have sporadic and distressing contacts or to have contacts when there is no prospect of returning home. For a review of fostering see Wolkind and Rushton (1994).

In-patient and day-patient care

Child psychiatric in-patient units require easy access to paediatric advice, adequate space for play, easy access to schooling, and an informal design that still allows close observation. There should be some provisions for mothers to stay with their children.

Admission for in-patient treatment is usually arranged for any of three reasons:

- *severity*: the disorder is too severe to treat in any other way, for example, extreme hyperactivity, severe pervasive developmental disorder, life-threatening anorexia nervosa, and school refusal resistant to out-patient treatment;
- *need for observation* when the diagnosis is uncertain;
- *separation*: in-patient treatment can provide a necessary period away from a severely disturbing home environment, for example, when there is child abuse or gross over-protection.

Sometimes the mother is admitted as well as the child, thus helping to maintain the bonds between the two. This arrangement also allows close observation of the ways in which the mother responds to the child, for example in cases of child abuse. It is also an opportunity for the mother to learn new parenting skills by taking an increasing part in the child's care while both remain in hospital. For a review of in-patient care, see Black *et al.* (1998).

Day-hospital treatment for children provides many of the advantages of in-patient care without removing them from home. Unless there is any danger that the child may be abused, remaining at home has the advantage that relationships with other family members are maintained. Day care can relieve the family from some of the stressful effects of managing an overactive or autistic child.

Review of syndromes

The review of syndromes begins with the problems encountered in pre-school children. Specific and pervasive developmental disorders are described next. An account is then given of the main psychiatric disorders of childhood, in the order in which they appear in the major systems of classification. Other psychiatric disorders of childhood appear next before a brief account of the disorders of adolescence (which are generally similar to those of either childhood or adult life). The chapter ends with the subject of child abuse. Table 24.3 shows the arrangement of the remaining sections of this

chapter and shows where to find three additional topics which occur in both childhood and adult life.

Problems of pre-school children and their families

It has already been noted that in the pre-school years children are learning several kinds of social behaviour. They are acquiring sphincter control. They are learning how to behave at mealtimes, to go to bed at an appropriate time, and to control angry feelings. They are also becoming less dependent. All these behaviours are learned within the family. The psychiatric problems of pre-school children centre around these behaviours and they often reflect factors in the family as well as factors in the child. Many psychological problems at this age are brief, and can be thought of as delays in normal development. Most of these problems are treated by general practitioners and paediatricians. The more serious problems may be referred to child psychiatrists.

Prevalence

Richman *et al.* (1982) studied a sample of 705 families with a 3-year-old child in a London borough. The most frequent abnormalities of behaviour in these children were bed-wetting at least three times a week (present in 37%), wetting by day at least once a week (17%), overactivity (14%), soiling at least once a week (13%), difficulty in settling at night (13%), fears (13%), disobedience (11%), attention seeking (10%), and temper tantrums (5%).

Whether these behaviours are reported as problems depends on the attitudes of the parents as well as on the nature, severity, and frequency of the behaviour. Richman *et al.* overcame this difficulty by making their own ratings of the extent of problems. They based this assessment on the effects on the child's well-being and the consequences for the other members of the family. They used common-sense criteria to decide whether the problems were mild, moderate, or severe. Seven per cent of 3-year-olds

Table 24.3 Arrangement of sections on disorder of children in this and other chapters

Problems of pre-school children and their families

Specific developmental disorders

    Specific reading disorder

    Mathematics disorder (specific arithmetic disorder)

    Communication disorders

    Motor skills disorder

Pervasive developmental disorders

    Childhood autism

    Rett's disorder

    Overactive disorder with mental retardation and stereotyped movements

    Childhood disintegrative disorder

    Asperger's syndrome

    Atypical autism and pervasive developmental disorder

Hyperkinetic disorder

Conduct disorders

    Truancy

(Juvenile delinquency)

Anxiety disorders

    Separation anxiety disorder

    Phobic anxiety disorder

    Social anxiety disorder of childhood

    Sibling rivalry disorder

    Post-traumatic stress disorder

    Obsessive-compulsive disorders

Somatoform disorders and other unexplained physical symptoms

    Conversion disorders

Mood disorders

(School refusal)

Other childhood psychiatric disorders

    Functional enuresis

    Faecal soiling

    Elective mutism

    Stammering

    Dementia

    Schizophrenia

Gender identity disorders

    Effeminacy in boys

    Tomboyishness in girls

Suicide and deliberate self-harm

Psychiatric aspects of physical illness in childhood

Psychiatric problems of adolescence

Child abuse

    Physical abuse (non-accidental injury)

    Emotional abuse

    Child neglect

    Non-organic failure to thrive and deprivation dwarfism

    Sexual abuse

Conditions considered in other chapters

    Tic disorders (p. 430)

    Suicide and deliberate self-harm (pp. 513 and 530)

    Factitious disorder by proxy (p. 475)

in their survey had behaviour problems of marked severity and 15% had mild problems. The behaviours most often rated as problems were temper tantrums, attention seeking, and disobedience.

Prognosis

As explained above, many psychological problems of pre-school children are brief. However, Richman *et al.* (1982) found that certain problems detected in 3-year-old children were still present at the age of 8. These problems were overactivity, difficulty in controlling the child, speech difficulty, effeminacy, and autism.

Aetiology

Aetiological factors are related to the stage of development, the child's temperament, and influences in the family. There are wide individual variations in the rate at which normal development proceeds, particularly in sphincter control and language acquisition. As noted above (p. 803), a child's temperamental characteristics are evident from the earliest weeks. These characteristics are capable of affecting the mother's response – how much time she spends with her child, how often she picks him up, and so on. These maternal responses may in turn affect the child's development. Behaviour problems at this age are also associated with poor marital relationships, maternal depression, rivalry with siblings, and inadequate parental behaviour. See Richman *et al.* (1982) and Campbell (1995) for further information.

Some common problems of pre-school children

Temper tantrums

Occasional temper tantrums are normal in toddlers, and only persistent or very severe tantrums are abnormal. The immediate cause is often unwitting reinforcement by excessive attention and inconsistent discipline on the part of the parents. When this arises it is often because the parents have emotional problems of their own or because the relationship between them is unsatisfactory. Temper tantrums usually respond to kind but firm and consistent setting of limits. In treatment it is first necessary to discover why the parents have been unable to set limits in this way. They should be helped with any problems of their own and advised how to respond to the tantrums.

Sleep problems

The most frequent sleep difficulty is wakefulness at night, which is most frequent between the ages of 1 and 4 years. About a fifth of children of this age take at least an hour to get to sleep or are wakeful for long periods during the night. When wakefulness is an isolated problem and not very distressing to the family, it is enough to reassure parents that it is likely to improve. When sleep disturbances are severe or persistent, two possible causes should be considered. First, the problems may have been made worse by physical illness or an emotional disorders. Second, they may have been exacerbated by the parents' excessive concern and inability to reassure the child. If no medical or psychiatric disorder is detected, the reasons for the parents' concerns should be sought and dealt with as far as possible. Some parents overstimulate their child in the evening, or condone crying in the night by taking the child into their own bed. A behavioural approach to these problems is generally helpful (Richman *et al.* 1985). The handbook by Douglas and Richman (1984) is useful for parents.

Hypnotic medication may be used occasionally for special occasions but should not be used in the long term.

Other sleep problems such as nightmares and night terrors are common among healthy toddlers but they seldom persist for long. They are discussed on p. 441.

For a review of sleep problems see France and Hudson (1993).

Feeding problems

Minor food fads or food refusal are common in pre-school children, but do not usually last long. In a minority the behaviour is severe or persistent, although not accompanied by signs of poor nourishment. When this happens it is often because the parents, who are often overattentive and perfectionistic, are unwittingly reinforcing the child's behaviour.

Treatment is directed to the parents' management of the problem. They should be encouraged to ignore the feeding problem and refrain from offering the child special foods or otherwise attempting to do anything unusual to persuade him to eat. Instead, he should be offered a normal meal and left to decide whether to eat it or not.

Pica

Pica is the eating of items generally regarded as inedible, for example soil, paint, and paper. It is often associated with other behaviour problems. Cases should be investigated carefully because some are due to brain damage, or autism, or mental retardation. Some are associated with emotional distress, which should be reduced if possible. Otherwise, treatment consists of common-sense precautions to keep the child away from the abnormal items of diet. Pica usually diminishes as the child grows older. For a review of the history of ideas about pica see Parry-Jones and Parry-Jones (1992).

Reactive attachment disorder of infancy and early childhood.

This term denotes a syndrome starting before the age of 5 years and associated with grossly abnormal care-giving. There are two subtypes: inhibited and disinhibited. Children in the first subgroup may show a combination of behavioural inhibition, vigilance, and fearfulness, which is sometimes called frozen watchfulness. These children are miserable, difficult to console, and sometimes aggressive. Some fail to thrive. Such behaviour is seen among children who have been abused (see p. 855).

Children with the disinhibited subtype of the disorder relate indiscriminately to people, irrespective of their closeness, and are excessively familiar with strangers. Such behaviour has been described most clearly in children raised in institutions. In DSM-IV, the diagnosis is made when the disturbance of relationships appears to be a direct result of abnormal care-giving. ICD-10 does not use this

criterion but requires that the behaviour is present in several situations.

Aetiology It seems that these syndromes are characteristic of the type of care-giving (abusive or institutional) rather than of the child. Insecure attachment in infancy is often followed by conflicts with care-givers and impulsive behaviour later in childhood. Nevertheless, considerable improvement can occur if the child experiences a secure attachment to a care-giver, for example, as a result of fostering or adoption. (These observations have not been made specifically in relation to attachment disorder as defined in ICD-10 and DSM-IV.)

Assessment and treatment of the problems of pre-school children

Usually the information is largely from the parents. The assessor seeks to discover whether the problem is primarily in the child or related difficulties in the mother or the entire family. The problem behaviour is assessed, together with the child's general level of development, and the functioning of the family.

Apart from particular points already mentioned under the specific disorders, *treatment* includes advice for the mother (and if necessary for other family members), about relevant aspects of child rearing. There is little evidence about the value of treatment. Behavioural methods are probably useful, and language delay may benefit from special teaching. Occasionally medication is needed to reduce extreme overactivity (see p. 833). It is often helpful to arrange for the child to spend part of the day away from the family in a playgroup or nursery school. For further information about the assessment of pre-school children see American Academy of Child and Adolescent Psychiatry (1998a).

For a general review of preschool problems see Campbell (1995).

Specific developmental disorders

Both DSM-IV and ICD-10 contain categories for specific developmental disorders, which are

Table 24.1 Specific disorders of psychological development

DSM-IV	ICD–10
Learning disorder	*Specific developmental disorders of scholastic skills*
Reading disorder	Specific reading disorder
Disorder of written expression	Specific spelling disorder
Mathematics disorder	Specific disorder of arithmetic skills
	Mixed disorder of scholastic skills
Communication disorders	*Specific developmental disorders of speech and language*
Phonological disorder	Specific speech articulation disorder
Expressive language disorder	Expressive language disorder
Mixed receptive-expressive language disorder	Receptive language disorder
– ⎤	Acquired aphasia with epilepsy*
Stuttering ⎦	(Stuttering†)
Motor skills disorder	
Developmental coordination disorder	Specific developmental disorder of motor function

* In DSM-IV acquired aphasia with epilepsy is classified as an (acquired) receptive-expressive language disorder.

circumscribed developmental delays that are not attributable to another disorder or to lack of opportunity to learn (Table 24.4). It is debatable whether these conditions should be classified as mental disorders at all, since many children meeting the criteria have no other signs of psychopathology. In ICD-10, these developmental disorders are divided into specific developmental disorders of scholastic skills, speech and language, and motor function. In DSM-IV, the same disorders are called learning disorder, communication disorders, and motor skill disorder, respectively.

Specific developmental disorders of scholastic skills are divided further into specific reading disorder, specific spelling disorder, and specific arithmetic disorder. In DSM-IV, these conditions are called reading disorder, disorder of written expression, and mathematics disorder, respectively.

Specific reading disorder

In DSM-IV, this condition is named reading disorder. It is defined by a reading age well below (usually 1.5–2 standard deviations) the level expected from the child's age and IQ (Yule 1967). Defined in this way, the disorder was found in about 4% of 10–11-year-olds in the Isle of Wight, and about twice that percentage in London (Yule and Rutter 1985).

Clinical features

Specific reading disorders should be clearly distinguished from general backwardness in scholastic achievement resulting from low intelligence or inadequate education. They should also be distinguished from poor reading due to lack of opportunity to learn at home or at school, or due to poor visual acuity. The child presents with a history of serious delay in learning to read, which has been evident from the early years of schooling and has sometimes been preceded by delayed acquisition of speech and language. Errors in reading include omissions, substitutions, or distortions of words, slow reading, long hesitations, and reversals of words or letters. There may also be poor comprehension. Writing and spelling are impaired, and in older children these problems may be more obvious than the reading problems. There may be associated emotional problems, but development in other areas is not affected. Compared with children with general backwardness at school, those with specific reading retardation are much more often boys; they are also more likely to have minor neurological abnormalities, and are likely to come from socially disadvantaged homes.

Specific reading retardation is associated with conduct disorder more often than would be expected through chance (Rutter *et al.* 1970a, 1970b). The association may arise in part because the two conditions have common neurodevelopmental or temperamental origins; in part because reading retardation leads to conduct problems at school when the child is frustrated by failures; and in part because conduct disorder gives rise to problems in learning to read.

Aetiology

Reading is a complex skill which depends on more than one psychological process and is learned in several stages. Therefore it is not surprising that no single cause has been identified for specific reading disorder. A widely held theory of the learning of reading is that children first use visual methods; they learn the appearance of whole words, and cannot decipher new words. The next stage of learning is alphabetical; children become able to decode new words from the sounds associated with the letters. In the final stage, reading becomes automatic and flexible in combining visual and alphabetical methods. (This model of reading, although not accepted by all, is useful in clinical practice.)

It has been suggested that a group of children with specific reading disorder have a neuropsychological syndrome with poor coordination, constructional difficulties, and left/right confusion. Many

children with specific disorders have one or two of these problems, but there is no evidence for a specific group, separate from others. Despite this, the term dyslexia is in common use and is useful in conveying to laymen the message that the reading problems are not due to laziness or stupidity and that the child needs help.

Genetic causes The frequent occurrence of reading disorder in family members suggests a genetic cause, and the family patterning suggests that there is not a single mode of inheritance (Rutter *et al.* 1990). A locus for dyslexia has been reported on chromosome 6 (for example, Gayan *et al.* 1999), but others have failed to replicate the finding (for example, Field and Kaplan 1998).

Neurological causes Children with cerebral palsy and epilepsy have increased rates of specific reading disorder. It has been suggested that children who have specific reading disorder, but no obvious neurological disease, may have minor neurological abnormalities. The evidence does not support this idea. The most likely cause appears to be a *disorder of brain maturation* affecting one or more of the perceptual and language skills required in reading. This explanation is consistent with the following findings: difficulties in verbal coding and sequencing in many cases, confusion between right and left, difficulty in visual scanning, and general improvement with age.

Social factors It seems that difficulties insufficient in themselves to cause reading retardation may do so when the child is brought up in an illiterate or otherwise disadvantaged family, receives little attention at school, or changes school frequently. As already noted, children with reading disorder have a high rate of conduct disorder.

For a review of the acquisition of reading skills and of reading disorder see Snowling (1991).

Assessment and treatment

It is important to identify the disorder early. *Assessment* is carried out by an educational or clinical psychologist using an individually administered standardized test of reading accuracy and comprehension. *Treatment* is educational unless there are additional medical or behavioural problems requiring separate intervention. Treatment should be started as early as possible before the child has a sense of failure. Several educational approaches are used but it is most important to reawaken the interest of a child with a long experience of failure. Parental interest and continued extra teaching seem to be helpful, but there is no evidence that any one method of teaching is better than others. If there are behavioural problems secondary to frustration caused by the reading difficulty, they may lessen as reading improves; others may need separate attention.

Prognosis

Prognosis varies with the severity of the condition. Among children with a mild problem in mid-childhood, only about a quarter achieve normal reading skills by adolescence. Very few with severe problems in mid-childhood overcome them by adolescence. Whilst there is insufficient evidence to be certain what happens to these people as adults, those with substantial difficulties in adolescence seem likely to retain them (Maughan *et al.* 1985). For a review of reading disorders see Beitchman and Young (1997).

Mathematics disorder (specific arithmetic disorder)

The first of these terms is used in DSM-IV; the term in parentheses is used in ICD-10. Difficulty with arithmetic is probably the second most common specific disorder. Problems include failure to understand simple mathematical concepts, failure to recognize numerical symbols or mathematical signs, difficulty in carrying out arithmetic manipulations, and inability to learn mathematical tables. These problems are not due simply to lack of opportunities to learn and are evident from the time of the child's first attempts to learn mathematics.

There has been no study of its *epidemiology*, although it is thought to be quite common.

Although it causes less severe handicap in everyday life than reading difficulties, it can lead to secondary emotional difficulties when the child is at school.

The *causes* are uncertain. Dyscalculia occurs in some adults with parietal lobe lesions, but no brain damage has been found in children with specific arithmetic disorder. It seems unlikely that there is a single cause. *Assessment* is usually based on the arithmetic subtests of the Wechsler Intelligence Scale for Children (WISC) and the Wechsler Adult Intelligence Scale (WAIS) and on specific tests. *Treatment* is by remedial teaching but it is not known whether it is effective. The *prognosis* is not known. For a review see O'Hare *et al.* (1991).

Communication disorders (developmental disorders of speech and language)

Children vary widely in their achievement of speech and language. Half of all children use words with meanings by 12.5 months and 97% do so by 21 months. Half form words into simple sentences by 23 months (Neligan and Prudham 1969). Vocabulary and complexity of language develop rapidly during the pre-school years. However, when children start school, 1% are seriously retarded in speech and 5% have difficulty in making themselves understood by strangers. The process by which language is acquired is complex and is still not fully understood.

Causes of speech and language disorder

No cause can be found in the majority of children with speech and language disorders. These cases are said to have specific developmental speech and language disorder. It is most important to detect the primary conditions that are present in the minority. The most common of these causes is *learning disability*. Other important causes are *deafness, cerebral palsy, and pervasive developmental disorder*. *Social deprivation* can cause mild delays in speaking or add to the effects of the other causes.

Classification

The classification differs in some ways between ICD-10 and DSM-IV. ICD-10 uses the title 'specific developmental disorders of speech and language', whereas DSM-IV has the wider title 'communication disorders'. Three disorders appear in both classifications, though with some differences in nomenclature:

◆ phonological disorder (DSM-IV) or specific speech articulation disorder (ICD-10);

◆ specific developmental expressive language disorder (the term used in both classifications);

◆ mixed receptive-expressive disorder (DSM-IV); here ICD-10 has the narrower term specific developmental receptive language disorder. (The reason for the difference is explained below.)

ICD-10 (but not DSM-IV) has a fourth category of acquired aphasia with epilepsy. In DSM-IV, the wider title of the group allows the inclusion of stuttering; The narrower title in ICD-10 does not cover stuttering, which is coded instead under behavioural disorders of childhood (see Table 24.4).

Phonological disorder (specific developmental speech articulation disorder)

In this condition, accuracy in the use of speech sound is below the level appropriate for the child's mental age but language skills are normal. Errors in making speech sounds are normal in children up to about the age of 4 years, but by age 7 most speech sounds should be normal. By age 12 years nearly all speech sounds should be made normally. Children with specific speech articulation disorder make errors of articulation so severe that it is difficult for others to understand their speech. Speech sounds may be omitted or distorted, or other sounds substituted. In assessing speech production, appropriate allowance should be made for regional accents and dialects. The sounds affected most often are those developing later in the normal sequence of development (l, r, s, z, th, and ch for English speakers).

Prevalence depends on the criteria used to determine when speech production is abnormal; a rate of 2–3% has been cited among 6- to 7-year-olds (American Psychiatric Association 1994a).

Specific developmental expressive language disorder

In this disorder, the ability to use expressive spoken language is markedly below the level appropriate for the child's mental age. Language comprehension is within normal limits but there may be abnormalities in articulation. Language development varies considerably among normal children, but the absence of single words by 2 years of age, and of two-word phrases by 3 years of age signifies abnormality. Signs at later ages include restricted vocabulary, difficulties in selecting appropriate words, and immature grammatical usage. Non-verbal communication, if impaired, is not affected as severely as spoken language, and the child makes efforts to communicate. Disorders of behaviour are often present.

Cluttering Some children speak rapidly and with an erratic rhythm such that the grouping of words does not reflect the grammatical structure of their speech. This abnormality, which is known as cluttering, is classified as an associated feature of expressive language disorder in DSM-IV but in ICD-10 it is classified (with stammering) among other behavioural disorders of childhood.

Prevalence of expressive language disorder depends on the method of assessment; a rate of 3–5% of children has been proposed (American Psychiatric Association 1994a).

Prognosis It is reported that about half of the children meeting DSM-IV criteria develop normal speech by adult life, while the rest have long-lasting difficulties (American Psychiatric Association 1994a). Prognosis is worse when the language disorder is severe, or there is a co-morbid condition, such as conduct disorder.

Treatment Treatment is mainly through special education. Psychiatrists are likely to be involved when there is a co-morbid disorder, and may need to advise the parents about the child's rights for special education.

For a review of expressive language disorder, see American Academy of Child and Adolescent Psychiatry (1998b).

Receptive-expressive (or receptive) developmental language disorder

In this disorder the understanding of language is below the level appropriate to the child's mental age. In almost all cases, expressive language is also disturbed (a fact recognized in DSM-IV by the term receptive-expressive language disorder).

The development of receptive language ability varies considerably among normal children. However, failure to respond to familiar names, in the absence of non-verbal cues, by the beginning of the second year of age, or failure to respond to simple instructions by the end of the second year, are significant signs suggesting receptive language disorder – provided that deafness, learning disability, and pervasive developmental disorder have been excluded. Associated social and behavioural problems are particularly frequent in this form of language disorder.

The *prevalence* depends on the criteria for diagnosis, but a frequency of up to 3% of school-age children has been suggested (American Psychiatric Association 1994a).

The *prognosis* is poor with around 75% continuing throughout childhood. The prognosis is worse when the language disorder is severe, or there is a co-morbid condition, such as conduct disorder.

Treatment is through special education. The psychiatrist's role is the same as in expressive language disorder (see above).

For a review of receptive language disorder see American Academy of Child and Adolescent Psychiatry (1998b).

Acquired aphasia with epilepsy (Landau–Kleffner syndrome)

In this disorder, a child whose language has so far developed normally loses both receptive and expressive language but retains general intelli-

gence. There are associated EEG abnormalities, nearly always bilateral and temporal, and often with more widespread disturbances. Most of the affected children develop seizures either before or after the change in expressive language. The disorder starts usually between 3 and 9 years of age. In most cases the loss of language occurs over several months but it may be more rapid. In the early stages the severity of the impairment may fluctuate.

The *aetiology* is unknown but an inflammatory encephalitis has been proposed. The prognosis is variable: about two-thirds are left with a receptive language deficit, but the other third recover completely.

Assessment Early investigation is essential both to determine the nature and severity of the speech and language disorder and to exclude mental retardation, deafness, cerebral palsy, and pervasive developmental disorder. The speech-producing organs should be examined. It is particularly important to detect deafness at an early stage.

Parents can give some indication of the child's speech and language skills, especially if they complete a standardized inventory. With younger children it may be necessary to rely on this information, but children from about the age of 3 years can be tested by a standard test of language appropriate to the child's age. If possible, such a test should be carried out by a speech therapist or a psychologist specializing in the subject.

Treatment Treatment depends partly on the cause but usually includes a programme of speech training carried out through play and social interaction. In milder cases this help is best provided at home by the parents who are given information on what to do. More severe difficulties are likely to require specialized help in a remedial class or a special school. Treatment should start early.

For a review the development of speech and language and of their disorders see Bishop (1994). For a review of the disorders of speech and language see Kolvin (2000).

Motor skills disorder

Some children have delayed motor development, which results in clumsiness in school work or play. In ICD-10, this condition is called specific developmental disorder of motor function. It is also known as clumsy child syndrome or specific motor dyspraxia. The children can carry out all normal movements, but their coordination is poor. They are late in developing skills such as dressing, walking, and feeding. They tend to break things and are poor at handicrafts and organized games. They may also have difficulty in writing, drawing, and copying. IQ testing usually shows good verbal but poor performance scores.

These children are sometimes referred to a psychiatrist because of secondary emotional disorder. An explanation of the nature of the problem should be given to the child, the family, and the teachers. Special teaching may improve confidence. It may be necessary to exempt the child from organized games or other school activities involving motor coordination. There is usually some improvement with time. Further information is given by Cantwell and Baker (1985) and Henderson (1987).

Pervasive developmental disorders

The term pervasive developmental disorder refers to a group of disorders characterized by abnormalities in communication and social interaction and by restricted repetitive activities and interests. These abnormalities occur in a wide range of situations. Usually, development is abnormal from infancy and most cases are manifest before the age of 5 years.

Six conditions are included under this rubric in ICD-10 (see Table 24.5); two of these do not appear in DSM-IV, namely atypical autism and overactive disorder with mental retardation and stereotyped movements.

Childhood autism (autistic disorder)

This condition was described by Kanner (1943) who suggested the name infantile autism. The term childhood autism is used in ICD-10 but autistic disorder is the term in DSM-IV.

Clinical features

In his original description, Kanner (1943) identified the main features, which are still used to make the diagnosis. In both DSM-IV and ICD-10, three kinds of abnormality are required to make the diagnosis of autism:

Table 24.5 Pervasive developmental disorders

DSM-IV	ICD–10
Autistic disorder	Childhood autism
Rett's syndrome	Rett's syndrome
Childhood disintegrative disorder	Other childhood disintegrative disorder
	Overactive disorder with mental retardation and stereotyped movements
Asperger's disorder	Asperger's syndrome
Pervasive developmental disorder not otherwise specified (including atypical autism)	Atypical autism
	Pervasive developmental disorder not otherwise specified

- abnormalities of social development;
- abnormalities of communication;
- restriction of interests and behaviour.

Of these, the abnormalities of social development are the most specific to autism. Abnormal development is usually apparent before the age of 3 years. There are reports that early signs of autism can be detected in infancy.

Abnormalities of social development The child is unable to make warm emotional relationships with people (autistic aloneness). Autistic children do not respond to their parents' affectionate behaviour by smiling or cuddling. Instead, they appear to dislike being picked up or kissed. They are no more responsive to their parents than to strangers and do not show interest in other children. There is little difference in their behaviour towards people and inanimate objects. A characteristic sign is gaze avoidance, that is, the absence of eye-to-eye contact.

Abnormalities of communication Speech may develop late or never appear. Occasionally, it develops normally until about the age of 2 years and then disappears in part or completely. This lack of speech is a manifestation of a severe cognitive defect. As autistic children grow up, about half acquire some useful speech, although serious impairments usually remain, such as the misuse of pronouns and the inappropriate repeating of words spoken by other people (echolalia). Some autistic children are talkative, but their speech is a repetitive monologue rather than a conversation with another person.

The cognitive defect also affects non-verbal communication and play; autistic children do not take part in the imitative games of the first year of life, and later they do not use toys in an appropriate way. They show little imagination or creative play.

Restriction of interests and behaviour Obsessive desire for sameness is a term applied to stereotyped behaviour together with evidence of distress if there is any change in the environment. For example, autistic children may prefer the same food repeat-edly, insist on wearing the same clothes, or engage in repetitive games. Some are fascinated by spinning toys.

Odd behaviour and mannerisms are common. Some autistic children engage in odd motor behaviour such as whirling round and round, twiddling their fingers repeatedly, flapping their hands, or rocking. Others do not differ obviously in motor behaviour from normal children.

Other features Autistic children may suddenly show anger or fear without apparent reason. They may be overactive and distractible, sleep badly, or soil or wet themselves. Some injure themselves deliberately. About 25% of autistic children develop *seizures*, usually about the time of adolescence.

Intelligence level Kanner originally believed that the intelligence of autistic children was normal. Later research has shown that three-quarters have IQ scores in the 'retarded' range, and this finding appears to represent true intellectual impairment (Rutter and Lockyer 1967). Some autistic children show areas of ability despite impairment of other intellectual functions, and in some cases they have exceptional but restricted powers of memory or mathematical skill (Hermelin and O'Connor 1983).

Epidemiology

The *prevalence* of autism is probably about 5.2 per 10 000 children. It is four times as common in boys as in girls (Fombonne 1999).

Aetiology

The cause of childhood autism is unknown. It is likely that the central abnormality is cognitive, affecting particularly symbolic thinking and language (Rutter 1983), and that the behavioural abnormalities are secondary to this cognitive defect.

Genetic influences have a major importance. The condition is 50 times more frequent in the siblings of affected persons than in the general population (Rutter *et al.* 1990). Several twin studies have shown a much higher concordance between monozygotic than between dizygotic twins (for example, Rutter *et al.* 1993; Bailey *et al.* 1995). Autism has been linked to a region on chromosome 7q (International Molecular Genetic Study of Autism Consortium 1998), but further replication is required. Cognitive abnormalities are more frequent among the siblings of autistic probands than in the general population, suggesting that the phenotype may be wider than the syndrome of autism as currently defined (Bailey *et al.* 1998).

Organic brain disorder has been suspected as a cause of autism because there is an increased frequency of complications in pregnancy and childbirth among these patients. Also, autism is associated with epilepsy (in 20% of cases). When an autistic patient has an unaffected identical twin, the autistic twin is more likely to have had obstetric complications at birth. However, the birth complications are of a kind strongly associated with minor congenital abnormalities. This finding suggests that the obstetric complications may have resulted from an abnormality in the fetus. If so, they may be a result rather than a cause of autism, or reflect a common risk factor (Bolton *et al.* 1997). Neuroimaging studies have so far been inconclusive. (Piven *et al.* 1996).

Other evidence for biological causes Autism is associated with fragile X syndrome (see p. 882). Gillberg (1992) estimated that up to a third of cases of autism are associated with a medical condition but Rutter *et al.* (1994a) consider that the proportion is about 1in 10. Possible biological causes of autism are reviewed by Volkmar and Klin (2000). Claims of an association with MMR vaccine have not been reliably confirmed.

Abnormal parenting In a much quoted paper, Kanner (1943) suggested that autism was a response to abnormal parents who were characterized as cold, detached, and obsessive. Kanner's idea has not been substantiated (see Koegel *et al.* 1983). It is now thought that any psychological abnormalities in the parents are likely to be either a response to the problems of bringing up the autistic child, or a manifestation in the parents of the genes that have produced autism in the child. Although unsupported by evidence, persistent lay beliefs about the role of parenting still cause distress among the parents who hear of it.

Other theories There is no evidence for a relationship between childhood autism and schizophrenia, and autistic children do not grow up to be schizophrenic.

Psychopathology

Theory of mind in autism This theory attempts to identify a basic psychological disorder in autism. By the age of 4 years, normal children are able to form an idea of what others are thinking. For example, if a normal child watches while another normal child is shown the location of a hidden object and is then sent out of the room while the object is moved to a new hiding place, the observer who has remained in the room will conclude that the other child will expect the object to be in the original position when he returns to the room. An autistic child tends to lack this appreciation of what another child is likely to be thinking; in this example, an autistic child is likely to say that the other child will think that the object has been moved to its new place. It is not certain how specific to autism is this difficulty in appreciating what others know and expect, or how central it is to the psychopathology. In any case, its cause is not known. For a review of the evidence for the theory of mind in autism, see Yirmiya *et al.* (1998).

Other possible 'core' psychological disorders in autism include impaired ability to relate to others, and impaired ability to extract high-level meaning from diverse sources of information. None of the proposed core disorders can account for more than a part of the clinical picture.

Differential diagnosis

It is more usual to encounter partial syndromes than the full syndrome of childhood autism. These partial syndromes must be distinguished from the *childhood disintegrative disorders* arising after the age of 30 months (see p. 830) and *Asperger's syndrome* (autistic psychopathy) (see p. 830).

Deafness should be excluded by appropriate tests of hearing. *Communication disorder* (see p. 823) differs from autism in that the child usually responds normally to people and has good non-verbal communication. *Learning disability* can be differentiated because, although the child has general intellectual retardation, responses to other people are more normal than those of an autistic child. Also, an autistic child has more impairment of language relative to other skills than is found in a learning disabled child of the same age.

Prognosis

Between 10 and 20% of children with childhood autism begin to improve between the ages of about 4 and 6 years, and are eventually able to attend an ordinary school and obtain work. A further 10–20% can live at home but cannot work and need to attend a special school or training centre. The remainder, at least 60%, improve little and are unable to lead an independent life; many need long-term residential care (Russell 1970). Those who improve may continue to show language problems, emotional coldness, and odd behaviour. As noted already, a substantial minority develop epilepsy in adolescence. Pointers to better prognosis are communicative speech by the age of about 6 years and higher IQ.

Assessment

Assessment should be concerned with more than the diagnosis of autism. The following additional factors need to be considered (Lord and Rutter 1994):

♦ cognitive level;

♦ language ability;

♦ communication skills, social skills and play, and repetitive or otherwise abnormal behaviour;

♦ stage of social development in relation to age, mental age, and stage of language development;

♦ associated medical conditions;

♦ psychosocial factors.

Treatment

In the absence of any specific treatment, management has three main aspects: management of the abnormal behaviour, education and social services, and help for the family.

Management of abnormal behaviour Contingency management (see p. 737) may control some of the abnormal behaviour of autistic children. Such treatment is often carried out at home by the parents, instructed and supervised by a clinical psychologist. It is not known whether this treatment has any lasting benefit, but in autism even temporary changes are often worthwhile for the patient and the family.

Education and social services Most autistic children require special schooling. It is generally thought better for them to live at home and to attend special day schools. If the condition is so severe that the child cannot stay in the family, residential schooling is necessary. Special care is needed to avoid an institutional atmosphere, since this can increase social withdrawal. In some cases, the educational and residential needs of autistic children can be provided through the services for the learning disabled. Older adolescents may need vocational training.

For a review of psychological and educational treatments see Howlin (1998).

Help for the family The family of an autistic child needs considerable help to cope with the child's behaviour, which is often bewildering and distressing. Although the doctor may be able to do little specifically to help the patient, he must not withdraw from the family, who need continuing support and encouragement in their efforts to help the child. Some parents request genetic counselling and it seems that the risk of a further autistic child is about 3% (Lord and Rutter 1994). Many parents find it helpful to join a voluntary organization in which they can meet other parents of autistic children and discuss common problems.

Other suggested treatments Individual psychotherapy has been used in the hope of effecting more fundamental changes but there is no evidence that it succeeds. Nor is there evidence that any form of medication is effective in childhood autism, except in the short-term management of behaviour problems when an antipsychotic drug may be used.

A general review of treatment is given by Volkmar and Klin (2000).

Rett's disorder

Rett's disorder (or Rett's syndrome) is a rare condition which has to date been reported only in girls. The reported prevalence is 0.8 per 10 000 girls (Kerr and Stevenson 1985). After a period of normal development in the first months of life, head growth slows and over the next 2 years there is arrest of cognitive development and loss of purposive skilled hand movements. Stereotyped movements develop with hand-clapping and hand-wringing movements. Ataxia of the legs and trunk may develop. Interest in the social environment diminishes in the first few years of the disorder, but may increase again later. Expressive and receptive language development is impaired severely and there is psychomotor retardation. Some patients develop severe learning disability. Pedigree studies show that there is rarely a family history of the disorder. See Olsson and Rett (1990) for a review.

Overactive disorder with mental retardation and stereotyped movements

This condition is included in ICD-10 but not in DSM-IV. It is an ill-defined syndrome which occurs in children with severe learning disability (IQ less than 50) who have hyperactivity, inattention, and stereotyped movements. In adolescence, overactivity may be replaced by reduced activity (an unusual outcome in hyperkinetic syndrome). It is not certain whether this combination of features defines a distinct entity.

Childhood disintegrative disorder

Childhood disintegrative disorder (also known as Heller's disease) begins after a period of normal development usually lasting for more than 2 years. It is unclear how far the childhood disintegrative disorder is distinct from childhood autism. It resembles childhood autism in the marked loss of cognitive functions, abnormalities of social behaviour and communication, and unfavourable outcome. It differs from childhood autism in the loss of motor skills and of bowel or bladder control. The condition may arrest after a time, or progress to a severe neurological condition. For a review see Harris (1996).

Asperger's syndrome

This condition, first described by Asperger (1944), is sometimes called autistic psychopathy. (Asperger's original paper in German has been translated into English – see Frith 1991.) The condition is characterized by severe and sustained abnormalities of social behaviour similar to those of childhood autism, with stereotyped and repetitive activities, and motor mannerisms such as hand and finger twisting, or whole body movements. It differs from autism in that there is no general delay or retardation of cognitive development or language. The disorder is more common in boys than girls. The children develop normally until about the third year when they begin to lack warmth in their relationships and speak in monotonous stilted ways. They are solitary, and embark on and spend much time in narrow interests. They may embark repeatedly on long monologues on the same subject. They are often clumsy and eccentric. They are more interested in others than are children with autism but they do not share interests or pleasures with others, and are without friends.

The *prevalence* of the syndrome is uncertain. Using ICD-10 criteria, a rate of about 39 per 10 000 was reported by Ehlers and Gillberg (1993), but only four cases were detected so that the confidence limits extend from 0.6 to 56 per 10 000 (see Fombonne 1999, p. 781). Reported rates depend on the definition used in the research.

The *cause* of Asperger's syndrome is unknown. It is uncertain whether the condition is a variant of childhood autism or a separate disorder. The *prognosis* is that the abnormalities usually persist into adult life. Most people with the disorder can work, but few form successful relationships and marry. For a review of Asperger's syndrome, see Volkmar and Klin (2000).

Atypical autism and pervasive developmental disorder NOS

The terms atypical autism (ICD-10) and pervasive developmental disorder, not otherwise specified (NOS) (DSM-IV) denote a residual category for pervasive developmental disorders that resemble autism but do not meet the diagnostic criteria for any of the syndromes within this group. The prevalence of these cases varies according to the criteria adopted but most investigations show that they are at least as common as autism (see Fombonne 1999). It is not known what is the relation between these cases and those which meet the criteria for the other syndromes within the group of pervasive developmental disorders.

Hyperkinetic disorder

About a third of children are described by their parents as overactive, and 5–20% of school children are so described by teachers. These reports encompass behaviour varying from normal high spirits to a severe and persistent disorder. This overactivity often varies in different situations. Hyperkinetic disorders are more severe forms of overactivity, associated with marked inattention, hence the widely used term attention-deficit hyperactivity disorder.

Hyperkinetic disorder (attention-deficit hyperactivity disorder)

Clinical features

The cardinal features of this disorder are:

- extreme and persistent restlessness;
- sustained and prolonged motor activity;
- difficulty in maintaining attention;
- impulsiveness and difficulty in withholding responses.

All these features vary with the situation so that parents and teachers may give different accounts of the child's behaviour.

Children with the disorder are often reckless, and prone to accidents. They may have learning difficulties, which result in part from poor attention and lack of persistence with tasks. Many develop minor forms of antisocial behaviour as the condition continues, particularly disobedience, temper tantrums, and aggression. These children are often socially disinhibited and unpopular with other children. Mood fluctuates, but low self-esteem and depressive mood are common.

Restlessness, overactivity, and related symptoms often start before school age. Sometimes the child was overactive as a baby, but more often significant problems begin when the child begins to walk; he is constantly on the move, interfering with objects and exhausting his parents.

Diagnostic criteria

In both ICD-10 and DSM-IV, the cardinal features for the diagnosis of the disorder are impaired attention, hyperactivity, and impulsiveness. However, the two systems differ in the details of the criteria for diagnosis. Both systems require that symptoms should have started in childhood: ICD-10 specifies before 6 years of age; DSM-IV specifies before 7 years of age. An important difference is that ICD-10 requires both hyperactivity and impaired attention, whereas for DSM-IV the diagnosis can be made if there is either inattention or hyperactivity and impulsiveness. ICD-10 requires that the criteria are met both at home and at school, whereas DSM-IV requires only that they be present in one situation with impairment (which does not have strict criteria) in the other. Thus children who meet ICD-10 criteria are more severely impaired than those who meet DSM-IV criteria.

In ICD-10 the disorder can be further classified as:

- disturbance of activity and attention and
- hyperkinetic conduct disorder.

The latter term is used when criteria for both hyperkinetic disorder and conduct disorder are met. (The division is made because the presence of associated aggression, delinquency, or antisocial behaviour is associated with a less good outcome – see below.)

Autistic children are often hyperactive and inattentive, but these features are regarded as part of the syndrome of childhood autism; hyperactivity disorder is not diagnosed in addition to autism.

Epidemiology

Estimates of the prevalence of hyperkinetic disorder vary according to the criteria for diagnosis. Using DSM-IV criteria, a prevalence of 3–5% is suggested (American Psychiatric Association 1994a). Using ICD-10 criteria, a prevalence of 1.7% was found among primary school boys (Taylor *et al.* 1991). Rates are three to four times higher in boys than in girls; also the rate among boys is highest during school age and declines in adolescence, whereas the (lower) rate in girls is the same in both age groups (Ross and Ross 1982; Szatmari *et al.* 1989).

Aetiology

It seems likely that the disorder is aetiologically heterogenous. Signs suggesting neurodevelopmental impairment or delay are found in children with hyperkinetic disorder, for example, clumsiness, language delay, and abnormalities of speech (Schachar 1991). Although these signs are generally associated with birth complications, they could result from factors acting at an earlier stage of development of the brain.

Genetic factors are suggested by the study of family members, twins and adopted children and by comparisons of monozygotic and dizygotic twins. Biederman *et al.* (1992), using DSM-IIIR criteria, found that, compared with controls, probands with attention-deficit hyperactivity disorder had more first-degree relatives with the same disorder. Twin studies show a much higher concordance for monozygotic than for dizygotic pairs (Eaves *et al.* 1997). Adoption studies show that the biological parents of children with the attention-deficit hyperactivity disorder are more likely to have the same or a related disorder than are the adoptive parents (van den Oord *et al.* 1994). For a review see Thapar *et al.* (1999).

Linkage has been reported between attention-deficit hyperactivity disorder and the dopamine D_4 receptor gene (Smalley *et al.* 1998), and with an allele of the dopamine transporter gene (Cook *et al.* 1995; Gill *et al.* 1997). These findings are consistent with evidence that drugs affecting the dopamine system lead to improvement in the disorder (see below), but further replication is required before their significance can be assessed.

Social factors It seems that social factors increase an innate tendency to hyperactivity since overactive behaviour is more frequent among young children living in poor social conditions (Richman *et al.* 1982). Also, studies of twins indicate that both shared and non-shared environmental effects contribute to aetiology (Eaves *et al.* 1997).

Other factors In the past, lead intoxication (Needleman *et al.* 1979) and food additives (Feingold 1975) have been suggested as causes of hyperkinetic syndrome, and more recently zinc deficiency has been suggested, but there is no convincing evidence for either of these suggested causes (see Schachar and Ickowicz 2000 for a review of this and other aspects of aetiology).

Prognosis

Overactivity usually lessens gradually as the child grows older, especially when it is mild and not present in every situation. It usually ceases by puberty. The prognosis for any associated learning difficulties is less good, whilst antisocial behaviour has the worst outcome. When the overactivity is severe, and is accompanied by learning failure or associated with low intelligence, the prognosis is poor and the conditions may persist into adult life, usually as antisocial disorder and drug abuse rather than continued hyperactivity. It is uncertain whether mood and anxiety disorders are increased in adult life; one study found that they were not (Mannuzza *et al.* 1993), whereas another report concluded that they were increased (McArdle *et al.* 1997).

Treatment

A hyperactive child exhausts his parents who need support from the start of treatment, particularly as it may be difficult to reduce the child's behaviour. The child's teachers need advice about management, which may include remedial teaching. Methods of *behaviour modification* may help to reduce the inadvertent reinforcement of overactivity by parents and teachers.

Stimulant drugs may be tried, especially when there is severe restlessness and attention deficit. These drugs increase dopamine and noradrenaline activity and it is thought that these actions underlie their therapeutic effects. The usual drugs are methylphenidate or dexamphetamine. Dosage should be related to body weight following the manufacturers' instructions. When methylphenidate is used, it is often appropriate to start with 2.5 mg in the morning, adding after 4 days a further 2.5 mg at midday, and, depending on the response and side-effects, increasing cautiously to a maximum of 10 mg in the morning and 10 mg at midday for a 5-year-old of average weight (or a lower dose for a younger child). The potential short-term benefits are decreased restlessness, aggressiveness, and sometimes improved attention. These effects do not usually diminish with time, but it has not been shown that they are associated with better long-term outcome. The *side-effects* include irritability, depression, insomnia, and poor appetite. High doses may provoke stereotyped behaviour, which disappears when the dose is reduced. With high doses, there may be some slowing of growth, but adult stature and weight do not seem to be affected (Taylor 1994; Spencer *et al.* 1996). The drug may be needed for many months and some children take it for years; careful monitoring is essential. The drug may be stopped from

time to time in an attempt to minimize side-effects and to confirm that medication is still needed. In clinical trials, short-term benefits of the drug have been shown in about two-thirds of children with hyperkinetic syndrome (Ottenbacher and Cooper 1983), but the long-term benefits are uncertain. It seems best to reserve drug treatment for more severe cases that have not responded to other treatment. Surprisingly, there is no report of children treated in this way becoming addicted to the drug.

For a review of the evidence about stimulants as a treatment of this disorder, see College Research Unit of the Royal College of Psychiatrists (1999). For a general review of management, see American Academy of Child and Adolescent Psychiatry (1997b) or Overmeyer and Taylor (1999).

Conduct disorders

Conduct disorders are characterized by severe and persistent antisocial behaviour. They form the largest single group of psychiatric disorders in older children and adolescents.

Clinical features

The essential feature of conduct disorder is persistent abnormal conduct which is more serious than ordinary childhood mischief. In the pre-school period, the disorder usually manifests as defiant and aggressive behaviour in the home, often with overactivity. The behaviours include disobedience, temper tantrums, physical aggression to siblings or adults, and destructiveness. In later childhood, conduct disorder is manifest in the home as stealing, lying, and disobedience, together with verbal or physical aggression. Later, the disturbance often becomes evident outside as well as inside the home, especially at school, or as truanting, delinquency, vandalism, and reckless behaviour, or as alcohol or drug abuse. Antisocial behaviour among teenage girls includes spitefulness, emotional bullying of peers, sexual promiscuity, and running away.

In children older than 7 years, persistent stealing is abnormal. Below that age, children seldom have a real appreciation of other people's property. Many children steal occasionally, so that minor or isolated instances need not be taken seriously. A small proportion of children with conduct disorder present with sexual behaviour that incurs the disapproval of adults. In younger children, masturbation and sexual curiosity may be frequent and obtrusive. Promiscuity may be a particular problem in adolescent girls. Fire-setting is rare, but obviously dangerous (see p. 915).

To constitute conduct disorders, these behaviours have to be more persistent that a reaction to changing circumstances such as adjusting to the arrival in the family of a new step-parent.

Classification

Both ICD-10 and DSM-IV require the presence of three symptoms from a list of 15, and a duration of at least 6 months. The criteria are closely similar in the two systems of classification.

Because conduct disorders vary widely in their clinical features, both systems divide conduct disorders. In DSM-IV, they are divided into childhood-onset type (onset before 10 years of age) and adolescent-onset type (with onset at 10 years of age or later). DSM-IV has an additional category, 'oppositional defiant disorder', for persistently hostile defiant provocative and disruptive behaviour outside the normal range but without aggressive or dyssocial behaviour. This disorder occurs mainly in children below 10 years of age. ICD-10 has four subdivisions of conduct disorder: socialized conduct disorder, unsocialized conduct disorder, conduct disorders confined to the family context, and oppositional defiant disorder.

Prevalence

The prevalence of conduct disorders is difficult to estimate because the dividing line between them and normal rebelliousness is arbitrary. Rates were established many years ago, and have not been revised by more recent evidence. Rutter *et al.* (1970a) found the prevalence of 'antisocial disorder' to be about 4% among 10–11 year olds on the Isle of Wight. In a subsequent study in London about twice this rate was found (Rutter *et al.* 1975a, 1976a). A subsequent study in a province

of Canada found a rate of 5.5% (Offord *et al.* 1987). Higher rates hae been reported in older adolescents (see Scott 2000). Studies in the community, in psychiatric practice, and in the juvenile courts all indicate that conduct disorders are about four times more common in boys than girls (Rutter *et al.* 1970a; Gath *et al.* 1977).

Aetiology

Environmental factors are important; conduct disorders are commonly found in children from unstable, insecure, and rejecting families living in deprived areas. Antisocial behaviour is frequent among children from broken homes, those from homes in which family relationships are poor, and those who have been in residential care in their early childhood. Conduct disorders are also related to adverse factors in the wider social environment of the neighbourhood and school (Rutter *et al.* 1975b; Gath *et al.* 1977).

Genetic factors Adoption studies suggests that genetic factors play a smaller part in the aetiology of conduct disorder (Rutter *et al.* 1990) than in adult antisocial behaviour. However, it seems that persistent cases originating in childhood have a stronger genetic aetiology than those starting in adolescence (Silberg *et al.* 1996). Alcoholism and personality disorder in the father is reported to be strongly associated with conduct disorder in the children (Earls *et al.* 1988); the association could be through genetic or environmental mechanisms.

Organic factors Children with brain damage and epilepsy are prone to conduct disorder, as they are to other psychiatric disorders. An important finding in the Isle of Wight survey was a strong association between antisocial behaviour and specific reading disorder (see p. 822). It is not known whether antisocial behaviour and reading disorder result from common predisposing factors, or whether one causes the other.

See Rutter *et al.* (1998) for a review of the aetiology of conduct disorder.

Prognosis

Conduct disorders usually run a prolonged course in childhood (Rutter *et al.* 1976a). The long-term outcome varies considerably with the nature and extent of the disorder. In an important study, Robins (1966) found that almost half of people who had attended a child guidance clinic for conduct disorder in adolescence showed some form of antisocial behaviour in adult life. No cases of sociopathic disorder were found in adult life among those with diagnoses other than conduct disorder in adolescence. Follow-up of conduct-disordered children cared for in children's homes and of controls led to similar conclusions: about 40% of the conduct-disordered children had DSM-III antisocial personality disorder in their twenties, and many of the rest had persistent and widespread social difficulties below the threshold for diagnosis of a personality disorder. Pervasive social difficulty in adult life was also related to upbringing in a children's home, but conduct disorder had an additional effect when this variable was controlled for (Zoccolillo *et al.* 1992).

There are no good indicators of the long-term outcome of individual cases. The best available predictors seem to be the extent of the childhood antisocial behaviour and the quality of relationships with other people (Robins 1978). Other research indicates that the presence of hyperactivity or inattention and poor peer relations predict a poor outcome of childhood conduct disorder (Farrington *et al.* 1990), although it is not certain whether these are specific factors or merely indices of the severity of the conduct disorder. In the study by Zoccolillo *et al.* (1992), there were few changes until adult life, when some people improved substantially following marriage to a supportive and non-deviant partner.

Treatment

Mild conduct disorders often subside without treatment other than common-sense advice to the parents. For more severe disorders, treatment for the child is often combined with treatment and social support for the family. There is no convincing evidence that any treatment affects the overall long-term prognosis. Nevertheless, some short-term benefits can often be achieved, and in some cases adverse family factors can be modified in a way that could improve prognosis. Some families are difficult to help by any means, especially where there is material deprivation, chaotic relationships, and poorly educated parents. See Borduin (1999) for a review of treatment, and American Academy of Child and Adolescent Psychiatry (1997c) for practice guidelines.

Parent training programmes These programmes use behavioural principles (see p. 814). Parents are taught how the child's antisocial behaviour may be reinforced unintentionally by their attention to it, and how it may be provoked by interactions with members of the family. Parents are also taught how to reinforce normal behaviour by praise or rewards and how to set limits on abnormal behaviour, for example, by removing the child's privileges such as an hour less time to play a game. As aids to learning, parents are provided with written information and videotapes showing other parents applying behavioural procedures. For a review of parent training programmes see Webster-Stratton (1991).

Anger management Young people who are habitually aggressive have been shown to misperceive hostile intentions in other people who are not in fact hostile. They also tend to underestimate the level of their own aggressive behaviour, and choose inappropriate behaviours rather than more appropriate verbal responses (Dodge *et al.* 1990). Anger management programmes seek to correct these ideas by teaching how to inhibit sudden inappropriate responses to angry feelings (for example, Stop! What should I do!), and how to reappraise the intentions of other people and use socially acceptable forms of self-assertion. Kazdin *et al.* (1987) showed that these methods reduce the problems of aggressive children who do not have conduct disorder. Similar benefits have been reported with conduct-disordered children (Kendall *et al.* 1991).

Other methods Group therapy is seldom helpful (Kazdin 1997). Remedial teaching should be arranged if there are associated reading difficulties. Medication is of little value.

Residential care Occasionally, residential placement may be necessary in a foster home, group home, or special school. This should be done only for compelling reasons. There is no evidence that institutional care improves the prognosis for conduct disorder.

Truancy

The treatment of truancy requires separate consideration. A direct and energetic approach is called for. Pressure should be brought to bear upon the child to return to school and, if possible, the support of the family should be enlisted. At the same time, an attempt should be made to resolve any educational or other problems at school. In all this, it is essential to maintain good communications between clinician, parents, and teachers. If other steps fail, court proceedings may need to be initiated.

Juvenile delinquency

A juvenile delinquent is a young person who has been found guilty of an offence that would be categorized as a crime if committed by an adult. In most countries, the term applies only to a young person who has attained the age of criminal responsibility – at present 10 years in the UK, but ranging widely in other countries. Thus delinquency is not a psychiatric diagnosis but a legal category. However, juvenile delinquency may be associated with psychiatric disorder, especially conduct disorder. For this reason, it is appropriate to interrupt this review of the syndromes of child psychiatry to consider juvenile delinquency.

The majority of adolescent boys, when asked to report their own behaviour, admit to offences against the law and a fifth are convicted at some time (West and Farrington 1973). Many fewer girls than boys are delinquent. About a quarter of the boys cautioned or convicted for indictable offences

in England and Wales in 1995 were aged 10–17. Also, almost half of males aged between 14 and 17 years were cautioned or convicted for shoplifting or other offences (see Bailey 2000). Similar rates have been reported in other countries (D. J. Smith 1995). Amongst boys who are convicted, only about half are convicted again and few juvenile delinquents continue to offend in adult life. The few who offend repeatedly are very difficult to manage. In considering these figures, it has to be remembered that crime statistics may be misleading. Nevertheless, there seems to be a substantial similarity in the characteristics of self-reported offenders and of convicted offenders (West and Farrington 1973).

Delinquency is sometimes equated with conduct disorder. This is wrong, for although the two categories overlap, they are not the same. Many delinquents do not have conduct disorder (or any other psychological disorder). Equally, many of those with conduct disorder do not offend. Nevertheless, in an important group, persistent law-breaking is preceded and accompanied by abnormalities of conduct, such as truancy, aggressiveness, and attention seeking, and by poor concentration.

Causes

The causes of juvenile delinquency are complex and overlap with the causes of conduct disorder. The causes are reviewed briefly here; for a fuller account see Rutter *et al.* (1998).

Social factors Delinquency is related to low social class, poverty, poor housing, and poor education. There are marked differences in delinquency rates between adjacent neighbourhoods, which differ in these respects. Rates also differ between schools. Many social theories have been put forward to explain the origins of crime, but none offers a completely adequate explanation. For a review see Farrington (2000).

Family factors Many studies have found that crime runs in families (Farrington *et al.* 1996). For example, about half of boys with criminal fathers are convicted, compared with a fifth of those with fathers who are not criminals (West and Farrington 1977). The reasons for this are poorly understood but they may include poor parenting and shared attitudes to the law.

In a much quoted retrospective study, Bowlby (1944) examined the characteristics of 'juvenile thieves' and argued that prolonged separation from the mother during childhood was a major cause of their problems. More recent work has not confirmed such a precise link (see p. 806). Although delinquency is particularly common among those who come from broken homes, this seems to be largely because separation often reflects family discord in early and middle childhood (Rutter and Madge 1976). Other family factors correlated with delinquency are large family size and child-rearing practices, including erratic discipline and harsh or neglecting care.

Factors in the child *Genetic factors* appear to be less significant among the causes of delinquency than in the more serious criminal behaviour of adult life (see p. 900). (The possible role of genetic factors in conduct disorder has already been considered – p. 834.) There are important relationships between delinquency and slightly below average IQ as well as *educational and reading difficulties* (Rutter *et al.* 1976a). There are at least two possible explanations for the latter finding. Temperament or social factors may predispose to both delinquency and reading failure. Alternatively, reading difficulties may result in frustration and loss of self-esteem at school, and these may in turn predispose to antisocial behaviour. *Physical abnormalities* probably play only a minor role among the causes of delinquency, even though brain damage and epilepsy predispose to conduct disorder.

Assessment

When the child is seen as part of an ordinary psychiatric referral and the delinquency is accompanied by a psychiatric syndrome, the latter should be assessed in the usual way. Sometimes the child psychiatrist is asked to see a delinquent specifically to prepare a court report. In these circumstances, as well as making enquiries among the parents and teachers, it is essential to consult any social worker or probation officer who has been involved with the child.

Psychological testing of intelligence and educational achievements can be useful. The form of the report is similar to that described in Chapter 26 (p. 928). It should include a summary of the history and present mental state together with recommendations about treatment.

Violence among adolescents

There is concern in the USA about increasing rates of violent offences by adolescents. The arrest rate for murder and manslaughter by people under the age of 18 years rose by 60% between 1981 and 1991, compared with a 5% rise for people over that age (Federal Bureau of Investigation 1992). Although the rates of murder and manslaughter among adolescents have not risen in the same way in the UK, there is concern about less extreme violent acts by young people (Shepherd and Farrington 1996).

The causes of violent behaviour among young people are not fully understood, although most violent offenders commit many other kinds of offence. In the UK, Bailey and Aulich (1997) studied 50 cases of the most extreme form of violence among juveniles – homicide. Many had pre-existing conduct or emotional disorders, and adverse family and social circumstances. A smaller number had learning difficulties. However, none of the 76 features studied separated these young people from other young offenders. Similar findings have been reported from the USA (Meyers and Kemph 1990). For a review see Bailey (1997).

Treatment

In this section we consider measures intended to reduce the chances of further offending. However, many of the children and adolescents who appear before juvenile courts have psychiatric disorders requiring treatments described elsewhere in this chapter. These disorders include conduct disorders, mood disorders, substance abuse, learning disability, and epilepsy.

When considering the treatment of delinquent children and adolescents, psychiatrists need to understand the legal system in the country in which they work. The legal responses include a fine, the requirement that the parent or guardian take proper control, supervision by a social worker, a period at a special centre, or an order committing the child to the care of the local authority. The exact provisions vary from one country to another, and readers should enquire about the arrangements in the places in which they work. Since delinquent behaviour is common, mainly not serious, and usually a passing phase, it is generally appropriate to treat first offences with minimal intervention coupled with firm disapproval. The same applies to minor offences that are repeated. A more vigorous response is required for more serious, recurrent delinquency. For this purpose a community-based programme is usually preferred, with the main emphasis on improving the family environment, reducing harmful peer group influences, helping the offender to develop better skills for solving problems, and improving educational and vocational accomplishments. When this approach fails, custodial care will be considered.

In recent years the main aim of the law as it applies to children and young persons has been treatment rather than punishment or even deterrence. There has been extensive criminological research to determine the effectiveness of the measures used. The general conclusions are not encouraging, though not surprising since delinquency is strongly related to factors external to the child, including family disorganization, antisocial behaviour among the parents, and poor living conditions. The risk of reconviction seems to be greater among children who have had any court appearance or period of detention than among children who have committed similar offences without any official action having been taken (West and Farrington 1977).

There have been many attempts to establish and evaluate treatments that might be effective. One of the earliest, the Highfields Project, compared group treatment in a small well-staffed unit with the usual custodial sentence. Modest benefits were found for the former. A larger study, the Pilot Intensive Counselling Organization (PICO) project, found some evidence that 9 months of counselling was of more benefit to 'amenable' boys in a medium-security unit than to more difficult and uncooperative ('non-amenable') boys. An elaborate investigation known as the Community Treatment Project of the Californian Youth Authority (Warren 1973) found that community treatment was generally at least as effective as institutional care.

These and subsequent studies suggest the need to match the type of treatment to the type of offender. Some delinquents seem to respond better to authoritative supervision, and others to more permissive counselling. Unfortunately, it is not yet possible to provide any satisfactory practical guidelines about the choice of treatment for the individual delinquent. See Mulvey *et al.* (1993) and Bailey (2000) for a review of research on the prevention and treatment of juvenile delinquency.

Anxiety disorders

In ICD-10, anxiety disorders in childhood are classified as emotional disorders with onset specific to childhood (Table 24.6). DSM-IV does not contain this category and with two exceptions classifies childhood anxiety disorders in the same way as anxiety disorders in adult life. The exceptions are separation anxiety disorder and reactive attachment disorder, which are listed under the heading 'other disorders of infancy, childhood or adolescence'. ICD-10 has a diagnosis of sibling rivalry disorder. DSM-IV does not have this diagnosis in the main classification, but sibling relationship problems can be coded under 'other conditions that may be the focus of clinical attention'.

Prevalence

The prevalence of anxiety disorders in childhood is uncertain because epidemiological studies have usually employed the wider category of emotional disorder, or asked about symptoms rather than syndromes of anxiety. In their survey of the Isle of

Table 24.6 Anxiety disorders in childhood	
DSM-IV	**ICD–10**
	F93 Emotional disorders with specific onset in childhood
Separation anxiety disorder	Separation anxiety disorder of childhood
Phobic anxiety disorder*	Phobic anxiety disorder of childhood
Social phobia*	Social anxiety disorder of childhood
Sibling relationship problems†	Sibling rivalry disorder
Post-traumatic stress disorder*	*Other anxiety disorders**
Obsessive-compulsive disorder*	Post-traumatic stress disorder
	Obsessive-compulsive disorder

* There is no separate category for these disorders in childhood; the adult categories are used (see text).

† Listed under 'other conditions that may be the focus of clinical attention'.

Wight, Rutter *et al.* (1970a) found a prevalence of emotional disorders of 2.5% in both boys and girls. In a London suburb, the corresponding figure was doubled (Rutter *et al.* 1975a). (In both places, the rate of conduct disorder was about twice that of emotional disorder.) More recent surveys of the general population suggest rates of anxiety disorders of 6–9% among 7- to 11-year-olds, of which about half was separation anxiety disorder (see below) (Anderson *et al.* 1987; Bird 1996).

Normal anxiety in childhood

Anxiety is common in childhood, but its nature changes as the child grows older: infants pass through a stage of fear of strangers; during pre-school years separation anxiety and fears of animals, imaginary creatures, and the dark are common; in early adolescence these fears are replaced by anxiety about social situations and personal adequacy. Anxiety disorders in childhood resemble these normal anxieties and follow the same developmental sequence though they are more severe and more prolonged. Phobias and separation anxiety disorder usually start in early childhood, and social anxiety disorder starts in adolescence.

There is no clear dividing line between normal anxiety and anxiety disorders in childhood. Also,

there is often overlap between disorders, i.e. an individual child's disorder may fulfil the criteria for more than one disorder listed in ICD-10 or DSM-IV, for example, phobic disorder and separation anxiety disorder.

Separation anxiety disorder

Separation anxiety disorder is a fear of separation from people to whom the child is attached which is clearly greater than normal separation anxiety of toddlers or pre-school children, or persists beyond the usual pre-school period, and is associated with significant problems of social functioning. The onset is before the age of 6 years. The diagnosis is not made when there is a generalized disturbance of personality development.

Clinical picture

Children with this disorder are excessively anxious when separated from parents or other attachment figures, and unrealistically concerned that harm may befall these persons or that they will leave the child. They may refuse to sleep away from these persons or, if they agree to separate, may have disturbed sleep with nightmares. They cling to their attachment figures by day, demanding attention. Anxiety is often manifested as physical symptoms of stomach ache, headache, nausea, and vomiting, and may be accompanied by crying, tantrums, or social withdrawal. Separation anxiety disorder is one cause of school refusal (see p. 845).

Epidemiology

Community surveys suggest that rates of separation anxiety disorder are about 3–4% among 7–11-year-olds (Anderson *et al.* 1987; Benjamin *et al.* 1990).

Aetiology

Separation anxiety disorder is sometimes precipitated by a frightening experience. This may be brief, for example, admission to hospital, or prolonged, for example, conflict between the parents. In some cases separation anxiety disorder develops in children who react with excessive anxiety to a large number of everyday stressors and who are therefore said to have an anxiety-prone temperament. Sometimes the condition appears to be a response to anxious or overprotective parents.

Course

The disorder often improves with time, but may worsen again when there is a change in the child's routine such as a move of school. Some cases may progress to panic disorder and agoraphobia in adult life (Silove *et al.* 1995).

Treatment

Account should be taken of the whole range of possible aetiological factors including stressful events, previous actual separation, an anxiety-prone temperament, and the behaviour of the parents. Stressors should be reduced if possible, and the children should be helped to talk about their worries. It is more important to involve the family, helping them to understand how their own concerns or overprotection effect the child. Anxiolytic drugs may be needed occasionally when anxiety is extremely severe, but they should be used for short periods only. When separation anxiety is worse in particular circumstances, the child may benefit from the behavioural techniques used for phobias as described in the next section.

Phobic anxiety disorder

This diagnosis for children corresponds to specific phobia for adults (see p. 227). Minor phobic symptoms are common in childhood. They usually concern animals, insects, the dark, school, and death. The prevalence of more severe phobias varies with age. Severe and persistent fears of animals usually begin before the age of 5, and nearly all have declined by the early teenage years. At age 11 a rate of only about 2% has been found (Anderson *et al.* 1987; Milne *et al.* 1995).

Course

Most improve but a minority, probably 10–15%, persist into adult life (Last *et al.* 1997).

Treatment

Most childhood phobias improve without specific treatment provided the parents adopt a firm and reassuring approach. For phobias that do not improve, simple behavioural treatment can be combined with reassurance and support. The child is encouraged to encounter feared situations in a graded way, as in the treatment of phobias in adult life. Dynamic psychotherapy has also been used, but it is not obviously more effective than simple behavioural treatment. For a review see Bernstein *et al.* (1996).

Social anxiety disorder of childhood

This term is used in ICD-10 to describe disorders starting before the age of 6 years in which there is anxiety with strangers greater or more prolonged than the fear of strangers, which normally occurs in the second half of the first year of life. Children with this condition tend to have an inhibited temperament in infancy (Schwartz *et al.* 1999).

These children are markedly anxious in the presence of strangers and avoid them. The fear, which may be mainly of adults or of other children, interferes with social functioning. It is not accompanied by severe anxiety on separation from the parents.

Aetiology and treatment resemble those of other anxiety disorders of childhood.

Sibling rivalry disorder

This category is listed in ICD-10 for children who show extreme jealousy or other signs of rivalry of a sibling, starting during the months following the birth of that sibling. The signs are clearly greater than the emotional upset and rivalry which is common in such circumstances, and they are persistent and cause social problems. When the disorder is severe there may be hostility and even physical harm to the sibling. The child may regress in behaviour, for example, losing previously learned control of bladder or bowels, or act in a way appropriate for a younger child. There is usually opposition to the parents and behaviour intended to obtain their attention, often with temper tantrums. There may be sleep disturbance and problems at bedtime.

In treatment, parents should be helped to divide their attention appropriately between the two children, to set limits for the older child, and to help him or her feel valued. For a review see Dunn and Kendrick (1982).

Post-traumatic stress disorder

Although not included in ICD-10 among the anxiety disorders with onset usually in childhood, post-traumatic stress disorder (PTSD) can occur in childhood life. The clinical picture resembles that of the same disorder in adult life (see p. 194) with disturbed sleep, nightmares, flashbacks, and avoidance of reminders of the traumatic events. Children with post-traumatic stress disorder often have irrational separation anxiety, and young children may show regressive behaviour.

Aetiology

As in adults, the cause is an encounter with exceptionally severe stressors, for example, those encountered by children caught up in war, civil unrest, or natural disasters. Physical and sexual abuse may also provoke post-traumatic stress disorder in children (Goodwin 1988). As with adults, cases after vehicle and other accidents are more common than those after the less frequent major disasters. One study found a rate of about 17% of PTSD lasting more than 3 months, among children involved in road accidents (Mirza *et al.* 1998).

Prognosis

The prognosis of the disorder has not been studied systematically in childhood, but severe reactions have been reported to last for 6 months to a year or longer (Yule 1994).

Treatment

Treatment resembles that for adults (see p. 198). As with adults, immediate counselling (debriefing) is often provided for all those involved in a disaster. At least for adults, the value of this procedure is doubtful, unless cognitive therapy procedures are incorporated to help the victim 'process' the memories of the events (see p. 198). It is likely that the same principles apply to the treatment of children but at the time of writing there are no controlled studies addressed to this question.

Obsessive–compulsive disorders

Obsessive–compulsive disorders are rare in childhood. However, several related forms of repetitive behaviour are common, particularly between the ages of 4 and 10 years. These repetitive behaviours include preoccupation with numbers and counting, the repeated handling of certain objects, and hoarding. Normal children commonly adopt rituals such as avoiding cracks in the pavement or touching lamp posts. These behaviours cannot be called compulsive because the child does not struggle against it (see p. 19 for the definition of obsessive and compulsive symptoms). The preoccupations and rituals of obsessive–compulsive disorder are more extreme than these behaviours of healthy children and take up an increasing amount of the child's time, for example, rechecking schoolwork many times or frequently repeated handwashing.

Clinical picture

Obsessional disorder rarely appears in full form before late childhood, though the first symptoms may appear earlier. The onset may be rapid or gradual.

Obsessional disorders in childhood generally resemble those in adult life (see p. 242). The presenting symptoms are more often rituals than obsessional thoughts. Washing rituals are the most frequent, followed by repetitive actions and checking. Obsessional thoughts are most often concerned with contamination, accidents or illness affecting the patient or another person, and concerns about orderliness and symmetry. The content of symptoms often change as the child grows older. The obsessional symptoms may be provoked by external cues such as unclean objects. Children with obsessional symptoms usually try to conceal them, especially outside the family. Obsessional children often involve their parents by asking them to take part in the rituals or give repeated reassurance about the obsessional thoughts.

Aetiology

Genetic factors are suggested by the observation that obsessive–compulsive disorder is more frequent among the first-degree relatives of children and adolescents with obsessive–compulsive disorder than among the general population (Lenane *et al.* 1990.) However, the probands in this study had been referred for treatment, and it is possible that this biased the sample since parents with obsessive–compulsive disorder may be more likely to seek treatment for their affected children. Also, familial aggregation of cases might indicate social learning rather than genetic inheritance.

Neurotransmitter disorders Studies with adults suggest the involvement of serotonin systems in the brain (see p. 245) and there is a report of decreased density of the platelet serotonin transporter in children and adolescents with obsessional-compulsive disorder (Sallee *et al.* 1996).

Neurological factors There is an association between obsessive–compulsive disorder in childhood and conditions thought to arise from dysfunction of the basal ganglia. Some children with obsessive–compulsive disorder have tics or choreiform movements. Conversely, children with Gilles de la Tourette syndrome have obsessional and compulsive symptoms, and these symptoms have also been described in children with Sydenham's chorea.

Autoimmune factors The association with Sydenham's chorea, which is thought to be an autoimmune disorder following streptococcal infection, has led to the description of a subtype of childhood-onset obsessive–compulsive disorder which has been named paediatric autoimmune neuropsychiatric disorder associated with streptococcal infection – PANDAS (Swedo and Pekar 2000).

Taken together, these observations linking childhood obsessive–compulsive disorder and neurological disorder suggest that the former may arise from a disorder in some part of the basal ganglia (see Flament and Chabane 2000 for a review).

Epidemiology

The prevalence of obsessive–compulsive disorder in childhood is between 1 and 4% (see Flament and Chabane 2000).

Associated disorders

Severe and persistent obsessional thoughts and compulsive rituals in childhood are often accompanied by anxiety and depressive symptoms. In some cases there is an associated anxiety or depressive disorder. As noted above, tics occur in between 17 and 40% of children with obsessive–compulsive disorder (Geller *et al.* 1996). Many of the children with Gilles de la Tourette syndrome have obsessional symptoms, and it is important to make the distinction between this condition (see p. 431) and obsessive–compulsive disorder.

Prognosis

Clinical observations suggest that less severe forms of the disorder have a generally good outcome, but severe forms have a poor prognosis. In a 2–7-year follow-up of patients initially treated in drug trials, 43% still met diagnostic criteria for obsessive–compulsive disorder and only 6% were in full remission (Leonard *et al.* 1993). Other studies broadly confirm these findings (see Flament and Chabane 2000).

Treatment

When obsessional symptoms occur as part of an anxiety or depressive disorder, treatment is directed to the primary disorder. True obsessional disorders of later childhood are treated along similar lines to an anxiety disorder with the addition of behavioural methods similar to those used with adults (see p. 247). It is important to involve the family in treatment.

Clomipramine has been found to be more effective than placebo in obsessive–compulsive disorder of children aged 10 and over (deVeaugh-Geiss *et al.* 1992). As in adults, the symptoms are reduced but not removed by this treatment (Leonard *et al.* 1991). In a large multicentre, randomized trial, sertaline was shown to be an effective treatment for children and adolescents with obsessive–compulsive disorder (March *et al.* 1998). For consensus guidelines on management, see March *et al.* (1997).

Somatoform disorders and other unexplained physical symptoms

Children with a psychiatric disorder often complain of somatic symptoms which do not have a physical cause (Campo and Fritsch 1994; Garralda 1996). These complaints include abdominal pain, headache, cough, and limb pains. Most of these children are treated by family doctors. The minority who are referred to specialists are more likely to be sent to paediatricians than to child psychiatrists. *Chronic fatigue syndrome* (see p. 469) occurs in older children and adolescents and is usually best treated jointly by a paediatrician and a psychiatrist or clinical psychologist (Vereker 1992).

Abdominal pain

Abdominal pain is the symptom that has been studied most thoroughly. It has been estimated to occur in between 4 and 17% of all children, and is a common reason for referral to a paediatrician. In most cases abdominal pain is associated with headache, limb pains, and sickness. Physical causes for the abdominal pain are seldom found and psychological causes are often suspected. Some of these unexplained abdominal pains are related to anxiety and, as discussed on p. 840, others have been ascribed to 'masked' depressive disorder. Some appear to be a direct symptomatic response to stressful events. Treatment is similar to that for other emotional disorders. Follow-up suggests that a quarter of cases severe enough to require investigation by a paediatrician develop psychiatric problems or unexplained physical symptoms in adult life.

Conversion disorders

Conversion disorders (or conversion and dissociative disorder in ICD terminology) are more common in adolescence than in childhood, both in individual patients and in the rare epidemic form of the disorders (see p. 257). In childhood, symptoms are usually mild and seldom last long. The most frequent symptoms include paralyses, abnormalities of gait, and inability to see or hear normally. As in adults, dissociative and conversion symptoms can occur in the course of organic illness as well as in a dissociative or conversion disorder. As with adults, organically determined physical symptoms are sometimes misdiagnosed as conversion disorder when the causation physical pathology is difficult to detect and stressful events coincide with the onset of the symptom (Rivinus *et al.* 1975). For this reason, the diagnosis of dissociative (and conversion) disorder should be made only after the most careful search for organic disease.

Epidemiology

Conversion disorders were encountered rarely in the Isle of Wight study of children in the community (Rutter *et al.* 1970a). Among children referred to paediatricians, these disorders have been reported in 3–13%. In a survey of prepubertal children referred to a psychiatric hospital, Caplan (1970) found that conversion disorder was diagnosed in about 2%. In almost half of this 2%, organic illness was eventually detected either near the time or during the 4–11-year follow-up. Amblyopia was the symptom of organic disorder most likely to be diagnosed as psychogenic.

Treatment

Conversion and other somatoform disorders should be treated as early as possible before secondary gains accumulate. The psychiatrist and paediatrician should work closely together. Thorough physical investigation is required before the psychiatric diagnosis is made but unnecessary physical investigation should be avoided. Treatment is directed mainly at reducing any stressful circumstances and encouraging the child to talk about the problem. Symptoms may subside with these measures, or may need management comparable to that used for conversion disorder in adults (see p. 256). Physiotherapy and behavioural methods may be valuable for motor symptoms. For a review of child psychiatric syndromes with somatic presentation see Garralda (2000).

Mood disorders

Mania is probably extremely uncommon before puberty although there have been recent claims that it is more frequent than this (see Biederman 1998). The following account is therefore concerned with depressive disorders. Mood disorders in adolescence are considered on p. 853.

Healthy children are understandably unhappy in distressing circumstances, for example, when a parent is seriously ill or a grandparent has died. Some of these children are tearful, lose interest and concentration, and may eat and sleep badly. This section is not concerned with these normal forms of unhappiness, but with depressive disorders.

Psychiatrists have disagreed about the boundaries of the syndromes of depressive disorder in childhood. Some believe that the condition resembles that in adult life with only minor modifications accounted for by age. Thus young children do not experience guilt in an adult form and may have difficulty in describing feelings as sadness or despair. Other psychiatrists maintained that in childhood depressive disorders present not only with symptoms seen in adults but also in a form with little or no depressed mood but with a variety of other symptoms including unexplained abdominal pains, headache, anorexia, and enuresis, as well as irritability and anxiety (Kovacs 1996). It is not unreasonable to suggest that in childhood, as in adult life, depressive symptoms can come to light because of associated physical or behavioural symptoms. However, in children, as in adults, further examination of such cases will reveal evidence of depressed mood and the diagnosis of depressive disorder should be made only when there is clear evidence of the principal features of the syndrome seen in adults (see p. 271).

Depressive disorder should be distinguished clearly from depressive symptoms occurring as a component of an emotional or conduct disorder.

Epidemiology

Although depressive symptoms are common in middle and late childhood, depressive disorders are infrequent. In their landmark survey, Rutter *et al.* (1970a) found depressive disorder in only three of the girls and none of the boys among 2000 10–11-year-olds, though depressive symptoms were common as part of other disorders. Among 14-year-olds, Rutter *et al.* (1976b) found a depressive disorder in 1.5%. More recent estimates give higher figures: 1% of children in middle childhood, and 2–5% in mid-adolescence (Harrington 1994). Rates of depressive disorders are about equal among males and females before puberty (Kashani and Simonds 1979), but the increase in rate of depression during adolescence is greater among girls. Between 50 and 80% of children who meet diagnostic criteria for depressive disorder also meet the criteria for another diagnosis, especially an anxiety disorder (see Goodyer 2000).

Aetiology

The causes of depressive disorder in childhood appear to be similar to those of depressive disorder in adult life (see p. 287).

Genetic factors The rates of depressive disorder among first-degree relatives of children with depressive disorder (Harrington *et al.* 1993) are greater than the rates in the general population, suggesting genetic factors. Also there are strong continuities between depressive disorders in childhood and adult life. Harrington *et al.* (1990) followed up people who, when children, had been treated for a depressive disorder diagnosed by criteria similar to those in use today. Of the index group, 58% had a depressive disorder in adult life compared with 31% of a control group. However, members of the index group were no more likely than controls to have other kinds of psychiatric disorder in adult life.

As noted above, bipolar disorders seem to be rare in childhood (the great majority, perhaps all, appear first in adolescence).

Other causes Negative *life events* often precede the onset of depressive disorder in children, as they do in adults (Goodyer *et al.* 1985). *Temperament* also seems important, especially the tendency to react intensely to environmental stimuli (Goodyer *et al.* 1993).

Treatment

Any distressing circumstances should be reduced, if this is possible, while the child is helped to talk about feelings. The nature of the disorder is explained to the child and to the parents (who are often surprised by the diagnosis). Clinical trials of antidepressant drugs have not shown significant benefits over placebo, although one trial found that of fluoxetine was effective (Emslie *et al.* 1997). Cognitive–behaviour therapy has been found to be effective in moderately severe depression in adolescents, and this treatment should usually be tried first unless depression is severe (Harrington *et al.* 1998a, 1998b).

For a clinical guidelines for the assessment and treatment of depressive disorders in childhood see American Academy of Child and Adolescent Psychiatry (1998c).

Suicide in childhood

Suicide in childhood is considered on p. 513.

School refusal

School refusal is not a psychiatric disorder but a pattern of behaviour that can have many causes. It is convenient to consider it at this point in the chapter because of its association with anxiety and depressive disorder. School refusal is one of many causes of repeated absence from school. Physical illness is the most common. A small number of children miss school repeatedly because they are deliberately kept at home by parents to help with domestic work or for company. Some are truants who could go to school but choose not to, often as a form of rebellion. An important group stay away from school because they are anxious or miserable when there. These are the school refusers. The important distinction between truancy and school refusal was first made by Broadwin (1932). Later, Hersov (1960) studied 50 school refusers and 50 truants, all referred to a child psychiatric clinic. Compared with the truants, the school refusers came from more neurotic families, were more depressed, passive, and overprotected, and had better records of schoolwork and behaviour.

Prevalence

Temporary absences from school are extremely common, but the prevalence of school refusal is uncertain. In the Isle of Wight study school refusal was reported in rather less than 3% of 10- and 11-year-olds with psychiatric disorder (Rutter *et al.* 1970a). It is most common at three periods of school life, between 5 and 7 years, at 11 years with the change of school, and especially at 14 years and older.

Clinical picture

At times, the first sign to the parents that something is wrong is the child's sudden and complete refusal to attend school. More often there is an increasing reluctance to set out, with signs of unhappiness and anxiety when it is time to go.

These children complain of somatic symptoms of anxiety such as headache, abdominal pain, diarrhoea, sickness, or vague complaints of feeling ill. These complaints occur on school days but not at other times. Some children appear to want to go to school but become increasingly distressed as they approach it. The final refusal can arise in several ways. It may follow a period of gradually increasing difficulty of the kind just described. It may appear after an enforced absence for another reason, such as a respiratory tract infection. It may follow an event at school such as a change of class. It may occur when there is a problem in the family such as the illness of a grandparent to whom the child is attached. Whatever the sequence of events, the children are extremely resistant to efforts to return them to school and their evident distress makes it hard for the parents to insist that they go.

Aetiology

Several causes have been suggested. Separation anxiety is particularly important in younger children. In older children there may be a true school phobia, i.e. a specific fear of certain aspects of school life including travel to school, bullying by other children, or failure to do well in class. Other children have no specific fears but feel inadequate and depressed. Some older children have a depressive disorder.

Prognosis

Clinical experience suggests that most younger children eventually return to school. However, a proportion of the most severely affected adolescents do not return before the time when their compulsory school attendance ceases. There have been few studies of the longer prognosis of school refusal. Berg and Jackson (1985) followed up 168 teenage school refusers who had been treated as in-patients. After 10 years, about half still suffered from emotional or social difficulties or had received further psychiatric care. This study was concerned with severe cases and the general prognosis may be rather better.

Treatment

Except in the most severe cases, arrangements should be made for an early return to school. There should be discussion with the schoolteachers, who should be given advice about any difficulties that are likely to be encountered. It is sometimes more satisfactory for someone other than the mother to accompany the child to school at first. In a few cases a more elaborate graded behavioural plan is necessary. In the most severe cases admission to hospital may be required to reduce anxiety before a return to school can be arranged. Occasionally a change of school is appropriate.

Any depressive disorder should be treated. It has been reported that antidepressants are effective for school refusal even when there is no depressive disorder, but this view is not generally accepted. In all cases the child should be encouraged to talk about his feelings and the parents given support.

See Elliot (1999) for a review of school refusal.

Other childhood psychiatric disorders

Functional enuresis

Functional enuresis is the repeated involuntary voiding of urine occurring after an age at which continence is usual (see below) in the absence of any identified physical disorder. Enuresis may be nocturnal (bed-wetting) or diurnal (daytime wetting) or both. Most children achieve daytime and night-time continence by 3 or 4 years of age. Nocturnal enuresis is often referred to as primary if there has been no preceding period of urinary continence. It is called secondary if there has been a preceding period of urinary continence.

Nocturnal enuresis can cause great unhappiness and distress, particularly if the parents blame or punish the child. This unhappiness may be made worse by limitations imposed by enuresis on activities such as staying with friends or going on holiday.

Epidemiology

In the UK, the prevalence of nocturnal enuresis is about 10% at 5 years of age, 4% at 8 years, and 1% at 14 years. Similar figures have been reported from the USA. Nocturnal enuresis occurs more frequently in boys. Daytime enuresis has a lower prevalence and is more common in girls than boys. About half of daytime wetters also wet their beds at night.

Aetiology

Nocturnal enuresis occasionally results from physical conditions but more often appears to be caused by delay in the maturation of the nervous system, either alone or in combination with environmental stressors. There is some evidence for a genetic cause; about 70% of children with enuresis have a first-degree relative who has been enuretic (Bakwin 1961). Also, concordance rates for enuresis are twice as high in monozygotic as in dizygotic twins (Hallgren 1960). Linkage has been reported to several different loci (see Super and Postlewaite 1997), but further research is required before the significance of the findings can be assessed.

Although most enuretic children are free from psychiatric disorder, the proportion with psychiatric disorder is greater than that of other children. Psychological factors can contribute to aetiology, for example, unduly rigid toilet training, negative or indifferent attitudes of parents, and stressful events leading to anxiety in the child.

Assessment

A careful history and appropriate physical examination is required to exclude undetected physical disorder, particularly urinary infection, diabetes, or epilepsy, and to assess possible precipitating factors and the child's motivation.

Psychiatric disorder should be sought. If none is found, an assessment should be made of any distressing circumstances affecting the child. An evaluation is made of the attitudes of the parents and siblings to the bed-wetting. Finally, the parents should be asked how they have tried to help the child.

Treatment

Any physical disorder should be treated. If the enuresis is functional, an explanation should be given to the child and the parents that the condition is common and the child is not to blame. It should be explained to the parents that punishment and disapproval are inappropriate and unlikely to be effective. The parents should be encouraged not to focus attention on the problem but to reward success without drawing attention to failure. Many younger enuretic children improve spontaneously soon after an explanation of this kind, but those over 6 years of age are likely to need more active measures.

The next step is usually advice about restricting fluid before bedtime, lifting the child during the night, and the use of star charts to reward success.

Enuresis alarms Children who do not improve with these simple measures may be treated with an *enuresis alarm*. In the original pad and bell method, two perforated metal plates, separated by a cotton sheet, were incorporated in a low-voltage circuit including a battery, a switch, and a bell or buzzer. The resistance of the cotton sheet prevented current from flowing in the circuit. When the bed was made, the plates were placed under the position in which the child's pelvis will rest. When the child began to pass urine, the circuit was complete and the bell or buzzer sounded. The child turned off the switch, and rose to complete the emptying of the bladder. The bed was remade and a dry sheet was put between the metal plates before the child returned. Although effective, this method was cumbersome and has now been largely replaced by a sensor which detects the voiding of urine when attached to the child's pyjama trousers, and an alarm is carried on the wrist or in a pocket (Schmitt 1986). Either method requires about 6–8 weeks of treatment and some families break off before this has been completed.

The enuresis alarm seldom succeeds with children under the age of 6, or those who are uncooperative. For the rest, the alarm method, carried to completion, is effective within a month in about

70–80% of cases, although about a third relapse within a year (Forsythe and Butler 1989; Butler *et al.* 1990). It has been suggested that children with associated psychiatric disorder do less well than the rest.

Medication The synthetic antidiuretic hormone des-amino-D-arginine vasopressin (desmopressin) has a more prolonged action than natural vasopressin. It has been used in the treatment of nocturnal enuresis, when it can be given intranasally or orally. In one clinical trial about half the enuretic children treated with intranasal hormone became dry (Miller and Klauber 1990), and good results have been reported for an oral preparation (Skoog *et al.* 1997). However, patients relapse when treatment is stopped. Side-effects of the oral preparation include rhinitis and nasal pain; other side-effects are nausea and abdominal pain.

Enuresis can be treated with imipramine in a dose related to the child's age in accordance with the manufacturer's instructions. Most bed-wetters improve initially, but most relapse when the drug is stopped. For this reason and because of their side-effects and the danger of accidental overdose, the tricyclics are seldom the first-choice treatment.

See Butler (1998) and von Gontard (1998) for reviews of enuresis.

Faecal soiling

At the age of 3 years, 6% of children are still soiling themselves with faeces at least once a week; at 7 years the figure is 1.5%. By the age of 11 years, the figure is only 1% once a month or more. Soiling is three times more frequent in boys than in girls.

The term *encopresis* is sometimes used but in two senses. In its wider sense it is a synonym for faecal soiling. In its narrower sense it denotes the repeated deposition of formed faeces in inappropriate places. Because of this ambiguity, the term faecal soiling is used here.

Children who soil their clothes for any reason may feel ashamed, deny what has happened, and try to hide the dirty clothing.

Aetiology

Faecal soiling has several causes:

◆ *Constipation with overflow* is a common cause. Constipation has many causes, but common ones are low-fibre diet, pain on defecation due, for example, to an anal fissure, or refusal to pass faeces as a form of rebellion. Hirschsprung's disease is an uncommon but important cause. Soiling results when, after prolonged constipation, liquid faeces leak round the plug of hard faeces in the rectum.

◆ *Fear of using the toilet* Occasionally children who have no pain on passing faeces fear sitting on the toilet for other reasons, for example, that some harmful creature lives there.

◆ *Failure to learn bowel control* This can occur in children with learning disability or children of normal intelligence whose training has been inconsistent or inadequate.

◆ *Stress-induced regression* Children who have recently learned control may lose it as a result of a highly stressful experience such as sexual abuse.

◆ *Rebellion* Some children appear to defecate deliberately in inappropriate places and some children smear faeces on walls or elsewhere. Usually the family has many social problems, and often the child has other emotional or behavioural difficulties. The act appears to be a form of aggression towards the parents, though this intention is usually denied by the child.

Treatment

Treatment depends on the cause. The first step is to check for chronic constipation, and if it is present, to treat the cause. For this, joint assessment with a paediatrician may be needed. Even when constipation is not the main cause, it may require treatment as a secondary problem. A child who is fearful of the toilet should be reassured sympathetically. Inadequate toilet training may be improved using behavioural techniques including achievable targets, and star charts or other rewards, together with help for the parents. Stress-induced regression usually disappears when the child has been helped to overcome the trauma. Soiling as rebellion is more difficult to treat since it is generally part of wider social and psychological difficulties which may require intensive and prolonged help. If outpatient treatment fails in these cases, or in those due to inadequate or unsuitable training, the child may respond to behavioural management in hospital. If the child is admitted, the parents need to be closely involved in the treatment to avoid relapse when the child returns home.

Prognosis

Whatever the cause, it is unusual for encopresis to persist beyond the middle teenage years, although associated problems may continue. When treated, most cases improve within a year.

For a review of faecal soiling see Hersov (1994), Kelly (1996). For clinical guidelines on the management of chronic constipation and soiling in children see Felt *et al.* (1999).

Elective mutism

In this condition, a child refuses to speak in certain circumstances, although he does so normally in others. Usually speech is normal in the home but lacking in school. There is no defect of speech or language, only a refusal to speak in certain situations. Often there is other negative behaviour such as refusing to sit down or to play when invited to do so. The condition usually begins between 3 and 5 years of age after normal speech has been acquired. Although reluctance to speak is not uncommon among children starting school, clinically significant elective mutism is rare, probably occurring in about 1 per 1000 children. Assessment is difficult because the child often refuses to speak to the psychiatrist so that diagnosis depends to a large extent on the parents' account. In questioning the parents, it is important to ask whether speech and comprehension are normal at home. Although psychotherapy, behaviour modification, and speech therapy have been tried, there is no evidence that any treatment is generally effective. In some cases, elective mutism lasts for months or years. A 5–10-year

follow-up of a small group showed that only about half had improved (Kolvin and Fundudis 1981).

For a review see Kolvin (2000).

Stammering

Stammering (or stuttering) is a disturbance of the rhythm and fluency of speech. It may take the form of repetitions of syllables or words, or of blocks in the production of speech. Stammering is four times more frequent in boys than in girls. It is usually a brief problem in the early stages of language development. However, 1% of children suffer from stammering after they have entered school.

The cause of stammering is not known, although many theories exist. It seems unlikely that all cases have the same causes; genetic factors, brain damage, and anxiety may all play a part in certain cases but do not seem to be general causes. Stammering is not usually associated with a psychiatric disorder even though it can cause embarrassment and distress. Most children improve whether treated or not. Many kinds of psychiatric treatment have been tried, including psychotherapy and behaviour therapy, but none has been shown to be effective. The usual treatment is speech therapy.

Tic disorders

Tic disorders including Gilles de la Tourette syndrome are considered on pp. 430–1.

Dementia

Dementing disorders are rare in childhood. They result from organic brain diseases such as lipidosis, leucodystrophy, or subcaudate sclerosing panencephalitis. Some of the causes are genetically determined and may affect other children in the family. The prognosis is variable. Many cases are fatal, others progress to profound mental retardation.

Schizophrenia

Schizophrenia is almost unknown before 7 years of age, and seldom begins before late adolescence. When it occurs in childhood, the onset may be acute or insidious. The whole range of symptoms that characterize schizophrenia in adult life may occur (see Chapter 12), and in both DSM-IV and ICD-10 the criteria for diagnosis in children are the same as those used with adults; there is no separate category of childhood schizophrenia. Before symptoms of schizophrenia appear, many of these children are odd, timid, or sensitive, and their speech development is delayed. Early diagnosis is difficult, particularly when these non-specific abnormalities precede the characteristic symptoms.

Treatment is with antipsychotic drugs as in the management of schizophrenia in adults, though with appropriate reductions in dosage. The child's educational needs should be met and support given to the family. See Jacobsen and Rappoport (1998) or Volkmar (1996) for a review of schizophrenia in childhood.

Gender identity disorders

Effeminacy in boys

Some boys prefer to dress in girls' clothes and to play with girls rather than boys. Some have an obvious effeminate manner and say that they want to be girls. The cause of this condition is unknown. There is no evidence of any endocrine basis for these behaviours. Various family influences have been suggested, including the encouragement of feminine behaviour by the parents, a lack of boys as companions in play, a girlish appearance, and a lack of an older male with whom the child can identify. However, many children experience these influences without being effeminate.

In *treatment* it is difficult to know how far intervention is appropriate. Associated emotional disturbance in the child may require help, and it may be useful to investigate and discuss any family behaviours that seem to be contributing to or maintaining the child's behaviour. The prognosis is uncertain. Adult males with transvestism and transsexualism frequently recall enjoying feminine play as children, but follow-up studies of effeminate behaviour in early childhood show that the condition is more likely to proceed to homosexuality or bisexuality in adult life than to transsexualism or transvestism (Zuger 1984; Green 1985).

Tomboyishness in girls

In girls, the significance of marked tomboyishness for future sexual orientation is not known. It is usually possible to reassure the parents, and sometimes necessary to discuss their attitudes to the child and their responses to her behaviour.

For a review of gender identity disorders see Green (2000b).

Suicide and deliberate self-harm

Both deliberate self-harm and suicide are rare amongst children less than 12 years of age (though more common in adolescence). These problems are discussed in the chapter on suicide and deliberate self-harm (pp. 513 and 530).

Psychiatric aspects of physical illness in childhood

The associations between physical and psychiatric disorders in children resemble those in adults (see Chapters 14 and 16). There are three main groups of association which are met at least as frequently in paediatric as in child psychiatric practice:

- psychological and social consequences of physical illness;
- psychiatric disorders presenting with physical symptoms without a physical cause, for example, abdominal pain;
- physical complications of psychiatric disorders; for example, eating disorders and faecal soiling.

Most medical disorders of children are discussed in the chapter on psychiatry and medicine (Chapter 16). In this section we consider only some special problems in childhood.

The consequences of childhood physical illness

Psychiatric disorder provoked by physical illness

When physically ill, children are more likely than adults to develop delirium. A familiar example is delirium caused by febrile illness.

Some chronic physical illnesses and their treatment have psychological consequences for the child. In the Isle of Wight study of children (Rutter *et al.* 1970a), the prevalence of psychiatric disorder was only slightly increased with physical illnesses that do not affect the brain (for example, asthma or diabetes); however, the prevalence was considerably higher with organic brain disorder or epilepsy. Chronic illness may impair reading ability and general intellectual development (Rutter *et al.* 1970a; Eiser 1986), and sometimes also self-esteem and the ability to form relationships. The effects of the social and education problems caused by childhood illness may persist into adult life.

Effect on parents

The effects on parents are particularly important when the child's physical illness is chronic. Parents are naturally distressed by learning that their child has a chronic, disabling physical illness. The effects on the parents depend on many factors including the nature of the physical disorder, the temperament of the child, the parents' emotional resources, and the circumstances of the family. The parents may experience a sequence of emotional reactions like those of bereavement, and their marital and social lives may be affected. Most parents eventually develop a warm, loving relationship with a handicapped child and cope successfully with the difficulties. A few manage less well and may have unrealistic expectations, or they may be rejecting or overprotective.

Effect on siblings

The brothers and sisters of children with physical problems may develop emotional or behavioural disturbances. They may feel neglected, irritated by restrictions on their social activities, or resentful of having to spend so much time helping in the case of the handicapped child. Although some studies have shown more emotional and behavioural disturbances in siblings than would be expected by chance (e.g. Breslau and Prabucki 1987), most siblings manage well and may even benefit through increased abilities to cope with stress and to show compassion for others.

Management

Everyone involved in the care of physically disabled children should be aware of the psychological difficulties commonly experienced by these children and their families. When giving distressing information to families, it is particularly important to take time. It may be necessary to see the family many times, providing continuing advice and support. There should be regular liaison between the paediatrician and the child psychiatrist. There is a need for good communication with teachers and any social workers or others involved with the welfare of the child. Short periods of relief care can enable a family to continue with the care of a handicapped child.

Advice on imparting to parents the diagnosis of life-threatening illness affecting their children is given by Wooley *et al.* (1989).

Children in hospital

The admission of a child to hospital has important psychological consequences for the child and family. In the past, most hospitals discouraged families from visiting children. Bowlby (1951) suggested that this separation could have adverse immediate and long-term psychological effects; he identified successive stages of protest, despair, and detachment in the child during admission to hospital. These ideas were influential and it has become general policy to encourage parents to visit and take part in the care of their child and, if the child is young, to sleep in the hospital if family circumstances allow this. It is also recognized as important to prepare children for admission by explaining in simple terms what will happen, and by introducing to them the members of staff who will care for them in hospital.

It has been shown that repeated admission to hospital in early or middle childhood is associated with behavioural and emotional disturbances in adolescence (Rutter 1981). It is possible that these long-term consequences may be less following the improvements in hospital care mentioned above (Shannon *et al.* 1984).

Psychiatric problems of adolescence

There are no specific disorders of adolescence. However, special experience and skill are required to apply the general principles of psychiatric diagnosis and treatment to patients at this time of transition between childhood and adult life. It is often particularly difficult to distinguish psychiatric disorder from the normal emotional reactions of the teenage years. For this reason, this section begins by discussing how far emotional disorder is an inevitable part of adolescence. For a general review of problems in adolescence and their treatment, the reader is referred to Graham *et al.* (1999), Chapter 5.

Psychological changes in adolescence

Considerable changes – physical, psychosexual, emotional, and social – take place in adolescence. In the 1950s and 1960s it was widely assumed that these changes were commonly accompanied by substantial emotional upset. Indeed, Anna Freud (1958) regarded 'disharmony within the psychic structure' as a 'basic fact' of adolescence. Others described alienation, inner turmoil, adjustment reactions, and identity crises as common features of this time of life. Recently, a more cautious view has prevailed. Rutter *et al.* (1976a) concluded that rebellion and parental alienation are uncommon in mid-adolescence, although inner turmoil, as indicated by reports of misery, self-depreciation, and ideas of reference, is present in about half of all adolescents. However, this turmoil seldom lasts for long and usually goes unnoticed by adults. Rebellious behaviour is more common among older adolescents and many become estranged from school during their last year of compulsory attendance. Other problems include excessive drinking of alcohol and the use of drugs and solvents (discussed in Chapter 18), problems in relationships and sexual difficulties, and irresponsible behaviour in driving cars and motorcycles.

Epidemiology of psychiatric disorder in adolescence

Although psychiatric disorders are only a little more common in adolescence than in the middle years of childhood, the pattern of disorder is markedly different, being closer to that of adults. In adolescence the sexes are affected equally, anxiety is less common than in earlier years, and depression and school refusal are more frequent. An epidemiological study of adolescents in the USA (Whitaker *et al.* 1990) has found that the most common disorders are dysthymic disorder, major depression, and generalized anxiety disorder, followed by bulimia and anorexia nervosa, obsessive–compulsive disorder, and panic disorder. The precise estimates are difficult to interpret in relation to DSM-IV criteria because DSM-III was used, the population was confined to school attenders, and the information was solely from self-report.

Clinical features of psychiatric disorders of adolescence

Anxiety disorders

School refusal is common between 14 years of age and the end of compulsory schooling, and at this age is often associated with other psychiatric disorders. Generalized anxiety states are less common in adolescence than in childhood. Social phobias begin to appear in early adolescence; agoraphobia appears in the later teenage years.

Conduct disorders

About half the cases of conduct disorder seen in adolescents have started in childhood. Those that begin in adolescence differ in being less strongly associated with reading retardation and family pathology. Among younger children, aggressive behaviour is generally more evident in the home or at school. Among adolescents, it is more likely to appear outside these settings as offences against property. Truancy also forms part of the conduct disorders occurring at this age.

Mood disorders

Depressive symptoms are more common in adolescence than in childhood. In the Isle of Wight study they were 10 times more frequent among 14-year-olds than among 10-year-olds. In depressive disorder of adolescence, depressive mood is often less immediately obvious than anger, alienation from parents, withdrawal from social contact with peers, and underachievement at school.

The classification and aetiology of mood disorder are the same for adolescents as for adults, as described in Chapter 11. Major depression in adolescents is more often associated with major depression in relatives than is depression in childhood (Klein *et al.* 2001). Contrary to early beliefs, bipolar affective disorder is now thought to occur in adolescence. From retrospective studies of the adolescent disorder of adults diagnosed as manic-depressive, it appears that the first episodes of these illnesses may manifest in adolescence as abnormal behaviour, which may be misdiagnosed because the associated mood disorder is not detected.

The treatment of affective disorder is as described in Chapter 11, but with appropriate reductions in drug doses. Lithium is usually an effective prophylactic when the illness is recurrent. See Ryan and Puig-Antich (1986) or Goodyer (2000) for a review of mood disorder in adolescence.

Schizophrenia

Schizophrenia in adolescence is more common in boys than in girls. Usually the diagnosis presents little difficulty. When there is difficulty it is usually in detecting characteristic symptoms, especially in patients whose main features are gradual deterioration of personality, social withdrawal, and decline in social performance. The prognosis may be good for a single acute episode with florid symptoms, but is poor when the onset is insidious.

Eating disorders

Problems with eating and weight are common in adolescence. They are discussed in Chapter 15 since they resemble closely the same conditions in adult life. It is particularly important to involve the parents and perhaps other family members in

the treatment of an adolescent patient with eating disorders. Formal family therapy has been shown to be of value for anorexia nervosa in adolescents. For a review see Steiner and Lock (1998).

Suicide and deliberate self-harm

In recent years there has been a marked increase in suicide and deliberate self-harm among adolescents. These subjects are discussed in Chapter 17 (pp. 513 and 530).

Alcohol and substance abuse

Problems of substance abuse in adolescence are similar to those in adults, as described in Chapter 18. Excessive drinking is common among adolescents. Most adolescent heavy drinkers seem to reduce their drinking as they grow older, but a few progress to more serious drinking problems in adult life. Prevention programmes have been developed but there is no evidence they are effective (Foxcroft *et al.* 1997).

Occasional drug taking is common in adolescence and is often a group activity. Cigarette smoking and the use of cannabis and 'Ecstacy' are especially frequent. Solvent abuse is largely confined to adolescence and is usually of short duration. Abuse of drugs such as amphetamines, barbiturates, opiates, and cocaine is less common but more serious, since most drug-dependent adults have experimented with these drugs during adolescence. There is a strong association between conduct disorder in childhood and drug-taking in adolescence (Robins 1966).

Most adolescents experiment with drugs for short periods and do not become regular users. Those who persist in taking drugs are more likely to come from discordant families or broken homes, to have failed at school, and to be members of a group of persistent drug users. Feelings of alienation and low self-esteem may also be important.

Since regular drug taking starts less often in adult life than in adolescence, the limitation of drug taking among adolescents is an important preventive measure, but there is no evidence that it can be achieved. Drug-dependency clinics specifically for adolescents have been provided in the

USA, for example, but their effectiveness has not been demonstrated convincingly.

See American Academy of Child and Adolescent Psychiatry (1998d) for advice about the assessment and treatment of adolescents with substance abuse problems.

Sexual problems

Concern about sexuality is normal in adolescence. Excessive worry about masturbation and sexual identity and orientation may lead to medical consultation. Sexual abuse is increasingly a cause of referral to psychiatrists (see p. 858).

Many teenage pregnancies are terminated and some of the remainder are unwanted. There is a raised incidence of prenatal complications as compared with older mothers. Very young mothers frequently have substantial difficulties as parents and there is a poor outlook for many teenage marriages. The psychological and social problems of teenage pregnancy show that there is a need for access to continuing medical and social services during and after pregnancy.

Assessment of adolescents

There are special skills in interviewing adolescents. In general, young adolescents require an approach similar to that used for children, while with older adolescents it is more appropriate to employ that used with adults. It must always be remembered that a large proportion of adolescents attending a psychiatrist do so somewhat unwillingly and also that most have difficulty in expressing their feelings in adult terms. Therefore the psychiatrist must be willing to spend considerable time establishing a relationship with an adolescent patient. To do this, he must show interest in the adolescent, respecting his point of view, and talking in terms that he can understand. As in adult psychiatry, it is important to collect systematic information and describe symptoms in detail, but with adolescents the psychiatrist must be prepared to adopt a more flexible approach to the interview.

It is usually better to see the adolescent before interviewing the parents. In this way, the psychia-trist makes it clear that he regards the adolescent as an independent person. Later, other members of the family may be interviewed and the family seen as a whole. As well as the usual psychiatric history, particular attention should be paid to information about the adolescent's functioning at home, in school, or at work, and about his relationship with peers. Relevant physical examination should be carried out unless it has been performed by the person who made the referral.

Such an assessment should allow allocation of the problem to one of three classes. In the first, no psychiatric diagnosis can be made and reassurance is all that is required. In the second, there is no psychiatric diagnosis but anxious parents or a disturbed family need additional help. In the third, there is a psychiatric disorder requiring treatment.

Treatment of adolescents

Treatment methods are intermediate between those employed in child and adult psychiatry. As in the former, it is important to work with relatives and teachers. It is necessary to help, reassure, and support the parents and sometimes extend this to other members of the family. This is especially important when the referral reflects the anxiety of the family about minor behavioural problems rather than the presence of a definite psychiatric disorder. However, it is also important to treat the adolescent as an individual who is gradually becoming independent of the family. In these circumstances, family therapy as practised in child psychiatry is usually inappropriate and may at times be harmful.

Services for adolescents

The proportion of adolescents in the population who are seen in psychiatric clinics is less than the proportion of other age groups. Of those referred, some of the less mature adolescents can be helped more in a child psychiatry clinic. Some of the older and more mature adolescents are better treated in a clinic for adults. Nevertheless, for the majority the care can be provided most appropriately by a specialized adolescent service provided that close links are maintained with child and adult psychiatry services and with paediatricians. There are variations in the organization of these units and the treatment they provide, but most combine individual and family psychological treatment with the possibility of drug treatment for severe disorders. Most units accept out-patient referrals not only from doctors but also from senior teachers, social workers, and the courts. When the referral is non-medical, the general practitioner should be informed and the case discussed with him. All adolescent units work with schools and social services. In-patient facilities are usually limited in extent, so that it is important to agree with social services what kinds of problems need admission to a health service unit and which should be cared for in residential facilities provided (in the UK) by social services. Reasons for admission to a health service in-patient unit include the following:

♦ severe or very unusual mental symptoms requiring that the person's mental state be observed carefully, investigations carried out, or treatment monitored closely;

♦ behaviour that is dangerous to the self or others and that is due to psychiatric disorder.

When dangerous behaviour relates to personality and circumstances and not to illness, a hospital unit is not more effective than secure residential accommodation, and the behaviour of such adolescents may be stressful for others with mental disorders.

Child abuse

In recent years, the concept of child abuse has been widened to include the overlapping categories of physical abuse (non-accidental injury), emotional abuse, sexual abuse, and neglect. Most of the literature on child abuse refers to developed countries, rather than to developing countries in which children commonly face poor nutrition, other hardships such as severe physical punishment, abandonment, and employment as beggars and prostitutes.

The term *fetal abuse* is sometimes applied to behaviours detrimental to the fetus, including physical assault and the taking by the mother of substances likely to cause fetal damage. *Factitious disorder (or Munchausen syndrome) by proxy* is the name given to apparent illness in children, which has been fabricated by the parents, and to conditions induced by parents, for example, by partly smothering the child. (See p.475).

For a review of child abuse and neglect the reader is referred to Jones (2000).

Physical abuse (non-accidental injury)

Estimates of the prevalence of physical abuse vary with the criteria used. In the United Kingdom the annual incidence of physical abuse has been estimated as 0.8 per thousand children. Higher rates are reported in the US. (See Jones 2000). Less severe injury is probably much more frequent, but often does not come to professional attention.

Clinical features

Parents may bring an abused child to the doctor with an injury said to have been caused accidentally. Alternatively, relatives, neighbours, or other people may become concerned and report the problem to police, social workers, or voluntary agencies. The most common forms of injury are multiple bruising, burns, abrasions, bites, torn upper lip, bone fractures, subdural haemorrhage, and retinal haemorrhage. Some infants are smothered, usually with a pillow, and the parents report an apnoeic attack. Suspicion of physical abuse should be aroused by the pattern of the injuries, a previous history of suspicious injury, unconvincing explanations, delay in seeking help, and incongruous parental reactions. The psychological characteristics of abused children vary but include fearful responses to the parents, other evidence of anxiety or unhappiness, and social withdrawal. Such children often have low self-esteem, may avoid adults and children who make friendly approaches, and may be aggressive.

Aetiology

Child abuse is more frequent in neighbourhoods in which family violence is common, schools, housing, and employment are unsatisfactory, and there is little feeling of community.

In parents, the factors associated with child abuse include youth, abnormal personality, psychiatric disorder, lower social class, social isolation, disharmony and breakdown in marriage, and a criminal record. When a parent has a psychiatric disorder, it is most often a personality disorder; only a few parents have disorders such as schizophrenia or affective disorder. Many parents give a history of having themselves suffered abuse or deprivation in childhood. In abusing families, relationships between the parents are harsher and colder than in matched controls (Jones and Alexander 1978). Although child abuse is much more common in families with other forms of social pathology, it is certainly not limited to such families.

In the children, risk factors include premature birth, early separation, need for special care in the neonatal period, congenital malformations, chronic illness, and a difficult temperament.

Management

Doctors and others involved in the care of children should always be alert to the possibility of child abuse. They need to be particularly aware of the risks to children who have some of the characteristics described above, or are cared for by parents with the predisposing factors listed.

Doctors who suspect abuse should refer the child to hospital and inform a paediatrician or casualty officer of their suspicions. In the hospital emergency department, in-patient admission should be arranged for all children in whom non-accidental injury is suspected. If possible, the doctor's concerns should be discussed with the parents, and in any case they should be told that admission is necessary to allow further investigations. If the parents refuse admission, it may be necessary in England and Wales to apply to a magistrate for a Place of Safety Order; similar action may be appropriate in other countries. During admission, assessment must be thorough and include photographs of injuries and skeletal radiography. Radiological examination may show evidence of previous injury or, occasionally, of bone abnormalities such as osteogenesis imperfecta. A CT scan may be needed if subdural haemorrhage is suspected. All findings must be fully documented.

Once it has been decided that non-accidental injury is probable, senior doctors should talk to the parents. Other children in the family should be seen and examined. In assessing the parents, the following points should be considered (Skuse and Bentovim (1994):

- ◆ Do they acknowledge their part in the abuse?
- ◆ Do they accept the need to change their behaviour?
- ◆ Do they show a willingness to try new approaches to the child?
- ◆ Will they accept help with their personal or relationship problems?

The subsequent procedure will vary according to the administrative arrangements in different countries. In the UK, the Social Services Department should be notified so that they can organize a case conference for the exchange of information and opinions between various representatives of hospital and community. It may be decided to put the child's name on a child abuse register, thereby making the Social Services Department responsible for visiting the home and checking the problem regularly.

In some cases, the risk of returning the child to the parents is too great and separation is required. If the parents do not agree to separation, a care order can be sought by the Social Services Department. When abuse is severe, prolonged, or permanent, separation may be necessary and parents may face criminal charges. Because there are known cases of injury or death in children returned to their parents, it is vitally important that most careful assessment be made before physically abused children are returned. Countries vary in the requirements and procedures for reporting and monitoring possible physical abuse in children, and readers should inform themselves of the arrangements in the area in which they work.

For further information about the assessment of children who may have been abused, see American Academy of Child and Adolescent Psychiatry (1997a).

Prognosis

Children who have been subjected to physical abuse are at high risk of further problems. For example, the risk of further severe injury is probably between 10 and 30%, and sometimes the injuries are fatal. Abused children are likely to have subsequent high rates of physical disorder, delayed development, and learning difficulties. There are also increased rates of behavioural and emotional problems in later childhood and adult life even when there has been earlier therapeutic intervention (Lynch and Roberts 1982; Cohn and Daro 1987). As adults, many former victims of abuse have difficulties in rearing their own children. The outcome is better for abused children who can establish a good relationship with an adult and can improve their self-esteem; and for those without brain damage (Lynch and Roberts 1982; Rutter 1985).

Emotional abuse

The term emotional abuse usually refers to persistent neglect or rejection sufficient to impair a child's development. However, the term is sometimes applied to gross degrees of overprotection, verbal abuse, or scapegoating, which impair development. Emotional abuse often accompanies other forms of child abuse.

Emotional abuse has various effects on the child, including failure to thrive physically, impaired psychological development, and emotional and conduct disorders (Rutter 1985). Diagnosis depends on observations of the parents' behaviour towards the child, which may include frequent belittling or sarcastic remarks about him during the interview. One or both parents may have a disorder of personality, or occasionally a psychiatric

disorder. The parents should be interviewed separately and together to discover any reasons for the abuse of this particular child; for example, he may fail to live up to their expectations, or may remind them of another person who has been abusive to one of them. The parents' mental state should be assessed. For a review see Hart *et al.* (1998).

Treatment

In treatment, the parents should be offered help with their own emotional problems and with the day-to-day interactions with the child. It is often difficult to persuade parents to accept such help. If they reject help and if the effects of emotional abuse are serious, it may be necessary to involve the social services and to consider the steps described above for the care of children suffering physical abuse. The child is likely to need individual help.

Child neglect

Child neglect may take several forms including emotional deprivation, neglect of education, physical neglect, lack of appropriate concern for physical safety, and denial of necessary medical or surgical treatment. These forms of neglect may lead to physical or psychological harm.

Child neglect is more common than physical abuse, and it may be detected by various people, including relatives, neighbours, teachers, doctors, or social workers. Child neglect is associated with adverse social circumstances, and is a common reason for a child to need foster care (Fanshel 1981).

Non-organic failure to thrive and deprivation dwarfism

Paediatricians recognize that some children fail to thrive for no apparent organic cause. In children under 3, this condition is called non-organic failure to thrive (**NOFT**); in older children it is called psychosocial **short** stature syndrome (PSSS) or deprivation **dwarfism**.

Clinical picture

Non-organic failure to thrive is caused by the deprivation of food and close affection. In the children seen in the psychiatric service, there is usually evidence of problems in the parent-child relationship since the child's early infancy; these include rejection and, in extreme cases, expressed hostility towards the child. There may be physical or sexual abuse as well. Community surveys reveal other children whose failure to thrive is related to abnormal chewing and swallowing mechanisms (Wilensky *et al.* 1996). The infant who is failing to thrive may present either with recent weight loss or a weight persistently below the third percentile for chronological age. Height (or length) may be reduced. Head circumference may eventually be affected, and there may be cognitive and developmental delay. The infant may be irritable and unhappy, or, in more severe cases, lethargic and resigned. There is a clinical spectrum ranging from infants with mild feeding problems to those with all the severe features described above (Skuse 1985). If food and care are provided, the infants usually grow and develop quickly (Kempe and Goldbloom 1987).

Psychosocial short stature or 'deprivation dwarfism' was first reported by Powell *et al.* (1967). They described 13 children with abnormally short stature, unusual eating patterns, retarded speech development, and temper tantrums. Since this original account, the syndrome has been widely recognized. Although short in stature, the children may be of normal weight when seen by the doctor or even slightly overweight for their height. Growth hormone secretion is abnormal, with diminished 24-hour circulating levels due to diminished pulse amplitude (Stanhope *et al.* 1988). In severe cases the head circumference is reduced. Emotional and behavioural disorders occur, and may include food searching, scavenging, hoarding, disturbed sleep, and sometimes urination or defecation in inappropriate places (McCarthy 1981). There is often cognitive and developmental delay with impairment of language skills. They have low self-esteem and are commonly depressed. There is usually a history of deprivation or of psychological maltreatment. Away from the deprived environment, these children eat ravenously, sometimes until they vomit through overindulgence.

Treatment

In treating either syndrome, the first essential is to ensure the child's safety, which often means admission to hospital. Subsequently, some children can be managed at home, but some need foster care. Some parents can be helped to understand their child's needs and to plan for them; other parents are too hostile to be helped. If help is feasible, it should be intensive and should probably focus on changing patterns of parenting. It is unusual for the parents to be psychiatrically ill, but some have severe post-partum depression or other psychiatric disorder.

Prognosis

With both syndromes, the prognosis for severe cases is poor for psychological development and physical growth. The mortality rate is significant (Oates *et al.* 1985). Some of the less severe cases improve when removed from the abusing environment. Some children have to be placed permanently in foster care because family patterns are resistant to change. The abnormal behaviour is usually lost quickly and mental development follows physical growth (Skuse 1989).

Factitious disorder by proxy

This condition, in which a parent brings a child for treatment of fabricated symptoms, is discussed on p. 475.

Sexual abuse

The term sexual abuse refers to the involvement of children in sexual activities which they do not fully comprehend and to which they cannot give informed consent, and which violate generally accepted cultural rules. The term covers various forms of sexual contact with or without varying degrees of violence. The term also covers some activities not involving physical contact, such as exhibitionism and posing for pornographic photographs or films. The abuser is commonly known to the child and is often a member of the family (incest). A minority of children are abused by groups of paedophiles (sex rings).

Epidemiology

The annual incidence is about 2 per 1000 children per year (Jones 2000). The prevalence of sexual abuse has been estimated from criminal statistics or from surveys, but differences in definition and thoroughness of reporting making it difficult to interpret published figures. It is agreed that children are more often female – probably about 2–3:1 (Finkelhor 1986). The offender is usually male. Much sexual abuse takes place within the family, and stepfathers are over-represented among abusers (Russell 1984). The extent of sexual abuse by women is not known. It has been suggested that women may carry out about 10% of the sexual abuse of children (Glaser 1991). Faller (1987) reported that four-fifths of the women involved were the mothers of at least one of their victims, and McCarty (1986) found that many of the women abusers reported having been sexually abused themselves as children.

Retrospective studies suggest that between 20 and 50% of women in populations surveyed recall some experience of abuse in childhood (Peters *et al.* 1986). These figures include a wide range of experiences, ranging from minor touching to repeated intercourse. Effects on adults of abuse in childhood are described below and on p. 211.

Clinical features

The presentation of child sexual abuse depends on the type of sexual act and the relationship of the offender to the child. Children are more likely to report abuse when the offender is a stranger. Sexual abuse may be reported directly by the child or a relative, or it may present indirectly with unexplained problems in the child, such as physical symptoms in the urogenital or anal area, pregnancy, behavioural or emotional disturbance, or precocious or otherwise inappropriate sexual behaviour. In adolescent girls, running away from home or unexplained suicide attempts should raise the suspicion of sexual abuse. When abuse occurs within the family, marital and other family problems are common (Furniss *et al.* 1984; Madonna *et al.* 1991).

Effects of sexual abuse

Early emotional consequences of sexual abuse include anxiety, fear, depression, anger, and inappropriate sexual behaviour, as well as reactions to any unwanted pregnancy. As noted above, there may be inappropriate sexual behaviour and aggressive acts. A sense of guilt and responsibility is common. Some children show signs of post-traumatic stress disorder (see p. 194).

It is not certain how common these reactions are, or how they relate to the nature and circumstances of the abuse. Long-term effects are said to include depressed mood, low self-esteem, self-harm, difficulties in relationships, and sexual maladjustment in the form of either hypersensitivity or sexual inhibition. Effects of abuse are generally greater when the abuse has involved physical violence and penetrative intercourse. Some of the long-term effects are probably related to the events surrounding the disclosure of the abuse, including any legal proceedings.

In assessing these long-term effects, it should be remembered that sexual abuse often occurs in families with severe and chronic problems which are likely to have their own adverse long-term consequences. Nevertheless, even when these other factors are controlled for, sexual abuse in childhood seems to be associated with psychiatric disorder in adult life, especially with depressive disorders (Fergusson *et al.* 1996).

See Stevenson (1999) for a review of the long-term consequences of sexual abuse in childhood.

Aetiology

There is little reliable information about sexual abuse of children. It occurs in all socioeconomic groups, but is more frequent among socially deprived families. Finkelhor (1984) suggests that there are several preconditions which make sexual abuse more likely: in the abuser, deviant sexual motivation, impulsivity, a lack of conscience, and a lack of external restraints (for example, cultural tolerance); in the child, a lack of resistance (through insecurity, ignorance, or other causes of vulnerability).

Assessment

It is important to be ready to detect sexual abuse and to give serious attention to any complaint by a child of being abused in this way. When abuse has been established, it is important to assess whether it is likely to continue if the child remains at home and, if so, how dangerous it is likely to be. It is also important not to make the diagnosis without adequate evidence, which requires social investigation of the family as well as psychological and physical examination of the child. The child should be interviewed sympathetically and encouraged to describe what has happened. Drawings or toys may help younger children to give a description, but great care must be taken to ensure that they are not used in a way that suggests to the child events that have not taken place. Young children can recall events accurately, but they are more suggestible than adults (see p. 812 and Jones 1992 for advice on interviewing).

At an appropriate time it is often necessary to arrange a physical examination, including inspection of the genitalia and anal region and, if intercourse may have taken place within 72 hours, the collection of specimens from the genital and other regions (Kingman and Jones 1987). Usually this physical examination should be carried out by a paediatrician or police surgeon with special experience in the problem (see Royal College of Physicians 1991 for advice about physical examination).

The final decision as to whether abuse has taken place should be made after collecting information from the child, the physical examination, and social enquiries about the family.

For further information about assessment see American Academy of Child and Adolescent Psychiatry (1997a).

Treatment

The initial management and the measures to protect the child are similar to those for physical abuse (see p. 856), including a decision about separating the child from the family. There are particular difficulties involved in intervening with families in which sexual abuse has occurred. These include a marked tendency to deny the seriousness of the abuse and of other family problems, and in some cases deviant sexual attitudes and behaviour of other family members, possibly including other children. Individual and group treatment has been used for the offenders with the general aim of enabling the person to reduce denial and consider the effects of the abuse on the child. If the mother has a history of abuse, this needs to be discussed to help her understand how this may have affected her response to her child's abuse.

Some sexually abused children have highly abnormal sexual development for which they require help. They also need counselling to help them to deal with the emotional impact of the abuse, to come to terms with it, and to improve low self-esteem. Help should be in the form of a staged programme of rehabilitation for the whole family rather than a brief intervention. For a review of the treatment of child sexual abuse see Jones (2000).

Ethical and legal problems in child and adolescent psychiatry

As well as the ethical and legal problems related to the treatment of adults and discussed in Chapter 3 and elsewhere, the following issues are particularly likely to arise in the care of children with psychiatric disorders.

Conflicts of interest

In general, the interests of the child take precedence over those of the parents. This principle is most obvious, and most easily followed, in cases of child abuse. In other cases, the decision is more difficult, for example, when a depressed mother is neglecting her child and is likely to become more depressed if substitute care is arranged. Such problems can usually be resolved by discussion with the parents, and between the professionals caring for the child and for the parent.

Confidentiality

The care of children often involves collaboration between medical and social services, and sometimes with teachers. Different agencies may have different policies about the confidentiality of records, and doctors should take account of these differences when deciding what information to disclose.

Consent

In each country, the law decides an age below which parents give consent on behalf of the child. Below this age, the child's agreement should be obtained, if possible, since this will aid treatment, but if the child refuses the parents can decide. This problem arises, for example, when an adolescent under the legal age of consent refuses treatment for anorexia nervosa. The parents can also refuse treatment; however, their right to do so is linked to their duty to protect the child. In cases in which the parents' refusal appears not to be in the interests of the child, countries generally have provisions for a decision by a court of law.

Some of the complexities of English law can be mentioned briefly to illustrate the problems that have to be resolved in all legal systems. A fuller account of these and other issues is given by Hope and Savelescu (2001). Readers should find out how these issues are dealt with in the country in which they are working before they undertake the care of patients under the age at which adult rules of consent apply.

In English law, the age from which people are judged legally capable of giving or refusing consent is 18 years. However, English law recognizes that most of those aged between 16 and 18 years have the capacity to give consent to treatment and allows them to do so without the need for consent by a parent. The position is less clear when a 16- or 17-year-old does not consent to treatment but it is probably the case that the parents' consent is sufficient. The decision in each case is likely to depend on the consequences of refusal; the more severe these are, the more likely is it that a court would accept that the child's refusal can be over-ridden by the parents. Further complexities arise with children under 16, some of whom are competent to give consent to certain treatments. There is no general assumption of competence at this age, and it has to be established in the individual case, but if it is established, the minor can give consent. The question arose most notably in respect to the provision of contraception without the additional consent of a parent. In the Gillick case, it was ruled that, in English law, the minor could consent without the need to obtain the consent of the parent. It is probable, however, that with certain more invasive and risky treatments, the consent of a parent could be legally necessary – as well as clinically desirable. If a minor under the age of 16 years refuses treatment, this can be over-ruled by the parents if refusal is likely to result in harm. A final complexity concerns the definition of a parent. This problem arises, for example, when the person accompanying the child is not the person recognized by the law as having parental responsibility. For example, in English law, a father who is not married to the mother does not automatically have legal responsibility.

Consent for research poses similar problems for subjects below the legal age of consent. In most countries, parents consent on behalf of their children, and they may find it difficult to balance the risks to the child against the benefits, which are usually not to their child but to other children who might be treated for the same condition in the future. It is important that they are able to discuss the issues fully, and generally with a person additional to the person who is requesting the consent (for example, a nurse). Guidelines have been published, for example, by the British Paediatric Association (1992).

Appendix History taking and examination in child psychiatry

The format and extent of an assessment will depend on the nature of the presenting problem. The following scheme is taken from the book by Graham (1991), which should be consulted for further information. Graham suggests that *clinicians with little time available should concentrate on the items in bold type.*

1 **Nature and severity of presenting problem(s). Frequency. Situations in which it occurs. Provoking and ameliorating factors. Stresses thought by parents to be important.**

2 Presence of other current problems or complaints.

   (a) Physical. Headaches, stomach ache. Hearing, vision. Seizures, faints, or other types of attacks.

   (b) Eating, sleeping, or elimination problems.

   (c) **Relationship with parents and siblings. Affection, compliance.**

   (d) Relationships with other children. Special friends.

   (e) Level of activity, attention span, concentration.

   (f) Mood, energy level, sadness, misery, depression, suicidal feelings. General anxiety level, specific fears.

   (g) Response to frustration. Temper tantrums.

   (h) Antisocial behaviour. Aggression, stealing, truancy.

   (i) **Educational attainments, attitude to school attendance.**

   (j) Sexual interest and behaviour.

   (k) Any other symptoms, tics, etc.

3 Current level of development.

   (a) Language: comprehension, complexity of speech.

   (b) Spatial ability.

   (c) Motor coordination, clumsiness.

4 Family structure.

   (a) **Parents. Ages, occupations. Current physical and emotional state. History of physical or psychiatric disorder. Whereabouts of grandparents.**

   (b) **Siblings. Ages, presence of problems.**

   (c) Home circumstances: sleeping arrangements.

5 Family function.

   (a) **Quality of parental relationship. Mutual affection. Capacity to communicate about and resolve problems. Sharing of attitudes over child's problems.**

   (b) **Quality of parent-child relationship. Positive interaction: mutual enjoyment. Parental level of criticism, hostility, rejection.**

   (c) Sibling relationships.

   (d) Overall pattern of family relationships. Alliance, communication. Exclusion, scapegoating. Intergenerational confusion.

6 Personal history.

   (a) Pregnancy complications. Medication. Infectious fevers.

   (b) Delivery and state at birth. Birth weight and gestation. Need for special care after birth.

   (c) Early mother-child relationship. Post-partum maternal depression. Early feeding patterns.

   (d) Early temperamental characteristics. Easy or difficult, irregular, restless baby and toddler.

   (e) Milestones. Obtain exact details only if outside range of normal.

Appendix *Continued*

(f) **Past illnesses and injuries. Hospitalizations.**

(g) Separations lasting a week or more. Nature of substitute care.

(h) Schooling history. Ease of attendance. Educational progress.

7 Observation of a child's behaviour and emotional state.

(a) **Appearance. Signs of dysmorphism. Nutritional state. Evidence of neglect, bruising, etc.**

(b) **Activity level. Involuntary movements. Capacity to concentrate.**

(c) **Mood. Expression of signs of sadness, misery, anxiety, tension.**

(d) **Rapport, capacity to relate to clinician. Eye contact. Spontaneous talk. Inhibition and disinhibition.**

(e) **Relationship with parents. Affection shown. Resentment. Ease of separation**

(f) Habits and mannerisms.

(g) Presence of delusions, hallucinations, thought disorder.

(h) Level of awareness. Evidence of minor epilepsy.

8 Observation of family relationships.

(a) Patterns of interaction – alliances, scapegoating.

(b) Clarity of boundaries between generations: enmeshment.

(c) Ease of communication between family members.

(d) Emotional atmosphere of family. Mutual warmth. Tension, criticism.

9 Physical examination of child.

10 Screening neurological examination.

(a) Note any facial asymmetry

(b) Eye movements. Ask the child to follow a moving finger and observe eye movement for jerkiness, incoordination.

(c) Finger-thumb apposition. Ask the child to press the tip of each finger against the thumb in rapid succession. Observe clumsiness, weakness.

(d) Copying patterns. Drawing a man.

(e) Observe grip and dexterity in drawing.

(g) Jumping up and down on the spot.

(h) Hopping.

(i) Hearing. Capacity of child to repeat numbers whispered two metres behind him.

Further reading

Black, D., Hendriks, J. H., and Wolkind, S. (eds) (1998). *Child psychiatry and the law*, 3rd edn. Gaskell, London. (Deals with all aspects of child psychiatry and the law, within the framework of English law. More directly relevant to those working in the UK, although the general issues apply more widely.)

Gelder, M. G., López-Ibor, J. J. Jr, and Andreasen, N. C. (eds) (2000). *New Oxford textbook of psychiatry*, Part 9: Child and adolescent psychiatry. Oxford University Press, Oxford. (The 33 chapters in this part of the textbook provide a comprehensive account of the subject written for the general psychiatrist.)

Goodman, R. and Scott, S. (1997). *Child psychiatry*. Blackwell Science, Oxford. (A brief, concise introduction to the subject.)

Graham, P., Turk, J., and Verhulst, F. C. (1999). *Child psychiatry: a developmental approach*, 3rd edn. Oxford University Press, Oxford. (A comprehensive text for trainees.)

Rutter, M., Taylor, E., and Hersov, L. (1994). *Child psychiatry: modern approaches*, 3rd edn. Blackwell, Oxford. (A comprehensive work of reference. Less recent than the other books in this list but still valuable).

CHAPTER 25

Learning disability (mental retardation)

Learning disability (mental retardation)

This chapter is concerned with a general outline of the features, epidemiology, and aetiology of learning disabilities (mental retardation), the organization of services and, more specifically, with the psychiatric disorders affecting these people. Many of the psychiatric problems of children with learning disabilities are similar to those of children of normal intelligence; an account of these problems is given in Chapter 24 on child psychiatry.

Terminology

Over the years, several terms have been applied to people with intellectual impairment from early life. In the nineteenth and early twentieth centuries, the word idiot was used for people with severe intellectual impairment, and imbecile for those with moderate impairment. The special study and care of such people was known as the field of mental deficiency. When these words came to carry stigma, they were replaced by the terms mental subnormality and mental retardation. The term mental handicap has also been widely used, but recently the term learning disability is generally preferred in the UK. However, the term mental retardation is still used in ICD-10 and DSM-IV and it is in use in the USA and many other countries. In previous editions of this book, we have used the term mental retardation; in this edition we have decided to adopt the term learning disability unless the historical or other context requires another term.

The concept of learning disability or mental retardation

A fundamental distinction has to be made between intellectual impairment starting in early childhood (learning disability or mental retardation) and intellectual impairment developing later in life (dementia). In 1845, Esquirol made this distinction when he wrote:

Idiocy is not a disease, but a condition in which the intellectual faculties are never manifested; or have never been developed sufficiently to enable the idiot to acquire such an amount of knowledge as persons of his own age and placed in similar circumstances with himself are capable of receiving. (Esquirol 1845, pp. 446–7)

Early in the twentieth century, Binet's tests of intelligence provided quantitative criteria for ascertaining the condition. These tests also made it possible to identify lesser degrees of the condition that might not be obvious otherwise (Binet and Simon 1905). Unfortunately, it was widely assumed that people with such lesser degrees of intellectual impairment were socially incompetent and required institutional care (Corbett 1978).

Similar views were reflected in the legislation of the time. For example, in England and Wales the Idiots Act of 1886 made a simple distinction between idiocy (more severe) and imbecility (less severe). In 1913, the Mental Deficiency Act added a third category for people who 'from an early age display some permanent mental defect coupled with strong vicious or criminal propensities in which punishment has had little or no effect'. As a result of this legislation, people of normal or near-normal intelligence were admitted to hospital for long periods simply because their behaviour offended against the values of society. Although some of these people had committed crimes, others had not, for example, girls whose repeated illegitimate pregnancies were interpreted as a sign of the 'criminal' propensities mentioned in the Act.

Although, in the past, the use of social criteria clearly led to abuse, it is unsatisfactory to define mental retardation in terms of intelligence alone. Social criteria must be included, since a distinction must be made between people who can lead a normal or near-normal life and those who cannot. A useful modern definition is the one of the American Association for Mental Deficiency (AAMD), which defines mental retardation (the term preferred in the USA) as 'sub-average general intellectual functioning which originated during the development period and is associated with impairment in adaptive behaviour' (Heber 1981).

DSM-IV defines mental retardation as a 'significantly sub-average general intellectual functioning, that is accompanied by significant limitations in adaptive functioning in at least two of the following skill areas: communication, self-care, home living, social/interpersonal skills used for community resources, self direction, functional academic skills, work, leisure, health and safety' and having an onset before the age of 18.

Both ICD-10 and DSM-IV have the following four subtypes: mild (IQ 50–70); moderate (IQ 35–49); severe (IQ 20–34); profound (IQ below 20).

The ICD classification of impairment, disability, and handicap is relevant to the problems of people with learning disability. The impairment is of the central nervous system; the disability is in learning and acquiring new skills. The extent to which disabilities lead to impairment depends, in part, on experiences in the family and at school, and on the correction of associated problems such as deafness. The final stage, handicap, depends on the degree of disability and on other factors including the support that is provided.

Educationalists use other terms and these differ between countries. In the UK, the term is *special needs*, whereas in the USA, three groups are recognized: educable mentally retarded (EMR), trainable mentally retarded (TMR), and severely mentally retarded (SMR).

Epidemiology

Epidemiology of learning disability

In 1929, in an important survey of schoolchildren in six areas of the UK, E. O. Lewis found that the total prevalence of mental retardation was 27 per 1000, and the prevalence of moderate and severe learning disability (IQ less than 50) was 3.7 per 1000. Subsequent studies in many countries have broadly confirmed these early findings. In the population aged 15–19, the prevalence of moderate and severe learning disabilities is between 3.0 and 4.0 per 1000. The prevalence of moderate and severe learning disability has changed little since the 1930s. However, *incidence* of severe learning disability has fallen substantially, because antenatal, natal, and neonatal care have improved. The reason that prevalence has not changed is because patients are living longer, particularly those with Down's syndrome. This change has also affected the age distribution of people with severe learning disability, so that the numbers of adults have increased (see Fryers 2000 for a review of epidemiology).

Tizard (1964) drew attention to the distinction between 'administrative' prevalence and 'true' prevalence. He defined administrative prevalence as 'the numbers for whom services would be required in a community which made provision for all who needed them'. If the true prevalence of all levels of learning disabilities (IQ less than 70) is 20–30 per 1000 of the population of all ages (Broman *et al.* 1987), then the administrative prevalence is about 10 per 1000 of all ages. In other words, less than half of all such people require special provision. Administrative prevalence is higher in lower socioeconomic groups and in childhood when more patients need services. It falls after the age of 16 (Richardson 1992) because there is continuing slow intellectual development and gradual social adjustment.

For a review of the epidemiology of learning disability see Roeleveld *et al.* (1997).

Epidemiology of psychiatric disorder among learning-disabled people

Because the definition of learning disability is imprecise and because it is difficult to identify psychiatric disorder among people with learning disabilities, estimates of the prevalence of dual diagnoses (i.e. learning disability plus another psychiatric disorder) are likely to be inaccurate. However, it is undoubtedly greater than in the general population and this applies in children and adolescents (Lindsey 1997), adults (Wilson 1997) and the elderly (Collacott 1997). Most good community-based studies have found prevalence rates of 30–40% for coexistent psychiatric disorder in people with learning disabilities.

In an important survey of all children aged 9–11 years with an IQ under 70, Rutter *et al.* (1970a) found that almost a third were rated as 'disturbed' by their parents, whilst about 40% were so rated by their teachers. These rates were three to four times higher than the rates among intellectually normal children. Among children with severe learning disabilities, most surveys using standardized instruments have found that about half have psychiatric disorder, with the highest rates among those with the most profound learning disabilities (see Scott 1994).

Among people with mild learning disability, the types of psychiatric syndromes are similar to those in people of normal intelligence. Among people with moderate and severe learning disability, however, certain kinds of disorder are especially frequent, notably hyperactivity, pervasive developmental disorders, stereotypies, and self-injury.

Clinical features of learning disability

General description

The most frequent manifestation of learning disability is uniformly low performance on all kinds of intellectual task including learning, short-term memory, the use of concepts, and problem solving. Specific abnormalities may lead to particular difficulties. For example, lack of visuospatial skills may cause practical difficulties, such as inability to dress, or there may be disproportionate difficulties with language or social interaction, both of which are strongly associated with behaviour disorder. Among learning-disabled children, the common behaviour problems of childhood tend to occur when they are older and more physically developed than normal children and the problems last longer. Such behaviour problems usually improve slowly as the child grows older but may be replaced by problems that start in adult life.

Mild learning disability (IQ 50–70)

People with mild learning disability account for about 85% of people with learning disability. Usually their appearance is unremarkable and any sensory or motor deficits are slight. Most people in this group develop more or less normal language abilities and social behaviour during the pre-school years, and their learning disability may never be formally identified. In adult life, most people with learning disability can live independently in ordinary surroundings, though they may need help in coping with family responsibilities, housing, and employment, or when under unusual stress.

Moderate learning disability (IQ 35–49)

People in this group account for about 10% of the learning disabled. Most have better receptive than expressive language skills, which is a potent cause of frustration and challenging behaviour. Speech is usually relatively simple and often better understood by people who know the patient well. Many make use of simplified signing systems such as Makaton sign language. Activities of daily living such as dressing, feeding, and attention to hygiene are usually acquired over time but extended activities of daily living including use of money and road sense generally require support. Similarly, supported employment and residential provision are the rule.

Severe learning disability (IQ 20–34)

People with severe learning disability account for about 3–4% of the learning disabled. In the pre-school years their development is usually greatly slowed. Eventually many of them can be helped to look after themselves under close supervision and to communicate in a simple way, for example, by using objects of reference. As adults they can undertake simple tasks and engage in limited social activities, but they need supervision and a clear structure to their lives.

Profound learning disability (IQ below 20)

People in this group account for 1–2% of the learning disabled. Development across a range of domains tends to be at the level expected of a 12-month-old infant. Accordingly, people with profound learning disability are a vulnerable and highly needy group who require support and supervision, even for simple activities of daily living.

Physical disorders among learning-disabled people

Physical disorders are common among people with learning disability but they are not always identified. A learning-disabled person may not complain of feeling ill, and conditions may be noticed only because of changes in behaviour. Relatives should be told of the possible significance of such changes and encouraged to seek help. Clinicians should be aware of associations between certain learning-disability syndromes and physical illness (see, for example, Down's syndrome, p. 881).

The most important physical disorders in the learning disabled are sensory and motor disabilities, epilepsy, and incontinence. Severely learning disabled people (especially children) usually have one or often several of these problems. Only a third are continent, ambulant, and without severe behaviour problems. A quarter are highly dependent on other people. Among the mildly learning disabled, similar problems occur, but less frequently. Nevertheless, they are important because they determine whether special educational programmes are needed. Any sensory disorders add an important additional obstacle to normal cognitive development. Motor disabilities are frequent, and include spasticity, ataxia, and athetosis. As children grow older, the likelihood of physical problems increases in both the mildly and severely disabled. (Cooper 1999). Ear infections and dental caries are particularly common in this population.

Epilepsy is common among the learning disabled, especially the severely disabled. Forsgren *et al.* (1990) surveyed all the severely learning-disabled children (in hospital and in the community) originating from one London suburb. One-third of these children had experienced seizures at some time, and one-fifth had had at least one seizure in the year before the enquiry. Epilepsy was most common when learning disability was due to gross cerebral damage. Some epilepsy syndromes tend to improve with age but others are associated with neurodegenerative disorders in patients.

The epilepsy syndromes encountered in the general population affect people with learning disability but there are some differences of emphasis, notably that severe and mixed epilepsy syndromes are relatively common in patients with significant CNS damage. There are also some syndromes particularly associated with learning disability. *West's syndrome* starts in the first year of life. The seizures are actually a form of myoclonus and are often referred to as 'infantile spasms' or 'salaam attacks' with simultaneous tonic flexion of the neck and movements of the upper arms outward and forward. The episodes last for a few seconds. The EEG is strikingly abnormal with continuous multifocal spikes and large-amplitude slow waves, known as hypsarrhythmia. Several syndromes causing learning disability have been associated with this epilepsy syndrome, including tuberose sclerosis complex, and autistic spectrum disorders. *Lennox-Gastaut syndrome* is also strongly associated with learning disability. A triad of seizure types occur: absences, myoclonic jerks, and drop attacks. The EEG shows frequent diffuse spikes and slow wave discharges (Laidlaw *et al.* 1993).

Psychiatric disorders among learning-disabled people

In the past, psychiatric disorder amongst the learning disabled was often viewed as different from that seen in people of normal intelligence. One view was that people with learning disability did not develop emotional disorders; another view was that they developed these disorders but that the causes were biological rather than psychosocial. It is now generally agreed that people with learning disability experience psychiatric disturbances similar to those affecting the general population. However, the symptoms are often greatly modified by low intelligence (Russell 1997). Delusions, hallucinations, and obsessions may not be easily recognized in people who have limited language development and cannot easily describe them. Hence in diagnosing psychiatric disorder among the learning disabled, more emphasis has to be given to behaviour and less to reports of mental phenomena than would be the case in people of normal intelligence.

The reported *prevalences of psychiatric disorders* among the learning disabled are higher than those in the general population, but because of methodological problems, the range of estimates is wide (Scott 1994). The problems include the definition and recognition both of the learning disability and of the psychiatric disorder, as well as problems of sampling. The lower the IQ, the greater the difficulty in diagnosing psychiatric syndromes. For a review see Enfield and Tonge (1996).

Schizophrenia

The point prevalence of schizophrenia in people with learning disability is about 3% compared with 1% in the general population. This excess is consistent with the neurodevelopmental hypothesis of schizophrenia (see p. 359). Also, key areas for the elaboration of some of the symptoms of schizophrenia may be implicated in the disorder causing the learning disability, notably the medial temporal lobe of the dominant cerebral hemisphere.

The clinical picture of schizophrenia in the learning disabled is characterized by poverty of thinking. Delusions are less elaborate than in schizophrenics of normal intelligence, and hallucinations have a simple and repetitive content. When IQ is less than 45, it may be difficult to distinguish between the motor disorders of schizophrenia and the motor disturbances common among the learning disabled. The diagnosis of schizophrenia should be considered whenever intellectual or social functioning worsens without evidence of an organic cause, and especially if any new behaviour is odd and out of keeping with the patient's previous behaviour. When there is continuing doubt, a trial of antipsychotic drugs is often appropriate. Although a response to such medication is helpful to the patients, it does not, of course, confirm the diagnosis of schizophrenia.

The principles of *treatment* of schizophrenia in learning disabled people are the same as in patients of normal intelligence (see Chapter 12).

Mood disorder

People with learning disability are less likely than those of normal intelligence to complain of mood changes or to express depressive ideas. Diagnosis has to be made mainly on an appearance of sadness, changes in appetite and sleep, and behavioural changes of retardation or agitation. Severely depressed patients with adequate verbal abilities may describe hallucinations or delusions.

The rate of *suicide* in people with moderate and more severe learning disabilities is lower than in the general population. There are no good studies of people with mild and borderline learning disability, their vulnerability and social disadvantage. The motivation of poorly planned suicidal attempts may be misinterpreted, since the patient's view of the lethality of the attempt is of paramount importance, and is likely to be influenced by cognitive impairment. Self-injurious behaviours in more severely disabled patients are particularly difficult to interpret.

The differential diagnosis of mood disorder includes thyroid dysfunction, which is especially prevalent in those with Down's syndrome. *Mania* has to be diagnosed mainly from overactivity and behavioural signs of excitement, irritability, or nervousness.

The principles of *treatment* of mood disorders among the mentally retarded are the same as among people of normal intelligence (see Chapter 11).

Anxiety disorders and related conditions

Adjustment disorders are common among people with learning disability, occurring when there are changes in the routine of their lives. Anxiety disorders are frequent, especially at times of stress. Phobic disorders also develop but are often overlooked. Post-traumatic stress disorders have been reported in people with learning disability who have suffered physical or sexual abuse (Ryan 1994). Obsessive–compulsive disorders are also more frequent than in the general population. Conversion and dissociative symptoms are sometimes florid, taking forms understandable in terms of the patient's understanding of illness. Somatoform disorders and other causes of functional somatic symptoms can result in persistent requests for medical attention. *Treatment* is usually directed more to bringing about adjustments in the patient's environment, though reassurance and counselling, put in appropriately simple terms, can be helpful.

Eating disorders

Overeating and unusual dietary preferences are frequent among people with learning disability. Anorexia and bulimia nervosa appear to be less common than in the general population. Overeating and obesity are features of the Prader–Willi syndrome, a genetic cause of learning disability.

Personality disorder

Personality disorder is common among learning-disabled people, but is difficult to diagnose. Sometimes it leads to greater problems in management than those caused by the learning disability itself. The general approach is as described on p. 180, though with more emphasis on finding an environment to match the patient's temperament and less on attempts to bring about self-understanding.

Delirium and dementia

With learning disability, *delirium* is relatively frequent, probably because underlying cerebral disorders predispose to this kind of response to infection, medication, and other precipitating factors. As in people of normal intelligence, delirium is more common in childhood and old age than at other ages. Disturbed behaviour due to delirium is sometimes the first indication of physical illness. Also, delirium is frequently due to side-effects of drugs (especially antiepileptic, antidepressants, and other psychotropic medication).

Dementia

A progressive decline in intellectual and social functioning may be the first indication of dementia. From the early twenties, age-related neuronal death affects the CNS. People with learning disability are at risk of surpassing the threshold for dementia at a relatively younger age than those who have higher levels of intellectual functioning to start with. A progressive decline in intellectual and social functioning may be the first indication of dementia. Care is necessary to distinguish dementia from conditions such as depression and delirium, which give the impression of loss of intellectual capacity. The syndrome known as *childhood disintegrative disorder* (p. 830) is a form of dementia occurring in early life, often associated with lipidoses or other progressive brain pathology. Despite exhaustive investigations, many cases are of unknown aetiology (Evan-Jones and Rosenbloom 1978). As the life expectation of people with learning disability is increasing, dementia in later life is becoming more common. There is a particular association between Alzheimer's disease and Down's syndrome (see p. 882).

Disorders that are usually first diagnosed in childhood and adolescence

Many of the disorders in this category are more frequent in children with learning disability than in the general population and they are more likely to continue into adult life. It is important to be aware that relatively specific developmental disorders of scholastic skills, speech, and language and motor function may occur alongside more global learning disability.

Autism and attention-deficit hyperkinetic disorder

Both autism and hyperkinetic disorder are more common among the learning disabled than among the general population. The decision whether overactivity is abnormal is more difficult in learning disabled people than others, and has to take account of developmental stage rather than age in years. These disorders are discussed on pp. 826 and 831 and are not considered further here.

Abnormal movements

Stereotypes, mannerisms, and rhythmic movement disorders (including head banging and rocking) are common in people with severe learning disability, being present in about 40% of children and 20% of adults. *Repeated self-injurious behaviours* are less common but important. There is a specific association with the X-linked recessive disorder and with Lesch–Nyhan syndrome in which the biting away of the corner of a lip is common. Prader–Willi syndrome is strongly associated with a pattern of self-injury where patients pick their skin, and sometimes the subcutaneous tissues. Such clinical

observations have given rise to the concept of 'behavioural phenotypes', in which a behaviour is linked with a specific genotype. For a review, see O'Brien and Yule (1966).

Challenging behaviours

The term challenging behaviour is often used to describe behaviours that are of an intensity or frequency sufficient to impair the physical safety of the learning disabled person, to pose a danger to others, or make difficult participation in the community. It is probable that around 20% of learning-disabled children and adolescents and 15% of learning-disabled adults have some form of challenging behaviour. The causes of such behaviour include pain and discomfort, understimulation and overstimulation, desire for tangible reward, desire to escape unpleasant situations, difficulties in communication, side-effects of medication, and psychiatric disorders. Behavioural treatment (see p. 891) carried out in the places in which the behaviour most often appears or, in severe cases, in a residential unit is sometimes helpful. For more information see Emerson (1995). When possible, the primary cause is treated.

Forensic problems

People with mild learning disability have higher rates of criminal behaviour than the general population (see also Chapter 26, p. 903). The causes of this excess are complex, although influences in the family and social environment are often of most importance. Impulsivity, suggestibility, exploitability, and desire to please are other important reasons for involvement in crime. Compared with the general population, learning-disabled people who commit offences are more likely to be detected and, once apprehended, may be more likely to confess. Among the more serious offences, arson and sexual offences (usually exhibitionism) are said to be particularly common.

Increased suggestibility, with the risk of false confessions (see also p. 921), requires special care in questioning a learning-disabled person about an alleged offence. In the UK, police interrogation should proceed according to the Police and Criminal Evidence Act with the presence of an appropriate adult to ensure that the learning-disabled person understands the situation and the questions. Suggestibility can be assessed clinically, although a formal rating scale is available (Gudjonsson 1992). Once convicted, psychiatric supervision and specialized education may be needed. See Holland (1997) for a review of forensic aspects of learning disability.

Sleep disorders

Serious sleep problems are common among people with learning disabilities and can be a source of considerable distress to them and their carers (Brylewski and Wiggs 1998). Furthermore, sleep disorders may be associated with subsequent challenging behaviours and a worsening of cognitive impairment. The high rate of sleep disorders in this population is accounted for by four factors. First, there may be coexistent damage to CNS structures important for the sleep-wake cycle. Second, there may be epileptic seizures starting during sleep. Third, there may be epilepsy-related sleep instability which disrupts sleep architecture without causing frank seizures. The fourth and most common factor is inadvertent reinforcement of waking, for example, by giving drinks, allowing the watching of television, and so on. *Treatment* is directed to the cause.

Sexual relationships, marriage, and parenthood

Most people with learning disability develop sexual interests as do other people. Although the learning disabled are encouraged to live as normally as possible in other ways, sexual expression is usually discouraged by parents and other carers, and sexual feelings may not even be discussed.

In the past, sexual activity by people with learning disability was discouraged because it was feared that they might produce disabled children. It is now known that many kinds of severe learning disability are not inherited and that those that are inherited are often associated with infertility. A second concern is that people with learning disability will not be good parents. A study in Norway found that 40% of 126 children born to parents with learning disability suffered from 'failures of care' (Morch *et al.* 1997). However, a report from the UK indicates that some people with learning disability can care for a child successfully provided they are strongly supported (Booth and Booth 1993).

These issues should be considered carefully in each case, and contraception made available where appropriate.

Sexual problems

Some people with learning disability have a child-like curiosity about other people's bodies, which can be misunderstood as sexual. Some expose themselves without fully understanding the significance of their actions.

Effects of learning disability on the family

When a newborn child is found to be disabled, the parents are inevitably distressed. Feelings of rejection are common, but seldom last long and are replaced by feeling of the loss of the hoped for normal child. Frequently, the diagnosis of learning disability is not made until after the first year of life, and the parents then have to make great changes in their hopes and expectations for the child. They often experience prolonged depression, guilt, shame, or anger, and have difficulty in coping with the many practical and financial problems. They too grieve for the intact child they had hoped and planned for. A few reject their children, others become overinvolved in their care, sacrificing other important aspects of family life (Floyd and Phillippe 1993). Most families eventually achieve a satisfactory adjustment, although the temptation to overindulge the child remains. However well they adjust psychologically, the parents are still faced with a long prospect of prolonged hard work, frustration, and social problems.

If the child also has a physical handicap, these problems are increased. See Benson and Gross (1989) for a review.

There have been several studies on the effect of a child's learning disability on the family. In an influential study, Ann Gath (1978) compared two groups of families, those with a Down's syndrome child at home and controls with a normal child of the same age. Gath concluded that:

despite the understandable emotional reactions to the fact of the baby's abnormality, most of the families in the study have adjusted well, and two years later are providing a home environment that is stable and enriching for both the normal and handicapped children. (Gath 1978, p. 116)

However, it seemed likely that siblings were often at some disadvantage because of the time and effort that had to be devoted to the disabled child. These findings have been supported by subsequent research (see Gath 2000).

More recent studies have found that mothers with a learning-disabled child at home received help from their husbands but little help from other people, and many professionals were seen by the parents as lacking interest and expertise. Many parents report difficulties in obtaining help in looking after the children in school holidays and during weekends or evenings. For a review of the effects of learning disability on the family see Gath (2000).

Maltreatment and abuse

Many learning disabled children and their families are characterized by factors known to be associated in the general population with maltreatment of children (see p. 856). Nevertheless, although it is often said that abuse of learning-disabled children is frequent, there is no convincing epidemiological evidence to support this assertion.

Aetiology of learning disability

Introduction

Lewis (1929) distinguished two kinds of mental retardation (as it was then called): subcultural, i.e. the lower end of the normal distribution curve of intelligence in the population, and pathological, i.e. retardation due to specific disease processes. In a study of the 1280 mentally retarded people living in the Colchester Asylum, Penrose (1938) found that most cases were due not to a single cause but to an interaction of inherited and environmental factors. Subsequent research has confirmed that learning disability has multiple causes. This is particularly true for mild learning disability which is usually due to a combination of genetic and adverse environmental factors, and which is more common in the lower social classes.

Among the *severely learning disabled*, physical causes are found in 55–75% of cases (Broman *et al.* 1987). Prenatal causes predominate, of which the most frequent are idiopathic cerebral palsy, Down's syndrome, and fragile X syndrome; the proportion with fragile X syndrome is increasing steadily, accounting for 10–15%. Another three causes – other chromosomal anomalies, single-gene disorders, and idiopathic epilepsy – each account for 5–10% of cases.

It should be noted that increasing success in identifying specific causes of severe learning disability does not remove the need to consider all the additional social and other factors in every case. Until recently, severe learning disability was thought to be evenly distributed in the population; now it is known to be more common in the lower socioeconomic groups, possibly because preventive measures have been less effective in this group.

Whilst the aetiology of learning disability in developed countries is predominantly due to genetic and perinatal causes, postnatal factors (hypothyroidism, infection, trauma, toxicity) are important in developing countries. For a review of aetiology see Scott (1994), Deb and Ahmed (2000), and Kaski (2000).

Genetic factors

There is good evidence from family, twin, and adoption studies that polygenic inheritance is important in determining intelligence within the normal range, and that much mild mental retardation represents the lower end of the distribution curve of intelligence (Plomin 1994, 1995; Thapar *et al.* 1994). Fragile X syndrome is the most common known inherited cause of learning disability, and is particularly associated with moderate and mild cases. In severe learning disability, many genetic abnormalities, including about 180 single-gene defects, are responsible for the metabolic disorders and other anomalies that cause the learning disability (see Tables 25.1 and 25.2).

Table 25.1 summarizes the most frequent causes, but it is not exhaustive. Many of these causes are rare, and they are not described in this chapter. Information about some of the less rare conditions is summarized in Table 25.2. These syndromes are more likely to be dealt with by paediatricians than by psychiatrists. If psychiatrists take over the care of a patient suffering from any of these rare syndromes, they should work closely with the paediatrician and family doctor, and should acquaint themselves with up-to-date knowledge of the particular syndrome by studying a textbook of paediatrics and discussing the case with the appropriate specialist.

Some specific genetic syndromes

Specific genetic syndromes require some separate comment. Five groups may be recognized:

♦ *Dominant conditions* These are rare; examples are the phakomatoses, including neurofibromatosis.

♦ *Recessive conditions* This is the largest group of specific gene disorders. It includes most of the inherited metabolic conditions such as phenylketonuria (the commonest inborn error of metabolism), homocystinuria, and galactosaemia.

♦ *Chromosomal abnormalities* These can be divided into two groups:

(a) *Sex-linked conditions* The prevalence of mental retardation is 25% greater in males than in females. Lehrke (1972) was the first to suggest that the excess among males might be due to X-chromosome-linked causes. Recent research suggests that up to a fifth of learning disability in males is due to X-linked causes. Many rare specific X-linked syndromes have been identified, for example, glucose dehydrogenase deficiency and the Lesch–Nyhan syndrome. However, in most cases there is no metabolic abnormality, for example, the 'fragile X syndrome' (see p. 882). Sex chromosome abnormalities, such as Klinefelter's syndrome (XXY) and Turner's syndrome (XO), may also cause retardation.

(b) *Autosomal chromosome abnormalities* The most common is Down's syndrome (see p. 881).

♦ *Conditions with partial and complex inheritance* such as anencephaly. This group is poorly understood.

Social factors

Studies of the general population suggest that factors in the social environment may account for variation in IQ of as much as 20 points. The evidence comes from two kinds of enquiry. The first is epidemiological. Low IQ is related to lower social class, poverty, poor housing, and an unstable family environment. Such social factors may be the effects of low intelligence and do not necessarily exclude a genetic cause. Thus learning-disabled people might drift into an adverse social environment and bring up their children there. Follow-up studies from birth to adolescence have found marked differences in measured IQ according to psychosocial predictors (Sameroff *et al.* 1987).

The second source of evidence comes from attempts to enrich the environment of deprived children in special residential care (O'Connor 1968) and to provide special education. In one early experiment, children from large and unsatisfactory institutions were transferred to small well-staffed children's homes or given more stimulating

Table 25.1 The aetiology of learning disability

Genetic

Chromosome abnormalities

Fragile site

    Fragile X syndrome

Trisomy 21

    Down's syndrome

Trisomy 13

    Patau's syndrome

Trisomy 18

    Edwards' syndrome

Terminal deletion 5

    Cri du chat

Microdeletions

    Williams' syndrome

    Prader–Willi syndrome

    Angelman's syndrome

Metabolic disorders affecting

Amino acids (e.g. phenylketonuria, homocystinuria, Hartnup disease)

The urea cycle (e.g. citrullinuria, aminosuccinic aciduria)

Lipids (Tay–Sachs, Gaucher's, and Niemann–Pick diseases)

Carbohydrate (galactosaemia)

Purines (Lesch-Nyhan syndrome)

Mucopolysaccharidoses (Hurler's, Hunter's, Sanfillipo's, and Morquio's syndromes)

With gross disease of the brain

Tuberose sclerosis

Neurofibromatosis

With brain malformations

Neural tube defects

Hydrocephalus

Microcephalus

Antenatal damage

Infections (rubella, cytomegalovirus, syphilis, toxoplasmosis)

Intoxications (lead, certain drugs, alcohol)

Physical damage (injury, radiation, hypoxia)

Placental dysfunction (toxaemia, nutritional growth retardation)

Endocrine disorders (hypothyroidism, hypoparathyroidism)

Perinatal damage

Birth asphyxia

Complications of prematurity

Kernicterus

Intraventricular haemorrhage

Postnatal damage

Injury (accidental, child abuse)

Intoxication (lead mercury)

Infections (encephalitis, meningitis)

Autism

Impoverished environment

Table 25.2 Notes on some causes of learning disability

Syndrome	Aetiology	Clinical features	Comments
Chromosome abnormalities (for Down's syndrome and X-linked learning disability, see text)			
Triple X	Trisomy X	No characteristic feature	Mild learning disability
Trisomy 18 (Edwards' syndrome)	Trisomy 18	Growth deficiency, abnormal skull shape and facial features, clenched hands, rocker bottom feet, cardiac and renal abnormalities	
Trisomy 13 (Patau's syndrome)	Trisomy 13	Structural abnormalities of the brain, lip, and palate, polydactyly	Most die within a few weeks of birth
Cri du chat	Deletion in chromosome 5	Microcephaly, hypertelorism, typical cat-like cry, failure to thrive	Most die in early childhood
Inborn errors of metabolism			
Phenylketonuria	Autosomal recessive causing lack of liver phenylalanine hydroxylase. Commonest inborn error of metabolism	Lack of pigment (fair hair, blue eyes); retarded growth; associated epilepsy, microcephaly, eczema, and hyperactivity	Detectable by postnatal screening of blood or urine; treated by controlling the intake of phenylalanine from the diet during early years of life
Homocystinuria	Autosomal recessive causing lack of cystathione synthetases	Ectopia lentis, fine and fair hair, joint enlargement, skeletal abnormalities similar to Marfan's syndrome; associated with thromboembolic episodes	Learning disability variable; sometimes treated by methionine restriction
Galactosaemia	Autosomal recessive causing lack of galactose 1-phosphate uridyl transferase	Presents following introduction of milk into diet; failure to thrive, hepatosplenomegaly, cataracts	Detectable by postnatal screening for the enzymic defect; treatable by galactose-free diet; toluidine blue test on urine
Tay–Sachs disease	Autosomal recessive resulting in increased lipid storage (the earliest form of the cerebro-macular degenerations)	Progressive loss of vision and hearing; spastic paralysis; cherry-red spot at macula of retina; epilepsy	Death at 2–4 years

Table 25.2 Continued

Syndrome	Aetiology	Clinical features	Comments
Hurler's syndrome	Autosomal recessive affecting mucopolysaccharide storage	Grotesque features; protuberant abdomen; hepatosplenomegaly; associated cardiac abnormalities	Death before adolescence
Lesch–Nyhan syndrome	X-linked recessive leading to enzyme defect affecting purine metabolism. Excessive uric acid production and excretion. Gene on short arm of chromosome q26–27	Almost all are normal at birth. Development of choreoathetoid movements, scissors position of legs, and self-mutilation of lips and fingers	Diagnosed prenatally, by sampling amniotic fluid and enzyme estimation. Postnatal diagnosis by enzyme estimation in hair roots. Death in early adult life. Self-mutilation may be reduced by treatment with hydroxytryptophan
Other inherited disorders			
Neurofibromatosis (von Recklinghausen's syndrome)	Autosomal dominant inheritance	Neurofibromata, café au lait spots, vitiligo; associated with symptoms determined by site of neurofibromata; astrocytomas, meningioma	Learning disability in a minority
Tuberose sclerosis (epiloia)	Autosomal dominant (very variable penetrance). Linkage to two genes, TSC1 and TSC2	Epilepsy, adenoma sebaceum on face, white skin patches, shagreen skin, retinal phakoma, subungual fibromata; associated multiple tumours in kidney, spleen, and lungs	Learning disability in about 70% (more frequent with TSC2 gene)
Lawrence–Moon–Biedl syndrome	Autosomal recessive	Retinitis pigmentosa, polydactyly, sometimes with obesity and impaired genital function	Learning disability usually not severe
Infection			
Rubella embryopathy	Viral infection of mother in first trimester	Cataract, microphthalmia, deafness, microcephaly, congenital heart disease	If mother infected in first trimester, 10–15% infants are affected (infection may be subclinical)
Toxoplasmosis	Protozoal infection of mother	Hydrocephaly, microcephaly, intracerebral calcification, retinal damage, hepatosplenomegaly, jaundice, epilepsy	Wide variation in severity

Table 25.2 Continued

Syndrome	Aetiology	Clinical features	Comments
Cytomegalovirus	Intrauterine infection	Brain damage; only severe cases are apparent at birth	60% of survivors have learning disability
Congenital syphilis	Syphilitic infection of mother	Many die at birth; variable neurological signs, 'stigmata' (Hutchinson teeth and rhagades often absent)	Uncommon since routine testing of pregnant women; infant's tests positive at first but may become negative
Cranial malformations			
Hydrocephalus	Sex-limited recessive; inherited developmental abnormality, e.g. atresia of aqueduct, Arnold–Chiari malformation, meningitis, spina bifida	Rapid enlargement of head. In early infancy, symptoms of raised CSF pressure; other features depend on aetiology	Mild cases may arrest spontaneously; may be symptomatically treated by CSF shunt; intelligence can be normal
Microcephaly	Recessive inheritance, irradiation in pregnancy, maternal infections	Features depend upon aetiology	Evident in up to a fifth of institutionalized patients with severe learning disability
Miscellaneous			
Spina bifida	Aetiology multiple and complex	Failure of vertebral fusion; *spina bifida cystica* is associated with meningocele or, in 15–20%, myelomeningocele; latter causes spinal cord damage with lower limb paralysis, incontinence, etc.	Hydrocephalus in four-fifths of those with myelomeningocele; retardation in this group
Cerebral palsy	Perinatal brain damage; strong association with prematurity	Spastic (common), athetoid and ataxic types; variable in severity	Majority are below average intelligence; athetoid are more likely to be of normal IQ
Hypothyroidism (cretinism)	Iodine deficiency or (rarely) atrophic thyroid	Appearance normal at birth; abnormalities appear at 6 months; growth failure, puffy skin, lethargy	Now rare in UK; responds to early replacement treatment
Hyperbilirubinaemia	Haemolysis, rhesus incompatibility, and prematurity	Kernicterus (choreoathetosis), opisthotonus, spasticity, convulsions	Prevention by anti-rhesus globulin; neonatal treatment by exchange transfusion

education. Twenty years later they were found to have higher IQs than those who, as children, had remained in their original institutions (Skeels 1966). More recent studies have confirmed that well-planned and prolonged intervention can be beneficial for socially deprived children (Garber 1988).

Other environmental factors

These include intrauterine infection (such as rubella), environmental pollutants (such as lead), maternal alcoholism in pregnancy (see pp. 545), severe malnutrition, iodine deficiency, and excessive irradiation to the womb. There may be vulnerable periods of brain development during which damage is particularly likely to follow exposure to such environmental hazards (Davison 1984; Holland 1994). Malnutrition in the first 2 years of life is probably the most common cause of learning disabilty in the world as a whole, but is much less frequent in developed countries. Iodine deficiency is an important cause in many developing countries.

There is no doubt that severe *lead intoxication* can cause an encephalopathy with consequent intellectual impairment. It is much less certain whether the moderate levels of lead found in some British children (in the past resulting in part from air pollution with lead additives in petrol) can cause intellectual retardation. It is known that children absorb lead more readily than adults, and therefore are at greater risk from environmental pollution. However, most of the studies have been of children from lower socioeconomic groups, and it is impossible to be certain how far findings of low intelligence (compared with children in other areas) are due to slightly raised lead levels in their blood and how far to social influences (see Pocock *et al.* 1994 for a review).

Birth injury

This is an important cause of learning disability. Early studies estimated that clinically recognizable birth injuries accounted for about 10% of learning disability. Pasamanick and Knobloch (1966) suggested a 'continuum of reproductive casualty' in which additional cases of mild intellectual retardation resulted from less obvious brain lesions sustained *in utero* or perinatally. Although prematurity and low birth weight are associated with learning disability (Lukeman and Melvin 1993; Hack *et al.* 1994), the theory of a continuum of reproductive casualty is not otherwise supported.

Some specific causes of mental handicap

Down's syndrome

In 1866, Langdon Down tried to relate the appearance of certain groups of patients to the physical features of ethnic groups. One of his groups had the condition originally called mongolism, and now generally known as Down's syndrome. This condition is a frequent cause of learning disability, occurring in 1 in every 650 live births. It is more frequent among older women, occurring in about 1 in 2000 live births for mothers aged 20–25 and 1 in 30 for those aged 45. The incidence of Down's syndrome has decreased because of reduced birth rates among older women, and increases in detection of the condition by amniocentesis and subsequent termination of pregnancy. Usually the learning disability is mild or moderate, but occasionally it is severe.

The clinical picture is made up of a number of features, any one of which can occur in a normal person. Four of these features together are generally accepted as strong evidence for the syndrome. The most characteristic signs are:

- a small mouth and teeth, furrowed tongue, and high-arched palate;
- oblique palpebral fissures and epicanthic folds;
- flat occiput;
- short and broad hands, a curved fifth finger and a single transverse palmar crease; and
- hyperextensibility or hyperflexibility of joints and hypotonia.

Clinical picture

There are often other associated abnormalities, and 10% are multiply handicapped. Congenital heart disease (especially septal defects) occurs in about 5%. Intestinal abnormalities are common, especially duodenal obstruction. Hearing may be impaired. An immunological defect predisposes to infections. There are also increased risks of acute leukaemia, hypothyroidism, and atlantoaxial instability.

There is considerable variation in the degree of learning disability; the IQ is generally between 20 and 50, and in 15% it is above 50. Mental abilities usually develop fairly quickly in the first 6 months to a year of life but then increase more slowly. The temperament of children with Down's syndrome has often been described as loveable and easygoing, but there is a wide individual variation. Emotional and behaviour problems are less frequent than in forms of retardation associated with clinically detectable brain damage.

In the past, the infant mortality of Down's syndrome was high, but with improved medical care survival into adult life is usual. About a quarter of people with Down's syndrome now live beyond 50 years of age. In middle life, people with Down's syndrome develop Alzheimer-like changes in the brain (Holland *et al.* 1998; Berg *et al.* 1995). However, clinical decline occurs in a smaller proportion of people and much later than would be expected from the neuropathological data (Wisniewski *et al.* 1994).

Many of the older people with Down's syndrome live with their families or in large residential groups and have led restricted lives. In the future, the social outlook may be better for those who have been involved in intensive early teaching and it is likely that most will require long-term support of a kind more vigorous than is currently available if the quality of their lives is to be maintained. See Carr (1994) for a review.

Aetiology

In 1959, Down's syndrome was found to be associated with the chromosomal disorder of trisomy (three chromosomes instead of the usual two). About 95% of cases are due to trisomy 21. These cases result from failure of disjunction during meiosis and are associated with increasing maternal age. The risk of recurrence in a subsequent child is about 1 in 100. The remaining 5% of cases of Down's syndrome are attributable either to translocation involving chromosome 21 or to mosaicism. The disorder leading to translocation is often inherited, and the risk of recurrence is about 1 in 10. Mosaicism occurs when non-disjunction takes place during any cell division after fertilization. Normal and trisomic cells occur in the same person, and the effects on cognitive development are particularly variable (Thapar *et al.* 1994). Down's pathology is presumed to be due to the increased 'dosage' of genes on chromosome 21. This could account for the excess of early-onset Alzheimer's (see p. 623).

Fragile X syndrome

Fragile X syndrome is the second most common specific cause of learning disability after Down's syndrome and is the most common inherited cause. It occurs in up to 1 in 1000 males and in a milder form in 1 in 200 females. It accounts overall for about 10% of those with learning disability, i.e. for about 7% of moderate and 4% of mild disability in males, and about 2.5% of moderate and 3% of mild learning disability in females.

There are a number of characteristic but somewhat variable clinical features, none of which is diagnostic. These features include enlarged testes, large ears, a long face, and flat feet. Psychological disturbances are said to include abnormalities of speech and language, autism and other social impairments, and disorders of attention and concentration. There are increased rates of several psychiatric disorders, including attention-deficit hyperactivity disorder. The inheritance of the condition is unusual and complex, and has been difficult to unravel. During recent years, there has been a major advance in understanding the molecular genetic basis of the condition, and a gene referred to as *FMR–1* has been identified. This gene contains an amplified CGG repeat sequence, which constitutes the fragile X anomaly.

The identification of the genetic abnormality makes it possible to identify affected heterozygous females who are clinically and even cytogenetically normal. These women can be advised of the high risk of affected offspring and the need for prenatal testing. Conversely, many women who are at risk of being carriers can be reassured they do not have the condition. Similarly, it is possible to determine whether men are transmitting carriers.

The psychological and psychiatric complications in the syndrome mean that there is a need for regular review of affected people. See Dykens *et al.* (1994), Margolis *et al.* (1999), and Pimentel (1999) for reviews of the fragile X syndrome.

Causes of psychiatric disorder and behaviour problems in the learning disabled

The diversity of psychiatric disorders among the learning disabled makes it unlikely that they have a single aetiology. As with mental disorder among people of normal intelligence, several causes have to be considered: biological, psychosocial, and developmental (Dosen 1993; Matson and Sevin 1994). Overall, there is no reason to expect that particular mental disorders co-morbid with learning disability have aetiologies which differ from those in people with normal intelligence.

Biological factors include specific associations such as those between the fragile X syndrome and attention-deficit hyperactivity disorder and anxiety disorder, between the Lesch–Nyhan syndrome and self-injury, and between Down's syndrome and Alzheimer's disease.

As already noted, people with severe learning disability have some organic brain pathology and so do a smaller number of those with moderate and mild learning disability. As mentioned in Chapter 24, psychiatric disorder is associated with brain damage in children of normal intelligence (Rutter *et al.* 1970a). There is also a known association

between cerebral pathology on the one hand and schizophrenia and affective disorders on the other (Davison and Bagley 1969; Davison 1983). Therefore, it is likely that some psychiatric disorders (including major psychiatric illnesses) in learning-disabled people are related to brain pathology. There is an especially close association between epilepsy and behaviour disorder in learning disabled people (see Matson and Sevin 1994). Such behaviour disorder may be due not only to the direct effects of epilepsy but also to the side-effects of anticonvulsant drugs (see p.437).

Psychosocial factors such as bereavement or a disrupted family may cause mental disorder and behaviour problems in the learning disabled as they do in people of normal intelligence. People with learning disability may develop adjustment reactions or mental disorder when the arrangements for their care are disrupted or if they are treated badly or exploited. Such factors have been seen as mediated, at least in part, through conditioning and social learning. Operant conditioning models point to the importance of inadequate environmental reinforcement of adaptive behaviours and the reinforcement of maladaptive behaviours.

Developmental factors include abnormalities of temperament, difficulty in acquiring language and social skills, low self-esteem, and educational failure. These difficulties may discourage the efforts of families and carers, so adding to the disadvantage.

It should not be forgotten that *iatrogenic factors* can contribute to the causes of psychiatric disorder among people with learning disability. As mentioned above, these include the side-effects of drugs, especially those used to treat epilepsy, and over- or understimulating environments in the community or within an institution.

The assessment of people with learning disability

Assessment of the learning disabled is directed towards four main areas:

- aetiology of the learning disability;
- associated biomedical conditions;
- intellectual and social skills development;
- associated psychiatric disorders and their causes and consequences.

Severe learning disability can usually be diagnosed in infancy, especially as it is often associated with detectable physical abnormalities or with delayed motor development. Some people with learning disability have specific developmental disorders, i.e. impairment of specific functions greater than would be expected from the general intellectual level.

The clinician should be cautious in diagnosing less severe learning disability on the basis of delays in development. Although routine examination of a child may reveal signs of developmental delay, suggesting possible learning disability, confident diagnosis often requires specialist assessment. Full assessment has several stages: history taking, physical examination, examination of the mental state, developmental testing, functional behavioural assessment, analysis of the interaction between the disabled person and the family and the social support systems, and other aspects of adjustment. These stages will be considered in turn. Although this section is concerned mainly with the assessment of children, similar principles apply in adolescence and adult life.

History taking

In the course of obtaining a full history, particular attention should be given to any family history suggesting an inherited disorder and to abnormalities in the pregnancy or the delivery of the child. Dates of passing developmental milestones should be ascertained (see p. 798). A full account of any behaviour disorders should be obtained. Details of any associated medical conditions, such as congenital heart disease, epilepsy, and cerebal palsy, should be documented.

Physical examination

A systematic physical examination should include the recording of head circumference. It is important to be alert for the physical signs suggesting one of the many specific syndromes (see Table 25.2). Neurological examination is important and should include particular attention to impairments of vision and hearing. Neuroimaging studies may be required to supplement the physical examination.

Mental state examination:

The approach to this should be flexible as poor attention and concentration may necessitate serial assessments to gather all the information needed. Similarly, the interviewer may have to accompany the patient in some activity he or she prefers, such as drawing or going for a walk, in that formal assessments are often resisted. Questioning should take into account the receptive language developmental level of the patient. Behavioural observations by family, friends, and carers are often most helpful. Clinical assessment by experienced psychiatrists may be supplemented by the use of standardized scales of assessment of psychopathology which have been adapted for use in patients with learning disability (see Sturmey *et al.* 1991 for a review).

Developmental assessment

This assessment is based on a combination of clinical experience and standardized methods of measuring intelligence, language, motor performance, and social skills. Although the IQ is the best general index of intellectual development, it is not reliable in the very young.

Tests used in developmental assessment

Standardized assessment instruments are widely used in screening, diagnosing, and assessing the severity of disorders of psychological development. Several do not require special training for their

Box 25.1 Commonly used instruments in developmental assessment

Vineland Social Maturity Scale

The Vineland Scale is useful in the assessment of children who do not cooperate in testing since it can be completed by interview with a reliable informant. An overall social age can be derived from the scale, which may be usefully compared with mental and chronological age.

The British Ability Scales and Differential Ability Scales

These scales measure a range of functions and educational attainments, and can be used to calculate an overall IQ.

The Adaptive Behaviour Scales

These scales are probably the most widely used method for the assessment of social functioning in learning disabled adults.

The Portage Guide to Early Education

This assessment has been adopted for use internationally. It provides a broad-based developmental assessment including socialization, language, self-help, and cognitive and motor domains. Only a brief period of

training is required for the assessor, together with the active involvement of the parent or other carer.

Autism Behaviour Check List

This questionnaire is completed by the parent or other carer. It is a reliable indicator of problems in the area of autism and delay in social development.

The Disability Assessment Scale

This scale focuses on autistic and related social developmental, language disorders, and behavioural problems.

British (Peabody) Picture Vocabulary Test

This is a test of language comprehension, suitable for non-speaking children. The test booklet is largely pictorial and the age range covered is 3–19 years. Although professional training is not required, the test is used by psychologists and speech therapists.

Reynell Scales of Language Development

These scales assess comprehension and expressive language in the age range 1 month to 6 years. The test is of particular use with non-verbal children.

correct administration. There are pronounced 'floor effects', with many neuropsychological tests which are too difficult for some people with learning disability. It is useful to bear in mind the classification of tests employed. There are norm-referenced tests (such as the WAIS and other IQ measures); tests of adaptive behaviour in social settings; criterion-referenced tests which apply to particular skills without reference to population norms; and assessments of behavioural functioning.

Some commonly used instruments are described briefly in Box 25.1. The first four provide a general assessment over a range of developmental domains. The second four focus, either entirely or principally, on specific aspects of development. All have good reliability and validity.

Functional behavioural assessment

This is based on accounts by family and carers and the observations by the clinical team of the person's ability to care for himself, his social abilities including his ability to communicate, his sensory motor skills, and his relationships with others.

Assessment of interactions and adjustment

This assessment is concerned with the interaction between the person with the learning disability and those who are closely involved in care. The assessor considers opportunities for learning new skills, making relationships, and achieving maximum choice about way of life. If the person with learning disability has reasonable language ability, it is usually possible to obtain much of the information from him. When language is less well developed, the account has to be obtained mainly from informants. It is particularly important to obtain a complete description of any change from the usual pattern of behaviour. It is often necessary to ask parents, teachers, or care staff to keep records of behaviours such as eating, sleeping, and general activity so that problems can be identified and quantified. The assessor should keep in mind the possible causes of psychiatric disorder outlined above, including unrecognized epilepsy. For more information see Dosen (1993).

The care of people with learning disability

A historical perspective

Current arrangements for care and the remaining unsolved problems can best be understood in relation to the history of the development of services for people with learning disabilities (see M. Thomson 1998 for further information.)

A review of services can begin usefully in the early years of the nineteenth century. At this time there were numerous reports of improved forms of care, notably by Itard, physician-in-chief at the Asylum for the Deaf and Dumb in Paris, who attempted to train a 'wild boy' found in Aveyron in 1801. This child was thought to have grown up in the wild, isolated from human beings. Itard made great efforts to educate the boy, but after persisting for 6 years he concluded the training had failed. Nevertheless, his work had important and lasting consequences, for it led others to try educational methods. These methods were developed, for example, by Seguin, director of the School for Idiots at the Bicêtre in Paris who, in 1842, published the *Theory and nature of the education of idiots*. Seguin believed that the mentally retarded had latent abilities which could be encouraged by special training, involving physical exercise, moral instruction, and graded tasks (Seguin 1864, 1866).

These ideas were taken up in other countries, particularly Switzerland and Germany. The Swiss physician Guggenbuhl founded the first special residential institution for the mentally retarded at Abendberg in 1841. Similar institutions were opened in other parts of Europe to provide a training that would enable their pupils to live as independently as possible. However, it was recognized that some people with learning disability needed long-term care.

At the end of the nineteenth century, several influences led to a more custodial approach to the care of people with learning disability. These influences included the development of the science of genetics, the measurement of intelligence, the beliefs embodied in the eugenics movement, and a general decrease in public tolerance of abnormal behaviour. In England and Wales, such ideas were reflected in the Mental Deficiency Act 1913, which empowered local authorities to provide for the confinement of the 'intellectually and morally defective' and imposed upon the authorities a responsibility to provide training and occupation. In the years that followed, the total number of people of this kind in institution rose from 6000 in 1916 to 50 000 in 1939 and remained at high levels well into the post-war period.

In the 1960s the need for reform was recognized in several developed countries. This was prompted in part by the changes that had already been effected in psychiatric hospitals (see pp. 769–70), and by improved psychological research. However, much of the impetus came from campaigning by groups of parents, and from public concern about the generally poor conditions in which people with learning disabilities were housed. Surveys of hospitals for the 'retarded' showed that the mean IQ of their patients was over 70. Many residents had only mild learning disability, and many did not need hospital care. About the same time, it was shown that simple training could help many patients, both the mildly and severely learning disabled (O'Connor 1968). Further research showed the advantages of residential care in small homely units (Tizard 1964). However, public concern in the UK and other countries was aroused less by the findings of research than by revelations about the scandalously poor conditions in some hospitals for people with learning disabilities.

It is now recognized in all developed countries that people with learning disability should be integrated as far as possible into society. However, there have been divergent views about the best way to achieve greater integration. In the UK, resources have been inadequate and progress slow. In the USA, deinstitutionalization was carried out more quickly, with both successes and failures.

The main current principle of care is 'normalization', an idea developed in Scandinavia in the 1960s. This term refers to the general approach of providing a pattern of life as near normal as possible (Nirje 1970). Normalization implies that almost all people with learning disability will live in the community, participating in normal activities and relationships, making choices, and having full social opportunities. Children are brought up whenever possible with their families, and adults are encouraged to live as independently as possible. For the few who need special social and health care, accommodation and activities are designed to be as close as possible to those of family life. The concept of normalization has been further developed in the USA and elsewhere, and includes specialist help to enable people to achieve their full potential. Increasingly, disabled people are organizing themselves into advocacy groups, and those who are unable to speak for themselves about the services have advocates to speak for them.

General provisions

The precise model for the care of people with learning disability in a community matters less than the detail in which it is planned and the enthusiasm with which it is carried out. Good planning requires both an estimate of the needs of the population to be served, and a summation of individual assessments of those identified, since each person has individual needs. To achieve this, local case registers and linked developmental records are needed.

The general approach to care is educational and psychosocial. The family doctor and paediatrician are mainly responsible for the early detection and assessment of learning disability. The team providing continuing health care includes also psychologists, speech therapists, nurses, occupational therapists, and physiotherapists. Volunteers can play a valuable part, and it is useful to encourage self-help groups for parents. In the UK, residential provisions for people with learning disability are from several sources: health service, social services, and charitable bodies.

Specific services

The main elements in a comprehensive service for people with learning disability and their families or carers are:

- the prevention and early detection of learning disability;
- regular assessment of the learning-disabled person's attainments and disabilities;
- advice, support, and practical measures for families;
- provision for education, training, occupation, or work appropriate for each person;
- housing and social support to maximize self-care;
- medical, nursing, and other services for those who require these forms of help as out-patients, day patients, or in-patients;
- psychiatric and psychological services.

Preventive services

Primary prevention depends largely on genetic counselling, early detection of fetal abnormalities during pregnancy, and safe childbirth. *Secondary prevention* aims to prevent the progression of disability by either medical or psychological means. The latter include 'enriching' education and early attempts to reduce behavioural problems.

In developed countries, there remains considerable scope for reduction of the genetic causes of severe learning disability, but it is unlikely that it will be possible to affect the incidence of mild learning disability significantly. In developing countries, the incidence of learning disability could be substantially reduced by general measures to improve the health of mothers during pregnancy, and by better perinatal care. See Murphy (1994) for a review.

Genetic screening and counselling

These measures begins with assessment of the risk that an abnormal child will be born. Such an assessment is based on study of the family history, on knowledge of the genetics of conditions that give rise to learning disability, and on awareness of the possibilities for genetic screening. The risks of screening are explained to the parents who are encouraged to discuss them. Most parents seek advice only after a first abnormal child has been born. Those who seek advice before starting to have children do so usually because there is a person with learning disability on one or other side of the family. A positive diagnosis of an abnormality leading to termination or indeed a false-positive result of screening causes considerable distress (Iles and Gath 1993; Marteau 1994). It is important, therefore, that those involved in screening are alert to psychological issues and have the appropriate counselling skills.

Prenatal care

Prenatal care begins even before conception, with immunization against rubella for girls who lack immunity, and advice on diet, alcohol, and smoking.

Prenatal diagnosis overlaps with genetic screening. It is becoming available for an increasing number of conditions with the aim of providing information to those at risk of having abnormal children, reassurance to others, and appropriate treatment of affected infants through early diagnosis. Amniocentesis, fetoscopy, and ultrasound scanning of the fetus in the second trimester can reveal chromosomal abnormalities, most open neural tube defects, and about 60% of inborn errors of metabolism. Amniocentesis carries a small but definite risk, and so is usually offered only to women who have carried a previous abnormal fetus, women with a family history of congenital disorder, and women over 35 years of age.

Rhesus incompatibility is now largely preventable. Sensitization of a rhesus-negative mother can usually be avoided by giving anti-D antibody. An affected fetus can be detected by amniocentesis and treated if necessary by exchange transfusion. For pregnant women with diabetes mellitus, special care can improve the outlook for the fetus. Further information about these aspects of care will be found in textbooks of obstetrics and paediatrics.

Postnatal prevention

In the UK, all infants are routinely tested for phenylketonuria, and routine testing for hypothyroidism and galactosaemia is becoming increasingly common. Universal screening for elevated levels of lead has been advocated, but recent evidence suggests that it is more appropriate to target screening in areas where lead levels are known to be high (Diermayer *et al.* 1994). Intensive care units and improved methods of treatment for premature and low-birth-weight infants can prevent learning disability in some who would previously have suffered brain damage. However, the methods also enable the survival of some disabled children who would otherwise have died.

Compensatory education

Compensatory education is intended to provide optimal conditions for the mental development of the disabled child. This was the aim of the Head Start programme in the USA, which provided extra education for deprived children. Its methods varied from nursery schooling to attempts to teach specific skills. Many of the results were disappointing (Rutter and Madge 1976). A more intensive programme with similar aims was carried out in Milwaukee (Garber 1988). Skilled teachers taught children living in slum areas with mothers who had a low IQ (under 75). This additional education started when the child was 3 months old and continued until school age. At the same time, the mothers were trained in a variety of domestic skills. These children were compared with control children of the same age who came from similar families but who had not received additional education and whose mothers had not been trained. At the age of four and a half, the trained children had a mean IQ 27 points higher than that of the controls. This study can be faulted because the selection of children was not strictly random, and because some of the changes in test scores could have been due to practice. Nevertheless, the main findings probably stand: substantial effort by trained staff can produce worthwhile improvement in children of low intelligence born to socially disadvantaged mothers. The findings indicate the need to train the parents as well as children. Overall, it seems that early interventions can be effective, especially if they are family centred. However, many uncertainties remain about the components and the delivery of such help (see Murphy 1994).

Assessment

Severe learning disability is usually obvious from an early stage. Lesser degrees may become apparent only when the child starts school. Family doctors and teachers should be able to detect possible learning disability, but a full assessment may require attendance at a special centre where the child can be observed in many different activities. The methods have been described earlier (pp. 884–6).

Once learning disability has been diagnosed, regular reviews are required. For children, these reviews are usually carried out by a disciplinary child health team in cooperation with teachers and social workers. The child psychiatrist liaises with the team and sees children referred to him with emotional, behavioural, and psychiatric problems.

It is important to arrange a thorough review before the child leaves school. This review should assess the need for further education, the prospects for employment, unpaid occupation, independent living, and the need for specialist physical and psychological health care. Adults with learning disability need to be assessed regularly to make sure that they are continuing to achieve their potential and still receiving appropriate care. This is usually carried out by a multidisciplinary community team which includes a psychiatrist specializing in the care of the learning disabled.

Help for families

Help for families is needed from the time that the diagnosis is first made. It is not enough to give worried parents an explanation on just one occasion. They may need to hear the explanation several times before they can absorb all its implications. Adequate time must be allowed to explain the prognosis, indicate what help can be provided, and discuss the part the parents can play in helping their child to achieve full potential. Paediatricians and health visitors are usually involved in this process.

Thereafter, the parents need continuing support. When the child starts school, parents should be kept informed about progress, and feel involved in the planning and provision of care. They should be given help with practical matters, such as day care for the child during school holidays, baby-sitting, or arrangements for family holidays. In addition to practical assistance, the parents need continuing psychological support, which may be provided as a programme for the whole family (Murphy 1994; Petronko et al. 1994).

Families are likely to need extra help when their child is approaching puberty or leaving school. Making the transition from child to adult services is often extremely stressful. Both day and overnight care are often required to relieve carers and to encourage the learning-disabled person to become more independent.

Education, training, and occupation

One aspect of the policy of normalization is that children with learning disability should be educated as far as possible within mainstream schools. The extent to which this is done varies in different countries and different regions of the same country.

Research has consistently shown the value of an early start to the education of children with learning disability, who should attend a play group or nursery class. When school age is reached, the least disabled children can attend remedial classes in ordinary schools. Others need to attend special educational programmes for children with learning disabilities. It is still not certain which learning-disabled children benefit from ordinary schooling. Education in an ordinary school offers the advantages of more normal social surroundings, social integration, and the expectation of progress, but it may have the disadvantage of a lack of special teaching skills and equipment. Also, the methods of teaching emphasizing self-expression are inappropriate for some children with learning disability who need special teaching of language and communication (Howlin 1994). Another advantage in having disabled children in ordinary schools is that other pupils learn to accept that their integration into society is the norm.

Before learning-disabled children leave school, they need reassessment and vocational guidance. Most young people with mild learning disability are able to take normal jobs or enter sheltered employment. The severely disabled are likely to transfer to adult day centres, which should provide a wide range of activities if the abilities of each attender are to be developed as much as possible.

Residential care

It is now widely accepted that parents should be supported in caring for their learning-disabled children at home. If care is too heavy a burden for the parents because of their other family commitments, the learning-disabled child should, if possible, be in another family. Adults should be supported in ordinary housing, or placed with a family, or lodgings, or in a small residential group home. Studies such as those of Landesman-Dyer (1981) confirmed that moving learning-disabled children to smaller living units is not itself beneficial. Staff need to encourage the residents to develop their social skills and to live as normally as possible. Also, challenging behaviour is not

necessarily reduced by a move to a smaller living unit.

Medical services

People with learning disability should have the same access to general and specialist medical services as other citizens, but they require extra support if they are to obtain full benefit. Children and adults with learning disability often have physical handicaps or epilepsy, for which continuing medical care is needed. This care is usually obtained from the ordinary medical services and this arrangement can work well, provided doctors and nurses are sufficiently aware of how to deal with a learning-disabled patient and have the time and resources to do so. Families and carers are helped when care is coordinated by a single person so that they do not receive conflicting advice. Specialist nurses have a special role in such coordination. Shared care between neurologists and psychiatrists can improve outcomes for some patients, for example, in the diagnosis and treatment of episodic attacks.

Psychiatric services

Psychiatric care is an essential part of a comprehensive community service for people with learning disability. In some countries this care is provided by the generic mental health services, but in the UK it is generally provided by staff who specialize in the care of people with learning disability.

Treatment of psychiatric disorder and behavioural problems

Treatment of psychiatric disorder in the learning disabled follows the principles described elsewhere in this book, taking account of their special problems.

Psychiatric disorder in people with learning disability usually comes to notice through changes in behaviour. It should be remembered, however, that behavioural change can also result from physical illness or from stressful events, both of which should be carefully excluded. In the most disabled, and especially those with sensory deficits, behavioural disturbance may be due to understimulation and frustration at the inability to communicate wishes and needs. Once the cause is clear, the treatment follows. Physical illness should be treated promptly, stressful events reduced if possible, or a more stimulating environment provided when appropriate. If the disturbed behaviour results from a psychiatric disorder, the treatment is similar in most ways to that for a patient of normal intelligence with the same disorder. Carers are often involved in behavioural assessment and treatment methods and it is important to support them adequately.

The most serious and persistent disorders may require hospital admission for more intensive behavioural management, which may be combined with pharmacotherapy. See Petronko *et al.* (1994) for a review of treatment in the community and Spreat and Behar (1994) for a review of in-patient treatment.

Medication

The indications for psychotropic drugs are generally the same as in patients of normal intelligence and the full range of such medication should be available for the learning disabled. However, the psychiatrist has particular responsibility for organizing effective ongoing monitoring, including regular physical examination. The latter is especially important for patients with severe communication impairments who cannot describe side-effects. Also, neurologically impaired patients may be develop side-effects at lower doses and suffer from oversedation, delirium, and extrapyramidal symptoms. Antipsychotic and benzodiazepine drugs are often useful in the short-term control of behaviour problems. There are few controlled trials of the efficacy and tolerability of antipsychotic drugs in the longer-term treatment of abnormal behaviour (see Brylewski and Duggan 1998). Nonetheless, clinical experience suggests that severely behaviourally disturbed patients who

do not respond to psychosocial interventions sometimes benefit from prolonged use of medication with frequent monitoring of its effects and adjustment of dosage.

About one-third of patients with learning disability have epilepsy and *antiepileptic drug treatment* is required when the seizures are a significant risk for health, safety, and quality of life. Special care is needed in selecting a drug and dosage that controls seizures without producing unwanted effects. The older antiepileptic drugs sometimes produce oversedation and cognitive blunting. Modern 'first-line' antiepileptic drugs are often carbamazepine and sodium valproate (see pp. 701 and 703). Some patients with epilepsy that is difficult to treat benefit from one of the 'add-on' antiepileptic drugs but vigilance should be maintained for side-effects. The choice of drug should usually be made by, or in conjunction with, a neurologist.

Psychological treatment

Although limited understanding of language sets obvious limitations to the use of psychotherapy, simple discussion is often helpful. Cognitive therapies can be attempted with some patients with higher verbal ability. Counselling for parents is an important part of treatment. If more formal family therapy is undertaken, families generally prefer structural approaches, which address the problems and solutions relevant for them. Some people with profound learning disability can be helped by the use of play and sensory stimulation to encourage developmental advances (Hewett and Nind 1998).

Behaviour modification

Behavioural methods are potentially helpful to people with severe learning disability since some of the methods do not require language. Such methods can be used to encourage basic skills such as washing, toilet training, and dressing. Often parents and teachers are taught to carry out the training so that it can be maintained in the patient's everyday environment (Petronko *et al.* 1994). If the problem is an undesired behaviour, a search is made for any environmental factors that seem regularly to provoke it or reinforce it (functional analysis). If possible, these environmental factors are changed and carers helped to avoid rewarding the behaviour. At the same time, alternative adaptive responses are reinforced. Aggressive behaviour is sometimes dealt with by so-called 'time-out' in which the patient is ignored or secluded until the behaviour subsides. Techniques using negative reinforcement raise important ethical issues, and should not be used (see Matson and Taras 1989). If the problem is an insufficiency of some socially desirable behaviour, attempts can be made to reinforce such behaviour with material or social rewards, if necessary by 'shaping' the final behaviour from simpler components. Reward should be given immediately after the desired behaviour has taken place (for example, using the toilet). For training in skills such as dressing, it is often necessary to provide modelling and prompting in the early stages, and to reduce them gradually later (Petronko *et al.* 1994; Spreat and Behar 1994).

Special problems

Growing old

Several problems arise more frequently as people with learning disability live longer. When the parents are the carers, they may find care increasingly burdensome as they grow old. Such parents are often concerned about the future of their learning-disabled child when they have died and yet are reluctant to arrange alternative care while they are still alive.

The older person with learning disability also faces special problems. If his parents die first, he faces problems of bereavement. The isolation felt by many bereaved people may be increased because other people are not sure how to offer comfort, and because the learning-disabled person may be excluded from the ritual of mourning. These bereaved people should be helped to come to terms with the loss, using the principles that apply generally to grief counselling (see p. 210), but choosing appropriately simple forms of communication

(see Cathcart 1995; Hollins and Esterhuyzen 1997).

A third problem for people with learning disability as they grow old is the onset of dementia. This problem is considered on p. 872.

Exploitation and abuse

People with learning disability are vulnerable to exploitation and to physical and sexual abuse. In the past these problems were associated with poorly managed large institutions, but they can occur also in small community units. Such units need regular supervision, and clinicians should consider abuse as an uncommon but important cause of disturbed behaviour among people with learning disability.

Ethical and legal problems in the care of learning-disabled people

Normalization, autonomy, and the conflict of interests

The policy of normalization encourages learning disabled people to live as near normal lives as possible. This policy can create conflicts between the interests of the learning-disabled person and those of other people. These conflicts arise because many learning-disabled people require support from carers in some ways, if they are to achieve autonomy in other ways. For example, they may need help with dressing if they are to live away from hospital. Many carers are members of the family of the disabled person and arrangements that are entered into willingly may become burdensome if the needs of the disabled person increase, as the needs of other children increase, or as the parents grow older. It may then be difficult to balance the interests of the disabled person, the carers, and other members of the carers' family. These difficulties can usually be resolved most equitably if they are discussed with the disabled person, the carers, and the other family members, and between the professionals responsible for each of these people.

Normalization can also produce conflicts between the interests of an individual learning-disabled person and those of learning-disabled people as a whole. For example, normalization requires that learning-disabled children should be educated in ordinary schools whenever possible. However, in secondary schools, children with special needs were found to be bullied three times more often than other children (Whitney *et al.* 1994). It could be argued that the immediate interests of an individual child are to be educated in a special school where he will not be stigmatized and therefore less likely to be bullied. However, the interests of learning-disabled children as a group may be advanced by continuing the policy of education in ordinary schools whilst making strenuous efforts to eradicate bullying – even though this may not be achieved quickly.

Normalization also leads to ethical questions about sexual activity, contraception, and possible conflicts of interest between a learning-disabled mother and her child (see p. 874).

Consent to treatment

The important general issues relating to informed consent for physical and psychiatric treatment are discussed on p. 78–80. Many of the more severely learning-disabled people are unable to give informed consent, and it is essential to be aware of local legislation and practice. In the UK, there is no provision for others to give proxy consent for an adult who is not competent in this regard, and the clinical team must proceed in the patient's best interests. If there is doubt and in-patient admission is being sought, it is good practice to discuss matters with an approved social worker. Seriously ill patients who refuse potentially life-saving treatments can prove difficult to deal with in general medical settings. If the patient is sufficiently intellectually impaired so as not to understand the nature of the choice he or she faces and there is a medical emergency, it may be appropriate to proceed with treatment under 'common law'. If there is time, it may be necessary to refer the case for review in court, for example when the question of termination of pregnancy has to be decided.

The reader should discover the legal requirements in the place he is working, and discuss best practice with an experienced practitioner.

Consent to research

Consent to research requires the ability to understand information, to use the information rationally, to appreciate the consequences of situations, and to between alternatives (see chapter 3). In general, these abilities should be greater as the ratio of risk to benefit of the proposed research increases. The assessment of these abilities among the learning disabled is described in American Psychiatric Association (1998). All people who have agreed to take part in research should understand that they can withdraw consent if they wish. This point should be explained with particular care to the learning disabled. In one study, half the learning-disabled people who understood the purpose of a research project did not understand that they could withdraw from it (Arscott *et al.* 1998).

Further reading

Bouras, N. (1994). *Mental health in mental retardation.* Cambridge University Press, Cambridge. (Reviews the psychiatric problems of learning disabled people).

Dosen, A. and Day, K. (eds) (2001). *Treating mental illness and behaviour disorders in children and adults with mental retardation.* American Psychiatric Publishing, Washington, DC. (Reviews the principal methods of treatment, with additional information on epidemiology and aetiology.)

Gelder, M. G., López-Ibor, J. J. Jr, and Andreasen, N. C. (eds) (2000). *The new Oxford textbook of psychiatry*, Part 10: Mental retardation. Oxford University Press, Oxford. (The 13 chapters in this part of the textbook provide a systematic account of the subject written for the general psychiatrist.)

Goh, S. and Holland, A. J. (1994). A framework for commissioning services for people with learning disability. *Journal of Public Health Medicine* 16, 279–85.

Russell, O. (ed.) (1997). *Seminars in the psychiatry of learning disabilities.* Gaskell, London. (Covers the main topics at a level intended for psychiatric trainees.)

CHAPTER 26

Forensic psychiatry

Forensic psychiatry

Chapter 4 covered general legal and ethical issues in the practice of medicine and psychiatry. This chapter is concerned with other aspects of psychiatry and the law covered by the term *forensic psychiatry*; this is used in two ways:

- Narrowly it is applied to the branch of psychiatry that deals with the assessment and treatment of mentally abnormal offenders.

- In its broad sense, the term is applied to all legal aspects of psychiatry including the civil law and laws regulating psychiatric practice as well as the subspecialty concerned with mentally abnormal offenders.

Forensic psychiatrists are concerned with both these issues. In addition, they also assess risk and treat people with violent behaviour who have not at the time committed an offence in law. They have a growing role in the assessment and treatment of victims.

Offenders with mental disorders constitute a minority of all offenders, but they present many difficult problems for psychiatry and the law. These include *legal issues*, such as the relationship between the mental disorder and the crime which may affect the court's determination of responsibility, and *practical clinical questions*, such as whether an offender needs psychiatric treatment and finding the appropriate location for that treatment.

The psychiatrist therefore needs knowledge not only of the law but also of the relationship between particular kinds of crime and particular kinds of psychiatric disorder. It is also important to be aware that mental health services form only a small part of the social and legal response to criminal deviance; the psychiatrist working with offenders

---

Box 26.1 Ethical issues in forensic psychiatry

The principal ethical issues relate to 'boundary problems' (see Chapter 3). The psychiatrist and others involved need to be clear about accountability to legal authorities, etc., rather than to the individual being assessed and treated:

- preparation of medico-legal reports
- voluntary treatment
- involuntary treatment
- assessment of dangerousness.

---

needs to be able to liaise with others in the criminal justice system, such as lawyers, prison staff, and probation officers. Concepts of deviance, guilt, and legality are influenced by legal, political, and social factors, as well as by clinical issues.

In reading this chapter it is important to be aware of the very large differences between countries and jurisdictions which mean great national variation in epidemiology, definitions of crime, legal practice, and the role of the psychiatrist. Readers need to be aware of legal issues and procedures in their jurisdiction. In the following account, the situations and procedures in the UK (and more especially England and Wales) are used as an example to illustrate general themes. Ethical issues are summarized in Box 26.1.

General criminology

There is a very large literature on criminology and many theories of the causes of crime; interested readers are referred to criminology textbooks (see Farrington 2000; Maguire 1997). Most theories have emphasized the sociological aspects of crime, deviance, and other types of rule breaking. Social studies have drawn attention to social and economic causes of crime in the family, peer group, and subculture, and in conditions of poverty, poor schooling, and unemployment. Since many of the proposed predisposing social and individual factors are inter-related, simple conclusions are not possible. However, it is widely held that such causes of crime are more important than individual psychological factors such as genetics and psychological traits. However, psychological risk factors for offending are the subject of most correctional and forensic mental health programmes (Gendreau *et al.* 1996).

Prevalence

Prevalence figures must be viewed cautiously because they depend on reporting and upon the definitions of crime. In most countries, property offences are the most common type of crime. Figure 26.1 shows all the crimes recorded by the police in England and Wales in 1992, and Figure 26.2 shows details of violent crime. By contrast, forensic mental health services are most likely to be involved with individuals who have committed crimes of interpersonal violence, apart from instances where repeated property crime may indicate a mental disorder.

Figures 26.1 and 26.2 show details of *recorded* crime but much criminal behaviour is unreported. This is especially true of violence within the home, such as rape, child abuse, or partner battering. Figure 26.3 shows changes in recorded crime and also in crime reported to the British Crime Survey 1997, which asks subjects about their experience of criminal victimization (Home Office 1998). Wounding and assaults constitute a significantly higher proportion of interpersonal violence than shown in Figure 26.1.

National differences

There are large national differences in the rates and patterns of crime. For example, rates of criminal activity are lower than those in the UK in Sweden but higher in the USA. Crimes of violence are especially common in the USA. Rates and patterns of national statistics are affected by local legislation, the recording of crimes, and by the conduct of legal proceedings.

Gender

In all cultures, crime is predominantly an activity of young men. In England and Wales half of all indictable offences are committed by males aged under 21, and a quarter by males aged under 17. Since the Second World War there has been a steady rise in the rates of both crimes against property and of violent crimes. There has been a sharp increase in the numbers of offences committed by women. However, there is no cultural group where men account for less than 80% of offenders (Monahan 1997). In most Western cultures, male prisoners outnumber female prisoners by 30:1. This gender difference is reflected in forensic

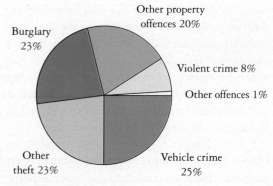

4.5 million crimes

Figure 26.1 Recorded crime. [After Home Office (1999). Information on the criminal justice system in England and Wales. Digest 4]

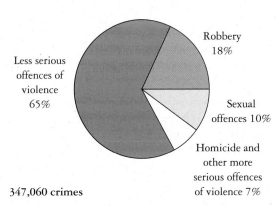

347,060 crimes

Figure 26.2 Violent crime. [After Home Office (1999). Information on the criminal justice system in England and Wales. Digest 4]

mental health services, where male patients make up the vast majority. Whether this is the same in non-Western cultures has not been reported.

Ethnicity

In most countries, ethnic minority groups are over-represented in prisoner populations. This is usually because minority groups are more likely to be poor, unemployed, and living in poor housing, all of which are risk factors for crime. Minority groups are therefore also more likely to be over-represented in forensic patient populations. (Fernando *et al.* 1998; Kaye and Lingiah 2000).

There is considerable concern in many countries as to the extent to which the high rates of arrests and convictions of members of minority groups are in part due to discrimination against them at all stages of the criminal justice system: suspicion, stopping and arresting in the street, cautioning and charging, prosecution and trial outcome, and sentencing.

Victims

Most property crime is committed against strangers. By contrast, most serious interpersonal violence (such as rape, homicide, or child abuse) is committed by offenders against people who are known to them.

In England and Wales in 1992, recorded offences of domestic violence (battering) exceeded recorded assaults on young men for the first time. Domestic

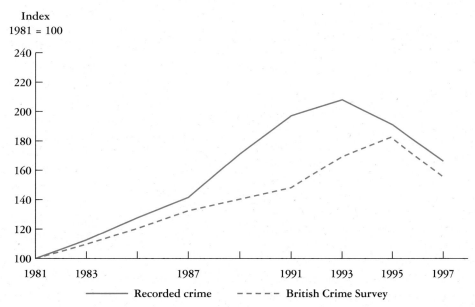

Figure 26.3 Trends in crime 1981–1997. [After Home Office (1999). Information on the criminal justice system in England and Wales. Digest 4.]

violence (assaults on partners) is considerably more common, but is less likely to be recorded. Both men and women can be victims of sexual assault, but the proportion of female victims greatly exceed the proportion of male victims.

Victims of crime tend to be disadvantaged groups living in poorer parts of urban communities; on this account we may expect that the mentally disordered are as likely to be victims of crime as perpetrators.

Causes of crime

It is important to distinguish several widely used terms with different meanings.

- *Criminal behaviour* (crime) needs to be distinguished from *delinquent or rule-breaking* behaviour; not all rule breaking, or socially unacceptable behaviour is criminal. Thus fire setting is a *behaviour*; the *crime* is called arson. Not all criminal behaviour is violent; in fact the vast majority is not; thus general theories of the causes of crime will not necessarily address the causes of violence.

- There is an important distinction between *aggression* and violence; aggressive behaviour is not always violent, it is constrained by social rules.

- *Violence* is aggressive behaviour that transgresses social norms. An example is street fighting, which transgresses the criminal law, in contrast to boxing, which conforms to social rules. Multiple factors determine whether an individual is aggressive in a particular situation: personality, the immediate social group, the behaviour of the victim, disinhibiting factors such as alcohol or drugs, general environmental factors such as noise and social pressure, physiological factors such as fatigue, hunger, and lack of sleep, and the presence of mental abnormality. Aggression is not a crime, but violent behaviour generally is because it results in harm defined by the law.

Genetic and physiological factors

Early *studies of twins* suggested that concordance rates for criminality were substantially greater in monozygotic twins than in dizygotic twins (Lange 1931). *Later adoption studies* in Sweden and in Denmark have confirmed the genetic influence but shown that it is more modest than Lange supposed. It is mainly significant for severe and persistent criminality. The relationship is stronger for crimes against property than for violent crimes (see Brennan and Mednick 1993). It is uncertain how genetic factors could lead to criminality. Prospective studies have shown a relationship between measures of physiological arousal at age 15 years and criminal acts at age 24 years. It is possible that genetic factors determine arousability, which is related to the speed of learning to inhibit antisocial behaviour (Brennan and Mednick 1993).

The gender difference in offending has raised the question of the influence of either the Y chromosome or testosterone on offending. However, there is little evidence that *chromosomal or hormonal abnormalities* are causally associated with criminal behaviour or aggression.

There is increasing evidence that abnormalities of *serotonin* may be relevant to commission of some types of impulsive violence, especially suicidal and self-harming behaviour (Virkkunen *et al.* 1996).

Psychosocial factors

Individual psychological development interacts with social factors and cultural values to make offending more likely (Table 26.1). Rule breaking and antisocial behaviour often start in childhood or early adulthood.

- Follow-up studies of delinquent youth show that early patterns of antisocial behaviour are likely to persist into adulthood (Farrington 1994).

- Delinquency is associated with harsh parenting and poverty.

- Other studies have showed an association between childhood adversity and later violence

(Maxfield and Widdom 1996). Exposure to physical abuse or neglect in childhood significantly increases the risk of violent offending in later life, for both men and women.

- Early childhood adversity is a risk factor for the later development of antisocial personality; perhaps by affecting the development of social attitudes (Weiler and Widom 1996).

The specific association between childhood adversity and violence may be mediated by a number of factors. First, abused and neglected children may have a heightened perception of threat from others (Dodge *et al.* 1997). Second, they may have decreased capacities to make successful interpersonal relationships; perhaps because they have decreased empathy for others, or because they lack the capacity for self-awareness (Fonagy *et al.* 1997). Individuals who become violent may have decreased capacity to manage arousal or regulate affects such as anger or anxiety; perhaps as a result of being exposed to fear experiences. Finally, it is important to consider the operation of resilience or vulnerability factors, such as temperament.

Table 26.1 **Psychosocial risk factors for offending (see Farrington 2000)**
Individual factors
Hyperactivity and impulsivity
Low intelligence
Child-rearing – poor supervision, harsh discipline, rejection, teenage mothers
Parental conflict – separations
Criminal parents
Large family size
Social factors
Socioeconomic deprivation
Peer influences
School influences
Community influences
Situational factors

Studies of offenders who are violent towards others frequently report that they describe cognitive distortions favouring violence and justifying their violence by blaming their victim. Cultural values of the social group may interact with such cognitive schemata to increase risk, for example, in relation to sexual violence. See Farrington (2000) for a review.

Psychiatric causes

There is a small but important group of offenders whose criminal behaviour seems to be partly explicable by specific psychological or psychiatric abnormalities. This group particularly concerns the psychiatrist and is discussed in the next section. (Chiswick 2000; Farrington 2000).

The association between mental disorder and crime

Frequency

One of the few studies of the association between mental disorder and violence in a large community sample, the Epidemiologic Catchment Area Study in the USA, found significant associations between subject's violent behaviour and mental disorder (Swanson *et al.* 1990). The relationships between crime and mental disorder are difficult to study in unselected populations. For practical reasons, research has focused on the prevalence and association of mental disorder in prisoners but:

- not all criminals are brought to trial and found guilty;

- not all criminals go to prison, so studies of prisoners may result in sampling bias;

- mentally disordered offenders may be diverted away from courts and prisons, or they may not be prosecuted.

Recent work has shown that a significant proportion of prisoners have mental disorders, and this proportion is higher than the general population. For example, in a widely quoted study Gunn *et al.*

(1991) described the prevalence of psychiatric disorder among male sentenced prisoners in England and Wales, and their treatment needs, on the basis of a 5% sample. Using standardized diagnostic instruments, they concluded that, overall, 37% had diagnosable disorder (with some having more than one type of disorder):

- 0.6% had mental retardation,
- 2% psychosis,
- 6% neurotic disorder,
- 10% personality disorder,
- 12% alcohol dependence,
- 12% drug dependence.

They considered that 3% of the prisoners required treatment in a psychiatric hospital and 5% could benefit from treatment in a prison therapeutic community. A further 10% were thought to require further psychiatric assessment treatment within prison. See Chiswick (2000), Gunn (2000) and Lamb and Weinburger (1998) for reviews of mental illness in prison populations.

The nature of the association

A causal relationship between mental disorder and crime is difficult to show empirically, especially if the type of crime is not defined. The finding that mentally disordered individuals are over-represented in prison does not mean that their mental disorder caused them to offend.

It must always be borne in mind that criminal law breaking is not an indicator of itself of mental disorder, no matter how heinous or bizarre the behaviour. For example, most sexual violence is not associated with mental disorder in the perpetrator; accounts of sexual violence by invading armies make it clear that some types of violence may have social rather than diagnostic meaning.

Overall, it is essential to emphasize that only a small minority of all people who commit violent acts have psychotic disorders. The vast majority of patients with psychotic illnesses are no more dangerous than members of the general population, and there is no evidence that homicidal behaviour is becoming more common in people with mental illness (Taylor and Gunn 1999).

Many, if not most, violent offenders are in a state of distress at the time of the violence, which is highly disturbing for them, even if it is not severe and persistent enough to meet criteria for a formal diagnosis. This may be hard to appreciate, especially since assessment of offenders often takes place many weeks or months after the offence, and in a setting where it may be difficult for the offender to express emotion. For a review of the association between psychiatric disorder and offending see Chiswick (2000).

Most criminological evidence has suggested that criminality and mental illness are only weakly associated, and that apparent relationships may be coincidental (Monahan and Steadman 1994; Wessely 1997). However, there are some exceptions:

- In certain circumstances, psychiatric disorder may be a risk factor for violent crime (Monahan and Steadman 1994). The psychiatric disorders most likely to be associated with violent crime are personality disorders, alcohol and drug dependence, and individuals with paranoid symptomatology (including delusions and hallucinations). The personality type most associated with violence is 'psychopathy' (Blackburn 1998). 'Psychopathy' is a psychological construct, and should not be confused with the legal term 'psychopathic disorder', or the tabloid press term, 'psychopath'. Recent evidence suggests an association between violence and psychotic disorders, especially those with paranoid ideation (Beck 1994). Risk factors for violence may be additive, so that an individual with a personality disorder and a history of substance abuse, who then becomes psychotic, may present a significantly increased risk of violence.

- Some types of psychiatric disorder, such as mental retardation, may be associated with non-violent crime. There is a sizeable group of recidivist offenders who are socially isolated, and often homeless and unemployed, who may be judged to be suffering from personality disorder. They are frequently of low intelligence, and some have chronic schizophrenia. In this group, criminality is just one manifestation of social incompetence.

Specific psychiatric disorders

Substance dependence and crime.

There are close relationships between substance abuse and crime which have substantially affected legislation, enforcement, and national policies (South 1994).

Alcohol and crime are related in three important ways:

- alcohol intoxication may lead to charges related to public drunkenness or to driving offences;
- intoxication reduces inhibitions and is strongly associated with crimes of violence, including murder;
- the neuropsychiatric complications of alcoholism (see Chapter 18) may also be linked with crime.

For example, offences may be committed during alcoholic amnesias or 'blackouts' (periods of several hours or days which the heavy drinker cannot subsequently recall, although at the time he appeared normally conscious to other people and was able to carry out complicated actions). However, the association is complex, and social factors related to drinking may be as important as alcohol itself. See Johns (2000).

Intoxication with drugs may lead to criminal behaviour including violent offences. Drug abusers, especially those dependent on heroin and cocaine, commit repeated offences against both property and people to pay for their drugs. Some of the offences involve violence. Rates of drug abuse are increased among prisoners, and many succeed in obtaining drugs in prison. Involvement in criminal activity and with other criminals may lead to drug usage. For a review of the relationship between drug dependence and crime see Johns (2000).

Learning disability

There is no evidence that most criminals are of markedly low intelligence. Recent surveys have shown that most delinquent youths are within the lower part of the normal range of intelligence and that only about 3% are learning disability (Lund 1990). There is no reason to suppose that the distribution of intelligence is any different amongst adult criminals. However, compared with other offenders, the mentally retarded are more likely to be caught.

People with learning disabilities may commit offences because they do not understand the implications of their behaviour, or because they are susceptible to exploitation by other people. The closest association between learning disability and crime is a high incidence of sexual offences, particularly indecent exposure by males. The exposer is often known to the victim and therefore the rate of detection is high. There is also said to be an association between mental retardation and arson. No other crimes are closely associated with learning disability.

Affective disorder

Depressive disorder is sometimes associated with shoplifting (see p. 915). Much more seriously, severe depressive disorder may lead to *homicide*. When this happens, the depressed person has usually experienced delusions, for example, that the world is too dreadful a place for him and his family to live in; he then kills his spouse or children to spare them from the horrors of the world. The killer often commits suicide afterwards. A mother suffering from post-partum disorder may sometimes kill her newborn child or her older children. Rarely, a person with severe depressive disorder may commit homicide because of a persecutory belief, for example, that the victim is conspiring against the patient. Occasionally, ideas of guilt and unworthiness lead depressed patients to confess to crimes that they did not commit.

Manic patients may spend excessively on expensive objects such as jewellery or cars that they cannot pay for. They may hire cars and fail to return them, or steal cars for their own use. They may be charged with fraud, theft, or false pretences. Manic patients are also prone to irritability and aggression, which may lead to offences of violence, though the violence is seldom severe.

Schizophrenia and related disorder

Psychotic illnesses may be associated with violence, especially when paranoid symptomatology is present, or the patient also has a substance abuse problem. Violence may occur because the offender is frightened, and cognitive awareness is reduced by the presence of the psychotic state. Any mental state or disorder in which paranoid psychotic symptoms feature may be associated with an increased risk of violent behaviour.

Epidemiology

There is conflicting evidence about the relationship between schizophrenia and crime, probably because of differences in the populations studied. Although most research has focused on homicide and other violent crimes, recent evidence suggests that schizophrenic patients are more likely to commit both non-violent and violent offences.

In a large study of mentally abnormal offenders in Germany, the risk of homicide was found to be moderately increased in schizophrenia compared with the general population (Böker and Häfner 1977). In Sweden, a study of 790 schizophrenic patients aged over 15 years found that although the overall crime rate of male schizophrenics was similar to that of the general population, the rate of violent offences was four times higher. However, the violence was almost always of minor severity (Lindqvist and Allebeck 1990). In the USA, the Epidemiological Catchment Area Study found that the 1-year prevalence of reported violence by schizophrenics was considerably higher than in the general population. By contrast, a recent study by Wessely did not find violence was associated with a diagnosis of schizophrenia; he notes the import-ance of confounding variables such as sex and ethnicity (Wessely 1997).

In some people with schizophrenia, violence results from delusions and hallucinations. According to a hospital case record study by Planansky and Johnston (1977), violence in schizophrenics may be associated with any of the following features:

- great fear and loss of self-control associated with non-systematized delusions;
- systematized paranoid delusions including the conviction that enemies must be defended against;
- irresistible urges;
- instructions from hallucinatory voices;
- unaccountable frenzy.

More recently, Buchanan *et al.* (1993) concluded that the risk of violence is greatest where delusions are accompanied by strong affect and when the person has made efforts to try and confirm the truth of the delusions. Taylor (1985) interviewed remanded psychotic men and concluded that psychiatric symptoms accounted for most of the very violent behaviour, and that in about 40% there was a direct psychiatric 'drive' to commit the offence.

Risk assessment is discussed on p. 924. However, it is essential to note here that violent threats made by psychotic patients should be taken very seriously (especially in those with a history of previous violence); most serious violence occurs in those already known to psychiatrists. This is especially true if there is an identifiable victim.

Post-traumatic stress disorder

Post-traumatic stress disorder (PTSD) may be related to offending in three ways:

- Patients with PTSD may abuse substances in ways which increase their risk of criminal behaviour.
- PTSD is associated with increased irritability and decreased affect regulation, which may make angry and aggressive behaviour more likely.

◆ Rarely, patients with PTSD may experience dissociative episodes in which violence can take place, especially in circumstances resembling their original trauma. This is often hard to determine retrospectively.

PTSD has been the basis for psychiatric defences to homicide, especially in cases where battered women have killed a battering partner. In circumstances where there has been prolonged trauma, then occasional acts of retaliatory violence are not uncommon.

Morbid jealousy

The syndrome of morbid jealousy (see p. 389) may be associated with several of the above diagnoses. It has been identified in 12% of 'insane' male murderers and 3% of 'insane' women murderers. It is particularly dangerous because of the risk of the offence being repeated with another partner. It may sometimes be hard to distinguish morbid jealousy from culturally accepted beliefs about women held by some subgroups of men. Extreme possessiveness or control of women's behaviour, which may be accompanied by violence, is acceptable in some cultures and may not be perceived as an indication of mental disorder.

Organic mental disorders

Delirium is occasionally associated with criminal behaviour; usually because of confusion or disinhibition caused by the disorder. Diagnostic problems may arise if the mental disturbance improves before the offender is examined by a doctor.

Dementia is sometimes associated with offences, though crime is otherwise uncommon among the elderly and violent offences are rare. Violent and disinhibited behaviour may also occur after traumatic damage to the brain following *head injury*. It may be hard to distinguish the effects of post-traumatic neurological difficulties from post-traumatic psychological disorder.

Epilepsy

The association between epilepsy and crime is complex and poorly understood. There are more people with epilepsy in prison than would be expected from the general population prevalence. However, there is little evidence that epilepsy itself is causally responsible for the crimes. It may be that having epilepsy causes difficulties for the individual which make criminal behaviour more likely. Violent behaviour is sometimes associated with EEG abnormalities in the absence of clinical epilepsy, but it is doubtful that this indicates a causal relationship.

Epileptic automatisms may be rarely associated with violent behaviour, and subsequent criminal proceedings.

Episodic dyscontrol syndrome

The alleged episodic dyscontrol syndrome has attracted considerable attention but remains controversial. It was described by Bach-y-Rita *et al.* (1971) in patients who had repeated unprovoked episodes of violence. These authors considered that the syndrome had more than one cause and their series included patients with epilepsy. Maletzky (1973) excluded patients with epilepsy, schizophrenia, pathological intoxication with alcohol, and acute intoxication with drugs, and described a residual group of patients whose unexplained episodes of violence were preceded by a sequence of aura, headache, and drowsiness. About half reported amnesia for the episode and half had EEG abnormalities, usually in the temporal lobes. Maletzky reported improvement with the antiepileptic drug phenytoin, but there was no placebo control group against which to assess this finding. These findings have not been confirmed by subsequent studies. The evidence for a distinct syndrome of episodic dyscontrol is not convincing.

Impulse control disorders

DSM-IV contains a rubric for 'impulse control disorders not otherwise classified' which brings together four speculative conditions relevant to forensic psychiatry: intermittent explosive disorder, pathological gambling, pyromania, and kleptomania. (The rubric also contains another condition, trichotillomania, hair pulling). In

ICD-10 these conditions are classified under abnormalities of adult personality and behaviour as 'habit and impulse disorders'. Whatever their clinical value, none of these conditions has been established as a separate diagnostic entity.

Intermittent explosive disorder

This term is used to describe repeated episodes of seriously aggressive behaviour directed to people or property that is out of proportion to any provoking events and is not accounted for by another psychiatric disorder (for example, antisocial personality disorder, substance abuse, or schizophrenia). The aggression may be preceded by tension and followed by relief of this tension. Later the person feels remorse. The clinical features clearly overlap with accounts of the episodic dyscontrol syndrome but without the associated physical symptoms and signs. If care is taken to exclude other causes, the condition is rare. Many psychiatrists doubt whether this behaviour indicates a distinct psychiatric disorder.

Pathological gambling

Pathological ('compulsive') gambling may lead to behaviours that bring the gambler to the attention of the courts, for example, fraud or stealing to obtain money to pay for the habit. Gambling is pathological when it is repeated frequently and dominates the person's life; the gambling persists when the person can no longer afford to pay his debts. The person lies, steals, or defrauds in order to obtain money or avoid repayment and to continue the habit. Family life may be damaged, other social relationships impaired, and employment put at risk. The pathological gambler has an intense urge to gamble, which is difficult to control. He is preoccupied with thoughts of gambling, much as a person dependent on alcohol is preoccupied with drink. Often, increasing sums of money are gambled, either to increase the excitement or in an attempt to recover previous losses. Gambling continues despite inability to repay debts and despite awareness of the resulting social and legal problems. If gambling is prevented, the person becomes irritable and even more preoccu-

pied with the behaviour. Similarities between patterns of behaviour and those of people dependent on drugs have led to the suggestion that pathological gambling is itself a form of addictive behaviour. The prevalence of pathological gambling is not known. It is probably more frequent among males. Most gamblers seen by psychiatrists are adults, but there is concern that young people are increasingly being involved, usually with gambling machines in amusement arcades and other places. The causes of pathological gambling are not known. For reviews of pathological gambling see Gunn and Taylor (1993, pp. 481–5) and Moran (2000).

Pyromania

Pyromania is one cause of fire-setting (see p. 915). The term pyromania refers to repeated episodes of deliberate fire-setting, which are not carried out for monetary gain, to conceal a crime, as an act of vengeance, for social or political motives, or as a consequence of hallucinations, delusions, or impaired judgement (resulting from intoxication, dementia, or mental retardation, for example). The diagnosis is not made when there is an associated antisocial personality disorder, a manic episode, or (among children or adolescents) a conduct disorder. In this rare condition, the act of fire-setting is preceded by tension or arousal, and is followed by relief of tension. People with pyromania have a preoccupation with fires and firefighting. They enjoy watching fires. They may plan the fire-setting in advance, taking no account of the danger to other people from their actions. When other causes listed above are excluded, pyromania is rare; indeed, some writers doubt its existence.

Kleptomania

The term kleptomania refers to repeated failure to resist impulses to steal objects that are not needed, either for use or for their monetary value. The impulses are not associated with delusions or hallucinations, or with motives of anger or vengeance. Before the act of stealing there is increased tension; after the act there is relief of tension. The diagnosis is not made when there is an associated antisocial personality disorder, a manic episode, or (among children or adolescents) a conduct disorder, nor when the stealing results from sexual fetishism. The objects stolen may be of little value and could have been afforded; they may be hoarded, thrown away, or returned later to the owner. The patient knows that the stealing is unlawful, and may feel guilty and depressed after the immediate pleasurable sensations that follow the act. The disorder occurs more often among women. Associations with anxiety and eating disorders have been described. The behaviour may be sporadic with long intervals of remission, or may persist for years despite repeated prosecutions. When other causes of repeated stealing are excluded, the condition is rare; indeed, some writers doubt its existence as a separate syndrome, pointing out that diagnosis depends on accused persons' descriptions of their own motives.

Specific offender groups

Females

Women are more law-abiding than men. The most common offence is stealing with shoplifting, accounting for half of all convictions of women for indictable offences. By contrast, violent and sexual offences are uncommon (Heidensohn 1997). Women are also responsible for forms of antisocial behaviour that are regarded less severely by the law than those for which men are prosecuted, such as soliciting and some forms of social security fraud.

There are differences in the way men and women are treated by the criminal justice system. Women are sentenced more leniently for similar offences and they are more likely to be seen as 'sick'. Psychiatric disorder is frequent amongst women admitted to prison (Maden *et al.* 1994), with personality disorder and drug abuse being especially common. Rates for self-harm before and during imprisonment are also high.

The 'premenstrual syndrome' is often suggested as a causative factor by defence lawyers and has occasionally been accepted as such in a number of recent court decisions. It is possible that premenstrual symptoms may complicate or exacerbate pre-existing social and psychological difficulties, but it is unlikely that they are ever a primary cause of offending (Gunn and Taylor 1993, pp. 598–623).

Young people

National crime statistics show that increasing numbers of young people (under 18) are becoming involved in criminal behaviour, including serious interpersonal violence. Where there has been interpersonal violence, the victim is often well known to the young person, and may be a family member. Homicide by young people is often associated with long histories of family violence before the killing. Serious violence by young people and children is rare.

Ethnic minorities

It is well established that some ethnic groups are over-represented in the criminal justice system as offenders, and there is some evidence to suggest that this may be so in forensic psychiatric services. Patients from non-Caucasian groups may be more likely to receive mental illness diagnoses, and individual personality difficulties may be overlooked. Different cultural beliefs may be relevant, especially within the family, or to the expression of symptoms of mental illness. As indicated above, people from ethnic minorities may be at risk of negative discrimination by the criminal justice system and also socially stigmatized by having a mental disorder (Fernando *et al.* 1998; Kaye and Lingiah 2000).

Psychiatric aspects of specific crimes

The following sections are concerned with the types of offences that are most likely to be associated with psychological factors: crimes of violence, sexual offences, and some offences against property.

Crimes of violence

Amongst mentally abnormal offenders, violence is more often associated with personality disorder than with psychiatric disorder. It is particularly common in people with antisocial personality traits who abuse alcohol or drugs, or who have marked paranoid or sadistic traits. It is often part of a persistent pattern of impulsive and aggressive behaviour, but it may be a sporadic response to stressful events in 'over-controlled' personalities (Megargee 1966).

Cultural norms are important determinants of the occurrence of violence. It is still uncertain whether depictions of violence in the media affect rates of violent behaviour in the general population. The assessment of dangerousness and the management of violence are discussed on p. 923.

Homicide

Most legal jurisdictions recognize different categories of homicide, depending on the degree of intention and responsibility shown by the perpetrator. For example, in the USA, defendants may be charged with different 'degrees' of murder; in England and Wales, there are three legal categories of homicide: murder, manslaughter, and infanticide.

In England and Wales murder and manslaughter are defined by historical precedent and not by statute. According to a widely quoted definition put forward by Lord Coke in 1797, murder occurs:

when a man of sound memory and of the age of discretion unlawfully killeth within any country of the realm any reasonable creature in rerum natura under the King's peace with malice aforethought, either expressed by the party or implied by law, so as the party wounded or hit, etc, die of the wound or hit within a year and a day after the same.

Manslaughter is a diverse crime covering all unlawful homicides that are not murder. Various types of homicide fall within this category, but it is customary and useful to divide manslaughter into two main groups, designated 'voluntary' and 'involuntary' manslaughter, respectively. In voluntary manslaughter, the defendant may have malice aforethought of murder but the presence of some defined mitigating circumstances reduces his crime to a less serious grade of criminal homicide. In involuntary manslaughter, there is no malice aforethought; it includes, for example, causing death by gross negligence.

Normal and abnormal homicide

Mental disorders may count as a form of mitigation when an individual is charged with murder, and thus the charge is reduced to manslaughter. It is common practice to divide homicide into 'normal' and 'abnormal' according to the legal outcome. Homicide is 'normal' if there is a conviction of murder or common law manslaughter; it is 'abnormal' if there is a finding of insane murder, suicide murder, diminished responsibility, or infanticide.

'Normal' homicide accounts for half to two-thirds of all homicides occurring in the UK, i.e. the majority of killings. The same is true of other Western countries, such as the USA, where the overall homicide rate is much higher than in the UK. 'Normal' homicide is most likely to be committed by young men of low social class. In the UK, the victims are mainly family members or close acquaintances. In countries with high homicide rates, a greater proportion of killings are associated with robbery or sexual offences. Sexual homicide may result from panic during a sexual offence or may be a feature of a sadistic killing, sometimes committed by a shy man with bizarre sadistic and other violent fantasies.

'Abnormal' homicide accounts for a third to half of all homicides in the UK. It is usually committed by older people. The victims of abnormal homicide are usually family members. In those who commit 'abnormal' homicide, the most common psychiatric diagnosis is depressive disorder, especially in those who kill themselves afterwards. Other associated diagnoses are schizophrenia, personality disorder, and alcoholism. Homicide by women is much less frequent than by men; when it occurs, it is nearly always 'abnormal' and the most common category is infanticide (Shaw *et al* 1999).

There is very considerable public concern about dangerousness and homicide amongst mentally ill people. There is no evidence that these problems are increasing or that there is any reason to doubt that, in general principle, the care of mental illness in the community is safe (Taylor and Gunn 1999). Nevertheless, better care is needed for the very small minority who are dangerous.

A large proportion of all murderers are under the influence of alcohol at the time of the crime. In a survey of 400 people charged with murder in Scotland, 58% of the men and 30% of the women were found to have been intoxicated at the time of the offence (Gillies 1976). Drug abuse is also an important factor (Tardiff *et al.* 1994).

Multiple homicide

Multiple murders are rare, although they attract great public attention. They include:

- those without mental illness who kill several people at once, sometimes a family killing which is often followed by suicide (Gaupp 1974; Cantor *et al* 2000);
- killings attributable to a psychotic illness in which the killer aims to save himself or his family from a perceived threat;
- serial killings taking place over a period of time. These may be 'normal' (for example, killings by terrorists), or abnormal (e.g. psychotic, or motivated by sexual sadism or necrophilia).

Homicide followed by suicide

Homicide is often followed by suicide, and English data suggest that this occurs in about 10% of cases. In the USA, murder followed by suicide presents 1.5% of all suicides and 5% of all homicides (Marzuk *et al.* 1992). In the UK, West (1965) studied 78 cases occurring in the London area over the years 1954–1961. The offenders were much more likely to be women, were of higher social class, and had fewer previous convictions than other convicted homicide offenders. The victims were usually children. Half the homicides were 'abnormal' in the sense defined above; in most cases

the offender was severely depressed at the time of the offence. In most of the 'normal' offences, the killer appeared to have felt driven to suicide by illness or distressing circumstances.

In Marzuk *et al.*'s study in the USA, the four most common clinical types were jealousy (50–75%), killing of elderly spouses in poor health, killing of a child often attributable to depression in the parent, and multiple murders by a depressed, paranoid, or intoxicated person. Approximately a quarter to a fifth of all jealous men who killed their spouses also committed suicide.

Parents who kill their children

A quarter of all victims of murder or manslaughter in the UK are under the age of 16. Most of them are killed by a parent who is mentally ill, usually the mother (Scott 1973; d'Orban 1979). The classification of child murder is difficult, but useful categories are mercy killing, psychotic murder, and killing as the end result of battering or neglect. This last category is most common, and is discussed further on p. 855.

Infanticide

A woman who kills her child may be charged with murder or manslaughter. Some jurisdictions (such as English law) recognize a special category of child killing called infanticide, which is treated as manslaughter and therefore attract less harsh penalties. The judge has the same freedom of sentencing for a conviction of infanticide as for a conviction of manslaughter. The English legal concept of infanticide is unusual in that the accused is required to show only that her mind was disturbed as a result of birth or lactation, but not that the killing was a consequence of her mental disturbance.

Resnick (1969) found that two types of infanticide could be discerned. When the killing occurred within the first 24 hours after birth, in most cases the child was unwanted, and the mother was young and unequipped to care for the child but not psychiatrically ill. When the killing occurred more than 24 hours after childbirth, in most cases the mother had a depressive disorder and killed the child to save it from the suffering she anticipated for it; about a third of the mothers also tried to take their own lives.

Marks and Kumar (1993) examined records of all infants aged under a year who were victims of homicide during 1982–1988. Infants were most at risk on the first day of life, and the relative risk decreased steadily thereafter until by the final quarter of the first year of life the risk of homicide was the same as that of the general population. Parents were the most frequent perpetrators, mothers on the first day and thereafter fathers were slightly more likely to be recorded as the prime suspect. Mothers received less severe sentences than fathers. Contrary to wide belief, puerperal psychotic illness was a relatively infrequent cause of homicide by the mother. Later infant homicides are usually fatal child abuse. Infanticide is strongly associated with motherhood at a young age (Overpeck *et al.* 1998).

Family homicide

Another useful way to distinguish homicides is in the context of the relationship between the perpetrator and the victim. Most serious violence takes place within the family. As noted above, a quarter of all homicide victims are aged under 16, and 80% of these are killed by their parents. Most homicide perpetrators know their victims well; half the female victims of homicide are wives or partners of the perpetrator; the rest are friends or relatives.

Domestic violence

This subject has received increasing attention in recent years (Eisenstat and Bancroft 1999). Family violence is very common. The targets are usually women (and their children). Most batterers do not have either a diagnosable mental disorder or a criminal history. It often takes women many years to escape from the relationship. Family violence is strongly associated with excessive drinking. Some people are violent only within their family, whilst others are also violent outside the family. Violence in the family can have long-term deleterious effects

Table 26.2 Ethical and legal issues – domestic violence
◆ Confidentiality is especially important because of the risk of retaliation by the abuser.
◆ Careful records are essential, including documentation of the injuries. Written comments should be obtained for photographs.
◆ Specialist advise should be sought about providing practical and other help to those who wish to end the relationship.
◆ Where the risk of serious violence is believed to be very high, disclosure to the police and other authorities and other persons to provide protection need to be carefully planned with the maximum collaboration with the victims.

on the psychological and social development of the children as well as on the mental health of the spouse (see Chapter 24).

Violence in the family may also be directed to children (child abuse is reviewed on p. 855) and to elderly relatives (violence to the elderly is referred to on p. 633). Any of these forms of violence may (rarely) result in homicide.

Particular alertness to possible domestic violence is required in emergency departments, but also in primary care and in obstetric and paediatric clinics. Intervention is difficult and raises ethical issues (Table 26.2).

Violence to partners

Violence by men towards their wives is much more frequent than violence to husbands, physically more serious, and more often reported. It appears that most of the perpetrators of wife battering are men with aggressive personalities, whilst a few are violent only when suffering from psychiatric illness, usually a depressive disorder. Other common features in the men are morbid jealousy and heavy drinking. Such men may have suffered violence in childhood, and often come from backgrounds in which violence is frequent and tolerated. Although behaviour by the victim may contribute to or provoke (but not justify) violence, this is often hard to assess if only the perpetrator is interviewed; when battering is seen as a 'joint' problem, the batterer may have less incentive to stop the violence. It is vital to bear in mind that repetitive battering, especially in the context of jealousy, is a risk factor for homicide.

Violence in the workplace

Violence is increasing in the workplace and receiving growing attention. As well as physical attacks, it is also being taken to include threats and various forms of harassment (Fletcher *et al.* 2000). Psychological consequences can be severe. Many organizations have guidelines and training programmes which aim to prevent such problems and to deal with the consequences.

Sexual offences

Sexually violent offences

In the UK, sexual offences account for less than 1% of all indictable offences recorded by the police. Sexual offenders make up a relatively large proportion of offenders referred to psychiatrists, though only a small proportion of people charged with sexual offences are assessed by psychiatrists. Most sexual offences are committed by men; they are rare among women, apart from soliciting for purposes of prostitution. See Mezey and King (2000) for a review of male victims of sexual assault.

As a group, sexual offenders are older than other offenders. Reconviction rates of sexual offenders are generally lower than those of other offenders, but a minority of recidivist sexual offenders are extremely difficult to manage. See Hanson (1998) for a review of recidivism.

The most common sexual offences are indecent assault against women, indecent exposure, and unlawful intercourse with girls aged under 16. Some sexual offences do not involve physical violence (for example, indecent exposure, voyeurism, and most sexual offences involving children); others may involve considerable violence (for example,

rape). The nature and treatment of non-violent sexual offences are discussed in Chapter 19, but their forensic aspects are considered here. For reviews see Hale *et al.* (2000) and White *et al.* (1998).

The psychological consequences for victims of sexual offences are discussed on p. 916, and sexual abuse of children is discussed on below.

Sexual abuse of children

The age of consent varies in different countries. In England and Wales it is illegal to have any heterosexual activity with a person aged under 16, or (at the time of writing) homosexual activity with people aged under 18. Sexual offences involving children are reported commonly, amounting to over half of all reported sexual offences in the UK. It is probable that many more offences are not reported, particularly those occurring within families. The offences vary in severity from mild indecency to seriously aggressive behaviour, but the large majority do not involve violence.

Adults who commit sexual offences against children may or may not be paedophilic. *Paedophiles* are defined as having a primary sexual interest in prepubertal children. They are almost always male. They may be homosexual or heterosexual, and usually abuse children not previously well known to them. They are rarely mentally ill. Victims are often prepared over a long period of time; some paedophiles may seek work in occupations where they will have access to children who will be left in their care. It is difficult to classify paedophiles, but the following groups have been recognized: the timid and sexually inexperienced, the learning disabled, those who have experienced normal sexual relationships but prefer sexual activity with children, and a predatory group who may use violence. In rare cases, paedophile sexual activities end in murder (see also p. 604).

However, not all child sex offenders are paedophiles as defined above, because a significant majority of child sex offenders do not have a primary sexual interest in children. Many child sex offenders have 'normal' heterosexual histories and may be involved in such relationships at the time that they offend. Paedophilic child sex offenders typically are strangers to children, or else have gained opportunistic access to children through their chosen work or social activities. However, the majority of child sex offending is carried out by men (usually) who have some familial relationship to the child. Most commonly these are stepfathers or other male members of the extended family circle. These men are typically not primary paedophiles, although it has been argued that some primary paedophiles do seek to marry adult women with children in order to access potential victims. Some researchers have also found that a proportion of men who appear to be primarily attracted to adult women also describe attraction to children. Some theorists have argued that what child sex offenders are excited by is the vulnerability of children and the discrepancy in power between adults and children, rather than the physical qualities of childhood.

Sexual abuse of children by family members is considered on p. 858.

The prognosis is difficult to determine. Among those who receive a prison sentence, the recidivism rate is about one in three. Although most offenders do not progress from less serious to more serious activities, an important minority do progress to violent sexual offences. For this reason psychiatrists may be asked to give an opinion on an offender's dangerousness.

Assessment

Usually, the perpetrator and the victim are assessed separately by different people. Interviewing children after sexual abuse is considered on p. 860; this section considers interviews with the adult. In trying to decide whether an offence is likely to be repeated and whether there is likely to be a progression to more serious offences, the psychiatrist should first consider:

♦ the duration and frequency of the particular sexual activity in the past, since paedophiles often deny their offending;

♦ the depositions and the victim's statement need careful review;

♦ the offender's predominant sexual preferences; exclusively paedophile inclinations and behaviour indicate greater risk of repetition. Older paedophiles are less likely to be aggressive.

The interview should determine:

♦ previous sexual history;

♦ whether alcohol or drugs played any part in the offence, and if so whether the person is likely to continue using them;

♦ regret or guilt;

♦ stressful circumstances associated with the offence (and the likelihood that these will continue);

♦ the degree of access to children;

♦ evidence of any psychiatric disorder or personality features such as lack of self-control.

In drawing conclusions it is important to be aware of the limitations of psychiatric knowledge of this form of behaviour.

Treatment

Treatment is directed towards any associated psychiatric disorder. Direct treatment of the sexual behaviour is difficult. Group therapy run jointly by mental health and probation services may be helpful. Behavioural treatment has been directed towards encouraging desirable sexual behaviour, but the evidence for effectiveness is unconvincing. The use of sex hormones or drugs to reduce sex drive has been advocated, but its value is uncertain and its use raises ethical issues.

Sexual abuse of children is discussed further on p. 858.

Indecent exposure

This is the legal term for the offence of indecently exposing the genitals to other people. It is applied to all forms of exposure; exhibitionism is by far the most frequent form, but exposure may also occur as an invitation to intercourse, as a prelude to sexual assault, or as an insulting gesture. Exhibitionism, (see also p. 605), is the medical name for the behaviour of those who gain sexual satisfaction from repeatedly exposing to the opposite sex. In England

and Wales, indecent exposure is one of the most frequent sexual offences. It is most common in men aged between 25 and 35. Indecent exposers rarely have a history of psychiatric disorder or other criminal behaviour. However, they may have other types of compulsive disorder, such as substance abuse. However, exhibitionism is listed as a psychiatric disorder in both DSM and ICD. Although many do not reoffend, a proportion of offenders are repeated recidivists, and may proceed to more serious sexual violence.

Indecent assault

The term indecent assault refers to a wide range of behaviour from attempting to touch a stranger's buttocks to sexual assault without attempted penetration. The psychiatrist is most commonly asked to give a psychiatric opinion on adolescent boys and on men who have assaulted children. Although many adolescent boys behave in ways that could be construed as 'indecent', more serious indecent behaviour is associated with aggressive personality, ignorance, and lack of social skills, personal unattractiveness, and occasionally subnormal intelligence. Treatment depends on the associated problems.

Stalking

The lay term 'stalking' is usually taken to mean the repeated, unwanted, and intrusive targeting of a particular victim with following and other harassment (see Mullen *et al.* 2000). It implies an intensive preoccupation with the victim. The scope of behaviour is wide:

- following;
- communication by telephone, mail, electronic communication;
- ordering goods and services in the victim's name;
- aggression and threats, including violence, damage to property and false accusations.

Most stalkers are men and victims women. The victims may suffer severe distress (Pathé and Mullen 1997). Management requires cooperation

between forensic psychiatrists and the criminal justice system in assessing risks, treating any associated psychiatric disorder and protecting and treating the victim. See Mullen (2000) for a review.

Rape

In English law, a man commits rape if:

- he has unlawful sexual intercourse (whether vaginal or anal) with a woman or man who at the time of the intercourse does not consent to it;
- at the time he knows that she does not consent to the intercourse or he is reckless as to whether she consents to it.

Most jurisdictions define rape in terms of the lack of consent of the victim. Not all jurisdictions recognize male rape or sexual assault. Some countries (such as the USA) additionally define lack of consent by age; so called 'statutory rape'. English law is among the few recognizing rape within marriage.

Rape is a violent act; offenders vary in the degree of aggression which is used, and the extent to which this is instrumental in exerting control, or exciting for its own sake. Most rapists are married or in partnerships; over half fail to perform sexually during the assault. Rapists frequently have previous convictions for non-sexual violent offences.

The act of rape varies in terms of the relationship between the rapist and his victim. Most rapists know their victims (Figure 26.4). In contrast to popular belief, stranger rape is a minority. Stranger rapes are more likely to be physically violent and involve the use of weapons; this may reflect the fact that rapists who know their victims may not need to use physical threats to control them. Instead, family members may be threatened. Most rapes take place in the home, another contrast to popular belief.

Epidemiology

Rape and other forms of sexual aggression towards women are probably much more frequent in the population than the number reported to the police (Lees 1999). Only one-third of reported rapes are

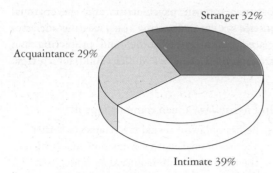

Figure 26.4 Relationship between rapist and victim 1988. [After Home Office (1993). Information on the criminal justice system in England and Wales. Digest 2]

proceeded with by the police, and only one-third of those proceeded with will be heard at a higher court. Even then, the alleged rapist has only a one in three chance of being convicted and this is most likely where the rape fits the stereotype of stranger rape. Victims of acquaintance rape (often rightly) assume they will not be believed.

The prevalence of male rape is unknown. It is likely that many male rapes go unreported, since male victims may be reluctant to come forward. As in rape of females, rape of males is associated with a wish to degrade or dominate the other person. Rapists of males tend to be violent heterosexual men; it is likely that they have anxieties about their masculine identity. Some studies have suggested that rape of either men or women is associated with gender identity problems in the rapist.

Causes

Most explanations of rape are sociocultural in terms of cultural attitudes to women, and social constructions of male and female gender roles. In psychological terms, men who are violent to women often have a rigid and conservative idealized view of the female role, coupled with denigration of any woman who transgresses that role. Rapists frequently blame their victims for the attack, by justifying the rape in terms of the woman's behaviour, e.g. 'she deserved to be raped because she was flirting with X'. Rape victims report more problems than victims of other kinds of assault, and

victims of assault describe more than those of robbery. Although in a third of cases the victim is an acquaintance of the rapist, and in a fifth there appears to have been some initial participation by the victim in events leading up to the offence, this should not be confused with voluntary participation in the rape itself. There is little evidence for the frequently expressed view that rape victims encourage the rape itself, or change their minds about having sex.

Lack of resistance is sometimes presented as evidence of consent. However, Amir (1971) found that half of rape victims were threatened with injury, either verbally or with weapons, and about third were handled roughly or violently. In such a dangerous situation submission without physical resistance is understandable and may indeed be the most usual reaction to such severe threat. The view that a lack of resistance indicated consent may reflect cultural attitudes to women and may be used as part of a legal strategy by defendants. Exposure to such attitudes may cause the rape victim further distress.

Rape is rarely associated with severe mental illness. In these cases it is usually sexual behaviour associated with disinhibition as part of a manic illness, or paranoid delusions in psychotic states. Evidence of current substance abuse is found in at least 50% of rapists. In many cases of rape, both rapists and victim will have been using drugs or alcohol; this may reflect the fact that many rape scenarios begin with both parties being in a social situation. Some men who commit rape, homicide, or other violent offences have considerable sexual problems or suffer sexual jealousy, and these may have contributed to their dangerousness. A small group of men obtain sexual pleasure from sadistic assaults on unwilling partners. Frequently, the only evidence of psychological abnormality is the deviant sexual desire itself.

Prognosis

In the UK, most rapists serve only half their sentence in prison, and are then released on license to be supervised by the probation service. The reconviction rate is 30%. The prison service offers psychological treatment to rapists as part of the Sex Offender Treatment Programme (SOTP) in prisons; the best available data to date suggest that rapists do not make much improvement on this programme, reflecting the significant social and cultural aspects of rape.

Child abduction

Child abduction is rare. A child may be abducted by one of the parents, by a man with a sexual motive, or by an older child. Babies are usually abducted by women who may have one of three kinds of motives: to achieve comfort, to manipulate another person, and on impulse by psychiatrically disturbed women. Fortunately, most stolen babies are well cared for and are found quickly (see Stephenson 1995).

Offences against property

Shoplifting

The vast majority of shoplifting, like other theft, is carried out by people without any mental disorder. Many adolescents admit occasional shoplifting. Both observational studies (Buckle and Farrington 1984) and the reports of huge losses from shops suggest that shoplifting is common among adults.

A minority of shoplifters suffer from psychiatric disorders. Apart from depressive disorders, various other psychiatric diagnoses may be associated at times with shoplifting (Gudjonsson 1990). Patients with all types of mental illness, especially those with 'substance abuse', may steal because of economic necessity. Patients with disinhibiting conditions may be more likely to steal impulsively, and patients with eating disorders may steal food. In other conditions, shoplifting may result from distractibility, for example, organic mental disorders, when the person is confused or forgetful, and panic attacks when the person may run out of the shop without paying.

The *assessment* of a person charged with shoplifting is similar to that for any other forensic problem. If the accused has a depressive disorder at the time of the examination, the psychiatrist should try to establish whether the disorder was present at the time of the offence or whether it developed after the charge was brought. The legal question most often posed is whether the accused had the intention to steal, and if a mental condition could have affected that intention.

Arson

This offence is regarded extremely seriously, not only because it can result in great damage to property, but also because it threatens life. Most arsonists are males. Although the courts refer many arsonists for psychiatric assessment, the psychiatric literature on arson is small. Certain groups can be recognized:

- fire-setters who are free from psychiatric disorder and who start fires for financial or political reasons or for revenge; they are sometimes referred to as motivated arsonists.

- so-called pathological fire-setters, who suffer from mental retardation, mental illness, or alcoholism. In a consecutive series of men remanded in custody, Taylor and Gunn (1984) found an association between psychotic disorder and arson. However, psychotic fire-setters are reported to account for only 10–15% of arsons.

- a third group that resembles the DSM criteria for pyromania (see p. 906), although the validity of this diagnostic criteria is unsubstantiated. These individuals (who sometimes join conspicuously in firefighting) obtain intense satisfaction and tension relief from fire-setting. Young men who set fires are often delinquent in other ways. Among female fire-setters, the behaviour often occurs in the context of other impulsive behaviours, such as deliberate self-harm. In this group, the behaviour may be associated with a diagnosis of borderline personality disorder.

The risks of further offences were assessed in a 20-year follow-up by Soothill and Pope (1973) who found that only 4% of arsonists were re-convicted for arson, but about half of them were charged with offences of other kinds. An important guideline is that a person convicted of arson a second time is at a much greater risk of further offences.

In addition, certain other factors point to an increased risk of a further offence: antisocial personality disorder, mental retardation, persistent social isolation, and evidence that fire-raising was done for sexual gratification or relief of tension.

The scope for psychiatric intervention is limited. Management of arsonists within hospital requires a secure setting and close observation.

Children also present with problems of fire-raising. Sometimes the behaviour represents extreme mischievousness in psychologically normal children, at times as a group activity, and sometimes it springs from psychiatric disturbance. Most of 104 child fire-setters referred to a child psychiatric clinic in London had shown marked antisocial and aggressive behaviour before the fire-setting. The most frequent diagnosis was conduct disorder (Jacobson 1985). Among children charged with fire-setting, the recurrence rate in the following 2 years is reported to be under 10%. For a review of arson see Prins (2000).

Psychiatric aspects of being a victim of crime

It is only relatively recently that criminology and society have paid attention to the role and needs of victims (see Zedner 1997; Mezey and Robbins 2000 for reviews). Surveys of general populations indicate that the experience of being a victim of crime is frequent and is related to geographical area, sex, age, and social habits. Much violence, especially sexual and domestic assaults, is unreported. There are differences between men and women in the experience as victims of crime. Young men are particularly at risk of personal violence by reason of their ways of life, whilst women are more likely to suffer domestic and sexual violence. In the UK, around a sixth of assaults on Asians and Afro-Caribbeans are believed to be racially motivated.

Women express greater fear of crime and are more likely to avoid areas that may be dangerous (Heidensohn 1997).

The response of the victim is important in determining whether an offence is reported to the police and whether charges are brought.

Psychological impact

Childhood abuse and experience of violence may have major consequences in adult life (see p. 854).

Adult crime victims are at risk of a variety of early and late psychological problems. These include the immediate distress following the crime and the subsequent distress associated with investigation and court hearings. Post-traumatic stress disorder (see p. 194) is frequently reported. These consequences are more common and severe immediately after the crime, but they may persist for many years. See also sections on PTSD (p. 194) and on accidents (p. 496).

Types of crime

Murder

Relatives of victims feel isolation and shame and an inability to share their distress greater than in other bereavement. The bureaucracy of legal processes increases anger and a feeling of being apart from the world (Rock 1998).

Rape

There is much evidence that rape victims may suffer long-term psychological effects (Mezey and Robbins 2000). Recent research has shown very high levels of intrusive thoughts and other post-traumatic symptoms in the week following rape. Serious distress may also be experienced by the partners and families of rape victims (see p. 914).

In the USA, many crisis intervention centres staffed by multidisciplinary teams have been set up for rape victims. Cognitive–behavioural treatment is helpful (Foa *et al.* 1999a).

Burglary and robbery

Although the consequences are less severe than those following violent crime, they include adjustment disorder and post-traumatic stress disorder. Victims may become preoccupied with security.

Terrorist crimes

There have been many published reports of terrorist crimes, including shootings, bombings, and hostage-taking. All have reported severe immediate distress with PTSD and other psychiatric consequences, in a minority being persistent.

Other Crimes

Victim distress is also prominent in a number of other offences including domestic violence, workplace violence, and stalking.

Witness competence

Although most of the evidence on competence as a witness and procedures for giving evidence relates to children, somewhat similar issues arise with adult victims who may be called on to give evidence in court. The issues and procedures have attracted more attention in the USA than elsewhere. This is because it has been argued in the US courts that the presence of a post-traumatic reaction could be evidence that a crime has occurred. Expert witnesses therefore have testified for the prosecution in such cases as rape trials or domestic violence where the defendant denies the charge. This type of *post hoc* reasoning is difficult to sustain, and is unlikely to be accepted in the British courts.

Management

The severity and persistence of psychological problems indicate the need for both routine and specialist help for victims. Critical incident debriefing in unhelpful (Raphael and Wilson 2000).

Support for victims of crime may be available within the community. For example, in the UK, the Home Office fund the national Victim Support scheme, who routinely contact victims of crime to offer support. A special service is also available to support crime victims who are appearing at the Crown Court. However, these services rely on volunteers who may not be able to offer long-term help and who cannot offer specialist psychiatric intervention. Voluntary groups, such as Rape Crisis, offer support to victims of sexual assault. Compensation is available to crime victims from the Criminal Injuries Compensation Board, and psychiatrists may be asked to provide reports in relation to claims for compensation for psychological distress.

Specialist services

There is a need for access to specialist psychiatric assessment and treatment services with particular experience of the problems suffered by victims. These may be provided within normal community services, within a specialized trauma clinic or, occasionally, in more narrowly defined units such as rape clinics.

Routine psychiatric care

It is important that assessment of routine consulters to psychiatric services includes enquiry about experiences of being a victim as this may be important in both aetiology and planning treatment.

The role of the psychiatrist in the criminal courts

Mental state, intention, and responsibility

Most jurisdictions require evidence of *guilty intention* for an offender to be convicted. Psychiatrists are therefore most often asked to provide opinions about how (and whether) psychiatric illness in the accused affected the intent to commit the crime. Underlying the need for psychiatric opinion is the principle that a person should not be regarded as culpable unless he was able to control his own behaviour and to choose whether to commit an unlawful act or not. It follows from this principle that, in determining whether or not a person is guilty, it is necessary to consider his mental state at the time of the act, and especially his intention.

In Anglo Saxon jurisdictions, *mens rea* is a technical term for intention, which covers many different states of mind. Intent has various meanings but the main principle is that the person perceives and intends that his act will produce unlawful consequences. Three other forms of intent need consideration:

♦ 'recklessness', which is defined as the deliberate taking of an unjustifiable risk. A man is reckless with respect to the consequence of his act, when he foresees it may occur but does not desire it.

♦ *negligence* acting negligently is defined as bringing about a consequence which a 'reasonable and prudent' man would have foreseen and avoided.

♦ *accident* (or 'blameless inadvertence').

The key issue in *responsibility* is whether the accused had the mental capacity to form the intention; or whether mental disorder might have affected that capacity. Sometimes it will be beyond psychiatric expertise or evidence to answer this question. A psychiatrist who has been asked to give an opinion on these matters should liaise closely with the lawyers as to the relevant psychiatric contribution.

Children

In most jurisdictions, the age of the accused may be thought to affect their capacity to form the intent to commit crime. Most jurisdictions exclude children under a certain age from criminal prosecution; for example, in English Law, children under 10 are excluded because they are deemed incapable of forming criminal intent (the Latin term for this being *doli incapax*). Children between the ages of 10 and 14 years may be convicted if there is evidence of *mens rea* and that the child knew that the offence was legally or morally wrong.

There are a number of issues affecting criminal proceedings about which psychiatric opinion may be obtained. *The discussion will be based on the law in England and Wales, but the principles apply more widely.* For further information on the criminal law of England and Wales, the reader is referred to standard legal texts.

Competence to stand trial

This issue may arise in relation to any charge. Most jurisdictions require that a defendant must be in a fit condition to defend himself. In English law, the issue is called 'fitness to plead' and may be raised by the defence, the prosecution, or the judge. It cannot be decided in a magistrates' court, but only by a jury.

It is necessary to determine how far the defendant can:

♦ understand the nature of the charge;

♦ understand the difference between pleading guilty and not guilty;

♦ instruct counsel;

♦ challenge jurors;

♦ follow the evidence presented in court.

A person may be suffering from severe mental disorder but still be fit to stand trial.

An individual may be found unfit to plead under the terms of the Criminal Procedures and Insanity (Unfitness to Plead) Act 1991. If an individual is found not fit to plead, then the court will hold a 'trial of the facts' to determine whether the individual carried out the offence. If the offence is not serious, then the court may make an order directing the offender to have treatment, often as an out-patient. In cases where the offence is serious, or carries a mandatory penalty (like murder), the court will direct the offender to be detained in hospital indefinitely. If he should become fit to plead, he may be returned to court for a trial. Detention after being found unfit to plead (or legally insane – see below) operates in the same way as detention accompanied by a restriction order. An American study of 85 people judged incompetent to stand trial showed that most had been charged with serious offences. Plans for psychiatric care after release were generally inadequate (Lamb 1987).

Legal insanity (not guilty by reason of insanity)

This defence may also be raised to any charge. Essentially, in raising the defence, it is argued that the defendant lacked *mens rea* for the charge because they were 'legally insane'. This term has nothing to do with diagnostic terms or classifications such as ICD-10 or DSM-IV. *Legal insanity is defined in different ways in different jurisdictions*, and a finding of insanity usually results in the defendant being admitted for treatment in hospital, as opposed to being sent to prison. In some jurisdictions, a 'not guilty by reason of insanity' verdict may result in more lenient sentencing.

In English Law, insanity is defined in law by the MacNaughten Rules, after the famous case of Daniel MacNaughten who, in 1843, shot and killed Edward Drummond, private secretary to the Prime Minister, Sir Robert Peel. In the trial at the Old Bailey, a defence of insanity was presented on the grounds that MacNaughten had suffered from delusions that he was persecuted by spies. His delusional system gradually focused on the Tory Party, and he decided to kill their leader, Sir Robert Peel (West 1974). MacNaughten was found not guilty on the grounds of insanity and was admitted to Bethlem Hospital. Because this was a contentious decision, the judges of the time drew up rules which were not enacted in the law but provided guidance. To establish a defence on the ground of insanity, it must be clearly proved that, at the time of committing the act, the party accused was:

labouring under such a defect of reason, from disease of the mind, as not to know the nature and quality of the act he was doing, or, if he did know it, that he did not know what he was doing was wrong.

Several other jurisdictions (some states in the USA and Australia) have used the MacNaughten Rules as a basis for their own definitions of legal insanity. Many critics have argued that the rules are much too narrow, and that few truly mentally ill offenders would fulfil these criteria. Indeed, it is doubtful whether MacNaughten himself fulfilled them. In some countries, the insanity defence is widely used whenever an individual with a mental illness is charged with an offence, especially crimes of violence like homicide. In English law, the insanity defence is rarely used, mainly because the alternative defence of diminished responsibility (see below) is available.

Diminished responsibility

Some jurisdictions include the concept of diminished responsibility, i.e. an individual's blameworthiness may be reduced by his having a mental illness. In English law, it is *only* available in relation to the charge of murder and is defined as:

where a person kills or is party to a killing of another, he shall not be convicted of murder if he was suffering from such abnormality of mind (whether arising from a condition of arrested or retarded development of mind or any inherent causes or induced by disease or injury) as substantially impaired his mental responsibility for his acts and omissions in doing or being party to the killing.

There are difficulties with this definition. 'Abnormality of mind' bears no resemblance to any diagnostic category; it is basically anything which the 'reasonable man' would call abnormal. It has been widely interpreted. Successful pleas have been based on conditions such as 'emotional immaturity', 'mental instability', 'psychopathic personality', 'reactive depressed state', 'mixed emotions of depression, disappointment, and exasperation', and 'premenstrual tension'.

The relationship between abnormality of mind and responsibility is not established empirically, and psychiatrists do not necessarily have expertise in this area. Most legal commentators argue that any finding of responsibility is for the jury to decide, and is not a matter of expert evidence. Nevertheless, psychiatrists may be asked to comment on this issue.

Assessment

Most defendants charged with murder undergo extensive psychiatric assessment. In England and Wales, a prison doctor carries out a psychiatric assessment of every person charged with murder. This doctor may ask for a second psychiatric opinion, often from a specialist in forensic psychiatry but sometimes from a general psychiatrist. The defence lawyers often seek independent psychiatric advice. It is good practice for the doctors involved, whether engaged by prosecution or defence lawyers, to discuss the case. Disagreement is unusual. Copies of the reports are distributed to the judge and to the prosecution and defence lawyers. Similar arrangements apply to other offences in which a psychiatric opinion is required.

If the psychiatric evidence is accepted by the court, supporting diminished responsibility, then the defendant will be convicted of manslaughter rather than murder. Whereas a murder conviction results in a mandatory life sentence, a manslaughter conviction can result in a range of sentences; from a suspended sentence to life imprisonment. In other jurisdictions, psychiatric evidence which supports diminished responsibility may affect whether the convicted offender receives the death penalty.

In the UK, offenders who are convicted of manslaughter in this way may be detained in hospital under the relevant mental health law. If the offence is particularly dangerous, and the offender presents a risk to the public, then the court may impose a restriction order, which will then require the Home Office to be involved in decisions about discharge.

Infanticide is a particular form of manslaughter charge, which can only be brought against women who have killed their newly born children (under a year old). If there is psychiatric evidence to show that the woman was mentally ill at the time of the killing, then she will be found guilty of infanticide rather than murder. The disposal options for infanticide are the same as for manslaughter. The court may make a hospital order as before; restriction orders are rarely applied. This is a rare example of the English law formally recognizing the existence of psychiatric illness as relevant to the commission of an offence; namely post-partum psychosis.

Absence of intention (automatism)

In some cases, it will be argued that the defendant lacked intention altogether for an offence (techni-cally, absence of *mens rea*) – 'automatism'. The paradigm example is acts committed while sleep walking. Automatism is hard to determine retrospectively, and the defence is rarely used. This issue may arise in relation to patients who abuse alcohol or drugs where it may be argued that they were 'intoxicated' and therefore had no intention to commit the crime. The law on intoxication is complicated and specialist legal advice should be sought.

Fitness to be punished

In those jurisdictions which have corporal or capital punishment, psychiatrists may be asked to assess offenders to determine whether they are mentally well enough to be punished. In addition to assessment, psychiatrists may be asked to treat offender patients in order to make them fit to be punished or executed. In countries where this is relevant, such as the USA, there has been considerable debate about the ethical dilemmas raised by this issue. Some authors have argued that it is unethical for psychiatrists to be involved in these procedures.

Other psychiatric issues that may be relevant to the criminal court

Amnesia

Over a third of those charged with serious offences, especially homicide, report some degree of amnesia for the offence and inadequate recall of what happened. It has sometimes been argued that loss of memory should be regarded as evidence of unfitness to plead, but such arguments have been unsuccessful. The factors most commonly associated with claims of amnesia are extreme emotional arousal, alcohol abuse and intoxication, and severe depression. Amnesia has to be distinguished from malingering in an attempt to avoid the consequences of the offence. However, there appear to be instances of true amnesias for offences, just as there is impaired recall by victims and witnesses of offences. Moreover, the factors associated with amnesia are similar in offenders and victims. In the absence of organic disease, the presence of amnesia is unlikely to be accepted as having any legal implications (see Gunn and Taylor 1993, pp. 291–9).

False confessions

Accounts of trials and other descriptive evidence indicate that false confessions to criminal deeds are sometimes made. However, the frequency of such confessions is unknown. Gudjonsson (1992) suggested that there are three main types of false confession:

◆ voluntary

◆ coerced-compliant

◆ coerced-internalized.

Voluntary confessions may arise from a morbid desire for notoriety, from difficulty in distinguishing fact from fantasy, from a wish to expiate guilt feelings, or from a desire to protect another person. Coerced-compliant confessions result from forceful interrogation and are usually retracted subsequently. Coerced-internalized confessions are made when the technique of interrogation undermines suspects' own memories and recollections so that they come to believe that they may have been responsible for the crime. Factors making a person more likely to make a false confession include a history of substance abuse, head injury, a bereavement, current anxiety, or guilt.

The assessment of possible false confessions is difficult. It requires a thorough review of the circumstances of arrest, custody, and interrogation, as well as an assessment of the personality and the current mental and physical state of the suspect. Usually the assistance of a clinical psychologist will be required to carry out a neuropsychological assessment and in some cases an assessment of suggestibility.

False accusations

Occasionally there are reports of individuals who claim to be the victims of a crime that has not occurred and who make false accusations. Examples are accusations of rape and also of stalking (Pathé

et al. 1999). Legal and clinical experience suggests such cases are uncommon and that accusers frequently have severe personality and other problems.

The treatment of offenders with mental disorder

General issues

The *assessment* needs to include as much information as possible from a variety of sources including, if possible, the general practice notes. In forensic cases relatives may not be the most reliable informants; particularly since they have often been victims of interpersonal violence. Careful attention must be paid to both mental illness and personality disorders, as well as histories of substance abuse, which are extremely common.

Forensic psychiatric treatment usually involves treating general psychiatric conditions in rather specialized settings, such as secure treatment units or hospitals. It may also involve involuntary out-patient care (Swanson *et al.* 2000). Treatment planning involves not only the appropriate medications, but also organization of appropriate psychological interventions (see Rice and Harris 1997 and J. Gunn 2000 for reviews). This is particularly true for forensic patients with severe personality disorders. Management of such patients requires specialist training for staff and support by forensic psychotherapists. It also depends upon introducing evidence-based psychiatric care into forensic practice (Lindquist and Skipworth 2000).

Many forensic patients suffer from personality disorder; the general principles of management are described in Chapter 7 (see also Hinshelwood 1999; Royal College of Psychiatrists 1999).

Treatability is an issue which is often discussed. Until recently, some patients with personality disorder have been excluded from treatment on the grounds of 'untreatability'. This reflects a lack of familiarity with treatment options available for personality disorder (Perry *et al.* 1999). The notion

Table 26.3 Assessment of treatability

- The severity of the patient's psychopathology
- Other aspects of the patient's psychological health: resilience of vulnerability factors
- Co-morbidity with other disorders
- The availability of appropriate therapy and therapists
- The experience and attitude of the assessor
- Time: patients may be more ready to engage in therapy at some time than at others

of 'untreatability' arguably applies equally to patients with severe psychotic illnesses who are 'treatment resistant' where there may be little evidence of improvement over time. Assessment of treatability is complex and affected by a number of factors (see Table 26.3). Like risk, treatability assessments may have to be repeated over time.

Settings of treatment

After conviction, an offender may be treated on a compulsory or a voluntary basis. In the UK, special treatment for mentally abnormal offenders is, in principle, provided by the Home Office (the prison medical service and the probation service) and by the Department of Health (special hospitals, specialist forensic services, and general psychiatry services). However, many mentally abnormal offenders do not receive the psychiatric treatment that they require (Gunn *et al.* 1991). The role of forensic psychiatric services in the UK is described by Stone *et al.* (2000). For a general review of the organization of services see Bluglass (2000).

Much work with offenders is carried out by general psychiatrists who assess patients and prepare court reports. General psychiatrists as well as forensic psychiatrists treat offenders given non-custodial sentences. Forensic psychiatrists work in separate units and undertake specialized assessment and court work. In many places there are community forensic services to provide assessment and treatment. Forensic psychiatrists may work to

provide care for patients needing security in ordinary psychiatric hospitals.

The mentally abnormal in prison

Surveys have shown that about a third of sentenced prisoners have a psychiatric disorder and 2% have a psychosis (see Lamb and Weinburger 1998). Most of these disorders can be treated in prison, but a few need transfer to a hospital. Reasons for transfer include unpredictable violence, life-threatening self-harm, and failure to improve with treatment in prison.

The medical services have to provide psychiatric care under extremely difficult conditions, and it has been argued that there should be a substantial increase in the contribution of psychiatrists to the provision of medical care within prisons. A few prisons offer psychiatric treatment, usually of personality disorders and sexual offences, as a main part of their work; one such prison is at Grendon Underwood in England. Although there is an undoubted need for psychiatric care within prisons, there would be disadvantages in a system which encouraged the courts to send the mentally abnormal to prison rather than to hospital services.

Offenders in hospital

Most jurisdictions allow for the detention of mentally abnormal offenders in secure psychiatric settings. In England and Wales, a convicted offender may be committed to hospital for compulsory psychiatric treatment under a Mental Health Act hospital order. There is also provision in law for a prisoner to be transferred from prison to a psychiatric hospital. One important point is that hospital orders may have no time limit, whilst most prison sentences are of fixed length. The length of stay in a psychiatric hospital may be shorter or longer than a prison sentence.

Special hospitals and secure units in the UK

In the UK, detention of mentally abnormal offenders may be in a local psychiatric hospital, a medium security unit, or a maximum secure hospital (or 'special hospital'). In England, the first special provision for the criminally insane was made in 1800. Following a trial in which Hadfield was found not guilty by reason of insanity for shooting at King George III, a special criminal wing was established at the Bethlem Hospital. In 1863, Broadmoor, the oldest of the special hospitals, opened under the management of the then Home Office. There are now four high-security special hospitals in England and Wales.

The detention of patients in special hospitals is for an indeterminate length of stay. For those with mental illness (mostly schizophrenia), length of detention is associated with the severity or chronicity of the psychiatric disorder rather than the nature of the offence. By contrast, for patients suffering from psychopathic disorder, the main determinant of length of stay was the nature of the offence.

The closure of the larger mental hospitals has had unforeseen consequences for the care of mentally abnormal offenders. There is less physical security in the new psychiatric hospitals and less willingness by hospital staff to tolerate severely disturbed behaviour. As a result, it has become increasingly difficult to arrange admission to hospital for offenders, particularly those who are severely disturbed. In addition, length of stay in hospital has shortened, making it more difficult to arrange treatment for patients with chronic disorders and severe behaviour disorder. Two alternative provisions have been developed:

- well-staffed *secure areas in ordinary psychiatric hospitals* in which the less dangerous of these patients can be treated;
- *special secure units* associated with psychiatric hospitals to provide a level of security between that of an ordinary hospital and a special hospital. Problems have arisen about the criteria for selecting patients for these special secure units, and about their role in relation to both ordinary psychiatric hospitals and the special hospitals.

Treatment in the community

Offender patients may not pose sufficient risk, or be sufficiently ill, to require treatment in hospital. Courts may also use non-custodial sentences in which the offender-patient may receive support from the probation service as well as psychiatric treatment. On occasions, psychiatric treatment as an in-patient or out-patient may be made a condition of probation, with which the offender must agree to comply.

The psychiatric treatment provided for a mentally abnormal offender is similar to that for a patient with the same psychiatric disorder who has not broken the law. It is often difficult to provide psychiatric care for offenders with chronic psychiatric disorders who commit repeated petty offences. In the past they would have been long-stay patients in a psychiatric hospital, but now they are treated in the community where they may be unwilling to cooperate with treatment and may be difficult to follow up because they change address or become homeless.

The management of violence in hospitals

Violent incidents are not confined to patients with forensic problems, but this is a convenient place to consider their management. Although not frequent, violent incidents in hospitals are increasing. The reasons for this increase appear to include:

- changes in mental health policies that have made dangerousness a relatively more common reason for an admission (since non-violent patients are more likely to be treated in the community);
- overcrowding;
- lack of experienced staff;
- an increased tolerance of violence in some hospitals.

All psychiatrists should be familiar with how to analyse and manage incidents of violence in in-patient settings. Prior education and training are valuable before the event; the Royal College of Psychiatrists has provided guidelines (Royal College of Psychiatrists 1996). It is important that the staff have a clear policy for managing incidents of violence and are trained to carry it out. Such a policy calls for attention to the design of wards, arrangements for summoning assistance, and suitable training of the staff.

When violence is threatened or occurs, staff should be available in adequate numbers, and emergency medication such as intramuscular haloperidol or droperidol should be unobtrusively available. The emphasis should be on the prevention of violence.

Dangerous people can often be calmed by sympathetic discussion or reassurance, preferably given by someone whom the patient knows and trusts. It is important not to challenge the patient. It is inappropriate to reward violent or threatening behaviour by making concessions in treatment or ward rules, but every effort should be made to allow the patient to withdraw from confrontation without loss of face.

After an incident has occurred, the clinical team should meet to consider:

◆ the future care of the patient. For mentally disordered patients, there should be a review of the drugs prescribed and their dosage. When violence occurs in a person with a personality disorder, medication may be required in an emergency, but it is usually best to avoid maintenance medication. Other measures include trying to reduce factors that provoke violence or to provide the patient with more constructive ways of managing tension, such as taking physical exercise or asking a member of staff for help.

◆ supportive psychological interventions for patients or staff who have been the victim of a violent assault (see victims of crime, above).

◆ It should not be forgotten than such assaults are forms of interpersonal violence, which may be criminal. It may be helpful for the police to

be notified so the offence is recorded, even if a prosecution is not proceeded with.

◆ The possible effect on the whole patient group, whether or not they were present at the incident.

◆ Any possible changes in the general policy of the ward.

Risk assessment

The change to community care has made both minor criminality and rare violent offences more conspicuous and has resulted in increased public disquiet. Psychiatric services need the resources to minimize difficulties and to identify and manage serious threats of violence. See Mullen (2000) for a review of dangerousness and risk. The psychiatrist may need to assess risk in everyday psychiatric practice and also in forensic work.

In everyday practice, both out-patients and in-patients may appear to be dangerous, and careful risk assessment may be required so that the most appropriate steps can be taken in the interests of the patient and of other people. Risk of serious harm to others is an important criterion for compulsory detention in hospital (see also Chapter 2).

In forensic work the court may ask for the psychiatrist's advice on the defendant's dangerousness so that a suitable sentence can be passed. The psychiatrist may also be asked to comment on offenders who are detained in institutions and who are being considered for release. In both kinds of circumstance there is an ethical dilemma between the need to protect the community from someone who might show violent behaviour and the obligation to respect the human rights of the offender.

There have been two broad approaches:

◆ *Clinical* Psychiatrists have tried to identify factors associated with dangerousness in an individual patient, but no reliable predictors of violence have been established (Dolan and Doyle 2000).

◆ *Actuarial* There is a large literature on the use of actuarial methods in predicting future crim-

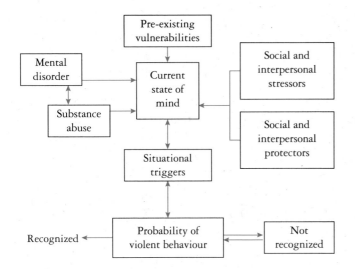

Figure 26.5 Schematic representation of the issues which should be considered in assessing the probability of violent behaviour. [After Mullen, P. (2000). Dangerousness, risk and the prediction of probabilty. In *The new Oxford textbook of psychiatry* (eds. M. G. Gelder, J. J. López-Ibor Jr, and N. C. Andreasen), Chapter 11.4.3. Oxford University Press, Oxford. Reproduced with permission]

inal behaviour amongst offenders and amongst other populations, such as psychiatric patients. However, in general, the low correlations between predicted and observed behaviour have meant they have been unhelpful in individual predictions. Although some recent instruments have a higher degree of accuracy, they are time-consuming to administer (Monahan *et al.* 2000).

There are no fixed clinical rules for assessing risk but there are a number of authoritative advisory publications. A thorough review should be made of the history of previous violence, the characteristics of the current offence and the circumstances in which it occurred, and the mental state (Figure 26.5). In making the review, it is helpful to consider certain key questions:

- whether any consistent pattern of behaviour can be discerned;
- whether any circumstances have provoked violence in the past and are likely to occur again in the future;
- whether there is any good evidence that the defendant is willing to change his behaviour;
- whether there is likely to be any response to treatment (Table 26.4).

Of these predictors, the most useful is a history of past violence (see Mullen 2000).

Particular difficulties may arise in the assessment of dangerousness in people of antisocial personality or with learning disabilities, both of whom may be poorly motivated to comply with care. Another difficult problem is presented by the person who threatens to commit a violent act such as homicide. Here the assessment is much the same as for suicide threats (Gunn and Taylor 1993, p. 632). The psychiatrist should ask the threatener about his intent, motivation, and the potential victim, and should make a full assessment of mental state. Some patients who make threats can be helped by out-patient support and treatment, but sometimes hospital admission is required if the risk is high. It may be necessary to warn potential victims.

It is a valuable principle for the psychiatrist not to rely entirely on his own evaluation of dangerousness, but to discuss the problem with other colleagues, including psychiatrists, general practitioners, social workers, and relatives (see Tardiff 1992; Mullen 2000).

Table 26.4 Factors associated with dangerousness

Male gender

History

- One or more previous episodes of violence
- Repeated impulsive behaviour
- Evidence of difficulty in coping with stress
- Previous unwillingness to delay gratification
- Antisocial traits and lack of social support

The offence

- Bizarre violence
- Lack of provocation
- Lack of regret
- Continuing major denial

Mental state

- Morbid jealousy
- Paranoid beliefs plus a wish to harm others
- Deceptiveness
- Lack of self-control
- Threats to repeat violence
- Attitude to treatment, poor compliance

Circumstances

- Provocation or precipitant likely to recur
- Alcohol or drug abuse
- Social difficulties and lack of support

Appendix: the psychiatric report

A psychiatric report prepared for a major criminal charge is an important document, and should be based on full psychiatric and social examination. It is essential that the psychiatrist read all the depositions by witnesses, statements by the accused, and any previous medical notes and social reports. Family members should be interviewed. When evidence about previous offences is not admissible (as

is the case in English Law) the psychiatrist's report should not include these facts. This may cause problems for the psychiatrist, whose opinion is often based in large part on the previous behaviour of the offender. The writing of the court report follows the usual format (see p. 928 and should include discussions of mental state at the time of the alleged offence and of fitness to plead. The involvement of the psychiatrist at various stages of the legal process in England and Wales is shown in Table 26.5.

The role of the psychiatrist in relation to the court

The psychiatrist's role is to draw on his special knowledge to help the court. He should not attempt to tell the court what to do. In the UK, the duty of the expert medical witness is to the court as a whole; he is not expected to be partisan. It is sometimes hard for psychiatrists to appreciate that they must remain neutral and not provide evidence to order that supports the party instructing them. This is particularly difficult because most psychiatrists use their clinical skills to establish rapport with individuals on whom they are preparing a report.

The psychiatrist should be aware that the court will see the report and that it may be read out in open court. Reports commissioned and paid for by lawyers are the property of the court.

The assessment

Psychiatrists should prepare themselves as thoroughly as possible before the interview. They should have a clear idea as to the purpose of the examination, and particularly as to any question of fitness to plead. They should have details of the present charge and past convictions, together with copies of any statements made by the defendant and witnesses. Psychiatrists should also study any available reports of the defendant's social history; during their subsequent interview they should go through this report with the defendant and check its accuracy. Psychiatrists should begin by explaining to the client the source of the referral and why the referral was made. They should explain that the

Table 26.5 **The involvement of psychiatrists in the stages of the UK legal process**

Stage 1 Arrest	Stage II Pre-trial	Stage III At the trial	Stage IV After the trial
Removal to a place of safety Assessment after arrest Court diversion schemes	Court report Remand for in-patient assessment or treatment Transfer from prison for assessment	Special problems: • fitness to plead • diminished responsibility Advice about disposal	Treatment under hospital orders or guardianship Transfer from prison Decisions about release Treatment in the community

psychiatrist's opinion may be given in court and that the defendant is under no obligation to answer any questions if he chooses not to. Detailed notes should be made, recording any significant comments in the defendant's own words.

At some stage in the interview (not necessarily at the start), the alleged crime should be discussed. The defendant may or may not admit guilt. The psychiatrist is not required to obtain a statement either way, although the defendant's views will be of interest.

A detailed history of physical illnesses should be taken; particular attention should be paid to neurological disorders including head injury and epilepsy. A careful history of previous psychiatric disorder and treatment should be obtained. If there has been a previous psychiatric opinion or treatment, further information should be sought. Full examination of the present mental state is made in the usual way. Special investigations should be requested if suitable. If the defendant's intelligence level is under question, an assessment should be made by a clinical psychologist who normally submits a separate report.

It is important to obtain further information from relatives and other informants. If the defendant is remanded in custody, the staff may have long periods of contact with the prisoner and may be able to give particularly useful information.

Preparing the report

The preparation of a court report will be affected by the circumstances of the case, and the instructions given by solicitors. Court reports for civil and criminal cases may be very different. A possible outline is given in Box 26.2. More detail is available in papers by Rix (1999a, 1999b).

In preparing a court report, the psychiatrist should remember that it will be read by non-medical people. Therefore the report should be written in simple English and should avoid jargon. If technical terms are used, they should be defined as accurately as possible. The report should be concise.

Advice on medical treatment

One of the psychiatrist's main functions is to give an opinion as to whether or not psychiatric treatment is indicated. The psychiatrist should make sure that any recommendations on treatment are feasible, if necessary by consulting colleagues, social workers, or others. If hospital treatment is recommended, the court should be informed whether or not a suitable placement is available.

Box 26.2 Some headings for a court report

- A statement of the *psychiatrist's full name, qualifications, present appointment* (and, in England and Wales, whether approved under Section 12 of the Mental Health Act).

- Where and when the interview was conducted and whether any third person was present.

- *Sources of information* including documents that have been examined.

- *Family and personal history of the defendant/plaintiff.* Usually this need not be given in great detail, particularly if a social report is available to the court. The focus should be on information relevant to the diagnosis and disposal.

- *The account of the events given by the defendant/plaintiff.* This will depend on whether the defendant is pleading guilty or not guilty. If the accused admits to the crime, comment may be made on his attitude to it such as degree of remorse. If he is pleading not guilty, any reference to the alleged crime is inadmissible.

- *Other behaviour* It may be relevant to mention other items of behaviour, even if not directly involved in the crime, such as alcohol or drug abuse, quality of relationships with other people, tolerance of frustration, and general social competence.

- *Present mental state* Only the salient positive findings should be stated and negative findings should be omitted. A general diagnosis should be given

in the terms of the Mental Health Act (mental illness, mental impairment, or psychopathic disorder). A more specific diagnosis can then be given, but the court will be interested in a categorical statement rather than the finer nuances of diagnosis.

- *Mental state at the time of the relevant events* This is often a highly important issue, especially in criminal cases, and yet it can be based only on retrospective speculation. The assessment can be helped by accounts given by eye witnesses who saw the offender at the time of the crime or soon after. A current psychiatric diagnosis may suggest the likely mental state at the time of the crime. For example, if the accused suffers from chronic schizophrenia or a chronic organic mental syndrome, the mental state may well have been the same at the time of the crime as at the examination. However, if the accused suffers from a depressive disorder (now or recently) or from an episodic disorder such as epilepsy, it is more difficult to infer what the mental state is likely to have been at the material time. To add to the difficulty, even if it is judged that the defendant was suffering from a mental disorder, a further judgement is needed as to his *mens rea* at the time of the crime.

- *Conclusions*

The assessment of risk is important here (see p. 924). The psychiatrist should not recommend any form of disposal other than treatment. However, the court often welcomes respectfully worded comments on the suitability of possible sentences, particularly in the case of young offenders.

The psychiatrist appearing in court

The psychiatrist appearing in court should be fully prepared and should have well-organized copies of all reports and necessary documents. It is helpful to speak to the lawyer involved beforehand, in order to clarify any points that may be raised in court. When replying to any questions in court, it is important to be brief and clear, to restrict the answers to the psychiatric evidence, and to avoid speculation. A number of expert witness training programmes are available, which may be useful for psychiatrists who often give expert evidence.

Further reading

Gelder, M. G., López-Ibor, J. J. Jr, and Andreasen, N. C. (eds) (2000). *The new Oxford textbook of psychiatry*, Part 11: Forensic psychiatry. Oxford University Press, Oxford.

Bluglass, R. S. and Bowden, P. (eds) (1990). *Principles and practice of forensic psychiatry.* Routledge, London. (Although now somewhat out-of-date still a major reference work.)

Gunn, J. and Taylor, P. (eds) (1993). *Forensic psychiatry: clinical, legal and ethical issues.* Butterworth Heinemann, London. (A readable reference work.)

Maguire, M. (1997) *The Oxford Textbook of Criminology* (2nd edn) Clarendon Press, Oxford. (An authoritative review of criminology with numerous chapers relevant to forensic psychiatry.)

Stone, J. H., Roberts, M., O'Grady, J., Taylor, A. U., and O'Shea, K. (2000). *Faulk's basic forensic psychiatry*, 3rd edn. Blackwell, Oxford. (A useful medium-length textbook.)

References

Abas, M. A., Sahakian, B. J., and Levy, R. (1990). Neuropsychological deficits and CT scan changes in elderly depressives. *Psychological Medicine* **20**, 507–20.

Abas, M., Broadhead, J .C., Mbape, P., and Khumalo-Satakukwa, G. (1994). Defeating depression in the developing world. *British Journal of Psychiatry* **164**, 293–6.

Abel, G. and Osborn, C. A. (2000). The paraphilias. In *The new Oxford textbook of psychiatry* (eds M. G. Gelder, J. J. López-Ibor Jr, and N. C. Andreasen), Chapter 4.11.3. Oxford University Press, Oxford.

Abel, G. G. and Rouleau, J. L. (2000). Behavioural therapy strategies for medical patients. In *Psychiatric care of the medical patient* (eds A. Stoudemire, B. S. Fogel, and D. B. Greenberg). Oxford University Press, New York.

Abelson, J. L., Glitz, D., Cameron, O. G., *et al.* (1991). Blunted growth hormone response to clonidine in patients with generalized anxiety disorder. *Archives of General Psychiatry* **48**, 157–62.

Abraham, H. D. (2000). Disorders relating to the use of phencyclidine and hallucinogens. In *The new Oxford textbook of psychiatry* (eds M. G. Gelder, J. J. López-Ibor Jr, and N. C. Andreasen), Chapter 4.2.3.4. Oxford University Press, Oxford.

Abraham, K. (1911). Notes on the psychoanalytic investigation and treatment of manic-depressive insanity and allied conditions. In *Selected papers on psychoanalysis*, pp. 137–56. Hogarth Press and Institute of Psychoanalysis, London (1927).

Acierno, R., Resnick, H. S., and Kilpatrick, D. G. (1997). Health impact of interpersonal violence 1: prevalence rates, case identification, and risk factors for sexual assault, physical assault, and domestic violence in men and women. *Behavioural Medicine* **23**, 53–64.

Ackerman, N. W. (1958). *The psychodynamics of family life.* Basic Books, New York.

Ackner, B. (1954a). Depersonalization: I. Aetiology and phenomenology. *Journal of Mental Science* **100**, 939–53.

Ackner, B. (1954b). Depersonalization: II. The clinical syndromes. *Journal of Mental Science* **100**, 954–72.

Ackner, B. and Oldham, A. J. (1962). Insulin treatment of schizophrenia. A three year follow up of a controlled study. *Lancet* **1**, 504–6.

Adams, I. B. and Martin, B. R. (1996). Cannabis: pharmacology and toxicology in animals and humans. *Addiction* **91**, 1585–614.

Ader, R., Felten, D. L., and Cohen, N. (2000). *Psychoneuroimmunology* (3rd ed). Academic Press, London.

Adler, A. (1943). Neuropsychiatric complications in victims of Boston's Coconut Grove disaster. *Journal of the American Medical Association* **123**, 1098–111.

Adolphs, R., Tranel, D., Damasio, H., and Damasio, A. (1994). Impaired recognition of emotion in facial expressions following bilateral damage to the human amygdala. *Nature* **372**, 669–72.

Agras, W. S., Walsh, B. T., Fairburn, C. G., Wilson, G. T., and Kraemer, H. C. (2000). A multicenter comparison of cognitive–behavioral therapy and interpersonal psychotherapy for bulimia nervosa. *Archives of General Psychiatry* **57**, 459–66.

Akiskal, H. (2000). Dysthymia, cyclothymia, and related chronic subthreshold mood disorders. In *The new Oxford textbook of psychiatry* (eds M. G. Gelder, J. J. López-Ibor Jr, and N. C. Andreasen), Chapter 4.5.8. Oxford University Press, Oxford.

Alexander, D. A. (1972). 'Senile dementia'. A changing perspective. *British Journal of Psychiatry* **121**, 207–14.

Alexander, F. (1950). *Psychosomatic medicine.* Norton, New York.

Alexander, P. C. and Lupfer, S. L. (1987). Family characteristics and long term consequences associated with sexual abuse. *Archives of Sexual Behaviour* **16**, 235–45.

Alexopoulos, G. S., Silver, J. M., Kahn, D. A., Frances, A., and Carpenter, D. (eds) (1998). Treatment of agitation in older persons with dementia. Expert Consensus Guideline Series; Postgraduate Medicine.

Alldridge, P. (1979). Hospitals, madhouses and asylums: cycles in the care of the insane. *British Journal of Psychiatry* 134, 321–4.

Allebeck, P. and Olsen, J. (1998). Alcohol and fetal damage. *'Alcoholism' Clinical and Experimental Research* 22 (Suppl 7), 329S–32S.

Allen, C. (1969). *A textbook of psychosexual disorders*, 2nd edn. Oxford University Press, London.

Allodi, F. A. (1991). Assessment and treatment of torture victims: a critical review. *Journal of Nervous and Mental Disease* 179, 4–11.

Alström, J. E., Nordlund, C. L., Persson, G., *et al.* (1984). Effects of four treatment methods on social phobic patients not suitable for insight-oriented psychotherapy. *Acta Psychiatrica Scandinavica* 70, 97–110.

Althof, S. E. and Seftel, A. D. (1995). The evaluation and management of erectile dysfunction. *Psychiatric Clinics of North America* 1,171–92.

American Academy of Child and Adolescent Psychiatry (1997a). Practice parameters for the forensic evaluation of children and adolescents who may have been physically or sexually abused. *Journal of the American Academy of Child and Adolescent Psychiatry* 36(10 suppl), 37S–56S.

American Academy of Child and Adolescent Psychiatry (1997b). Practice parameters for the assessment and treatment of children, adolescents, and adults with attention deficit/hyperactivity disorder. *Journal of the American Academy of Child and Adolescent Psychiatry* 36(10 suppl), 85S–121S.

American Academy of Child and Adolescent Psychiatry (1997c). Practice parameters for the assessment and treatment of children, adolescents, and adults with conduct disorder. *Journal of the American Academy of Child and Adolescent Psychiatry* 36(10 suppl), 122S–39S.

American Academy of Child and Adolescent Psychiatry (1998a). Summary of the practice parameters for the psychiatric assessment of infants and toddlers (0–36 months). *Journal of the American Academy of Child and Adolescent Psychiatry* 37, 127–32.

American Academy of Child and Adolescent Psychiatry (1998b). Practice parameters for the assessment and treatment of children and adolescents with language and learning disorders. *Journal of the American Academy of Child and Adolescent Psychiatry*, 37(10 suppl), 46S–62S.

American Academy of Child and Adolescent Psychiatry (1998c). Practice guidelines for the assessment and treatment of children and adolescents with depressive disorders. *Journal of the American Academy of Child and Adolescent Psychiatry* 37(10 suppl), 63S–83S.

American Academy of Child and Adolescent Psychiatry (1998d). Practice parameters for the assessment and treatment of children and adolescents with substance misuse disorders. *Journal of the American Academy of Child and Adolescent Psychiatry* 36(10 suppl), 140S–56S.

American Psychiatric Association (1980). *Diagnostic and statistical manual of mental disorders*, 3rd edn, revised. American Psychiatric Association, Washington, DC.

American Psychiatric Association (1987). *Diagnostic and statistical manual of mental disorders*, 3rd edn. American Psychiatric Association, Washington, DC.

American Psychiatric Association (1994a). *Diagnostic and statistical manual of mental disorders*, 4th edn. American Psychiatric Association, Washington, DC.

American Psychiatric Association (1994b). Practice guideline for the treatment of patients with bipolar disorder. *American Journal of Psychiatry* 151(12 suppl), 1–36.

American Psychiatric Association (1995). *Principles of medical ethics with annotations especially for psychiatry.* American Psychiatric Association, Washington, DC.

American Psychiatric Association (1998). Guidelines for assessing the decision-making capacities of potential research subjects with cognitive impairment. *American Journal of Psychiatry* 155, 1649–50.

American Psychiatric Association (1999). Practice guidelines for the treatment of patients with delirium. *American Journal of Psychiatry* 156, Suppl to Issue 5.

American Psychiatric Association (2000). *Diagnostic and statistical manual of mental disorders*, 4th edn, *Text revision.* American Psychiatric Association, Washington, DC.

American Psychiatric Association (2000). Practice guidelines for the treatment of patients with HIV/AIDS. *American Journal of Psychiatry* 157 (suppl).

Amies, P. L., Gelder, M. G., and Shaw, P. M. (1983). Social phobia: a comparative clinical study. *British Journal of Psychiatry* 142, 174–9.

Amir, M. (1971). *Patterns in forcible rape*. Chicago University Press, Chicago, IL.

Ammerman, R. T., Van Hasselt, V. B., and Herson, M. (1986). Psychological adjustment of visually handicapped children and youth. *Clinical Psychological Review* 6, 67–85.

Amsel, L. and Mann, J. J. (2000). Biological aspects of suicidal behaviour. In *The new Oxford textbook of psychiatry* (eds M. G. Gelder, J. J. López-Ibor Jr, and N. C. Andreasen), Chapter 4.15.3. Oxford University Press, Oxford.

Anand, A. and Charney, D. S. (2000). Norepinephrine dysfunction in depression. *Journal of Clinical Psychiatry* 61(suppl 10), 16–24.

Anand, A., Verhoeff, P., Seneca, N., *et al.* (2000). Brain SPECT imaging of amphetamine-induced dopamine release in euthymic bipolar disorder patients. *American Journal of Psychiatry* 157, 1108–14.

Anderson, I. M. (1999). Lessons to be learnt from meta-analyses of newer versus older antidepressants. In *Recent topics for advances in psychiatric treatment* (ed. A. Lee), Vol. 2, pp. 45–51. Royal College of Psychiatrists, Gaskill Press, London.

Anderson, I. M. (2000). Selective serotonin reuptake inhibitors versus tricyclic antidepressants: a meta-analysis of efficacy and tolerability. *Journal of Affective Disorders* 58, 19–36.

Anderson, I. M., Parry-Billings, M., Newsholme, E. A., *et al.* (1990). Decreased plasma tryptophan concentration in major depression: relationship to melancholia and weight loss. *Journal of Affective Disorders* 20, 185–191.

Anderson, I. M., Nutt, D. J., and Deakin, J. F. W. (2000). Evidence-based guidelines for treating depressive disorders with antidepressants: a revision of the 1993 British Association for Psychopharmacology guidelines. *Journal of Psychopharmacology* 14, 3–20.

Anderson, J. C., Williams, S., McGee, R., and Silva, P. A. (1987). DSMIII disorder in pre-adolescent children; prevalence from a large sample in the general population. *Archives of General Psychiatry* 44, 69–76.

Andreasen, N. C. and Hoenck, P. R. (1982). The predictive value of adjustment disorders: a follow-up study. *American Journal of Psychiatry* 139, 584–590.

Andreasen, N. C. and Wasek, P. (1980). Adjustment disorder in adolescents and adults. *Archives of General Psychiatry* 37, 1166–70.

Andreasen, N. J. C. (1985). Post-traumatic stress disorder. In *Comprehensive textbook of psychiatry*, 4th edn, Vol.3 (eds H. I. Kaplan and B. J. Sadock). Williams and Wilkins, Baltimore, MD.

Andreasson, S., Allebeck, P., Engstrom, A., *et al.* (1987). Cannabis and schizophrenia: a longitudinal study of Swedish conscripts. *Lancet* 2, 1483–5.

Andrews, G., Crino, R., Hunt, C. I. (1994). *The treatment of anxiety disorders: clinician's guide and patient manuals*. Cambridge University Press, Cambridge.

Andrews, G., Slade, T., and Peters, L. (1999). Classification in psychiatry: ICD-10 versus DSM-IV. *British Journal of Psychiatry* 174, 3–5.

Angst, J. (1992). How recurrent and predictable is depressive illness? In *Long-term treatment of depression* (eds S. Montgomery and F. Rouillon), pp. 1–13. Wiley, Chichester.

Angst, J. (2000). Course and prognosis of mood disorders. In *The new Oxford textbook of psychiatry* (eds M. G. Gelder, J. J. López-Ibor Jr, and N. C. Andreasen), Chapter 4.5.6. Oxford University Press, Oxford.

Angst, J. and Dobler-Mikola, A. (1985). The Zurich Study. VI A continuum from depression to anxiety disorders? *European Archives of Psychiatry and Neurological Sciences* 235, 179–86.

Ansbacher, H. and Ansbacher, R. (1964). *The individual psychotherapy of Alfred Adler*. Basic Books, New York.

Appleby, L. (1993). Parasuicide: features of repetition and the implications for intervention. *Psychological Medicine,* 23 13–16.

Appleby, L., Cooper, J., Amos, T., and Faragher, B. (1999). Psychological autopsy of suicides by people aged under 35. *British Journal of Psychiatry* 175, 168–74.

Appleton, K., House, A., and Dowell, A. (1998). A survey of job satisfaction, sources of stress and psychological symptoms among general practitioners in Leeds. *British Journal of General Practice* 48, 1059–63.

Armor, D. J., Polich, J. M., and Stambul, H. B. (1976). *Alcoholism and treatment*. Rand Corporation and Interscience, Santa Monica, CA.

Arnulf, I., Bonnet, A.M., Damier, P. *et al.* (2000). Hallucinations, REM sleep and Parkinson's disease: a medical hypothesis. *Neurology* 55, 281–8.

Aronson, R., Offman, H. J., Joffe, R. T., and Naylor, C. D. (1996). Triiodothyronine augmentation in the treatment of refractory depression. a meta-analysis. *Archives of General Psychiatry* 53, 842–8.

Arriageda, P. V., Growdon, J. H., Hedley Whyte, E. T., and Hyman, R. T. (1992). Neurofibrillary tangles but not senile plaque parallel the duration and severity of Alzheimer's disease. *Neurology* **42**, 63–5.

Arscott, K., Dagnan, D., and Kroese, B. (1998). Consent to psychological research by people with an intellectual disability. *Journal of Applied Research in Intellectual Disability* **11**, 77–83.

Asher, R. (1951). Munchausen's syndrome. *Lancet* **1**, 339–41.

Ashworth, M. and Gerada, C. (1997). Addiction and dependence-II: Alcohol. *British Medical Journal* **315**, 358–60.

Asperger, H. (1944). Die 'Autistischen Psychopathien' Kindesalter. *Archiv für Psychiatrie und Nervenkrankheiten* **117**, 76–136.

Audini, B., Marks, I. M., Lawrence, R. E., *et al.* (1994). Home-based versus out-patient/in-patient care for people with serious mental illness. Phase II of a controlled trial. *British Journal of Psychiatry* **165**, 204–10.

Austin, M.-P., Ross, M., Murray, C., *et al.* (1992). Cognitive function in major depression. *Journal of Affective Disorders* **25**, 21–30.

Austoker, J. (1994). Reducing alcohol intake. *British Medical Journal* **308**, 1549–52.

Avery, D. H. (1998). A turning point for seasonal affective disorder and light therapy research. *Archives of General Psychiatry* **55**, 863–4.

Bach-y-Rita, G., Lion, J. R., Climent, C. E., and Ervin, F. R. (1971). Episodic dyscontrol: a study of 130 violent patients. *American Journal of Psychiatry* **127**, 1473–8.

Bailey, A., Le Couteur, A., Gottesman, I., *et al.* (1995). Autism as a strongly genetic disorder: evidence from a British twin study. *Psychological Medicine* **25**, 63–77.

Bailey, J. M. and Pillard, R. C. (1991). A genetic study of male sexual orientation. *Archives of General Psychiatry* **48**, 1089–96.

Bailey, S. (1997). Review: sadistic and violent acts in the young. *Child Psychology and Psychiatry Review* **2**, 92–102.

Bailey, S. (2000). Juvenile delinquency and serious antisocial behaviour. In *The new Oxford textbook of psychiatry* (eds M. G. Gelder, J. J. López-Ibor Jr, and N. C. Andreasen), Chapter 9.4.1. Oxford University Press, Oxford.

Bailey, S. and Aulich, L. (1997). Understanding murderous 'youth'. In *Forensic psychotherapy* (eds E. Welldon and C. van Leeson). Jessica Kingsley, London.

Bailey, V., Graham, P., and Boniface, D. (1978). How much child psychiatry does a general practitioner do? *Journal of the Royal College of General Practitioners* **28**, 621–6.

Bakish, D., Hooper, C. L., and Filtreau, M. J. (1996). A double-blind, placebo-controlled trial comparing fluvoxamine and imipramine in the treatment of panic disorder with and without agoraphobia. *Psychopharmacology Bulletin* **32**, 135–141.

Bakwin, H. (1961). Enuresis in children. *Journal of Paediatrics* **58**, 806–19.

Bal, S. S. (1987). Psychological symptomatology and health beliefs of Asian patients. In *Clinical psychology: research and development* (ed. H. Dent), pp.101–10. Croom Helm, London.

Baldessarini, R. J. and Tarazi, F. I. (1996). Brain dopamine receptors: a trial on their current status, basic and clinical. *Harvard Review of Psychiatry* **3**, 301–25.

Baldwin, R. (2000). Mood disorders in the elderly. In *The new Oxford textbook of psychiatry* (eds M. G. Gelder, J. J. López-Ibor Jr, and N. C. Andreasen), Chapter 8.5.4. Oxford University Press, Oxford.

Baldwin, R. C. (2001). Depressive Illness. In *Psychiatry in the elderly*, 3rd edn (eds R. Jacoby and C. Oppenheimer). Oxford University Press, Oxford.

Ball, D. M. and Murray, R. M. (1994). Genetics of alcohol misuse. *British Medical Bulletin* **50**, 18–35.

Ball, J. R. B. and Kiloh, L. G. (1959). A controlled trial of imipramine in the treatment of depressive states. *British Medical Journal* **2**, 1052–5.

Ballenger, J. C. (2000). Panic disorder and agoraphobia. In *The new Oxford textbook of psychiatry* (eds M. G. Gelder, J. J. López-Ibor Jr, and N. C. Andreasen), Chapter 4.7.3. Oxford University Press, Oxford.

Bancroft, J. H. J. (1989). *Human sexuality and its problems*, 2nd edn. Churchill Livingstone, Edinburgh.

Bancroft, J. H. J., Skrimshire, A. M., Casson, J., *et al.* (1977). People who deliberately poison or injure themselves: their problems and their contacts with helping agencies. *Psychological Medicine* **7**, 289–303.

Bandura, A. (1969). *Principles of behaviour modification*. Holt, Rinehart and Winston, New York.

Barber, T. X. (1962). Towards a theory of hypnosis: posthypnotic behaviour. *Archives of General Psychiatry* 1, 321–42.

Barker, J. C. and Barker, A. A. (1959). Deaths associated with electroplexy. *Journal of Mental Science* 105, 339–48.

Barker, P. (1988). *Basic child psychiatry*, 3rd edn. Blackwell Scientific Publications, Oxford.

Barker, P. (1992). *Basic family therapy*, 5th edn. Blackwell Scientific Publications, Oxford.

Barker, W. A., Scott, J., and Eccelston, D. (1987). The Newcastle chronic depression study: results of a treatment regime. *International Clinical Psychopharmacology* 2, 261–72.

Barlow, D. H., Esler, J. L., and Vitali, B. A. (1997). Psychosocial treatments for panic disorder, phobias and generalized anxiety disorder. In *A guide to treatments that work* (eds P. E. Nathan and J. M. Gorman), pp. 288–318. Oxford University Press, New York.

Barlow, D. H., Shear, K., Woods, S., and Gorman, J. A. (2000). A multicenter trial comparing cognitive–behaviour therapy, imipramine, their combination and placebo in the treatment of panic disorder Presented at the Anxiety Disorders Association.

Barnes, T. R. and Spence, S. A. (2000). Movement disorders associated with antipsychotic drugs: clinical and biological implications. In *The psychopharmacology of schizophrenia* (eds M. A. Reveley and J. F. W. Deakin), pp. 178–210. Oxford University Press, New York.

Barnett, R. J., Docherty, J. P., and Frommelt, S. M. (1991). A review of child psychotherapy research since 1963. *Journal of the American Academy of Child and Adolescent Psychiatry* 30, 1–14.

Baron, M. (1993). Genetic linkage and male homosexual orientation. *British Medical Journal* 307, 337–8.

Baron, M., Gruen, R., and Ranier, J. D. (1985). A family study of schizophrenic and normal control probands: implications for the spectrum concept of schizophrenia. *American Journal of Psychiatry* 142, 447–55.

Barr, L. C., Goodman, W. K., Price, L. H., McDougle, C. J., and Charney, D. S. (1992). The serotonin hypothesis of obsessive compulsive disorder: implications of pharmacologic challenge studies. *Journal of Clinical Psychiatry* 53(suppl), 17–28.

Barraclough, B. M. (1973). Differences between national suicide rates. *British Journal of Psychiatry* 122, 95–6.

Barraclough, B. M. and Shea, M. (1970). Suicide and Samaritan clients. *Lancet* 2, 868–70.

Barraclough, B. M. and Shepherd, D. M. (1976). Public interest: private grief. *British Journal of Psychiatry* 129, 109–13.

Barraclough, B. M., Bunch, J., Nelson, B., and Sainsbury, P. (1974). A hundred cases of suicide: clinical aspects. *British Journal of Psychiatry* 125, 355–73.

Barrett, C. J. (1978). Effectiveness of widow's groups in facilitating change. *Journal of Consulting and Clinical Psychology* 46, 20–31.

Barrowclough, C., Johnston, M., and Tarrier, N. (1994). Attributions, expressed emotion, and patient relapse: an attributional model of relatives' response to schizophrenic illness. *Behaviour Therapy* 25, 67–88.

Barsky, A. J., Fanta, J. M., Bailey, E. D., and Ahem, D. K. (1998). A prospective 4- to 5-year study of DSM-III-R hypochondriasis. *Archives of General Psychiatry* 55, 737–44.

Baruk, H. (1959). Delusions of passion. Reprinted in *Themes and variations in European psychiatry* (eds S. R. Hirsch and M. Shepherd), pp. 375–84. Wright, Bristol (1974).

Basmajian, J. V. (ed.) (1983). *Biofeedback: principles and practice for clinicians*. Williams and Wilkins, Baltimore, MD.

Bass, C. and Gill, D. (2000). Factitious disorder and malingering. In *The new Oxford textbook of psychiatry* (eds M. G. Gelder, J. J. López-Ibor Jr, and N. C. Andreasen), Chapter 5.2.9. Oxford University Press, Oxford.

Bassuk, E. L. (1984). Is homelessness a mental health problem? *American Journal of Psychiatry* 141, 1546–50.

Bateson, G., Jackson, D., Haley, J., and Weakland, J. (1956). Towards a theory of schizophrenia. *Behavioral Science* 1, 251–64.

Baucom, D. H., Shoham, V., Muester, K. T., *et al.* (1998). Empirically supported couple and family interventions for marital distress and adult mental health problems. *Journal of Consulting and Clinical Psychology* 66, 53–8.

Bauer, M. and Döpfmer, S. (1999). Lithium augmentation in treatment-resistant depression: meta-analysis of placebo-controlled studies. *Journal of Clinical Psychopharmacology* 19, 427–34.

Baumgarten, M., Hanley, J. A., Infante-Rivard, C., *et al.* (1994). Health of family members caring for elderly persons with dementia. *Annals of Internal Medicine* 120, 126–32.

Baxter, L. R., Schwartz, J. M., Bergman, K. S., *et al.* (1992). Caudate glucose metabolic rate changes with both drug and behavior therapy for obsessive–compulsive disorder. *Archives of General Psychiatry* 49, 681.

Bearn, J., Gossop, M., and Strang, J. (1996). Randomised double blind comparison of lofexidine and methadone in the in-patient treatment of opiate withdrawal. *Drugs and Alcohol Dependence* 43, 87–91.

Beasley, C. M., Dellva, M. A., Tamura, R. N., *et al.* (1999). Randomised double-blind comparison of the incidence of tardive dyskinesia in patients with schizophrenia during long-term treatment with olanzapine or haloperidol. *British Journal of Psychiatry* 174, 23–30.

Beauchamp, T. L. and Childress, J. F. (1994). *Principles of Biomedical Ethics* (4edn), Oxford University Press.

Bebbington, P., Wilkins, S., Jones, P., *et al.* (1993). Life events and psychosis. *British Journal of Psychiatry* 162, 72–9.

Beck, A. (1988). *Love is never enough*. Harper and Row, New York.

Beck, A., Croudace, T. J., Singh, S., and Harrison, G. (1997). The Nottingham Acute Bed Study: alternatives to acute psychiatric care. *British Journal of Psychiatry* 170, 247–52.

Beck, A. T. (1967). *Depression: clinical experimental and theoretical aspects*. Harper and Row, New York.

Beck, A. T. (1976). *Cognitive therapy and the emotional disorders*. International Universities Press, New York.

Beck, A. T. and Freeman, A. (1990). *Cognitive therapy for personality disorders*. Guilford Press, New York.

Beck, A. T., Ward, C. H., Mendelson, M., *et al* (1961). An inventory for measuring depression. *Archives of General Psychiatry* 4, 561–85.

Beck, A. T., Schuyler, D., and Herman, I. (1974). Development of suicide intent scales. In *The prediction of suicide* (eds A. T. Beck, H. L. P. Resaik, and D. J. Lettie). Charles Press, Philadelphia.

Beck, A. T., Steer, R. A., Kovacs, M., and Garrison, B. (1985). Hopelessness and eventual suicide: a 10-year prospective study of patients hospitalized with suicidal ideation. *American Journal of Psychiatry* 145, 559–63.

Beck, J. C. M. (1994). Epidemiology of mental disorder and violence: beliefs and research findings. *Harvard Review of Psychiatry* 2(1), 1–6.

Beekman, A. T. F., Copeland, J. R. M., and Prince, M. J. (1999). Review of community prevalence of depression in later life. *British Journal of Psychiatry* 174, 307–11.

Beitchman, J. H. and Young, A. R., (1997). Learning disorders with a special emphasis on reading disorders: a review of the past 10 years. *Journal of American Academy of Child and Adolescent Psychiatry* 36, 1020–32.

Beitchman, J. H., Zucker, K. J., and Hood, J. E. (1992). A review of the long term effects of child sexual abuse. *Child Abuse and Neglect* 16, 101–18.

Bell, C., Bulik, C., Clayton, P., Crow, S., *et al.* (2000). Practice guideline for the treatment of patients with eating disorders (revision). *American Journal of Psychiatry* 157,

Bender, D. A. (1982). Biochemistry of tryptophan in health and disease. *Molecular Aspects of Medicine* 6, 101–97.

Bendz, H., Aurell, M., Balldin, J., *et al.* (1994). Kidney damage in long-term lithium patients: a cross-sectional study of patients with 15 years or more on lithium. *Nephrology Dialysis Transplantation* 9, 1250–4.

Benedetti, G. (1952). *Die Alkoholhalluzinosen*. Thieme, Stuttgart.

Benjamin, H. (1966). *The transsexual phenomenon*. Julian Press, New York.

Benjamin, J., Li, L., Greenberg, B. D., Murphy, D. L., and Hamer, D. H. (1996). Population and familial association between the D4 dopamine receptor gene and measures of novelty seeking. *Nature Genetics* 12, 81–4.

Benjamin, R. S., Costello, E. J., and Warren, M. (1990). Anxiety disorders in a pediatric sample. *Journal of Anxiety Disorders* 4, 293–316.

Benjamin, S. (2000). Pain disorder. In *The new Oxford textbook of psychiatry* (eds M. G. Gelder, J. J. López-Ibor Jr, and N. C. Andreasen), Chapter 5.2.6. Oxford University Press, Oxford.

Bennett, D. H. (1983). The historical development of rehabilitation services. In *The theory and practice of rehabilitation* (eds F. N. Watts and D. H. Bennett). Wiley, Chichester.

Benson, B. A. and Gross, A. M. (1989). The effect of a congenitally handicapped child upon the marital dyad: a review of the literature. *Clinical Psychology Review* 9, 747–58.

Berelowicz, M. and Tarnopolsky, A. (1993). Borderline personality disorder. In *Personality disorder reviewed* (eds P. Tyrer and G. Stein), pp. 90–112. Gaskell, London.

Berg, I. and Jackson, A. (1985). Teenage school refusers grow up: a follow-up study of 168 subjects, ten years on average after in-patient treatment. *British Journal of Psychiatry* 147, 366–70.

Berg, J. M., Karlinsky, H., and Holland, A. J. (eds) (1995). *Alzheimer disease, Down syndrome and their relationship*. Oxford University Press, Oxford.

Bergen, A. L. M., Dahl, A. A., Guldberg, C., and Hansen, H. (1990). Langfeldt's schizophreniform psychoses fifty years later. *British Journal of Psychiatry* 157, 351–4.

Berger, M. (1985). Temperament and individual differences. In *Child and adolescent psychiatry: modern approaches*, 2nd edn (eds M. Rutter and L. Hersov). Blackwell Scientific, Oxford.

Bergmann, K., Foster, E. M., Justice, A. W., and Matthews, V. (1978). Management of the demented patient in the community. *British Journal of Psychiatry* 132, 441–9.

Berlin, R. M. (1984). Sleep disorders in a psychiatric consultation service. Often complicated by physical illness and common but frequently overlooked in liaison psychiatry. *American Journal of Psychiatry* 141, 582–4.

Berman, K. F., Torrey, E. F., Daniel, D. G., and Weinberger, D. R. (1992). Regional cerebral blood flow in monozygotic twins discordant and concordant for schizophrenia. *Archives of General Psychiatry* 49, 927–34.

Berman, R. M., Narasimhan, M., Miller, H. L., *et al.* (1999). Transient depressive relapse induced by catecholamine depletion: potential phenotypic vulnerability marker? *Archives of General Psychiatry* 56, 395–403.

Berman, S. M. and Noble, E. P. (1993). Childhood antecedents of substance misuse. *Current Opinion in Psychiatry* 6, 382–7.

Berman, K. F and Weinberger, D. R (1999). Neuroimaging studies of schizophrenia. In *Neurobiology of mental illness* (eds D.S. Charney, E. J. Nestle and B. S. Bunney), pp. 246–57. Oxford University Press, Oxford.

Bernheim (1890). *Suggestive therapeutics*, 2nd edn. Young J. Pentland, Edinburgh and London.

Bernstein, D. A. and Borkovec, T. D. (1973). *Progressive, relaxation training: a manual for the helpful professions*. Research Press, Champaign, IL.

Bernstein, G. A., Borchardt, C. M., and Perwein, A. R. (1996). Anxiety disorders in children and adolescents: a review of the past ten years. *Journal of the American Academy of Child and Adolescent Psychiatry* 35, 1110–19.

Bernstein, L. F. (2000). Burn trauma. In *Psychiatric care of the medical patient* (eds A. Stoudemire, B. S. Fogel, and D. B. Greenberg). Oxford University Press, New York.

Berrios, G. E. and Hodges, J. R. (2000). *Memory disorders in psychiatric practice*. Cambridge University Press, Cambridge.

Besson, J. A. O. (1993). Structural and functional brain imaging in alcoholism and drug misuse. *Current Opinion in Psychiatry* 6, 403–10.

Bhopal, R. S. (1986). The inter-relationship of folk, traditional and Western medicine within an Asian community in Britain. *Social Scientific Medicine* 22, 99–105.

Bialer, P. A., Wallack, J. J., and McDaniel, J. S. (2000). Human immunodeficiency virus and AIDS. In *Psychiatric Care of the Medical Patient* (eds A. Stoudemire, B. S. Fogel, and D. B. Greenberg). Oxford University Press, New York.

Bibring, E. (1953). The mechanism of depression. In *Affective disorders* (ed. P. Greenacre), pp. 14–47. International Universities Press, New York.

Biederman, J. (1998). Resolved: mania is mistaken for ADHD in prepubertal children. *Journal of the American Academy of Child and Adolescent Psychiatry* 37, 1091–9.

Biederman, J., Faraone, S. V., Keenan, K., *et al.* (1992). Further evidence for family-genetic risk factors in attention deficit hyperactivity disorder. *Archives of General Psychiatry* 49, 728–38.

Biggins, C. A., Boyd, J. L., Harrop, F. M., *et al.* (1992). A controlled, longitudinal study of dementia in Parkinson's disease. *Journal of Neurology, Neurosurgery and Psychiatry* 55, 566–71.

Bilder, R. M., Goldman, R. S., Robinson, D., *et al.* (2000). Neuropsychology of first-episode schizophrenia: initial characterization and clinical correlates. *American Journal of Psychiatry* 157, 549–59.

Billiad, M. (2000). Excessive sleepiness. In *New Oxford Textbook of Psychiatry* (eds M. G. Gelder, J. J. López-Ibor, N. C. Andreasen). Oxford University Press.

Binet, A. (1877). Le fetishisme dans l'amour. *Revue Philosophique* 24, 143.

Binet, A. and Simon, T. (1905). Méthodes nouvelles pour le diagnostic du niveau intellectuel des normaux. *L'Année Psychologique* 11, 193–244.

Bion, W. R. (1961). *Experiences in groups*. Tavistock Publications, London.

Birchwood, M. and Spencer, E. (2000). Cognitive–behaviour therapy for schizophrenia. In *The new Oxford textbook of psychiatry* (eds M. G. Gelder, J. J. López-Ibor Jr, and N. C. Andreasen), Chapter 6.3.2.4. Oxford University Press, Oxford.

Bird, H. R. (1996). Epidemiology of childhood disorders in a cross-cultural context. *Journal of Child Psychology and Psychiatry* 37, 35–49.

Birnbaum, K. (1908). *Psychosen mit Wahnbildung und wahnhafte Einbildungen bei Degenerativen*. Marhold, Halle.

Bishop, D. V. M. (1994). Developmental disorders of speech and language. In *Child and Adolescent Psychiatry. Modern Approaches*, 3rd edn (eds M. Rutter, E. Taylor, and L. Hersov). Oxford: Blackwell.

Bisserbe, J. C., Lane, R. M., Flament, M. F., *et al.* (1997). A double-blind comparison of sertraline and clomipramine in outpatients with obsessive–compulsive disorder. *European Psychiatry* 153, 1450–4.

Bisson, J. I., Jenkins, P. L., Alexander, J., and Bannister, C. (1997). Randomized controlled trial of psychological debriefing for victims of acute burns trauma. *British Journal of Psychiatry* 171, 78–81.

Black, D. (2000). The effects of bereavement in childhood. In *The new Oxford textbook of psychiatry* (eds M. G. Gelder, J. J. López-Ibor Jr, and N. C. Andreasen), Chapter 9.3.5. Oxford University Press, Oxford.

Black, D., Harris-Hendriks, J., and Wolkind, S. (1998). *Child psychiatry and the law*, 3rd edn. Gaskell, London.

Blackburn, R. (1998). Psychopathy and the contribution of personality to violence. In *Psychopathy: antisocial, criminal and violent behaviour* (eds T. Millon *et al.*). pp. 50–68. Guilford Press, New York.

Blackwood, D. (2000). P300, a state and a trait marker in schizophrenia. *Lancet* 355, 771–2.

Blackwood, D. and Muir, W. (1998). Genetics. In *Companion to psychiatric studies* (eds E. C. Johnson, C. P. L. Freeman, and A. K. Zealley), pp. 219–31. Churchill Livingstone, Edinburgh.

Blake, F., Gath, D., and Salkovskis, P. M. (1995). Psychological aspects of the premenstrual syndrome: developing a cognitive approach. In *Treatment of functional somatic symptoms* (eds R. Mayou, C. Bass, and M. Sharpe). Oxford University Press, Oxford.

Blanchard, E. B. (1992). Psychological treatment of benign headache disorders. *Journal of Consulting and Clinical Psychology* 60(4), 537–51.

Blanchard, B. (2001). *Irritable bowel syndrome. Psychosocial assessment and treatment*. American Psychological Association. Washington, D.C.

Blanchard, R. and Hucker, S. J. (1991). Age, transvestism, bondage, and concurrent paraphilic activities in 117 fatal cases of autoerotic asphyxia. *British Journal of Psychiatry* 159, 371–7.

Blank, A. S. (1992). The longitudinal course of posttraumatic stress disorder. In *Posttraumatic stress disorder: DSMIV and beyond* (eds J. R. T. Davidson and E. B. Foa), pp. 3–22. American Psychiatric Press, Washington, DC.

Blazer, D. G., Hughes, D., George L. K., Schwartz, M., and Boyer, R. (1991). Generalized anxiety disorder. In *Psychiatric disorders in America: the epidemiological catchment area study* (eds L. N. Robbins and D. A. Regier), pp.180–203. The Free Press, New York.

Bleuler, E. (1906). *Affektivität, Suggestibilität, und Paranoia*. Marhold, Halle.

Bleuler, E. (1911). (English edn 1950). *Dementia praecox or the group of schizophrenias*. International University Press, New York.

Bleuler, M. (1972). (English edn 1978). *The schizophrenic disorders: long term patient and family studies*. Yale Universities Press, New Haven, CT.

Bleuler, M. (1974). The long term course of the schizophrenic psychoses. *Psychological Medicine* 4, 244–54.

Blier, P. and de Montigny, C. (1994). Current advances and trends in the treatment of depression. *Trends in Pharmacological Sciences* 15, 220–6.

Bloch, S. (1986). Supportive psychotherapy. In *An introduction to the psychotherapies*, 2nd edn (ed. S. Bloch). Oxford University Press, Oxford.

Bloch, S. and Chodoff, P. (1981). *Psychiatric ethics*. Oxford University Press, Oxford.

Bloch, S. and Aveline, M. (1996). Group Psychotherapy. Ch 4 in: Block, S. (ed.) *An introduction to the psychotherapies*. 3rd edn. Oxford University Press, Oxford.

Bloch, S. and Harari, E. (2000). Family therapy. In *The new Oxford textbook of psychiatry* (eds M. G. Gelder, J. J. López-Ibor Jr, and N. C. Andreasen), Chapter 6.3.8. Oxford University Press, Oxford.

Block, G. J. (1980). *Mesmerism*. William Kaufmann, Los Altos, CA.

Block, S. D. (2000). Assessing and managing depression in the terminally ill patient: ACP-ASIM End of Life Consensus Panel. *Annals of Internal Medicine* **132**, 209–18

Bluglass, R. (2000). Organization of services. In *The new Oxford textbook of psychiatry* (eds M. G. Gelder, J. J. López-Ibor Jr, and N. C Andreasen), Chapter 11.9. Oxford University Press, Oxford.

Bogovsstavsley and Cummings (2000)

Böker, W. and Häfner, H. (1977). Crimes of violence by mentally disordered offenders in Germany. *Psychological Medicine* **7**, 733–6.

Boland, R. J., Goldstein, M. G., and Haltzman, S. D. (2000). Psychiatric management of behavioural syndromes in intensive care units. In *Psychiatric care of the medical patient* (eds A. Stoudemire, B. S. Fogel, and D. B. Greenberg). Oxford University Press, New York.

Bollini, P. and Mollica, R. F. (1989). Surviving without the asylum: an overview of the studies on the Italian Reform Movement. *Journal of Nervous and Mental Disease* **177**, 607–15.

Bolton, P., Murphy, M., MacDonald, H., Whitlock, B., Pickles, A., and Rutter, M. (1997). Obstetric complications in autism: consequences or causes of the condition? *Journal of the American Academy of Child and Adolescent Psychiatry* **36**, 272–81.

Bools, C. N., Neale, B. A., and Meadow, S. R. (1993). Follow up of victims of fabricated illness (Munchausen syndrome by proxy). *Archives of Disease in Childhood* **69**, 625–30.

Boot, D., Gillies, P., Fenelon, J., *et al.* (1994). Evaluation of the short-term impact of counselling in general practice. *Patient Education and Counselling* **24**, 79–89.

Booth, T. And Booth, W. (1993). Parents with learning difficulties: lessons for practitioners. *British Journal of Social Work* **23**, 459–80.

Borduin, C. M. (1999). Multi-systemic treatment of criminality and violence in adolescents. *Journal of the American Academy of Child and Adolescent Psychiatry* **38**, 242–9.

Bosinski, H. A., Peter, M., Bonatz, G., *et al.* (1997). A higher rate of hyperandrogenic disorders in female to male transsexuals. *Psychoneuroendocrinology* **22**, 361–80.

Bostwick, J. M. and Pankratz, V. S. (2000). Affective disorders and suicide risk: a re-examination. *American Journal of Psychiatry* **157**, 1925–32.

Boutros, N. and Braff, D. (1999). Clinical electrophysiology. In *Neurobiology of mental illness,* (eds D. S. Charney, E. J. Nestler, and B. S. Bunney), pp. 121–131. Oxford University Press, Oxford.

Bowden, C. L. (1996). Dosing strategies and time course of response to antimanic drugs. *Journal of Clinical Psychiatry* **57**(suppl 13), 4–9.

Bowden, C. L. (1998). New concepts in mood stabilization: evidence for the effectiveness of valproate and lamotrigine. *Neuropsychopharmacology* **19**, 194–9.

Bowden, C. L., Brugger, A. M., Swann, A. C., *et al.* (1994). Efficacy of divalproex vs lithium and placebo in the treatment of mania. *Journal of the American Medical Association* **271**, 918–24.

Bowden, C. L., Calabrese, J. R., McElroy, S. L., *et al.* (2000). A randomized, placebo-controlled 12-month trial of divalproex and lithium in treatment of outpatients with bipolar I disorder. *Archives of General Psychiatry* **57**, 481–9.

Bowlby, J. (1944). Forty-four juvenile thieves. Their characters and home life. *International Journal of Psychoanalysis* **25**, 19–53.

Bowlby, J. (1946). *Forty-four juvenile thieves: their characters and home-life*. Baillière, Tindall and Cox, London.

Bowlby, J. (1951). *Maternal care and maternal health.* World Health Organization, Geneva.

Bowlby, J. (1969). Psychopathology of anxiety: the role of affectional bonds. In Studies in Anxiety (ed. M. H. Lader). *British Journal of Psychiatry, Special Publication No. 3*.

Bowlby, J. (1973). *Attachment and loss.* Vol.2, *Separation, anxiety and anger.* Hogarth Press, London.

Bowlby, J. (1980). *Attachment and loss.* Vol.3, *Loss, sadness and depression.* Basic Books, New York.

Boyer, W. (1995). Serotonin uptake inhibitors are superior to imipramine and alprazolam in alleviating panic attacks: a meta-analysis. *International Clinical Pharmacology* **10**, 45–9.

Bradwejn, J., Koszcki, D., and Shriqui, C. (1991). Enhanced sensitivity to cholecystokinin tetrapeptide in panic disorder. *Archives of General Psychiatry* **48**, 603.

Braid, J. (1843). *Neurohypnology: or the rationale of nervous sleep, considered in relation with animal magnetism.* Churchill, London.

Brandon, S. (1991). The psychological aftermath of war. *British Medical Journal* 302, 305–6.

Brandon, S., Cowley, P., McDonald, C., *et al.* (1984). Electroconvulsive therapy: results in depressive illness from the Leicestershire Trial. *British Medical Journal* 288, 22–5.

Brandon, S., Cowley, P., McDonald, C. *et al.* (1985). Leicester ECT trial: results in schizophrenia. *British Journal of Psychiatry* 146, 177–83.

Brandon, S., Boakes, J, Glaser, D., and Green, R. (1998). Recovered memories of childhood sexual abuse. *British Journal of Psychiatry* 172, 296–307.

Brauer, A., Horlick, L. F., Nelson, E., *et al.* (1979). Relaxation therapy for essential hypertension: a Veterans Administration out-patient study. *Journal of Behavioural Medicine* 2, 21–9.

Brawman-Mintzer, O., Lydiard, R. B., Emmanuel, N., *et al.* (1993). Psychiatric comorbidity in patients with generalized anxiety disorder. *American Journal of Psychiatry* 150, 1216–18.

Breakey, W. R. (2000). Service needs of individuals and populations. In *The new Oxford textbook of psychiatry* (eds M. G. Gelder, J. J. López-Ibor Jr, and N. C. Andreasen), Chapter 7.2. Oxford University Press, Oxford.

Breen, N., Caine, D. and Coltheart, M. (2000). Models of face recognition and delusional misidentification: a critical review. *Cognitive Neuropsychology* 17, 55–71.

Brennan, P. A. and Mednick, S. A. (1993). Genetic perspectives on crime. *Acta Psychiatrica Scandinavica* 70(suppl), 19–36.

Breslau, N. and Prabucki, M. A. (1987). Siblings of disabled children: effects of chronic stress in the family. *Archives of General Psychiatry* 44, 1040–6.

Breslau, N., Davis, G. C., Andrewski, P., *et al.* (1997a). Sex differences in post-traumatic stress disorder. *Archives of General Psychiatry* 54,1044–8.

Breslau, N., Davis, G. C., Peterson, E., and Schultz, L. (1997b). Psychiatric sequelae of post-traumatic stress disorder in women. *Archives of General Psychiatry,* 54, 81–87.

Breslau, N., Kessler, R. C., Chilcoat, H. D., *et al.* (1998). Trauma and post-traumatic stress disorder in the community. *Archives of General Psychiatry* 55, 626–632.

Breuer, J. and Freud, S. (1893). Studies on hysteria. In *The standard edition of the complete psychological works*, Vol.2. Hogarth Press, London (1955).

Brewin, C. (2000). Recovered memories and false memories. In *The new Oxford textbook of psychiatry* (eds M. G. Gelder, J. J. López-Ibor Jr, and N. C. Andreasen), Chapter 4.6.3. Oxford University Press, Oxford.

Brewin, C. R., Andrews, B., Rose, S., and Kirk, M. (1999). Acute stress disorder and post-traumatic stress disorder in victims of violent crime. *American Journal of Psychiatry* 156, 360–6.

Brewin, C. R., Wing, J. K., Mangen, S. P. *et al.* (1987). Principles and practice of measuring needs in the care of the mentally ill: the MRC Needs for Care Assessment. *Psychological Medicine* 17, 971–81.

Briere, J. (1988). The long-term correlates of childhood sexual victimization. *Annals of the New York Academy of Sciences* 528, 327–34.

British Paediatric Association (1992). *Guidelines for the ethical conduct of medical research involving children.* Royal College of Paediatrics and Child Health, London.

Broadhead, J. and Jacoby, R. J. (1990). Mania in old age: a first prospective study. *International Journal of Geriatric Psychiatry* 5, 215–22.

Broadwin, I. T. (1932). A contribution to the study of truancy. *American Journal of Orthopsychiatry* 2, 253–9.

Brockington, I. (1998). *Motherhood and mental health.* Oxford University Press, Oxford.

Brockington, I. (2000). Obstetric and gynaecological conditions associated with psychiatric disorder. In *The new Oxford textbook of psychiatry* (eds M. G. Gelder, J. J. López-Ibor Jr, and N. C. Andreasen), Chapter 5.4. Oxford University Press, Oxford.

Brockington, I. F., Kendell, R. E., Kellett, J. M., *et al.* (1978). Trials of lithium, chlorpromazine and amitriptyline on schizoaffective patients. *British Journal of Psychiatry* 133, 162–8.

Broman, S., Nichols, P. L., Shaughnessy, P., and Kennedy, W. (1987). *Retardation in young children: a developmental study of cognitive deficit.* Lawrence Erlbaum, Hillsdale, NJ.

Brown and Marsden (1998).

Brown and Trimble (2000).

Brown, E. S., Rush, A. J., and McEwen, B. S. (1999). Hippocampal remodeling and damage by corticosteroids: implications for mood disorders. *Neuropsychopharmacology* 21, 474–84.

Brown, F. W. (1942). Heredity in the psychoneuroses. *Proceedings of the Royal Society of Medicine* 35, 785–90.

Brown, G. L. and Linnoila, M. I. (1990). CSF serotonin metabolite (5-HIAA) studies in depression, impulsivity, and violence. *Journal of Clinical Psychiatry* **51(suppl 4)**, 31–41.

Brown, G. R. (1994). Women in relationships with cross-dressing men: a descriptive study from a non-clinical setting. *Archives of Sexual Behaviour* **23**, 515–30.

Brown, G. W. and Birley, J. L. T. (1968). Crisis and life change at the onset of schizophrenia. *Journal of Health and Social Behaviour* **9**, 203–24.

Brown, G. W. and Harris, T. O. (1978). *Social origins of depression*. Tavistock, London.

Brown, G. W. and Harris, T. O. (1993). Aetiology of anxiety and depressive disorders in an inner-city population. 1 Early adversity. *Psychological Medicine* **23**, 143–54.

Brown, G. W., Carstairs, G. M. and Topping, G. G. (1958). *Lancet* **2**, 685–9.

Brown, G. W., Monck, E. M., Carstairs, G. M., and Wing, J. K. (1962). Influence of family life on the cause of schizophrenic illness. *British Journal of Preventive and Social Medicine* **16**, 55–68.

Brown, G. W., Bone, M., Dalison, B., and Wing, J. K. (1966). *Schizophrenia and social care*. Maudsley Monograph 17. Oxford University Press, London.

Brown, G. W., Harris, T. O., and Hepworth, C. (1995). Loss, humiliation and entrapment among women developing depression: a patient and non-patient comparison. *Psychological Medicine* **25**, 7–21.

Brown, P. and Pantelis, C. (1999). Ethical aspects of drug treatment. In *Psychiatric Ethics*, 3rd edn (ed. S. Bloch, P. Chodoff, and S. A. Green), pp. 245–73. Oxford University Press, Oxford.

Brown, P. and Marsden, C.D. (1998) What do the basal ganglia do? *Lancet* **351**, 1801–4.

Brown, R.J. and Trimble, M.R. (2000). Editorial. Dissociative psychopathology, non-epileptic seizures, and neurology. *Journal of Neurology, Neurosurgery and Psychiatry* **69**, 285–91.

Brown, W. (1934). *Psychology and psychotherapy*, 3rd edn. Edward Arnold, London.

Browne, K. and Saqui, S. (1987). Parent child interaction in abusing families and its possible causes and consequences. In *Child abuse: the educational perspective* (ed. P. Maher). Blackwell, Oxford.

Bruce, M. (2000). Managing amphetamine dependence. *Advances in Psychiatric Treatment* **6**, 33–40.

Bruce, M., Scott, N., Shine, P., and Lader, M. (1992). Anxiogenic effects of caffeine in patients with anxiety disorders. *Archives of General Psychiatry* **49**, 867–9.

Bruch, H. (1974). *Eating disorders: anorexia nervosa and the person within*. Routledge & Kegan Paul, London.

Brudny, J., Korein, J., Levidow, A., and Friedman, L. W. (1974). Sensory feedback therapy as a modality of treatment in central nervous system disorders of voluntary movement. *Neurology* **24**, 925–32.

Brugha, T., Wing, J. K., and Smith, B. L. (1989). Physical health of the long-term mentally ill in the community: is there unmet need? *British Journal of Psychiatry* **155**, 777–81.

Bryant, R. A., Harvey, A. G., Dang, S. T., Sackville, T., and Basten, C. (1998). Treatment of acute stress disorder: a comparison of cognitive–behaviour therapy and supportive counselling. *Journal of Consulting and Clinical Psychology* **66**, 862–6.

Bryer, J. B., Nelson, B. A., Miller, J. B., and Krol, P. A. (1987). Childhood sexual and physical abuse as factors in adult psychiatric illness. *American Journal of Psychiatry* **144**, 1426–30.

Brylewski, J. and Duggan, L. (1998). Antipsychotic medication for challenging behaviour in people with learning disability (Cochrane Review). In *The Cochrane Library*, Issue 4, Oxford.

Brylewski, J. and Wiggs, L. (1998). A questionnaire survey of sleep and night-time behaviour in a community-based sample of adults with intellectual disability. *Journal of Intellectual Disability Research* **42**, 154–62.

Buchan, H., Johnstone, E., McPherson, K., et al. (1992). Who benefits from electroconvulsive therapy? Combined results of the Leicester and Northwick Park Trials. *British Journal of Psychiatry* **160**, 355–9.

Buchanan, A., Reed, A., Wessely, S., et al. (1993). The phenomenological correlates of acting on delusions. *British Journal of Psychiatry* **163**, 77–81.

Buchsbaum, M. S. and Siegel, B. V. (1994). Neuroimaging and the aging process in psychiatry. *International Review of Psychiatry* **6**, 109–18.

Buchsbaum, M. S., Kesslak, J. P., Lynch, G., et al. (1991). Temporal and hippocampal metabolic rate during an olefactory memory task assessed by positron emission tomography in patients with dementia of the Alzheimer type and controls. *Archives of General Psychiatry* **48**, 840–7.

Buckle, A. and Farrington, D. P. (1984). An observational study of shop-lifting. *British Journal of Criminology* 24, 63–73.

Bucknill, J. C. and Tuke, D. H. (1858). *A manual of psychological medicine.* John Churchill, London.

Buglass, D., Clarke, J., Henderson, A. S., *et al.* (1977). A study of agoraphobic housewives. *Psychological Medicine* 7, 73–86.

Bunch, J. (1972). Recent bereavement in relation to suicide. *Journal of Psychosomatic Research* 16, 361–6.

Burgess, A. and Holmstrom, L. (1979a). Rape: sexual disruption and recovery. *American Journal of Orthopsychiatry* 49, 648–57.

Burgess, A. and Holmstrom, L. (1979b). Adaptive strategies and recovery from rape. *American Journal of Psychiatry* 136, 1278–82.

Burke, M. J. and Preskorn, S. H. (1999). Therapeutic drug monitoring of antidepressants – cost implications and relevance to clinical practice. *Clinical Pharmacokinetics* 37(2), 147–65.

Burns, T., Beardsmoore, A., Ashok, V. B., *et al.* (1993). A controlled trial of home-based acute psychiatric services. I: Clinical and social outcome. *British Journal of Psychiatry* 163, 49–54.

Burns, T., Paykell, E. S., and Lemon, S. (1991). Care of chronic neurotic out-patients by community psychiatric nurses. *British Journal of Psychiatry* 158, 685–90.

Burrow, T. (1927). The group method of analysis. *Psychoanalytic Review* 14, 268–80.

Burrows, G. D., Maguire, K. P. and Norman, T. R. (1998). Antidepressant efficacy and tolerability of the selective norepinephrine reuptake inhibitor reboxetine: a review. *Journal of Clinical Psychiatry* 59(suppl 14), 4–7.

Bushnell, J. A., Wells, J. E., and Oakley Browne, M. (1993). Long term effects of intrafamilial sexual abuse in childhood. *Acta Psychiatrica Scandinavica* 85, 136–42.

Butler, G., Cullington, A., Munby, M., *et al.* (1984). Exposure and anxiety management in the treatment of social phobia. *Journal of Consulting and Clinical Psychology* 52, 642–50.

Butler, R. J. (1998). Annotation: night wetting in children: psychological aspects. *Journal of Child Psychology and Psychiatry* 39, 453–63.

Butler, R. J., Forsythe, W. I., and Robertson, J. (1990). The body worn alarm in treatment of childhood enuresis. *British Journal of Child Psychiatry* 44, 237–41.

Bynum, W. F. (1985). The nervous patient in eighteenth- and nineteenth-century Britain: the psychiatric origins of British neurology. In *The anatomy of madness.* Vol. I, *People and ideas* (eds W. F. Bynum, R. Porter, and M. Shepherd). Tavistock Publications, London.

Byrne, W. and Parsons, B. (1993). Human sexual orientation. *Archives of General Psychiatry* 50, 228–39.

Cade, J. F. (1949). Lithium salts in the treatment of psychotic excitement. *Medical Journal of Australia* 2, 349–52.

Cadenhead, K. S., Light, G. A., Geyer, M. A., and Braff, D. L. (2000). Sensory gating deficits assessed by the P50 event-related potential in subjects with schizotypal personality disorder. *American Journal of Psychiatry* 157, 55–9.

Cadoret, R. J. (1978). Psychopathology in adopted-away offspring of biologic parents with antisocial behaviour. *Archives of General Psychiatry* 35, 176–84.

Cadoret, R. J., Yates, W. R., Troughton, E., *et al.* (1995). Genetic/environmental interaction in the genesis of aggressivity and conduct disorders. *Archives of General Psychiatry* 52, 916–24.

Calabrese, J. R., Bowden, C. L., Sachs, G. S. *et al.* (1999). A double-blind placebo-controlled study of lamotrigine monotherapy in outpatients with bipolar I depression. *Journal of Clinical Psychiatry* 60, 79–88.

Calhoun, K. S. and Atkeson, B. M. (1991). *Treatment of rape victims. Facilitating psychosocial adjustment.* Pergamon Press, New York.

Cameron, N. (1963). *Personality development and psychopathology: a dynamic approach.* Houghton Mifflin, Boston, MA.

Campana, A., Gambini, O., and Scarone, S. (1998). Delusional disorder and eye tracking dysfunction: preliminary evidence of biological and clinical heterogeneity. *Schizophrenia Research* 30, 51–8.

Campbell, S. B., (1995). Behaviour problems in preschool children: a review of recent research. *Journal of Child Psychology and Psychiatry* 36, 113–49.

Campo, J. V. and Fritsch, S. (1994). Somatization in children and adolescents. *Journal of the American Academy of Child and Adolescent Psychiatry* 33, 1223–35.

Cantor, C. H. (2000). Suicide in the western world. In *The International Handbook of Suicide and Attempted Suicide* (eds K. Hawton and K. van Heeringen). John Wiley and Sons, Chichester.

Cantor, C. H., Mullen, P. E., Alpers, P. A. (2000). Mass homicide: the civil massacre. *Journal of American Academy Psychiatry and the Law* **28**, 55–63.

Cantwell, D. P. and Baker, L. (1985). Coordination disorder. In *Comprehensive textbook of psychiatry*, 4th edn (eds H. I. Kaplan and B. J. Sadock). Williams and Wilkins, Baltimore, MD.

Cantwell, D. P. and Rutter, M. (1994). Classification: conceptual issues and substantive findings. In: *Child and adolescent psychiatry; modern approaches*, 3rd edn (eds M. Rutter, E. Taylor, and L. Hersov. Blackwell Science , Oxford.

Capgras, J. and Reboul-Lachaux, J. (1923). L'Illusion des sosies dans un délire systématisé chronique. *Bulletin de la Société Clinique de Médicine Mentale* **11**, 6–16.

Caplan, G. (1961). *An approach to community mental health.* Tavistock Publications, London.

Caplan, H. L. (1970). Hysterical conversion symptoms in childhood. M. Phil. Dissertation, University of London. (See the account in *Child psychiatry modern approaches*, 2nd edn (ed. M. L. Rutter and L. Hersov). Blackwell, Oxford (1985).

Carlier, I. V. E., Lamberts, R. D., van Uchelen, A. J., and Gersons, B. P. R. (1998). Disaster-related post-traumatic stress in police officers: a field study of the impact of debriefing. *Stress Medicine* **14**, 143–8.

Carlsson, A., Hansson, L. O., Waters, N., and Carlsson, M. L. (1999). A glutamatergic deficiency model of schizophrenia. *British Journal of Psychiatry* **174** (suppl 37), 2–6.

Carney, M. W. P., Roth, M., and Garside, R. F. (1965). The diagnosis of depressive syndromes and the prediction of ECT response. *British Journal of Psychiatry* **111**, 659–74.

Carone, B. J., Harrow, N., and Westermeyer, J. F. (1991). Posthospital course and outcome in schizophrenia. *Archives of General Psychiatry* **48**, 247–53.

Carr, A. (1991). Milan systemic family therapy: a review of ten empirical investigations. *Journal of Family Therapy* **13**, 237–63.

Carr, J. (1994). Annotation: long term outcome for people with Down's syndrome. *Journal of Child Psychology and Psychiatry* **35**, 425–39.

Carson, A. J., MacHale, S., Allen, K., *et al.* (2000). Depression after stroke and lesion location: a systematic review. *Lancet* **356**, 122–6.

Casey, P. R. and Tyrer, P. J. (1986). Personality functioning and symptomatology. *Journal of Psychiatric Research* **20**, 363–74.

Casey, P. R., Tyrer, P. J., and Dillon, S. (1984). The diagnostic status of patients with conspicuous psychiatric morbidity in primary care. *Psychological Medicine* **14**, 673–81.

Casey, R. and Berman, J. (1985). The outcome of psychotherapy with children. *Psychological Bulletin* **98**, 388–400.

Cassano, G. B., Petracca, A., Perugi, G., *et al.* (1988). Clomipramine for panic disorder: the first 10 weeks of a long-term comparison with imipramine. *Journal of Affective Disorders* **14**, 123–7.

Castle, D. J., Scott, K., Wessely, S., and Murray, R. M. (1993). Does social deprivation during gestation and early life predispose to later schizophrenia. *Social Psychiatry in Psychiatric Epidemiology* **28**, 1–4.

Catalan, J., Gath, D. H., Anastasiades, P., *et al.* (1991). Evaluation of a brief psychological treatment for emotional disorders in primary care. *Psychological Medicine* **21**, 1013–19.

Cathcart, F. (1995). Death and people with learning disabilities: interventions to support clients and carers. *Journal of Intellectual Disability Research* **41**, 331–8.

Caton, C. L. M., Wyatt, R. J., Felix, A., *et al.* (1993). Follow-up of chronically homeless mentally ill men. *American Journal of Psychiatry* **150**, 1639–42.

Cattell, R. B. (1963). *The sixteen personality factor questionnaire.* Institute for personality and Ability Testing, Chicago, Ill.

Cerletti, U. and Bini, I. (1938). Un nuovo metodo di shokterapia; 'Tettroshock'. *Bulletin Accademia Medica di Roma* **64**, 136–8.

Chalkley, A. J. and Powell, G. (1983). The clinical description of forty-eight cases of sexual fetishism. *British Journal of Psychiatry* **142**, 292–5.

Chalmers, J. S. and Cowen, P. J. (1990). Drug treatment of tricyclic resistant depression. *International Review of Psychiatry* **2**, 239–48.

Chamberlain, A. S. (1966). Early mental hospitals in Spain. *American Journal of Psychiatry* **123**, 143–9.

Chambers, J., Bass, C., and Mayou, R. (1999). Non-cardiac chest pain: assessment and management. *Heart* **82**, 656–7.

Chambers, R. A. and Druss, B. G. (1999). Droperidol: efficacy and side effects in psychiatric emergencies. *Journal of Clinical Psychiatry* **60**, 664–7.

Charlton, J., Kelly, S., Dunnell, K., Evans, B., Jenkins, R., and Wallis, R. (1992). Trends in suicide deaths in England and Wales. *Population Trends* 69, 10–16.

Charlton, J., Kelly, S., Dunnell, K., Evans, B., and Jenkins, R. (1993). Suicide deaths in England and Wales: trends in factors associated with suicide deaths. *Population Trends* 71, 34–42.

Charney, D. S., Heninger, G. R., and Breier, A. (1984). Nor-adrenergic function in panic patients. *Archives of General Psychiatry* 41, 751–62.

Charney, D. S., Woods, S. W., Heninger, G. R. *et al.* (1989). Noradrenergic function in generalized anxiety disorder: effects of yohimbine in healthy subjects and patients with generalized anxiety disorder. *Psychiatry Research* 27, 173–82.

Charney, D. S., Deutch, A. Y., Krystal, J. H., *et al.* (1993). Psychobiologic mechanisms of posttraumatic stress disorder. *Archives of General Psychiatry* 50, 294.

Checkley, S. A. (1992). Neuroendocrinology. In *Handbook of affective disorders* (ed. E. S. Paykel), pp. 255–66. Churchill Livingstone, Edinburgh.

Cheng, A. T. A. and Lee, C. S. (2000). Suicide in Asia and the Far East. In *The international handbook of suicide and attempted suicide* (eds K. Hawton and K. van Heeringen). John Wiley and Sons, Chichester.

Cheng, A. T.-A. and Chang, J.-C. (1999). Mental health aspects of culture and migration. *Current Opinion in Psychiatry* 12, 217–22.

Chevalier, H., Los, F., Boichut, D., *et al.* (1999). Evaluation of severe insomnia in the general population: results of a European multinational survey. *Journal of Psychopharmacology* 13(4)(Suppl 1), S21–4.

Chick, J. (1992). Doctors with emotional problems: how can they be helped. In *Practical problems in clinical psychiatry* (eds K. Hawton and P. Cowen), pp. 242–52. Oxford University Press, Oxford.

Chick, J. (1994). Alcohol problems in the general hospital. *British Medical Bulletin* 50, 200–10.

Chick, J. (1997). Alcohol and the brain. *Current Opinion in Psychiatry* 10, 205–10.

Chick, J. (2000). Treatment of alcohol dependence. In *The new Oxford textbook of psychiatry* (eds M. G. Gelder, J. J. López-Ibor Jr, and N. C. Andreasen), Chapter 4.2.2.4. Oxford University Press, Oxford.

Chick, J., Ritson, B., Connaughton, J., *et al.* (1988). Advice versus extended treatment for alcoholism: a controlled study. *British Journal of Addiction* 83, 159–70.

Chiswick, D. (2000). Associations between psychiatric disorder and offending. In *The new Oxford textbook of psychiatry* (eds M. G. Gelder, J. J. López-Ibor Jr, and N. C. Andreasen), Chapter 11.3. Oxford University Press, Oxford.

Chochinov, H. M., Wilson, K. G., Enns, M., Lander, S. (1994). Prevalence of depression in the terminally ill: effects of diagnostic criteria and symptoms threshold judgements. *American Journal of Psychiatry* 151, 537–540.

Chou, J. C. (1991). Recent advances in the treatment of mania. *Journal of Clinical Psychopharmacology* 11, 3–21.

Chou, J. C., Zito, J. M., Vitrai, J. *et al.* (1996). Neuroleptics in acute mania: a pharmacoepidemiologic study. *Annals of Pharmacotherapy* 30, 1396–8

Chouinard, G., Ross-Chouinard, A. Annable. L., and Jones, B. D. (1980). Extrapyramidal symptom rating scale. *Canadian Journal of Neurological Science* 7(3), 233.

Christensen, H., Henderson, A. S., Jorm, A. F., Mackinnon, A. J., Scott, R., and Korten, A. E. (1995). ICD-10 mild cognitive disorder: epidemiological evidence on its validity. *Psychological Medicine* 25, 105–20.

Ciompi, L. (1980). The natural history of schizophrenia in the long term. *British Journal of Psychiatry* 136, 413–20.

Citrome, L. and Volavka, J. (1999). Schizophrenia: violence and comorbidity. *Current Opinion in Psychiatry* 12, 47–51.

Clancy, J., Noyes, R., Noenk, P. R., and Slymen, D. J. (1978). Secondary depression in anxiety neurosis. *Journal of Nervous and Mental Disease* 166, 846–50.

Clare, A. W. (1997). The disease concept in psychiatry. In *The essentials of postgraduate psychiatry* (eds R. Murray, P. Hill, and P. McGuffin). Cambridge University Press, Cambridge.

Claridge, G. and Hewitt, J. K. (1987). A biometrical study of schizotypy in a normal population. *Personality and Individual Differences* 8, 303–12.

Clark, D. B. and Agras, W. S. (1991). The assessment and treatment of performance anxiety in musicians. *American Journal of Psychiatry* 148, 598–605.

Clark, D. M. (1986). A cognitive approach to panic. *Behaviour Research and Therapy* 24, 461–70.

Clark, D. M. (2000). Cognitive–behaviour therapy for anxiety disorders. In *The new Oxford textbook of psychiatry* (eds M. G. Gelder, J. J. López-Ibor Jr, and N. C. Andreasen), Chapter 6.3.2.1. Oxford University Press, Oxford.

Clark, D. M. (2001). A cognitive perspective on social phobia. In W. R Crozier and L. Alden (eds) *International handbook of social anxiety: concepts, research and interventions related to self and shyness*. John Wiley. New York.

Clark, D. M. and Teasdale, J. D. (1982). Diurnal variation in clinical depression and accessibility of memories of positive and negative experiences. *Journal of Abnormal Psychology* 91, 87–95.

Clark, D. M., Salkovskis, P. M., Hackmann, A., *et al.* (1994). A comparison of cognitive therapy, applied relaxation and imipramine in the treatment of panic disorder. *British Journal of Psychiatry* 164, 759–69.

Clark, D. M., Salkovskis, P. M., Hackmann, A., *et al.* (1998). Two psychological treatments for hypochondriasis. A randomised controlled trial. *British Journal of Psychiatry* 173, 218–25.

Clarkin, J. F., Marziali, E., and Munroe-Blum, H. (1991). Group and family treatments for borderline personality disorder. *Hospital and Community Psychiatry* 42(10), 1038–42.

Classen, C., Koopman, C., Hales, R., and Spiegel, D. (1998). Acute stress disorder as a predictor of post-traumatic stress symptoms. *American Journal of Psychiatry* 155, 620–4.

Clayton, P. J. (1979). The sequelae and non-sequelae of conjugal bereavement. *American Journal of Psychiatry* 136, 1530–4.

Clayton P. J. (1990). The comorbidity factor: establishing the primary diagnosis in patients with mixed symptoms of anxiety and depression. *Journal of Clinical Psychiatry* 51(suppl), 35–9.

Clayton, P. J. and Darvish, H. S. (1979). Course of depressive symptoms following the stress of bereavement. In *Stress and mental disorder* (eds J. Bartlett, R. M. Rose, and G. L. Klerman), pp.121–39. Raven Press, New York.

Clayton, P. J., Herjanic, M., and Murphy, G. E. (1974). Mourning and depression: their similarities and differences. *Canadian Psychiatric Association Journal* 19, 309–13.

Cleckley, H. M. (1964). *The mask of sanity: an attempt to clarify issues about the so-called psychopathic personality*, 4th edn. Mosby, St Louis, MO.

Clerc, G. E., Ruimy, P., and Verdeac-Pailles, J. (1994). A double-blind comparison of venlafaxine and fluoxetine in patients hospitalised for major depression and melancholia. *International Clinical Psychopharmacology* 9, 139–43.

Clinical Psychiatry Committee (1965). Clinical trials of the treatment of depressive illness: report to the Medical Research Council. *British Medical Journal* 1, 881–6.

Clinical Research Centre (Division of Psychiatry) (1984). The Northwick Park ECT trial: predictors of response to real and simulated ECT. *British Journal of Psychiatry* 144, 227–37.

Clomipramine Collaborative Study Group (1991). Clomipramine and the treatment of patients with obsessive–compulsive disorder. *Archives of General Psychiatry* 48, 730–8.

Cloninger, C. R. (1986). A unified biosocial theory of personality and its role in the development of anxiety states. *Psychiatric Developments* 3, 167–226.

Cloninger, C. R., Svrakic, D. M., and Przybeck, T. R. (1993). A psychobiological model of temperament and character. *Archives of General Psychiatry* 50, 975–90.

Coccaro, E. F. and Kavoussi, R. J. (1997). Fluoxetine and impulsive aggressive behaviour in personality-disordered subjects. *Archives of General Psychiatry* 54, 1081–8.

Coccaro, E. F., Siever, L. J., Clar, H. M., *et al.* (1989). Serotonergic studies in patients with affective and personality disorders. *Archives of General Psychiatry* 46, 587–99.

Cockerham, W. C. (1997). The social determinants of the decline of life expectancy in Russia and eastern Europe: a lifestyle explanation. *Journal of Health and Social Behavior* 38(2), 117–30.

Cody, M. (1990). Depression and the use of antidepressants in patients with cancer. *Palliative Medicine* 4, 271–8.

Cohen, H. W., Gibson, G., and Alderman, M. H. (2000). Excess risk of myocardial infarction in patients treated with antidepressant medications: association with use of tricyclic agents. *American Journal of Medicine* 108, 2–8.

Cohen, L. S. and Rosenbaum, J. F. (1998). Psychotropic drug use during pregnancy: weighing the risks. *Journal of Clinical Psychiatry* 59(suppl 2), 18–28.

Cohen, S. D., Monteiro, W., and Marks, I. M. (1984). Two-year follow-up of agoraphobics after exposure and imipramine. *British Journal of Psychiatry* 144, 276–81.

Cohn, A. H. And Daro, D. (1987). Is treatment too late: what 10 years of evaluative research tells us. *Child Abuse and Neglect* 11, 433–42.

Cole, C. M., O'Boyle, M., Emory, L. E., and Meyer, W. J. 3rd (1997). Comorbidity of gender dysphoria and other major psychiatric diagnoses. *Archives of Sexual Behaviour* 26, 13–26.

Cole, J. D., Goldberg, S. C. and Klerman, G. L. (1964). Phenothiazine treatment in acute schizophrenia. *Archives of General Psychiatry* 10, 246–61.

Collacott, R. (1997). Psychiatric problems in elderly people with learning disabilities. In *The psychiatry of learning disabilities* (ed. O. Russell), pp.136–47. Gaskell, London.

College Research Unit of the Royal College of Psychiatrists (1999). *Focus on the use of stimulants in children with attention deficit hyperactivity disorder.* Gaskell, London.

Collinge, J. (2000). Prion disease. In *The new Oxford textbook of psychiatry* (eds M. G. Gelder, J. J. López-Ibor Jr, and N. C. Andreasen), Chapter 4.1.5. Oxford University Press, Oxford.

Collins, R., Peto, R., Gray, R., and Parish, S. (1996). Large-scale randomized evidence: trials and overviews. In *Oxford Textbook of Medicine*, 3rd edn (eds D. J. Weatherall, J. G. G. Ledingham, and D. A. Warrell), pp. 21–32. Oxford University Press, Oxford.

Committee on the Review of Medicines (1980). Systematic review of the benzodiazepines: guidelines for data sheets on diazepam, chlordiazepoxide, medazepam, temazepam, triazolam, nitrazepam and flurazepam. *British Medical Journal* 1, 910–12.

Committee on the Safety of Medicines (1995). Cardiac arrhythmias with pimozide. *Current Problems in Pharmacovigilance* 21, 2.

Compton, M. T. and Nemeroff, C. B. (2000). The treatment of bipolar depression. *Journal of Clinical Psychiatry* 61(**suppl** 9), 57–67.

Connell, P. H. (1958). *Amphetamine psychosis.* Maudsley Monograph No. 5. Oxford University Press, Oxford.

Conolly, J. (1856). *The treatment of the insane without mechanical restraints.* Reprinted 1973. Dawson, London.

Cook, E. H. Jr, Stein, M .A., Krasowski, M. D., *et al.* (1995). Association of attention deficit disorder and the dopamine transporter gene. *American Journal of Human Genetics* 56, 993–8.

Cookson, J. (1998). Lithium and other drug treatments for recurrent affective disorder. In *The management of depression* (ed. S. Checkley), pp. 275–306. Blackwell Science, Oxford.

Coons, P. M. (1998). The dissociative disorders. Rarely considered and underdiagnosed. *Psychiatric Clinics of North America* 21, 637–48.

Cooper, A. F., Kay, D. W. K., Curry, A. R., Garside, R. F., and Roth, M. (1974). Hearing loss in paranoid and affective psychoses of the elderly. *Lancet* 2, 851–61.

Cooper, B. (1986). Mental disorder as reaction: the history of a psychiatric concept. In *Life events and psychiatric disorder: controversial issues* (ed. H. Katchnig). Cambridge University Press, Cambridge.

Cooper, B. and Singh, B. (2000). Population research and mental health policy. Bridging the gap. *British Journal of Psychiatry* 176, 407–11.

Cooper, J. E. and Oates, M. (2000). The principles of clinical assessment in psychiatry. In *The new Oxford textbook of psychiatry* (eds M. G. Gelder, J. J. López-Ibor Jr, and N. C. Andreasen), Chapter 1.10.1. Oxford University Press, Oxford.

Cooper, J. E., Kendell, R. E., Gurland, B. J., *et al.* (1972). *Psychiatric diagnosis in New York and London.* Maudsley Monograph No.20. Oxford University Press, London.

Cooper, P. J. and Murray, L. (1998). Fortnightly review. Postnatal depression. *British Medical Journal* 316, 1884–6.

Cooper, S.-A. (1999). The relationship between psychiatric and physical health in elderly people with intellectual disabilities. *Journal of Intellectual Disability Research* 43, 54–60.

Copeland, J. R. M., Kelleher, M. J., Kellett, J. M., *et al.* (1975). Evaluation of a psychogeriatric service: the distinction between psychogeriatric and geriatric patients. *British Journal of Psychiatry* 126, 21–9.

Copeland, J. R., Dewey, M. E., Scott, A., *et al.* (1998). Schizophrenia and delusional disorder in older age: community prevalence, incidence, comorbidity, and outcome. *Schizophrenia Bulletin* 24, 153–61.

Corbett, J. A. (1978). The development of services for the mentally handicapped: a historical and national review.

In *The care of the handicapped child* (ed. J. Apley). Heinemann, London.

Corsellis, J. A. N., Bruton, C. J., and Freeman-Browne, D. (1973). The aftermath of boxing. *Psychological Medicine* 3, 270–303.

Coryell, W. and Zimmerman, M. (1989). Personality disorder in the families of depressed schizophrenic and never-ill probands. *American Journal of Psychiatry* 146, 469–502.

Coryell, W., Noyes, R., and Clancy, J. (1982). Excess mortality in panic disorder: comparison with primary unipolar depression. *Archives of General Psychiatry* 39, 701–3.

Costa, P. T. and McCrae, R. R. (1992). *Revised NEO Personality Inventory (NEO PI-P) and NEO Five Factor Inventory Professional Manual*. Psychological Assessment Resources Odessa, FL.

Cotard, M. (1882). Du délire de négations. *Archives de Neurologie, Paris* 4, 152–70, 282–96. [Trans. by M. Rohde in Hirsch, S. R. and Shepherd, M. (eds), *Themes and variations in European psychiatry*, pp. 353–73. Wright, Bristol.]

Courbon, P. and Fail, G. (1927). Sydrome 'd'illusion de Frégoli' et schizophrénie. *Bulletin de la Société Clinique de Médicine Mentale* 15, 121–4.

Cowen, P. J. (1992). New antidepressants: have they superseded tricyclics? In *Practical problems in clinical psychiatry* (eds K. Hawton and P. J. Cowen), pp.22–32. Oxford University Press, Oxford.

Cowen, P. J. (1997). Pharmacotherapy for anxiety disorders: drugs available. *Advances in Psychiatric Treatment* 3, 66–71.

Cowen, P. J. (1998a). Efficacy of treatments for resistant depression. In *The Management of Depression* (ed. S. Checkley), pp. 234–51. Blackwell Science, Oxford.

Cowen, P. J. (1998b). Neuroendocrine challenge tests: what can we learn from them? In *Methods in neuroendocrinology* (ed. L. D. Van de Kar), pp. 205–23, CRC Press, Boca Raton, FL.

Cowen, P. J. (1999). Pharmacological management of treatment-resistant depression. In *Recent topics for advances in psychiatric treatment* (ed. A. Lee), Vol. 2, pp. 52–9. Royal College of Psychiatrists, Gaskill Press, London.

Cowie, V. (1961). The incidence of neurosis in the children of psychotics. *Acta Psychiatrica Scandinavica* 37, 37–71.

Cox, B. J., Swinson, R. P., Morrison, B., *et al.* (1993). Clomipramine, fluoxetine, and behaviour therapy in the treatment of OCD: a meta-analysis. *Journal of Behaviour Therapy and Experimental Psychiatry* 24, 149–53.

Craddock, N. and Jones, I. (1999). Genetics of bipolar disorder. *Journal of Medical Genetics* 36, 585–94.

Craig, T. K. J. (2000). Mental health services for homeless mentally ill people. In *The new Oxford textbook of psychiatry* (eds M. G. Gelder, J. J. López-Ibor Jr, and N. C. Andreasen), Chapter 7.10.2. Oxford University Press, Oxford.

Craig. T. K. J., Boardman, A. P., Mills, K., Daly-Jones, O., Drake, H. (1993). The South London somatisation study I: longitudinal course and the influence of early life experiences. *British Journal of Psychiatry* 163, 579–588.

Crammer, J. (1990). *Asylum history: Buckinghamshire County Pauper Lunatic Asylum – St Johns*. Gaskell, London.

Crawford, M. and Wessely, S. (1998). The changing epidemiology of deliberate self-harm – implications for service provision. *Health Trends* 30, 66–8.

Creed, F. (1999). The relationship between psychosocial parameters and outcome in irritable bowel syndrome. *American Journal of Medicine* 107(5A), 74S–80S.

Creed, F., Black, D., Anthony, P., *et al.* (1990). Randomized controlled trial of day patient versus inpatient psychiatric treatment. *British Medical Journal* 300, 1033–7.

Creed, F., Mbaya, P., Lancashire, S., *et al.* (1997). Cost effectiveness of day and inpatient psychiatric treatment. *British Medical Journal* 314, 1381–5.

Creighton, F. J., Hyde, C. E., and Farragher, B. (1991). Douglas House: Seven years' experience of a community hostel ward. *British Journal of Psychiatry* 159, 500–4.

Crimlisk, H. L., Bhatia, K., Cope, H., David, A., Marsden, C. D., and Ron, M. A. (1998). Slater revisited: 6 year follow up study of patients with medically unexplained motor symptoms. *British Medical Journal* 316, 582–6.

Crisp, A. H. (1977). Diagnosis and outcome of anorexia nervosa: the St George's view. *Proceedings of the Royal Society of Medicine* 70, 464–70.

Cross-National Collaborative Panic Study (1992). Drug treatment of panic disorder: comparative efficacy of alprazolam, imipramine, and placebo. *British Journal of Psychiatry* 160, 191–202.

Crott, R. and Gilis, P. (1998). Economic comparisons of the pharmacotherapy of depression: an overview. *Acta Psychiatrica Scandinavica* 97, 241–52.

Crow, T. J. (1985). The two-syndrome concept: origins and current status. *Schizophrenia Bulletin* 11, 471–85.

Crow, T. J. (1994). Aetiology of schizophrenia. *Current Opinion in Psychiatry* 7, 39–42.

Crow, T. J. (2000). Do obstetric complications really cause psychosis? Why it matters. *British Journal of Psychiatry* 176, 527–30.

Crowe, M. (1998). Sexual therapy and the couple. In *Psychosexual disorders* (eds H. Freeman, I. Pullen, G. Stein, and G. Wilkinson), Chapter 4. Gaskell, London.

Crowe, M. (2000). Psychotherapy with couples. In *The new Oxford textbook of psychiatry* (eds M. G. Gelder, J. J. López-Ibor Jr, and N. C. Andreasen), Chapter 6.3.7. Oxford University Press, Oxford.

Crowe, M. and Ridley, J. (1990). *Therapy with couples: a behavioural-systems approach to marital and sexual problems.* Blackwells, Oxford.

Crowe, M. J. (1973). Conjoint marital therapy: advice or interpretation. *Journal of Psychosomatic Research* 17, 309–15.

Crowe, R. R. (1974). An adoption study of antisocial personality. *Archives of General Psychiatry* 31, 785–91.

Crowe, R. R., Noyes, R., Pauls, D. L., and Slymen, D. (1983). A family study of panic disorder. *Archives of General Psychiatry* 40, 1065–9.

Csernansky, J. G., Mahmoud, R. and Brenner, R. (2002). Comparison of risperidone and haloperidol for the prevention of relapse in patients with schizophrenia. *The New England Journal of Medicine* 346, 16–22.

Cummings, J. L. (2000). Cholinesterase inhibitors: a new class of psychotropic compounds. *American Journal of Psychiatry* 157, 4–15.

Cummings, J. L. and Frankel, M. (1985). Gilles de la Tourette syndrome and the neurological basis of obsessions and compulsions. *Biological Psychiatry* 20, 1117–26.

Cunningham Owens, D. G. (1998). Clinical psychopharmacology. In *Companion to Psychiatric Studies* (eds E. C. Johnstone, C. P. L. Freeman and A. K. Zeally), pp. 81–148. Churchill Livingstone, Edinburgh.

Cunningham Owens, D. G. and Johnstone, E. C. (2000). Treatment and management of schizophrenia. In *The new Oxford textbook of psychiatry* (eds M. G. Gelder, J. J. López-Ibor Jr, and N. C. Andreasen), Chapter 4.3.7. Oxford University Press, Oxford.

Curran, S. and de Pauw, K. (1998). Selecting an antidepressant for use in a patient with epilepsy: safety considerations. *Drug Safety* 18(2), 125–33.

Curran, V. and Travill, R. A. (1997). Mood and cognitive effects of 3,4-methylene dioxymethamphetamine (MDMA, 'ecstasy'): weekend high followed by midweek low. *Addiction* 92, 821–31.

Da Costa, J. M. (1871). An irritable heart: a clinical study of functional cardiac disorder and its consequences. *American Journal of Medical Science* 61, 17–52. (See extracts in S. Jarcho (1959). On irritable heart. *American Journal of Cardiology* 4, 809–17.)

Da Prada, M., Pieri, L., Cesura, A., and Kettler, R. (1994). The pharmacology of moclobemide. *Reviews in Contemporary Pharmacotherapy* 5, 1–80.

Dahabra, S., Ashton, C. H., Bahrainian, M., *et al.* (1998). Structural and functional abnormalities in elderly patients clinically recovered from early- and late-onset depression. *Biological Psychiatry* 44, 34–46.

Dahl, A. A. (1993). The personality disorders: a critical review of family, twin and adoption studies. *Journal of Personality Disorders* **Supplement**, 86–99.

Daniels, N. and Sabin, J. E. (1997). Limits to health care: fair procedures, democratic deliberation, and the legitimacy problem for insurers. *Philosophy and Public Affairs* 26, 303–50.

Danish University Antidepressant Group (1990). Paroxetine: a selective serotonin reuptake inhibitor showing better tolerance but weaker antidepressant effect than clomipramine in a controlled multicentre study. *Journal of Affective Disorders* 18, 289–99.

Dardennes, R., Even, C., Bange, F., and Heim, A. (1995). Comparison of carbamazepine and lithium in the prophylaxis of bipolar disorders. A meta-analysis. *British Journal of Psychiatry* 166, 378–81.

Davanloo, H. (1980). *Short-term dynamic psychotherapy.* Aronson, New York.

David, A. S. (2000). Neuropsychological features of schizophrenia. In *The new Oxford textbook of psychiatry* (eds M. G. Gelder, J. J. López-Ibor Jr, and N. C. Andreasen), Chapter 4.3.3. Oxford University Press, Oxford.

David, A. S. and Busatto, G. (1999). The hallucination: a disorder of brain and mind. In *Disorders of brain and mind* (eds M. A. Ron and A. S. David), pp. 336–62. Cambridge University Press, Cambridge.

Davidson, J. R. T. (1992). Monoamine oxidase inhibitors. In *Handbook of affective disorders* (ed. E. S. Paykel), pp. 345–58. Churchill Livingstone, Edinburgh.

Davidson, J. R. T. (1997). Biological therapies for post-traumatic stress disorder. *Journal of Clinical Psychiatry* **58(suppl 9)**, 29–32.

Davidson, J., Turnbull, C. D., and Miller, R. D. (1980). A comparison of inpatients with primary unipolar depression and depression secondary to anxiety. *Acta Psychiatrica Scandinavica* **61**, 377–86.

Davidson, J., Kudler, H., Smith, R., *et al.* (1990). Treatment of post-traumatic stress disorder with amitriptyline and placebo. *Archives of General Psychiatry* **47**, 259–66.

Davidson, J. R. T., Hughes, D., Blazer, D. G., and George, L. K. (1991). Post-traumatic stress disorder in the community: an epidemiological study. *British Journal of Psychiatry* **21**, 713–21.

Davidson, J. R. T., Hughes, D. C., George, L. K. *et al.* (1993a). The epidemiology of social phobia: findings from the Duke Epidemiological Catchment Area Study. *Psychological Medicine* **23**, 709–18.

Davidson, J .R. T., Potts, N., Richichi, E., *et al.* (1993b). Treatment of social phobia with clonazepam and placebo. *Journal of Clinical Psychopharmacology* **13**, 423–8.

Davidson, K. and Ritson, E. B. (1993). The relationship between alcohol dependence and depression. *Alcohol and Alcoholism* **28**, 147–55.

Davidson, M., Reichenberg, A., Rabinowitz, J., *et al.* (1999). Behavioral and intellectual markers of schizophrenia in apparently healthy male adolescents. *American Journal of Psychiatry* **156**, 1328–35.

Davies, A. M. (1986). *Epidemiological data on the health of the elderly: a review of the present state of research* (eds H. Häfner, G. Moschel, and N. Sartorius). Springer-Verlag, Berlin.

Davies, A. M. and Fleischman, R. (1981). Health status and the use of health services as reported by older residents of the Baka neighbourhood, Jerusalem. *Israeli Medical Sciences* **17**, 138–44.

Davies, B. M. and Morgenstern, F. S. (1960). A case of cysticercosis, temporal lobe epilepsy and transvestism. *Journal of Neurology, Neurosurgery and Psychology* **23**, 247–9.

Davis, J. M., Metalon, L., Watanabe, M., and Blake, L. (1993). Depot antipsychotic drugs: place in therapy. *Drugs* **47**, 741–73.

Davis, R. and Markham, A. (1997). Ziprasidone. *CNS Drugs* **8(2)**, 153–9.

Davison, A. N. (1984). Neurobiology and neurochemistry of the developing brain. In *Scientific studies in mental retardation* (eds J. Dobbing, A. D. B. Clarke, J. A. Corbett, and R. O. Robinson). Royal Society of Medicine and Macmillan, London.

Davison, K. (1983). Schizophrenia-like psychoses associated with cerebral disorders: a review. *Psychiatric Developments* **1**, 1–34.

Davison, K. and Bagley, C. R. (1969). Schizophrenia-like psychoses associated with organic disorders of the central nervous system: a review of the literature. In *British Journal of Psychiatry Special Publication No.4, Current problems in neuropsychiatry* (ed. R. N. Herrington). Headley, Ashford, Kent.

Dawkins, S. (1961). Non-consummation of marriage. *Lancet* **2**, 1029–33.

De Amicis, L. A., Goldberg D. C., LoPiccolo, J., *et al.* (1985). Clinical follow-up of couples treated for sexual dysfunction. *Archives of Sexual Behaviour* **14**, 467–89.

De Clérambault, G. (1921). Les délires passionels. Erotomanie, revendication, jalousie. *Bulletin de la Société Clinique de Médicine Mentale* **61**–7.

De Clérambault, G. G. (1987). Psychoses of passion (English translation). In *The clinical roots of the schizophrenia concept* (ed. J. Cutting and M. Shepherd). Cambridge University Press, Cambridge.

de Girolamo, G. and Dotto, P. (2000). Epidemiology of personality disorders. In *The new Oxford textbook of psychiatry* (eds M. G. Gelder, J. J. López-Ibor Jr, and N. C. Andreasen), Chapter 4.12.5. Oxford University Press, Oxford.

De Hert, N. and Peuskens, J. (2000). Psychiatric aspects of suicidal behaviour: schizophrenia. In *The international handbook of suicide and attempted suicide* (eds K. Hawton and K. van Heeringen), pp. 121–34. John Wiley & Sons, Chichester.

De Jesus Mari, J. and Streiner, D. L. (1994). An overview of family interventions and relapse on schizophrenia: meta-analysis of research findings. *Psychological Medicine* **24**, 565–78.

de Lima, M. S., Hotoph, M., and Wessely, S. (1999). The efficacy of drug treatments for dysthymia: a systematic review and meta-analysis. *Psychological Medicine* **29**, 1273–89.

de Pauw, K. (2000). Depersonalization disorder. In *The new Oxford textbook of psychiatry* (eds M. G. Gelder, J. J. López-Ibor Jr, and N. C. Andreasen), Chapter 4.9. Oxford University Press, Oxford.

De Veaugh-Geiss, J., Moroz, G., Biederman, J., *et al.* (1992). Clomipramine hydrochloride in childhood and adolescent obsessive–compulsive disorder: a multicenter trial. *Journal of the American Academy of Child and Adolescent Psychiatry* **31**, 45–9.

de Wilde, E. J. (2000). Adolescent suicidal behaviour: a general population perspective. In *The international handbook of suicide and attempted suicide* (eds K. Hawton and K. van Heeringen), John Wiley & Sons, Chichester.

Deb, S. and Ahmed, Z. (2000). Specific conditions leading to mental retardation. In *The new Oxford textbook of psychiatry* (eds M. G. Gelder, J. J. López-Ibor Jr, and N. C. Andreasen), Chapter 10.4. Oxford University Press, Oxford.

Dedman, P. (1993). Home treatment for acute psychiatric disorder. *British Medical Journal* **306**, 1359–60.

Déjerine, J. and Gauckler, E. (1913). *Psychoneurosis and psychotherapy* (trans. S. E. Jelliffe and J. B. Lippincott). Reissued by Arno Press, New York.

Delacourte, A., Buée, L. (2000). Tau pathology: a marker of neurodegenerative disorders. *Current Opinion in Neurology* **13**, 371–6.

DeLisi, L. E. (1999). A critical overview of recent investigations into the genetics of schizophrenia. *Current Opinion in Psychiatry* **12**, 29–39.

Den Boer, J. A. (1997). Social phobia; epidemiology, recognition and treatment. *British Medical Journal* **315**, 796–800.

Den Boer, J. A. and Westenberg, H. G. M. (1988). Effect of a serotonin and nor-adrenalin uptake inhibitor in panic disorder: a double blind comparative study with fluvoxamine and maprotiline. *International Clinical Psychopharmacology* **3**, 59–74.

Department of Health (1996). *Health and personal social services statistics for England.* The Stationary Office, London.

Department of Health (1999a). *A national service framework for mental health.* Department of Health, London.

Department of Health (1999b). *Drug misuse and dependence – Guidelines on clinical management.* HM Stationery Office, London.

Department of Health (1999c). *Saving lives: our healthier nation.* The Stationary Office, London.

Department of Health and Social Security (1984). *The management of deliberate self harm.* HM (84) 25. DHSS, London.

Depression Guideline Panel (1993). *Depression in primary care,* Vol. 2. *Treatment of major depression.* Clinical Practice Guideline, No 5. pp. 71–86. Department of Health and Human Services, Rockville, MD.

DeQuardo, J. R. (1998). Pharmacologic treatment of first-episode schizophrenia: early intervention is key to outcome. *Journal of Clinical Psychiatry* **59(suppl 19)**, 9–17.

Derby, I. M. (1933). Manic-depressive 'exhaustion' deaths. *Psychiatric Quarterly* **7**, 435–9.

DeRubeis, R. J., Gelfand, L. A., Tang, T. Z., and Simons, A. D. (1999). Medications versus cognitive behavior therapy for severely depressed outpatients: mega-analysis of four randomized comparisons. *American Journal of Psychiatry* **156**, 1007–13.

Devanand, D. P., Dwork, A. J., Hutchinson, E. R., *et al.* (1994). Does ECT alter brain structure? *American Journal of Psychiatry* **151**, 957–70.

Devilly, G. J. and Spence, S. H. (1999). The relative efficacy and treatment distress of EMDR and a cognitive–behavior trauma protocol in the amelioration of posttraumatic stress disorder. *Journal of Anxiety Disorders* **13**, 131–57.

Devlin, M. J.. Yanovski, S. Z., and Wilson, G. T. (2000). Obesity: what mental health professionals need to know. *American Journal of Psychiatry* **157**, 854–66.

Deykin, E. Y. and Buka, S. L. (1994). Suicidal ideation and attempts among chemically dependent adolescents. *American Journal of Public Health* **84**, 634–9.

Diehl, D. L. and Eisenberg, D. (2000). Complementary and alternative medicine (CAM): epidemiology and implications for research. *Progress in Brain Research* **122**, 445–55.

Diermayer, M., Hedberg, K., and Fleming, D. (1994). Backing off universal childhood lead screening in the USA: opportunity or pitfall? *Lancet* **344**, 1587–8.

DiMatteo, M. R., Lepper, H. S., and Croghan, T. W. (2000). Depression is a risk factor for noncompliance with medical treatment – meta-analysis of the effects of anxiety and depression on patient adherence. *Achives of Internal Medicine* **160**, 2101–7.

Dinan, T. G. (1994). Glucocorticoids and the genesis of depressive illness: a psychobiological model. *British Journal of Psychiatry* **164**, 365–71.

Dingemanse, J. (1993). An update of recent moclobemide interaction data. *International Clinical Psychopharmacology* 7, 167–80.

Dinwiddie, S. H. (1994). Abuse of inhalants: a review. *Addiction* 89, 925–39.

Dodge, K. A., Price, J. M., Bachorowski, J., and Newman, J. P. (1990). Hostile attributional biases in severely aggressive adolescents. *Journal of Abnormal Psychology* 99, 385–92.

Dodge, K., Pettit, G., and Bates, J. E. (1997). How the experience of early physical abuse leads children to become chronically aggressive. In *Developmental perspective on trauma: theory research and intervention* (eds D. Cichetti and S. Toth), pp. 263–88. University of Rochester Press, NJ.

Dolan, R. J. (1999). On the neurology of morals. *Nature Neuroscience* 2, 927–9.

Dolan, M. and Bishay, N. (1996). The effectiveness of cognitive therapy in the treatment of non-psychotic morbid jealousy. *British Journal of Psychiatry* 168, 588–93.

Dolan, M. and Doyle, M. (2000). Violence risk prediction. Clinical and actuarial measures and the role of the Psychopathy Checklist. *British Journal of Psychiatry* 177, 303–311.

Done, D. J., Johnstone, E. C., Frith, C. D., *et al.* (1991). Complications of pregnancy and delivery in relation to psychosis in adult life: data from the British perinatal mortality survey sample. *British Medical Journal* 302, 1576–80.

Done, D. J., Crow, T. J., Johnstone, E. C., and Sacker, A. (1994). Childhood antecedence of schizophrenia and affective illness: social adjustment at ages 7 and 11. *British Medical Journal* 309, 699–703.

d'Orban, P. T. (1979). Women who kill their children. *British Journal of Psychiatry* 134, 560–71.

Dosen, A. (1993). Diagnosis and treatment of psychiatric and behavioural disorders in mentally retarded individuals: the state of the art. *Journal of Intellectual Disability Research* 37, 1–7.

Douglas, J. and Richman, N. (1984). *My child won't sleep: a handbook for management for parents*. Penguin, Harmondsworth.

Drake, R. E., Mercer-McFadden, C., Muesser, K. T., *et al.* (1998). Review of integrated mental health and substance abuse treatments for patients with dual disorders. *Schizophrenia Bulletin* 24, 589–608.

Dreifuss, F. E., Bancaud, J., Henricksen, O., *et al.* (1981). Proposal for a revised clinical and electroencephalographic classification of epileptic seizures. *Epilepsia* 22, 489–503.

Drevets, W. C. (1998). Functional neuroimaging studies of depression: the anatomy of melancholia. *Annual Review of Medicine* 49, 341–61.

Drevets, W. C., Ongur, D., and Price, J. L. (1998). Neuroimaging abnormalities in the subgenual prefrontal cortex: implications for the pathophysiology of familial mood disorders. *Molecular Psychiatry* 3, 220–6.

Drossman, D. A. (1998). Presidential address: Gastrointestinal illness and the biopsychosocial model. *Psychosomatic Medicine* 60, 258–67.

Druss, B. and Pincus, H. (2000). Suicidal ideation and suicide attempts in general medical illnesses. *Archives of Internal Medicine* 160, 1522–1526.

Dubini, A., Bosc, M., and Pollin, V. (1997). Do noradrenaline and serotonin differentially affect social motivation and behaviour. *European Neuropsychopharmacology* 7(suppl 1), S49–55.

Dubois P. (1909). *The psychic treatment of nervous disorders*, 6th edn. Funk and Wagnalls Company, New York and London.

Duffy, J. D. and Coffey, C.E. (1997). The neurobiology of depression. In: *Contemporary Behavioral Neurology* (eds. M.R. Trimble, J.L. Cummings), Butterworth-Heinemann: Boston.

Dugbartey, A. T. (1998). Neurocognitive aspects of hypothyroidism. *Archives of Internal Medicine* 158, 1413–18.

Duman, R. S., Heninger, G. R., and Nestler, E. J. (1997). A molecular and cellular theory of depression. *Archives of General Psychiatry* 54, 597–606.

Dunbar, H. F. (1954). *Emotions and bodily changes*. Columbia University Press, New York.

Dunlap, K. (1932). *Habits: their making and unmaking*. Liverheight, New York.

Dunn, J. and Fahy, T. A. (1990). Police admissions to a psychiatric hospital: demographic and clinical differences between ethnic groups. *British Journal of Psychiatry* 156, 373–8.

Dunn, J. and Kendrick, C. (1982). *Siblings: love, envy and understanding*. Cambridge University Press, Cambridge.

Dunn, K. M., Croft, P. R., and Hackett, T. I. (1998). Sexual problems: a study of the prevalence and need for health care in the general population. *Good Family Practice* 15, 519–24.

Dunner, D. L., Ishiki, D., Avery, D. H., *et al.* (1986). Effect of alprazolam and diazepam on anxiety and panic attacks in panic disorder: a controlled trial. *Journal of Clinical Psychiatry* 47, 458–60.

Durkheim, E. (1951). *Suicide: a study in sociology* (trans. J. A. Spaulding and G. Simpson). Free Press, Glencoe, IL.

Dykens, E. M., Hodapp, R., and Leckman, J. F. (1994). Behaviour and development in fragile X syndrome. *Developmental Clinical Psychology and Psychiatry* 28.

Eagles, J. M. and Whalley, L. J. (1985). Decline in the diagnosis of schizophrenia among first admissions to Scottish mental hospitals from 1969 to 1978. *British Journal of Psychiatry* 146, 151–4.

Earls, F., Reich, W., Jung, K., and Cloninger, C. R. (1988). Psychopathology in children of alcoholic and antisocial parents. *Alcoholism: Clinical and Experimental Research* 12, 481–7.

Eaton, W. W. and Keyl, P. M. (1990). Risk factors for the onset of diagnostic interview schedule/DSM-III agoraphobia in a prospecctive population-based study. *Archives of General Psychiatry* 47, 819.

Eaton, W. W., Mortenson, P. B., Herrman, H., *et al.* (1992). Long-term course of hospitalisation for schizophrenia: (1) risk for hospitalisation. *Schizophrenia Bulletin* 18, 217–28.

Eaves, L. J., Silberg, J. L., Meyer, J. M., *et al.* (1997). Genetics and developmental psychopathology: 2. The main effects of genes and environment on behavioural problems in the Virginia Twin Study of Adolescent Behavioural Development. *Journal of Child Psychology and Psychiatry and Allied Disciplines* 38, 965–80.

Ebbage, J., Farr, C., Skinner, D. V., and White, P. D. (1994). The psychosocial assessment of patients discharged from accident and emergency departments after deliberate self poisoning. *Journal of the Royal Society of Medicine* 87, 515–16.

Ebstein, R. P., Novick, O., Umansky, R., *et al.* (1996). Dopamine D4 receptor (D4DR) exon III polymorphism associated with the human personality trait of novelty seeking. *Nature Genetics* 12, 78–80.

Eckhert, E. D., Bouchard, T. J., Bohlen, J., and Heston, L. L. (1986). Homosexuality in monozygotic twins reared apart. *British Journal of Psychiatry* 148, 421–5.

Edelstyn, N. M. J. and Oyebode, F. (1999). A review of the phenomenology and cognitive neuropsychological origins of the Capgras syndrome. *International Journal of Geriatric Psychiatry* 14, 48–59.

Edwards, G. (1994). *Alcohol policy and the public good.* Oxford University Press, Oxford.

Edwards, G., Orford, J., Egert, S., *et al.* (1977). Alcoholism: a controlled trial of 'treatment' and 'advice'. *Journal of Studies on Alcohol* 38, 1004–31.

Edwards, J. G. (1999). Prevention of relapse and recurrence of depression: newer versus older antidepressants. In *Recent topics from advances in psychiatric treatment*, Vol. 2 (ed. A. Lee), pp. 60–5. Gaskill Press, London.

Edwards, J. G. and Anderson, I. (1999). Systematic review and guide to selection of selective serotonin reuptake inhibitors. *Drugs* 57(4), 507–33.

Egger, M., Davey Smith, G., Schneider, M., and Minder, C. (1997). Bias in meta-analysis detected by a simple, graphical test. *British Medical Journal* 315, 629–34.

Ehlers, A., (2000). Post-traumatic stress disorder. In *The new Oxford textbook of psychiatry* (eds M. G. Gelder, J. J. López-Ibor Jr, and N. C. Andreasen), Chapter 4.6.2. Oxford University Press, Oxford.

Ehlers, A. and Clark, D. M. (2000). A cognitive model of post-traumatic stress disoder. *Behaviour Research and Therapy* 38, 319–45.

Ehlers, A., Mayou, R. A., and Bryant, B. (1998). Psychological predictors of chronic post-traumatic stress disorder after motor vehicle accidents. *Journal of Abnormal Psychology* 107, 508–19.

Ehlers, S. and Gillberg, C. (1993). The epidemiology of Asperger syndrome. A total population study. *Journal of Child Psychology and Psychiatry* 34, 1327–50.

Ehrhardt, A. A., Epstein, R., and Money, J. (1968). Fetal androgens and female gender identity in the early-treated adrenogenital syndrome. *Johns Hopkins Medical Journal* 122, 160–7.

Eisenberg, L. (1986). Does bad news about suicide beget bad news? *New England Journal of Medicine* 315, 705–7.

Eisenstat, S. A. and Bancroft, L. (1999). Domestic violence. *New England Journal of Medicine* 341, 886–91.

Eiser, C. (1986). Effects of chronic illness on the child's intellectual development. *Journal of the Royal Society of Medicine* 79, 2–3.

Eitinger, L. (1960). The symptomatology of mental disease among refugees in Norway. *Journal of Mental Science* 106, 947–66.

Elkin, I., Shea, T., Watkins, J. T., *et al.* (1989). National Institute of Mental Health Treatment of Depression Collaborative Research Programme: general effectiveness of treatments. *Archives of General Psychiatry* 46, 971–82.

Elliot, J. G. (1999). Practitioner review: school refusal: issues of conceptualisation, assessment and treatment. *Journal of Child Psychology and Psychiatry* 40, 1011–12.

Elliott, R. (1998). The neuropsychological profile in unipolar depression. *Trends in Cognitive Sciences* 2, 447–54.

Emanuel, E. J. (1994). Euthanasia: historical, ethical, and empiric perspectives. *Archives of Internal Medicine* 154, 1890–901.

Emanuel. L. L. (1998). Facing requests for physician assisted suicide: toward a practical and principled clinical skill set. *Journal of the American Medical Association* 280, 643–7.

Emerson, E. (1995). *Challenging behaviour: analysis and intervention in people with learning disabilities.* Cambridge University Press, Cambridge.

Emilien, G., Beyreuther, K., Masters, C. L., Maloteaux, J-M. (2000). Prospects for pharmacological intervention in Alzheimer disease. *Archives of Neurology* 57, 454–459.

Emslie, G., Rush, A., Weinberg, W., *et al.* (1997). A double-blind, randomized placebo-controlled trial of fluoxetine in depressed children and adolescents. *Archives of General Psychiatry* 54, 1031–7.

Endicott, J. and Spitzer, R. L. (1978). A diagnostic interview: the schedule for affective disorders and schizophrenia. *Archives of General Psychiatry* 35, 837–44.

Enfield, S. L. and Tonge, B. J. (1996). Population prevalence of psychopathology in children and adolescents with intellectual disability. II Epidemiological findings. *Journal of Intellectual Disability Research*, 40, 99–109.

Engel, G. and Romano, J. (1959). Delirium, a syndrome of cerebral insufficiency. *Journal of Chronic Diseases* 9, 260–77.

Enoch, M. D. and Trethowan, W. H. (1979). *Uncommon psychiatric syndromes.* Wright, Bristol.

Epstein, A. W. (1960). Fetishism: a study of its psychopathology with particular reference to a proposed disorder in brain mechanisms as an etiological factor. *Journal of Nervous and Mental Disease* 130, 107–19.

Epstein, A. W. (1961). Relationship of fetishism and transvestism to brain and particularly to temporal lobe dysfunction. *Journal of Nervous and Mental Disease* 133, 247–53.

Epstein, L., Valoski, A., Wing, R. R., and McCurley, J. (1994). Ten-year outcomes of behavioral family-based treatment for childhood obesity. Health Psychology 13(5), 373–83.

Erkinjuntti, T. (2000). Vascular dementia. In *The new Oxford textbook of psychiatry* (eds. M. G. Gelder, J. J. López-Ibor Jr, and N. C. Andreasen), Chapter 4.1.9. Oxford University Press, Oxford.

Ernst, A. and Zibrak, J. D. (1998). Carbon monoxide poisoning. *New England Journal of Medicine* 339, 1603–8.

Ernst, E. (1999). Second thoughts about safety of St John's wort. *Lancet* 354, 2014–15.

Errera, P. (1962). Some historical aspects of the concept, phobia. *Psychiatric Quarterly* 36, 325–36.

Escobar, J.I,, Waitzkin, H., Silver, R. C., Gara, M., and Holman, A. (1998). Abridged somatization: a study in primary care. *Psychosomatic Medicine* 60(4), 466–72.

Esiri, M. and Nagy, Z. (2002). Neuropathology. In *Psychiatry in the elderly*, 3rd edn (eds R. Jacoby and C. Oppenheimer). Oxford University Press, Oxford.

Espie, C. A. (2000). Insomnias. In *The new Oxford textbook of psychiatry* (eds M. G. Gelder, J. J. López-Ibor Jr, and N. C. Andreasen), Chapter 4.14.2. Oxford University Press, Oxford.

Esquirol, E. (1838). *Des maladies mentales.* Baillière, Paris. (Reprinted in 1976 by Arno Press, New York.)

Esquirol, E. (1845). *Mental maladies, a treatise on insanity* (transl. E. K. Hunt). Lea and Blanchard, Philadelphia, PA.

Essau, C. A. and Wittchen, H. U. (1993). An overview of the Composite International Diagnostic Interview (CIDI). *International Journal of Methods in Psychiatric Research* 3, 79–85.

Essen-Møller, E. (1971). Suggestions for further improvement of the international classification of mental disorders. *Psychological Medicine* 1, 308–11.

Evan-Jones, L. G. and Rosenbloom, L. (1978). Disintegrative psychosis in childhood. *Developmental Medicine and Child Neurology* 20, 462–70.

Evans, D. L., Staab, J. P., Petitto, J. M. *et al.* (1999). Depression in the medical setting: biopsychological interactions and treatment considerations. *Journal of Clinical Psychiatry* 60(suppl 4), 40–55.

Evans, M. D., Hollon, S. D., DeRubeis, R. J., *et al.* (1992). Differential relapse following cognitive therapy and pharmacotherapy for depression. *Archives of General Psychiatry* 49, 802–8.

Evans, M. O., Morgan, H. G., Hayward, A., and Gunnell, D. J. (1999). Crisis telephone consultation for deliberate self-harm patients: effects on repetition. *British Journal of Psychiatry* 175, 23–7.

Eysenck, H. J. (1970a). *Crime and personality.* Paladin Press, London.

Eysenck, H. J. (1970b). *The structure of human personality*. Methuen, London.

Eysenck, H. J. (1970c). A dimensional system of psycho-diagnosis. In *New approaches to personality classification* (ed. A. R. Mahrer), pp.169–207. Columbia University Press, New York.

Eysenck, H. J. and Eysenck, S. B. G. (1976). *Psychoticism as a dimension of personality*. Hodder and Stoughton, London.

Faedda, G. L., Tondo, L., Baldessarini, R. J., *et al.* (1993). Outcome after rapid versus gradual discontinuation of lithium treatment in bipolar disorders. *Archives of General Psychiatry* 50, 448–58.

Faergeman, P. M. (1963). *Psychogenic psychoses.* Butterworths, London.

Fairburn, C. G. (2000). Bulimia nervosa. In *The new Oxford textbook of psychiatry* (eds M. G. Gelder, J. J. López-Ibor Jr, and N. C. Andreasen), Chapter 4.10.2. Oxford University Press, Oxford.

Fairburn, C. G. and Carter, J. C. (1997). Self-help and guided self-help for binge eating. In *Eating disorders*, 2nd edn (eds D. M. Garner and P. E. Garfinkel). Guildford Press, New York and London.

Fairburn, C. G. and Wilson, G. T. (1993). Binge eating: definition and classification. In *Binge eating: nature, assessment and treatment* (eds C. G. Fairburn and G. T. Wilson), pp. 3–14. Guilford Press, New York.

Fairburn, C. G., Marcus, M. D. and Wilson, G. T. (1993). Cognitive–behavioural therapy for binge eating and bulimia nervosa: a comprehensive treatment manual. In *Binge eating: nature, assessment and treatment* (eds C. G. Fairburn and G. T. Wilson), pp. 361–404. Guilford Press, New York.

Fairburn, C. G., Doll, H. A., Welch, S. L., Hay, P. J., *et al.* (1998). Risk factors for binge eating disorder.

A community-based, case-control study. *Archives of General Psychiatry* 55, 425–32.

Fairburn, C. G., Cooper, Z., Doll, H. A., and Welch, S. L. (1999). Risk factors for anorexia nervosa. Three integrated case-control comparisons. *Archives of General Psychiatry* 56, 468–76.

Fairweather, S. and Stewart, N. (2001). Delirium – the physican's perspective. In *Psychiatry in the elderly*, 3rd edn (eds R. Jacoby and C. Oppenheimer). Oxford University Press, Oxford.

Falkai, P. and Bogerts, S. (1993). Brain development and schizophrenia. In *Neurobiology and psychiatry* (ed. R. Kerwin), Vol. 2, pp. 43–70. Cambridge University Press, Cambridge.

Faller, K. C. (1987). Women who sexually abuse children. *Violence and Victims* 2, 263–76.

Falloon, I. R. H., Kydd, R. R., Coverdale, J. H., *et al.* (1996). Early detection and intervention for initial episodes of schizophrenia. *Schizophrenia Bulletin* 22, 271–82.

Falret, J. P. (1854). Mémoire sur la folie circulaire. *Bulletin de l'Academie de Médicine* 19, 382–415. [Trans. into English in M. J. Sedler and E. C. Dessain (1983). Falret's discovery: the origin of the concept of bipolar affective illness. *American Journal of Psychiatry* 140, 1227–33.]

Fann, J. R. (1997). Traumatic brain injury and psychiatry. *Journal of Psychosomatic Research* 43, 335–43.

Fanshel, D. (1981). Decision-making under uncertainty: foster care for abused or neglected children? *American Journal of Public Health* 71, 685–6.

Farde, L., Wiesel, F. A., Nordstrom, A. L., and Sedvall, G. (1989). D_1- and D_2-dopamine receptor occupancy during treatment with conventional and atypical neuroleptics. *Psychopharmacology* 99, S28–31.

Faris, R. E. L. and Dunham, H. W. (1939). *Mental disorders in urban areas*. Chicago University Press, Chicago, IL.

Farmer, R., Tranah, T., O'Donnell, I., and Catalan, J. (1992). Railway suicide: the psychological effect on drivers. *Psychological Medicine* 22, 407–14.

Farrell, B. A. (1981). *The standing of psychoanalysis*. Oxford University Press, Oxford.

Farrington, D. P. (2000). Psychosocial causes of offending. In *The new Oxford textbook of psychiatry*. (eds M. G. Gelder, J. J. López-Ibor Jr, and N. C. Andreasen), Chapter 11.2. Oxford University Press, Oxford.

Farrington, D. P. (1994). Human development and criminal careers. In *The Oxford handbook of criminology* (ed. M. Maguire), pp.511–84. Clarendon Press, Oxford.

Farrington, D. P., Loeber, R., and VanLammen, W. B. (1990). Long-term criminal outcomes of hyperactivity-impulsivity-attention deficit and conduct problems in childhood. In *Straight and devious pathways from childhood to adulthood* (eds L. N. Robins and M. Rutter), pp.62–81. Cambridge University Press, New York.

Farrington, D., Barnes, G., and Lamberst, S. (1996). The concentration of offending in families. *Legal and Criminal Psychology* 1, 47–63.

Fawcett, J. and Barkin, R. L. (1998). Review of the results from clinical studies on the efficacy, safety and tolerability of mirtazapine for the treatment of patients with major depression. *Journal of Affective Disorders* 51, 267–85.

Fawcett, J., Scheftner, W. A., Fogg, L., Clark, D. C., Young, M. A., Hedeker, D., and Gibbons, R. (1990). Time-related predictors of suicide in major affective disorder. *American Journal of Psychiatry* 147, 1189–94.

Fawzy, F. I. and Fawzy, N. W. (1998). Group therapy in the cancer setting. *Journal of Psychosomatic Research* 45, 191–200.

Fawzy, F. I., Fawzy, N. W., Arndt, L. A., and Pasnau, R. O. (1995). Critical review of psychosocial interventions in cancer care. *Archives of General Psychiatry* 52, 100–13.

Fazel, S. and Jacoby, R. (2001). Psychiatric aspects of crime and the elderly. In *Psychiatry in the elderly*, 3rd edn (eds R. Jacoby and C. Oppenheimer). Oxford University Press, Oxford.

Federal Bureau of Investigation (1992). *Uniform crime reports for the United States, 1991*. US Government Printing Office, Washington, DC.

Feighner, J. P., Robins, E., Guze, S. B., *et al.* (1972). Diagnostic criteria for use in psychiatric research. *Archives of General Psychiatry* 26, 57–63.

Feighner, J., Targum, S. D., Bennett, M. E. *et al.* (1998). A double-blind, placebo-controlled trial of nefazodone in the treatment of patients hospitalized for major depression. *Journal of Clinical Psychiatry* 59, 246–53.

Feingold, B. F. (1975). Hyperkinesis and learning difficulties linked to artificial food and colors. *American Journal of Nursing* 75, 797–803.

Feinmann, C. (1999). *The mouth, the face and the mind*. Oxford University Press, Oxford.

Felderman, H. A., Goldstein, I., Hatzichristoudg, A., *et al.* (1994). Impotence and its medical and psychological correlates: results of the Massachusetts male ageing study. *Journal of Urology* 151, 54–61.

Felt, B., Wise, C. G., Olson, A., *et al.* (1999). Guideline for the management of paediatric idiopathic constipation and soiling. *Archives of Paediatric and Adolescent Medicine* 153, 380–5.

Fenelon, G., Mahieux, F., Huon, R. and Ziegler, M. (2000). Hallucinations in Parkinson's disease. Prevalence, phenomenology and risk factors. *Brain* 123, 733–45.

Fenichel, O. (1945). *The psychoanalytic theory of neurosis*. Kegan Paul, Trench and Trubner, London.

Fennel, M. J. V (2000). Depression. In *Cognitive behaviour therapy for psychiatric problem: a practical guide*, 2nd edn (eds K. Hawton, P. M. Salkovskis, J. Kirk, and D. M. Clark). Oxford University Press.

Fennell, M. (1993). Depression. In *Cognitive behaviour therapy for psychiatric problems* (ed. K. Hawton, P. M. Salkovskis, J. Kirk, and D. M. Clark), pp. 169–234. Oxford University Press, Oxford.

Fenton, G. W. (1986). Epilepsy and hysteria. *British Journal of Psychiatry* 149, 28–37.

Fenton, G. W. (1999). Neurosurgery for mental disorder: past and present. *Advances in Psychiatric Treatment* 5, 261–70.

Fenton, W. S. and McGlashan, T. H. (1991). Natural history of schizophrenia subtypes. (1) Longitudinal study of paranoid, hebephrenic and undifferentiated schizophrenia. *Archives of General Psychiatry* 48, 969–77.

Fergusson, D. M., Horwood, L. J., Lynskey, M. T., *et al.* (1996). Childhood sexual abuse and psychiatric disorder in young adulthood: II. Psychiatric outcomes of childhood sexual abuse. *Journal of the American Academy of Child and Adolescent Psychiatry* 35, 1365–74.

Fernando, S., Ndegwa, D., and Wilson, M. (1998). *Forensic psychiatry, race and culture*. Routledge, London.

Ferrey, G. and Zebdi, S. (1999). Acute psychotic episode or bouffée délirante polymorphe, an evolutive diagnosis. *Encephale* 25, 26–32.

Ferrier, I. N., Stanton, B. R., Kelly, T. P., and Scott, J. (1999a). Neuropsychological function in euthymic patients with bipolar disorder. *British Journal of Psychiatry* 175, 246–51.

Ferrier, I. N., Tyrer, S. P., and Bell, A. J. (1999b). Lithium therapy. *Recent Topics from Advances in Psychiatric Treatment* 2, 76–83.

Feske, U. and Chambless, D. L. (1995). Cognitive behavioral versus exposure only treatment for social phobia: a meta-analysis. *Behavior Therapy* 26, 695–720.

Field, L. L. and Kaplan, B. J. (1998). Absence of linkage of phonological coding dyslexia to chromosome 6p23–21.3 in a large family data set. *American Journal of Human Genetics* 63, 1448–56.

Fineberg, N. (1999). Evidence-based pharmacotherapy for obsessive–compulsive disorder. *Advances in Psychiatric Treatment* 5, 357–65.

Fink, P. (2000). Somatization disorder and related disorders. In *The new Oxford textbook of psychiatry* (eds M. G. Gelder, J. J. López-Ibor Jr, and N. C. Andreasen.), Chapter 5.2.3. Oxford University Press, Oxford.

Finkelhor, D. (1984). *Child sexual abuse: new theory and research*, pp.53–68. Free Press, London.

Finkelhor, D. (1986). *A sourcebook of child sexual abuse.* Sage, Beverley Hills, CA.

Finlay-Jones, R. and Brown, G. W. (1981). Types of stressful life event and the onset of anxiety and depressive disorders. *Psychological Medicine* 11, 803–16.

First, M. B., Spitzer, R .L., Gibbon, M., *et al.* (1995). The Structured Clinical Interview for DSMIII-R Personality Disorders (SCID-II), 1: description. *Journal of Personality Disorders* 9, 83–91.

Fisher, J. E. and Carstensen, L. L. (1990). Behavior management of the dementias. *Clinical Psychology Review* 10, 611–29.

Fitzgerald, R. G. and Parkes, C. M. (1998). Blindness and loss of other sensory and cognitive functions. *British Medical Journal* 316, 1160–3.

Fitzpatrick, R., Fletcher, A., Gore, S., *et al.* (1992). Quality of life measures in health care. I: Applications and issues in assessment. *British Medical Journal* 305, 1074–7.

Flament, M. F. and Chabane, N. (2000). Obsessive–compulsive disorder and tics in children and adolescents. In *The new Oxford textbook of psychiatry* (eds M. G. Gelder, J. J. López-Ibor Jr, and N. C. Andreasen), Chapter 9.2.6. Oxford University Press, Oxford.

Flaskerud, J. H. and Hu, L. T. (1992). Relationship of ethnicity to psychiatric diagnosis. *Journal of Nervous and Mental Disease* 180, 296–303.

Fleminger, S. (2000). The management of dementia. In *The new Oxford textbook of psychiatry* (eds M. G. Gelder, J. J. López-Ibor Jr, and N. C. Andreasen), Chapter 4.1.14. Oxford University Press, Oxford.

Fletcher, A., Gore, S., Jones, D., *et al.* (1992). Quality of life measures in health care. II Design, analysis and interpretation. *British Medical Journal* 305, 1145–8.

Fletcher, T. A., Jan Brakel, S., and Cavanaugh, J. L. (2000). Violence in the workplace: new perspectives in forensic mental health services in the USA. *British Journal of Psychiatry* 176, 339–44.

Flint, J., Carley, R., DeFries, J. C., *et al.* (1995). A simple genetic basis for a complex psychological trait in laboratory mice. *Science* 268, 1432–5.

Flor-Henry, P. (1969). Psychosis and temporal lobe epilepsy: a controlled investigation. *Epilepsia* 10, 363–95.

Floyd, F. and Phillippe, K. (1993). Parental interactions with children with and without mental retardation: behavior, management, coerciveness, and positive exchange. *American Journal of Mental Retardation* 97, 673–84.

Foa, E. B., Steketee, G., Kozak, M. J., and Dugger, D. (1987). Imipramine and placebo in the treatment of obsessive compulsives: their effect on depression and on obsessional symptoms. *Psychopharmacology Bulletin* 23, 8–11.

Foa, E. B., Rothbaum, B. O., Riggs, D. S., and Murdock, T. B. (1991). Treatment of posttraumatic stress disorder in rape victims: a comparison between cognitive–behavioural procedures and counselling. *Journal of Consulting and Clinical Psychology* 59, 715–23.

Foa, E. B., Riggs, D. S., and Gershvny, B. S. (1995). Arousal, numbing and intrusion: Symptom structure of PTSD following assault. *American Journal of Psychiatry* 152, 116–20.

Foa, E. B., Dancu, C. V., Hembree, E. A., Jaycox, L. H., Meadows, E. A., and Street. G. P. (1999a). A comparison of exposure therapy, stress inoculation training, and their combination for reducing posttraumatic stress disorder in female assault victims. *Journal of Consulting and Clinical Psychology* 67, 194–200.

Foa, E. B., Davidson, J. R. T. And Frances, A. J. (1999b). Treatment of post-traumatic stress disorder. *Journal of Clinical Psychiatry* 60, suppl 10.

Foa, E. B., Keane, T. M., and Friedman, M. J. (2000). *Effective treatments for PTSD*. Guilford, New York.

Folstein, S. (2000). Dementia due to Huntingdon's Disease. In *New Oxford Textbook of Psychiatry* (eds M. G. Gelder, J. J. López-Ibor, N. C. Andreasen). Oxford University Press.

Fombonne, E. (1999). The epidemiology of autism: a review. *Psychological Medicine* 29, 769–86.

Fonagy, P. (2000). Psychoanalysis and other long-term dynamic psycotherapies. In *The new Oxford textbook of psychiatry* (eds M. G. Gelder, J. J. López-Ibor Jr, and N. C. Andreasen), Chapter 6.3.5. Oxford University Press, Oxford.

Fonagy, P. and Target, M. (2000). Child psychoanalysis. In *The new Oxford textbook of psychiatry* (eds M. G. Gelder, J. J. López-Ibor Jr, and N. C. Andreasen), Chapter 9.5.2. Oxford University Press, Oxford.

Fonagy, P. *et al.* (1997). Morality, disruptive behavior, BPD, crime and their relationships to security of attachment. In *Attachment and Psychopathology* (eds L. Atkinson and K. Zucker), pp. 223–74. Guilford, New York.

Ford, D. E. and Kamerow, D. B. (1989). Epidemiologic study of sleep disturbances and psychiatric disorders. *Journal of the American Medical Association* 262, 1479–84.

Ford, R., Durcan, G., Warner, L., *et al.* (1998). One day survey by the Mental Health Act Commission of acute adult psychiatric inpatient wards in England and Wales. *British Medical Journal* 317, 1279–83.

Fordham, F. (1990). *An introduction to Jung's psychology.* Penguin, Harmondsworth.

Forrest, G. C. and Standish, E. (1984). Supporting bereaved parents after perinatal death. In *Recent research in developmental psychopathology* (ed. J. E. Stevenson). Pergamon Press, Oxford.

Forsgren, L., Edvinsson, S. O., Blomqvist, H. K., *et al.* (1990). Epilepsy in a population of mentally retarded children and adults. *Epilepsy Research* 6, 234–48..

Förstl, H., Burns, A., Levy, R., *et al.* (1993). Neuropathological correlates of behavioural disturbance in confirmed Alzheimer's disease. *British Journal of Psychiatry* 163, 364–8.

Forsythe, W. I. and Butler, R. J. (1989). Fifty years of enuretic alarms. *Archives of Disease in Childhood* 64, 879–85.

Fossey, M. D. and Lydiard, R. B. (1990). Placebo responses in patients with anxiety disorders. In *Handbook of anxiety* (eds R Noyes, M. Roth, and G. D. Burrows), Vol. 4, pp. 27–56. Elsevier, Amsterdam.

Foster, E. M., Kay, D. W. K., and Bergmann, K. (1976). The characteristics of old people receiving and needing domiciliary services. *Age and Ageing* 5, 345–55.

Foster, T., Gillespie, K., and McClelland, R. (1997). Mental disorders and suicide in Northern Ireland. *British Journal of Psychiatry* 170, 447–52.

Foulkes, S. H. (1948). *Introduction to group-analytic psychotherapy.* Heinemann, London.

Foulkes, S. H. and Lewis, E. (1944). Group analysis: a study in the treatment of groups on psychoanalytic lines. *British Journal of Medical Psychology* 20, 175–82.

Fox, N. C., Freeborough, P. A., and Rosser, M. N. (1996). Visualisation and quantification of rates of atrophy in Alzheimer's disease. *Lancet* 348, 94–7.

Foxcroft, D. R., Lister-Sharp, D., and Lowe, G. (1997). Alcohol misuse prevention for young people: a systematic review reveals methodological concerns and lack of reliable evidence for effectiveness. *Addiction* 92, 531–7.

France, K. G. and Hudson, S. M. (1993). Management of infant sleep disturbance: a review. *Clinical Psychology Review* 13, 635–47.

Francis, P. T., Palmer, A. M., Snape, M., Wilcock, G. K. (1999). The cholinergic hypothesis of Alzheimer;s disease. A review of progress. *Journal of Neurology, Neurosurgery and Psychiatry* 66, 137–147.

Frank, E., Kupfer, D. J., Perel, J. M., *et al.* (1990). Three year outcomes of maintenance therapies in recurrent depression. *Archives of General Psychiatry* 47, 1093–9.

Frank, E., Kupfer, D. J., Wagner, E. F., *et al.* (1991). Efficacy of interpersonal therapy as a maintenance treatment of recurrent depression. *Archives of General Psychiatry* 48, 1053–9.

Frank, E., Kupfer, D. J., Perel, J. M., *et al.* (1993). Comparison of full dose versus half dose pharmacotherapy in the maintenance treatment of recurrent depression. *Journal of Affective Disorders* 27, 139–41.

Frank, J. D. (1967). *Persuasion and healing.* Johns Hopkins Press, Baltimore, MD.

Frasure-Smith, N. and Lespérance, F. (2000). Coronary artery disease, depression and social support: only the beginning. *European Heart Journal* 21, 1043–5.

Frasure-Smith, N., Lesperance, F., Gravel, G. *et al.* (2000). Social support, depression and mortality during the first year after myocardial infarction. *Circulation* 101, 1919–1924.

Frasure-Smith, N., Lespérance, F., and Talajic, M. (1995). Depression and 18 month prognosis after myocardial infarction. *Circulation* 91, 999–1005.

Fredrikson, M., Wik, G., Greitz, T., *et al.* (1993). Regional cerebral blood flow during experimental phobic fear. *Psychophysiology* 30, 126–30.

Freeman, C. (1999). Anaesthesia for electroconvulsive therapy. *Psychiatric Bulletin* 23, 740–1.

Freeman, C. P. L. (1998). Neurotic disorders. In *Companion to psychiatric studies* (eds E. C. Johnstone, C. P. L. Freeman, and A. K. Zealley), pp. 465–507. Churchill Livingstone, London.

Freeman, C. P. L., Weeks, D., and Kendell, R. E. (1980). ECT: II Patients who complain. *British Journal of Psychiatry* 137, 17–25.

Freeman, C. P. L., Trimble, M. R., Deakin, J. F. W., *et al.* (1994). Fluvoxamine versus clomipramine in the treatment of obsessive compulsive disorder: a multi-center, randomized, double-blind parallel group comparison. *Journal of Clinical Psychiatry* 55, 301–5.

Freeman, W. and Watts, J. W. (1942). *Psychosurgery.* Thomas, Springfield, IL.

Freemantle, N. and Geddes, J. (1998). Understanding and interpreting systematic reviews and meta-analyses. Part 2: meta-analyses. *Evidence-based Mental Health* 1, 102–4.

French, S. A. and Jeffery, R. W. (1994). Consequences of dieting to lose weight: effects on physical and mental health. *Health Psychology* 13(3), 195–212.

Freud, A. (1936). *The ego and the mechanisms of defence.* Hogarth Press, London.

Freud, A. (1958). Adolescence. I. Adolescence in the psychoanalytic theory. In *The psychoanalytic study of the child* (ed. A. Freud), Vol. XIII. International University Press, New York.

Freud, A. (1966). *Normality and pathology in childhood: assessments of development.* Hogarth Press and Institute of Psychoanalysis, London.

Freud, S. (1892). *The standard edition of the complete psychological works* (ed. J. Strachey), Vol. 1. Hogarth Press, London.

Freud, S. (1893). On the psychical mechanisms of hysterical phenomena. In *The standard edition of the complete psychological works* (ed. J. Strachey), Vol. 3, pp. 25–42. Hogarth Press, London.

Freud, S. (1895a). Obsessions and phobias, their psychical mechanisms and their aetiology. In *The standard edition of the complete psychological works* (ed. J. Strachey), Vol. 3. Hogarth Press, London.

Freud, S. (1895b). The justification for detaching from neurasthenia a particular syndrome: the anxiety of neurosis. *Neurologisches Zentralblatt* 14, 50–66. [Reprinted (transl. J. Riviere) in *Collected papers* 1, 76–106 (1940)].

Freud, S. (1911). Psychoanalytic notes upon an autobiographic account of cases of paranoia. (Schreber). In *The standard edition of the complete psychological works*, Vol. 12, pp. 1–82. Hogarth Press, London.

Freud, S. (1914). On narcissism: an introduction. In *Collected papers*, Vol. 4 (1925), pp. 30–59 (transl. J. Riviere). Hogarth Press and Institute of Psychoanalysis, London.

Freud, S. (1917). Mourning and melancholia. In *The standard edition of the complete psychological works*, Vol. 14, pp. 243–58. Hogarth Press, London.

Freud, S. (1923). Psychoanalysis. In *The standard edition of the complete psychological works*, Vol. 18, pp. 235–54. Hogarth Press, London.

Freud, S. (1924a). *Neurosis and psychosis.* Reprinted in Penguin Freud Library, Vol. 10, pp. 209–18. Penguin, Harmondsworth.

Freud, S. (1924b). *The loss of reality in neurosis and psychosis.* Reprinted in Penguin Freud Library, Vol. 10, pp. 219–29. Penguin, Harmondsworth.

Freud, S. (1927). Fetishism. *International Journal of Psychoanalysis* 9, 161–6. Also in *The standard edition of the complete psychological works*, Vol. 21, pp. 147–57. Hogarth Press, London.

Freud, S. (1935). *An autobiographic study.* Hogarth Press, London.

Friedli, K., King, M. B., Lloyd, M., and Horder, J. (1997). Randomized controlled assessment of non-directive psychotherapy versus routine general practitioner care. *Lancet* 350, 1662–5.

Friedman, L. J. (1962). *Virgin wives: a study of unconsummated marriage.* Tavistock Publications, London.

Friedman, M. and Rosenman, R. H. (1959). Association of specific behaviour pattern with blood and cardiovascular findings. *Journal of the American Medical Association* 169, 1286–96.

Friedman, M., Thorensen, C. E., and Gill, J. J. (1986). Alteration of Type A behaviour and its effect on cardiac recurrences in postmyocardial infarction patients: summary results of the recurrent coronary prevention project. *American Heart Journal* 112, 653–65.

Friedman, T. and Gath, D. (1989). The psychiatric consequences of spontaneous abortion. *British Journal of Psychiatry* 155, 810–30.

Frisch, A., Postilnick, D., Rockah, R., *et al.* (1999). Association of unipolar major depressive disorder with genes of the serotonergic and dopaminergic pathways. *Molecular Psychiatry* 4, 389–92.

Frith, C. (1996). Neuropsychology of schizophrenia. What are the implications of intellectual and experiential abnormalities for the neurobiology of schizophrenia? *British Medical Bulletin* 52, 618–26.

Frith, U. (1991). Autistic psychopathy in childhood. In *Autism and Asperger syndrome* (ed. U. Frith), pp. 37–92. Cambridge University Press, Cambridge.

Fromm-Reichmann, F. (1948). Notes on the development of treatment of schizophrenia by psychoanalytic psychotherapy. *Psychiatry* 11, 263–73.

Frucht, S., Fahn, S., Ford, B. (1999). French horn embouchure dystonia. *Movement Disorders* 14, 171–3.

Frye, M. A., Ketter, T. A., Leverich, G. S., *et al.* (2000). The increasing use of polypharmacotherapy for refractory mood disorders: 22 years of study. *Journal of Clinical Psychiatry* 61, 9–15.

Fryers, T. (2000). Epidemiology of mental retardation. In *The new Oxford textbook of psychiatry.* (eds M. G. Gelder, J. J. López-Ibor Jr, and N. C. Andreasen), Chapter 10.2. Oxford University Press, Oxford.

Fukuda, K., Straus, S. E., Hickie, I. B., Sharpe, M., Dobbins, J. G., and Komaroff, A. L. (1994). Chronic fatigue syndrome: a comprehensive approach to its definitions and management. *Annals of Internal Medicine* 121, 953–9.

Fullerton, C. S., and Ursano, R. J. (eds) (1997). *Post-traumatic stress disorder: acute and long term responses to trauma and disaster.* American Psychiatric Press, Washington and London.

Fulton, M. and Winokur, G. (1993). A comparative study of paranoid and schizoid personality disorders. *British Journal of Psychiatry* 150, 1363–7.

Fundudis, T. (1997). Young child's memory: how good is it? How much do we know about it? *Child Psychology and Child Psychiatry Review* 2, 150–8.

Furlong, R. A., Ho, L., Walsh, C., *et al.* (1998). Analysis and meta-analysis of two serotonin transporter gene polymorphisms in bipolar and unipolar affective disorders. *American Journal of Medical Genetics (Neuropsychiatric Genetics)* 81, 58–63.

Furniss, T., Bingley-Miller, L., and Bentovim, A. (1984). Therapeutic approach to sexual abuse. *Archives of Disease in Childhood* 59, 865–70.

Furukawa, T. A. (1999). From effect size into number needed to treat. *Lancet* 353, 1680.

Fyer, A. J., Mannuzza, S., Chapman, T. F., *et al.* (1993). A direct interview family study of social phobia. *Archives of General Psychiatry* 50, 286.

Fyer, A. J., Mannuzza, S., Chapman, T. F., *et al.* (1995). Specificity in familial aggregation of phobic disorders. *Archives of General Psychiatry* 52, 564–73.

Fyer, M. R., Frances, A. J., Sullivan, T., *et al.* (1988). Co-morbidity of borderline personality disorder. *Archives of General Psychiatry* 45, 348–52.

Gabbard, G. O. (2000). A neurobiologically informed perspective on psychotherapy. *British Journal of Psychiatry* 177, 117–22.

Gagnon, J. and Simon, W. (1973). *Sexual conduct: the social sources of human sexuality.* Aldine, Chicago, IL.

Gale, E. and Ayer, W. A. (1969). Treatment of dental phobias. *Journal of the American Dental Association* 78, 1304–7.

Ganser, S. J. (1898). Über einen eigenartigen hysterischen Dämmerzustand. *Archiv für Psychiatrie und Nervenkrankheiten* 30, 633–40. [Transl. C. E. Schorer in *British Journal of Criminology* 5, 120–6 (1965)].

Garber, H. L. (1988). *The Milwaukee Project: preventing mental retardation in children at risk.* American Association on Mental Retardation, Washington, DC.

Garbutt, J. C., West, S. L., Carey, T. S., *et al.* (1999). Pharmacological treatment of alcohol dependence: a review of the evidence. *Journal of the American Medical Association* 281(14), 1318–25.

Garety, P. and Morris, I. (1984). A new unit for psychiatric patients: organization, attitudes and quality of care. *Psychological Medicine* 14, 183–92.

Garmezy, N. and Mastern, A. S. (1994). Chronic adversities. In *Child and adolescent psychiatry: modern approaches*, 3rd edn (eds M. Rutter, E. Taylor, and L. Hersov), pp.191–208. Blackwell Scientific Publications, Oxford.

Garralda, M. E. (1994). Primary care psychiatry. In *Child and adolescent psychiatry*, 3rd edn (ed M. Rutter, L. Hersov and E. Taylor), pp.1055–70. Blackwell Science, Oxford.

Garralda, E. (2000). The relationship between physical and mental health in children and adolescents. In *The new Oxford textbook of psychiatry* (eds M. G. Gelder, J. J. López-Ibor Jr, and N. C. Andreasen), Chapter 9.3.2. Oxford University Press, Oxford.

Garralda, M. E. (1996). Somatization in children. *Journal of Child Psychiatry and Psychology* 37, 13–33.

Garralda, M. E. and Bailey, D. (1986). Children with psychiatric disorders in primary care. *Journal of Child Psychology and Psychiatry* 27, 611–24.

Garrard, P. and Hodges, J.R. (2000). Semantic dementia: clinical, radiological and pathological perspectives. J Neurol 247, 409–22.

Gask, L. (1992). Training general practitioners to detect and manage emotional disorders. *International Review of Psychiatry* 4, 293–300.

Gastaut, M. (1969). Clinical and electroencephalographic classification of epileptic seizures. *Epilepsia* 10(suppl), 2–21.

Gath, A. (1978). *Down's syndrome and the family*. Academic Press, London.

Gath, A. (2000). Families with a mentally retarded member and their needs. In *The new Oxford textbook of psychiatry* (eds M. G. Gelder, J. J. López-Ibor Jr, and N. C. Andreasen), Chapter 10.8. Oxford University Press, Oxford.

Gath, D., Hassal, C., and Cross, K. W. (1973). Whither psychotic day patients? A study of day patients in Birmingham. *British Medical Journal* 1, 94–8.

Gath, D., Cooper, P., Gattoni, F., and Rockett, D. (1977). *Child guidance and delinquency in a London Borough*. Maudsley Monograph No.24. Oxford University Press, London.

Gath, D., Cooper, P., Bond, A., and Edmonds, G. (1982a). Hysterectomy and psychiatric disorder: II. Demographic psychiatric and physical factors in relation to psychiatric outcome. *British Journal of Psychiatry* 140, 343–50.

Gath, D., Cooper, P., and Day, A. (1982b). Hysterectomy and psychiatric disorder: 1. Levels of psychiatric morbidity before and after hysterectomy. *British Journal of Psychiatry* 140, 335–42.

Gaupp, R. (1974). The scientific significance of the case of Ernst Wagner. In *Themes and variations in European psychiatry*. S. R. Hirsch, and M. Shepherd (eds). John Wright and Sons, Bristol.

Gayan, J., Smith, S. D., Cherny, S. S., *et al.* (1999). Quantitative-trait locus for specific language and reading deficits on chromosome 6p. *American Journal of Human Genetics* 64, 157–64.

Gayford, J. J. (1981). Indecent exposure: a review of the literature. *Medicine, Science and the Law* 21, 233–42.

Gazzaniga, M.S. (2000). Cerebral specialization and interhemispheric communication. Does the corpus callosum enable the human condition? *Brain* 123, 1293–1326.

Geaney, D. P., Ellis, P. M., Soper, N., *et al.* (1992). Single photon emission tomography assessment of cerebral dopamine D_2 receptor blockade in schizophrenia. *Biological Psychiatry* 32, 293–5.

Gebhard, P. H., Raboch, J., and Giese, H. (1970). *The sexuality of women* (transl. C. Bearne). Andre Deutsch, London.

Geddes, J. (1999). Asking structured and focused clinical questions: essential first step of evidence-based practice. *Evidence-based Mental Health* 2, 35–6.

Geddes, J. (2000). From science to practice. In *The new Oxford textbook of psychiatry* (eds M. G. Gelder, J. J. López-Ibor Jr, and N. C. Andreasen), Chapter 1.12. Oxford University Press, Oxford.

Geddes, J. Freemantle, N. Harrison, P. Bebbington, P. (2000). Atypical antipsychotics in the treatment of schizophrenia: systematic overview and meta-regression analysis. *British Medical Journal* 321, 1371–6.

Geddes, J. R. and Harrison, P. J. (1997). Closing the gap between research and practice. *British Journal of Psychiatry* 171, 220–5.

Geddes, J. R. and Lawrie, S. M. (1995). Obstetric complications and schizophrenia: a meta-analysis. *British Journal of Psychiatry* 167, 786–93.

Gelder, M. G. (1991). Adolf Meyer and his influence on British psychiatry. In *150 Years of British psychiatry 1841–1991* (eds G. E. Berrios and H. Freeman), pp. 419–35. Gaskell, London.

Gelder, M. G., Marks, I. M., and Wolff, H. (1978). Desensitization and psychotherapy in phobic states: a controlled enquiry. *British Journal of Psychiatry*, 113, 53–73.

Gelernter, C. S., Uhde, T. W., Cimbolic, P., *et al.* (1991). Cognitive–behavioural and pharmacological treatments of social phobia – a controlled study. *Archives of General Psychiatry* 49, 938.

Gelernter, J. (1999). Clinical molecular genetics. In *Neurobiology of mental illness* (eds D. S. Charney, E. J. Nestler, and B. S. Bunney), pp. 108–20. Oxford University Press, Oxford.

Geller, D. A., Biederman, J., Griffin, S., *et al.* (1996). Comorbidity of obsessive compulsive disorder with disruptive behaviour disorders. *Journal of the American Academy of Child and Adolescent Psychiatry* 35, 1637–46.

Gendreau, P., Little, T., and Goggin, C. (1996). A meta analysis of the predictors of adult offender recidivism: what works. *Criminology* 34, 575–607.

General Medical Council (2000). *Confidentiality: protecting, providing information.* General Medical Council, London.

General Register Office (1968). A glossary of mental disorders. *Studies on medical and population subjects 22.* HMSO, London.

Gentil, V., Lotufo-Neto, F., Andrade, L., *et al.* (1993). Clomipramine, a better reference drug for panic/agoraphobia. I. Effectiveness comparison with imipramine. *Journal of Pharmacology* 7(4), 316–24.

George, M. S., Lisanby, S. H., and Sackheim, H. A. (1999). Transcranial magnetic stimulation: applications in neuropsychiatry. *Archives of General Psychiatry* 56, 300–11.

Geroldi, C., Akkawi, N.M., Galluzzi, S., *et al.* (2000). Temporal lobe asymmetry in patients with Alzheimer's disease with delusions. *Journal of Neurology, Neurosurgery and Psychiatry* 69, 187–91.

Gersons, B. P. R. and Carlier, I. V. E. (1992). Post-traumatic stress disorder: the history of a recent concept. *British Journal of Psychiatry* 161, 742–8.

Geschwind, N. (1965). Disconnexion syndromes in animals and man. *Brain* 88, 237–94, 585–644.

Gibb, W. R. (1989). Dementia and Parkinson's disease. *British Journal of Psychiatry* 154, 596–614.

Gijs, L. and Gooren, L. (1996). Hormonal and psychopharmacological interventions in the treatment of paraphilias. *Journal of Sex Research* 33, 273–90.

Gill, B., Meltzer, H., Hinds, K., and Petticrew, M. (1996). *Psychiatric morbidity among homeless people.* OPCS Surveys of Psychiatric Morbidity in Great Britain. HMSO, London.

Gill, M., Daly, G., Heron, S., *et al.* (1997). Confirmation of association between attention deficit hyperactivity disorder and a dopamine transporter polymorphism. *Molecular Psychiatry* 2, 311–13.

Gillam, S. J., Jarman, B., White, P., and Law, R. (1989). Ethnic differences in consultation rates in urban general practice. *British Medical Journal* 299, 958–60.

Gillberg C. L. (1992). Autism and autistic-like conditions; subclasses among disorders of empathy. *Journal of Child Psychology and Psychiatry* 33, 813–42.

Gilles de la Tourette (1885). Etude sur une affection nerveuse characterisée par l'incoordination motrice accompagnee d'écholalie et de coprolalie. *Archives de Neurologie* 9, 19–42.

Gillies, N. (1976). Homicide in the west of Scotland. *British Journal of Psychiatry* 128, 105–27.

Girela, E., Villanueva, E., Hernandez-Cueto, C., and Luna, J. D. (1994). Comparison of the CAGE questionnaire versus some biochemical markers in the diagnosis of alcoholism. *Alcohol and Alcoholism* 29, 337–43.

Gitlin, M. J. (1993). Lithium-induced renal insufficiency. *Journal of Clinical Psychopharmacology* 13, 276–9.

Gjessing, R. (1947). Biological investigations in endogenous psychoses. *Acta Psychiatrica Scandinavica* (Kbh). Suppl. 47.

Glaister, B. (1982). Muscle relaxation training for fear reduction of patients with psychological problems: a review on controlled studies. *Behaviour Research and Therapy* 20, 493–504.

Glaser, D. (1991). Treatment issues in child sexual abuse. *British Journal of Psychiatry*, 159, 769–82.

Glover, G. R. (1992). *CAPSE–10. Computer assisted PSE10.* World Health Organization, Geneva.

Glover, L. and Pearce, S. (1995). Chronic pelvic pain. In *Treatment of functional somatic symptoms* (eds R. A. Mayou, C. Bass, and M. Sharpe), pp. 313–27. Oxford University Press, Oxford.

Goffman, E. (1961). *Asylums: essays on the social situation of mental patients and other inmates.* Doubleday, New York.

Goktepe, E. O., Young, L. B., and Bridges, P. K. (1975). A further review of the results of stereotactic tractotomy. *British Journal of Psychiatry* 126, 270–81.

Gold, J. N. and Weinberger, D. R. (1991). Frontal lobe structure, function, and connectivity in schizophrenia. In *Neurobiology in psychiatry* (ed. R. Kerwin), Vol. 1, pp. 39–59. Cambridge University Press, Cambridge.

Goldberg, D. (1972). *The detection of psychiatric illness by questionnaire.* Maudsley Monograph No.21. Oxford University Press, London.

Goldberg, D. (ed.) (1997). *The Maudsley handbook of practical psychiatry.* Oxford Medical Publications, Oxford.

Goldberg, D. and Hillier, V. P. (1979). A scaled version of the General Health Questionnaire. *Psychological Medicine* 9, 139–45.

Goldberg, D. and Huxley, P. (1980). *Mental illness in the community*. Tavistock Publications, London.

Goldberg, D. and Huxley, P. (1992). *Common mental disorders: a biosocial model*. Routledge, London.

Goldberg, D., Richels, J., Downing, R., and Hesbacher, P. (1976). A comparison of two psychiatric screening tests. *British Journal of Psychiatry* **129**, 61–7.

Goldberg, D., Steele, J., and Smith, J. (1980). Teaching psychiatric interview techniques to family doctors. *Acta Psychiatrica Scandinavica* **62(suppl 285)**, 41–7.

Goldberg, D., Mann, A., and Tylee, A. (2000). Psychiatry in primary care. In *The new Oxford textbook of psychiatry* (eds M. G. Gelder, J. J. López-Ibor Jr, and N. C. Andreasen), Chapter 7.8. Oxford University Press, Oxford.

Goldberg, D. M., Soleas, G. J., and Levesque, M. (1999). Moderate alcohol consumption: the gentle face of Janus. *Clinical Biochemistry* **32(7)**, 505–18.

Goldberg, E. M. and Morrison, S. L. (1963). Schizophrenia and social class. *British Journal of Psychiatry* **109**, 785–802.

Goldman, E. and Morrison, D. (1984). *Psychodrama: experience and process*. Kendall/Hunt, IA.

Goldman, H. and Morrissey, J. P. (1985). The alchemy of mental health policy: homelessness and the fourth cycle of reform. *American Journal of Public Health* **75**, 727–31.

Goldstein, I. (1986). Arterial revascularisation procedures. *Seminars in Urology* **4**, 252–8.

Goldstein, I., Lue, T. F., Padma-Nathan, H., *et al.* (1998). Oral sildenafil in the treatment of erectile dysfunction. *New England Journal of Medicine* **338**,1397–404.

Goldstein, R. B., Black, D. W., Nasrallah, A., and Winokur, G. (1991). The prediction of suicide-sensitivity, specificity, and predictive value of a multivariate model applied to suicide among 1906 patients with affective disorders. *Archives of General Psychiatry* **48**, 418–22.

Goodman, R. (1987). The developmental neurobiology of language. In *Language development and disorders* (eds W. Yule and M. Rutter), pp. 129–45. MacKeith Press, London.

Goodman, R., and Scott, S. (1997). *Child psychiatry*. Blackwell, Oxford.

Goodman, W. K., Price, L. H., and Rasmussen, S. A. (1989a). The Yale-Brown Obsessive Compulsive Scale. *Archives of General Psychiatry* **46**, 1006–11.

Goodman, W. K., Price, L. H., Rasmussen, S. A., *et al.* (1989b). Efficacy of fluvoxamine in obsessive–compulsive disorder. *Archives of General Psychiatry* **46**, 36–44.

Goodwin, F. K. and Jamison, K. R. (1990). Medical treatment of acute bipolar depression. In *Manic depressive illness* (eds F. K. Goodwin and K. R. Jamison), pp. 630–64. Oxford University Press, Oxford.

Goodwin, G. M. (1999). Prophylaxis of bipolar disorder: how and who should we treat in the long term? *European Neuropsychopharmacology* **9(suppl 4)**, S125–9.

Goodwin, J. (1988). Post-traumatic symptoms in abused children. *Journal of Traumatic Stress* **4**, 475–88.

Goodyer, I. (2000). Emotional disorders with their onset in childhood. In *The new Oxford textbook of psychiatry* (eds M. G. Gelder, J. J. López-Ibor Jr, and N. C. Andreasen), Chapter 9.2.5. Oxford University Press, Oxford.

Goodyer, I., Kolvin, I., and Gatzanis, S. (1985). Recent undesirable life events and psychiatric disorder in childhood and adolescence. *British Journal of Psychiatry* **147**, 517–23.

Goodyer, I. M., Kolvin, I., and Gatzanis, S. (1987). The impact of recent undesirable life events on psychiatric disorders in childhood and adolescence. *British Journal of Psychiatry* **151**, 179–84.

Goodyer, I., Ashby, L., Altham, P. M. E. and Vize, P. J. C. (1993). Temperament and major depression in 11–16 year olds. *Journal of Child psychology and Psychiatry* **34**, 1409–23.

Gordon, D., Burge, D., Hammen, C., *et al.* (1989). Observations of interactions of depressed women with their children. *American Journal of Psychiatry* **146**, 50–5.

Gould, M. S., Wallenstein, S., and Kleinman, M. (1990). Time-space clustering of teenage suicide. *American Journal of Epidemiology* **131**, 71–8.

Gould, R. A., Buckminster, S., Pollack, M. H., *et al.* (1997). Cognitive–behavioral and pharmacological treatment for social phobia: a meta-analysis. *Clinical Psychology: Science and Practice* **4**, 291–306.

Gournay, K. (2000). Role of the community psychiatric nurse in the management of schizophrenia. *Advances in Psychiatric Treatment* **6**, 243–51.

Gournay, K. and Brooking, J. (1994). Community psychiatric nurses in primary health care. *British Journal of Psychiatry* **165**, 231–8.

Grabowski, J. and Schmitz, J. M. (1998). Psychologic treatment of substance abuse. *Current Opinion in Psychiatry* 11, 289–93.

Graham, P. (1991). *Child psychiatry: a developmental approach*, 2nd edn. Oxford University Press, Oxford.

Graham, P. and Rutter, M. (1968). Organic brain dysfunction and child psychiatric disorder. *British Medical Journal* 3, 695–700.

Graham, P. and Stevenson, J. (1987). Temperament and psychiatric disorder: the genetic contribution to behaviour in childhood. *Australian and New Zealand Journal of Psychiatry* 21, 267–74.

Graham, P., Turk, J., and Verhulst, F. (1999). *Child Psychiatry, a developmental approach*, 3rd edn. Oxford University Press, Oxford.

Grahame-Smith, D. G. and Aronson, J. K. (2001). *Oxford textbook of clinical pharmacology and drug therapy*, 3rd edn. Oxford University Press, Oxford.

Grant, I. and Atkinson, J. H. (2000). Neuropsychiatric aspects of HIV infection nd AIDS. In *Comprehensive textbook of psychiatry*, 7th edn (eds B. J. Sadock and V. A. Sadock). Lippincott, Williams & Wilkins, Philadelphia.

Green, R. (1974). *Sexual identity conflict in children and adults*. Duckworth, London.

Green, R. (1985). Atypical psychosexual development. In *Child and adolescent psychiatry*, 2nd edn (eds M. Rutter and L. Hersov). Blackwell Scientific Publications, Oxford.

Green, R. (1998). Transsexual's children. *International Journal of Transgenderism* 2, 1–7.

Green, R. (2000a). Gender identity disorder in adults. In *The new Oxford textbook of psychiatry* (eds M. G. Gelder, J. J. López-Ibor Jr, and N. C. Andreasen), Chapter 4.11.4. Oxford University Press, Oxford.

Green, R. (2000b). Gender identity disorder in children and adolescents. In *The new Oxford textbook of psychiatry* (eds M. G. Gelder, J. J. López-Ibor Jr, and N. C. Andreasen), Chapter 9.2.12. Oxford University Press, Oxford.

Green, R. and Fleming, D (1991). Transsexual surgery follow-up: status in the 1990s. In *Annual review of sex research* (eds J. Bancroft, C. Davis, and D. Weinstein). Society for Scientific Study of Sex, Mt Vernon, IA.

Greenhalgh, T. (1997). Papers that summarise other papers (systematic reviews and meta-analyses). *British Medical Journal* 315, 672–5.

Greenson, R. R. (1967). *The techniques and practice of psychoanalysis*. Hogarth Press, London.

Greer, S. (1969). The prognosis of anxiety states. In *Studies in anxiety* (ed. M. H. Lader), pp.151–7. Royal Medicopsychological Association, London.

Greist, J. H. and Greist, G. L. (1981). *Fearless flying: a passenger guide to modern airline travel*. Nelson Hall, Chicago.

Griesinger, W. (1867). *Mental pathology and therapeutics*, 2nd edn (transl. C. Lockhart Robertson and J. Rutherford). New Sydenham Society, London.

Griffiths, J., Ravindran, A. V., Merali, Z., and Anisman, H. (2000). Dysthymia: a review of pharmacological and behavioral factors. *Molecular Psychiatry* 5, 242–61.

Growden, J. H. and Rosser, M. N. (eds) (1998). *The dementias*.Blue Books of Practical Neurology (Vol 19). Butterworth-Heinemann, Oxford.

Grundy, E. (1987). Community care for the elderly 1976–84. *British Medical Journal* 294, 626–9.

Grundy, E (1996). Population review: (5). The population aged 60 and over. *Population Trends* 84, 14–20.

Gual, A. and Colom, J. (1997). Why has alcohol consumption declined in countries of southern Europe? *Addiction* 92(**suppl** 1), S21–31.

Gudjonsson, G. H. (1990). Psychological and psychiatric aspects of shoplifting. *Medicine, Science and Law* 30, 45–51.

Gudjonsson, G. H. (1992). *The psychology of interrogations, confessions and testimony*. Wiley, Chichester.

Gunn, J. (2000). Future directions for treatment in forensic psychiatry. *British Journal of Psychiatry* 176, 332–8.

Gunn, J. and Taylor, P. J. (1993). *Forensic psychiatry: clinical, legal and ethical issues*. Butterworth-Heinemann, London.

Gunn, J., Maden, A., and Swinton, M. (1991). Treatment needs of prisoners with psychiatric disorders. *British Medical Journal* 303, 338–41.

Gunn, M. and Wheat, K. (2000). General principles of law relating to people with mental disorders. In *The new Oxford textbook of psychiatry* (eds M. G. Gelder, J. J. López-Ibor Jr, and N. C Andreasen), Chapter 11.1. Oxford University Press, Oxford.

Gunnell, D. G., Peters, T. J., Kammerling, R. M., and Brooks, J. (1995). Relation between parasuicide, suicide, psychiatric admissions, and socio-economic deprivation. *British Medical Journal* 311, 226–30.

Guo, Z., Cupples, L.A., Kurz, A. *et al.* (2000). Head injury and the risk of AD in the MIRAGE study. *Neurology* 54, 1316–23.

Gureje, O., Üstün, T. B., and Simon, G. E. (1997). The syndrome of hypochondriasis: a cross-national study in primary care. *Psychological Medicine,* 27, 1001–10.

Gureje, O., Von Korff, M., Simon, G. E., and Gater, R. (1998). Persistent pain and well being: a World Health Organization Study in Primary Care. *Journal of the American Medical Association* 280, 147–51.

Gurling, H. M. D. and Cook, C. C. H. (1999). The genetic predisposition to alcohol dependence. *Current Opinion in Psychiatry* 12, 269–75.

Gurman, A. S. (1979). Research on marital and family therapy: progress, perspective and prospect. In *Handbook of psychotherapy and behaviour change*, 2nd edn (eds S. L. Garfield and A. E. Bergin). Wiley, New York.

Gurman, A. S. and Kriskern, D. P. (1991). *Handbook of family therapy*. Brunner-Mazel, New York.

Gustafson, L. (2000). Frontotemporal dementias. In *The new Oxford textbook of psychiatry* (eds M. G. Gelder, J. J. López-Ibor Jr, and N. C. Andreasen), Chapter 4.1.4. Oxford University Press, Oxford.

Guthrie, E., Creed, F., Dawson, D., and Tomenson, B. (1991). A controlled trial of psychological treatment for the irritable bowel syndrome. *Gastroenterology* 100, 450–7.

Guthrie, E., Creed, F., Dawson, D., Tomenson, B. (1993). A randomised controlled trila of psychotherapy in patients with refractory irritable bowel syndrome. *British Journal of Psychiatry* 163, 315–321.

Guze, S. (1989). Biological psychiatry: is there any other kind? *Psychological Medicine* 19, 315–23.

Haaga, D. A. F. and Beck, A. T. (1992). Cognitive therapy. In *Handbook of affective disorders* (ed. E. S. Paykel), pp. 511–23. Churchill Livingstone, Edinburgh.

Hachinski, V. (1999). Stalin's last years: delusions or dementia? *European Journal of Neurology* 6, 129–32.

Hachinski, V., Lassen, N. A., and Marshall, J. (1974). Multi-infarct dementia. *Lancet* 2, 207–9.

Hack, M., Taylor, H. G., Klein, N., *et al.* (1994). School-age outcomes in children with birth weights under 750 g. *New England Journal of Medicine* 331, 753–9.

Hackett, T. P. and Weissman, A. (1962). The treatment of the dying. *Current Psychiatric Therapy* 2, 121–6.

Hacking, I. (1998). *Mad travellers. Reflections on the reality of transient mental illnesses.* Free Association Books, London.

Häfner, H., Maurer, K., Loffler, W., and Riecher-Rossler, A. (1993). The influence of age and sex on the onset and early course of schizophrenia. *British Journal of Psychiatry* 162, 80–6.

Haig, R. A. (1992). Management of depression in patients with advanced cancer. *Medical Journal of Australia* 156, 499–503.

Hale, R., Minn, C., and Zachary, A. (2000). Assessment and management of sexual offenders. In *The new Oxford textbook of psychiatry* (eds M. G. Gelder, J. J. López-Ibor Jr, and N. C Andreasen), Chapter 11.4.2. Oxford University Press, Oxford.

Haley, J. (1963). *Strategies of psychotherapy*. Grune and Stratton, New York.

Hall, W. and Solowij, N. (1998). Adverse effects of cannabis. *Lancet* 352, 1611–16.

Hallgren, B. (1960). Nocturnal enuresis in twins. *Acta Psychiatrica Scandinavica* 35, 73–90.

Halligan P, Bass C, Marshall J (eds). (2001). *Contemporary approaches to the study of hysteria. Clinical and theoretical perspectives* . Oxford Medical Publications, Oxford University Press.

Hamburg, D. A., Artz, P., Reiss, E., *et al.* (1953). Clinical importance of emotional problems in the care of patients with burns. *New England Journal of Medicine* 248, 355–9.

Hamer, D. H., Hu, S., Magnuson, V. L., *et al.* (1993). A linkage between DNA markers on the X chromosome and male sexual orientation. *Science* 261, 321–7.

Hamilton, M. (1959). The assessment of anxiety states by rating. *British Journal of Medical Psychology* 32, 50–5.

Hamilton, M. (1967). Development of a rating scale for primary depressive illness. *British Journal of Social and Clinical Psychology* 6, 278–96.

Hamilton, M. (ed.) (1984). *Fish's schizophrenia*, 3rd edn. Wright, Bristol

Hanson, K (1998). Predicting relapse: a meta analysis of sexual offender recidivism studies. *Journal of Consulting and Clinical Psychology* 66, 348–62.

Hare, E. H. (1959). The origin and spread of dementia paralytica. *Journal of Mental Science* 105, 594–626.

Hare, E. H. (1973). A short note on pseudo-hallucinations. *British Journal of Psychiatry* 122, 469–76.

Hare, E. H. and Shaw, G. K. (1965). *Mental health on a new housing estate: a comparative study of two districts of Croydon*. Maudsley Monograph No. 12. Oxford University Press, London.

Harper, P. S. (1993). Clinical consequences of isolating the gene for Huntington's disease. *British Medical Journal* 307, 397–8.

Harrington, R. (1994). Affective disorders. In *Child and adolescent psychiatry: modern approaches* (eds M. Rutter, E. Taylor, and L. Hersov), pp.330–50. Blackwell Scientific Publications, Oxford.

Harrington, R. C., Fudge, H., Rutter, M., Pickles, A., and Hill, J. (1990). Adult outcomes of childhood and adolescent depression in psychiatric status. *Archives of General Psychiatry* 47, 465–73.

Harrington, R. C., Fudge, H., Rutter, M. L., *et al.* (1993). Child and adult depression: a test of continuities with data from a family study. *British Journal of Psychiatry* 162, 627–33.

Harrington, R. C., Whittaker, J., and Shoebridge, P. (1998a). Psychological treatment of depression in children and adolescents: a review of treatment research. *British Journal of Psychiatry*, 173, 291–8.

Harrington, R., Whittaker, J., Shoebridge, P., *et al.* (1998b). Systematic review of the efficacy of cognitive–behaviour therapies in childhood and adolescent depressive disorder. *British Medical Journal* 316, 1559–63.

Harris, E. C. and Barraclough, B. M. (1995). Suicide as an outcome for medical disorders. *Medicine* 73, 281–96.

Harris, E. C. and Barraclough, B. (1997). Suicide as an outcome for mental disorders: a meta-analysis. *British Journal of Psychiatry* 170, 205–28.

Harris, E. C. and Barraclough, B. (1998). Excess mortality of mental disorder. *British Journal of Psychiatry* 173, 11–53.

Harris, J. C. (1996). Childhood disintegrative disorder. *Developmental Neuropsychiatry* 2, 239–43.

Harrison, F. (1991). The Children's Act 1989. *Journal of the Medical Defence Union* 4, 82–3.

Harrison, G., Owens, D., Holton, A. *et al.* (1988). A prospective study of severe mental disorder in Afro-Caribbean patients. *Psychological Medicine* 18, 643–57.

Harrison, G., Mason, P., Glazebrook, C., *et al.* (1994). Residence of incident cohort of psychotic patients after 13 years of follow-up. *British Medical Journal* 308, 813–19.

Harrison, P. J. (2000a). The neurobiology of schizophrenia. In *The new Oxford textbook of psychiatry* (eds M. G. Gelder, J. J. López-Ibor Jr, and N. C. Andreasen), Chapter 4.3.5.2. Oxford University Press, Oxford, Oxford.

Harrison, P. J. (2000b). Dopamine and schizophrenia – proof at last? *Lancet* 356, 958–9.

Hart, S., Binggeli, N., And Brassard, M. (1998). Evidence for the effects of psychological maltreatment. *Journal of Emotional Abuse* 1, 27–58.

Harvey, A. G. and Bryant, R. A. (1998). The relationship between acute stress disorder and post-traumatic stress disorder: a prospective evaluation of motor vehicle accident survivors. *Journal of Consulting and Clinical Psychology* 66, 507–12.

Harvey, P. D. and Keefe, R. S. (2001). Studies of cognitive changes in patients with schizophrenia following novel antipsychotic treatment. *American Journal of Psychiatry* 158, 176–84.

Harvey, I., Nelson, S. J., Lyons, R. A., *et al.* (1998). A randomized controlled trial and economic evaluation of counselling in primary care. *British Journal of General Practice* 48, 1043–8.

Harwood, D. and Jacoby, R. (2000). Suicidal behaviour among the elderly. In *The international handbook of suicide and attempted suicide* (eds K. Hawton and K. van Heeringen). John Wiley & Sons, Chichester.

Haug, J. O. (1962). Pneumoencephalographic studies in mental disease. *Acta Psychiatrica Scandinavica Suppl* 165, 1–114.

Hawton, K. E. (1985). *Sex therapy: a practical guide*. Oxford University Press, Oxford.

Hawton, K. (1990). Self-cutting: can it be prevented? In *Dilemmas and difficulties in the management of psychiatric patients* (eds K. Hawton and P. Cowen). Oxford University Press, Oxford.

Hawton, K. (2000a). Treatment of suicide attempters and prevention of suicide and attempted suicide. In *The new Oxford textbook of psychiatry* (eds M. G. Gelder, J. J. López-Ibor Jr, and N. C. Andreasen), Chapter 4.15.4. Oxford University Press, Oxford.

Hawton, K. (2000b). General hospital management of suicide attempters. In *The international handbook of suicide and attempted suicide* (eds K. Hawton and K. van Heeringen), John Wiley & Sons, Chichester.

Hawton, K. and Fagg, J. (1988). Suicide and other causes of death following attempted suicide. *British Journal of Psychiatry* **152**, 359–66.

Hawton, K. and van Heeringen, K. (eds) (2000). *The international handbook of suicide and attempted suicide.* John Wiley & Sons, Chichester.

Hawton, K. E. and Oppenheimer, C. (1983). Women's sexual problems. In *Women's problems in general practice* (eds A. Anderson and A. McPherson). Oxford University Press, Oxford.

Hawton, K. E., Catalan, J., Martin, P., and Fagg, J. (1986). Long term outcome of sex therapy. *Behaviour Research and Therapy* **24**, 377–85.

Hawton, K. E., McKeown, S., Day, A., *et al.* (1987). Evaluation of out-patient counselling compared with general practitioner care following overdoses. *Psychological Medicine* **17**, 751–62.

Hawton, K., Fagg, J., and McKeown, P. (1989). Alcoholism, alcohol and attempted suicide. *Alcohol and Alcoholism* **24**, 3–9.

Hawton, K., Arensman, E., Townsend, E., *et al.* (1998). Deliberate self harm: systematic review of efficacy of psychosocial and pharmacological treatments in preventing repetition. *British Medical Journal* **317**, 441–7.

Hawton, K. E., Simkin, S,. Deeks, J. J., *et al* (1999). Effects of a drug overdose in a television drama on presentations to hospital for self poisoning: time series and questionnaire study. *British Medical Journal* **318**, 972–7.

Hay, G. G. (1970). Dysmorphophobia. *British Journal of Psychiatry* **116**, 399–406.

Hay, P. J., Sachdev, P. S., Cummings, S., *et al.* (1993). Treatment of obsessive–compulsive disorder by psychosurgery. *Acta Psychiatrica Scandinavica* **87**, 197–207.

Haynes, B. (1999). Can it work? Does it work? Is it worth it? The testing of healthcare interventions is evolving. *British Medical Journal* **319**, 652–3.

Heath, A. C., Bucholz, K. K., Madden, P. A., *et al.* (1997). Genetic and environmental contributions to alcohol dependence risk in a national twin sample: consistency of findings in women and men. *Psychological Medicine* **27**(6), 1381–96.

Heath, A. C., Madden, P. A., Bucholz, K. K., *et al.* (1999). Genetic differences in alcohol sensitivity and the inheritance of alcoholism risk. *Psychological Medicine* **29** (5), 1069–81.

Heber, R. (1981). A manual on terminology and classification in mental retardation. *American Journal of Mental Deficiency* **Suppl. 64**.

Hecker, E. (1871). Die Hebephrenie. *Virchows Archiv für Pathologie and Anatomie* **52**, 394–429. (See *American Journal of Psychiatry* **142**, 1265–71).

Heidensohn, F. (1994a). Women as perpetrators and victims of crime: a sociological perspective. *British Journal of Psychiatry* **158**(suppl 10), 50–4.

Heidensohn, F. (1994b). Gender and crime. In *The Oxford handbook of criminology* (ed. M. Maguire), pp.997–1040. Clarendon Press, Oxford.

Heim, C. and Nemeroff, C. B. (2000). The impact of early adverse experiences on brain systems involved in the pathophysiology of anxiety and affective disorders. *Biological Psychiatry* **46**, 1509–22.

Heim, C., Newport, J. D., Heit, S., *et al.* (2000). Pituitary-adrenal and autonomic responses to stress in women after sexual and physical abuse in childhood. *Journal of the American Medical Association* **284**, 592–7.

Heimberg, R. G., Liebowitz, M. R., Hope, D. A., *et al.* (1998). Cognitive–behavioral group therapy versus phenelzine in social phobia: 12 week outcome. *Archives of General Psychiatry* **55**, 1133–41.

Heinman, J. R. and LoPiccolo, J. (1983). Clinical outcome of sex therapy. *Archives of General Psychiatry* **40**, 443–9.

Helzer, J. E. and Canino, G. J. (1992). Comparative analysis of alcoholism in ten cultural regions. In *Alcoholism in North America, Europe and Asia* (eds J. E. Helzer and G. J. Canino), pp. 289–308. Oxford University Press, Oxford.

Hemingway, H. and Marmot, M. (1999). Psychosocial factors in the aetiology and prognosis of coronary heart disease: systematic review of prospective cohort studies. *British Medical Journal* **318**, 1460–7.

Hemmings, A. (1997). Counselling in primary care: a randomized controlled trial. *Patient Education and Counselling* **32**, 219–30.

Hemsley, D. R. (1993). A simple (or simplistic?) cognitive model for schizophrenia. *Behaviour Research Therapeutics* **31**, 633–45.

Henderson, A. S. (1990). The social psychiatry of later life. *British Journal of Psychiatry* **156**, 645–53.

Henderson, A. S. (1994). *Dementia*. World Health Organization, Geneva.

Henderson, A. S. and Blackwood, D. H. R. (1999). Molecular genetics in psychiatric epidemiology: the promise and challenge. *Psychological Medicine* **29**, 1265–71.

Henderson, D. C., Cagliero, E., Gray, C., *et al.* (2000). Clozapine, diabetes mellitus, weight gain, and lipid abnormalities: a five-year naturalistic study. *American Journal of Psychiatry* **157**, 975–81.

Henderson, D. K. (1939). *Psychopathic states*. Chapman & Hall, London.

Henderson, D. K. and Gillespie, R. D. (1930*). Textbook of psychiatry for students and practitioners*, 2nd edn. Oxford University Press, London.

Henderson, S. E. (1987). The assessment of 'clumsy' children: old and new approaches. *Journal of Child Psychology and Psychiatry* **28**, 511–27.

Hendin, H. and Haas, A. P. (1991). Suicide and guilt as manifestations of PTSD in Vietnam combat veterans. *American Journal of Psychiatry* **148**, 586–91.

Heninger, G. R. (1999). Psychiatric research in the 21st century: opportunities and limitations. *Molecular Psychiatry* **4**, 429–36.

Hennessy, S., Bilker, W. B., Knauss, J. S., Margolis, D. J., Kimmel, S. E., Reynolds, R. E., Glasser, D. B., Morrison, M. F. and Strom, B. L. (2002) Cardiac arrest and ventricular arrhythmia in patients taking antipsychotic drugs: cohort study using administrative data. *British Medical Journal* **235**, 1070–1072

Henretta, J. C. (1994). Recent trends in retirement. *Reviews in Clinical Gerontology* **4**, 71–81.

Herbert, J. (1997). Stress, the brain, and mental illness. *British Medical Journal* **315**, 530–5.

Herbert, T. B. and Cohen, S. (1993). Depression and immunity: a meta-analytic review. *Psychological Bulletin* **113**, 472–86.

Heresco-Levy, U., Javitt, D. C., Ermilov, M., *et al.* (1999). Efficacy of high-dose glycine in the treatment of enduring negative symptoms of schizophrenia. *Archives of General Psychiatry* **56**, 29–36.

Hermelin, B. and O'Connor, N. (1983). The idiot savant: flawed genius or clever Hans? *Psychological Medicine* **13**, 479–81.

Herrman, H., McGorry, P., Bennett, P., *et al.* (1989). Prevalence of severe mental disorders in disaffiliated and homeless people in inner Melbourne. *American Journal of Psychiatry* **146**, 1179–84.

Hersov, L. (1960). Refusal to go to school. *Journal of Child Psychology and Psychiatry* **1**, 137–45.

Hersov, L. (1994). Faecal soiling. In *Child and adolescent psychiatry: modern approaches*, 3rd edn (eds M. Rutter, E. Taylor, and L. Hersov.), pp. 520–8. Blackwell Science, Oxford.

Heston, L. J. (1966). Psychiatric disorders in foster home reared children of schizophrenic mothers. *British Journal of Psychiatry* **112**, 819–25.

Hetherington, E. M., Cox, M., and Cox, R. (1985). Long-term effects of divorce on the adjustments of children. *Journal of the American Academy of Child Psychiatry* **24**, 518–30.

Hewett, D. and Nind, M. (eds) (1998). Interaction in action: reflections on the use of intensive interaction. David Fulton, London.

Hewett, S. H. and Ryan, P. J. (1975). Alternatives to living in psychiatric hospitals – a pilot study. *British Journal of Hospital Medicine* **14**, 65–70.

Hibbert, G. A. (1984a). Ideational components of anxiety, their origin and content. *British Journal of Psychiatry* **144**, 618–24.

Hibbert, G. A. (1984b). Hyperventilation as a cause of panic attacks. *British Medical Journal* **288**, 263–4.

Hickling, E. J. and Blanchard, E. B. (1999). Current understanding, treatment and law. In *The international handbook of road traffic accidents and psychological trauma*. Pergamon, Oxford.

Higgins, S. R., Budney, A. J., Bickel, W. K. *et al.* (1993). Achieving cocaine abstinence with a behavioural approach. *American Journal of Psychiatry* **150**, 763–9.

Higgitt, A. and Fonagy, P. (1993). Psychotherapy in borderline and narcissistic personality disorder. In *Personality disorder review* (eds P. Tyrer and G. Stein), pp.225–61. Gaskell, London.

Hill, D. (1952). EEG in episodic psychotic and psychopathic behaviour: a classification of data. *Electroencephalography and Clinical Neurophysiology* **4**, 419–42.

Hiller, W., Zaudig, M., and Bose, M. V. (1989). The overlap between depression and anxiety on different levels of psychopathology. *Journal of Affective Disorders* **16**, 223–31.

Himmelhoch, J. M., Thase, M. E., Mallinger, A. G., and Houck, P. (1991). Tranylcypromine versus imipramine in anergic bipolar depression. *American Journal of Psychiatry* **148**, 910–16.

Hindley, P. and Kitson, N. (1999). *Mental health and deafness*. Whurr, London.

Hinshelwood, R. (1999). The difficult patient. *British Journal of Psychiatry*, **174**, 187–90.

Hirono, N., Mega, M.S., Dinov, I.D., Mishkin, F. and Cummings, J.L. (2000). Left frontotemporal hypoperfusion is associated with aggression in patients with dementia. *Archives of Neurology* 57, 861–6.

Hirsch, S. and Leff, J. (1975). *Abnormalities in parents of schizophrenics*. Maudsley Monograph No 22. Oxford University Press, London.

Hirsch, S. R. (1987). Planning for bed needs and resource requirements in acute psychiatry. *Bulletin of the Royal College of Psychiatrists* 11, 398–407.

Hirsch, R. D. and Vollhardt, B. R.. (2000). Elder maltreatment. In *New Oxford Textbook of Psychiatry* (eds M. G. Gelder, J. J. López-Ibor, N. C. Andreasen). Oxford University Press.

Hirschfeld, M. (1944). *Sexual anomalies and perversions: physical and psychological development and treatment*. Aldor, London.

Hirschfeld, R. M. A., Allen, M. H., McEvoy, J. P., *et al.* (1999). Safety and tolerability of oral loading divalproex sodium in acutely manic bipolar patients. *Journal of Clinical Psychiatry* 60, 815–18.

Hoag, M. J. and Burlingame, G. M. (1997). Evaluating the effectiveness of child and adolescent group treatment: a meta-analytic review. *Journal of Clinical Child Psychology*, 26, 234–46.

Hobbs, M., Mayou, R., Harrison, B., and Worlock, P. (1996). A randomized controlled trial of psychological debriefing for road traffic accidents *British Medical Journal* 7, 1438–9.

Hobbs, N. (1994). Childhood sexual abuse: how women can be helped to overcome its long-term effects. In *Dilemmas and difficulties in the management of psychiatric patients* (eds K. Hawton and P. Cowen), pp.183–96. Oxford University Press, Oxford.

Hodges, J. R. (1994). *Cognitive assessment for clinicians*. Oxford University Press, Oxford.

Hoehn-Saric, R., Pearlson, G. D., Harris, G. J., *et al.* (1991). Effects of fluoxetine on regional cerebral blood flow in obsessive–compulsive patients. *American Journal of Psychiatry* 148, 1243–5.

Hofman, A., Rocca, W. A., Brayne, C., *et al.* (1991). The prevalence of dementia in Europe: a collaborative study of 1980–1990 findings. *International Journal of Epidemiology* 20, 736–48.

Hogan, D. M. (1998). Annotation: the psychological development and welfare of children of opiate and cocaine users: review and research needs. *Journal of Child Psychology and Psychiatry* 39, 609–20.

Holden, N. (1987). Late paraphrenia or the paraphrenias? *British Journal of Psychiatry* 150, 635–9.

Holden, U. and Woods R. T. (1995). *Positive approaches to dementia care*. Churchill Livingstone, Edinburgh.

Holland, A. J. (1994). Down's syndrome and Alzheimer's disease. In *Mental health in mental retardation: recent advances and practices* (ed. N. Bouras), pp.154–67. Cambridge University Press, Cambridge.

Holland, A. J. (1997). Forensic psychiatry and learning disability. In *The psychiatry of learning disabilities* (ed. O. Russell), pp. 259–73. Gaskell, London.

Holland, A. J., Hon. J., Huppert, F. A., *et al.* (1998). Population-based study of the prevalence and presentation of dementia in individuals with mental retardation. *Journal of Intellectual Disability Research* 41, 152–64.

Holland, J. C. (1998). *Psycho-oncology*. Oxford University Press, Oxford.

Holland, J. C. (1999). Update: NCCN practice guidelines for the management of psychosocial distress. *Oncology* 13(11A), 459–507,

Hollander, E., Liebowicz, M. R., DeCaria, C., *et al.* (1990). Treatment of depersonalization with serotonin reuptake blockers. *Journal of Clinical Psychopharmacology* 32, 468–9.

Hollander, E., Neville, D., Frenkel, M., *et al.* (1992). Body dysmorphic disorder. Diagnostic issues and related disorders. *Psychosomatics* 33, 156–65.

Hollingshead, A. B. and Redlich, F. C. (1958). *Social class and mental illness: a community study*. Wiley, New York.

Hollins, S., and Esterhayzen, A. (1997). Bereavement and grief in adults with learning disabilities: interventions to support clients and carers. *Journal of Intellectual Disability Research* 41, 331–8.

Hollister, J. M. and Cannon, T. D. (1999). Neurodevelopmental disturbances in the aetiology of schizophrenia. In *Disorders of brain and mind*. (eds M. A. Ron and A. S. David), pp. 280–302. Cambridge University Press, Cambridge.

Holmes, J. (2000). Object relations, attachment theory, self-psychology, and interpersonal psychoanalysis. In *The new Oxford textbook of psychiatry* (eds M. G. Gelder, J. J. López-Ibor Jr, and N. C. Andreasen), Chapter 3.3.2. Oxford University Press, Oxford.

Holmes, P. and Karp, M. (1991). *Psychodrama, inspiration and technique*. Tavistock Publications and Routledge, London.

Holmes, T. and Rahe, R. H. (1967). The social adjustment rating scale. *Journal of Psychosomatic Research* 11, 213–18.

Holroyd, S. (2000). Personality disorders in the elderly. In *The new Oxford textbook of psychiatry* (eds. M. G. Gelder, J. J. López-Ibor Jr, and N. C. Andreasen), Chapter 8.5.6. Oxford University Press, Oxford.

Holsboer, F. (1992). The hypothalamic-pituitary-adrenocortical system. In *Handbook of affective disorders* (ed. E. S. Paykel), pp. 267–87. Churchill Livingstone, Edinburgh.

Holzman, P. S. (2000). Eye movements and the search for the essence of schizophrenia. *Brain Research Reviews* 31, 350–6.

Home Office (1998). Research, Development and Statistics Directorate. Information on the criminal justice system in England and Wales. *Digest 4*. Home Office, London.

Hope, T. (1994). The structure of wandering in dementia. *International Journal of Geriatric Psychiatry* 9, 149–55.

Hope, T., Hicks, N., Reynolds, D. J. M., *et al.* (1998). Rationing and the Health Authority. *British Medical Journal* 317, 1067–9.

Hopkins, A., Shorvan, S., Cascino, G. (1999). *Epilpsey* (2nd ed) Chapman and Hall Medical, London.

Hopkins, A. (1992). The management of patients with chronic headache not due to obvious structural disease. In *Medical symptoms not explained by organic disease* (ed. F. Creed), pp. 34–46. Royal College of Psychiatrists, London.

Horney, K. (1939). *New ways in psychoanalysis*. Kegan Paul, London.

Horowitz, M. J. (1986). *Stress response systems*, 2nd edn. Jason Aronson, NJ.

Horst, W. D. and Preskorn, S. H. (1998). Mechanisms of action and clinical characteristics of three atypical antidepressants: venlafaxine, nefazodone, bupropion. *Journal of Affective Disorders* 51, 237–54.

Horton, R. W. (1992). The neurochemistry of depression: evidence derived from studies of post-mortem brain tissue. *Molecular Aspects of Medicine* 13, 191–203.

Horwath, E., Lish, J., Johnson, J., *et al.* (1993). Agoraphobia without panic: clinical reappraisal of an epidemiologic finding. *American Journal of Psychiatry* 150, 1496–501.

Hotopf, M., Churchill, R., and Lewis, G. (1999). Pragmatic randomised controlled trials in psychiatry. *British Journal of Psychiatry* 175, 217–23.

Hotopf, M. H., Noah, N. Wessely, S. (1996). Chronic fatigue and psychiatric morbidity following viral meningitis: a controlled study. *Journal of Neurology, Neurosurgery, and Psychiatry* 60, 504–509.

Hotopf, M., Wilson-Jones, C., Mayou, R., Wadsworth, M., and Wessely, S. (2000). Childhood predictors of adult medically unexplained hospitalisations. *British Journal of Psychiatry* 176, 273–80.

Hoult, J., Reynolds, I., Charbonneau-Powis, M., *et al.* (1983). Psychiatric hospital versus community treatment: the results of a randomised trial. *Australia and New Zealand Journal of Psychiatry* 17, 160–7.

House, A. (1988). Mood disorders in the physically ill – problems of definition and measurement. *Journal of Psychosomatic Research* 32, 345–353.

House, A., Dennis, M., Molyneux, A., *et al.* (1989). Emotionalism after stroke. *British Medical Journal* 298, 991–4.

House, A., Dennis, M., Mogridge, L., *et al.* (1991). Mood disorders in the year after first stroke. *British Journal of Psychiatry* 158, 83–92.

House, R. M. (2000). Transplantation surgery. In *Psychiatric care of the medical patient* (eds A. Stoudemire, B. S. Fogel, and D. B. Greenberg). Oxford University Press, New York.

Housekamp, B. M. and Foy, D. W. (1991). The assessment of posttraumatic stress disorder in battered women. *Journal of Interpersonal Violence* 6(3), 367–75.

Houston, F. and Royse, A. B. (1954). Relationship between deafness and psychotic illness. *Journal of Mental Science* 100, 900–3.

Howard, R. (2000). Schizophrenia and paranoid disorders of late life. In *The new Oxford textbook of psychiatry* (eds. M. G. Gelder, J. J. López-Ibor Jr, and N. C. Andreasen), Chapter 8.5.3. Oxford University Press, Oxford.

Howard, R. and Levy, R. (2001). Late-onset schizophrenia and very late onset schizophrenia-like psychosis. In *Psychiatry in the elderly*, 3rd edn (eds R. Jacoby and C. Oppenheimer). Oxford University Press, Oxford.

Howard, R., Mellers, J., Petty, R., *et al.* (1995). Magnetic resonance imaging volumetric measurements of the superior temporal gyrus, hippocampus, parahippocampal gyrus, frontal and temporal lobes in late paraphrenia. *Psychological Medicine* 25, 495–503.

Howard, R., Rabins, P. V., Seeman, M. V., and Jeste, D. V. (2000). Late onset schizophrenia and very-late-onset-schizophrenia-like-psychosis: an international consensus. *American Journal of Psychiatry* 157, 172–8.

Howlin, P. (1994). Special educational treatment. In *Child and adolescent psychiatry: modern approaches*, 3rd edn (eds M. Rutter, E. Taylor, and L. Hersov), pp. 1071–88. Blackwell Scientific Publications, Oxford.

Howlin, P. (1998). Practitioner review: psychological and educational treatments for autism. *Journal of Child Psychology and Psychiatry and Allied Disciplines* 39, 307–22.

Hsiao, M. C., Liu, C. Y., Yang, Y. Y., and Yeh, E. K. (1999). Delusional disorder: retrospective analysis of 86 Chinese outpatients. *Psychiatry and Clinical Neurosciences* 53, 673–6.

Hucker, S. J. (1990). Sexual asphyxia. In *Principles and practice of forensic psychiatry* (eds P. Boeden and R. Bluglass). Churchill Livingston, Edinburgh.

Hughes, J. R. (1995). The EEG in psychiatry: an outline with summarised points and references. *Clinical EEG* 26, 92–101.

Hull, C. L. (1943). *Principles of behaviour*. Appleton, New York.

Humphreys, M. S., Johnstone, E. C., MacMillan, J. F., and Taylor, P. J. (1992). Dangerous behaviour preceding first admissions for schizophrenia. *British Journal of Psychiatry* 161, 501–5.

Hunter, R. and MacAlpine, I. (eds) (1963). *Three hundred years of psychiatry 1535–1860*, pp.441–4. Oxford University Press, London.

Huntington's Disease Collaborative Research Group (1993). A novel gene containing a trinucleotide repeat that is expanded and unstable on Huntington's disease chromosomes. *Cell* 72, 971–83.

Iancu, I., Dannon, P. N., and Zohar, J. (2000). Obsessive–compulsive disorder. In *The new Oxford textbook of psychiatry* (eds M. G. Gelder, J. J. López-Ibor Jr, and N. C. Andreasen), Chapter 4.8. Oxford University Press, Oxford.

Ichim, L., Berk, M. and Brook, S. (2000). Lamotrigine compared with lithium in mania: a double-blind randomized controlled trial. *Annals of Clinical Psychiatry* 12, 5–10.

Iles, S. and Gath, D. (1993). Psychiatric outcome of termination of pregnancy for foetal abnormality. *Psychological Medicine* 23, 407–13.

Imboden, J. B., Canter, A., and Cluff, L. E. (1961). Convalescence from influenza: a study of the psychological and clinical determinants. *Archives of Internal Medicine* 108, 393–9.

Insel, T. R. (1991). Serotonin in obsessive compulsive disorder: a causal connection or more monomania about a major monoamine. In *5-Hydroxytryptamine in psychiatry: a spectrum of ideas* (eds M. Sandler, A. Coppen, and S. Harnett), pp. 228–57. Oxford University Press, Oxford.

Insel, T. R. (1992). Towards a neuroanatomy of obsessive compulsive disorder. *Archives of General Psychiatry* 49, 739–44.

Inskip, H. M., Harris, E. C., and Barraclough, B. (1998). Lifetime risk of suicide for affective disorder, alcoholism and schizophrenia. *British Journal of Psychiatry* 172, 35–7.

International Gender Dysphoria Association (1985). Standards of care: the hormonal and surgical sex reassignment of gender dysphoric persons. *Archives of Sexual Behaviour* 14, 79–90.

International Molecular Genetic Study of Autism Consortium (1998). A full genome scan for autism with evidence for linkage to a region on chromosome 7q. *Human Molecular Genetics* 7, 571–8.

International Multicenter Trial Group on Moclobemide in Social Phobia (1997). Moclobemide in social phobia: a double-blind, placebo-controlled clinical study. *European Archives of Psychiatry and Clinical Neuroscience* 247, 71–80.

Isacsson, G., Holmgren, P., Wasserman, D., and Bergman, U. (1994). Use of antidepressants among people committing suicide in Sweden. *British Medical Journal* 8, 506–9.

Iversen, L. (2000). Drugs for cognitive disorders. In *The new Oxford textbook of psychiatry* (eds M. G. Gelder, J. J. López-Ibor Jr, and N. C. Andreasen), Chapter 6.2.7. Oxford University Press, Oxford.

Ives, R. (2000). Disorders relating to the use of volatile substances. In *The new Oxford textbook of psychiatry* (eds M. G. Gelder, J. J. López-Ibor Jr, and N. C. Andreasen), Chapter 4.2.3.7. Oxford University Press, Oxford.

Jaber, M., Robinson, S. W., Missale, C., and Caron, M. G. (1996). Dopamine receptors and brain function. *Neuropharmacology* 35, 1503–19.

Jablensky, A. (2000a). Course and outcome of schizophrenia and their prediciton. In *The new Oxford textbook of psychiatry* (eds M. G. Gelder, J. J. López-Ibor Jr, and N. C. Andreasen), Chapter 4.3.6. Oxford University Press, Oxford.

Jablensky, A. (2000b). Epidemiology of schizophrenia. In *The new Oxford textbook of psychiatry* (eds M. G. Gelder, J. J. López-Ibor Jr, and N. C. Andreasen), Chapter 4.3.4. Oxford University Press, Oxford.

Jackson, M. and Cawley, R. (1992). Psychodynamics and psychotherapy on an acute psychiatric ward. *British Journal of Psychiatry* 160, 41–50.

Jacobs, D. and Silverstone, T. (1986). Dextroamphetamine-induced arousal in human subjects as a model for mania. *Psychological Medicine* 16, 323–9.

Jacobs, M. (1988). *Psychodynamic counselling in action*. Sage, London.

Jacobs, P. A., Brunton, M., Melville, M. M., *et al.* (1965). Aggressive behaviour and subnormality. *Nature* 208, 1351–2.

Jacobs, S. (1993). *Pathological grief – maladaption to loss*. American Psychiatric Press, Washington, DC.

Jacobs, S. C., Hansen, F., and Berkman, L. (1989). Depressions of bereavement. *Comprehensive Psychiatry* 30, 218–24.

Jacobsen, L. K., and Rapoport, J. L. (1998). Research update: childhood-onset schizophrenia: implications of clinical and neurobiological research. *Journal of Child Psychology and Psychiatry* 39, 101–13.

Jacobson, A. M. (1996). The psychological care of patients with insulin-dependent diabetes mellitus. *New England Journal of Medicine* 334, 1249–53.

Jacobson, E. (1938). *Progressive relaxation*. Chicago University Press, Chicago.

Jacobson, E. (1953). Contribution to the metapsychology of cyclothymic depression. In *Affective disorders* (ed. P. Greenacre). International Universities Press, New York.

Jacobson, R. R. (1985). Child firesetters: a clinical investigation. *Journal of Child Psychology and Psychiatry* 26, 759–68.

Jacobson, R. R. (1995). The post-concussional syndrome: physiogenesis, psychogenesis and malingering: an integrative model. *Journal of Psychosomatic Research* 39, 675–93.

Jacoby, R. (2000a). Suicide and deliberate self-harm in elderly people. In *The new Oxford textbook of psychiatry* (eds. M. G. Gelder, J. J. López-Ibor Jr, and

N. C. Andreasen), Chapter 8.5.7. Oxford University Press, Oxford.

Jacoby, R. (2000b). Assessment of mental disorder in older patients and of the treatment needs of patients and their carers. In *The new Oxford textbook of psychiatry* (eds. M. G. Gelder, J. J. López-Ibor Jr, and N. C. Andreasen), Chapter 8.4. Oxford University Press, Oxford.

Jacoby, R. and Oppenheimer, C. (eds) (2001). *Psychiatry in the elderly*, 3rd edn. Oxford University Press, Oxford.

Jamison, K. R. (1992). Manic-depressive illness: what role does psychotherapy have in management? In *Practical problems in clinical psychiatry* (eds K. Hawton and P. J. Cowen), pp. 33–50. Oxford University Press, Oxford.

Janca, A., Üstür, T. B., and Sartorius, N. (1994). New versions of World Health Organization instruments for the assessment of mental disorders. *Acta Psychiatrica Scandinavica* 90, 73–83.

Janet, P. (1925). *Psychological healing*. Allen and Unwin, London.

Janoff-Bulman, R. (1985). The aftermath of victimization: rebuilding shattered assumptions. In *Trauma and its wake: the study and treatment of posttraumatic stress disorder* (ed. C. R. Figley), pp.15–25. Brunner-Mazel, New York.

Janoff-Bulman, R. and Frieze, I. H. (1983). A theoretical perspective for understanding reactions to victimization. *Journal of Social Issues* 39, 1–17.

Janssen, H. J. E. M., Cuisinier, M. C. J., Hoogduin, K. A. L., and De Graauw, K. P. H. M. (1996). Controlled prospective study on the mental health of women following pregnancy loss. *American Journal of Psychiatry* 153, 226–30.

Januzzi, J. L., Stern, T. A., Pasternak, R. C., and DeSanctis, R. W. (2000). The influence of anxiety and depression on outcomes of patients with coronary artery disease. *Archives of Internal Medicine* 160, 1913–21.

Jarman PR, Bhatia KP, Davie C *et al.* (2000). Paroxysmal dystonic choreoathetosis: clinical features and investigation of pathophysiology in a large family. *Movement Disorders*; 15, 648–57.

Jaspers, K. (1913). *Allgemeine Psychopathologie*. Springer, Berlin.

Jaspers, K. (1963). *General psychopathology* (*Allgemeine Psychopathologie*, 7th edn, 1959, trans. J. Hoenig and M. W. Hamilton). Manchester University Press, Manchester.

Jenike, M. A., Hyman, S., Baer, L., *et al.* (1990). A controlled trial of fluvoxamine in obsessive–compulsive disorder: implications for a serotonergic theory. *American Journal of Psychiatry* 147, 1209–15.

Jenike, M. A., Baer, L., Ballantine, H. T., *et al.* (1991). Cingulotomy for refractive obsessive–compulsive disorder. *Archives of General Psychiatry* 48, 548.

Jenkins, J. M. and Smith, M. A. (1990). Factors protecting children living in disharmonious homes: maternal reports. *Journal of the American Academy of Child and Adolescent Psychiatry* 29, 60–9.

Jenkins, R., Lewis, G., Bebbington, P., *et al.* (1997). The National Psychiatric Morbidity Surveys of Great Britain – initial findings from the Household Survey. *Psychological Medicine* 27, 775–89.

Jenkins, R., Bebbington, P., Brugha, T. S., *et al.* (1998). British psychiatric morbidity survey. *British Journal of Psychiatry* 173, 4–7.

Jennings, C., Barraclough, B. M., and Moss, J. R. (1978). Have the Samaritans lowered the suicide rate? A controlled study. *Psychological Medicine* 8, 413–22.

Jerremalm, A., Jansson, L. and Öst, L. G. (1986). Cognitive and physiological reactivity and the effects of different behavioural methods in the treatment of social phobia. *Behaviour Research and Therapy* 24, 171–80.

Jeste, D. V., Lacro, J. P., Bailey, A., *et al.* (1999). Lower incidence of tardive dyskinesia with risperidone compared with haloperidol in older patients. *Journal of American Geriatric Society* 47(6), 716–19.

Jilek, W. G. (2000). Traditional non-Western folk healing as relevant to psychiatry. In *The new Oxford textbook of psychiatry* (eds M. G. Gelder, J. J. López-Ibor Jr, and N. C. Andreasen), Chapter 6.5. Oxford University Press, Oxford.

Jobst, K. A., Smith, A. D., Barker, D. S., *et al.* (1992). Association of atrophy of the medical temporal lobe with reduced blood blow in the posterior parietotemporal cortex in patients with a clinical and pathological diagnosis of Alzheimer's disease. *Journal of Neurology, Neurosurgery and Psychiatry* 55, 190–4.

Joffe, R. T., Singer, W., Levitt, A. J., and MacDonald, C. (1993). A placebo-controlled comparison of lithium and triiodothyronine augmentation of tricyclic antidepressants in unipolar refractory depression. *Archives of General Psychiatry* 50, 387–93.

Johns, A. (2000). Forensic aspects of alcohol and drug disorders. In *The new Oxford textbook of psychiatry* (ed.

M. G. Gelder, J. J. López-Ibor Jr, and N. C Andreasen), Chapter 11.4. Oxford University Press, Oxford.

Johnson, M.A., Krauss, G.L., Miller, N.R., Medura, M., Paul, S.R. (2000). Visual function loss from vigabatrin: effect of stopping the drug. *Neurology* 55, 40–5.

Johnson, G. (1998). Lithium – early development, toxicity, and renal function. *Neuropsychopharmacology* 19, 200–5.

Johnson, S. (1997). Dual diagnosis of severe mental illness in substance misuse: a case for specialist services? *British Journal of Psychiatry* 171, 205–8.

Johnstone, E. C. (1991). Disabilities and circumstances of schizophrenic patients: a follow-up study. *British Journal of Psychiatry* 159(**suppl 13**), 5–46.

Johnstone, E. C., Crow, T. J., Frith, C. D., *et al.* (1976). Cerebral ventricular size in cognitive impairment in chronic schizophrenia. *Lancet* 2, 924–6.

Johnstone, E. C., Cunningham-Owens, D. G., Rith, C. D., *et al.* (1980). Neurotic illness and its response to anxiolytic and antidepressant treatment. *Psychological Medicine* 10, 321–8.

Johnstone, E., Crow, T., Ferrier, I. *et al.* (1983). Adverse effects of anticholinergic medication on positive schizophrenic symptoms. *Psychological Medicine* 13, 513–27.

Johnstone, E. C., Crow, T. J., Frith, C. D., and Owens, D. G. C. (1988). The Northwick Park 'functional' psychosis study: diagnosis and treatment response. *Lancet* 2, 120–5.

Jolley, A. G., Hirch, S. R., Morrison, E., *et al.* (1990). Trial of brief intermittent neuroleptic prophylaxis for selected schizophrenic outpatients: clinical and social outcome at two years. *British Medical Journal* 301, 837–41.

Jones, D. (1992). *Interviewing children who have been sexually abused*, 4th edn. Gaskell Press, London.

Jones, D. P. H. (2000). Child abuse and neglect. In *The new Oxford textbook of psychiatry* (eds M. G. Gelder, J. J. López-Ibor Jr, and N. C. Andreasen), Chapter 9.3.1. Oxford University Press, Oxford.

Jones, D. P. H. and Alexander, H. (1978). Treating the abusive family within the family care system. In: *The battered child*, 4th edn (eds R. E. Helfer and R. S. Kempe). University of Chicago Press, London.

Jones, K. (1972). *A history of the mental health services*. Routledge & Kegan Paul, London.

Jones, M. (1952). *Social psychiatry: a study of therapeutic communities*. Tavistock, London.

Jones, M. (1968). *Social psychiatry in practice*, p. 105. Penguin Books, Harmondsworth.

Jones, P., Rodgers, B., Murray, R., and Marmot, M. (1994). Child developmental risk factors for adult schizophrenia in the British 1946 birth cohort. *Lancet* 344, 1398–402.

Jönson, E. G., Nöthen, M. M., Gustavsson, J. P., *et al.* (1997). Lack of evidence for allelic association between personality traits and the dopamine D4 receptor gene polymorphism. *American Journal of Psychiatry* 154, 697–9.

Jordan, B.D. (2000). Chronic traumatic brain injury associated with boxing. *Seminars in Neurology* 20, 179–85.

Jorge, R. E., Robinson, R. G., and Arndt, S. (1993). Are there symptoms that are specific for depressed mood in patients with traumatic brain injury? *Journal of Nervous and Mental Disease* 181, 91.

Jorm, A. F. (2000). The ageing population and the epidemiology of mental disorders among the elderly. In *The new Oxford textbook of psychiatry* (eds M. G. Gelder, J. J. López-Ibor Jr, and N. C. Andreasen), Chapter 8.3. Oxford University Press, Oxford.

Jorm, A. (2001).

Jorm, A. F., Korten, A. E., and Henderson, A. F. (1987). The prevalence of dementia: a quantitative integration of the literature. *Acta Psychiatrica Scandinavica* 76, 465–79.

Jorm, A. F., Christensen, H., Henderson, A. S., *et al.* (1994). Complaints of cognitive decline in the elderly: a comparison of reports by subjects and informants in a community survey. *Psychological Medicine* 24, 365–74.

Joy, C. B., Adams, C. E., Rice, K., *et al.* (1999). Crisis intervention for people with severe mental illnesses (Cochrane Review). *Cochrane Library* 1. Update Software, Oxford.

Joyce, P. R. (2000). Epidemiology of mood disorders. In *The new Oxford textbook of psychiatry* (eds M. G. Gelder, J. J. López-Ibor Jr, and N. C. Andreasen), Chapter 4.5.4. Oxford University Press, Oxford.

Judd, L. L., Akiskal, H. S., Maser, J. D., *et al.* (1998). A prospective 12-year study of subsyndromal and syndromal depressive symptoms in unipolar major depressive disorders. *Archives of General Psychiatry* 55, 694–700.

Kahlbaum, K. (1863). *Die Gruppirung der psychichen Krankheiten*. Kafemann, Danzig.

Kahn, E. (1928). Die psychopathischen Personlichkeiten. In *Handbuch der Geisteskrankheiten*, Vol. 5, p. 227. Springer, Berlin.

Kahn, R. J., McNair, D. M., Lipman, R. S., *et al.* (1986). Imipramine and chlordiazepoxide in depressive and anxiety disorders. II Efficacy in anxious outpatients. *Archives of General Psychiatry* 43, 79–85.

Kallmann, F. J. (1952). Study on the genetic affects of male homosexuality. *Journal of Nervous and Mental Disease* 115, 1283–98.

Kalucy, R. S., Crisp, A. H., and Harding, B. (1977). A study of 56 families with anorexia nervosa. *British Journal of Medical Psychology* 50, 381–95.

Kaminski, M., Rumeau-Rouquette, C., and Schwartz, D. (1976). Consommation d'alcool chez les femmes enceintes et issue de la grossesse. *Revue d'Epidemiologie et de Santé Publique* 24, 27–40.

Kamphuis, J. H. and Emmelkamp, P. M. G. (2000). Stalking – a contemporary challenge for forensic and clinical psychiatry. *British Journal of Psychiatry* 176, 206–9.

Kandel, E. R. (1998). A new intellectual framework for psychiatry. *American Journal of Psychiatry* 155, 457–69.

Kandel, E. R. (1999). Biology and the future of psychoanalysis: a new intellectual framework for psychiatry revisited. *American Journal of Psychiatry* 156, 505–24.

Kane, J., Honigfeld, G., Singer, J., and Meltzer, H. Y. (1988). Clozapine for the treatment-resistant schizophrenic: a double blind comparison with chlorpromazine. *Archives of General Psychiatry* 45, 789–96.

Kane, J. M. (1999). Tardive dyskinesia in affective disorders. *Journal of Clinical Psychiatry* 60(suppl 5), 43–7.

Kane, R. L. (1985). Special needs of the elderly. In *Oxford textbook of public health* (ed. W. W. Holland), Vol.4. Oxford University Press, Oxford.

Kanner, L. (1943). Autistic disturbance of affective contact. *Nervous Child* 2, 217–50.

Kantor, J. S., Zitrin, C. M., and Zeldis, S. M. (1980). Mitral valve prolapse in agoraphobic patients. *American Journal of Psychiatry* 137, 467–9.

Kaplan, H. I., Sadock, B. J., and Grebb, J. A. (1994). Substance related disorders. In *Synopsis of psychiatry*, pp. 383–456. Williams & Wilkins, Baltimore, MD.

Kapur, N., House, A., Creed, F., Feldman, E., Friedman, T., and Guthrie, E. (1998). Management of deliberate self-poisoning in adults in four teaching hospitals: descriptive study. *British Medical Journal* 316, 831–2.

Kapur, S., Zipursky, R. B., and Remington, G. (1999). Clinical and theoretical implications of 5-HT$_2$ and D$_2$ receptor occupancy of clozapine, risperidone, and olanzapine in schizophrenia. *American Journal of Psychiatry* 156, 286–93.

Karkowski, L. M. and Kendler, K. S. (1997). An examination of the genetic relationship between bipolar and unipolar illness in an epidemiological sample. *Psychiatric Genetics* 7, 159–63.

Kasanin, J. (1933). The acute schizoaffective psychoses. *American Journal of Psychiatry* 13, 97–126.

Kashani, J. H. and Simonds, J. F. (1979). The incidence of depression in children. *American Journal of Psychiatry* 136, 1203–5.

Kaski, M. (2000). Aetiology of mental retardation: general issues and prevention. In *The new Oxford textbook of psychiatry* (eds M. G. Gelder, J. J. López-Ibor Jr, and N. C. Andreasen), Chapter 10.3. Oxford University Press, Oxford.

Kasl-Godley, J. and Gatz, M. (2000). Psychosocial interventions for individuals with dementia: an intergration of theory, therapy, and a clinical understanding of dementia. *Clinical Psychology Review* 20, 755–782.

Katerndahl, D. A. (1993). Lifetime prevalence of panic states. *American Journal of Psychiatry* 150, 246–9.

Katon, W., von Korff, M., Lin, E., *et al.* (1990). Distressed high utilizers of medical care: DSMIII-R diagnoses and treatment needs. *General Hospital Psychiatry* 12, 355–62.

Katz, I. R., Jeste, D. V., Mintzer, J. E., Clyde, C., Napolitano, J., and Brecher, M. (1999). Comparison of Risperdone and placebo for psychosis and behavioral disturbances associated with dementia: a randomized, double-blind trial. *Journal of Clinical Psychiatry* 60, 107–15.

Katz, M., Abbey, S., Rydall, A., and Lowy, F. (1995). Psychiatric consultation for competency to refuse medical treatment. A retrospective study of patient characteristics and outcome. *Psychosomatics* 36, 33–41.

Katzelnick, D. J., Kobak, K. A., Greist, J. H., *et al.* (1995). Sertraline for social phobia: a double blind, placebo-controlled crossover study. *American Journal of Psychiatry* 152, 1368–71.

Kavanagh, D. J. (1992). Recent developments in expressed emotion in schizophrenia. *British Journal of Psychiatry* 160, 601–20.

Kavka, J. (1949). Pinel's conception of the psychopathic state. *Bulletin of the History of Medicine* 23, 461–8.

Kay, D. W. K. (1972). Schizophrenia and schizophrenia-like states in the elderly. *British Journal of Hospital Medicine* 8, 369–76.

Kay, D. W. K. and Bergmann, K. (1980). Epidemiology of mental disorder among the aged in the community. In *Handbook of mental health and ageing* (eds J. E. Birren and R. B. Sloane). Prentice-Hall, Englewood Cliffs, NJ.

Kay, D. W. K. and Roth, M. (1961). Environmental and hereditary factors in the schizophrenias of old age ('late paraphrenia') and their bearing on the general problem of causation in schizophrenia. *Journal of Mental Science* 107, 649–86.

Kay, D. W. K., Beamish, P. and Roth, M. (1964). Old age mental disorders in Newcastle-upon-Tyne: 1: a study in prevalence. *British Journal of Psychiatry* 110, 146–58.

Kay, S. R., Fiszbeim, A., and Opler, L. A. (1987). Positive and Negative Symptom Scale (PANSS) for schizophrenia. *Schizophrenia Bulletin* 13, 261–76.

Kaye, C. and Lingiah, T. (2000). *Culture and ethnicity in secure psychiatric practice: working with difference.* Jessica Kingsley, London.

Kazdin, A. E. (1997). Practitioner review: psychosocial treatments for conduct disorder in children. *Journal of Child Psychology and Psychiatry* 38, 161–78.

Kazdin, A. E., Esveldt-Dawson, K., French, N. H., and Unis, A. S. (1987). Problem solving skills and relationship therapy in the treatment of antisocial child behaviour. *Journal of Consulting and Clinical Psychology* 55, 76–85.

Keck, P. E., McElroy, S. L., and Strakowski, S. M. (1998). Anticonvulsants and antipsychotics in the treatment of bipolar disorder. *Journal of Clinical Psychiatry* 59(**suppl** 6), 74–81.

Kedward, H. B. and Cooper, B. (1966). Neurotic disorders in urban practice: a 3 year follow-up. *Journal of the Royal College of General Practitioners* 12, 148–63.

Kelly, J.P. (2000). Concussion in sports and recreation. *Seminars in Neurology* 20, 165–71.

Kelly, C. P. (1996). Chronic constipation and soiling: a review of the psychological and family literature. *Child Psychology and Psychiatry Review*, 1, 59–66.

Kelly, W. F. (1996). Psychiatric aspects of Cushing's syndrome. *Quarterly Journal of Medicine* 89, 543–51.

Kemp, R., Hayward, P., Applewhaite, G., *et al.* (1996). Compliance therapy in psychotic patients: randomised controlled trial. *British Medical Journal* 312, 345–9.

Kempe, R. S. and Goldbloom, R. B. (1987). Malnutrition and growth retardation (failure to thrive) in the context of child abuse and neglect. In *The battered child* (eds R. E. Helfer and R. S. Kempe), pp.315–35. University of Chicago Press, London.

Kendall, P. C., Ronan, K. R., and Epps, J. (1991). Aggression in children and adolescents: cognitive behavioural treatment perspective. In *The development of treatment of childhood aggression* (eds D. J. Pepler and K. H. Rubin), pp.341–60. Lawrence Erlbaum, Hillsdale, NJ.

Kendell, R. E. (1968). *The classification of depressive illness*. Maudsley Monograph No. 18. Oxford University Press, London.

Kendell, R. E. (1975). *The role of diagnosis in psychiatry*. Blackwell, Oxford.

Kendell, R. E., Chalmers, J. C., and Platz, C. (1987). Epidemiology of puerperal psychoses. *British Journal of Psychiatry* 150, 662–73.

Kendell, R. E., Malcolm, D. E., and Adams, W. (1993). The problem of detecting changes in the incidence of schizophrenia. *British Journal of Psychiatry* 162, 212–18.

Kendell, R. E., McInneny, K., Juszczak, E., and Bain, M. (2000). Obstetric complications and schizophrenia. *British Journal of Psychiatry* 176, 516–22.

Kendler, K. S. (1996). Major depression and generalised anxiety disorder. Same genes (partly) different environments – revisited. *British Journal of Psychiatry* 168, 68–75.

Kendler, K. S. (1997). The diagnostic validity of melancholic major depression in a population-based sample of female twins. *Archives of General Psychiatry* 54, 299–304.

Kendler, K. S. and Gruenberg, A. M. (1984). An independent analysis of the Danish adoption study of schizophrenia. VI. The relationship between psychiatric disorders as defined by DSMIII in the relatives and adoptees. *Archives of General Psychiatry* 41, 555–64.

Kendler, K. S. and Walsh, D. (1995). Schizophreniform disorder, delusional disorder and psychotic disorder not otherwise specified: clinical features, outcome and familial psychopathology. *Acta Psychiatrica Scandinavica* 91, 370–8.

Kendler, K. S., Gruenberg, A. M., and Strauss, J. S. (1981). An independent analysis of the Copenhagen sample for the Danish adoption study of schizophrenia. The relationship between schizotypal personality disorder and schizophrenia. *Archives of General Psychiatry* 38, 982–7.

Kendler, K. S., Gruenberg, A. M., and Tsuang, M. T. (1985a). Psychiatric illness in first degree relatives of schizophrenic and surgical control patients: a family study using DSMIII criteria. *Archives of General Psychiatry* 42, 770–9.

Kendler, K. S., Masterson, C. C., and Davis, K. L. (1985b). Psychiatric illness in first-degree relatives of patients with paranoid psychosis, schizophrenia and medical illness. *British Journal of Psychiatry* 47, 524–31.

Kendler, K. S., MacLean, C., Neale, M., Kessler, R., Heath, A., and Eaves, L. (1991). The genetic epidemiology of bulimia nervosa. *American Journal of Psychiatry* 148, 1627–37.

Kendler, K. S., Neale, M. C., Kessler, R. C., Heath, A. C., and Eaves, L. J. (1992a). Major depression and generalized anxiety disorder: same genes(partly) different environments? *Archives of General Psychiatry* 49,716–722.

Kendler, K. S., Neale, M. C., Kessler, R. C., *et al.* (1992b). Childhood parental loss and adult psychopathology in women: a twin study perspective. *Archives of General Psychiatry* 49, 109–116.

Kendler, K. S., Neale, M. C., Kessler, R. C., *et al.* (1992c). A population-based twin study of major depression in women: the impact of varying definitions of illness. *Archives of General Psychiatry* 49, 257–66.

Kendler, K. S., McGuire, M., Gruenberg, A. M., *et al.* (1993a). The Roscommon family study: (3) Schizophrenia-related personality disorders in relatives. *Archives of General Psychiatry* 50, 781–8.

Kendler, K. S., McGuire, M., Gruenberg, A. M., *et al.* (1993b). The Roscommon family study: (1) Methods, diagnosis of probands and risk of schizophrenia in relatives. *Archives of General Psychiatry* 50, 527–40.

Kendler, K. S., McGuire, M., Gruenberg, A. M., *et al.* (1993c). The Roscommon family study: (2) The risk of non-schizophrenic non-affective psychosis in relatives. *Archives of General Psychiatry* 50, 645–52.

Kendler, K. S., McGuire, M., Gruenberg, A. M., *et al.* (1993d). The Roscommon family study: (4) Affective illness, anxiety disorders and alcoholism in relatives. *Archives of General Psychiatry* 50, 781–8.

Kendler, K. S., Neale, M. C., Kessler, R. C., *et al.* (1993e). Panic disorder in women: a population- based twin study. *Psychological Medicine* 23, 397–406.

Kendler, K. S., Neale, M. C., Heath, A. C., *et al.* (1994). A twin-family study of alcoholism in women. *American Journal of Psychiatry* 151, 707–15.

Kendler, K. S., Karkowski, L. M. and Prescott, C. A. (1999). Causal relationship between stressful life events and the onset of major depression. *American Journal of Psychiatry* 156, 837–841.

Kendrick T., Burns, T., and Freeling, P. (1995). Randomised controlled trial of teaching general practitioners to carry out structured assessments of their long term mentally ill patients. *British Medical Journal* 311, 93–8.

Kendrick, T. (1999). Primary care options to prevent mental illness. *Annals of Medicine* 31, 359–63.

Kennard, D. (1998). *An introduction to therapeutic communities*, 2nd edn. Jessica Kingsley, London.

Kerkhof, A. (2000). Attempted suicide; patterns and trends. In *The international handbook of suicide and attempted suicide* (eds K. Hawton and K. van Heeringen), John Wiley & Sons, Chichester.

Kernberg, O .F. (1975). *Borderline conditions and pathological narcissism*. Jason Aronson, New York.

Kernberg, O. F. (1993). *Severe personality disorders: psychotherapeutic strategies*. 2nd edn. Yale University Press, New Haven CT.

Kerr, A. M. and Stevenson, J. B. P. (1985). Rett's syndrome in the West of Scotland. *British Medical Journal* 291, 579–82.

Kerr, T. A., Roth, M., and Shapira, K. (1974). Prediction of outcome in anxiety states and depressive illness. *British Journal of Psychiatry* 124, 125–31.

Kessel, N. and Grossman, G. (1965). Suicide in alcoholics. *British Medical Journal* 2, 1671–2.

Kessler, R. C. and Walters, E. E. (1998). Epidemiology of DSM-III-R major depression and minor depression among adolescents and young adults in the National Comorbidity Survey. *Depression and Anxiety* 7, 3–14.

Kessler, R. C., McGonagle, K. A., Zhao, S., *et al.* (1994). Lifetime and 12-month prevalence of DSM-III-R psychiatric disorders in the United States: results from the National Comorbidity Survey. *Archives of General Psychiatry* 51, 8–20.

Kessler, R. C., Rubinow, D. R., Holmes, C., *et al.* (1997). The epidemiology of DSM-III-R Bipolar I disorder in a general population survey. *Psychological Medicine* 27, 1079–89.

Kesteren,P., Gooren, L., and Megers, J. (1996). An epidemiological and demographic study of transsexuals in the Netherlands. *Archives of Sexual Behaviour* 25, 589–600.

Kety, S. S., Wender, P. A., Jacobsen, B., *et al.* (1994). Mental illness in the biological and adoptive relatives of schizophrenic adoptees. *Archives of General Psychiatry* 51, 442–55.

Kety, S., Rosenthal, D., Wender, P. H., *et al.* (1975). Mental illness in the biological and adoptive families of adopted individuals who have become schizophrenic. In *Genetic research in psychiatry* (eds R. R. Fieve, D. Rosenthal, and H. Bull). Johns Hopkins University Press, Baltimore, MD.

Kilbourne, E. M., Philen, R. M., Kamb, M. L., and Falk, H. (1996). Tryptophan produced by Showa Denko and epidemic eosinophilic-myalgia syndrome. *Journal of Rheumatology Supplement* 46, 81–8.

Kilian, J. G., Kerr, K., Lawrence, C., and Celermajer, D. S. (1999). Myocarditis and cardiomyopathy associated with clozapine. *Lancet* 354, 1841–5.

Kiloh, L. G. and Garside, R. F. (1963). The independence of neurotic depression and endogenous depression. *British Journal of Psychiatry* 109, 451–63.

Kiloh, L. G., Smith, J. S., and Johnson, G. F. (1988). *Physical treatments in psychiatry*. Blackwell Scientific Publications, Oxford.

Kilpatrick, D. G., Resnick, H. S., and Acierno, R. (1997). Health impact of interpersonal violence 3: implications for clinical practice and public policy. *Behavioural Medicine* 23, 79–85

Kilzieh, N. and Akiskal, H. S. (1999). Rapid-cycling bipolar disorder: an overview of research and clinical experience. *Psychiatric Clinics of North America* 22, 585–607.

Kim, K. I., Li, D., and Kim, D. H. (1999). Depressive symptoms in Koreans, Korean-Chinese and Chinese: a transcultural study. *Transcultural Psychiatry* 36, 303–16.

King, D. W., King, L. A., Foy, D. W., and Gudanowski, D. M. (1996). Pre-war factors in combat related post-traumatic stress disorder: structural equation modelling with a national sample of female and male Vietnam veterans. *Journal of Consulting and Clinical Psychology* 64, 520–31.

King, M. and McDonald, E. (1992). Homosexuals who are twins: a study of 46 probands. *British Journal of Psychiatry* 160, 407–9.

Kingman, R. and Jones, D. P. H. (1987). Incest and other forms of sexual abuse. In *The battered child*, 4th edn (eds R. E. Helfer and R. S. Kempe). University of Chicago Press, London.

Kinsey, A. C., Pomeroy, W. B., and Martin, C. E. (1948). *Sexual behavior in the human male*. Saunders, Philadelphia, PA.

Kinsey, A. C., Pomeroy, W. B., Martin, C. E., and Gebhard, P. H. (1953). *Sexual behavior in the human female*. Saunders, Philadelphia, PA.

Kiraly, S. J., Gibson, R. E., Ancill, R. J., and Holliday, S. G. (1998). Risperidone: treatment response in adult and geriatric patients. *International Journal of Psychiatry in Medicine* 28, 255–63.

Kirby, R. S. (1994). Impotence: diagnosis and management of male erectile dysfunction. *British Medical Journal* 308, 957–61.

Kirby, R. S., Carson, C., and Webster, G. D. (1991). *Impotence: diagnosis and management*. Butterworth Heinemann, Oxford.

Kirli, S. and Caliskan, M. (1998). A comparative study of sertraline versus imipramine in postpsychotic depressive disorder of schizophrenia. *Schizophrenia Research* 33, 103–11.

Kirmayer, L. J. and Robbins, J. M. (1991). Three forms of somatization in primary care: prevalence, co-occurrence, and sociodemographic characteristics. *Journal of Nervous and Mental Disease* 179, 647–55.

Kisely, S. R. and Goldberg, D. P. (1996). Physical and psychiatric comorbidity in general practice. *British Journal of Psychiatry* 169, 236–42.

Kisely, S., Goldberg, D., and Simon, G. (1997). A comparison between somatic symptoms with and without clear organic cause: results of an international study. *Psychological Medicine* 27, 1011–19.

Kitwood, T. (1997). *Dementia reconsidered*. Open University Press, Milton Keynes.

Klaf, F. S. and Hamilton, J. G. (1961). Schizophrenia – a hundred years ago and today. *Journal of Mental Science* 107, 819–28.

Klein, D. F. (1964). Delineation of two drug-responsive anxiety syndromes. *Psychopharmacologia* 5, 397–408.

Klein, D. F. (1993). False suffocation alarms, spontaneous panics, and related conditions: an integrative hypothesis. *Archives of General Psychiatry* 50, 306.

Klein, D. N., Lewinsohn, P. M., Seeley, J. R. and Rohde, P. (2001). A family study of major depressive disorder in a community sample of adolescents. *Archives of General Psychiatry* 58, 13–20.

Klein, E., Kreinen, I., Chistyakov, A., *et al.* (1999). Therapeutic efficacy of right prefrontal slow repetitive transcranial magnetic stimulation in major depression: a double-blind controlled study. *Archives of General Psychiatry* 56, 315–20.

Klein, F., Sepekoff, B., and Wolf, T. J. (1985). Sexual orientation: a multiple variable, dynamic process. *Journal of Homosexuality* 11, 35–49.

Klein, M. (1934). A contribution to the psychogenesis of manic-depressive states. Reprinted in *Contributions to psychoanalysis 1921–1945: developments in child and adolescent psychology*, pp. 282–310. Hogarth Press, London (1948).

Klein, M. (1952). Notes on some schizoid mechanisms. In *Developments in psychoanalysis* (eds J. Jacobs and J. Riviere). Hogarth Press, London.

Klein, M. (1963). *The psychoanalysis of children* (translated by A. Strachey). Hogarth Press and Institute of Psychoanalysis, London.

Kleinknecht, R. A., Klepac, R. K., and Alexander, L. D. (1973). Origin and characteristics of fear of dentistry. *Journal of the American Dental Association* 86, 842–8.

Kleinman, A. (1982). Neurasthenia and depression: a study of somatization and culture in China. *Culture, Medicine and Psychiatry* 6, 117–96.

Kleinman, A. (1986). *Social origins of distress and disease: depression, neurosthenia and pain in modern China*. Yale University Press, New Haven, CT.

Kleist, K. (1928). Cycloid paranoid and epileptoid psychoses and the problem of the degenerative psychosis. Reprinted in *Themes and variations in European psychiatry* (eds S. R. Hirsch and M. Shepherd). Wright, Bristol (1974).

Kleist, K. (1930). Alogical thought disorder: an organic manifestation of the schizophrenic psychological deficit. In *The clinical roots of the schizophrenic concept* (eds

J. Cutting and M. Shepherd). Cambridge University Press, Cambridge (1987).

Klerman, G. L., Weissman, M. M., Rounsaville, B. J., and Chevron, E. S. (1984). *Interpersonal psychotherapy of depression*. Basic Books, New York.

Klerman, G. L., Budman, S., Weissman, M. M., *et al.* (1987). Efficacy of a brief psychosocial intervention for symptoms of stress and distress among patients in primary care. *Medical Care* 25,1078–88.

Knapp, M. and Chisholm, D. (2000). Economic analysis of psychiatric services. In *The new Oxford textbook of psychiatry* (eds M. G. Gelder, J. J. López-Ibor Jr, and N. C. Andreasen), Chapter 7.7. Oxford University Press, Oxford.

Koch, J. L. A. (1891). *Die Psychopathischen Minderwertigkeiter*. Dorn, Ravensburg.

Kocsis, J. H., Croughan, J. L., Katz, M. N., *et al.* (1990). Response to treatment with antidepressants of patients with severe or moderate non-psychotic depression and of patients with psychotic depression. *American Journal of Psychiatry* 147, 621–4.

Koegel, R., Schreibman, L., O'Neil, R. E., and Burke, J. C. (1983). The personality and family interaction characteristics of parents with autistic children. *Journal of Consulting and Clinical Psychology* 51, 683–92.

Koenig, H. G. and Blazer, D. G. (1992). Epidemiology of geriatric affective disorders. *Clinics in Geriatric Medicine* 8, 235–51.

Kohen, D. and Bristow, M. (1996). Neuroleptic malignant syndrome. *Advances in Psychiatric Treatment* 2, 151–7.

Kolle, K. (1931). *Die primare Verrucktheit: psychopathologische, klinische und genealogische Untersuchungen*. Thieme, Leipzig.

Kolvin, I. (2000). Speech and language disorders of childhood and psychological mutism. In *The new Oxford textbook of psychiatry* (eds M. G. Gelder, J. J. López-Ibor Jr, and N. C. Andreasen), Chapter 9.2.11. Oxford University Press, Oxford.

Kolvin, I. and Fundudis, T. (1981). Elective mute children: psychological development and background factors. *Journal of Child Psychology and Psychiatry,* 22, 219–32.

Kopelman, M. D. (1986). Clinical tests of memory. *British Journal of Psychiatry* 148, 517–625.

Kopelman, M. D. (2000). Amnesic syndromes. In *The new Oxford textbook of psychiatry* (eds. M. G. Gelder, J. J. López-Ibor Jr, and N. C. Andreasen), Chapter 4.1.13. Oxford University Press, Oxford.

Kornstein, S. G., Sholare, E. F., and Gardner, D. F. (2000). Endocrine disorders. In *Psychiatric care of the medical patient* (eds A. Stoudemire, B. S. Fogel, and D. B. Greenberg). Oxford University Press, New York.

Koro, C. E., Fedder, D. O., L'Italien, G. J., Weiss, S., Magder, L. S., Kreyenbuhl, J., Revicki, D. and Buchanan R. W. (2002). Assessment of independent effect of olanzapine and risperidone on risk of diabetes among patients with schizophrenia: population based nested case-control study. *British Medical Journal* 325. 243–245.

Kovacs, M. (1996). Presentation and course of major depression during childhood and later years of the lifespan. *Journal of the American Academy of Child and Adolescent Psychiatry* 35, 705–15.

Kraepelin, E. (1897). Dementia praecox. In *The clinical roots of the schizophrenic concept* (eds J. Cutting and M. Shepherd). Cambridge University Press, Cambridge (1981).

Kraepelin, E. (1904). *Clinical psychiatry: a textbook for students and physicians* (edited and translated from 7th edition of Kraepelin's *Textbook* by A. R. Diefendof). Macmillan, New York.

Kraepelin, E. (1915). Der Verfolgungswahn der Schwerhörigen. *Psychiatrie*, Vol. 8, Part 4. Barth, Leipzig.

Kraepelin, E. (1919). *Dementia praecox and paraphrenia*. Livingstone, Edinburgh.

Kraepelin, E. (1921). Manic depressive insanity and paranoia (translated by R. M. Barclay from the 8th edition of *Lehrbuch der Psychiatrie*, Vols III and IV). Livingstone, Edinburgh.

Krafft-Ebing, R. (1888). *Lehrbuch der Psychiatrie*. Enke, Stuttgart.

Krafft-Ebing, R. (1924). *Psychopathic sexuality with special reference to contrary sexual instinct*. Authorized translation of the 7th German edition by C. G. Chaddock. F. A. Davis, Philadelphia, PA.

Kreitman, N. (ed.) (1977). *Parasuicide*. Wiley, London.

Kreitman, N. and Foster, J. (1991). The construction and selection of predictive scales, with special reference to parasuicide. *British Journal of Psychiatry* 159, 185–92.

Kretschmer, E. (1927). Der sensitive Beziehungswahn. Reprinted and translated as Chapter 8 in *Themes and variations in European psychiatry* (eds S. R. Hirsh and M. Shepherd). Wright, Bristol (1974).

Kretschmer, E. (1936). *Physique and character,* 2nd edn (transl. W. J. H. Sprott and K. P. Trench). Trubner, New York.

Kringlen, E. (1965). Obsessional neurosis: a long term follow up. *British Journal of Psychiatry* 111, 709–22.

Krishnamoorthy, E.S. and Trimble, M.R. (1999). Forced normalization: clinical and therapeutic relevance. *Epilepsia* 40 Suppl 10, S57–64.

Kroenke, K. and Price, R. K. (1993). Symptoms in the community. Prevalence, classification, and psychiatric comorbidity. *Archives of Internal Medicine* 153, 2474–80.

Kroenke, K. and Swindle, R. (2000). Cognitive–behavioral therapy for somatization and symptom syndromes: a critical review of controlled clinical trials. *Psychotherapy and Psychosomatics* 69, 205–215.

Kroenke, K., Spitzer, R. L., deGruy III, F. V., *et al.* (1997). Multisomatoform disorder. An alternative to undifferentiated somatoform disorder for the somatizing patient in primary care. *Archives of General Psychiatry*, 54, 352–358.

Krystal, J. H., Belger, A., D'Souza, C., *et al.* (1999). Therapeutic implications of the hyperglutamatergic effects of NMDA antagonists. *Neuropsychopharmacology* 22, S143–57.

Kubler-Ross, E. (1969). *On death and dying.* Macmillan, New York.

Kushner, D. (1998). Mild traumatic brain injury. Toward understanding manifestations and treatment. *Archives of Internal Medicine* 158, 1617–24.

Lader, M. (1994). Anxiolytic drugs: dependence, addiction and abuse. *European Neuropsychopharmacology* 4, 85–91.

Lader, M. H. (1969). Psychophysiological aspects of anxiety. In *Studies of anxiety* (ed. M. H. Lader). *British Journal of Psychiatry Special Publication*, No. 3.

Laidlaw, J., Richens, A., and Chadwick, D. (1993). *A textbook of epilepsy*, 4th edn. Churchill Livingstone, Edinburgh.

Lamb, H. R. (1987). Incompetency to stand trial: appropriateness and outcome. *Archives of General Psychiatry* 44, 754.

Lamb, H. R. and Weinburger, L. (1998). Persons with severe mental illness in jails and prisons: a review. *Psychiatric Services*, 49, 483–92.

Landesmann-Dyer, S. (1981). Living in the community. *American Journal of Mental Deficiency* 86, 223–34.

Lange, J. (1931). *Crime as destiny* (transl. C. Haldane). George Allen, London.

Langfeldt, G. (1961). The erotic jealousy syndrome. A clinical study. *Acta Psychiatrica Scandinavica* 36 (suppl 151), 7–68.

Laruelle, M. (1998). Imaging dopamine transmission in schizophrenia: A review and meta-analysis. *Quarterly Journal of Nuclear Medicine* 42, 211–21.

Lasègue, C. (1877). Les exhibitionnistes. *Union Medicale* 23, 709–14.

Last, C. G., Hansen, C., and Franco, N. (1997). Anxious children in adulthood; a prospective study of adjustment. *Journal of the American Academy of Child and Adolescent Psychiatry* 36, 645–52.

Laumann, E. O., Gagnon, J. H., Michaels R. T., and Michaels, S. (1994). *The social organization of sexuality.* University of Chicago Press, Chicago.

Lavori, P. W. (2000). Placebo control groups in randomized treatment trials: a statistician's perspective. *Biological Psychiatry* 47, 717–23.

Lawrie, S. M., Whalley, H., Kestelman, J. N., *et al.* (1999). Magnetic resonance imaging of brain in people at high risk of developing schizophrenia. *Lancet* 353, 30–3.

Layden, M. A., Newman, C. F., Freeman, A., and Morse, S. B. (1993). *Cognitive therapy of borderline personality.* Allyn & Bacon, Boston, MA.

Lazarus, R. S. (1993). Coping theory and research: past, present and future. *Psychosomatic Medicine* 55, 234–47.

Ledermann, S. (1956). *Alcool, alcoolisme, alcoolisation.* Presses Universitaires de Paris, Paris.

LeDoux, J. (1998). *The emotional brain.* Weidenfeld & Nicolson, London.

Lee, L. M., Stevenson, R. W., and Szasz, G. (1988). Prostaglandin E1 versus phentolamine/papaverine for the treatment of erectile impotence: a double-blind comparison. *Journal of Urology* 141, 54–7.

Lee, S. (1994). Neurasthenia and Chinese psychiatry in the 1990's. *Journal of Psychosomatic Research* 38, 487–91

Lees, A.J. (1988). Facial mannerisms and tics. *Advances in Neurology* 49, 255–61.

Lees, S. (1999). *Carnal knowledge: rape on trial.* Hamish Hamilton, London.

Leff, J. (1981). *Psychiatry around the globe: a transcultural view.* Dekker, New York.

Leff, J. (1993a). All the homeless people – where do they all come from? *British Medical Journal* 306, 669–70.

Leff, J. (1993b). The Taps Project: evaluating community placement of long-stay psychiatric patients. *British Journal of Psychiatry* 164(Suppl 19), 1–56.

Leff, J. (1998). Needs of the families of people with schizophrenia. *Advances in Psychiatric Treatment* 4, 277–84.

Leff, J. and Vaughn, C. (1981). The role of maintenance therapy and relative expressed emotion in relapse of schizophrenia: a two year follow up. *British Journal of Psychiatry* 139, 102–4.

Leff, J. P., Kuipers, L., Berkowitz, R., and Sturgeon, D. (1985). A controlled trial of intervention in the families of schizophrenic patients: two year follow-up. *British Journal of Psychiatry* 146, 594–600.

Lehman, A. F. and Steinwachs, D. M. (1998). Patterns of usual care for schizophrenia: initial result from the Schizophrenia Patient Outcomes Research Team (PORT) Client Survey. *Schizophrenia Bulletin* 24, 11–20.

Lehrke, R. (1972). A theory of X-linkage of major intellectual traits. *American Journal of Mental Deficiency* 76, 611–19.

Lelliott, P. T., Noshirvani, H. F., Basoglu, M., *et al.* (1988). Obsessive–compulsive beliefs and treatment outcome. *Psychological Medicine* 18, 697–702.

Lemoine, P., Harousseau, H., Borteyru, J.-P., and Menuet, J.-C. (1968). Les enfants de parents alcooliques: anomalies observées à propos de 127 cas. *Quest Médical* 25, 477–82.

Lenane, M. C., Swedo, S. E., Leonard, H., *et al.* (1990). Psychiatric disorders in first degree relatives of children and adolescents with obsessive compulsive disorder. *Journal of the American Academy of Child and Adolescent Psychiatry* 29, 407–12.

Lenox, R. H. and Hahn, C-G. (2000). Overview of the mechanism of action of lithium in the brain: fifty-year update. *Journal of Clinical Psychiatry* 61(suppl 9), 5–15.

Leon, A. C., Keller, M. B., Warshaw, M. G., *et al.* (1999). Prospective study of fluoxetine treatment and suicidal behaviour in affectively ill subjects. *American Journal of Psychiatry* 156, 195–201.

Leonard, H. L., Swedo, S. E., Lenane, M. C., *et al.* (1991). A double-blind desipramine substitution during long-term clomipramine treatment in children and adolescents with obsessive–compulsive disorder. *Archives of General Psychiatry* 48, 922–7.

Leonard, H. L., Swedo, S., Lenane, M. C., *et al.* (1993). A 2- to 7-year follow-up study of 54 obsessive–compulsive children and adolescents. *Archives of General Psychiatry* 50, 429.

Leonhard, K. (1957). *The classification of endogenous psychoses*. English translation of the 8th German edition of *Aufteilung der Endogenen Psychosen* by R Berman. Irvington, New York (1979).

Leonhard, K., Korff, I. and Schultz, H. (1962). Die Temperamente und den Familien der monopolaren und bipolaren phasishen Psychosen. *Psychiatrie und Neurologie* 143, 416–34.

Lesch, K. P., Bengel, D., Heils, A., Sabol, S. Z., *et al.* (1996). Association of anxiety related traits with a polymorphism in the serotonin transporter gene regulatory region. *Science* 274,1527–31.

Lespérance, F. and Frasure Smith, N. (2000). Depression in patients with cardiac disease: a practical review. *Journal of Psychosomatic Research* 48, 379–91.

LeVay, S. (1991). A difference in hypothalamic structure between heterosexual and homosexual men. *Science* 253, 1034–7.

Leventhal, J. (1998). Epidemiology of child sexual abuse. *Child Abuse and Neglect,* 22, 481–91.

Levin, E. (1997). Carers. In *Psychiatry in the elderly* (eds R. Jacoby and C. Oppenheimer), pp. 392–402. Oxford University Press, Oxford.

Levin, R. J. (2000). Normal sexual function. In *The new Oxford textbook of psychiatry* (eds M. G. Gelder, J. J. López-Ibor Jr, and N. C. Andreasen), Chapter 4.11.1. Oxford University Press, Oxford.

Lewin, B. (1999). Improving quality of life in patients with angina. *Heart* 82, 654–55.

Lewin, B., Robertson, I. H., Cay, E. L., *et al.* (1992). Effects of self-help post-myocardial-infarction rehabilitation on psychological adjustment and use of health services. *Lancet* 339, 1036–40.

Lewis, A. J. (1934). Melancholia: a clinical survey of depressive states. *Journal of Mental Science* 80, 277–8.

Lewis, A. J. (1936). Problems of obsessional neurosis. *Proceedings of the Royal Society of Medicine* 29, 325–36.

Lewis, A. J. (1953). Health as a social concept. *British Journal of Sociology* 4, 109–24.

Lewis, A. J. (1956). Psychological Medicine. In *Price's textbook of the practice of medicine*, 9th edn (ed. D. Hunter). Oxford University Press, London.

Lewis, A. J. (1970). Paranoia and paranoid: a historical perspective. *Psychological Medicine* 1, 2–12.

Lewis, E. O. (1929). Report on an investigation into the incidence of mental deficiency in six areas 1925–27. In *Report of the Mental Deficiency Committee*, Part IV. HMSO, London.

Lewis, G., Hawton, K., and Jones, P. (1997). Strategies for preventing suicide. *British Journal of Psychiatry* 171, 351–4.

Lhermitte, J. (1951). Visual hallucinations of the self. *British Medical Journal* 1, 431–4.

Liakos, A. (1967). Familial transvestism. *British Journal of Psychiatry* 113, 49–51.

Liberman, R. P., Mueser, K. T., Wallace, C. J., *et al.* (1986). Training skills in the psychiatrically disabled: learning coping and competence. *Schizophrenia Bulletin* 12, 631–47.

Liddell, M. B., Lovestone, S., Owen, M. J. (2001). Genetic risk of Alzheimer's disease: advising relatives. *British Journal of Psychiatry* 178, 7–11.

Liddle, P. F. (1987). The symptoms of chronic schizophrenia: a re-examination of the positive and negative dichotomy. *British Journal of Psychiatry* 151, 145–51.

Liddle, P. F. (2000). Functional brain imaging of schizophrenia. In *The psychopharmacology of schizophrenia* (eds M. A. Reveley and J. F. W. Deakin), pp. 109–130. Oxford University Press, London.

Liddle, P. F., Friston, K. J., Frith, C. D., *et al.* (1992). Patterns of cerebral blood flow in schizophrenia. *British Journal of Psychiatry* 160, 179–86.

Lidz, T., Fleck, S., and Cornelison, A. (1965). *Schizophrenia and the family*. International Universities Press, New York.

Lieberman, J. A. and Sobel, S. N. (1993). Predictors of treatment response in course of schizophrenia. *Current Opinion in Psychiatry* 6, 63–9.

Lieberman, M. A. (1990). A group therapist perspective on self-help groups. *International Journal of Group Psychotherapy* 40, 251–77.

Lieberman, M. A. and Yalom, I. (1992). Brief group psychotherapy for the spousally bereaved: a controlled study. *International Journal of Group Psychotherapy* 42, 117–32.

Lieberman, M. A., Yalom, I. D., and Miles, M. B. (1973). *Encounter groups: first facts*. Basic Books, New York.

Liebowitz, M. R., Gorman, J. M., and Fyer, A. J. (1988). Pharmacotherapy of social phobia: an interim report of a placebo controlled comparison of phenelzine and atenolol. *Journal of Clinical Psychiatry* 49, 252–7.

Liebowitz, M. R., Schneier, F. R., and Campeas, R. (1992). Phenelzine versus atenolol in social phobia: a placebo controlled comparison. *Archives of General Psychiatry* 49, 290.

Lilenfeld, L. R. and Kaye, W. H. (1998). Genetic studies of anorexia and bulimia nervosa in *Neurobiology in the treatment of eating disorders* (eds H. W. Hoek, J. L. Treasure, and M. A. Katzman). John Wiley, Chichester.

Linde, K., Ramirez, G., Mulrow, C. D., *et al.* (1996). St John's Wort for depression – an overview and meta-analysis of randomised clinical trials. *British Medical Journal* 313, 253–8.

Lindemann, E. (1944). Symptomatology and management of acute grief. *American Journal of Psychiatry* 101, 141–8.

Lindesay, J. (2000a). Delirium in the elderly. In *The new Oxford textbook of psychiatry* (eds M. G. Gelder, J. J. López-Ibor Jr, and N. C. Andreasen), Chapter 8.5.1. Oxford University Press, Oxford.

Lindesay, J. (2000b). Stress-related, anxiety, and obsessional disorders in elderly people. In *The new Oxford textbook of psychiatry* (eds M. G. Gelder, J. J. López-Ibor Jr, and N. C. Andreasen), Chapter 8.5.5. Oxford University Press, Oxford.

Lindesay, J. (2001). Neurotic disorders in the elderly. In *Psychiatry in the elderly*, 3rd edn (eds R. Jacoby and C. Oppenheimer). Oxford University Press, Oxford.

Lindqvist, P. and Allebeck, P. (1990). Schizophrenia and crime. *British Medical Journal* 157, 345–50.

Lindqvist, P. and Skipworth, J. (2000). Evidence-based rehabilitation in forensic psychiatry. *British Journal of Psychiatry* 176, 320–3.

Lindsay, D. S. and Reed, J. D. (1995). 'Memory work' and recovered memories of childhood sexual abuse: scientific evidence and public, professional and personal issues. *Psychology, Public Policy and the Law* 1, 846–908.

Lindsey, M. (1997). Emotional, behavioural and psychiatric disorders in children. In *The psychiatry of learning disabilities* (ed. O. Russell), pp. 81–104. Gaskell, London.

Linehan, M. M. (1993). *Cognitive–behavioral treatment of borderline personality disorder*. Guilford, New York.

Linehan, M. M., Armstrong, H. E., Suarez, A., Allmon, D., and Heard, H. L. (1991). Cognitive–behavioral treatment of chronically parasuicidal borderline patients. *Archives of General Psychiatry* 48, 1060–4.

Linehan, M. M., Heard, H. L., and Armstrong, H. E. (1993). Naturalistic follow-up of a behavioral treatment for chronically parasuicidal borderline patients. *Archives of General Psychiatry* 50, 971–4.

Linehan, M. M., Tutek, D. A., Heard, H. L., and Armstrong, H. E. (1994). Interpersonal outcome of cognitive behavioral treatment for chronically suicidal borderline patients. *American Journal of Psychiatry* 151(12), 1771–6.

Linet, O. I. and Ogrinc, F. G. (1996). Efficacy and safety of intracavernosal alprostadil in men with erectile dysfunction. *New England Journal of Medicine* 334, 873–7.

Links, P. (2000). A lower minimum legal drinking age was associated with increased suicide in youths 18–23 years of age. *Evidence-Based Mental Health* 3, 59.

Linnoila, M. and Charney, D. S. (1999). The neurobiology of aggression. In *Neurobiology of mental illness* (eds D. S. Charney, E. J. Nestler, and B. S. Bunney), pp. 855–72. Oxford University Press, Oxford.

Linnoila, M. I. and Virkkunen, M. (1992). Aggression, suicidality and serotonin. *Journal of Clinical Psychiatry* 53(suppl. 10), 46–51.

Linton, S. J. (2000). A review of psychological risk factors in back and neck pain. *Spine* 25, 1148–56.

Lipowski, Z. J. (1980). Organic mental disorders: introduction and review of syndromes. In *Comprehensive textbook of psychiatry*, 3rd edn (eds H. I. Kaplan, A. M. Freedman, and B. J. Sadock). Williams & Wilkins, Baltimore, MD.

Lipowski, Z. J. (1988). Somatization: the concept and its clinical application. *American Journal of Psychiatry* 145, 1358–68.

Lipowski, Z. J. (1990). *Delirium: acute confusional states.* Oxford University Press, New York.

Liptzin, B. (2000). Clinical diagnosis and management of delirium. In *Psychiatric care of the medical patient* (eds A. Stoudemire, B. S. Fogel, and D. B. Greenberg). Oxford University Press, New York.

Liptzin, B., Levkoff, S. E., Gottlieb, G. L., and Johnson, J. C. (1994). Delirium. In *DSMIV sourcebook* (eds T. A. Widiger, A. J. Frances, H. A. Pincus, *et al.*), Vol. 1, pp. 199–212. American Psychiatric Association, Washington, DC.

Lisanby, S. H., Maddox, J. H., Prudic, J., *et al.* (2000). The effects of electroconvulsive therapy on memory of autobiographical and public events. *Archives of General Psychiatry* 57, 581–90.

Lishman, W. A. (1968). Brain damage in relation to psychiatric disability after head injury. *British Journal of Psychiatry* 114, 373–410.

Lishman, W. A. (1988). Physiogenesis and psychogenesis in the post-concussional syndrome. *British Journal of Psychiatry* 153, 460–9.

Lishman, W. A. (1998). *Organic psychiatry: the psychological consequences of cerebral disorder.* 3rd edn. Blackwell Scientific Publications, Oxford.

Llewellyn, A. and Stowe, Z. N. (1998). Psychotropic medications in lactation. *Journal of Clinical Psychiatry* 59(suppl 2), 41–52.

Lloyd, K. R., Jenkins, R., and Mann, A. H. (1996). Long-term outcome of patients with neurotic illness in general practice. *British Medical Journal* 313, 26–8.

Lock, T. (1999). Advances in the practice of electroconvulsive therapy. In *Recent topics and advances in psychiatric treatment* (ed. A. Lee), Vol. 2, pp. 66–75. Royal College of Psychiatrists, Gaskill Press, London.

Lohr, J. B. and Lavori, P. (1998). Wither vitamin E and tardive dyskinesia? *Biological Psychiatry* 43, 861–2.

Longworth, C., Honey, G., and Sharma, T. (1999). Functional magnetic resonance imaging in neuropsychiatry. *British Medical Journal* 319, 1551–4.

Loranger, A. W., Sartorius, N., Andreoli, A., *et al.* (1994). The International personality Disorder Examination: the World Health Organization/Alcohol, Drug Abuse and Mental Health Administration International Pilot Study of Personality Disorders. *Archives of General Psychiatry* 51, 215–24.

Lord, C. and Rutter, M. (1994). Autism and pervasive developmental disorder. In *Child and adolescent psychiatry: modern approaches*, 3rd edn (eds M. Rutter, E. Taylor, and L. Hersov), pp. 569–93. Blackwell Scientific Publications, Oxford.

Lovestone, S. (2000). Dementia: Alzheimer's disease. In *The new Oxford textbook of psychiatry* (eds. M. G. Gelder, J. J. López-Ibor Jr, and N. C. Andreasen), Chapter 4.1.3. Oxford University Press, Oxford.

Lovestone, S. (2000). Dementia: Alzheimers Disease. In *New Oxford Textbook of Psychiatry* (eds M. G. Gelder, J. J. López-Ibor, N. C. Andreasen). Oxford University Press.

Lowe, A. (1999). Drug abuse and psychiatric comorbidity. *Current Opinion in Psychiatry* 12, 291–95.

Lowman, R. L. and Richardson, L. M. (1987). Pseudoepileptic seizures of psychogenic origin: a review of the literature. *Clinical Psychology Review* 7, 363–89.

Lukeman, D. and Melvin, D. (1993). Annotation: the preterm infant: psychological issues in childhood. *Journal of Child Psychology and Psychiatry* 34(6), 837–49.

Lukianowicz, N. (1958). Autoscopic phenomena. *Archives of Neurology and Psychiatry* 80, 199–220.

Lund, J. (1990). Mentally retarded criminal offenders in Denmark. *British Journal of Psychiatry* 156, 726–31.

Luxenberger, H. (1928). Vorläufiger Bericht über psychiatrische Serienuntersuchungen an Zwillingen. *Zeitschrift für die gesamte Neurologie und Psychiatrie* 116, 297–326.

Lynch, M. and Roberts, J. (1982). *Consequences of child abuse*. Academic Press, London.

Lyons, M. J., True, W. R., Eisen, S. A., *et al.* (1995). Differential hereditability of adult and juvenile antisocial traits. *Archives of General Psychiatry* 52, 906–15.

McAllister-Williams, R. H., Ferrier, I. N., and Young, A. H. (1998). Mood and neuropsychological function in depression: the role of corticosteroids and serotonin. *Psychological Medicine* 28, 573–84.

McArdle, P., O'Brien, G., and Kolvin, I. (1997). Is there a comorbid relationship between hyperactivity and emotional psychopathology? *European Child and Adolescent Psychiatry* 6, 142–50.

McBeth, J. and Silman, A. J. (1999). Unraveling the association between chronic widespread pain and psychological distress: an epidemiological approach. *Journal of Psychosomatic Research* 47, 109–14.

McCall, W. V., Reboussin, D. M., Weiner, R. D., and Sackheim, H. A. (2000). Titrated moderately suprathreshold vs fixed high-dose right unilateral electroconvulsive therapy. *Archives of General Psychiatry* 57, 438–44.

McCann, U. D., Szabo, Z., Scheffel, U., *et al.* (1998). Positron emission tomographic evidence of toxic effect of MDMA ('ecstasy') on brain serotonin neurones in human beings. *Lancet* 352, 1433–7.

McCarthy, D. (1981). The effects of emotional disturbance and deprivation and somatic growth. In *Scientific foundations of paediatrics* (eds J. A. Davis and J. Dobbing), pp. 54–73. Heinemann, London.

McCarty, L. M. (1986). Mother-child incest: characteristics of the offender. *Child Welfare*, 65, 447–59.

McClure, G. M. G. (2000). Changes in suicide in England and Wales 1960–1997. *British Journal of Psychiatry* 176, 64–7.

McConaghy, N. (1998). Paedophilia; a review of the evidence. *Australian and New Zealand Journal of Psychiatry* 32, 252–65.

McDonald, A. S. and Davey, G. C. L. (1996). Psychiatric disorders and accidental injury. *Clinical Psychology Review* 16, 105–27.

McDougall, W. (1926). *An outline of abnormal psychology*. Methuen, London.

McDougle, C. J., Goodman, W. C., Price, L. H., *et al.* (1990). Neuroleptic addition in fluvoxamine refractory obsessive compulsive disorder. *American Journal of Psychiatry* 147, 652–4.

McElroy, S. L., Keck, P. E., and Strakowski, S. M. (1996). Mania, psychosis, and antipsychotics. *Journal of Clinical Psychiatry* 57(suppl 3), 14–26.

McEvoy, J. P. (2000). Schizophrenia, substance misuse, and smoking. *Current Opinion in Psychiatry* 13, 15–19.

McEwen, B. S., Biron, C. A., Brunson, K. W., *et al.* (1997). The role of adrenocorticoids as modulators of immune function in health and disease: neural, endocrine and immune interactions. *Brain Research Reviews* 23, 79–133.

MacFarlane, A. B. (1985). Medical evidence in the Court of Protection. *Bulletin of the Royal College of Psychiatrists* 9, 26–8.

McFarlane, A. C. (1988). The longitudinal course of posttraumatic morbidity. *Journal of Nervous and Mental Disease* 176, 30–9.

McFarlane, A. C. (1989). The aetiology of post-traumatic morbidity: predisposing, precipitating and perpetuating factors. *British Journal of Psychiatry* 154, 221–8.

McGorry, P. D., Singh, B. S., Connell, S., *et al.* (1992). Diagnostic concordance in functional psychosis revisited: a study of inter-relationships between alternative concepts of psychotic disorder. *Psychological Medicine* 22, 367–78.

McGorry, P. D., Krstev, H., and Harrigan, S. (2000). Early detection and treatment delay: implications for outcome in early psychosis. *Current Opinion in Psychiatry* 13, 37–43.

McGrath, J. and Emmerson, W. B. (1999). Treatment of schizophrenia. *British Medical Journal* 319, 1045–8.

McGuffin, P. (1988). Genetics of schizophrenia. In *Schizophrenia. The major issues* (eds P. Bebbington and P. McGuffin), pp. 107–26. Heinemann, Oxford.

McGuffin, P., and Thapar, A. (1992). The genetics of personality disorder. *British Journal of Psychiatry* 160, 12–23.

McGuffin, P., Farmer, A. E., Gottesman, I. I., *et al.* (1984). Twin concordance for operationally defined schizophrenia. Confirmation of familiarity and heritability. *Archives of General Psychiatry* 41, 541–5.

McGuffin, P., Asherson, P., Owen, M., and Farmer, A. (1994). The strength of the genetic effect: is there room for an environmental influence in the aetiology of schizophrenia. *British Journal of Psychiatry* 164, 593–9.

McGuffin, P., Katz, R., Watkins, S., and Rutherford, J. (1996). A hospital-based twin register of the heritability of DSM-IV unipolar depression. *Archives of General Psychiatry* 53, 129–36.

McGuire, P. K. and Frith, C. D. (1996). Disordered functional connectivity in schizophrenia. *Psychological Medicine* 26, 663–7.

McHugh, P. R. and Slavney, P. R. (1986). *The perspectives of psychiatry*. John Hopkins University Press, Baltimore, MD.

McKeith, I. G. (2000). Lewy body dementia. In *The new Oxford textbook of psychiatry* (eds M. G. Gelder, J. J. López-Ibor Jr, and N. C. Andreasen), Chapter 4.1.6. Oxford University Press, Oxford.

McKeith, I. G., Galasko, D., Korsaka, K., *et al.* (1996). Consensus guidelines for the clinical and pathologic diagnosis of dementia with Lewy bodies (DLB). *Neurology* 47, 1113–24.

McKenna, P. J. (1984). Disorders with overvalued ideas. *British Journal of Psychiatry* 145, 579–85.

MacMahon, B. and Pugh, T. F. (1965). Suicide in the widowed. *American Journal of Epidemiology* 81, 23–31.

McNally, R. J. (1994). Choking phobia: a review of the literature. *Comprehensive Psychiatry* 35, 83–9.

McNeil, T. F., Cantor-Graae, E., and Weinberger, D. R. (2000). Relationship of obstetric complications and differences in size of brain structures in monozygotic twin pairs discordant for schizophrenia. *American Journal of Psychiatry* 157, 203–12.

McPherson, H., Herbison, P., and Romans, S. (1993). Life events and relapse in established bipolar affective disorder. *British Journal of Psychiatry* 163, 381–5.

Machlin, S., Harris, G., Pearlson, G., *et al.* (1991). Elevated medical frontal cerebral blood flow in obsessive äcompulsive patients: a SPECT study. *American Journal of Psychiatry* 148, 1240–2.

Maden, T., Swinlon, M., and Gonn, J. (1994). Psychiatric disorder in women serving a prison sentence. *British Journal of Psychiatry* 164, 44–54.

Madonna, P., van Scoyk, S., and Jones, D. P. H. (1991). Family interactions with incest and non-incest families. *American Journal of Psychiatry* 148, 46–9.

Maes, H. H., Woodard, C. E., Murrelle, L., *et al.* (1999). Tobacco, alcohol and drug use in eight- to sixteen-year-old twins: the Virginia Twin Study of Adolescent Behavioral Development. *Journal of Studies on Alcohol* 60(3), 293–305.

Maguire, M. (1997) *The Oxford Textbook of Criminology* (2nd ed) Clarendon Press, Oxford.

Maier, W., Lichtermann, D., Meyer, A., *et al.* (1993a). A controlled family study in panic disorder. *Journal of Psychiatric Research* 27(suppl. 1), 79–87.

Maier, W., Lichtermann, D., Minges, J., *et al.* (1993b). Continuity and discontinuity of affective disorders and schizophrenia. *Archives of General Psychiatry* 50, 871–83.

Maier, W., Schwab, S. and Rieştschel, M. (2000). The genetics of schizophrenia. *Current Opinion in Psychiatry* 13, 3–9.

Maj, M. (2000). Dementia due to HIV disease. In *The new Oxford textbook of psychiatry* (eds M. G. Gelder, J. J. López-Ibor Jr, and N. C. Andreasen), Chapter 4.1.10. Oxford University Press, Oxford.

Major, B., Cozzarelli, C., Cooper, M. L., *et al.* (2000). Psychological responses of women after first-trimester abortion. *Archives of General Psychiatry* 57, 777–84.

Makanjuola, R. O. A. (1982). Manic disorder in Nigerians. *British Journal of Psychiatry* 141, 459–63.

Maletzky, B. M. (1973). The episode dyscontrol syndrome. *Diseases of the Nervous System* 34, 178–84.

Malison, R. T., Price, L. H., Berman, R., *et al.* (1998). Reduced brain serotonin transporter availability in major depression as measured by $[^{123}I]$–2 beta-carbomethoxy–3 beta -(4-iodophenyl)tropane and single photon emission computed tomography. *Biological Psychiatry* 44, 1090–8.

Malmberg, A., Simkin, S., and Hawton, K. (1999). Suicide in farmers. *British Journal of Psychiatry* 175, 103–5.

Malmberg, L. and Fenton, M. (2000). Individual psychodynamic psychotherapy and psychoanalysis for schizophrenia and severe mental illness. *Cochrane Database Systematic Review* 2, CD001360.

Malt, U. F. (2000). Psychiatric aspects of accidents, burns and other trauma. In *The new Oxford textbook of psychiatry* (eds M. G. Gelder, J. J. López-Ibor Jr, and N. C. Andreasen), Chapter 5.3.8. Oxford University Press, Oxford.

Mander, A. J. and Loudon, J. B. (1988). Rapid recurrence of mania following abrupt discontinuation of lithium. *Lancet* 2, 15–17.

Mann (2001)

Mann, A. H., Jenkins, R., and Belsey, E. (1981). The twelve-month outcome of patients with neurotic illness in general practice. *Psychological Medicine* 11, 535–50.

Mann, K., Batra, A., Gunther, A., and Schroth, G. (1992). Do women develop alcoholic brain damage more readily than men? *Alcohol: Clinical and Experimental Research* 16, 1052–6.

Mannuzza, S., Klein, R. G., Bessler, A., *et al.* (1993). Adult outcome of hyperactive boys. *Archives of General Psychiatry* 50, 565–76.

Manu, P. (ed.) (1998). *Functional somatic syndromes. Etiology, diagnosis and treatment.* Cambridge University Press, Cambridge.

March, J. S., Biederman, J., Wolkow, R., *et al.* (1998). Sertraline in children and adolescents with obsessive–compulsive disorder: a multi-centre randomized controlled trial. *Journal of the American Medical Association* 280, 1752–6.

March, J., Frances, A., Carpenter, D., *et al.* (1997). The expert consensus guidelines series: treatment of obsessive–compulsive disorder. *Journal of Clinical Psychiatry* 4(**suppl.**), 2–72.

Marder, S. R., Wirshing, W. C., and Wirshing, D. A. (2000). New strategies with conventional antipsychotics. In *The psychopharmacology of schizophrenia* (eds M. A. Reveley and J. F. W. Deakin), pp. 211–24. Oxford University Press, New York.

Margolis, R. L., McInnes, M. G., Rosenblatt, A., and Ross, C. A. (1999). Trinucleotide repeat expansion and neuropsychiatric disease. *Archives of General Psychiatry* 56, 1019–31.

Marino, R. and Cosgrove, G. R. (1997). Neurosurgical treatment of neuropsychiatric illness. *Psychiatric Clinics of North America* 20(4), 933–43.

Marks, I. M. (1969). *Fears and phobias.* Heinemann, London.

Marks, I. M. (1988). Blood-injury phobia: a review. *American Journal of Psychiatry* 145, 1207–14.

Marks, I. M. and Gelder, M. G. (1966). Different ages of onset of varieties of phobia. *American Journal of Psychiatry* 123, 218–21.

Marks, I. M., Swinson, R. P., and Basoglu, M. (1993a). Alprazolam and exposure alone and combined in panic disorder and agoraphobia: a controlled study in London and Toronto. *British Journal of Psychiatry* 162, 776–87.

Marks, I. M., Swinson, R. P., Basoglu, M., *et al.* (1993b). Reply to comment on the London/Toronto study. *British Journal of Psychiatry* 162, 790–4.

Marks, I. M., Connolly, J., Muijen, M., *et al.* (1994). Home-based versus hospital based care for people with serious mental illness. *British Journal of Psychiatry* 165, 179–94.

Marks, M. N. and Kumar, R. (1993). Infanticide in England and Wales. *Medical Scientific Law* 33(3), 329–39.

Markus, E., Lange, A., and Pettigrew, T. F. (1990). Effectiveness of family therapy: a meta-analysis. *Journal of Family Therapy* 12, 205–21.

Marmar, C. R. (1991). Brief dynamic psychotherapy of post-traumatic stress disorder. *Psychiatric Annals* 21, 405–14.

Marmar, C. R., Horowitz, M. J., Weiss, D. S., *et al.* (1988). A controlled trial of brief psychotherapy and mutual help group treatment of conjugal bereavement. *American Journal of Psychiatry* 145, 203–9.

Marmor, J. (1953). Orality in the hysterical personality. *Journal of the American Psychoanalytic Association* 1 527–31.

Marriott, A., Donaldson, C., Tarrier, N., and Burns, A. (2000). Effectiveness of cognitive–behavioural family intervention in reducing the burden of care in carers of patients with Alzheimer's disease. *British Journal of Psychiatry* 176, 557–62.

Marsh, L. (2000). Neuropsychiatric aspects of Parkinson's Disease. *Psychosomatics* 41, 15–23.

Marshall, E. J. and Reed, J. L. (1992). Psychiatric morbidity in homeless women. *British Journal of Psychiatry* 160, 761–8.

Marshall, E. J., Edwards, G., and Taylor, C. (1994). Mortality in men with drinking problems: a 20-year follow-up. *Addiction* 89, 1293–8.

Marshall, M. (1989). Collected and neglected: are Oxford hostels for the homeless filling up with disabled psychiatric patients. *British Medical Journal* 299, 706–9.

Marshall, M. (1994). How should we measure need? Concept and practice in the development of a standardized assessment of need. *Philosophy Psychology and Psychiatry* 1, 27–36.

Marshall, M. and Gath, D. (1992). What happens to homeless mentally ill people? Follow-up of residents of Oxford hostels for the homeless. *British Medical Journal* 304, 79–80.

Marshall, M., and Lockwood, A. (1998). Assertive community treatment for people with psychiatric disorders. In *The Cochrane Library Issue 2*. Update Software, Oxford.

Marshall, M. and Lockwood, A. (2000). Assertive community treatment for people with severe mental disorders (Cochrane Review). In *The Cochrane Library, Issue 2*. Update Software, Oxford.

Marshall, M., Hogg, L., Lockwood, A., *et al.* (1995). The Cardinal Needs schedule: a modified version of the MRC Needs for Care Schedule. *Psychological Medicine* 25, 605–17.

Marshall M., Gray, A., Lockwood, A., *et al.* (1998). Case management of people with severe mental disorders. *Cochrane Library Issue 2*. Update Software, Oxford.

Marteau, R. M. (1994). Psychology and screening: narrowing the gap between efficacy and effectiveness. *British Journal of Clinical Psychology* 33, 1–10.

Marteau, T. M. and Croyle, R. T. (1998). Psychological responses to genetic testing. *British Medical Journal* 316, 693–6.

Martin, J., Shochat, T., Ancoli-Israel, S. (2000). Assessment and treatment of sleep disturbances in older adults. *Clinical Psychology Review* 20, 783–805.

Mart'nez-Arán, A., Vieta, E., Colom, F., *et al.* (2000). Cognitive dysfunctions in bipolar disorder: evidence of neuropsychological disturbances. *Psychotherapy and Psychosomatics* 69, 2–18.

Martucci, M., Balestrieri, M., Bisoffi, G. *et al.* (1999). Evaluating psychiatric morbidity in a general hospital: a two-phase epidemiological survey. *Psychological Medicine* 29, 823–832.

Marzuk, P. M., Tardiff, K., and Hirsch, C. S. (1992). The epidemiology of murder-suicide. *Journal of the American Medical Association* 267, 3179–81.

Masters, W. H. and Johnson, V. E. (1970). *Human sexual inadequacy*. Churchill, London.

Mate-Kole, C., Freschi, M., and Robin, A. (1990). A controlled study of psychological and social change after surgical gender reassignment in selected male transsexuals. *British Journal of Psychiatry* 157, 261–4.

Mathews, A., Gelder, M. G., and Johnson, D. (1981). *Agoraphobia: nature and treatment*. Tavistock Publications, London.

Matson, J. L. and Sevin, J. A. (1994). Theories of dual diagnosis in mental retardation. *Journal of Consulting and Clinical Psychology* 62(1), 6–16.

Matson, J. L. and Taras, M. E. (1989). A 20 year review of punishment and alternative methods to treat problem behaviors in developmentally delayed persons. *Research in Developmental Disabilities* 10, 85–104.

Mattick, R. P. and Peters, L. (1988). Treatment of severe social phobia: effects of guided exposure with and without cognitive restructuring. *Journal of Clinical Psychology* 56, 251–60.

Maudsley, H. (1879). *The pathology of mind*. Macmillan, London.

Maudsley, H. (1885). *Responsibility in mental disease*. Kegan Paul and Trench, London.

Maughan, B., Gray, G., and Rutter, M. (1985). Reading retardation and antisocial behaviour: a follow-up into employment. *Journal of Child Psychology and Psychiatry* 25, 741–58.

Mavissakalian, M. and Perel, J. M. (1992). Clinical experiments in maintenance and discontinuation of imipramine therapy in panic disorder with agoraphobia. *Archives of General Psychiatry* 49, 318–23.

Mawson, D., Marks, I. M., and Ramm, L. (1981). Guided mourning for morbid grief: a controlled study. *British Journal of Psychiatry* 138, 185–93.

Maxfield, M. and Widdom, C. (1996). The cycle of violence. *Archives of Paediatric and Adolescent Medicine* 150, 390–5.

May, P. R. A. (1968). *Treatment of schizophrenia*. Science House, New York.

Mayer, W. (1921). Über paraphrene psychosen. *Zentralblatt für die gesamte Neurologie und Psychiatrie* 71, 187–206.

Mayer-Gross, W. (1932). Die Schizophrenie. In *Bumke's Handbuch der Geisteskrankheiten*, Vol 9. Springer, Berlin.

Mayo-Smith, M. F. for the American Society for Addiction Medicine Working Group (1997). Pharmacological management of alcohol withdrawal: a meta-analysis and evidence-based practice guideline. *Journal of the American Medical Association* 278, 144–61.

Mayou, R. A. (1992). Psychiatric aspects of road traffic accidents. *International Review of Psychiatry* 4, 45–54.

Mayou, R. and Sharpe, M. C. (1995). Psychiatric illnesses associated with physical disease. *Baillière's Clinical Psychiatry* 1(2), 201–23.

Mayou, R., Bass, C., and Sharpe, M. (eds) (1995). *Treatment of functional somatic symptoms.* Oxford University Press, Oxford.

Mayou, R. A., Ehlers, A., and Hobbs, M. (2000). Psychological debriefing for road traffic accident victims. Three year follow-up of a randomised controlled trial. *British Journal of Psychiatry,* 176, 590–4.

Meadow, R. (1985). Management of Munchausen syndrome by proxy. *Archives of Diseases of Childhood* 60, 385–93.

Meagher, D. J. (2001). Delirium: optimising management. *British Medical Journal* 322, 144–149.

Mechanic, D. (1978). *Medical sociology*, 2nd edn. Free Press, Glencoe.

Meduna, L. (1938). General discussion of cardiazol therapy. *American Journal of Psychiatry* 94, Suppl 40.

Megargee, E. I. (1966). Uncontrolled and overcontrolled personality type in extreme antisocial aggression. *Psychological Monographs* 80, No.3.

Mehlum, L., Friis, S., Irion, T., *et al.* (1991). Personality disorders 2–5 years after treatment: a prospective follow-up study. *Acta Psychiatrica Scandinavica* 84, 72–7.

Meichenbaum, D. H. (1977). *Cognitive–behaviour modification.* Plenum, New York.

Meloy, J. R. (1998). *The psychology of stalking: clinical and forensic perspectives.* Academic Press, San Diego, CA.

Meltzer, H. Y. and Okayli, G. (1995). Reduction of suicidality during clozapine treatment of neuroleptic-resistant schizophrenia: impact on risk-benefit assessment. *American Journal of Psychiatry* 152, 183–90.

Meltzer, H., Gill, B., and Petticrew, M. (1994). *The prevalence of psychiatric morbidity among adults aged 16–64, living in private households, in Great Britain.* OPCS Surveys of Psychiatric Morbidity in Great Britain. HMSO, London.

Meltzer, H. Y., Alphs, L., Green, A. L., Altamura, A. C., Anand, R., Bertoldi, A., Bourgeois, M., Choimnard, G., Islam, Z., Kane, J., Krishnan, R., Linenmeyer, J-P. and Potkin, S. (2003). Clozapine treatment for suicidality in schizophrenia. *Archives of General Psychiatry* 60, 82–91.

Mendelson, G. (1995). 'Compensation neurosis' revisited: outcome studies of the effects of litigation. *Journal of Psychosomatic Research* 39, 695–706.

Mendelson, M. (1992). Psychodynamics. In *Handbook of affective disorders* (ed. E. S. Paykel), pp. 195–207. Churchill Livingstone, Edinburgh.

Mendelson, W. B. (1991). Neurotransmitters, sleep and affective disorder. In *Serotonin, sleep and mental disorder* (eds P. J. Cowen and C. Idzikowski), pp. 277–88. Wrightson Biomedical Publishing, Petersfield.

Mendelwicz, J., Papadimitiou, G., and Wilmotte, J. (1993). Family study of panic disorder: comparison of generalized anxiety disorder, major depression, and normal subjects. *Psychiatric Genetics* 3, 73–8.

Mendlewicz, J. (1976). The age factor in depressive illness: some genetic considerations. *Journal of Gerontology* 31, 300–3.

Mercier-Guidez, E. and Loas, G. (1998). Polydipsia and water intoxication in psychiatric inpatients: review of the literature. *Encephale* 24, 223–9.

Merskey, H. (1999). Ethical aspects of the physical manipulation of the brain. In *Ethical aspects of drug treatment*, 3rd edn (eds S. Bloch, P. Chodoff, and S. A. Green), pp. 275–99. Oxford University Press, Oxford.

Merskey, H. (2000). Conversion and dissociation. In *The new Oxford textbook of psychiatry* (eds M. G. Gelder, J. J. López-Ibor Jr, and N. C. Andreasen), Chapter 5.2.4. Oxford University Press, Oxford.

Merson, S., Tyrer, P., Oynett, S., *et al.* (1992). Early intervention in psychiatric emergencies: a clinical trial. *Lancet* 339, 1311–13.

Mesulam, M.M. (1998). From sensation to cognition. *Brain* 121, 1013–52.

Meyer, J. K. and Reter, D. J. (1979). Sex reassignment: follow up. *Archives of General Psychiatry* 36, 1010–15.

Meyers, W. C. and Kemph, J. P. (1990). DSMIII-R classification of homicidal youth: help or hindrance? *Journal of Clinical Psychiatry* 5, 239–42.

Mezey, G. C. and King, M. B (1989). The effects of sexual assault on men: a survey of 22 victims. *Psychological Medicine* 19, 205–209.

Mezey, G. and King, M. (eds) (2000). *Male victims of sexual assault*. Oxford University Press

Mezey, G. C. and Robbins, I. (2000). The impact of criminal victimisation. In *The new Oxford textbook of psychiatry* (eds M. G. Gelder, J. J. López-Ibor Jr, and N. C Andreasen), Chapter 11.5. Oxford University Press, Oxford.

Mezzich, J. E., Kirmayer, L. J., Kleinman, A., *et al.* (1999). The place of culture in DSM-IV. *Journal of Nervous and Mental Disease* 187, 457–64.

Mezzich, J. E., Olero-Ojeda, A. A., and Lee, S. (2000). International psychiatric diagnosis. In *The comprehensive textbook of psychiatry*, 7th edn (eds B. J. Sadock and V. A. Sadock). Lippincott, Williams & Wilkins, Philadelphia.

Michael, R. T., Gagnon, J. H., Laumann, E. O., and Kolata, G. (1994). *Sex in America; a definitive survey*. Little Brown and Company, London.

Miller, F. G. (2000). Placebo-controlled trials in psychiatric research: an ethical perspective. *Biological Psychiatry* 47, 707–16.

Miller, H. (1961). Accident neurosis. *British Medical Journal* 1, 919–25, 992–8.

Miller, K. and Klauber, G. T. (1990). Desmopressin acetate in children with severe primary nocturnal enuresis. *Clinical Therapeutics* 12, 357–66.

Miller, P. M. and Plant, M. (1996). Drinking, smoking and illicit drug use among 15- and 16-year olds in the United Kingdom. *British Medical Journal* 313, 394–7.

Miller, W. R. and Rollnick, S. (1991). *Motivational interviewing: preparing people to change addictive behaviour*. Guildford Press, London.

Milne, J. M., Garrison, C. Z., Addy, C. L., *et al.* (1995). Frequency of phobic disorder in a community sample of young adolescents. *Journal of the American Academy of Child and Adolescent Psychiatry* 34, 1202–11.

Mindham, R. H. S. (2000). Dementia in Parkinson's disease. In *The new Oxford textbook of psychiatry* (eds M. G. Gelder, J. J. López-Ibor Jr, and N. C Andreasen), Chapter 4.1.7. Oxford University Press, Oxford.

Minuchin, S., Rosman, B., and Baker, L. (1978*). Psychosomatic families: anorexia nervosa in context*. Harvard University Press, Cambridge, MA.

Mir, S. and Taylor, D. (1999). Serotonin syndrome. *Psychiatric Bulletin* 23, 742–7.

Mirza, K. A., Bhadrinath, B. R., Goodyer, I. M., and Gilmour, C. (1998). Post-traumatic stress reactions in children and adolescents following road traffic accidents. *British Journal of Psychiatry* 172, 443–7.

Mitchell, J . (1983). When disaster strikes: the critical incident debriefing process. *Journal of Emergency Medical Services* 8, 36–9.

Mitchell, W., Falconer, M. A., and Hill, D. (1954). Epilepsy with fetishism relieved by temporal lobectomy. *Lancet* 2, 626–30.

Mitchell-Heggs, N., Kelly, D., and Richardson, A. (1976). Stereotactic limbic leucotomy – a follow-up after 16 months. *British Journal of Psychiatry* 128, 226–41.

Modell, S., Lauer, C. J., Schreiber, W., *et al.* (1998). Hormonal response pattern in the combined DEX-CRH test is stable over time in subjects at high familial risk for affective disorders. *Neuropsychopharmacology* 18, 253–62.

Modigh, K., Wetenberg, P., and Eriksson, E. (1992). Superiority of clomipramine over imipramine in the treatment of panic disorder: a placebo controlled trial. *Journal of Clinical Psychopharmacology* 12, 251–61.

Mollica, R. (2000). The special psychiatric problems of refugees. In *The new Oxford textbook of psychiatry* (eds M. G. Gelder, J. J. López-Ibor Jr, and N. C. Andreasen), Chapter 7.10.1. Oxford University Press, Oxford.

Monahan, J. (1997). Clinical and actuarial predictions of violence. In *Modern scientific evidence: the law and science of expert testimony* (eds D. Faigman, D. Kaye, M. Saks, and J. Sanders), Vol. 1, p. 309. West Publishing, St Paul, MN.

Monahan, J. and Steadman, H. (1994). *Violence and mental disorder: developments in risk assessment*. Chicago University Press, Chicago.

Monahan, J., Steadman, H. J., Appelbaum, P. S., *et al.* (2000). Developing a clinically useful actuarial tool for assessing violence risk. *British Journal of Psychiatry* 176, 312–19.

Moncrieff, J. and Goodwin, G. M. (1995). Lithium revisited. A re-examination of the placebo-controlled trials of lithium prophylaxis in manic-depressive disorder. *British Journal of Psychiatry* 167, 569–74.

Money, J., Schwartz, M., and Lewis, V. G. (1984). Adult herotosexual status and fetal hormonal masculinization and demasculinization: 46 XX congenital virilizing adrenal hyperplasia and 46 XY androgen-insensitivity syndrome compared. *Psychoneuroendocrinology* 9, 405–14.

Monteiro, W., Marks, I. M., and Ramm, E. (1985). Marital adjustment and treatment outcome in agoraphobia. *British Journal of Psychiatry* 146, 383–90.

Montgomery, S. A. and Asberg, M. (1979). A new depression rating scale designed to be sensitive to change. *British Journal of Psychiatry* 134, 382–9.

Moorey, S. and Greer, S. (1989). *Psychological therapy for patients with cancer: a new approach.* Heinemann Medical, Oxford.

Moran, E. (2000). Special psychiatric problems relating to gambling. In *The new Oxford textbook of psychiatry* (eds M. G. Gelder, J. J. López-Ibor Jr, and N. C. Andreasen), Chapter 4.13.3. Oxford University Press, Oxford.

Morch, W. T., Skar, J., and Andersgard, A. B. (1997). Mentally retarded persons as parents: prevalence and the situation of their children. *Scandinavian Journal of Psychology* 38, 343–8.

Morel, B. A. (1860). *Traité des malades mentales.* Masson, Paris.

Morgagni, G. B. (1769). *The seats and causes of diseases investigated by anatomy* (transl. B. Alexander). Millar, London.

Morin, C. M., Colecchi, C., Stone, J., *et al.* (1999). Behavioral and pharmacological therapies for late-life insomnia. *Journal of the American Medical Association* 281, 991–9.

Morley, S., Eccleston, C., and Williams, A. (1999). Systematic review and meta-analysis of randomized controlled trials of cognitive behaviour therapy and behaviour therapy for chronic pain in adults, excluding headache. *Pain* 80, 1–13.

Morris, J. B. and Beck, A. T. (1974). The efficacy of antidepressant drugs. A review of research (1958–1972). *Archives of General Psychiatry* 30, 667–74.

Morris, R. G. (1997). Cognition and ageing. In *Psychiatry in the elderly* (eds R. Jacoby and C. Oppenheimer), pp. 37–62. Oxford University Press, Oxford.

Morris, R. G., Morris, L. W., and Britton, P. G. (1988). Factors affecting the emotional wellbeing of the caregivers of dementia sufferers. *British Journal of Psychiatry* 153, 147–56.

Morrison, J. (1989). Childhood sexual histories of women with somatization disorder. *American Journal of Psychiatry* 146, 239–41.

Morselli, E. (1886). Sulla dismorfofobia e sulla tabefobia. *Bolletin Academica Medica* VI, 110–19.

Mortensen, P. B., Cantor-Graae, E. and McNeil, T. F. (1997). Increased rates of schizophrenia among immigrants: some methodological concerns raised by Danish findings. *Psychological Medicine* 27, 813–20.

Mortimer, A. M. (2000). The neuropsychology of schizophrenia. In *The psychopharmacology of schizophrenia* (eds M. A. Reveley and J. F. W. Deakin), pp. 153–77. Oxford University Press, London.

Mueser, K. T. and Bond, G. R. (2000). Psychosocial treatment approaches for schizophrenia. *Current Opinion in Psychiatry* 13, 27–35.

Mukherjee, S., Sackheim, H. A., and Lee, C. (1988). Unilateral ECT in the treatment of manic episodes. *Convulsive Therapy* 4, 74–80.

Mukherjee, S., Sackheim, H. A. and Schnur, D. B. (1994). Electroconvulsive therapy of acute manic episodes: a review of fifty years experience. *American Journal of Psychiatry* 151, 169–76.

Mulholland, C. and Cooper, S. (2000). The symptom of depression in schizophrenia and its management. *Advances in Psychiatric Treatment* 6, 169–77.

Mullen, P. D. (1997). Compliance becomes concordance. *British Medical Journal* 314, 691–2.

Mullen, P. E. (2000). Dangerousness, risk and the prediction of probability. In *The new Oxford textbook of psychiatry* (eds M. G. Gelder, J. J. López-Ibor Jr, and N. C. Andreason), Chapter 11.4.3. Oxford University Press, Oxford.

Mullen, P. E. and Maack, L. H. (1985). Jealousy, pathological jealousy and aggression. In *Aggression and dangerousness* (eds D. P. Farington and J. Gunn). Wiley, Chichester.

Mullen, P. E. and Martin, J. (1994). Jealousy: a community study. *British Journal of Psychiatry* 164, 35–43.

Mullen, P. E., Martin, J. L., Anderson, J. C., *et al.* (1993). Childhood sexual abuse and mental health in adult life. *British Journal of Psychiatry* 163, 721–32.

Mullen, P., Pathé, M., and Purcell, R. (2000). *Stalkers and their victims.* Cambridge University Press, Cambridge.

Mulvey, E. P., Arthur, M. W., and Reppucci, A. (1993). The prevention and treatment of juvenile delinquency:

a review of the research. *Clinical Psychology Review* 13, 133–67.

Munro, A. and Mok, H. (1995). An overview of treatment in paranoia/delusional disorder. *Canadian Journal of Psychiatry* 40, 616–22.

Munroe, R. L. (1955). *Schools of psychoanalytic thought.* Hutchinson Medical, London.

Murphy, E., Smith, R., Lindesay, J., and Slatter, J. (1988). Increased mortality rates in late-life depression. *British Journal of Psychiatry* 152, 347–53.

Murphy, G. (1994). Services for children and adolescents with severe learning difficulties (mental retardation). In *Child and adolescent psychiatry: modern approaches*, 3rd edn (eds M. Rutter, E. Taylor, and L. Hersov), pp.1023–39. Blackwell Scientific Publications, Oxford.

Murphy, G. E. (1982). Social origins of depression in old age. *British Journal of Psychiatry* 141, 135–42.

Murphy, G. E., Wetzel, R. D., Robins, E., and McEvoy, L. (1992). Multiple risk factors predict suicide and alcoholism. *Archives of General Psychiatry* 49, 459–63.

Murphy, H. B. M. and Raman, A. C. (1971). The chronicity of schizophrenia in indigenous tropical people. *British Journal of Psychiatry* 118, 489–97.

Murray R. M. and Reveley, A. (1981). The genetic contribution to the neuroses. *British Journal of Hospital Medicine* 25, 185–90.

Murray, J. and Williams, P. (1986). Self-reported illness and general practice consultations in Asian born and British born residents of West London. *Social Psychiatry* 21, 139–45.

Murray, J. B. (1998). Pharmacological therapy of deviant sexual behaviour. *Journal of General Psychology* 115, 101–10.

Murray, L. and Cooper, P. J. (1997). Postpartum depression and child development. *Psychological Medicine* 27, 253–60.

Murray, R. M. and Castle, D. J. (2000). Genetic and environmental risk factors for schizophrenia. In *The new Oxford textbook of psychiatry* (eds M. G. Gelder, J. J. López-Ibor Jr, and N. C. Andreasen), Chapter 4.3.5.1. Oxford University Press, Oxford.

Mynors-Wallace, L. M., Gath, D. H., Lloyd-Thomas, A. R., and Tomlinson, D. (1995). Randomized controlled trial comparing problem solving treatment with amitriptyline and placebo for major depression in primary care. *British Medical Journal* 310, 441–5.

Nadelson, C. (1989). Consequences of rape: clinical treatment and aspects. *Psychotherapy and psychosomatics* 51, 187–92.

Naguib, M. and Levy, R. (1987). Late paraphrenia – neuropsychological impairment and structural brain abnormalities on computed tomography. *International Journal of Geriatric Psychiatry* 2, 83–90.

Näslund, J., Haroutunian, V., Mohs, R., Davis, K. L., Davies, P., Greengard, P., Buxbaum, J. D. (2000). Correlation between elevated levels of amyloid β-peptide in the brain and cognitive decline. *Journal of the American Medical Association* 283, 1571–1577

Nassir-Ghaemi, S. and Gaughan, S. (2000). Novel anticonvulsants: a new generation of mood stabilizers? *Harvard Review of Psychiatry* 8, 1–7.

Nathan, P. E. and Gorman, J. M. (eds) (1998). *A guide to treatments that work*, Chapters 15–18. Oxford University Press, New York.

Nathan, P. J. (1999). The experimental and clinical pharmacology of St John's Wort (*Hypericum perforatum* L.). *Molecular Psychiatry* 4, 333–8.

National Institute for Clinical Excellence (2002). Schizophrenia: Core interventions in the treatment and management of schizophrenia in primary and secondary care. *Clinincal Guidline* 1.

National Institutes of Health Consensus Development Panel (1999). Rehabilitation of persons with traumatic brain injury. *Journal of the American Medical Association* 282, 974–83.

National Institute of Mental Health (1985). Consensus Development Conference Statement. Mood disorders: pharmacological prevention of recurrences. *American Journal of Psychiatry* 142, 469–76.

National Institute on Drug Abuse (1991). *National Household Survey on Drug Abuse: highlights.* US Government Printing Office, Washington, DC.

National Schizophrenia Guideline Group (1999). *The early management of schizophrenia: Part 1. Pharmacological treatments, evidence based clinical practice guideline.* Royal College of Psychiatrists Research Unit; The British Psychological Society; Medicines Evaluation Group, Centre for Health Economics, University of York, York.

Naylor, C. D. (1997). Meta-analysis and the meta-epidemiology of clinical research. *British Medical Journal* 315, 617–19.

Needleman, H., Gunnoe, C., Leviton, A., *et al.* (1979). Deficits in psychologic and classroom performances of children with elevated dentine lead levels. *New England Journal of Medicine* 300, 689–95.

Neeleman, J. and Wessely, S. (1997). Changes in classification of suicide in England and Wales: time trends and associations with coroners' professional backgrounds. *Psychological Medicine* 21, 467–72.

Neligan, G. and Prudham, D. (1969). Norms for four standard developmental milestones by sex, social class and place in the family. *Developmental Medicine and Child Neurology* 11, 413–22.

Nelson, E. and Rice, J. (1997). Stability of diagnosis of obsessive–compulsive disorder in the epidemiological catchment area study. *American Journal of Psychiatry* 154, 826–31.

Nemiah, J. C. and Sifneos, P. E. (1970). Psychosomatic illness: a problem of communication. *Psychotherapy and Psychosomatics* 18, 154–60.

Nestadt, G., Romanoski, A. J., Samuels, J. F., *et al.* (1992). The relationship between personality and DSMIII axis I disorders in the population: results from an epidemiological survey. *American Journal of Psychiatry* 149, 1228–33.

Neumann, D., Housekamp, B., Pollock, V. and Briere, J. (1996). The long-term sequellae of child sexual abuse in women: a meta-analytic study *Child Maltreatment 1*, 6–16.

Neuropathology Group of the Medical Research Council Cognitive Function and Ageing Study (MRC CFAS). Pathological correlates of late-onset dementia in a multicentre, community-based population in England and Wales. *Lancet* 357, 169–175.

Newman, S. and Stygall, J. (1999). Changes in cognition following cardiac surgery. *Heart* 82, 541–2.

Newport, D. J. and Nemeroff, C. B. (1998). Assessment and treatment of depression in the cancer patient. *Journal of Psychosomatic Research* 45, 215–37.

Ngan, E. T. C., Yatham, L. N., Ruth, T. J., and Liddle, P. F. (2000). Decreased serotonin 2A receptor densities in neuroleptic-naive patients with schizophrenia: A PET study using [18F] setoperone. *American Journal of Psychiatry* 157, 1016–18.

NHS Centre for Reviews and Dissemination (1999). Drug treatments for schizophrenia. *Effective Health Care* 5, 1–12.

NICHD Early Child Care Research Network (1997). The effects of infant care on infant-mother attachment security: results of the NICHD Study of Early Child Care. *Child Development* 68, 860–79.

Nillson, A. (1993). The anti-aggressive actions of lithium. *Reviews in Contemporary Psychopharmacology* 4, 269–85.

Nimgaonkar, V. L., Fujiwara, T. M., Dutta, M., *et al.* (2000). Low prevalence of psychoses among the Hutterites, an isolated religious community. *American Journal of Psychiatry* 157, 1065–70.

Nirje, B. (1970). Normalisation. *Journal of Mental Subnormality* 31, 62–70.

Nock, M. K. and Marzuk, P. M. (2000). Suicide and violence. In *The international handbook of suicide and attempted suicide* (eds K. Hawton and K. van Heeringen). John Wiley & Sons, Chichester.

Nofzinger, E. A., Keshavan, M., Buysse, D. J., *et al.* (1999). The neurobiology of sleep in relation to mental illness. In *Neurobiology of mental illness* (eds D. S. Charney, E. J. Nestler, and B. S. Bunney), pp. 915–29. Oxford University Press, Oxford.

Nolen, W. A., Van de Putte, J. J., Dijken, W. A., *et al.* (1988). Treatment strategy in depression. 2. MAO inhibitors in depression resistant tricyclic antidepressants: two controlled cross-over studies with tranylcypromine versus 1,5-hydroxytryptophan and nomifensine. *Acta Psychiatrica Scandinavica* 78, 676–83.

Nordentoft, M. and Rubin, P. (1993). Mental illness and social integration among suicide attempters in Copenhagen. *Acta Psychiatrica Scandinavica* 88, 278–85.

Norman, R. M. G. and Malla, A. K. (1993). Stressful life events and schizophrenia. (1) A review of research. *British Journal of Psychiatry* 162, 161–6.

Nowell, P. D., Mazumdar, S., Buysse, D. J., *et al.* (1997). Benzodiazepines and zolpidem for chronic insomnia: a meta-analysis of treatment efficacy. *Journal of the American Medical Association* 278, 2170–7.

Noyes, R. (2000). Hypochondriasis. In *The new Oxford textbook of psychiatry* (eds M. G. Gelder, J. J. López-Ibor Jr, and N. C. Andreasen), Chapter 5.2.5. Oxford University Press, Oxford.

Noyes, R. and Hoehn-Saric, R. (1998). *The anxiety disorders*. Cambridge University Press, Cambridge.

Noyes, R. and Kletti, R. (1977). Depersonalization in response to life-threatening danger. *Comprehensive Psychiatry* 18, 375–84.

Nutt, D. (1999). Alcohol and the brain. *British Journal of Psychiatry* 175, 114–19.

Nutt, D. and Lawson, C. (1992). Panic attacks: a neurochemical overview of models and mechanisms. *British Journal of Psychiatry* 160, 165–78.

Nutt, D. J. (1996). Addiction: brain mechanisms and their treatment implications. *Lancet* 347, 31–6.

Nutt, D. J. and Bell, C. (1997). Advances in practical pharmacotherapy for anxiety. *Advances in Psychiatric Treatment* 3, 79–85.

Nyberg, S. and Farde, L. (2000). Non-equipotent doses partly explain differences among antipsychotics – implications of PET studies. *Psychopharmacology* 148, 22–3.

Oates, R. K., Peacock, A., and Forrest, D. (1985). Long-term effects of non-organic failure to thrive. *Paediatrics* 75, 36–40.

O'Brien, G. and Yule, W. (eds) (1996). Behavioural phenotypes. *Clinics in developmental medicine*. McKeith Press, Cambridge.

O'Brien, J. T. (1997). The glucocorticoid cascade hypothesis in man. *British Journal of Psychiatry* 170, 199–201.

Ochberg, S., Christiansen, P. E., Benke, K., *et al.* (1995). Paroxetine in the treatment of panic disorder: a randomized, double-blind controlled study. *British Journal of Psychiatry* 167, 374–9.

O'Connor, N. (1968). Psychology and intelligence. In *Studies in psychiatry* (eds M. Shepherd and D. L. Davis). Oxford University Press, London.

Ødegaard, Ø. (1932). Emigration and insanity. *Acta Psychiatrica Scandinavica* Suppl 4.

Offord, D. (2000). Epidemiology of psychiatric disorder in childhood and adolescence. In *The new Oxford textbook of psychiatry* (eds M. G. Gelder, J. J. López-Ibor Jr, and N. C. Andreasen), Chapter 9.1.3. Oxford University Press, Oxford.

Offord, D. R., Boyle, M. H., Szatmari, P., and Rae-Grant, N. I. (1987). Ontario Child Health Study. I Six month prevalence of disorder and service utilization. *Archives of General Psychiatry* 44, 832–6.

O'Hare, A. E., Brown, J. K., and Aitken, K. (1991). Dyscalculia in children. *Developmental Medicine and Child Neurology* 33, 356–61.

Old Age Depression Interest Group (1993). How long should the elderly take antidepressants? A double-blind placebo controlled study of continuation/prophylaxis therapy with dothiepin. *British Journal of Psychiatry* 162, 175–82.

Oldham, J. M., Skodol, A. E., Kellman, H. D., *et al.* (1992). Diagnosis of DSMIIIR personality disorders by two structured interviews: patterns of co-morbidity. *American Journal of Psychiatry* 149, 213–20.

O'Leary, K. D. and Beach, S. R. H. (1990). Marital therapy: a viable treatment for depression and marital discord. *American Journal of Psychiatry* 147, 183–6.

Olin, J. and Masand, P. (1996). Psychostimulants for depression in hospitalized cancer patients. *Psychosomatics* 37(1), 57–62.

Oliver, J. E. (1970). Huntington's chorea in Northamptonshire. *British Journal of Psychiatry* 116, 241–53.

Olsson, B. and Rett, A. (1990). A review of the Rett syndrome with a theory of autism. *Brain and Development* 12, 11–15.

Olweus, D. (1994). Bullying at school: basic facts and effects of a school based intervention programme. *Journal of Child Psychology and Psychiatry* 35, 1171–90.

O'Malley, S. S. and Krishnan-Sarin, S. (1998). Alcohol and neuropsychiatric disorders. *Current Opinion in Psychiatry* 11, 253–7.

O'Malley, P. G., Jackson, J. L., Santoro, J., Tomkins, G., Balden, E., Kroenke, K. (1999). Antidepressant therapy for unexplained symptoms and symptom syndromes. *Journal of Family Practice* 48, 980–990.

OPCS (Office of Population Censuses and Surveys) (1993). *Mortality statistics 1991: England and Wales, General*, Table 15. HMSO, London.

Oppenheimer, C. (2000). Special features of psychiatric treatment for the elderly. In *The new Oxford textbook of psychiatry* (eds M. G. Gelder, J. J. López-Ibor Jr, and N. C. Andreasen), Chapter 8.6. Oxford University Press, Oxford.

Orford, J. and Edwards, G. (1977). *Alcoholism*. Maudsley Monograph No. 26. Oxford University Press, London.

Ornish, D., Brown, S., Scherwitz, L. W., *et al.* (1990). Can lifestyle changes reverse coronary heart disease? *Lancet* 336, 129–33.

Orvaschel, H. (1983). Maternal depression and child dysfunction: children at risk. In *Advances in clinical psychology* (eds B. B. Lahey and A. E. Kazdun), Vol. 6, pp.167–97. Plenum Press, New York.

Öst, L. G. (1987a). Age of onset of different phobias. *Journal of Abnormal Psychology* 96, 223–9.

Öst, L. G. (1987b). Applied relaxation: description of a coping technique and review of controlled studies. *Behaviour Research and Therapy* 25, 397–409.

Ottenbacher, K. J. and Cooper, H. M. (1983). Drug treatment of hyperactivity in children. *Developmental Medicine and Child Neurology* 25, 358–66.

Overall, J. E. and Gorham, D. R. (1962). The Brief Psychiatric Rating Scale. *Psychological Reports* **10**, 799–812.

Overmeyer, S. and Taylor, E. (1999). Annotation: principles of treatment for hyperkinetic disorder; practical approaches for the UK. *Journal of Child Psychology and Psychiatry* **40**, 1147–57.

Overpeck, M. D., Brenner, R. A., Trumbe, A. C., *et al.* (1998). Risk factors for infant homicide in the United States. *New England Journal of Medicine* **339**, 1211–16.

Owen, M., Liddell, M., and McGuffin, P. (1994). Alzheimer's disease. *British Medical Journal* **308**, 672–3.

Owen, M. J., Cardno, A. G., and O'Donovan, M. C. (2000). Psychiatric genetics: back to the future. *Molecular Psychiatry* **5**, 22–31.

Owen, R. R., Gutierrez-Esteinou, R., Hsiao, J., *et al.* (1993). Effects of clozapine and fluphenazine treatment on responses to m-chlorophenylpiperazine infusions in schizophrenia. *Archives of General Psychiatry* **50**, 636–44.

Owens, M. J. and Ritchie, J. C. (1999). Clinical Neurochemistry. In *Neurobiology of mental illness*, (eds D. S. Charney, E. J. Nestler, and B. S. Bunney), pp. 132–48. Oxford University Press, Oxford.

Oyefeso, A., Ghodse, H., Clancy, C., *et al.* (1999). Suicide among drug addicts in the UK. *British Journal of Psychiatry* **175**, 277–82.

Paddison, P. (1993). *Treatment of adult survivors of incest*. American Psychiatric Press, Washington, DC.

Padma-Nathan, H., Goldstein, I., Payton, T., and Krane, R. J. (1987). Intracavernosal pharmacotherapy: the pharmacological erection program. *World Journal of Urology* **5**, 160–5.

Padma-Nathan, H., Hellstrom, W. G., Kaiser, F .E., *et al.* 1997). Treatment of men with erectile dysfunction with transurethral alprostadil. *New England Journal of Medicine* **336**, 1–7.

Paikoff, R. L. and Brooks-Gunn, J. (1995). Psychosexual development across the lifespan. In

Palazzoli, M., Boscolo, L., Cecchin, G., and Prata, G. (1978). *Paradox and counterparadox*. Aronson, New York.

Palmer, B. (2000). *Helping people with eating disorders. A clinical guide to assessment and treatment*. John Wiley, Chichester.

Palmer, M. S. and Collinge, J. (1992). Human prion diseases. In *Baillière's clinical neurology*, pp.627–47. Baillière Tindall, London.

Pantev, C., Oostenveld, R., Engelien, A., *et al.* (1998). Increased auditory cortical representation in musicians. *Nature* **392**, 811–14.

Paris, J. (1994). *Borderline personality disorder: a multidimensional approach*. American Psychiatric Press, Washington, DC.

Parker, G. (2000). Diagnosis, classification and differential diagnosis of the mood disorders. In *The new Oxford textbook of psychiatry* (eds M. G. Gelder, J. J. López-Ibor Jr, and N. C. Andreasen), Chapter 4.5.3. Oxford University Press, Oxford.

Parker, G., Hadzi-Pavlovic, D., Greenwald, S., and Weissman, M. (1995a). Low parental care as a risk factor to lifetime depression in a community sample. *Journal of Affective Disorders* **33**, 173–80.

Parker, G., Hadzi-Pavlovic, D., Hickie, I., *et al.* (1995b). Sub-typing depression, III. Development of a clinical algorithm for melancholia and comparison with other diagnostic measures. *Psychological Medicine* **25**, 833–40.

Parkes, C. M. (1996). *Bereavement: studies of grief in adult life*, 3rd edn. Tavistock/Routledge, London.

Parkes, C. M. (1971). The first year of bereavement: a longitudinal study of the reaction of London widows. *Psychiatry* **33**, 444–6.

Parkes, C. M. and Brown, R. J. (1972). Health after bereavement: a controlled study of young Boston widows and widowers. *Psychosomatic Medicine* **34**, 449–61.

Parkes, C. M., Benjamin, B., and Fitzgerald, R. G. (1969). Broken heart: a statistical study of increased mortality among widowers. *British Medical Journal* **1**, 740–3.

Parkes, J. D. (1985). *Sleep and its disorders*. Saunders, London.

Parnas, J., Schulsinger, F., Teasdale, T. W., *et al.* (1982). Perinatal complications and clinical outcome within the schizophrenia spectrum. *British Journal of Psychiatry* **140**, 416–20.

Parnas, J., Cannon, T. D., Jacobsen, B., *et al.* (1993). Lifetime DSM-III-R diagnostic outcomes in the off-spring of schizophrenic mothers. *Archives of General Psychiatry* **50**, 707–14.

Parry-Jones, B. and Parry-Jones, W. L. (1992). Pica: symptom or eating disorder? A historical assessment. *British Journal of Psychiatry* **160**, 341–54.

Parry-Jones, W. L. (1972). *The trade in lunacy*. Routledge & Kegan Paul, London.

Parsons, T. (1951). *The social system*. Free Press, Glencoe.

Pasamanick, B. and Knobloch, H. (1966). Retrospective studies on the epidemiology of reproductive casualty: old and new. *Merril-Palmer Quarterly of Behavioral Development* 12, 7–26.

Pasmanick, B., Scarpitti, F. R., and Lefton, M. (1964). Home versus hospital care for schizophrenics. *Journal of the American Medical Association* 187, 177–81.

Pathé, M. and Mullen, P. E. (1997). The impact of stalkers on their victims. *British Journal of Psychiatry* 170, 12–17.

Pathé, M., Mullen, P. E., and Purcell, R. (1999). Stalking: false claims of victimisation. *British Journal of Psychiatry* 174, 170–2.

Pato, M. T., Zohar-Kadouch, R., Zohar, J., *et al.* (1988). Return of symptoms after discontinuation of clomipramine in patients with obsessive compulsive disorder. *American Journal of Psychiatry* 145, 1521–5.

Patterson, G. R. (1982). *Coercive family process*. Castalia Eugene, OR.

Paykel, E. S. (1978). Contribution of life events to causation of psychiatric illness. *Psychological Medicine* 8, 245–53.

Paykel, E. S. (1989). Treatment of depression: the relevance of research to clinical practice. *British Journal of Psychiatry* 155, 754–63.

Paykel, E. S. (1990). Monoamine oxidase inhibitors: when should they be used. In *Dilemmas and difficulties in the management of psychiatric patients* (eds K. Hawton and P. Cowen), pp. 17–30. Oxford University Press, Oxford.

Paykel, E. S. (2000). Not an age of depression after all? Incidence rates may be stable over time. *Psychological Medicine* 30, 489–90.

Paykel, E. S. and Cooper, Z. (1992). Life events and social stress. In *Handbook of affective disorders* (ed. E. S. Paykel), pp. 149–70. Churchill Livingstone, Edinburgh.

Paykel, E. S., Myers, J. K., Dienelt, M. N., *et al.* (1969). Life events and depression: a controlled study. *Archives of General Psychiatry* 21, 753–60.

Paykel, E. S., Prusoff, B. A., and Myers, J. K. (1975). Suicide attempts and recent life events: a controlled comparison. *Archives of General Psychiatry* 32, 327–33.

Paykel, E. S., Scott, J., Teasdale, J. D., *et al.* (1999). Prevention of relapse in residual depression by cognitive therapy. *Archives of General Psychiatry* 56, 829–35.

Pearce, J., Hawton, K., and Blake, F. (1995). Psychological and sexual symptoms associated with the menopause and the effects of hormone replacement therapy. *British Journal of Psychiatry* 167, 163–73.

Pedersen, N. L., Plomin, R., McLearn, G. E., and Friberg, L. (1988). Neuroticism, extroversion and related traits in adult twins reared apart and reared together. *Journal of Personality and Social Psychology* 55, 950–7.

Penrose, L. (1938). *A clinical and genetic study of 1280 cases of mental deficiency*. HMSO, London.

Perez, V., Soler, J., Puigdemont, D., *et al.* (1999). A double-blind, randomized, placebo-controlled trial of pindolol augmentation in depressive patients resistant to serotonin reuptake inhibitors. *Archives of General Psychiatry* 56, 375–9.

Perley, M. J. and Guze, S. B. (1962). Hysteria – the stability and usefulness of clinical criteria. *New England Journal of Medicine* 266, 421–6.

Perry, A., Tarrier, N., Morriss, R., *et al.* (1999). Randomised controlled trial of efficacy of teaching patients with bipolar disorder to identify early symptoms of relapse and obtain treatment. *British Medical Journal* 318, 149–53.

Perry, J. C., Bannon, E., and Ianni, F. (1999). Effectiveness of psychotherapy for personality disorders. *American Journal of Psychiatry* 156, 1312–21.

Perry, R., McKeith, I., and Perry, E. (1997). Dementia with Lewy bodies. *Clinical, pathological, and treatment issues*. Oxford University Press, Oxford.

Persons, J. B. (1999). Most patients with a first episode of major depressive disorder experienced multiple levels of depressive symptoms over time. *Evidence-Based Mental Health* 2, 23.

Peselow, E. D., Robins, C., Bloch, P., *et al.* (1990). Dysfunctional attitudes in depressed patients before and after clinical treatment and in normal control subjects. *American Journal of Psychiatry* 147, 439–44.

Peselow, E. D., Fieve, R. R., Difiglia, C., and Sanfilipo, M. P. (1994). Lithium prophylaxis of bipolar illness: the value of combination treatment. *British Journal of Psychiatry* 164, 208–14.

Peters, S. D., Wyatt, G. E., and Finkelhor, D. (1986). Prevalence. In *A source book on child sexual abuse* (ed. D. Finkelhor). Sage, London.

Petrie, K. J. and Weinmann, J. A. (eds) (1997). *Perceptions of health and illness*. Harwood Academic Publishers, The Netherlands.

Petronko, M. R., Harris, S. L., and Kormann, R. J. (1994). Community based behavioral training approaches for people with mental retardation and mental illness. *Journal of Consulting and Clinical Psychology* 62(1), 49–54.

Petursson, H. and Lader, M. H. (1984). *Dependence on tranquillizers*. Oxford University Press, Oxford.

Peyser, C. E. and Folstein, S. E. (1993). Depression in Huntington disease. In *Depression in neurologic disease* (eds S. E. Starkstein and R. G. Robinson), pp.117–38. Johns Hopkins University Press, Baltimore, MD.

Pfeffer, C. R. (2000). Suicidal behaviour in children: an emphasis on developmental influences. In *The international handbook of suicide and attempted suicide* (eds K. Hawton and K. van Heeringen). John Wiley & Sons, Chichester.

Pfohl, B., Blum, N., and Zimmerman M. (1997). *Structured interview for DSMIV personality*. American Psychiatric Association, Washington, DC.

Pharoah, F. M., Mari, J. J., and Steiner, D. (2000). Family intervention for schizophrenia (Cochrane Review). In *The Cochrane Library, Issue 2*. Update Software, Oxford.

Phelan, M., Slade, M., Thornicroft, G., et al. (1995). The Camberwell Assessment of Need: the validity and reliability of an instrument to assess the needs of people with severe mental illness. *British Journal of Psychiatry* 167, 589–95.

Philipp, M., Kohnen, R., and Hiller, K.-O. (1999). Hypericum extract versus imipramine or placebo in patients with moderate depression: radomised multicentre study of treatment for eight weeks. *British Medical Journal* 319, 1534–8.

Phillips, K. A. (1996). *The broken mirror. Understanding and treating body dysmorphic disorder*. Oxford University Press, New York.

Phillips, K. A. (2000). Body dysmorphic disorder. In *The new Oxford textbook of psychiatry* (eds M. G. Gelder, J. J. López-Ibor Jr, and N. C. Andreasen), Chapter 5.2.8. Oxford University Press, Oxford.

Phillips, K. A., Dwight, M. M., and McElroy, S. L. (1998). Efficacy and safety of fluvoxamine in body dysmorphic disorder. *Journal of Clinical Psychiatry* 59, 165–71.

Piccinelli, M. and Simon, G. (1997). Gender and cross-cultural differences in somatic symptoms associated with emotional distress. An international study in primary care. *Psychological Medicine* 27, 433–44.

Pichot, P. (1982). The diagnosis and classification of mental disorders in French speaking countries: background, current view and comparison with other nomenclature. *Psychological Medicine* 12, 475–92.

Pichot, P. (1984). The French approach to classification. *British Journal of Psychiatry* 144, 113–18.

Pichot, P. (1994). Nosological models in psychiatry. *British Journal of Psychiatry* 164, 232–40.

Pimentel, M. M. (1999). Fragile X syndrome. *International Journal of Molecular Medicine* 3, 639–45.

Pincus, H. A., Wakefield Davis, W., and McQueen, L. E. (1999). 'Subthreshold' mental disorders. *British Journal of Psychiatry* 174, 288–96.

Pines, M. and Schlapobersky, J. (2000). G roup methods in adult psychiatry. In *The new Oxford textbook of psychiatry* (eds M. G. Gelder, J. J. López-Ibor Jr, and N. C. Andreasen), Chapter 6.3.6. Oxford University Press, Oxford.

Pippard, J. (1992). Audit of electroconvulsive treatment in two National Health Service regions. *British Journal of Psychiatry* 160, 621–37.

Pitman, R. K., Orr, S. P., Altman, B., et al. (1996). Emotional processing during eye movement desensitization and reprocessing therapy of Vietnam veterans with chronic post-traumatic stress disorder. *Comprehensive Psychiatry* 37, 419–29.

Pitta, J. C. N. and Blay, S. L. (1997). Psychogenic (reactive) and hysterical psychoses: a cross-system reliability study. *Acta Psychiatrica Scandinavica* 95, 112–18.

Pitts, F. N. and McClure, J. N. (1967). Lacate metabolism in anxiety neurosis. *New England Journal of Medicine* 25, 1329–36.

Piven, J., Arndt, S., Bailey, J., et al. (1996). Regional brain enlargement in autism: a magnetic resonance study. *Journal of the American Academy of Child and Adolescent Psychiatry* 35, 530–6.

Planansky, K. and Johnston, R. (1977). Homicidal aggression in schizophrenic men. *Acta Psychiatrica Scandinavica* 55, 65–73.

Plant, M. and Miller, P. (2000). Drug use has declined among teenagers in United Kingdom. *British Medical Journal* 320, 1536.

Plasky, P. (1991). Antidepressant usage in schizophrenia. *Schizophrenia Bulletin* 17, 649–57.

Plomin, R. (1994). *Genetics and experience*. Sage, Thousand Oaks, CA.

Plomin, R. (1995). Genetics and children's experiences in the family. *Journal of Child Psychology and Psychiatry* 36(1), 33–68.

Pocock, S. J., Smith, M., and Baghurst, M. (1994). Environmental lead and children's intelligence: a systematic review of the epidemiological evidence. *British Medical Journal* 309, 1189–97.

Poirier, M.-F. and Boyer, P. (1999). Venlafaxine and paroxetine in treatment-resistant depression. Double-blind, randomised comparison. *British Journal of Psychiatry* 175, 12–16.

Polak, P. B., Egan, D., and Bandenbergh, R. (1975). Prevention in mental health: a controlled study. *American Journal of Psychiatry* 132, 146–9.

Pollitt, J. (1960). Natural history studies in mental illness: a discussion based upon a pilot study of obsessional states. *Journal of Mental Science* 106, 93–113.

Pope, H. G., Jonas, J. M., Hudson, J. I., *et al.* (1983). The validity of DSM III borderline personality disorder: a phenomenological, family history, treatment response, and long term follow-up study. *Archives of General Psychiatry* 40, 23–30.

Porter, R., Ferrier, N. and Ashton, H. (1999). Anticonvulsants as mood stabilisers. *Advances in Psychiatric Treatment* 5, 96–103.

Portwich, Ph. and Barocka, A. (1998). Capgras' syndrome and other delusional misidentification syndrome (DMS). *Nervenheilkunde* 17, 296–300.

Posener, H. and Jacoby, R. (2001). Testamentary capacity. In *Psychiatry in the elderly*, 3rd edn (eds R. Jacoby and C. Oppenheimer). Oxford University Press, Oxford.

Post, F. (1971). Schizo-affective symptomatology in late life. *British Journal of Psychiatry* 118, 437–45.

Post, F. (1972). The management and nature of depressive illnesses in late life: a follow-through study. *British Journal of Psychiatry* 121, 393–404.

Post, R. M. (1991). Anticonvulsants as adjuncts or alternatives to lithium in refractory bipolar illness. In *Advances in neuropsychiatry and psychopharmacology. Vol. 2: Refractory depression* (ed. J. D. Amsterdam), pp. 155–65. Raven Press, New York.

Post, R. M., Leverich, G. S., Rosoff, A. S., and Altschuler, L. L. (1990). Carbamazepine prophylaxis in refractory affective disorders: a focus on long-term follow-up. *Journal of Clinical Psychopharmacology* 10, 318–22.

Post, R. M., Denicoff, K. D., Frye, M. A. and Leverich, G. S. (1997). Re-evaluating carbamazepine prophylaxis in bipolar disorder. *British Journal of Psychiatry* 170, 202–4.

Post, R. M., Frye, M. A., Denicoff, K. D., Leverich, G. S., Kimbrell, T. A., and Dunn, R. T. (1998). Beyond lithium in the treatment of bipolar illness. *Neuropsychopharmacology* 19, 206–19.

Powell, G. F., Brasel, J. A., and Blizzard, R. M. (1967). Emotional deprivation and growth retardation simulating idiopathic hypopituitarism. *New England Journal of Medicine*, 276, 1271–83.

Power, A. C. and Cowen, P. J. (1992). Fluoxetine and suicidal behaviour: some clinical and theoretical aspects of a controversy. *British Journal of Psychiatry* 161, 735–41.

Power, D. J., Benn, R. T., and Homes, J. N. (1972). Neighbourhood, school and juveniles before courts. *British Journal of Criminology* 12, 111–32.

Poynton, A. M., Kartsounis, L. D., and Bridges, P. K. (1995). A prospective clinical study of stereotactic subcaudate tractotomy. *Psychological Medicine* 25, 763–70.

Prakash, A. and Lamb, H. M. (1998). Zotepine. *CNS Drugs* 9(2), 153–75.

Pratt, J. H. (1908). Results obtained in treatment of pulmonary tuberculosis by the class method. *British Medical Journal* 2, 1070–1.

Preisig, M., Bellivier, F., Fenton, B. T., *et al.* (2000). Association between bipolar disorder and monoamine oxidase A gene polymorphisms: results of a multi-center study. *American Journal of Psychiatry* 157, 948–55.

Price, J. R. (2000). Managing physical symptoms: the clinical assessment as treatment. *Journal of Psychosomatic Research* 48, 1–10.

Price, L. H., Charney, D. S., and Heninger, G. R. (1985). Efficacy of lithium-tranylcypromine treatment in refractory depression. *American Journal of Psychiatry* 142, 619–23.

Prichard, J. C. (1835). *A treatise on insanity*. Sherwood Gilbert and Piper, London.

Prien, R. F. (1992). Maintenance treatment. In *Handbook of affective disorders* (ed. E. S. Paykel), pp. 419–35. Churchill Livingstone, Edinburgh.

Prien, R. F. and Kupfer, D. J. (1986). Continuation drug therapy for major depressive episodes: how long should it be maintained? *American Journal of Psychiatry* 143, 18–23.

Priest, R. G. (1976). The homeless person and the psychiatric services: an Edinburgh survey. *British Journal of Psychiatry* 128, 128–36.

Prigatano, G. P. (1999). *Principles of neuropsychological rehabilitation*. Oxford University Press, New York.

Primm, A. B. (1996). Assertive Community Treatment. In: *Integrated mental health services* (ed. W. R. Breakey) pp 222–37. Oxford University Press, New York.

Prince, M. (2000). Epidemiology. In *New Oxford Textbook of Psychiatry* (eds M. G. Gelder, J. J. López-Ibor, N. C. Andreasen). Oxford University Press.

Prins, H. (2000). The special problems of arson (fire-raising). In *The new Oxford textbook of psychiatry* (eds M. G. Gelder, J. J. López-Ibor Jr, and N. C Andreasen), Chapter 11.4.1. Oxford University Press, Oxford.

Prochaska, J. O. and Diclemente, C. C. (1986). Towards a comprehensive model of change. In *Treating addictive behaviors: processes of change* (eds W. R. Miller and N. Heather), pp. 3–27. Plenum Press, New York.

Project MATCH Research Group (1997). Matching alcoholism treatments to client heterogeneity: Project MATCH post-treatment drinking outcomes. *Journal of Studies on Alcohol* 58, 7–29.

Protheroe, C. (1969). Puerperal psychoses: a long term study, 1927–1961. *British Journal of Psychiatry* 115, 9–30.

Prudic, J., Sackheim, H. A. and Devanand, D. P. (1990). Medication resistance and clinical response to electroconvulsive therapy. *Psychiatry Research* 31, 287–96.

Pugh, R., Jerath, B. K., Schmidt, W. M., and Reed, R. B. (1963). Rates of mental disease related to child rearing. *New England Journal of Medicine* 22, 1224–8.

Putnam, F. W. (1991). Dissociative phenomena. In *Review of psychiatry* (eds A. Tasman and S. M. Goldfinger), pp 145–60. American Psychiatric Press, Washington, DC.

Putnam, F. W. and Loewenstein, R. J. (2000). Dissociative identity disorder. In *Comprehensive textbook of psychiatry*, 7th edn (eds B. J. Sadock and V. A. Sadock). Lippincott, Williams & Wilkins, Philadelphia.

Putnam, F. W., Guroff, J. J., and Silberman, E. K. (1986). The clinical phenomenology of multiple personality disorder: review of 100 recent cases. *Journal of Clinical Psychiatry* 47, 285–93.

Quay, H. C. and Werry, J. S. (1986). *Psychopathological disorders of childhood*, 3rd edn. Wiley, New York.

Quinn, J. and Twomey, P. (1998). A case of auto-erotic asphyxia in a long-term psychiatric setting. *Psychopathology* 31, 169–73.

Quitkin, F. M., McGrath, P. J., Stewart, J. W., *et al.* (1989). Phenelzine and imipramine in mood reactive depressives. *Archives of General Psychiatry* 46, 787–93.

Rabiner, E. A., Gunn, R. N., Castro, M. E., *et al.* (2000). β-Blocker binding to human 5-HT_{1A} receptors *in vivo* and *in vitro* implications for antidepressant therapy. *Neuropsychopharmacology* 23, 285–93.

Rabins, P. V., Lyketsos, C. G., and Steele, C. D. (1999). *Practical dementia care*. Oxford University Press, New York.

Rachman, S. (1974). Primary obsessional slowness. *Behaviour Research and Therapy* 11, 463–71.

Rachman, S. and Hodgson, R. J. (1980). *Obsessions and compulsions*. Prentice-Hall, Englewood Cliffs, NJ.

Radke-Yarrow, M., Nottelmann, E., Martinez, P., and Fox, M. B. (1993). Young children of affectively ill parents: a longitudinal study of social development. *Journal of the American Academy of Child and Adolescent Psychiatry* 31, 68–77.

Radnitz, C. L., Broderick, C. P., Perez-Strumolo, L., *et al.* (1996). The prevalence of psychiatric disorders in veterans with spinal cord injury: a controlled comparison. *Journal of Nervous and Mental Disease* 184, 431–33.

Raine, A., Lencz, T., Bihrle, S., La Casse, L., and Colletti, P. (2000). Reduced prefontal gray matter and reduced autonomic activity in antisocial personality disorder. *Archives of General Psychiatry* 57, 119–27.

Ralph, D. and McNicolas, T. (2000). UK Management guidelines for erectile dysfunction. *British Medical Journal* 321, 499–503.

Ramirez, A. J., Westcombe, A. M., Burgess, C. C., Sutton, S., Littlejohns, P., and Richards, M. A. (1999). Factors predicting delayed presentation of symptomatic breast cancer: a systematic review. *Lancet* 353, 1127–31.

Ramsay, N. (1992). Referral to a liaison psychiatrist from a palliative care unit. *Palliative Medicine* 6, 54–60.

Ramsay, R., Gorst-Unsworth, C., and Turner, S. (1993). Psychiatric morbidity in survivors of organised state violence including torture. *British Journal of Psychiatry* 162, 55–9.

Raphael, B. (1977). Preventive intervention with the recently bereaved. *Archives of General Psychiatry* 34, 1450–4.

Raphael, B. (1986). The problems of mental health and adjustment. In *When disaster strikes: a handbook for the caring profession* (ed. B. Raphael). Hutchinson, London.

Raphael, B. and Wilson, J. (eds) (2000). *Psychological debriefing. Theory, practice and evidence.* Cambridge University Press, Cambridge.

Rapoport, R. N. (1960). *Community as doctor.* Tavistock Publications, London.

Rasmussen, S. A. and Tsuang, M. T. (1986). Clinical characteristics and family history in DSMIII obsessive–compulsive disorder. *American Journal of Psychiatry* 143, 317–22.

Rauch, S. L., Savage, C. R., Alpert, N. M. *et al.* (1995). A positron emission tomography study of simple phobic symptom provocation. *Archives of General Psychiatry* 52, 20–8.

Ravizza, L., Maina, G., and Bogetto, F. (1997). Episodic and chronic OCD. *Depression and Anxiety* 6, 154–8.

Rawaf, S. (1998). Public health and addiction,: prevention. *Current Opinion in Psychiatry* 11, 273–8.

Regier, D. A. (2000). Community diagnosis counts. *Archives of General Psychiatry* 57, 223–4.

Regier, D. A., Kaelber, C. T., Roper, M. T., Rae, D. S., and Sartorius, N. (1994a). The ICD-10 Clinical Field Trial for Mental and Behavioral Disorders: results in Canada and the United States. *American Journal of Psychiatry* 151, 1340–50.

Regier, D. A., Narrow, W. E., Rae, D. S., *et al.* (1994b). The *de facto* US Mental and Addictive Disorders Service System. *Archives of General Psychiatry* 50, 85–94.

Regier, D. A., Kaelber, C. T., Rae D. S., *et al.* (1998). Limitations of diagnostic criteria and assessment instruments for mental disorders. Implications for research and policy. *Archives of General Psychiatry* 55, 109–15.

Reich, J., Goldenberg, I., Goisman, R., and Vasile, R. A. (1994). A prospective follow-along study of the course of social phobia. *Psychiatry Research* 54, 249–58.

Reid, S., Chalder, T., Cleare, A., Hotopf, M. Wessely, S. (2000). Chronic fatigue syndrome. *British Medical Journal* 320, 292–296.

Reilly, J. G., Ayis, S. A., Ferrier, I. N., *et al.* (2000). QTc-interval abnormalities and psychotropic drug therapy in psychiatric patients. *Lancet* 355, 1048–52.

Reite, M., Teale, P., and Rojas, D. C. (1999). Magnetoencephalography: applications in psychiatry. *Biological Psychiatry* 45, 1553–63.

Remafedi, G., French, S., Story, M., *et al.* (1998). The relationship between suicide risk and sexual orientation: results of a population based study. *American Journal of Public Health* 88, 57–60.

Resnick, H. S., Acierno, R., and Kilpatrick, D. G. (1997). Health impact of interpersonal violence 2: medical and mental health outcomes. *Behavioural Medicine* 23, 65–78.

Resnick, P. J. (1969). Child murder by parents. *American Journal of Psychiatry* 126, 325–34.

Reynolds III, C. F., Frank, E., Perel, J. M., *et al.* (1999). Nortriptyline and interpersonal psychotherapy as maintenance therapies for recurrent major depression. A randomised controlled trial in patients older than 59 years. *Journal of the American Medical Association* 281, 39–45.

Ribeiro, S. C. M., Tandon, R., Grunhaus, L., and Greden, J. F. (1993). The DST as a predictor of outcome in depression: a meta-analysis. *American Journal of Psychiatry* 150, 1618–29.

Rice, G., Anderson, C., Risch, N., and Ebers, G (1999). Male homosexuality: absence of linkage to microsatellite markets at Xq28. *Science* 284, 665–7.

Rice, M. and Harris, G. T. (1997). The treatment of mentally disordered offenders. *Psychology, Public Policy and Law* 3, 126–83.

Richardson, S. K. and Koller, H. (1992). Vulnerability and resilience in adults who were classified as mildly mentally handicapped in childhood. In *Vulnerability and resilience in human development* (eds B. Tizard and V. Varma), pp.102–23. JKP, London.

Richelson, E. (1998). Pharmacokinetic interactions of antidepressants. *Journal of Clinical Psychiatry* 59 (suppl 10), 22–6.

Richelson, E. (1999). Receptor pharmacology of neuroleptics: relation to clinical effects. *Journal of Clinical Psychiatry* 60(suppl 10), 5–14.

Richman, N., Stevenson, J., and Graham, P. (1982). *Preschool to school: a behavioural study.* Academic Press, London.

Richman, N., Douglas, J., Hunt, H., *et al.* (1985). Behavioural methods in the treatment of sleep disorders – a pilot study. *Journal of Child Psychology and Psychiatry* 26, 581–90.

Rickels, K., Csanalosi, I., and Chung, H. R. (1974). Amitriptyline in anxious-depressed outpatients: a controlled study. *American Journal of Psychiatry* **130**, 25–30.

Rickels, K., Downing, R., Schweizer, E., and Hassman, H. (1993). Antidepressants for the treatment of generalized anxiety disorder. *Archives of General Psychiatry* **50**, 884–95.

Rickels, K., Schweizer, E., Clary, C., *et al.* (1994). Nefazodone and imipramine in major depression: a placebo-controlled trial. *British Journal of Psychiatry* **164**, 802–5.

Rickles, N. K. (1950). *Exhibitionism*. Lippincott, Philadelphia, PA.

Riley, A. J. and Riley, E. J. (1978). A controlled study to evaluate directed masturbation in the management of primary orgasmic failure in women. *British Journal of Psychiatry* **133**, 404–9.

Rimes, K. and Salkovskis, P. M. (2000). Health screening programmes. In *The new Oxford textbook of psychiatry* (eds. M. G. Gelder, J. J. López-Ibor Jr, and N. C. Andreasen), Chapter 5.5. Oxford University Press, Oxford.

Rimm, D. C. and Masters, J. C. (1979). *Behavior therapy: techniques and empirical findings*. Academic Press, New York.

Ring, H. (1993). Psychological and social problems of Parkinson's disease. *British Journal of Hospital Medicine* **49**, 111–16.

Rivers, W. H. (1920). *Instinct and the unconscious*. Cambridge University Press, Cambridge.

Rivinus, T. M., Jamison, D. L., and Graham, P. J. (1975). Childhood organic neurological disease presenting as psychiatric disorder. *Developmental Medicine and Child Neurology* **23**, 747–60.

Rix, K. (1999a). Expert evidence and the Courts, paper 1: The history of expert evidence. *Advances in Psychiatry Treatment* **5**, 71–7.

Rix, K. (1999b). Expert evidence and the Courts, paper 2: Advances in psychiatric treatment. *Advances in Psychiatry Treatment* **5**, 154–60.

Robbins, T. W. and Everitt, B. J. (1999). Drug addiction: bad habits add up. *Nature* **398**, 567–70.

Roberts, A. H. (1969). *Brain damage in boxers*. Pitman, London.

Roberts, R. E., Attkisson, C., and Rosenblatt, A. (1998). Prevalence of psychopathology among children and adolescents. *American Journal of Psychiatry* **155**, 715–25.

Roberts, S. B. and Kendler, K. S. (1999). Neuroticism and self-esteem as indices of the vulnerability to major depression in women. *Psychological Medicine* **29**, 1101–9.

Robertson, M.M. (2000). Tourette syndrome, associated conditions and the complexities of treatment. *Brain* **123**, 425–62.

Robertson, M. M., Trimble, M. R., and Lees, A. J. (1988). The psychopathology of the Gilles de la Tourette syndrome. *British Journal of Psychiatry* **152**, 383–90.

Robins, L. N. (1966). *Deviant children grown up*. Williams & Wilkins, Baltimore, MD.

Robins, L. N. (1978). Sturdy childhood predictors of adult antisocial behaviour: replications from longitudinal studies. *Psychological Medicine* **8**, 611–22.

Robins, L. N. (1993). Vietnam veterans' rapid recovery from heroin addiction: a fluke or normal expectation? *Addiction* **88**, 1041–54.

Robins, L. N. and Regier, D. A. (1991). *Psychiatric disorder in America: the epidemiological catchment area study*. Free Press, New York.

Robins, L. N., Helzer, J. E., Croughan, J., and Ratcliff, K. S. (1981). National Institutes of Mental Health Diagnostic Interview Schedule. *Archives of General Psychiatry* **38**, 381–9.

Robinson, G. E. (2000). General overview of obstetrics, gynecology and reproductive issues. In *Psychiatric care of the medical patient* (eds A. Stoudemire, B. S. Fogel, and D. B. Greenberg). Oxford University Press, New York.

Robling, S. A., Paykel, E. S., Dunn, V. J., Abbott, R., Katona, C. (2000). Long-term outcome of severe puerperal psychiatric illness: a 23 year follow-up study. *Psychological Medicine* **30**, 1263–1271.

Robson, P. (1992). Opiate misusers: are treatments effective? In *Practical problems in clinical psychiatry* (eds K. Hawton and P. Cowen), pp. 141–58. Oxford University Press, Oxford.

Robson, P. (2000). Introduction to substance use disorders. In *The new Oxford texbook of psychiatry* (eds M. G. Gelder, J. J. López-Ibor Jr, and N. C. Andreasen), Chapter 4.2.3.1. Oxford University Press, Oxford.

Rock, P. (1998). *After homicide: practical and political responses to bereavement*. Clarendon Studies in Criminology. Oxford University Press, Oxford.

Rodin, G. and Abbey, S. (2000). Psychiatric aspects of surgery (including transplantation). In *The new Oxford textbook of psychiatry* (eds. M. G. Gelder, J. J. López-Ibor Jr, and N. C. Andreasen), Chapter 5.3.6. Oxford University Press, Oxford.

Rodin, I. and Thompson, C. (1997). Seasonal affective disorder. *Advances in Psychiatric Treatment* 3, 352–9.

Roeleveld, N., Zielhuis, G. A., and Gabreëls, F. (1997). The prevalence of mental retardation: a critical review of recent literature. *Developmental Medicine and Child Neurology* 39, 125–32.

Roman, G. C., Tatemichi, T. K., Erkinjuntti, T., Cummings, J. L., Masdeu, J. C., and Garcia, J. H. (1993). Vascular dementia: diagnostic criteria for research studies. *Neurology* 43, 250–60.

Ron, M. A. (1989). Psychiatric manifestations of frontal lobe tumours. *British Journal of Psychiatry* 155, 735–8.

Ron, M. A. (2000). Psychiatric aspects of neurological disease. In *The new Oxford textbook of psychiatry* (eds M. G. Gelder, J. J. López-Ibor Jr, and N. C. Andreasen), Chapter 5.3.2. Oxford University Press, Oxford.

Ron, M. A. and Logsdail, S. J. (1989). Psychiatric morbidity in multiple sclerosis: a clinical and MRI study. *Psychological Medicine* 19, 887–95.

Rooth, F. G. (1973). Exhibitionism, sexual violence and paedophilia. *British Journal of Psychiatry* 122, 705–10.

Rosanoff, A. J., Handy, L. M., and Rosanoff, I. A. (1934). Criminality and delinquency in twins. *Journal of Criminal Law and Criminology* 24, 923–34.

Rose, S. and Bisson, J. I. (1998). Brief early psychological interventions following trauma: a systematic review of the literature. *Journal of Traumatic Stress* 11, 697–710.

Rose, S., Brewin, C., Andrews, B., and Kirk, M. (1999). A randomized controlled trial of individual psychological debriefing for victims of violent crime. *Psychological Medicine* 29, 793–9.

Rosen, I. (1979). Exhibitionism, scopophilia and voyeurism. In *Sexual deviations*, 2nd edn (ed. I. Rosen). Oxford University Press, Oxford.

Rosen, R. C. and Leiblum, S. R. (1987). Current approaches to the evaluation of sexual desire disorders. *Journal of Sex Research* 23, 141–62.

Rosenbaum, J. F., Fava, M., Hoog, S. L., *et al.* (1998). Selective serotonin reuptake inhibitor discontinuation syndrome: a randomized clinical trial. *Biological Psychiatry* 44, 77–87.

Rosenblatt, A. and Leroi, I. (2000). Neuropsychiatry of Huntington's disease and other basal ganglia disorders. *Psychosomatics* 41, 24–30.

Rosenthal, N. E., Sack, D. A., Gillin, J. C., *et al.* (1984). Seasonal affective disorder: a description of the syndrome and preliminary findings with light therapy. *Archives of General Psychiatry* 41, 72–80.

Ross, C. A., McInnis, M. G., Margolis, R. L., and Li, S.-H. (1993). Genes with triplet repeats: candidate mediators of neuropsychiatric disorders. *Trends in Neurosciences* 254–60.

Ross, D. M. and Ross, S. A. (1982). *Hyperactivity: current issues, research and theory.* Wiley, New York.

Rossler, W., Loffler, W., Falkenheuer, B., *et al.* (1992). Does case management reduce rehospitalization rate? *Acta Psychiatrica Scandinavica* 86, 445–9.

Roth, A. J., McClear, K. Z., and Massie, M. J. (2000). Oncology. In *Psychiatric care of the medical patient* (eds A. Stoudemire, B. S. Fogel, and D. B. Greenberg). Oxford University Press, New York.

Roth, M. (1955). The natural history of mental disorder in old age. *Journal of Mental Science* 101, 281–301.

Roth, M. (1959). The phobic anxiety-depersonalization syndrome. *Proceedings of the Royal Society of Medicine* 52, 587–95.

Roth, M. and Ball, J. R. B. (1964). Psychiatric aspects of intersexuality. In *Intersexuality in vertebrates including man* (eds C. N. Armstrong and A. J. Marshall). Academic Press, London.

Rothbaum, B. O. (1997). A controlled study of eye movement desensitization and reprocessing in the treatment of posttraumatic stress disordered sexual assault victims. *Bulletin of the Meninger Clinic* 61, 317–34.

Rothbaum, B. O., Foa, E. B., Riggs, D. S., Murdock, T., and Walsh, W. (1992). A prospective examination of post-traumatic stress disorder in rape victims. *Journal of Traumatic Stress* 5(3), 455–76.

Rothlind, J. C., Bylsma, F. W., Peyser, C., *et al.* (1993). Cognitive and motor correlates of everyday functioning in early Huntington's disease. *Journal of Nervous and Mental Disease* 181, 194–8.

Rothman, D. (1971). *The discovery of the asylum.* Little Brown, Boston, MA.

Rouhani, M. and Holland, J. C. (2000). Psychiatric aspects of cancer. In *The new Oxford textbook of psychiatry* (eds. M. G. Gelder, J. J. López-Ibor Jr, and

N. C. Andreasen), Chapter 5.3.7. Oxford University Press, Oxford.

Roy, A., Nielsen, D. Rylander, G., *et al* (2000). The genetics of suicidal behaviour. In *The international handbook of suicide and attempted suicide* (eds K. Hawton and K. van Heeringen). John Wiley & Sons, Chichester.

Royal College of Physicians (1991). *Physical signs of sexual abuse in children*. Royal College of Physicians, London.

Royal College of Psychiatrists (1993). *Consensus statement on the use of high dose antipsychotic medication*. Council Report 26. Royal College of Psychiatrists, London.

Royal College of Psychiatrists (1995). *ECT handbook*. Royal College of Psychiatrists, London.

Royal College of Psychiatrists (1996). *Assessment and clinical management of risk of harm to other people*. Royal College of Psychiatrists Guidelines on Risk Assessment. Council Report 53. Royal College of Psychiatrists, Gaskell, London.

Royal College of Psychiatrists. (1999). *Offenders with personality disorder*. Council Report 71. Royal College of Psychiatrists, London.

Royal College of Psychiatrists (2000). *Good psychiatric practice*. Royal College of Psychiatrists, London.

Royal Commission on Long Term Care (1999). *With respect to old age: long term care – rights and responsibilities*. HMSO, London.

Roy-Byrne, P. P. and Cowley, D. S. (1995). Course and outcome of panic disorder: a review of recent studies. *Anxiety* 1, 151–160.

Roy-Byrne P. P., Milgrom, P., Khoon-May, T., *et al*. (1994). Psychopathology and psychiatric diagnosis in subjects with dental phobia. *Journal of Anxiety Disorders* 8, 19–31.

Rozanski, A., Blumenthal, J. A., Kaplan, J. (1999). Impact of psychological factors on the pathogenesis of cardiovascular disease and implications for therapy. *Circulation* 99, 2192–2217.

Rubin, R. T., Villanueva-Meyer, J., Ananth, J., *et al*. (1992). Regional xenon 133 cerebral blood flow and cerebral technetium Tc99m-HMPAO uptake in unmedicated patients with obsessive compulsive disorder and match normal control subjects. *Archives of General Psychiatry* 49, 695–702.

Rüdin, E. (1916). Studien über Vererbung und Entstehung geistiger Störungen: I. *Zur Vererbung und Neuentstehung der Dementia Praecox*. Springer, Berlin.

Rüdin, E. (1953). Ein Beitrag zur Frage der Zwangskrankäheit, unsbesondere ihrer hereditaren Beziehungen. *Archiv fur Psychiatrie und Nervenkrankheiten* 191, 14–54.

Rudorfer, M. V. and Potter, W. Z. (1989). Antidepressants: a comparative review of the clinical pharmacology and therapeutic use of the 'newer' versus the 'older' drugs. *Drugs* 37, 713–38.

Rundell, J. R., Ursano, R. J., Holloway, H. C., and Silberman, E. K. (1989). Psychiatric responses to trauma. *Hospital and Community Psychiatry* 40(1), 68–73.

Russell, D. E. H. (1984). The prevalence and seriousness of incestuous abuse: stepfathers versus biological fathers. *Child Abuse and Neglect* 8, 15–22.

Russell, G. F. M. (1979). Bulimia nervosa: an ominous variant of anorexia nervosa. *Psychological Medicine* 9, 429–48.

Russell, G. F. M. (2000). Anorexia nervosa. In *The new Oxford textbook of psychiatry* (eds M. G. Gelder, J. J López-Ibor Jr, and N. C. Andreasen), Chapter 4.10.1. Oxford University Press, Oxford.

Russell, G. F. M., Szmulker, G., Dare, C., and Eisler, I. (1987). An evaluation of family therapy in anorexia nervosa and bulimia nervosa. *Archives of General Psychiatry* 44, 1047–56.

Russell, O. (1970). Autistic children: infancy to adulthood. *Seminars in Psychiatry* 2, 435–40.

Russell, O. (ed.) (1997). *The psychiatry of learning disabilities*. Gaskell, London.

Rutter, M. (1966). *Children of sick parents: an environmental and psychiatric study*. Institute of Psychiatry, Maudsley Monographs No. 16. Oxford University Press, Oxford.

Rutter, M. (1972). Relationships between child and adult psychiatric disorders. *Acta Psychiatrica Scandinavica* 48, 3–21.

Rutter, M. (1981). *Maternal deprivation reassessed*. Penguin, Harmondsworth.

Rutter, M. (1983). Cognitive deficits in the pathogenesis of autism. *Journal of Child Psychology and Psychiatry* 24, 513–32.

Rutter, M. (1985). Resilience in the face of adversity: protective factors and resistance to psychiatric disorder. *British Journal of Psychiatry* 147, 598–611.

Rutter, M. (1995). Clinical implications of attachment concepts: retrospect and prospect. *Journal of Child Psychology and Psychiatry* 36, 549–71.

Rutter, M. (1996). Connections between child and adult psychopathology. *European Child and Adolescent Psychiatry* **5(suppl 1)**, 4–7.

Rutter, M. L. (1999). Psychosocial adversity and child psychopathology. *British Journal of Psychiatry* **174**, 480–93.

Rutter, M. and Lockyer, L. (1967). A five to fifteen year follow-up study of infantile psychosis: I. Description of sample. *British Journal of Psychiatry* **113**, 1169–82.

Rutter, M. and Madge, N. (1976). *Cycles of disadvantage: a review of research.* Heinemann, London.

Rutter, M. and Plomin, R. (1997). Opportunities for psychiatry from genetic findings. *British Journal of Psychiatry* **171**, 209–19.

Rutter, M., Graham, P., and Birch, H. G. (1970a). A neuropsychiatric study of childhood. *Clinics in developmental medicine*, No.35/36. Heinemann, London.

Rutter, M., Tizard, J., and Whitmore, K. (eds) (1970b). *Education, health and behaviour.* Longmans, London.

Rutter, M., Yule, W., Berger, M., *et al.* (1974). Children of West Indian immigrants. I. Rates of behavioural deviance and of psychiatric disorder. *Journal of Child Psychology and Psychiatry* **15**, 241–62.

Rutter, M., Cox, A., Tupling, C., Berger, M., and Yule, W. (1975a). Attainment and adjustment in two geographical areas: I. Prevalence of psychiatric disorders. *British Journal of Psychiatry* **126**, 493–509.

Rutter, M., Yule, B., Quinton, D., *et al.* (1975b). Attainment and adjustment in two geographical areas III: Some factors accounting for area differences. *British Journal of Psychiatry* **126**, 520–33.

Rutter, M., Graham, P., Chadwick, O., and Yule, W. (1976a). Adolescent turmoil: fact or fiction. *Journal of Child Psychology and Psychiatry* **17**, 35–56.

Rutter, M., Tizard, J., Yule, W., *et al.* (1976b). Isle of Wight Studies 1964–1974. *Psychological Medicine* **6**, 313–32.

Rutter, M., Chadwick, O., and Shaffer, D. (1983). Head injury. In *Developmental neuropsychiatry* (ed. M. Rutter), pp. 83–111. Churchill Livingstone, Edinburgh.

Rutter, M. L., MacDonald, H., LeCouteur, A., *et al.* (1990). Genetic factors in child psychiatric disorder. II Empirical findings. *Journal of Child Psychology and Psychiatry* **31**, 39–83.

Rutter, M., Bailey, A., Bolton, P., and Le Couter, A. (1993). Autism: syndrome definition and possible genetic mechanisms. In: *Nature, nurture and psychology*

(eds R. Plomin, and G. E. McClearn), pp. 269–84. American Psychiatric Association, Washington, DC.

Rutter, M., Bailey, A., Bolton, P., and Le Couteur, A. (1994a). Autism and known medical conditions: myth and substance. *Journal of Child Psychology and Psychiatry* **35**, 311–22.

Rutter, M., Taylor, E., and Hersov, L. (ed.) (1994b). *Child and adolescent psychiatry: modern approaches*, 3rd edn. Blackwell Scientific Publications, Oxford.

Rutter, M., Giller, H., and Hagell, A. (1998). *Antisocial behaviour by young people.* Cambridge University Press, Cambridge.

Rutter, M., Silberg, J., O'Connor, T., and Simonoff, E. (1999). Genetics and child psychiatry: II Empirical research finding. *Journal of Child Psychology and Psychiatry* **40**, 19–55.

Rutz, W., von Knorring, L., and Walinder, J. (1992). Long-term effects of an educational program for general practitioners given by the Swedish Committee for the prevention and treatment of depression. *Acta Psychiatrica Scandinavica* **85**, 83–8.

Ryan, N. D. and Puig-Antich, J. (1986). Affective illness in adolescence. In *American Psychiatric Association Annual Review* (eds A. J. Frances and R. E. Hales), Vol. 5. American Psychiatric Association, Washington, DC.

Ryan, R. (1994). Post-traumatic stress disorder in persons with developmental disabilities. *Community Mental Health Journal* **30**, 45–54.

Ryle, A. (1990). *Cognitive analytic therapy: active participation in change.* Wiley, Chichester.

Ryle, A. (1997). The structure and development of borderline personality disorder: a proposed model. *British Journal of Psychiatry* **170**, 82–7.

Sachdev, P. and Sachdev, J. (1997). Sixty years of psychosurgery: its present status and its future. *Australian and New Zealand Journal of Psychiatry* **31**, 457–64.

Sackett, D. L. (1996). Evaluation of clinical method. In *Oxford Textbook of Medicine*, 3rd edn (eds D. J. Weatherall, J. G. G. Ledingham, and D. A.Warrell), pp. 15–21. Oxford University Press, Oxford.

Sackett, D. L., Richardson, W. S., Rosenberg, W., and Haynes, R. B. (1997). *Evidence-based medicine. How to practise and teach EBM.* Churchill Livingstone, Edinburgh.

Sackheim, H. A., Prudic, J., Devanand, D. P., *et al.* (1990). The impact of medication resistance and continuation of pharmacotherapy on relapse following response to electroconvulsive therapy in major depression. *Journal of Clinical Psychopharmacology* 10, 96–104.

Sackheim, H. A., Prudic, J., Devanand, D. P. *et al.* (1993). Effects of stimulus intensity and electrode placement on the efficacy and cognitive effects of electroconvulsive therapy. *New England Journal of Medicine* 328, 839–46.

Sackheim, H. A., Prudic, J., Devanand, D. P., *et al.* (2000). A prospective, randomized, double-blind comparison of bilateral and right unilateral electroconvulsive therapy at different stimulus intensities. *Archives of General Psychiatry* 57, 425–434.

Sacks, O. (1973). *Awakenings*. Duckworth, London

Sainsbury, P. and Barraclough, B. (1968). Differences between suicide rates. *Nature* 220, 1252–3.

Sakel, M. (1938). *The pharmacological shock treatment of schizophrenia.* Nervous and Mental Diseases Monograph Series No. 62. Nervous and Mental Disease Publications, New York.

Saletu, B. and Anderer, P. (1999). EEG in psychiatry. *Neuropsychiatrie* 13, 161–77.

Salkovskis, P. (1997). Obsessive–compulsive disorder. In *Science and practice of cognitive behaviour therapy* (eds D. M. Clark and C. G. Fairburn), Chapter 8. Oxford University Press, Oxford.

Salkovskis, P. and Bass, C. (1997). Hypochondriasis. In *Science and practice of cognitive behaviour therapy* (eds D. M. Clark and C. G. Fairburn), Chapter 13. Oxford University Press, Oxford.

Salkovskis, P. M. and Campbell, P. (1994). Thought suppression in naturally occurring negative intrusive thoughts. *Behaviour Research and Therapy* 32, 1–8.

Salkovskis, P. M. and Clark, D. M. (1993). Panic disorder and hypochondriasis. *Advances in Behaviour Research and Therapy* 15, 24–48.

Salkovskis, P. M. and Warwick, H. M. C. (1986). Morbid preoccupations, health anxiety and reassurance: a cognitive–behavioural approach to hypochondriasis. *Behaviour Research and Therapy* 24, 597–602.

Sallee F. R., Richman, H., Beach, K., *et al.* (1996). Platelet serotonin transporter in children and adolescents with obsessive–compulsive disorder or Tourette's syndrome. *Journal of the American Academy of Child and Adolescent Psychiatry* 35, 1647–56.

Salminen, J. K., Saarijarvi, S., and Aarela, E. (1995). Two decades of alexithymia. *Journal of Psychosomatic Research* 39, 803–7.

Salmon, G. and West, A. (2000). Physical and mental health issues related to bullying in schools. *Current Opinion in Psychiatry* 13, 381–8.

Salzmann, J., Wolfson, A. N., Schatzenberg, A., *et al.* (1995). Effect of fluoxetine on anger in symptomatic volunteers with borderline personality disorder. *Journal of Clinical Psychopharmacology* 15, 23–9.

Sameroff, A., Seifer, R., Barocas, R., *et al.* (1987). IQ scores of 4-year-old children: social-environmental risk factors. *Pediatrics* 79, 343–50.

Sanders, A. R., Detera-Wadleigh, S. D., and Gershon, E. S. (1999). Molecular genetics of mood disorders. In *Neurobiology of mental illness* (eds D. S. Charney, E. J. Nestler, and B. S. Bunney), pp. 299–316. Oxford University Press, New York.

Sandifer, M. G., Hordern, A., Timbury, G. C., and Green, L. M. (1968). Psychiatric diagnosis: a comparative study in North Carolina. *British Journal of Psychiatry* 114, 1–9.

Sargant, W. and Dally, P. (1962). Treatment of anxiety state by antidepressant drugs. *British Medical Journal* 1, 6–9.

Sargant, W. and Slater, E. (1940). Acute war neuroses. *Lancet* 2, 1–2.

Sargant, W. and Slater, E. (1963). *An introduction to physical methods of treatment in psychiatry.* Livingstone, Edinburgh.

Sargent, P. A., Quested, D. J. and Cowen, P. J. (1998). Clomipramine enhances the cortisol response to 5-HTP: implications for the therapeutic role of 5-HT$_2$ receptors. *Psychopharmacology* 140, 120–2.

Sargent, P. A., Kjaer, K. H., Bench, C. J., *et al.* (2000). Brain serotonin$_{1A}$ receptor binding measured by positron emission tomography with [^{11}C] WAY–100635: effects of depression and antidepressant treatment. *Archives of General Psychiatry* 57, 174–80.

Sartorius, N., Kaelber, C. T., Cooper, J. E., *et al.* (1993). Progress toward achieving a common language in psychiatry: results from the field trial of the clinical guidelines accompanying the WHO classification of mental and behavioral disorders in ICD-10. *Archives of General Psychiatry* 50, 115.

Sartorius, N., Ustun, T. B., and Korton, A. (1995). Progress toward achieving a common language in psychiatry II: results from the International Field Trials of the ICD-10 Diagnostic Criteria for Research for Mental and Behavioral Disorders. *American Journal of Psychiatry* 152, 1427–37.

Sarwer, D. B., Wadden, T. A., Pertschuk, M. J., and Whitaker, L. A. (1998). The psychology of cosmetic surgery: a review and reconceptualization. *Clinical Psychology Review* 18, 1–22.

Sasson,Y. And Yohar, J. (1996). New developments in obsessive–compulsive disorder research: implications for clinical management. *International Journal of Psychopharmacology* 11(suppl 5), 3–12.

Saunders, A. M. (2000). Apolipoprotein E and Alzheimer disease: an update on genetic and functional analyses. *Journal of Neuropathology and Experimental Neurology* 59, 751–758.

Saxena, S., Brody, A. L., Schwartz, J. M., and Baxter, L. R. (1998). Neuroimaging and frontal-subcortical circuitry in obsessive–compulsive disorder. *British Journal of Psychiatry* 173(suppl 35), 26–37.

Saywitz, K. and Camparo, L. (1998). Interviewing child witnesses: a developmental perspective. *Child Abuse and Neglect* 22, 825–43.

Schachar, R. (1991). Childhood hyperactivity. *Journal of Child Psychology and Psychiatry* 32, 155–91.

Schachar, R. and Ickowicz, A. (2000). Attention deficit hyperkinetic disorders in childhood and adolescence. In *The new Oxford textbook of psychiatry* (eds M. G. Gelder, J. J. López-Ibor Jr, and N. C. Andreasen), Chapter 9.2.3. Oxford University Press, Oxford.

Schenck, C. H. and Mahowald, M. W. (2000). Parasomnias. In *The new Oxford textbook of psychiatry* (eds. M. G. Gelder, J. J. López-Ibor Jr, and N. C. Andreasen), Chapter 4.14.4. Oxford University Press, Oxford.

Schenk, D. B., Seubert, P., Lieberburg, I., Wallace, J. (2000). β-peptide immunization. A possible new treatment for Alzheimer disease. *Archives of Neurology* 57, 934–936.

Schmideberg, M. (1947). The treatment of psychopaths and borderline patients. *American Journal of Psychotherapy* 1, 45–70.

Schmitt, B. D. (1986). New enuresis alarms: safe successful and child operable. *Archives of Disease in Childhood* 43, 665–71.

Schneider, K. (1959). *Clinical psychopathology*. Grune and Stratton, New York.

Schneier, F. R., Johnson, J., Hornig, C. D., *et al.* (1992). Social phobia: comorbidity and morbidity in an epidemiological sample. *Archives of General Psychiatry* 49, 282–8.

Schneier, F. R., Marshall, R. D., Street, L., *et al.* (1995). Social phobia and specific phobias. In *Treatments of psychiatric disorders* (ed. G. O. Gabbard). American Psychiatric Press, Washington, DC.

Schneier, F. R., Goetz, D., Campeas, R., Fallon, B., Marshall, R., and Liebowitz, M. R. (1998) Placebo-controlled trial of moclobemide in social phobia. *British Journal of Psychiatry* 172, 70–7.

Schrenck-Notzing, A. von (1895). *The use of hypnosis in psychopathia sexualis with special reference to contrary sexual instinct* (trans. C. G. Chaddock). Institute of Research in Hypnosis Publication Society and the Julian Press, New York (1956).

Schuchter, S. R. and Zisook, S. (1993). The normal course of grief. In: *Handbook of bereavement* (eds M. S. Stroebe, W. Stroebe, and R. O. Hansson). Cambridge University Press, Cambridge.

Schuckit, M. A., Smith, T. L., Anthenellic, R. A., and Irwin, M. (1993). A clinical course of alcoholism in 636 male inpatients. *American Journal of Psychiatry* 150, 786–92.

Schulsinger, F. (1982). Psychopathy: heredity and environment. *International Journal of Mental Health* 1, 190–206.

Schultz, J. H. (1932). *Das autogene training*. Thieme, Liepzig.

Schultz, J. H. and Luthe, W. (1959). *Autogenic training: a psychophysiological approach*. Grune and Stratton, New York.

Schulz, P. M., Schulz, S. C., Golberg, S. C., Ettigi, P., Resnick, R. J., and Friedel, R. O. (1986). Diagnoses of relatives of schizotypal outpatients. *Journal of Nervous and Mental Disease* 174, 457–63.

Schwartz, C. E., Snidman, N., and Kagan, J. (1999). Adolescent social anxiety as an outcome of inhibited temperament in childhood. *Journal of the American Academy of Child and Adolescent Psychiatry* 38, 1008–15.

Schwartz, J. M. (1998). Neuroanatomical aspects of cognitive behavioural therapy response in obsessive compulsive disorder. *British Journal of Psychiatry* 173 supp 35, 26–37.

Schweizer, E. and Rickels, K. (1998). Benzodiazepine dependence and withdrawal: a review of the syndrome and its clinical management. *Acta Psychiatrica Scandinavica* 393, 95–101.

Scott, A. I. F., Weeks, D. J., and McDonald, C. F. (1991). Continuation of electroconvulsive therapy: preliminary guidelines and an illustrative case report. *British Journal of Psychiatry* 159, 867–70.

Scott, J. (1995). Psychotherapy for bipolar disorder. *British Journal of Psychiatry* 167, 581–8.

Scott, P. D. (1960). The treatment of psychopaths. *British Medical Journal* 1, 1641–6.

Scott, P. D. (1973). Parents who kill their children. *Medicine, Science and Law* 13, 120–126

Scott, S. (1994). Mental retardation. In *Child and adolescent psychiatry: modern approaches*, 3rd edn (eds M. Rutter, E. Taylor, and L. Hersov), pp. 616–46. Blackwell Scientific Publications, Oxford.

Scott, S. (2000). Conduct disorders in childhood and adolesence. Ch 9.2.4. In *New Oxford textbook of psychiatry.* (eds M. G. Gelder, J. J. Lopez-Ibor and N. C. Andreasen. Oxford University Press, Oxford.

Sedler, M. J. (1985). The legacy of Ewald Hecker: a new translation of 'Die Hebephrenie'. *American Journal of Psychiatry* 142, 1265–71.

Sedman, G. (1966). A phenomenological study of pseudo-hallucinations and related experiences. *British Journal of Psychiatry* 113, 1115–21.

Sedman, G. (1970). Theories of depersonalization: a reappraisal. *British Journal of Psychiatry* 117, 1–14.

Sedvall, G. C., Farde, L., and Pauli, S. (2000). Neurochemical imaging in schizophrenia. In *The psychopharmacology of schizophrenia* (eds M. A. Reveley and J. F. W. Deakin), pp. 131–52. Oxford University Press, London.

Segal, H. (1963). *Introduction to the work of Melanie Klein.* Heinemann Medical, London.

Segal, J., Berk, M., and Brook, S. (1998). Risperidone compared with both lithium and haloperidol in mania: a double-blind randomized controlled trial. *Clinical Neuropharmacology* 21, 176–80.

Seguin, E. (1864). Origin of the treatment and training of idiots. In *History of mental retardation* (eds M. Rosen, G. R. Clark, and M. S. Kivitz), Vol.1. University Park Press, Baltimore, MD (1976).

Seguin, E. (1866). *Idiocy and its treatment by the physiological method.* Brandown, Albany, NY.

Seibyl, J. P., Scanley, E., Krystal, J. H., and Innis, R. B. (1999). *Neuroimaging methodologies.* In *Neurobiology of mental illness* (ed. D. S. Charney, E. J. Nestler, and B. S. Bunney), pp. 170–94. Oxford University Press, Oxford.

Seiner, S, J. and Mallya, G. (1999). Treating depression in patients with cardiovascular disorder. *Harvard Review of Psychiatry* 7, 85–93.

Seivewright, N. and McMahon, C. (1996). Misuse of amphetamines and related drugs. *Advances in Psychiatric Treatment* 2, 211–18.

Selnes, O. A. and McKann, G. M. (2001). Coronary artery bypass surgery and the brain. *New England Journal of Medicine* 344, 451–2.

Sensky, T., Turkington, D., Kingdon, D., *et al.* (2000). A randomized controlled trial of cognitive–behavioral therapy for persistent symptoms in schizophrenia resistant to medication. *Archives of General Psychiatry* 57, 165–72.

Shadish, W. R., Ragsdaly, K., Glaser, R. R., *et al.* (1995). The efficacy and effectiveness of marital and family therapy: a perspective from meta-analysis. *Journal of Marital and Family Therapy* 21, 345–60.

Shaffer, D. (1974). Suicide in childhood and early adolescence. *Journal of Child Psychology and Psychiatry* 15, 275–91.

Shaffer, D., Pfeffer, C. R., and Gutstein, J. (2000). Suicide and attempted suicide in children and adolescents. In *The new Oxford textbook of psychiatry* (eds M. G. Gelder, J. J. López-Ibor Jr, and N. C. Andreasen), Chapter 9.2.10. Oxford University Press, Oxford.

Shannon, F. T., Fergusson, D. M., and Dimond, M. E. (1984). Early hospital admissions and subsequent behaviour problems in six-year-olds. *Archives of Disease in Childhood* 59, 815–19.

Shapiro, F. (1995). *Movement desensitization and reprocessing: basic principles, protocols and procedures.* Guilford, New York.

Sharma, T. (1999). Cognitive effects of conventional and atypical antipsychotics in schizophrenia. *British Journal of Psychiatry* 174(**suppl 38**), 44–51.

Sharp, C. W. and Freeman, P. L. (1993). The medical complications of anorexia. *British Journal of Psychiatry* 162, 452–62.

Sharpe, M. and Wessely, S. (2000). Chronic fatigue syndrome. In *The new Oxford textbook of psychiatry* (eds M. G. Gelder, J. J. López-Ibor Jr, and N. C. Andreasen), Chapter 5.2.7. Oxford University Press, Oxford.

Sharpe, M., Hawton, K., Seagroatt, V., *et al.* (1994). Depressive disorders in long-term survivors of stroke. Associations with demographic and social factors, functional status, and brain lesion volume. *British Journal of Psychiatry* **164**, 380–6.

Sharpe, M., Hawton, K., Simkin, S., *et al* (1996). Cognitive behaviour therapy for the chronic fatigue syndrome: a randomized controlled trial. *British Medical Journal* **312**, 22–6.

Sharpley, A. L. and Cowen, P. J. (1995). Effect of pharmacologic treatments on the sleep of depressed patients. *Biological Psychiatry* **37**, 85–98.

Sharpley, A. L., Vassallo, C. M., and Cowen, P. J. (2000). Olanzapine increases slow wave sleep: evidence for blockade of central 5-HT$_{2C}$ receptors in vivo. *Biological Psychiatry* **47**, 468–70.

Shaw, C., Abrams, K., and Marteau, T. M. (1999). Psychological impact of predicting individuals' risks of illness: a systematic review. *Social Science and Medicine* **49**, 1571–98.

Shaw, J., Appleby, L., Amos, T. *et al.* (1999). Mental disorder and clinical care in people convicted of homicide: national clinical survey. *British Medical Journal* **318**, 1240–1244.

Sheard, M. H., Marini, J. L., Bridges, C. I., and Wagner, E. (1976). The effect of lithium on impulsive aggressive behavior in man. *American Journal of Psychiatry* **133**, 1409–13.

Sheldon, W. H., Stevens, S. S., and Tucker, W. B. (1940). *The varieties of human physique*. Harper, London.

Shelton, R. C. (1999). Mood-stabilizing drugs in depression. *Journal of Clinical Psychiatry* **60(suppl 5)**, 37–40.

Shepherd, J. P. and Farrington, D. P. (1996). The prevention of delinquency, with particular reference to violent crime. *Medicine, Science and the Law* **36**, 331–6.

Shepherd, M. (1961). Morbid jealousy: some clinical and social aspects of a psychiatric symptom. *Journal of Mental Science* **107**, 687–753.

Shepherd, J., Stein, K. and Milne, R. (2000). Eye movement desensitization and reprocessing in the treatment of post-traumatic stress disorder: a review of an emerging therapy. *Psychological Medicine* **30**, 863–71.

Shepherd, M., Cooper, B., Brown, A. C and Katon, G. (1966). *Psychiatric illness in general practice*. Oxford University Press, Oxford.

Sherman, D. I. N., Ward, R. J., Warren-Perry, M., *et al.* (1993). Association of restriction fragment length polymorphism in alcohol dehydrogenase 2 gene with alcohol induced liver damage. *British Medical Journal* **307**, 1388–90.

Shibuya, A. and Yoshida, A. (1988). The genotypes of alcohol-metabolising enzymes in Japanese with alcohol liver disease. *American Journal of Human Genetics* **43**, 744–8.

Shields, J. (1962). *Monozygotic twins brought up apart and brought up together*. Oxford University press, London.

Shillito, F. H., Drinker, C. K., and Shaughnessy, T. J. (1936). The problem of nervous and mental sequelae of carbon monoxide poisoning. *Journal of the American Medical Association* **106**, 669–74.

Shneerson, J. M. (1999). *Drugs and sleep*. Blackwell Science, Oxford.

Shore, J. H., Vollmer, W. M., and Tatum, E. L. (1989). Community patterns of post-traumatic stress disorder. *Journal of Nervous and Mental Disease* **177**, 681–5.

Shorter, E. (1992). *From paralysis to fatigue. A history of psychosomatic illness in the modern era*. The Free Press, New York.

Shorvon, H. J., Hill, J. D. N., Burkitt, E., and Hastead, H. (1946). The depersonalization syndrome. *Proceedings of the Royal Society of Medicine* **39**, 779–92.

Shulman, K. (2001). Manic illness. In *Psychiatry in the elderly*, 3rd edn (eds R. Jacoby and C. Oppenheimer). Oxford University Press, Oxford.

Sibbald , B., Addington-Hall, J., Brenneman, D., and Freeling, P. (1996a). The role of counsellors in general practice: a qualitative study. *Occasional Papers of the Royal College of General Practitioners* **74**, 1–19.

Sibbald, B., Addington-Hall, J., Brenneman, D., and Freeling, P. (1996b). Investigation of whether on-site general practice counsellors have an impact on psychotropic drug prescribing rates and costs. *British Journal of General Practice* **46**, 63–67.

Sifneos, P. (1979). *Short term dynamic therapy*. Plenum Medical, New York.

Silberg, J., Meyer, J., Pickles, A., *et al.* (1996). Heterogeneity among juvenile antisocial behaviours: findings from the Virginia Twin Study of Adolescent Behavioural Development. In *Genetics of criminal and antisocial behaviour* (eds G. Bock and J. Goode). CIBA Foundation Symposium 194. Wiley, Chichester.

Silove, D., Harris, M., Morgan, A., *et al.* (1995). Is early separation anxiety a specific precursor of panic disorder-agoraphobia? A community study. *Psychological Medicine* **25**, 405–11.

Silva, A. J., Ferrari, M. M., Leong, G. B., and Penny, G. (1998). The dangerousness of persons with delusional jealousy. *Journal of the American Academy of Psychiatry and the Law* 26, 607–23.

Silva, H., Jerez, S., Ramirez, A., *et al.* (1998). Effects of pimozide on the psychopathology of delusional disorder. *Progress in Neuropsychopharmacology and Biological Psychiatry* 22, 331–40.

Silva, J. A., Derecho, D. V., Leong, G. B., and Ferrari, M. M. (2000). Stalking behavior in delusional jealousy. *Journal of Forensic Science* 45, 77–82.

Silveira, J. M. and Seeman, M. V. (1995). Shared psychotic disorder: a critical review of the literature. *Canadian Journal of Psychiatry* 40, 389–95.

Silverstone, T. and Cookson, J. (1982). The biology of mania. In *Recent advances in clinical psychiatry* (ed. K. Granville-Grassman), pp. 201–41. Churchill Livingstone, Edinburgh.

Simon, G. (2000). Epidemiology of somatoform disorders and other causes of unexplained medical symptoms. In *The new Oxford textbook of psychiatry* (eds. M. G. Gelder, J. J. López-Ibor Jr, and N. C. Andreasen), Chapter 5.2.2. Oxford University Press, Oxford.

Simon, G., Vonkorff, M., Heiligstein, J., *et al.* (1995). Initial antidepressant choice in primary care: effectiveness and cost effectiveness of fluoxetine vs. tricyclic antidepressants. *Journal of the American Medical Association* 275, 1897–902.

Simon, G. E., Von Korff, M., Piccinelli, M., Fullerton, C., Ormel, J. (1999). An international study of the relation between somatic symptoms and depression. *New England Journal of Medicine* 341, 1329–1335.

Simon, G., Gater, R., Kisely, S., and Piccinelli, M. (1996). Somatic symptoms of distress: an international primary care study. *Psychosomatic Medicine* 58, 481–8.

Simon, R. I. (1997). Video voyeurs and covert videotaping of unsuspecting victims: psychological and legal consequences. *Journal of Forensic Science* 42, 884–9.

Simon, R. I. (2000). Legal issues in psychiatry. In *Comprehensive textbook of psychiatry*, 7th edn (eds B. J. Sadock and V. A. Sadock). Lippincott, Williams & Wilkins, Philadelphia.

Simpson, L. (1990). The comparative efficacy of Milan Family Therapy for disturbed children and their families. *Journal of Family Therapy* 13, 267–84.

Sinclair, I. (2000). Residential care for social reasons. In *The new Oxford textbook of psychiatry* (eds M. G. Gelder, J. J. López-Ibor Jr, and N. C. Andreasen), Chapter 9.5.6. Oxford University Press, Oxford.

Singer, M. T. and Wynne, L. C. (1965). Thought disorder and family relations of schizophrenics: IV. Results and implications. *Archives of General Psychiatry* 12, 201–12.

Singh, S. P. and Lee, A. S. (1997). Conversion disorders in Nottingham: alive, but not kicking. *Journal of Psychosomatic Research* 43, 425–30.

Singleton, N., Meltzer, H., Gatward, R., *et al.* (1997). *Psychiatric morbidity among prisoners in England and Wales.* OPCS Surveys of Psychiatric Morbidity in Great Britain. HMSO, London.

Siris, S. G., Morgan, V., Fagerstrom, R., *et al.* (1987). Adjunctive imipramine in the treatment of post-psychotic depression. *Archives of General Psychiatry* 42, 533–9.

Siris, S. G., Bermanzohn, P. C., Gonzales, A., *et al.* (1991). Use of antidepressants for negative symptoms in a subset of schizophrenic patients. *Psychopharmacology Bulletin* 27, 331–5.

Skeels, H. (1966). Adult status of children with contrasting life experiences: a follow-up study. *Monograph of the Society for Research into Child Development* 31(3).

Skinner, B. F. (1953). *Science and human behaviour.* Macmillan, New York.

Skodol, A. E. and Oldham, J. M. (1991). Assessment and diagnosis of borderline personality disorder. *Hospital and Community Psychiatry* 42, 1021–8.

Skoog, G. and Skoog, I. (1999). A 40 year follow-up of patients with obsessive–compulsive disorder. *Archives of General Psychiatry* 56, 121–7.

Skoog, S. J., Stokes, A., and Turner, K. L. (1997). Oral desmopressin: a randomized double-blind placebo controlled study of effectiveness in children with primary nocturnal enuresis. *Journal of Urology* 158, 1035–40.

Skre, I., Onstad, S., Torgersen, S., *et al.* (1993). A twin study of DSMIIIR anxiety disorders. *Acta Psychiatrica Scandinavica* 88, 85–92.

Skuse, D. (1985). Non-organic failure to thrive. *Archives of Disease in Childhood* 60, 173–8.

Skuse, D. (1989). Emotional abuse and delay in growth. In *ABC of child abuse* (ed. R. Meadow), pp. 23–5. British Medical Association, London.

Skuse, D. and Bentovim, A. (1994). Physical and emotional maltreatment. In *Child and adolescent psychiatry: modern approaches*, 3rd edn (eds M. Rutter, E. Taylor, and L. Hersov), pp. 209–29. Blackwell Scientific Publications, Oxford.

Skynner, A. C. R. (1991). Open-systems group-analytic approach to family therapy. In *Handbook of family therapy* (eds A. S. Gurman and D. P. Kriskern). Brunner Mazel, New York.

Slater, E., Beard, A. W., Glithero, E. (1963). The Schizophrenia-like psychoses of epilepsy. *British Journal of Psychiatry* 109, 95–150.

Slater, E. (1951). Evaluation of electric convulsion therapy as compared with conservative methods in depressive states. *Journal of Mental Science* 97, 567–9.

Slater, E. (1965). The diagnosis of hysteria. *British Medical Journal* 1, 1395–9.

Slater, E. and Shields, J. (1969). Genetical aspects of anxiety. In *Studies of anxiety* (ed. M. H. Lader). *British Journal of Psychiatry Special Publication* No. 3.

Sledge, W. H., Tebes, J., Rakfeld, J., *et al.* (1996). Day hospital/crisis respite care versus inpatient care part 1: clinical outcomes. *American Journal of Psychiatry* 153, 1065–73.

Small, J. G., Klapper, M. H., Kellams, J. J., *et al.* (1988). Electroconvulsive treatment compared with lithium in the management of manic states. *Archives of General Psychiatry* 45, 727–32.

Small, J. G., Klapper, M. H., Milstein, V., *et al.* (1996). Comparison of therapeutic modalities for mania. *Psychopharmacology Bulletin* 32(4), 623–7.

Small, R., Lumley, J., Donohue, L., Potter, A., Waldenström, U. (2000). Randomised controlled trial of midwife led debriefing to reduce maternal depression after operative childbirth. *British Medical Journal* 321, 1043–1047.

Smalley, S. L., Bailey, J. G., Cantwell, D. P., *et al.* (1998). Evidence that the dopamine D4 receptor is a susceptibility gene in attention deficit hyperactivity disorder. *Molecular Psychiatry* 3, 427–30.

Smith, D., Dempster, C., Glanville, J., Freemantle, N., and Anderson, I. (2002). Efficacy and tolerability of venlafaxine compared wih selective serotonin re-uptake inhibitors and other antidepressants: a meta-analysis. *British Journal of Psychiatry*, 180, 396–404.

Smith, D. J. (1995). Youth crime and conduct disorders: trends, patterns and causal explanations. In *Psychosocial disorders in young people: time trends and their causes* (eds M. Rutter and D. J. Smith). Wiley, Chichester.

Smith, E. M., North, C. S., McCool, R. E., and Shea, J. M. (1990). Acute postdisaster psychiatric disorders: identification of persons at risk. *American Journal of Psychiatry* 147, 202–6.

Smith, G. R. (1995). Treatment of patients with multiple symptoms. In *Treatment of functional somatic symptoms* (eds R. A. Mayou, C. Bass, and M. Sharpe), pp.175–87. Oxford University Press, Oxford.

Smith, G. R., Hanson, R. A., and Ray, D. C. (1986). Patients with multiple unexplained symptoms. *Archives of Internal Medicine* 146, 69–72.

Smith, J. S. and Brandon, S. (1973). Morbidity from acute carbon monoxide poisoning at 3 year follow up. *British Medical Journal* 1, 318–21.

Smith, K. A. and Cowen, P. J. (1997). Serotonin and depression. In *Depression: neurobiological, psychopathological and therapeutic advances* (eds A. Honig and H. M. van Praag), pp. 129–46. John Wiley & Sons Ltd, Chichester.

Smith, K. A., Fairburn, C. G., and Cowen, P. J. (1997). Relapse of depression after rapid depletion of tryptophan. *Lancet* 349, 915–19.

Smith, K. A., Morris, J. S., Friston, K. J., *et al.* (1999). Brain mechanisms associated with depressive relapse and associated cognitive impairment following acute tryptophan depletion. *British Journal of Psychiatry* 174, 525–9.

Smith, K. A., Williams, C., and Cowen, P. J. (2000). Impaired regulation of brain serotonin function during dieting in women recovered from depression. *British Journal of Psychiatry* 176, 72–5.

Smith, S. E., Acton, L., and Sharp, T. (1997). Enhancement of dopamine-mediated behaviour by the NMDA antagonists MK–801 and CPP: similarities with repeated electroconvulsive shock. *Psychopharmacology* 133, 85–94.

Snaith, R. P., Baugh, S. J., Clayden, A. D., *et al.* (1982). The clinical anxiety scale: an instrument derived from the Hamilton Anxiety Scale. *British Journal of Psychiatry* 141, 518–523

Snowling, M. J. (1991). Developmental reading disorders. *Journal of Child Psychology and Psychiatry* 32, 49–77.

Snyder, D. K. and Wills, R. M. (1989). Behavioral versus insight orientated marital therapy: effects on individual and interpersonal functioning. *Journal of Consulting and Clinical Psychology* 57, 39–46.

Soares, J. C. and Gershon, S. (1998). The lithium ion: a foundation for psychopharmacological specificity. *Neuropsychopharmacology* 19, 167–82.

Soloff, P. H. (1994). Is there a drug treatment of choice for borderline personality disorder? *Acta Psychiatrica Scandinavica* 89(suppl 379), 50–5.

Soloff, P. H. and Millward, J. W. (1983). Psychiatric disorders in families of borderline patients. *Archives of General Psychiatry* 40, 37–44.

Soloff, P. H., George, A., Nathan, R. S., *et al.* (1986). Progress in psychopharmacology of personality disorders: a double blind study of amitriptyline, haloperidol and placebo. *Archives of General Psychiatry* **43**, 691–7.

Solowij, N. (1993). Ecstasy (3,4-methylenedioxymethanphetamine). *Current Opinion in Psychiatry* **6**, 411–15.

Sonino, N. and Fava, G. A. (1998). Psychosomatic aspects of Cushing's disease. *Psychotherapy and Psychosomatics* **67**, 140–6.

Soothill, K. L. and Pope, P. J. (1973). Arson: a twenty-year cohort study. *Medicine, Science and the Law* **13**, 127–38.

South, N. (1994). Drugs: control, crime, and criminological studies. In *The Oxford handbook of criminology* (eds M. Maguire, R. Morgan, and R. Reiner), pp. 393–440. Clarendon Press, Oxford.

Southwick, S. M., Krystal, J. H., Bremner, J .D., *et al.* (1997). Noradrenergic and serotonergic function in post-traumatic stress disorder. *Archives of General Psychiatry* **54**, 749–58.

Souza, F. G. and Goodwin, G. M. (1991). Lithium treatment and prophylaxis in unipolar depression: a meta-analysis. *British Journal of Psychiatry* **158**, 666–75.

Soyka, M., Naber, G., and Volcker, A. (1991). Prevalence of delusional jealousy in different psychiatric disorders. *British Journal of Psychiatry* **158**, 549–53.

Spanagel, R. (1999). Is there a pharmacological basis for therapy with rapid opioid detoxification? *Lancet* **354**, 2017–18.

Speilberger, C. D., Gorsuch, R. L., and Lushene, R. (1970). *State Trait Anxiety Inventory manual*. Consulting Psychologists Press, Palo Alto, CA.

Spence, S. A. (1999). Hysterical paralyses as disorders of action. *Cognitive Neuropsychiatry* **4**, 203–26.

Spencer, T. J., Biederman, J., Harding, M., *et al.* (1996). Growth deficits in ADHD children revisited: evidence for disorder-associated growth delays? *Journal of the American Academy of Child and Adolescent Psychiatry* **35**, 1460–9.

Spiegel, D. (1991). Dissociation and trauma. In *Review of psychiatry* (eds A. Tasman and S. M. Goldfinger), pp. 262–75. American Psychiatric Press, Washington DC.

Spiegel, D. and Barlow, D. H. (2000). Generalized anxiety disorders. In *The new Oxford textbook of psychiatry*

(eds M. G. Gelder, J. J. López-Ibor Jr, and N. C. Andreasen), Chapter 4.7.1. Oxford University Press, Oxford.

Spiegel, D. and Classen, C. (2000). *Group therapy for cancer patients: a research-based handbook of psychosocial care*. Basic Books, New York.

Spiegel, D. and Kato, P. M. (1996). Psychosocial influences on cancer incidence and progression. *Harvard Review of Psychiatry* **4**, 10–26.

Spiker, D. G., Weiss, J. C., Dealy, R. S., *et al.* (1985). The pharmacological treatment of delusional depression. *American Journal of Psychiatry* **142**, 430–6.

Spitzer, R. L. and Endicott, J. (1968). DIAGNO: a computer programme for psychiatric diagnosis utilizing the differential diagnostic procedures. *Archives of General Psychiatry* **18**, 746–56.

Spitzer, R. L. and Wakefield, J. C. (1999). DSM-IV diagnostic criterion for clinical significance: does it help solve the false positives problem? *American Journal of Psychiatry* **156**, 1856–64.

Spitzer, R. L. and Williams, J. B. W. (1985). Classification in psychiatry. In *Comprehensive textbook of psychiatry*, 4th edn (eds H. I. Kaplan and B. J. Sadock). Williams & Wilkins, Baltimore, MD.

Spitzer, R. L., Endicott, J., and Robins, E. (1978). Research and diagnostic criteria: rationale and reliability. *Archives of General Psychiatry* **35**, 773–82.

Spitzer, R. L., Williams, J. B. D., and Gibbon, M. (1987). *Structured clinical interview for DSMIV (SCID)*. Biometrics Research, New York State Psychiatric Institute, New York.

Spitzer, R. L., Williams, J. B. W., Gibbon, M., and First, M. B. (1990). *User's guide to the structured clinical interview for DSMIIIR*. American Psychiatric Press, Washington, DC.

Spitzer, R., First, M. B., Williams, J. B. W., *et al.* (1992). Now is the time to retire the term 'organic mental disorders'. *American Journal of Psychiatry* **149**(2), 240–4.

Spohr, H. L., Willms, J., and Steinhausen, H.-C. (1993). Prenatal alcohol exposure and long-term developmental consequences. *Lancet* **341**, 907–10.

Spreat, S. and Behar, D. (1994). Trends in the residential (inpatient) treatment of individuals with a dual diagnosis. *Journal of Consulting and Clinical Psychology* **62**(1), 43–8.

Squire, L. R., Slater, P. C., and Miller, P. L. (1981). Retrograde amnesia and bilateral electroconvulsive therapy. Long-term follow-up. *Archives of General Psychiatry* 38, 89–95.

Stahl, S. M. (1999). Selecting an atypical antipsychotic by combining clinical experience with guidelines from clinical trials. *Journal of Clinical Psychiatry* 60 (suppl 10), 31–41.

Stanhope, R., Adlard, P., Hamill, G., *et al.* (1988). Psychological growth hormone secretion during the recovery from psychosocial dwarfism: a case report. *Clinical Endocrinology,* 28, 335–9.

Stanley, M. A. and Beck, J. G. (2000). Anxiety disorders. *Clinical Psychology Review* 20, 731–754.

Starkstein, S. E. and Robinson, R. G. (eds) (1993). *Depression in neurologic disease.* The Johns Hopkins University Press, Baltimore, MD.

Statham, D. J., Heath, A. C., Madden, P. A., *et al.* (1998). Suicidal behaviour: an epidemiological and genetic study. *Psychological Medicine* 28, 839–55.

Stedeford, A. and Bloch, S. (1979). The psychiatrist in the terminal care unit. *British Journal of Psychiatry* 135, 7–14.

Stedeford, A. and Regnard, C. (1991). Confusional states in advanced cancer – a flow diagram. *Palliative Medicine* 5, 256–61.

Steffens, D. C. and Krishnan, K. R. R. (1998). Structural neuroimaging and mood disorders: recent findings, implications for classification, and future directions. *Biological Psychiatry* 43, 705–12.

Stein, A., Gath, D. H., Bucher, J., *et al.* (1991). The relationship between post-natal depression and mother child interaction. *British Journal of Psychiatry* 158, 46–52.

Stein, A., Stein, J., Walters, E. A., and Fairburn, C. G. (1995). Eating habits and attitudes among mothers of children with feeding disorders. *British Medical Journal* 310, 228.

Stein, D. J., Hollander, E. and Josephson, S. C. (1994). Serotonin reuptake blockers for the treatment of obsessional jealousy. *Journal of Clinical Psychiatry* 55, 30–3.

Stein, L. J. and Test, M. A. (1980). Alternative to mental hospital treatment. 1. Conceptual model, treatment program and clinical evaluation. *Archives of General Psychiatry* 37, 392–7.

Stein, M. B., Forde, D. R., Anderson, G. and Walker, J. R. (1997a). Obsessive–compulsive disorder in the community: an epidemiological survey with clinical reappraisal. *American Journal of Psychiatry* 154, 1120–6.

Stein, M. B., Walker, J. R., Hazen, A. L., and Forde, D. R. (1997b). Full and partial post-traumatic stress disorder: findings from a community survey. *American Journal of Psychiatry* 154, 1114–19.

Stein, M. B., Chartier, M. J., Hazen, A. L. *et al.* (1998a). A direct-interview family study of generalized social phobia. *American Journal of Psychiatry* 155, 90–7.

Stein, M. B., Liebowitz, M. R., Lydiard, R. B., *et al.* (1998b). Paroxetine treatment of generalized social phobia (social anxiety disorder): a randomized controlled trial. *Journal of the American Medical Association* 280, 708–13.

Stein, Z. and Susser, M. (1969). Widowhood and mental illness. *British Journal of Preventative and Social Medicine* 23, 106–10.

Steiner, H. and Lock, J. (1998). Anorexia nervosa and bulimia nervosa in children and adolescents: a review of the past 10 years. *Journal of the American Academy of Child and Adolescent psychiatry* 37, 352–9.

Stekel, W. (1953). *Sadism and masochism,* Vols 1 and 2. Liveright, London.

Stenager, E. N. and Stenager, E. (2000). Physical illness and suicidal behaviour. In *The international handbook of suicide and attempted suicide* (eds K. Hawton and K. van Heeringen). John Wiley & Sons, Chichester.

Stenager, E. N., Stenager, E., Koch-Henriksen, N., *et al.* (1992). Suicide in MS: an epidemiological investigation. *Journal of Neurology, Neurosurgery and Psychiatry* 55, 542–5.

Stenager, E, N., Madsen, C., Stenager, E., and Boldsen, J. (1998). Suicide in patients with stroke: epidemiological study. *British Medical Journal* 316, 1206.

Stengel, E. (1952). Enquiries into attempted sucide. *Proceedings of the Royal Society of Medicine* 45, 613–20.

Stengel, E. (1959). Classification of mental disorders. *Bulletin of the World Health Organization* 21, 601–63.

Stengel, E. and Cook, N. G. (1958). *Attempted suicide: its social significance and effects.* Maudsley Monograph No.4. Chapman & Hall, London.

Stephenson, T. (1995). Abduction of infants from hospital. *British Medical Journal* 310, 754–5.

Steptoe, A. and Wardle, J. (1994). *Psychosocial processes and health: a reader.* Cambridge University Press, Cambridge.

Stern, E., Silbersweig, D. A., Chee, K.-Y., *et al.* (2000). A functional neuroanatomy of tics in Tourette syndrome. *Archives of General Psychiatry* 57, 741–8.

Stern, R. S., Lipsedge, M. A., and Marks, L. M. (1973). Thought-stopping of neutral and obsessional thoughts: a controlled trial. *Behaviour Research and Therapy* 11, 659–62.

Sternbach, H. (1991). The serotonin syndrome. *American Journal of Psychiatry* 148, 705–13.

Stevenson, J. (1999). The treatment of the long-term sequelae of sexual abuse. *Journal of Child Psychology and Psychiatry* 40, 89–112.

Stober, G. (1999). The alcoholic hallucinosis. *Medizinische Welt* 50, 384–91.

Stoddard, F. J., Sheridan, R. L., Selter, L. F., and Greenberg, D. B. (2000). General surgery: basic principles of patient assessment. In *Psychiatric care of the medical patient* (eds A. Stoudemire, B. S. Fogel, and D. B. Greenberg). Oxford University Press, New York.

Stone, J. H., Roberts, M., O'Grady, J., *et al.* (eds) (2000). *Faulk's basic forensic psychiatry*, 3rd edn. Blackwell, Oxford.

Stone, M. (1985). Shellshock and the psychologists. In *The anatomy of madness, Vol.2, Institutions and society* (eds W. F. Bynum, R. Porter, and M. Shepherd), pp. 242–71. Tavistock Publications, London.

Stone, M. H. (1980). *The borderline syndromes: constitution, personality and adaptation.* McGraw-Hill, New York.

Stone, M. H. (1993). Long-term outcome in personality disorders. *British Journal of Psychiatry* 162, 299–313.

Stone, M. H., Hurt, S. W., and Stone, D. K. (1987). The PI–500: long term follow-up of borderline inpatients meeting DSMIII criteria. I: global outcome. *Journal of Personality Disorders* 1, 291–8.

Stores, G. (2000). Introduction to sleep-wake disorders. In *The new Oxford textbook of psychiatry* (eds M. G. Gelder, J. J. López-Ibor Jr, and N. C. Andreasen), Chapter 4.14.1. Oxford University Press, Oxford.

Storr, A. (2000). Analytical psychology (Jung). In *The new Oxford textbook of psychiatry* (eds M. G. Gelder, J. J. López-Ibor Jr, and N. C. Andreasen), Chapter 3.3.1. Oxford University Press, Oxford.

Stotland, N. L. and Stewart, D. E. (eds). 2001. *Psychological aspects of women's health care. The interface between psychiatry and obstetrics and gynecology.* (2nd ed). American Psychiatric Association.

Stoudemire, A., Fogel, B. S., and Greenberg, D. B. (2000). *Psychiatric care of the medical patient*, 2nd edn. Oxford University Press, New York.

Strain, E. C., Bigelow, G. E., Liebson, I. A., and Stitzer, M. L. (1999). Moderate- vs high-dose methadone in the treatment of opioid dependence: a randomized trial. *Journal of the American Medical Association* 281, 1000–5.

Strain, J. J., Rhodes, R., and Moros, D. A. (2000). Ethical issues in the care of the medically ill. In *Psychiatric care of the medical patient* (eds A. Stoudemire, B. S. Fogel, and D. B. Greenberg). Oxford University Press, New York.

Strang, J. (1993). Drug use and harm reduction: responding to the challenge. In *Psychoactive drugs and harm reduction* (eds N. Heather, A. Wodak, E. Nadelmann, and P. O'Hare P), pp. 3–20. Whurr Publishers, London.

Strathdee, G. and Jenkins, R. (1996). Purchasing mental health care for primary care. In *Commissioning mental health services* (eds G. Thornicroft and G. Strathdee), pp. 71–83. HMSO, London.

Strathdee, G. and Thornicroft, G, (1992). Community sectors of needs led mental health services. In *Measuring mental health needs* (eds G. Thornicroft, C. Brewin, and J. K. Wing), pp. 140–62. Gaskell, London.

Stroebe, M. S. and Stroebe, W. (1993). The mortality of bereavement: a review. In *Handbook of bereavement* (eds M. S. Stroebe and R. O Hansson), pp. 175–95. Cambridge University Press, Cambridge.

Stroebel, C. F. (1985). Biofeedback and behavioural medicine. In *Comprehensive textbook of psychiatry*, 4th edn (eds H. I. Kaplan and B. J. Sadock), pp. 1467–73. Williams & Wilkins, Baltimore, MD.

Strömgren, E. (1985). World-wide issues in psychiatric diagnosis and classification and the Scandinavian point of view. In *Mental disorders, alcohol and drug related problems*. Excerpta Medica, Amsterdam.

Stuart, R. B. (1980). *Helping couples change: a social learning approach to marital therapy.* Guilford Press, New York.

Stunkard, A. and Wadden, T. A. (2000). Obesity. In *The new Oxford textbook of psychiatry* (eds M. G. Gelder, J. J López-Ibor Jr, and N. C. Andreasen), Chapter 4.10.3. Oxford University Press, Oxford.

Sturmey, P., Reed, J., and Corbett, J. (1991). Psychometric assessment of psychiatric disorders in people with learning difficulties (mental handicap): a review of measures. *Psychological Medicine* 21, 143–55.

Sugarman, P. A. and Crawford, D. (1994). Schizophrenia in the Afro-Caribbean community. *British Journal of Psychiatry* 164, 474–80.

Sullivan, H. (1953). *The interpersonal theory of psychiatry.* Norton, New York.

Sulloway, F. J. (1979). *Freud: biologist of the mind.* Fontana, London.

Super, M. and Postlethwaite, R. J. (1997). Genes, familial enuresis and clinical management. *Lancet* 350, 159–60.

Susser, E., Struening, E. L., and Conover, S. (1989). Psychiatric problems in homeless men. *Archives of General Psychiatry* 46, 845–50.

Susser, M. (1990). Disease, illness, sickness; impairment, disability and handicap. *Psychological Medicine* 20, 471–3.

Svenson, S. and Folstein, S. E. (2000). Psychological aspects and risks of testing for genetic disorders. In *Psychiatric care of the medical patient* (eds A. Stoudemire, B. S. Fogel, and D. B. Greenberg). Oxford University Press, New York.

Swaab, D. F. and Hoffman, M. A. (1990). An enlarged suprachiasmatic nucleus in homosexual men. *Brain Research* 537, 141–8.

Swan, W. and Wilson, L. J. (1979). Sexual and marital problems in a psychiatric outpatient population. *British Journal of Psychiatry* 135, 310–15.

Swanson, J. W., Holzer, C. E., Ganju, V. K., and Jono, R. T. (1990). Violence and psychiatric disorder in the community: evidence from the Epidemiologic Catchment Area surveys. *Hospital and Community Psychiatry,* 41, 761–70 [published erratum appears in *Hospital and Community Psychiatry* 1991; 42(9) 954–5]

Swanson, J. W., Swartz, M. S., Borum, R., Hiday, V. A., Ryan Wagner, H., and Burns, B. J. (2000). Involuntary out-patient commitment and reduction of violent behaviour in persons with severe mental illness. *British Journal of Psychiatry* 176, 324–31.

Swedo, S. E. and Pekar, M. (2000). PANDAS: a new species of childhood-onset obsessive compulsive disorder? In *Childhood onset of 'adult' psychopathology. Clinical and research advances* (ed. J. L. Rappoport), pp. 103–19. American Psychiatric Association, Washington, DC.

Swedo, S. E., Pietrini, P., Leonard, H. L., *et al.* (1992). Cerebral glucose metabolism in childhood-onset obsessive–compulsive disorder: revisualization during pharmacotherapy. *Archives of General Psychiatry* 49, 690–4.

Swedo, S. E., Leonard, H. L., and Kiessling, L. S. (1994). Speculations on antineuronal antibody-mediated neuropsychiatric disorders in childhood. *Pediatrics* 93, 323–6.

Symmers, W. St C. (1968). Carcinoma of breast in transsexual individuals after surgical and hormonal interference with primary and secondary sex characteristics. *British Medical Journal* 2, 83–5.

Szasz, T. S. (1960). The myth of mental illness. *American Psychology* 15, 113–18.

Szatmari, P., Offord, D. R., and Boyle, M. H. (1989). Correlates, associated impairments and patterns of service utilization of children with attention deficit disorder: findings from the Ontario Child Health Study. *Journal of Child Psychology and Psychiatry and Allied Disciplines* 30, 205–17.

Szmuckler, G. and Holloway, F. (2001). In patient Treatment. Ch. 28. In *Textbook of Community Psychiatry* (eds G. Thornicroft, G. Szmuckler). Oxford University Press, Oxford.

Tan, E., Marks, I. M., and Marset, P. (1971). Bimedial leucotomy in obsessive compulsive neurosis: a controlled serial enquiry. *British Journal of Psychiatry* 118, 155–64.

Tansella, M. (1991). Community based psychiatry: long-term patterns of care in South Verona. *Psychological Medicine* 19 Suppl.

Tardiff, K. (1992). The current state of psychiatry in the treatment of violent patients. *Archives of General Psychiatry* 49, 493–9.

Tardiff, K., Marzule, P. M., Leon, A. C., *et al.* (1994). Homicide in New York City: cocaine use and firearms. *Journal of the American Medical Association* 272, 43–6.

Tarrier, N., Yusupoff, L., Kinney, C., *et al.* (1998). Randomised controlled trial of intensive cognitive behaviour therapy for patients with chronic schizophrenia. *British Medical Journal* 317, 303–7.

Task Force for Psychiatric Measures (2000). *Handbook of psychiatric measures.* American Psychiatric Association, Washington, DC.

Taylor, D. (1999). Depot antipsychotics revisited. *Psychiatric Bulletin* 23, 551–3.

Taylor, D., McConnell, D., McConnell, H., *et al.* (1999). *The Bethlem and Maudsley NHS Trust prescribing guidelines,* 5th edn, pp. 146–7. Martin Dunitz, London.

Taylor, E. (1991). *Biological risk factors for psychosocial disorders*. Cambridge University Press, Cambridge.

Taylor, E. (1994). Physical treatments. In *Child and adolescent psychiatry*, 3rd edn (eds M. Rutter, E. Taylor, and L. Hersov). Blackwell Scientific Publications, Oxford.

Taylor, E., Sandberg, S., Thorley, G., and Giles, S. (1991). *The epidemiology of childhood hyperactivity*. Maudsley Monograph No. 3. Oxford University Press, Oxford.

Taylor, F. H. (1966). The Henderson therapeutic community. In *Psychopathic disorders* (ed. M. Craft). Pergamon Press, Oxford.

Taylor, F. K. (1981). On pseudo-hallucinations. *Psychological Medicine* 11, 265–72.

Taylor, H. A. Jr (1999). Sexual activity and the cardiovascular patient: guidelines. *American Journal of Cardiology* 84, 6N–10N.

Taylor, P. J. (1985). Motives for offending among violent and psychotic men. *British Journal of Psychiatry* 147, 491–8.

Taylor, P. J. and Fleminger, J. J. (1980). ECT for schizophrenia. *Lancet* 1, 1380–2.

Taylor, P. J. and Gunn, J. (1984). Violence and psychosis. 1 – Risk of violence among psychotic men. *British Medical Journal* 288, 1945–9.

Taylor, P. J. and Gunn, J. (1999). Homicides by people with mental illness: myth and reality. *British Journal of Psychiatry*, 174, 9–14.

Taylor, P. J., Mahandra, B., and Gunn, J. (1983). Erotomania in males. *Psychological Medicine* 13, 645–50.

Taylor, S. (1996). Meta-analysis of cognitive–behavioral treatment for social phobia. *Journal of Behavior Therapy and Experimental Psychiatry* 27, 1–9.

Taylor, S. J. L. and Chave, S. (1964). *Mental health and environment*. Longman, London.

Teague, G. B., Bond, G. R., and Drake, R. E. (1998). Program fidelity in assertive community treatment: development and use of a measure. *American Journal of Orthopsychiatry* 68, 216–32.

Teasdale, J. D. (1983). Negative thinking in depression: cause, effect or reciprocal relationship. *Advances in Behaviour Research and Therapy* 5, 3–25.

Teasdale, J. D., Lloyd, C. A., and Hutton, J. M. (1998). Depressive thinking and dysfunctional schematic mental models. *British Journal of Clinical Psychology* 37, 247–57.

Tennant, C. (1988). Parental loss in childhood: its effect in adult life. *Archives of General Psychiatry* 45, 1045–50.

Thapar, A., Irving, I., Gottesman, I., *et al.* (1994). The genetics of mental retardation. *British Journal of Psychiatry* 164, 747–58.

Thapar, A., Holmes, J., Poulton, K., and Harrington, R. C. (1999). Genetic basis of attention deficit and hyperactivity. *British Journal of Psychiatry*. 174, 105–11.

Thase, M. E. and Friedman, E. S. (1999). Is psychotherapy an effective treatment for melancholia and other severe depressive states? *Journal of Affective Disorders* 54, 1–19.

Thies-Flechtner, K., Muller-Oerlinghausen, B., Seibert, W., *et al.* (1996). Effect of prophylactic treatment on suicide risk in patients with major affective disorders. *Pharmacopsychiatry* 29, 103–7.

Thomas, A., Chess, S., and Birch, H. G. (1968). *Temperament and behaviour disorders in children*. University Press, New York.

Thompson, A. and Pearce, J. (2000). The child as witness. In *The new Oxford textbook of psychiatry* (eds M. G. Gelder, J. J. López-Ibor Jr, and N. C. Andreasen), Chapter 9.4.2. Oxford University Press, Oxford.

Thompson, C. (1989). *The instruments of psychiatric research*. Wiley, Chichester.

Thompson, C., Franey, C., Arendt, J., and Checkley, S. A. (1988). A comparison of melatonin secretion in depressed patients and normal subjects. *British Journal of Psychiatry* 152, 260–5.

Thompson, L. W., Gallagher, D., and Breckenridge, J. S. (1987). Comparative effectiveness of psychotherapies for depressed elders. *Journal of Consulting and Clinical Psychology* 55, 385–90.

Thomson, L. D. G. (1998). Paranoid disorder and related syndromes. In *Companion to psychiatric studies* (eds E. C. Johnson, C. P. L. Freeman, and A. K. Zealley), pp. 431–45. Churchill Livingstone, Edinburgh.

Thomson, M. (1998). *The problem of mental deficiency. eugenics, democracy, and social policy in Britain, c.1870–1959*. Oxford University Press, Oxford.

Thoren, P., Asberg, M., Gronholm, B., *et al.* (1980). Clomipramine treatment of obsessive compulsive disorder. II biochemical aspects. *Archives of General Psychiatry* 27, 1289–94.

Thornicroft, G. and Tansella, M. (2000). Planning and providing mental health services for a community. In *The new Oxford textbook of psychiatry* (eds M. G. Gelder,

J. J López-Ibor Jr, and N. C. Andreasen), Chapter 7.5. Oxford University Press, Oxford.

Thornley, B., Adams, C. E., and Awad, G. (1997). Chlorpromazine versus placebo for those with schizophrenia (Cochrane Review). In *The Cochrane Library*. Update Software, Oxford.

Tizard, J. (1964). *Community services for the mentally handicapped*. Oxford University Press, London.

Tohen, M., Sanger, T. M., McElroy, S. L., *et al.* (1999). Olanzapine versus placebo in the treatment of acute mania. *American Journal of Psychiatry* 156, 702–9.

Tollison, C. D. and Adams, H. E. (1979). *Sexual disorders: treatment, theory and research*. Gardner Press, New York.

Tondo, L., Baldessarini, R. J., Floris, G., and Rudas, N. (1997). Effectiveness of restarting lithium treatment after its discontinuation in bipolar I and bipolar II disorders. *American Journal of Psychiatry* 154, 548–50.

Tondo, L., Baldessarini, R. J., Hennen, J., *et al.* (1998). Lithium treatment and risk of suicidal behavior in bipolar disorder patients. *Journal of Clinical Psychiatry* 59, 405–14.

Toone, B. (2000). Epilepsy. In *The new Oxford textbook of psychiatry* (eds M. G. Gelder, J. J. López-Ibor Jr, and N. C. Andreasen), Chapter 5.3.3. Oxford University Press, Oxford.

Torgersen, S. (1984). Genetic and sociological aspects of schizotypal and borderline personality disorders: a twin study. *Archives of General Psychiatry* 41, 546–54.

Trimble, M.R. (1997). Temporolimbic syndromes. In: *Contemporary Behavioral Neurology* (eds. M.R. Trimble, J.L. Cummings), Butterworth-Heinemann: Boston.

Trimble, M. R. (1999). A neurobiological perspective of the behaviour disorders of epilepsy. In *Disorders of brain and mind* (eds M. A. Ron and A. S. David), pp. 233–51. Cambridge University Press, Cambridge.

True, W. R., Rice, J., Eisen, S. A., *et al.* (1993). A twin study of genetic and environmental contributions to liability of posttraumatic stress symptoms. *Archives of General Psychiatry* 50, 257.

Trull, T. J. and Widiger, T. A. (1997). *Structured Interview for the Five-Factor Model of Personality. (SIFFM): professional manual*. Psychological Assessment Resources, Odessa, FL.

Trzepacz, P. and Dimartini, A. (2000). *The transplant patient. Biological, psychiatric and ethical issues in organ transplantation*. Cambridge University Press, Cambridge.

Trzepacz, P. T. (1994). The neuropathogenesis of delirium: a need to focus our research. *Psychosomatics* 35, 374–91.

Tsai, S. J., Hwang, J. P., Yang, C. H., and Liu, K. M. (1997). Delusional jealousy in dementia. *Journal of Clinical Psychiatry* 58, 492–4.

Tseng, W.-S., Kan-Ming, M., Hsu, J., *et al.* (1988). A sociocultural study of koro epidemics in Guangdong, China. *American Journal of Psychiatry* 145, 1538–43.

Tseng, W.-S., Asai, M., Kitanishi, K., *et al.* (1992). Diagnostic patterns of social phobia: comparisons in Tokyo and Hawaii. *Journal of Nervous and Mental Disease* 180, 380–5.

Tsoi, W. F. and Wong, K. E. (1991). A fifteen-year follow-up study of Chinese schizophrenic patients. *Acta Psychiatrica Scandinavica* 84, 217–20.

Tsuang, M. T., Stone, W. S., and Faraone, S. V. (2000). Schizoaffective and schizotypal disorders. In *The new Oxford textbook of psychiatry* (eds M. G. Gelder, J. J. López-Ibor Jr, and N. C. Andreasen), Chapter 4.3.8. Oxford University Press, Oxford.

Tuke, S. (1813). *A description of the Retreat*. Dawson, London (1964).

Turk, D. C. (1999). The role of psychological factors in chronic pain. *Acta Anaesthesiologica Scandinavica* 43, 885–8.

Turner, S. M., Beidel, D. C., and Jacob, R. G. (1994). Social phobia: comparison of behavior therapy and atenolol. *Journal of Consulting and Clinical Psychology* 62, 350–8.

Tyrer, P. and Davidson, K. (2000). Management of personality disorder. In *The new Oxford textbook of psychiatry* (eds M. G. Gelder, J. J. López-Ibor Jr, and N. C. Andreasen), Chapter 4.12.7. Oxford University Press, Oxford.

Tyrer, P. and Steinberg, D. (1975). Symptomatic treatment of agoraphobia and social phobias: a follow-up study. *British Journal of Psychiatry* 127, 163–8.

United Nations (1988). *United Nations world population chart*. United Nations, New York. [Quoted in Jacoby and Oppenheimer 1997, p. 63].

United Nations (1993). *United Nations demographic year book*. United Nations, New York. [Quoted in Jacoby and Oppenheimer 1997, p. 63].

Ursano, R. J. and Ursano, A. M. (2000). Brief individual dynamic pyschotherapy. In *The new Oxford textbood of psychiatry* (eds M. G. Gelder, J. J. López-Ibor Jr, and N. C Andreasen), Chapter 6.3.4. Oxford University Press, Oxford.

Üstün, T. B. and Sartorius, N. (1995). *Mental illness in general health care; an international study*. John Wiley, Chichester.

Vaillant, G. E. (1988). What can long-term follow-up teach us about relapse and prevention in addiction? *British Journal of Addiction* 83, 1147–57.

Valmaña, A. (1999). Nonmethadone pharmacotherapies in opioid addiction. *Current Opinion in Psychiatry* 12, 307–10.

Van Ameringen, M., Mancini, C., and Streiner, D. L. (1993). Fluoxetine efficacy in social phobia. *Journal of Clinical Psychiatry* 54, 27–32.

Van Bolkom, A. J. L., de Haan, E., van Oppen, P., *et al.* (1998). Cognitive and behavioural therapies alone versus in combination with fluvoxamine in the treatment of obsessive compulsive disorder *Journal of Nervous and Mental Disorder* 186, 492–9.

van den Hout, M., Arntz, A., and Merckelbach, H. (2000). Contributions of psychology to the understanding of psychiatric disorders. In *The new Oxford textbook of psychiatry* (eds M. G. Gelder, J. J. López-Ibor Jr, and N. C. Andreasen), Chapter 2.5.3. Oxford University Press, Oxford.

Van den Oord, E. J., Boomsma, D. I., and Verhulst, F. C. (1994). A study of problem behaviours in 10–15 year old biologically related and unrelated international adoptees. *Behaviour Genetics* 24, 193–205.

van der Kolk, B. A. and van der Hart, O. (1989). Pierre Janet and the breakdown of adaptation in psychological trauma. *American Journal of Psychiatry* 146, 1530–40.

Van Etten, M. L. and Taylor, S. (1998). Comparative efficacy of treatments for post-traumatic stress disorder: a meta-analysis. *Clinical Psychology and Psychotherapy* 5, 126–44.

Van Hoeken, D., Lucas, A. R., and Hoek, H. W. (1998). Epidemiology. In *Neurobiology in the treatment of eating disorders* (ed H. W. Hoek, J. L. Treasure, and M. A. Katzman). John Wiley, Chichester.

Van Kesteren, P. J., Asscheman, H., Megens, J. A., and Gooren, L. J. (1997). Mortality and morbidity of transsexual subjects treated with cross-sex hormones. *Clinical Endocrinology (Oxford)* 47, 337–42.

Van Kolk, B. A. and Fisler, R. (1995). Dissociation and the fragmentary nature of traumatic memories: overview and exploratory study. *Journal of Traumatic Stress* 8, 505–25.

Vanneste, J.A.L. (1994). Editorial. Three decades of normal pressure hydrocephalus: are we wiser now? *Journal of Neurology, Neurosurgery and Psychiatry* 57, 1021–5.

Van Loon, F. H. G. (1927). Amok and latah. *Journal of Abnormal and Social Psychology* 21 434–44.

van Vliet, I. M., den Boer, J. A., and Westenberg, H. G. M. (1994). Psychopharmacological treatment of social phobia: a double-blind placebo controlled study with fluvoxamine. *Psychopharmacology* 115, 128–34.

Van't Spijker, A., Trijsburg, R. W., and Duivenvoorden, H. J. (1997). Psychological sequelae of cancer diagnosis: a meta-analytical review of 58 studies after 1980. *Psychosomatic Medicine* 59, 280–93.

Varma, A.R. and Trimble, M.R. (1997) Subcortical neurologic syndromes. In: *Contemporary Behavioral Neurology* (eds. M.R. Trimble, J.L. Cummings), Butterworth-Heinemann: Boston.

Vaughn, C. E. and Leff, J. P. (1976). The influence of family and social factors as the course of psychiatric illness. *British Journal of Psychiatry* 129, 125–37.

Vauhkonen, K. (1968). On the pathogenesis of morbid jealousy with special reference to the personality traits of an interaction between jealous patients and their spouses. *Acta Psychiatrica Scandinavica Supplement* 202, 2–261.

Veith, I. (1965). *Hysteria: the case history of a disease*. University of Chicago Press, Chicago.

Vereker, M. (1992). Chronic fatigue syndrome: a joint paediatric-psychiatric approach. *Archives of Diseases of Childhood*, 67, 550–5.

Verhoeff, N. P. L. G. (1999). Radiotracer imaging of dopaminergic transmission in neuropsychiatric disorders. *Psychopharmacology* 147, 217–49.

Versiani, M., Nardi, A. E., and Mundim, F. D. (1992). Pharmacology of social phobia: a controlled study of moclobemide and phenelzine. *British Journal of Psychiatry* 161, 353–60.

Victor, M. and Adams, R. D. (1953). The effect of alcohol on the nervous system. *Proceedings of the Association of Research in Nervous and Mental Diseases* 32, 526–73.

Victor, M., Adams, R. D., and Collins, G. H. (1971). *The Wernicke-Korsakoff syndrome*. Blackwell, Oxford.

Viguera, A. C. and Cohen, L. S. (2000). Psychopharmacology during pregnancy, the post-partum period, and lactation. In *Psychiatric care of the medical patient* (eds A. Stoudemire, B. S. Fogel, and D. B. Greenberg). Oxford University Press, New York.

Vinogradov, S. and Yalom, I. D. (1989). *Concise guide to group psychotherapy*. American Psychiatric Press, Washington, DC.

Virag, R. (1982). Intracavernosus injection of papaverine for erectile failure. *Lancet* 2, 938.

Virkkunen, M., Goldman, D., and Linnoila, M. (1996). Serotonin in alcoholic violent offenders. In *Genetics of criminal and antisocial behaviour*. (eds G. R. Bock and J. A. Goode), pp. 168–82. CIBA Foundation Symposium 194. Wiley, Chichester.

Vitousek, K. and Manke, F. (1994). Personality variables and disorders in anorexia nervosa and bulimia nervosa. *Journal of Abnormal Psychology* 101, 137–47.

Vogeley, K. and Falkai, P. (1999). Brain imaging in schizophrenia. *Current Opinion in Psychiatry* 12, 41–6.

Volkmar, F. R. (1996). Childhood and adolescent psychosis: a review of the past ten years. *Journal of the American Academy of Child and Adolescent Psychiatry* 35, 843–51.

Volkmar, F. R. and Klin A. (2000). Autism and pervasive developmental disorders. In *The new Oxford textbook of psychiatry* (eds M. G. Gelder, J. J. López-Ibor Jr, and N. C. Andreasen), Chapter 9.2.2. Oxford University Press, Oxford.

Von Economo, C. (1929). *Encephalitis lethargica: its sequelae and treatment* (trans. K. O. Newman). Oxford University Press, Oxford (1931).

von Gontard, A. (1998). Annotation: day and night wetting in children – a paediatric perspective. *Journal of Child Psychology and Psychiatry* 39, 439–51.

Von Korff, M. and Simon, G. (1996). The relationship between pain and depression. *British Journal of Psychiatry* 168, 101–8.

Von Korff, M., Dworkin, S., LeResche, L., and Kruger, A. (1988). An epidemiologic comparison of pain complaints. *Pain* 32, 173–83.

Von Korff, M., Barlow, W., Charkin, D., and Deyo, R. A. (1994). Effects of practice style in managing back pain. *Annals of Internal Medicine* 121, 187–95.

Von Korff, R., Eaton, W. W., and Keyl, P. M. (1985). The epidemiology of panic attacks and panic disorder: results in three community surveys. *American Journal of Epidemiology* 122, 970–81.

Von Korff, M., Gruman, J., Schaefer, J., Curry, S. J., Wagner, E. H. (1997). Collaborative management of chronic illness. *Annals of Internal Medicine* 127, 1097–102.

Wacker, H. R., Mullejans, R., Klein, K. H., *et al.* (1992). Identification of cases of anxiety disorder and affective disorders in the community according to CD–10 and DSM-III-R using the Composite International Diagnostic Interview (CIDI). *International Journal of Methods of Psychiatric Research* 2, 91–100.

Wade, S. L., Monroe, S. M., and Michelson, L. K. (1993). Chronic life stress and treatment outcome in agoraphobia with panic attacks. *American Journal of Psychiatry* 150, 1491–5.

Wahlbeck, K., Cheine, M., Essali, A., and Adams, C. (1999). Evidence of clozapine's effectiveness in schizophrenia: a systematic review and meta-analysis of randomized trials. *American Journal of Psychiatry* 156, 990–9.

Walker, L. E. and Meloy, J. R. (1998). Stalking and domestic violence. In *The psychology of stalking: clinical and forensic perspectives* (ed. J. R. Meloy), pp. 139–61. Academic Press, San Diego, CA.

Walker, V. and Beech, H. R. (1969). Mood state and the ritualistic behaviour of obsessional patients. *British Journal of Psychiatry* 115, 1261–3.

Wallach, J. (1994). Laboratory diagnosis of factitious disorders. *Archives of Internal Medicine* 154, 1690–6.

Wallerstein, J. A. (1991). The long-term effects of divorce on children: a review. *Journal of the American Academy of Child and Adolescent Psychiatry* 30, 349–60.

Ward, C. H., Beck, A. T., Mendelson, M., *et al.* (1962). The psychiatric nomenclature. *Archives of General Psychiatry* 7, 198–205.

Ward, J., Hall, W., and Mattick, R. P. (1999). Role of maintenance treatment in opioid dependence. *Lancet* 353, 221–6.

Warner, R. W., Gater, R., Jackson, M. G., and Goldberg, D. P. (1993). Effects of a community mental health service on the practice and attitudes of general practitioners. *British Journal of General Practice* 43, 507–11.

Warren, M. Q. (1973). Correctional treatment in community settings. *Proceedings of the International Congress of Criminology, Madrid*.

Watson, J. B. and Rayner, R. (1920). Conditioned emotional reactions. *Journal of Experimental Psychology* 3, 1–14.

Watson, M., Haviland, J. S., Greer, S., Davidson, J., Bliss, J. M. (1999). Influence of psychological response on survival in breast cancer: a population based case control study. *Lancet* 354, 1331–1336.

Weatherall, D., Ledingham, J. G. G., and Warrell, D. A. (1995). *Oxford textbook of medicine*. Oxford University Press, Oxford.

Webster, L. (1994). Management of sexual problems in diabetic patients. *British Journal of Hospital Medicine* 51, 465–8.

Webster-Stratton, C. (1991). Annotation strategies for helping families with conduct disordered children. *Journal of Child Psychology and Psychiatry* 32, 1047–61.

Wechsler, D. (1945). A standardized memory scale for clinical use. *Journal of Psychology* 19, 87–95.

Weeks, D., Freeman, C. P. L., and Kendell, R. E. (1980). ECT: III Enduring cognitive deficits. *British Journal of Psychiatry* 137, 26–37.

Wegner, D. M. (1989). *White bears and other unwanted thoughts: suppression, obsession and the psychology of mental control*. Viking, New York.

Weiler, B. L. and Widom, C. S. (1996). Psychopathy and violent behaviour among abused and neglected young adults. *Criminal Behaviour and Mental Health* 6, 263–81.

Weinberg, M. S., Williams, C. J., and Calhan, C. (1994). Homosexual foot fetishism. *Archives of Sexual Behaviour* 23, 611–26.

Weinberger, D. R. (1995). From neuropathology to neurodevelopment. *Lancet* 346, 552–7.

Weinmann, J. and Petrie, K. J. (2000). Health psychology. In *The new Oxford textbook of psychiatry* (eds M. G. Gelder, J. J. López-Ibor Jr, and N. C. Andreasen), Chapter 5.7. Oxford University Press, Oxford.

Weisbrod, B. A., Test, M., and Stein, I. (1980). An alternative to mental hospital treatment. 2 Economic cost-benefit analysis. *Archives of General Psychiatry* 37, 400–5.

Weissman, M. M. and Merikangas, K. R. (1986). The epidemiology of anxiety and panic disorders. *Journal of Clinical Psychiatry* 47(**suppl**), 11–17.

Weissman, M. M., Prusoff, B. A., Dimascio, A., Neu, C., Goklaney, M., and Klerman, G. L. (1979). The efficacy of drugs and psychotherapy in the treatment of acute depressive episodes. *American Journal of Psychiatry* 136, 555–8.

Weissman, M. M., Bland, R. C., Canino, G. J., *et al.* (1994). The gross national epidemiology of obsessive compulsive disorder. *Journal of Clinical Psychiatry* 55, 5–11.

Weissman, M. M., Bland, R. C., Canino, G. J., *et al.* (1996). Cross-national epidemiology of major depression and bipolar disorder. *Journal of the American Medical Association* 276, 293–9.

Weissman, M. M., Markowitz, J. C., and Klerman, G. L. (1999). *Comprehensive guide to interpersonal therapy*. Basic Books, New York

Weisz, J. R., Weiss, B., Hann, S. S., *et al.* (1995). Effects of psychotherapy with children and adolescents revisited: meta-analysis of treatment outcome studies. *Psychological Bulletin* 117, 450–68.

Wellings, K., Field, J., Johnson, A. M., and Wadsworth, J. (1994). *Sexual behaviour in Britain*. Penguin Books, London.

Wells, A. and Butler, G. (1997). Generalized anxiety disorder. In *Science and practice of cognitive behaviour therapy* (eds D. M. Clark and C. G. Fairburn), Chapter 7. Oxford University Press, Oxford.

Wells, K. B., Golding, J. M., and Burnam, M. A. (1988). Psychiatric disorder in a sample of the general population with and without chronic medical conditions. *American Journal of Psychiatry* 145, 976–81.

Werner, E. E. and Smith, R. S. (1982). *Vulnerable but invincible: a study of resilient children*. McGraw-Hill, New York.

Wernicke, C. (1900). *Grundriss der Psychiatrie*. Thieme, Leipzig.

Wertheimer, A. (1992). *A special scar. The experiences of people bereaved by suicide*, 2nd edn. Routledge, London.

Wessely, S. (1987). Mass hysteria: two syndromes? *Psychological Medicine* 17, 109–20.

Wessely, S. (1997). The epidemiology of crime, violence and schizophrenia. *British Journal of Psychiatry* 170(**suppl 32**), 8–11.

Wessely, S., Hotopf, M., and Sharpe, M. (1998). *Chronic fatigue and its syndromes*. Oxford University Press, Oxford.

Wessely, S. and Hotopf, M. (1999). Is fibromyalgia a distinct clinical entity? Historical and epidemiological evidence. *Balliére's Clinical Rheumatology* 13, 427–36.

Wessely, S., Nimnuan, C., and Sharpe, M. (1999). Functional somatic syndromes: one or many? *Lancet* 354, 936–9.

West, D. (1965). *Murder followed by suicide*. Heinemann, London.

West, D. (1974). Criminology, deviant behaviour and mental disorder. *Psychological Medicine* 4, 1–3.

West, D. and Farrington, D. P. (1973). *Who becomes delinquent?* Heinemann Educational, London.

West, D. and Farrington, D. P. (1977). *The delinquent way of life.* Heinemann, London.

West, M. A. (1990). *The psychology of meditation.* Clarendon Press, Oxford.

Westen, D. (1997). Divergences between clinical and other research methods for assessing personality disorders: implications for research and the evolution of Axis II. *American Journal of Psychiatry* 154, 895–903.

Westphal, C. (1872). Die agoraphobie, eine neuropatische Erscheinung. *Archiv fur Psychiatrie und Nervenkrankheiten* 3, 209–37.

Wheeler, E. O., White, P. D., Reed, E. W., and Cohen, M. E. (1950). Neurocirculatory asthenia (anxiety neurosis, effort syndrome, neurasthenia). A twenty year follow up of one hundred and seventy three patients. *Journal of the American Medical Association* 142, 878–89.

Whitaker, A., Johnson, J., Shaffer, D., *et al.* (1990). Uncommon troubles in young people: prevalence estimates of selected psychiatric disorders in a nonreferred adolescent population. *Archives of General Psychiatry* 47, 487–96.

White, P., Bradley, C., Ferriter, M., and Hatzipetrou, L. (1998). Managements for people with disorders of sexual preference and for convicted sexual offenders. *The Cochrane Library, Issue 4.* Update Software, Oxford.

White, P. D., Thomas, J. M., Amess, J. *et al.* (1998). Incidence, risk and prognosis of acute and chronic fatigue syndromes and psychiatric disorders after glandular fever. *British Journal of Psychiatry* 173, 475–481.

Whitley, E., Gunnell, D., Dorling, D., and Smith, G. D. (1999). Ecological study of social fragmentation, poverty, and suicide. *British Medical Journal* 319, 1034–7.

Whitney, I. Smith, P. K., and Thompson, D. (1994). Bullying and children with special needs. In *School bullying: insights and perspectives* (eds P. K. Smith and S. Sharp), pp. 213–40. Routledge, London.

WHO Brief Intervention Group (1996). A cross-national trial of brief intervention with heavy drinkers. *American Journal of Public Health* 86, 948–55.

Widiger, T. A. and Costa, P. T. (1994). Personality and personality disorders. *Journal of Abnormal Psychology* 103, 78–91.

Widiger, T. A. and Clark, L. A. (2000). Toward DSM-V and the classification of psychopathology. *Psychological Bulletin* 126, 946–963.

Wieck, A., Kumar, R., Hirst, A. D., *et al.* (1991). Increased sensitivity of dopamine receptors and recurrence of affective psychosis after childbirth. *British Medical Journal* 303, 613–16.

Wiener, I., Breitbart, W., and Holland, J. (1996). Psychiatric issues in the care of dying patients. In *Textbook of consultation-liaison psychiatry* (eds J. R. Rundell and M. G. Wise). American Psychiatric Press, Washington, DC.

Wilcock, G. K., Bucks, R. S., and Rockwood, K. (eds) (1999). *Diagnosis and management of dementia.* Oxford University Press, Oxford.

Wilensky, D. S., Ginsberg, G., Altman, M., *et al.* (1996). A community study of failure to thrive in Israel. *Archives of Disease in Childhood* 75, 145–8.

Wilkinson, G., Allen, P., Marshall, E., *et al.* (1993). The role of the practice nurse in the management of depression in general practice: treatment adherence to antidepressant medication. *Psychological Medicine* 23, 229–37.

Williams, D. (1969). Neural factors related to habitual aggression: consideration of the differences between those habitual aggressive and others who have committed crimes of violence. *Brain* 92, 503–20.

Williams, J., Spurlock, G., McGuffin, P., *et al.* (1996). Association between schizophrenia and T102C polymorphism of the 5-hydroxytryptamine type 2a-receptor. *Lancet* 347, 1294–6.

Williams, J., McGuffin, P., Nothen, M., and Owen, M. J. (1997). A meta analysis of association between the 5-HT$_{2A}$ receptor T102C polymorphism and schizophrenia. *Lancet* 349, 1221.

Williams, J. H. (1998). Using behavioural ecology to understand depression. *British Journal of Psychiatry* 173, 453–4.

Williams, J. H., Wellman, N. A., Geaney, D. P., Cowen, P. J., Feldon, J., and Rawlins, J. N. (1998). Reduced latent inhibition in people with schizophrenia: an effect of psychosis or of its treatment. *British Journal of Psychiatry* 172, 243–9.

Williams, J. M. G. (1992). Autobiographical memory and emotional disorders. In *The handbook of emotion and memory, research and theory* (ed. S. A. Christianson), pp. 451–77. Lawrence Erlbaum Associates, Hillsdale, NJ.

Williams, J. M. G. and Pollock, L. R. (2000). The psychology of suicidal behaviour. In *The international handbook of suicide and attempted suicide* (eds K. Hawton and K. van Heeringen). John Wiley & Sons, Chichester.

Wilson, B. A. (1999). *Case studies in neuropsychologial rehabilitation.* Oxford University Press, New York.

Wilson, D. N. (1997). Psychiatric disorders and mild learning disability. In *The psychiatry of learning disabilities* (ed. O. Russell), pp.125–35. Gaskell, London.

Wilson, G. T. (1993). Behavioral treatment of obesity: thirty years and counting. *Advances in Behaviour Research and Therapy* 16, 31–75.

Wilson, G. T. (1994). Behavioral treatment of childhood obesity: theoretical and practical implications. *Health Psychology* 13, 371–2.

Wilson, M. (1993). DSM-III and the transformation of American psychiatry: a history. *American Journal of Psychiatry* 150, 399–410.

Wing, J. K. (1994). Mental illness. In *Health care needs assessment* (eds A. Stevens and J. Raferty). Radcliffe Medical Press, Abingdon, Oxfordshire.

Wing, J. K. and Brown, G. W. (1970). *Institutionalism and schizophrenia.* Cambridge University Press, London.

Wing, J. K. and Furlong, R. (1986). A haven for the severely disabled within the context of a comprehensive psychiatric community service. *British Journal of Psychiatry* 149, 449–57.

Wing, J. K. and Hailey, A. M. (eds) (1972). *Evaluating a community psychiatric service.* Oxford University Press, London.

Wing, J. K., Bennett, D. H., and Denham, J. (1964). The industrial rehabilitation of long stay psychiatric patients. *Medical Research Council Memorandum No. 42.* HMSO, London.

Wing, J. K., Cooper, J. E. and Sartorius, N. (1974). *Measurement and classification of psychiatric symptoms; and instruction manual for the PSE and the CATEGO programme.* Cambridge University Press, Cambridge.

Winnick, C. and Evans, J. T. (1996). The relationship between non-enforcement of state pornography laws and rates of sex crime arrest. *Archives of Sexual Behaviour* 25, 439–53.

Winston, A., Pollack, J., MacCulloch, L., *et al.* (1991). Brief psychotherapy for personality disorders. *Journal of Nervous and Mental Disease* 179, 188–93.

Wirz-Justice, A. and Van den Hoofdakker, R. H. (1999). Sleep deprivation in depression: what do we know, where do we go? *Biological Psychiatry* 46, 445–53.

Wisner, K. L., Gelenberg, A. J., Leonard, H., *et al.* (1999). Pharmacologic treatment of depression during pregnancy. *Journal of the American Medical Association* 282, 1264–9.

Wisniewski, H. M., Silverman, J., and Wegiel, J. (1994). Ageing, Alzheimer disease and mental retardation. *Journal of Intellectual Disability Research* 38, 233–9.

Witherington, R. (1989). Vacuum constriction device for the management of erectile impotence. *Journal of Urology* 141, 320–2.

Withers, N. W., Pulvirenti, L., Koob, G. F., and Gillin, J. C. (1995). Cocaine abuse and dependence. *Journal of Clinical Psychopharmacology* 15, 63–78.

Wittchen, H-U., Zhao, S., Kessler, R. C., and Eaton, W. W. (1994). DSM-III-R generalized anxiety disorder in the National Comorbidity Survey. *Archives of General Psychiatry* 51, 355–64.

Wolberg, L. R. (1977). *The techniques of psychotherapy.* Grune and Stratton, New York.

Wolf, S. and Wolff, H. G. (1947). *Human gastric function.* Oxford University Press, New York.

Wolff, C. (1971). *Love between women.* Duckworth, London.

Wolff, H. G. (1962). A concept of disease in man. *Psychosomatic Medicine* 24, 25–30.

Wolff, K., Welch, S., and Strang, J. (1999). Specific laboratory investigations for assessments and management of drug problems. *Advances in Psychiatric Treatment* 5, 180–91.

Wolkind, S. (1994). Legal aspects of child care. In *Child and adolescent psychiatry: modern approaches*, 3rd edn (eds M. Rutter, E. Taylor, and L. Hersov). Blackwell Scientific Publications, Oxford.

Wolkind, S. N. and Rushton, A. (1994). Residential and foster family care. In *Child and adolescent psychiatry: modern approaches*, 3rd edn (eds M. Rutter, E. Taylor, and L. Hersov), pp. 252–66. Blackwell Scientific Publications, Oxford.

Wolozin, B., and Behl, C. (2000). Mechanisms of neurodegenerative disorders. *Archives of Neurology* 57, 793–6, 801–4.

Wolpe, J. (1958). *Psychotherapy by reciprocal inhibition.* Stanford University Press, Stanford, CA.

Wolpert, L. (1999). *Malignant sadness: the anatomy of depression.* Faber, London.

Wood, P. (1941). Da Costa's syndrome (or effort syndrome). *British Medical Journal* 1, 767–74, 805–11, 846–51.

Woods, B. and Charlesworth, G. (2001). Psychological assessment and treatment. In *Psychiatry in the elderly*, 3rd edn (eds R. Jacoby and C. Oppenheimer). Oxford University Press, Oxford.

Wooff, K. and Goldberg, D. (1988). Further observations on the practice of community care in Salford: differences between community psychiatric nurses and mental health social workers. *British Journal of Psychiatry* 163, 30–7.

Wooley, H., Stein, A., Forrest, G. C., and Baum, J. D. (1989). Imparting the diagnosis of life threatening illness in children. *British Medical Journal* 298, 1623–6.

Worden, J. W. (1996). *Children and grief: when a parent dies*. Guilford Press, New York.

Worden, J. W. (1991). *Grief counselling and grief therapy: a handbook for the mental health practitioner*, 2nd edn. Routledge, London.

World Health Organization (1973). *Report of the International Pilot Study of Schizophrenia*, Vol.1. World Health Organization, Geneva.

World Health Organization (1978a). *Mental disorders: glossary and guide to their classification in accordance with the ninth revision of the International Classification of Diseases*. World Health Organization, Geneva.

World Health Organization (1978b). *Alma-Ata 1978: primary health care*. World Health Organization, Geneva.

World Health Organization (1984). *Mental health care in developing countries: a critical appraisal of research findings*. Technical Report Series 698. World Health Organization, Geneva.

World Health Organization (1988). *Psychiatric disability assessment schedule*. World Health Organization, Geneva.

World Health Organization (1989). *Composite International Diagnostic Interview (CIDI)*. World Health Organization, Geneva.

World Health Organization (1990). *International classification of mental health settings*. World Health Organization, Geneva.

World Health Organization (1992a). *Glossary: differential definitions of SCAN items and commentary on the SCAN text*. World Health Organization, Geneva.

World Health Organization (1992b). *The ICD-10 classification of mental and behavioural disorders*. World Health Organization, Geneva.

World Health Organization (1998). *Primary prevention of mental, neurological and psychosocial disorders*. World Health Organization, Geneva.

Wright, I. C., Rabe-Hesketh, S., Woodruff, P. W. R., et al. (2000). Meta-analysis of regional brain volumes in schizophrenia. *American Journal of Psychiatry* 157, 16–25.

Wrightson, P. and Gronwall, D. (1999). *Mild head injury*. Oxford University Press, Oxford.

Wroblewska, A. M. (1997). Androgenic-anabolic steroids and body dysmorphia in young men. *Journal of Psychosomatic Research* 42, 225–34.

Wu, J. C. and Bunney, W. E. (1990). The biological basis of an antidepressant response to sleep deprivation and relapse: review and hypothesis. *American Journal of Psychiatry* 147, 14–21.

Wulsin, L. R., Vaillant, G. E., Wells, V. E. (1999). A systematic review of the mortality of depression. *Psychosomatic Medicine* 61, 6–17.

Wylie, K. (1994). New approaches to paraphilias. *British Journal of Sexual Medicine* 21, 18–21.

Wylie, K. (1998). Physical treatments for sexual dysfunctions. In *Psychosexual disorders* (eds H. Freeman, I. Pullen, G. Stein, and G. Wilkinson), pp.59–83. Gaskell, London.

Yalom, I. D. (1985). *The theory and practice of group psychotherapy*, 3rd edn. Basic Books, New York.

Yalom, I., Lieberman, M. A., and Miles, M. B. (1973). *Encounter groups: first facts*. Basic Books, New York.

Yap, P. M. (1965). Koro – a culture-bond depersonalization syndrome. *British Journal of Psychiatry* 111, 43–50.

Yates, W. R. and Bowers, W. A. (2000). Cognitive therapy in the medical-psychiatric patient. In *Psychiatric care of the medical patient* (eds A. Stoudemire, B. S. Fogel, and D. B. Greenberg). Oxford University Press, New York.

Yatham, L. N., Steiner, M., Liddle, P. F., et al. (2000). A PET study of brain 5-HT$_2$ receptors and their correlation with platelet 5-HT$_2$ receptors in healthy humans. *Psychopharmacology* 151, 424–7.

Yehuda, R., Southwick, S. M., Nussbaum, G., et al. (1990). Low urinary cortisol excretion in patients with post-traumatic stress disorder. *Journal of Nervous and Mental Disease* 178, 366–9.

Yehuda, R., McFarlane, A. C., and Shaler, A. Y. (1998). Predicting the development of post-traumatic stress disorder from the acute response to a traumatic event. *Biological Psychiatry* 4A, 1305–13.

Yirmiya, N., Erel, O., Shaked, M., *et al.* (1998). Meta-analyses comparing theory of mind abilities of individuals with autism, individuals with mental retardation and normally developing individuals. *Psychological Bulletin* 124, 283–307.

Yonkers, K. A., Warshaw, M. G., Massion, A. O., and Keller, M. B. (1996). Phenomenology and course of generalized anxiety disorder. *British Journal of Psychiatry* 168, 308–13.

Young, L. T., Robb, J. C., Hasey, G. M., *et al.* (1999). Gabapentin as an adjunctive treatment in bipolar disorder. *Journal of Affective Disorders* 55, 73–7.

Young, W., Goy, R., and Phoenix, C. (1964). Hormones and sexual behaviour. *Science* 143, 212–18.

Yule, W. (1967). Predicting reading ages on Neale's analysis of reading ability. *British Journal of Educational Psychology* 37, 252–5.

Yule, W. (1994). Post-traumatic stress disorders. In *Child and adolescent psychiatry: modern approaches*, 3rd edn (eds M. Rutter, E. Taylor, and L. Hersov). Blackwell Scientific Publications, Oxford.

Yule, W. and Rutter, M. (1985). Reading and other learning difficulties. In *Child and adolescent psychiatry: modern approaches*, 2nd edn (eds M. Rutter and L. Hersov). Blackwell, Oxford.

Zedner, L. (1994). Victims. In *The Oxford handbook of criminology* (eds M. Maguire, R. Morgan, and R. Reiner). Clarendon Press, Oxford.

Zeitlin, H. (1986). *The natural history of psychiatric disorder in children*. Maudsley Monograph No. 29. Oxford University Press, Oxford.

Zenner, M. T., Nobile, M., Henningsen, R., *et al.* (1998). Expression and characterization of a dopamine D4R variant associated with delusional disorder. *FEBS Letters* 422, 146–50.

Zhou, J. N., Hofman, M. A., Gooren, L. J., and Schwaab, D. F. (1995). A sex difference in the human brain and its relation to transsexuality. *Nature* 378, 68–70.

Zisook, S. and Shichter, S. R. (1993). Uncomplicated bereavement. *Journal of Clinical Psychiatry* 54(10), 365–72.

Zitrin, C. M., Klein, D. F., and Woerner, M. G. (1978). Behaviour therapy, supportive psychotherapy, imipramine and phobias. *Archives of General Psychiatry* 35, 307–16.

Zitrin, C. M., Klein, D. F., Woerner, M. G., and Ross, D. C. (1983). Treatment of phobias: I. Comparison of imipramine hydrochloride and placebo. *Archives of General Psychiatry* 40, 125–38.

Zobeck, T. S., Grant, B. F., Stinson, F. S., and Bertolucci, D. (1994). Alcohol involvement in fatal traffic crashes in the United States: 1979–1990. *Addiction* 89, 227–31.

Zoccolillo, M., Pickles, A., Quinton, D., and Rutter, M. (1992). The outcome of childhood conduct disorder: implications for defining adult personality disorder and conduct disorder. *Psychological Medicine* 22, 971–86.

Zohar, J. and Judge, R. (1996). Paroxetine versus clomipramine in the treatment of obsessive compulsive disorder. *British Journal of Psychiatry* 169, 468–74.

Zuger, B. (1984). Early effeminate behaviour in boys: outcome and significance for homosexuality. *Journal of Nervous and Mental Diseases* 172, 90–7.

Index

The index is arranged in letter-by-letter alphabetical order. Page numbers in *italic* refer to tables, figures and boxes. *vs* denotes differential diagnosis or comparisons.